Educational Review Manual in Neurology

2nd Edition—2008

Editors-in-Chief:

Morris Levin, MD
Associate Professor of Medicine (Neurology)
and Psychiatry, Dartmouth Medical School
Director, Dartmouth Neurology Residency Program
Dartmouth-Hitchcock Medical Center, Lebanon, New Hampshire

Gregory L. Holmes, MD
Professor of Medicine (Neurology) and Pediatrics,
Dartmouth Medical School
Chief, Section of Neurology
Dartmouth-Hitchcock Medical Center, Lebanon, New Hampshire

Jeffrey A. Cohen, MD
Professor of Medicine (Neurology), Dartmouth Medical School
Associate Chief, Section of Neurology
Director, Clinical Neurophysiology Fellowship
Dartmouth-Hitchcock Medical Center, Lebanon, New Hampshire

Castle Connolly Graduate Medical Publishing, Ltd.
New York, NY

CCGMP
Castle Connolly Graduate Medical Publishing

Castle Connolly Graduate Medical Publishing, Ltd.

17 Battery Place, Suite 643 • New York, NY 10004 • Tel: 212.644.9696 • Fax: 646.827.6443 • www.ccgmp.com • e-mail: info@ccgmp.com

Castle Connolly Graduate Medical Publishing, Ltd. publishes review manuals in 14 medical specialties and subspecialties and in pharmacy.

NOTICE

This book is intended for use by licensed physicians wishing to review and update their skills in neurology. It is not intended for use in the delivery of health care services, and cannot replace sound clinical judgment or individualized patient care for such purposes.

The authors, publishers, distributors, and sponsors of this book expressly disclaim all warranties, express or implied, with respect to this book and its contents, including any warranties as to the quality, accuracy, completeness or suitability of the information contained in this book for any particular purpose.

The authors, publishers, distributors and sponsors of this book expressly disclaim any liability to any person or organization for any loss or damage caused by any errors or omissions in this book.

ISBN 978-0-9816948-0-1

Our thanks to Copy Editor Bob McCann

Contents

ORTHO-McNEIL NEUROLOGICS®
Division of Ortho-McNeil-Janssen Pharmaceuticals, Inc.

1125 Trenton-Harbourton Rd.
Titusville, NJ 08560
Telephone: 609-730-2000

May 15, 2008

Dear Neurology Resident:

Ortho-McNeil Neurologics®, Division of Ortho-McNeil-Janssen Pharmaceuticals, Inc., is proud to sponsor *The Educational Review Manual in Neurology*, a thorough and up-to-the-minute review of the field.

This manual is a tool to assist you through the completion of residency training. It was prepared under the expert guidance of editors-in-chief Morris Levin, MD, Director of the Dartmouth Neurology Residency Program, Gregory L. Holmes, MD, Section Chief, Neurology at Dartmouth-Hitchcock Medical Center and Professor of Medicine and Pediatrics at Dartmouth University, and Jeffrey A. Cohen, MD, Professor of Medicine at Dartmouth and Director of the Clinical Neurophysiology Fellowship at Dartmouth-Hitchcock Medical Center. Written by a superb faculty of specialists and educators from medical centers around the U.S., the manual will be an invaluable tool for you in the months and years ahead.

When a neurological disorder enters a life, it changes a life. We honor your devotion and commitment to addressing the needs of each patient. Ortho-McNeil Neurologics® is dedicated to helping you provide better solutions that will help your patients today and in the future.

Ortho-McNeil Neurologics® commends the authors and the editors for an outstanding effort in developing this review. We hope that the wealth of information presented herein will enrich your understanding of neurology and help you to confidently complete your training.

Regards,

Ortho-McNeil Neurologics®

Chapter 1: Introduction to the Second Edition

This book was written in an attempt to help neurology residents assess their knowledge base as they complete their training. Neurology is growing dramatically, driven by the exponential growth in neuroscience knowledge. As a result, the task for clinicians to stay current becomes more challenging. We had hoped that this review manual would aid the trainee in mastering the clinical neurological sciences. Based on the positive feedback we received after the publication of the first edition, it seems our goal was reached. This new edition allowed us the opportunity to update and expand our chapters. It also allowed us to incorporate specific suggestions made by a number of our colleagues in other institutions. We felt these suggestions were very helpful and make for a better text. For instance, two entirely new chapters were commissioned and written—one concerning psychiatric disease in neurology and another covering the borderland between neurosurgery and neurology.

Many resources are available to assist busy neurologists in their continuing education, from traditional texts to case-based approaches, to Internet or CD-ROM training modules. We attempted to use a traditional approach, presenting information in an organized fashion, broken down into chapters. We made a serious attempt to make these presentations concise, clear, and thorough. Tables are used liberally to improve clarity and to make the review process as efficient as possible. Authors consist of experts in their subspecialty fields, as well as in medical education.

There are 34 chapters organized as follows:

I.) Two initial chapters on the neurological examination (adult and child).

II.) Four chapters on practical neuroscience – neuroanatomy, neurochemistry, neuroradiology and neuropathology.

III.) Twenty-six chapters on the various areas of neurological disease.

IV.) Two new chapters covering psychiatry and neurosurgery.

The material presented here is succinct, focused, accurate, and hopefully helpful to you, the reader. We have attempted to cover most of the important scientific and clinical information that the competent neurologist should have at their disposal. However, this book is not intended to serve as a complete text for the enormous field of the clinical neurosciences. Rather, there are selected references at the end of each chapter directing the reader to appropriate resources. We hope this review will motivate readers to search out the original source.

This new edition includes more case-based questions at the end of each chapter, with over 650 examination-type questions in this text.

While some readers will read the book from cover to cover, we suspect that many will pick chapters based on their individual needs. For that reason we asked each author to prepare their chapters so as to serve as a stand-alone reference review.

We hope this book will not only serve its purpose–to review basic neuroscience and clinical neurology–but will also be an "enjoyable read." To this end, the authors have tried to make these chapters readable and thought provoking. We sincerely hope this goal is achieved. Again, as you have done, please feel free to send any comments to us.

We wish to thank all of the contributing authors for their hard work. We would also like to thank our students and residents who continue to stimulate our creative processes.

Morris Levin, MD

Gregory L. Holmes, MD

Jeffrey A. Cohen, MD

Dartmouth Medical School
Hanover, New Hampshire

Chapter 2: The Neurological Examination: Adults

James L. Bernat, MD

Contents

Acknowledgement

This chapter was modified from Chapter 1 in: Bernat JL, Vincent FM. *Neurology: Problems in Primary Care*. 2nd ed. Los Angeles, Calif: Practice Management Information Corp.; 1995. (With permission.)

Neurology may be distinguished from other branches of medicine by its reliance upon a skillful physical examination for diagnosis. The brain and spinal cord cannot be inspected, palpated, auscultated, or percussed. The clinician must learn and perfect techniques to inferentially measure nervous system function.

1. Neurological Assessment

The assessment of the patient with nervous system disease differs from assessment in other branches of medicine. Before a differential diagnosis can be constructed on the basis of history, physical examination, and laboratory data, the clinician must localize the lesion to the affected area of the nervous system.

Consider the patient whose chief complaint is left arm weakness. Lesions of the right hemisphere, brain stem, spinal cord, cervical nerve roots, brachial plexus, peripheral nerve, neuromuscular junction, and muscle all can produce left arm weakness. But, it would be absurd for the clinician to generate a differential diagnosis that includes hemispheric stroke, brain stem tumor, transverse myelitis, herniated cervical disc, brachial plexus neuropathy, diabetic mononeuropathy, myasthenia gravis, and polymyositis. The function of the history, and to a greater extent, of the neurological examination, is to localize the lesion in the nervous system. If the examination reveals a spastic left hemiparisis, left-sided multimodality sensory loss, mild lower-left facial weakness, and left homonymous hemianopia, the clinician can localize the lesion to the right hemisphere. This localization permits the clinician to exclude diseases in other parts of the nervous system from the differential diagnosis. The differential diagnosis is then constructed on the basis of the history, physical, and laboratory findings of disorders affecting that portion of the nervous system. In neurological assessment, the clinician must localize the lesion before making a differential diagnosis.

2. History

In neurology, as in all of medicine, history is 90% of diagnosis. In paroxysmal disorders of the nervous system, including migraine and epilepsy, history may be 100% of diagnosis. Neurological histories include chief complaint, present illness, medical history, family history, social history, and review of systems.

When recording the chief complaint and present illness, it is particularly important to clarify the meaning of words used by the patient to describe his symptoms. Words such as "weak," "numb," "seizure," "dizziness," and "double vision" may mean different experiences to different patients. It is most helpful for the clinician to obtain a chronological history of the illness, its course, previous testing, the effects of previous treatment, and the presence of exacerbating and ameliorating factors. In nervous system disorders that affect consciousness and cognition, it is necessary to obtain corroborating history from the spouse, relatives, fellow workers, and friends. In cases of paroxysmal disorders that affect consciousness, such as seizures and syncope, it is necessary to contact eyewitnesses to describe precisely what happened. Clinicians should not rely on second-hand information because it may be inaccurate.

The medical history sets the stage for the present illness. In the patient with a presumptive diagnosis of stroke, it is necessary to inquire about past hypertension, angina, myocardial infarction, intermittent claudication, smoking, hyperlipidemia, and diabetes. Past major illnesses, operations, injuries, and hospitalizations should be reviewed.

Family history is particularly important. Hereditary transmission is seen in many diseases of the nervous system. Many otherwise undiagnosed polyneuropathy and other neuromuscular disease syndromes can be shown to be hereditary if a careful family history is obtained and if family members are interviewed and examined.

The social history should contain questions about tobacco, alcohol, and drug use; occupational traumas; toxin exposure; the patient's living arrangements and financial status; allergies; and current medications. The review of systems in the neurological patient should include questions about headache, dizziness, loss of consciousness, memory loss, confusion, visual and hearing disturbances, difficulty in speaking and swallowing, bowel, bladder, and sexual dysfunction, weakness, numbness, clumsiness, imbalance, falling, and trouble walking.

The handedness of the patient must be determined. Right-handed patients must be asked if they have always been right-handed or if they were forced to switch in childhood. The extent of handedness can be determined by inquiring with which hand the patient writes, eats, throws a ball, and threads a needle.

3. Neurological Examination: General Remarks

Conduct of the neurological examination is designed to answer the question: "From which part of the nervous system does the patient's complaints originate?" The examination includes both "horizontal" and "vertical" components. Horizontally, the physician screens for abnormalities in mental status, cranial nerves, motor and sensory functions, coordination, gait and station, and reflexes. In the vertical dimension, the examiner can assess each system at a variable depth, using more refined tests, depending upon the findings and the nature of the problem.

In practice, most experienced clinicians have evolved a "screening" neurological examination: a brief overview of the complete exam that can be performed in five minutes. Any abnormalities found on screening can be pursued in more depth (vertically) by more sensitive supplementary methods of examination. The screening neurological examination should include:

Mental status: level of consciousness, attention, immediate memory, and language.

Cranial nerves: pupillary reflexes, visual acuity, visual fields, eye movements, facial movements, hearing, swallowing, phonation, shoulder shrug, and tongue movements.

Motor: sample of upper and lower limb tone, strength, and appearance.

Sensory: pain and vibration sensation in all four limbs.

Coordination: finger-to-nose and heel-to-shin tests.

Gait and station: ordinary walking and tandem gait.

Reflexes: deep-tendon reflexes of biceps, triceps, brachioradialis, knees, and ankles.

The order of the components of the neurological examination is not critical. It is, however, necessary for the clinician to learn and follow one particular order so that parts of the exam are not omitted inadvertently. The above listed order of the screening exam has a logical pattern. Mental status is assessed first. The interpretation of the remainder of the examination findings will be affected if the patient is confused or aphasic. Coordination testing follows testing of mental status, cranial nerves, motor, and sensory function because coordination requires all these primary functions in addition to cerebellar function. Similarly, normal gait and station require all the preceding functions. Reflexes, the most objective part of the examination, may be performed following the motor exam or at the end of the exam.

The patient generally should be disrobed and wearing a hospital gown. The examining room should be warm and quiet. The clinician should try to relax the patient by gentle reassurance that the exam will be painless.

4. Physical Examination Pertinent Features

The neurological examination does not exist in isolation from the general physical examination. Certain features of the general physical examination are performed as part of every neurological assessment. They include the examination of: vital signs; optic fundi; facies; head, neck, and extremity pulses; color; and evidence of limb trophic changes.

Other portions of the general examination may be performed, depending on the presenting problem. For the patient in whom cerebrovascular disease is in the differential diagnosis, a neurovascular examination is performed, including the palpation of carotid and facial arteries; listening for carotid, orbital, and subclavian bruits; detailed examination of the heart; and blood pressure determination in both arms. For the patient with acute sciatica, the clinician should examine the back for tenderness, range of movements, and muscle spasm; straight leg raising and inverse straight leg raising; lower extremity joint range of movements; and often rectal examination.

5. Mental Status

A complete mental status examination should assess level of consciousness, orientation, attention, language, recent and remote memory, higher integrative functions, thought, and behavior. Examiners vary greatly in mental status questionnaires. Experienced clinicians have evolved certain questions that they have validated internally on the basis of examinations of hundreds of patients, but few routine mental status questions in general use have been validated statistically, ie, specific answers correlated with specific proved diagnoses.

Level of consciousness is assessed first. Normally, patients are "alert," showing full wakefulness and quick responsiveness to verbal questions and commands. The "lethargic" patient exhibits blunted wakefulness and impaired responsiveness to verbal questions and commands. The "stuporous" patient exhibits a pathological state of sleep-like unawareness and unresponsiveness from which he can be aroused to temporary responsiveness only by noxious stimuli. The "comatose" patient exhibits a pathological state of sleep-like unawareness and unresponsiveness from which he cannot be aroused despite the use of noxious stimuli. More subtle impairments of the level of consciousness are manifest by inability to maintain attention.

Orientation testing is performed next. Normal patients are oriented properly to name, age, birth date, home address, location of examination, and exact day, date, season, and general time of day of the examination. In confusional states, disorientation for time usually appears earliest followed by disorientation for place.

Attention is next assessed—the ability to continue to respond to and continue thinking about a specific stimulus without distraction by intervening stimuli. Attention for at least 30 seconds is considered normal. Attention is assessed both by behavioral observations throughout the examination and by specific tests. In the digit repetition test, patients are asked to repeat a string of random integers of increasing length. Normally, patients should be able to accurately repeat 6 integers. The serial sevens test requires patients to subtract 7 from 100, then 7 from the remainder, and so on. (Subtraction of serial threes from 20 is an alternative test if arithmetic ability or education is in question.) Normal patients should make no more than two errors in eight serial subtractions. Patients can be described as normally attentive, or with grades of inattentiveness.

Memory assessment is a crucial component of the mental status exam. The clinician tests both new short-term memory recording and the intactness of long-term memory traces. (So-called "immediate memory" is merely attention, as discussed above.) The ability to record and recall new memory traces over the short term is tested by asking the patient to repeat and remember three unrelated words (eg, "table," "red," and "53 Broadway"), distracting him, then asking him to say the words after five or ten minutes. Normally, at least two of the words should be remembered without cues, and all three with cues (eg, "Remember, one was a street address").

More detailed, individual assessments of verbal and visual short-term memory can be made. For verbal memory, a short detailed story can be read to the patient; afterward the patient is asked to repeat the story. He is scored on the percentage of individual parts of the story that he can recount. Visual memory can be tested by showing the patient a series of geometric designs, then hiding them and asking the patient to draw them from memory.

Remote memory is tested by asking the patient to recall the dates of significant life events, but the answers must be corroborated by a spouse or other family member. Alternatively, the patient can be quizzed about dates and facts in history that most people are expected to remember (eg, in the United States, recent Presidents, dates of recent wars, details of the World Trade Center catastrophe).

Higher integrative functions are assessed following the assessment of the fundamental mental skills of attention, orientation, language, and memory. These tests are highly education-biased, hence must be interpreted in light of the patient's formal educational level and employment history. Tests of fund of knowledge and proverb interpretation are particularly education-biased and must be interpreted cautiously. Better are tests of similarities and differences. For example, the patient is asked to name as many ways in which an apple and an orange are similar and are different. The question is repeated for chair and table, then for painting and statue. The patient is asked the difference between a child and a midget, and between a river and a canal.

Tests of calculation should be given. The patient can be asked: "How many nickels are there in $1.35?" or, "If apples cost 35 cents each, how much change should I get if I buy a dozen apples and pay five dollars?"

Thought and behavior should be assessed. The examiner should first make an assessment of the patient's mood. Is he apathetic, depressed, euphoric, or manic? Behavior should be assessed. Is there evidence for restlessness or agitation? Thought should be assessed. Is there anxiety? Are there morbid thoughts, illusions, hallucinations, delusions, obsessions, or compulsions?

The Language Examination

Aphasia is an acquired disturbance of language function, usually the result of a language-dominant hemispheric lesion. The aphasic patient requires a detailed assessment of language function. The language examination includes tests for spontaneous speech, repetition, naming, comprehension of written and spoken words, reading, writing, and praxis. Each phase of language function is tested first with common, easy tasks. If the patient completes them successfully, she is given more difficult language tasks until the threshold of error for each task is reached.

Spontaneous Speech

Eight characteristics of spontaneous speech can be assessed: 1) rate of output; 2) rhythm, inflection, and prosody (emotional expression or "sing-songiness"); 3) pronunciation; 4) effort; 5) press of speech; 6) phrase length; 7) paraphasias; and 8) word content. Nonfluent aphasias are characterized by sparse output (fewer than 50 words per minute), much effort, poor articulation, dysprosody, short phrase length, and use of substantive words. Fluent aphasias feature normal or increased word output (100 to 200 words per minute), often with press of speech, normal pronunciation, prosody, and phrase length, but with paraphasias, idiosyncratic, newly created words substitute for the intended word by the aphasic patient.

Repetition

The ability to correctly repeat spoken phrases is impaired in most aphasias. Patients are asked to repeat phrases of increasing difficulty, beginning with "hello," "today is Tuesday," and "down to earth." They are then challenged with more improbable phrases, such as "the fox slept on the bush." Finally, they are given the most difficult phrase of all: "no ifs, ands, or buts." Mildly aphasic patients may correctly repeat the simple phrases but fail to repeat the low-probability phrases. The phrase "no ifs, ands, or buts" is difficult for aphasic patients to repeat because it uses as nouns three words ordinarily used as conjunctions.

Naming

The ability to name common objects (word-finding) is almost universally impaired in aphasia. Patients are asked to name common articles of clothing worn by the examiner, body parts, or common objects. If a patient can name common objects, the examiner asks her to name less common objects, such as parts of a wristwatch (crystal, face, band, stem). An inability to name (dysnomia) may be seen in nonaphasic disorders, particularly in acute delirium.

Comprehension

Posterior aphasias impair the comprehension of spoken or written words to varying degrees. Comprehension is difficult to test in the aphasic patient because verbal and performance measures of successful comprehension may be impaired even when comprehension is intact. The nonfluently aphasic patient with intact comprehension cannot respond verbally to the examiner's questions, leading the unwary examiner to suspect a comprehension disturbance. The apraxic aphasic patient with intact comprehension may not be able to follow the examiner's commands, producing similar conclusions in the unwary. Spoken comprehension is properly tested by having the patient respond to the question with a nonverbal simple gesture. She can be asked to point to the object named by the examiner in a group of assembled common objects (safety pin, rubber band, paper clip, key, thumb tack, penny, nickel, dime, quarter) or asked to point to objects in the room (window, door, ceiling, floor). Written comprehension can be tested by telling the patient to follow a command that the examiner has written on a card—without reading it aloud first. The examiner can write "close your eyes," "raise your hands," or "open your mouth."

Reading

The patient is asked to read aloud sentences in a magazine after the examiner ascertains that she can see the letters with proper refraction. If the patient can read the sentences aloud, she can then be asked to explain their meaning. Inability to read is termed alexia.

Writing

Agraphia, the inability to write, is just as common in aphasia as is the inability to speak. Written word output usually follows speech word output. Verbally nonfluent patients with anterior lesions write with poorly formed letters, reduced output, and retained substantive words—in short, graphical nonfluency. Similarly, verbally fluent patients are also graphically fluent with lengthy, wordy sentences and frequent paraphasias. The examiner can dictate simple sentences for the patient to print or write, allowing for clumsiness if the nondominant hand is used because of paresis of the dominant hand. Patients should not be asked to sign their name because this overlearned act frequently survives the aphasic insult and is not diagnostically useful.

Praxis

The patient is asked to use his left hand to "show me how you brush your teeth, ...comb your hair, ...salute, ...wave good-bye." Inability to perform these learned acts properly despite intact hearing, comprehension, strength, and coordination is termed apraxia. Left hemiapraxia if often seen in anterior aphasias.

Screening Mental Status Testing

The preceding tests are time consuming and subject to varied interpretations. A statistically validated rapid screening mental status examination, called the Mini-Mental State, has been devised by Marshall Folstein and colleagues. It can sensitively assess mental status in only five to ten minutes, and its results have been correlated with diagnostic syndromes. It is useful in assessing patients with cognitive impairment except those with severe aphasia. The format for the Mini-Mental State examination is presented in Table 1.

The highest possible total score on the Mini-Mental State examination is 30. Its originators found that normal patients, including the elderly, scored 25 to 30; depressed or neurotic patients, 20 to 30; and demented patients, usually below 20. The test is useful for rapid dementia screening and for serial use in a delirious patient.

Table 1

Mini Mental State Examination

Maximum Score	Score	
Orientation		
5	( )	What is the (year) (season) (date) (day) (month)?
5	( )	Where are we (state) (town) (country) (hospital floor)?
Registration		
3	( )	Name 3 objects (1 second to say each). Then ask the patient all 3 after you have said them. Give one point for each correct answer. Then repeat them until he learns all three.
Attention and Calculation		
5	( )	Serial 7s. One point for each correct. Stop after 5 answers. Alternatively, spell "world" backwards.
Recall		
3	( )	Ask for the three objects repeated above. Give 1 point for each correct.
Language		
9	( )	Name a pencil and watch (2 points) Repeat: "No ifs, ands, or buts" (1 point) Follow a three-stage command: "Take a paper in your right hand, fold it in half, and put it on the floor." (3 points) Read and obey: "Close your eyes." (1 point) Write a sentence. (1 point) Copy a design. (1 point)
Total Score	____	

Folstein MF, Folstein FE, McHugh PR. Mini mental state. J Psychiatr Res. *1975;12:189-198.*

6. Cranial Nerves

Olfactory Nerve (I)

The olfactory nerves subserve the sense of smell and are a direct extension of the central nervous system (CNS) from the limbic region to the olfactory mucosa. Olfaction is tested by presenting an odoriferous substance to the patient with eyes closed—testing each nostril separately—and asking if he or she can smell and recognize the substance. The best test substances have an aroma but are not pungent. A bottle of oil of wintergreen or one containing solid cloves is a useful test substance. Pungent substances (eg, ammonia) irritate the nasal mucosa, stimulating the trigeminal nerve, which makes them inadequate tests of olfaction. Commercial olfactory tests using scratch-and-sniff cards are widely available.

The most common causes of anosmia are obstructive, and include occluded nasal passages from upper respiratory infection and deviated septum. Nonobstructive causes include occipital head trauma in which anosmia is often bilateral and permanent, vitamin B_{12} deficiency, and tabes dorsalis. Unilateral nonobstructive, nontraumatic anosmia suggests an olfactory groove meningioma. Olfaction is reduced in Alzheimer disease, Parkinson disease, and other neurodegenerative disorders.

Optic Nerve (II)

The visual system, including eyes, optic nerves, optic tracts, optic radiations, and visual cortex are usually tested as a whole. A lesion of any one anatomic component produces a predictable pattern of impairment of visual acuity or visual fields, as shown in Figure 1.

The examiner begins by inspecting the surface of the visual apparatus and continues inspection by funduscopic examination. The lens is examined for opacities by setting the ophthalmoscope at positive 5 or 6 diopters and holding it several inches from the patient's cornea. Then the optic fundus is examined with the ophthalmoscope set at 0 to negative 4 diopters, depending upon the refraction of patient and physician.

The examiner should inspect the optic disc and optic cup. The disc is normally a pale pink color and the cup is a paler pink. The cup is 1 or 2 diopters in depth, the disc margins are normally sharp, and the temporal border more well-defined than the nasal. Arteries and veins can be inspected as they cross the disc margin. Normally, 16 to 22 vascular structures can be counted, with an artery-to-vein ratio of 3:5.

Figure 1

Visual field defects resulting from lesions in different regions of the visual system

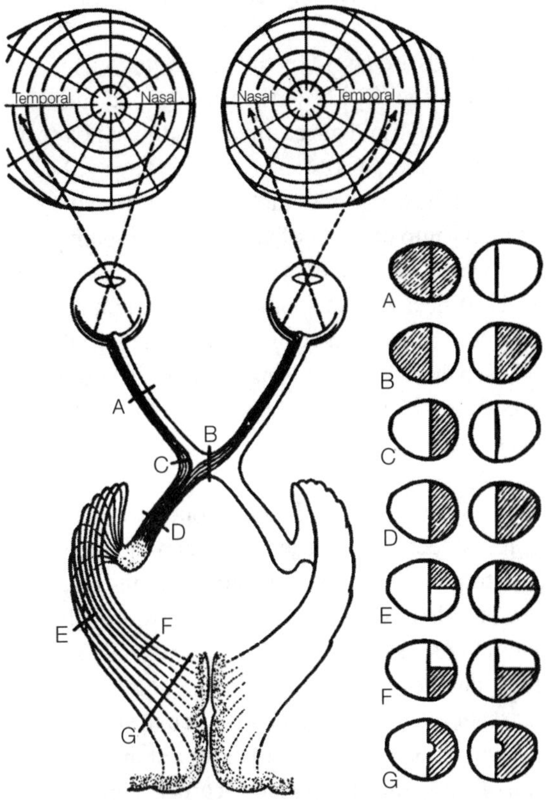

Homans JA. A Textbook of Surgery. *4th ed. Springfield, Ill: Chas. C. Thomas; 1932.*

Papilledema is said to be present when the disc margin is blurred, the normal spontaneous pulsations of the retinal veins are no longer seen, the vessel count across the disc margin exceeds 22, and the disc itself is raised above the surrounding retina by more than 1 diopter. Normal ophthalmic conditions, including drusen and myelinated nerve fibers, can be mistaken for papilledema. Optic atrophy is present when the disc is pale, slightly smaller than usual, has a very sharply defined outline, and has a smaller vessel count than normal.

Visual acuity is best tested with a standard Snellen chart at 20 feet, with each eye tested individually, using the best possible refractive correction. The patient may gaze through a pinhole if uncorrected myopia is present. A less adequate test is near visual acuity with a 14-inch pocket visual acuity card.

Visual fields are tested by the confrontation technique with each eye tested separately. The patient covers one eye and gazes directly at the opposite eye of the examiner, who stands 2 to 3 feet away. The examiner slowly moves the test object from the periphery into the field of vision and compares the point where the patient first acknowledges seeing the test object with the point that the examiner sees it. A small red test object (eg, a red match head) is most sensitive for disclosing subtle visual field defects. It is difficult but possible to plot the blind spots similarly.

For stuporous, confused, or uncooperative patients, the threat technique is used. The examiner makes a rapid flicking finger movement toward the patient's eye, quickly advancing sequentially from each quadrant of vision. A blink response usually signifies that the visual field is grossly intact. The examiner must take care to not touch the patient's eyelash or cornea, and not to move a standing column of air against the patient's cornea, thereby inducing a corneal blink reflex. Using another technique, the examiner stands behind the seated patient and quietly moves his hand from behind the patient's head into the periphery of his vision. The patient usually moves his eyes or head to gaze at the examiner's hand as soon as he can see it.

Visual fields are tested most accurately by formal means using a tangent screen or perimeter. The tangent screen examines the fields out to 30 degrees and is sufficiently sensitive to disclose field defects due to CNS disease. The perimeter examines fields to 90 degrees; it can additionally disclose ocular abnormalities, such as constricted fields from glaucoma. Blind spots can be measured accurately with both techniques. Many machines eliminate poor visual fixation as a source of error. These machines also allow fields to be tested using different test object sizes and colors, to detect the subtlest abnormalities.

Oculomotor Nerve (III), Trochlear Nerve (IV), Abducens Nerve (VI)

Tests of cranial nerves III, IV, and VI are commonly performed together. These nerves leave the rostral brain stem, traverse the cavernous sinus, and enter the orbit through the superior orbital fissure to innervate the eyelid and the ocular muscles. Dysfunction of the III, IV, and VI nerve system can occur at the nuclear level in the brain stem by infarction, hemorrhage, or tumor; at the peripheral nerve level by nerve compression or infarction; at the neuromuscular junction level in myasthenia gravis; or at the muscle level in myopathic disorders, such as from thyroid disease. Complete assessment of III, IV, and VI nerve function includes testing pupillary reflexes, eye movements, and presence of ptosis and nystagmus.

Normal pupillary size is determined by the resting equilibrium between the sympathetic pupillodilating fibers and the parasympathetic pupilloconstricting fibers. The pupillary light reflex has the optic nerve as the afferent limb and the oculomotor nerve as efferent limb. The pupillary dark reflex has the optic nerve as the afferent limb and the eye sympathetics as the efferent limb. The anatomy of the system and sites of common defects are shown in Figure 2.

Pupillary size, roundness and symmetry are first observed. The pupil is usually 3.0 to 7.0 mm in diameter. It constricts to bright light, to accommodation, and with advancing age. Ordinarily, both pupils constrict consensually, even when a stimulus is applied to only one eye. Pupillary size is graded as follows:

<1.0 mm	Pinpoint
1.0 to 3.0mm	Small
3.0 to 7.0mm	Mid-position
>7.0 mm	Large

Physiologic anisocoria is a pupillary difference of less than 1.0 mm. True anisocoria is a pupillary difference greater than 1.0 mm.

Figure 2

Anatomy of papillary innervation

A. The parasympathetic pupilloconstrictor pathway. B. The sympathetic pupillodilator pathway

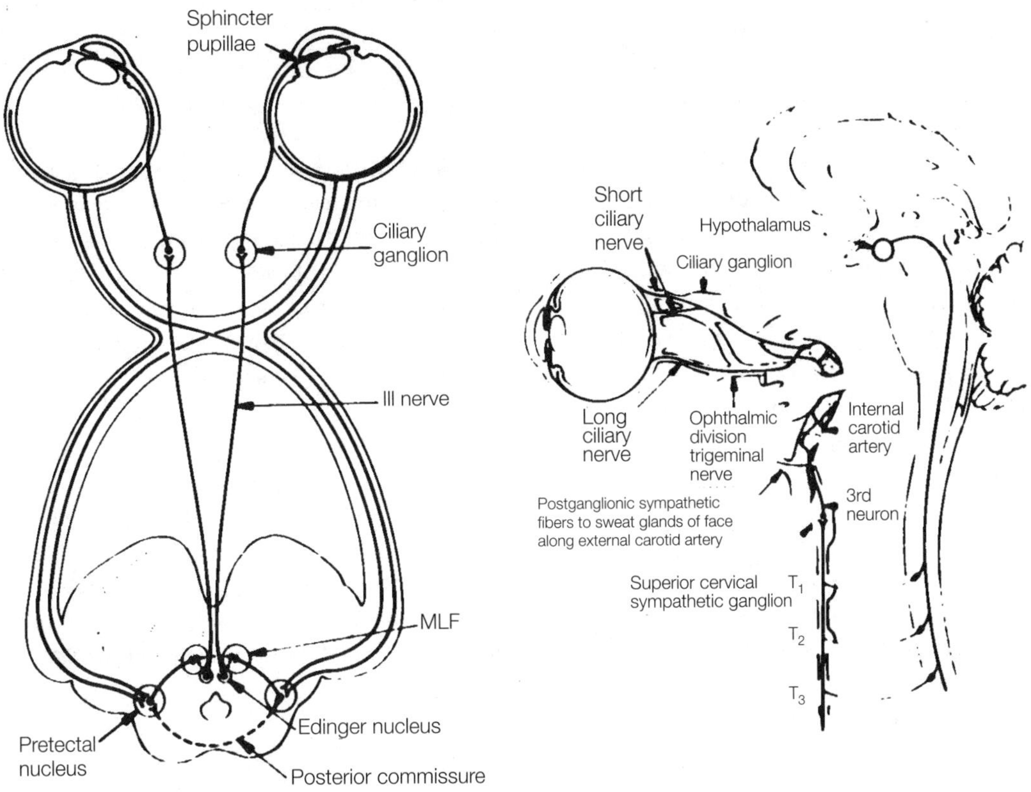

Plum F, Posner JB. The Diagnosis of Stupor and Coma. *3rd ed. Philadelphia, Pa: FA Davis; 1980:41.*

Pupillary light reflexes are tested by shining a point light source obliquely into one pupil and observing the rapidity and magnitude of the direct and consensual constriction. The light is not shined into the pupil from the direct front because the patient may attempt to focus on the flashlight, perhaps producing an accommodation response. Both the direct and consensual reactions should be assessed in each eye. Pupillary dark reflexes are tested in a darkened room to see if the pupils normally dilate. If anisocoria is present, the ambient light should be dimmed or the patient moved to a dark room, where it can be reassessed. In Horner syndrome, the small pupil will not dilate in darkness, while the normal pupil will dilate; thus, the anisocoria of Horner syndrome is amplified in darkness.

Pupillary reflex impairment can be the result of an afferent optic nerve lesion or to an efferent oculomotor nerve lesion. In the afferent optic nerve lesion caused by, say, optic neuritis, there is a loss or delay in both the direct and consensual light reflexes from that eye. There is a normal direct and consensual pupillary light reflex when light is shined into the unaffected eye. In an efferent oculomotor nerve lesion, the direct pupillary reflex is absent, but the consensual reflex persists. Shining the light in the unaffected pupil produces a direct but not a consensual reflex.

Pupillary reflexes to accommodation are part of the near reflex triad of convergence, pupilloconstriction, and change in lens shape for near vision. The patient is asked to look into the distance, then suddenly to focus on the examiner's finger, which is placed 10 to 15 inches from the patient's face. Detectable pupilloconstriction should be present during accommodation.

Several stereotyped pupillary abnormalities have been recognized in addition to the afferent and efferent pupillary lesions already described. The Argyll Robertson pupil is a small, slightly irregular pupil that constricts to accommodation but not to light. Tertiary syphilis was formerly the most common cause of Argyll Robertson pupils but now diabetes is a more common cause. Adie's, or tonic, pupil is a midposition pupil that constricts incompletely and very slowly to sustained light or accommodation stimuli. Generalized hyporeflexia commonly accompanies Adie's pupil(s). Horner's pupil is part of the miosis, ptosis, anhidrosis, and enophthalmos of Horner syndrome; it is caused by sympathetic denervation. Horner's pupil is small and reactive to light and accommodation but does not enlarge in darkness.

The presence of ptosis should be ascertained. There are two eyelid elevating muscles: 1) the levator palpebra, innervated by the oculomotor nerve, which is responsible for 90%-95% of eyelid elevation; and 2) Müller's muscle, innervated by the sympathetic nervous system, which is responsible for 5%-10% of elevation. Ptosis from a complete third nerve lesion is severe, with the eyelid drooped, completely covering the eye. Ptosis from a sympathetic nervous system lesion (ie, Horner syndrome) is mild, with a slight droop of the upper lid that covers more of the pupil than usual. Ptosis in myasthenia gravis and in ocular myopathies is usually of intermediate severity. Occasionally, ptosis can occur solely from a cerebral lesion.

Assessment of extraocular movements sensitively tests most functions of the third nerve and all functions of the fourth and sixth nerves. Each eye is moved horizontally, vertically, or in rotation by the action of the six extraocular muscles. The functions of the extraocular muscles are listed in Table 2; their anatomic relationships are shown in Figure 3.

Eye movements are tested best by having the patient gaze at a point light source about 3 feet away. The examiner can see the reflection of the light as a bright dot in the exact center of the patient's pupils during normal conjugate-gaze "fovealization" of an image. If the least dysconjugation occurs, the examiner can see the dot move off center in the affected eye.

Table 2

Functions of the Extraocular Muscles

Muscle	Cranial Nerve	Primary Function	Secondary Function
Lateral rectus	IV	Abduction	--
Medial rectus	III	Adduction	--
Inferior rectus	III	Depresses when eye abducted	Extorts when eye adducted
Superior rectus	III	Elevates when eye abducted	Intorts when eye adducted
Inferior oblique	III	Elevates when eye abducted	Extorts when eye abducted
Superior oblique	IV	Depresses when eye adducted	Intorts when eye abducted

Figure 3

Anatomy of the extraocular muscles

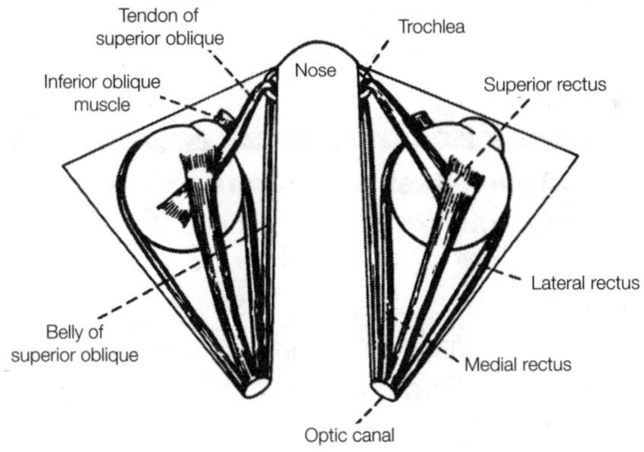

Joynt RJ. Clinical Neurology. *Philadelphia, Pa: Lippincott Harper & Row; 1989.*

Primary gaze is tested first, the examiner noting any ocular dysconjugation or nystagmus. Horizontal gaze is tested next by having the patient look laterally to his extreme right and then to his extreme left. Vertical gaze is tested by asking the patient to look up and then down with eyes laterally deviated to the right; the test is repeated with eyes deviated to the left. These maneuvers are illustrated in Figure 4.

In a complete left sixth nerve palsy, the affected eye is slightly adducted on primary gaze because of the loss of lateral rectus function. Right lateral gaze is normal. Left lateral gaze reveals normal adduction of the right eye, and failure of abduction of the left eye. Vertical gaze is normal. The patient experiences horizontal diplopia that is worse on left lateral gaze.

In a complete left third nerve palsy, the eye is abducted and depressed ("down and out") on primary gaze. This position is achieved because of the resulting vector of the resting tone of the two remaining innervated muscles, the lateral rectus (VI nerve) abducting the eye, and the superior oblique (IV nerve) depressing the eye. There is a failure of adduction because of medial rectus paresis, a loss of upward gaze because of superior rectus and inferior oblique paresis, and a loss of most downward gaze because of inferior rectus paresis. Additionally, there is profound ptosis because of loss of levator palpebra function, and a dilated, unreactive pupil because of parasympathetic denervation and unapposed sympathetic stimulation. With the eyelid held open, the patient has profound vertical and horizontal diplopia that is worse on attempted upward gaze and looking to the right.

In a complete left fourth nerve palsy, there is inability to depress the eye in the adducted position. Patients develop vertical diplopia, worst on attempted reading, which they learn can be compensated for somewhat by tilting (laterally flexing) their heads ("Bielchowsky's sign"). On testing, if the examiner asks them to tilt their head to the opposite side, the diplopia is worsened.

Figure 4

Actions of the extraocular muscles

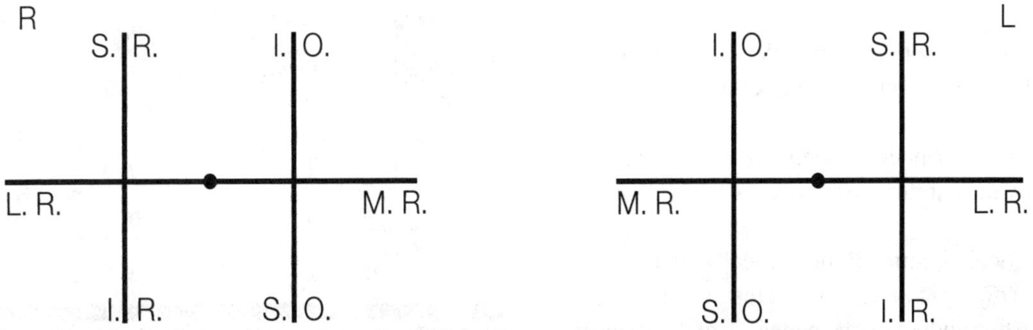

Mayo Clinic. Clinical Examinations in Neurology. *5th ed. Philadelphia Pa: Saunders; 1981.*

For the patient who complains of diplopia, the history itself may be diagnostic. The examiner should ask if the diplopia is horizontal, vertical, or both (diagonal). Is it worse on gaze to the left, right, up, or down? Is it worse for near vision (eg, reading) or far vision? Does it change character with changes in direction of gaze?

In the case of a left sixth nerve palsy, the patient should report that the diplopia is horizontal, worse on attempted left lateral gaze, and worse for far vision. Purely horizontal diplopia limits the dysfunction to the left or right medial or lateral rectus muscles. The fact that the diplopia is worse on left lateral gaze further limits the dysfunction to the left lateral rectus or right medial rectus muscles. If the diplopia is worse on far gaze, the left lateral rectus muscle must be involved because it is more necessary for far gaze, while the medial rectus is more necessary for near gaze. Thus, is some cases, the weak muscle can be adduced merely by a careful history.

The examination for diplopia is directed toward the identification of the weak extraocular muscle(s). If the examiner cannot be confident which muscle is weak by the flashlight following test, the red glass test is performed. The examiner covers one of the patient's eyes with a red transparent glass or plastic cover and asks him to look at a flashlight point light source. Ordinarily, one red-and-white image is seen. In diplopia, the images are separated; one red and one white. Using the red glass test, the examiner can determine from which eye each image is produced. The examiner tests all nine cardinal fields of gaze, with results as shown in Figure 5.

There are several rules of thumb for identifying the affected eye and muscle:

1. The distance between diplopic images increases in the direction of action of the paretic muscle.

2. The more peripherally-lying image is that produced by the paretic eye.

3. In vertical diplopia, if the vertical distance between diplopic images is greatest with the affected eye abducted, the paresis is of the inferior or superior rectus; if the vertical distance between diplopic images is greatest with the eye adducted, the paresis is of inferior or superior oblique muscles.

Figure 5

The red glass test to evaluate extraocular muscle paralysis

A. Right lateral rectus palsy; B. Right medial rectus palsy; C. Right inferior rectus palsy; D. Right superior rectus palsy; E. Right superior oblique palsy; F. Right inferior oblique palsy.

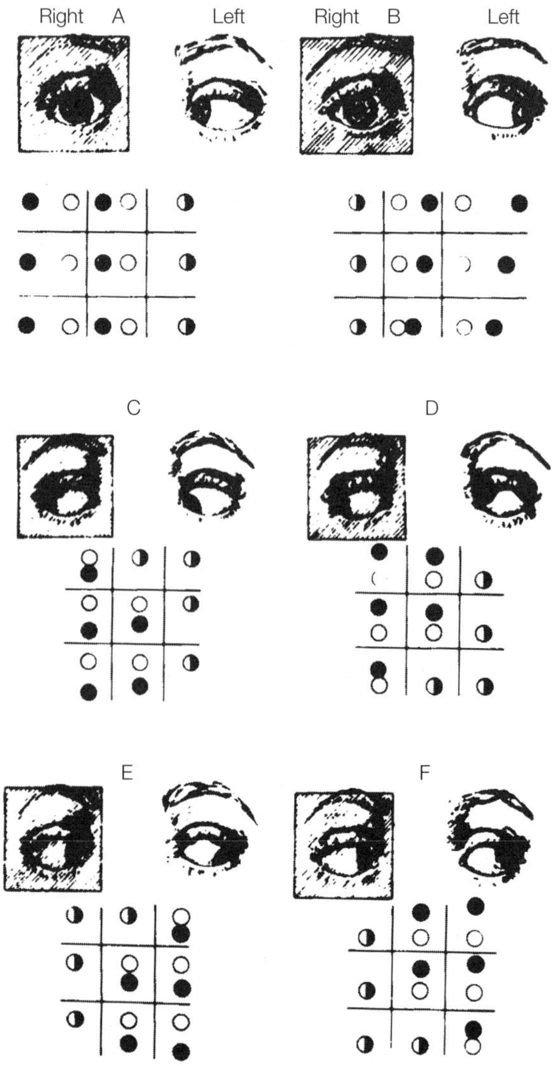

Cogan DG. Neurology of the Ocular Muscles. *2nd ed. Springfield, Ill: Charles C. Thomas; 1978.*

Table 3

Nystagmus

Category	Characteristics	Cause
Peripheral vestibular imbalance	Horizontal or rotary; suppressed by fixation; worsened by head movement; impaired caloric response	Labyrinth
Central vestibular	Vertical, horizontal or rotary; poorly suppressed by fixation; smooth pursuit impaired	Central vestibular dysfunction
Gaze-evoked	Induced by eccentric eye positions; seen best in darkness; pursuit deficit; rebound nystagmus	Seen in myesthenia gravis and eye paresis
Rebound	Evoked by sustained eccentric gaze	Neural mechanism
Disassociated	Nystagmus different in each eye (eg, internuclear ophthalmoplegia)	Unknown
Congenital	Horizontal, conjugate, variable amplitude; accompanied by head shaking; worse with attention and arousal	Blindness in some cases
Latent	Conjugate; evoked by covering one eye; the other eye drifts towards the nose	Unknown
Acquired pendular	No fast or slow component; has both	Cerebellar dysfunction in multiple sclerosis and palatal myoclonus
Voluntary	Rapid oscillation at 15-25 Hz; tending to coverage	Voluntary
Pursuit	Solely horizontal or vertical; low velocity drift	Lesions of parietal lobes or cerebellum
Rare forms	Consult Leigh and Zee	

Leigh RJ, Zee DS. The Neurology of Eye Movements. *Philadelphia, Pa: Davis; 1983:192-193.*

4. If the primary function of an eye muscle cannot be assessed, the examiner should try to assess its secondary function. For example, the detection of a fourth nerve paresis in the setting of a third nerve paresis is difficult because the eye cannot be adducted (due to medial rectus paresis) to permit testing depression, the primary action of the superior oblique muscle. But because the fourth nerve is secondarily an intorter in the abducted position, attempted adduction-depression movements intort the eye in the presence of intact fourth nerve function.

Nystagmus should be assessed. By convention, the direction of the nystagmus is said to be in the direction of the fast component. Nystagmus may be purely horizontal, purely vertical, or rotatory. Types and causes of nystagmus are listed in Table 3.

The patient with a congenital strabismus may confound the examination of extraocular muscle function. Ordinarily, despite marked ocular dysconjugation, such patients do not complain of diplopia, because long ago they have suppressed the superfluous image. A fixed eye muscle imbalance (tropia) is usually obvious to the examiner. More vexing is the phoria ("lazy eye"), a latent imbalance that becomes manifest when visual loss or states of generalized illness interrupt the fusion mechanism promoting conjugate binocular vision and, as a result, ocular disconjugation and diplopia become present.

The patient with strabsimus has normal eye movements when each eye is tested individually. Only when the eyes are tested together is the dysconjugate gaze observed. Phorias can be detected by the cover test. The patient looks at an object on the wall and the examiner covers one eye, then the other. The phoria is made manifest when binocular vision is interrupted by covering the eye. The patient's affected eye is seen to move quickly from its abnormal resting position to look directly at the object, once it is uncovered.

Trigeminal Nerve (V)

The trigeminal nerve has both motor and somatic sensory functions. It arises from the pons, wherein the motor nuclei lie, whereas the sensory nuclei reside in the Gasserian ganglion. The trigeminal nerve divides into ophthalmic (first), maxillary (second), and mandibular (third) divisions (Figure 6). The first division supplies sensation to the cornea and to the forehead and frontal scalp to the vertex of the head. The second division supplies sensation to the cheeks, nose, upper teeth, and palate. The third division supplies sensation to the lower teeth, mandible, tongue, and ear, and provides innervation to the muscles of mastication.

Figure 6

Trigeminal nerve sensory distribution

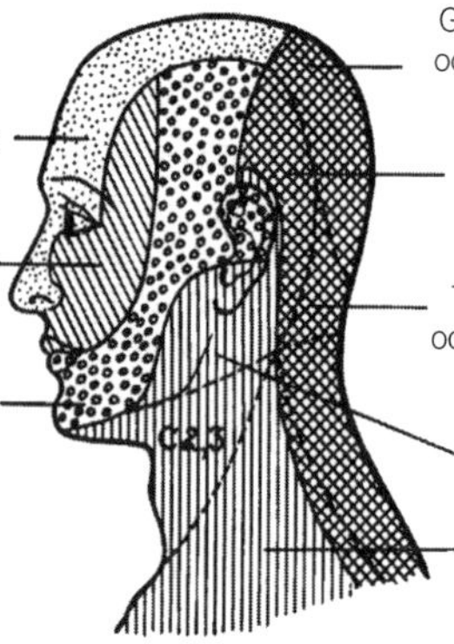

Brash JC. Cunningham's Textbook of Anatomy. *9th ed. New York, NY: Oxford; 1956.*

Examination of the motor function of the trigeminal nerve begins with observation of the temporalis muscles for evidence of hollowing. Palpation of the masseter muscle bulk can be performed with the patient clenching his teeth. The strength of the bite can be tested by having the patient bite down unilaterally on a tongue depressor placed between the molar teeth. The patient then slowly opens his jaw and the examiner looks for evidence of jaw deviation. In unilateral pterygoid weakness, the jaw deviates toward the side of the weak muscle. The examiner can then push laterally against the jaw as the patient opposes the force.

Sensation is tested with pin, light touch, vibration, position, and temperature stimuli, as discussed in the section "Sensory Examination." The corneal reflex has the trigeminal nerve as the afferent limit and the facial nerve as the efferent limb. A light wisp of cotton is used as a stimulus. The tapered end of a sterile cotton-tipped applicator, twisted to a cotton point, is an ideal stimulus. The patient is asked to gaze to his left. The examiner then approaches the right eye from the right side and briefly touches the cotton tip on the right conjunctiva. This serves as a control stimulus because some people are so sensitive to touch anywhere about the eye that they blink even in response to this stimulus. Ordinarily there should be no blink because conjunctival stimulation does not elicit the reflex. The examiner then touches the right cornea and assesses the strength of the blink reflex. The process is repeated on the left with the eyes directed to the right and the examiner approaching from the left. The patient can be asked to compare the perceived sensations of the two stimuli.

Facial Nerve (VII)

The facial nerve has motor, parasympathetic, somatic sensory, and special sensory functions. The nerve arises from the pons, travels with the eighth nerve through the internal auditory canal, then through the facial canal in the temporal bone, and exits the skull through the stylomastoid foramen. The motor portion innervates the muscles of facial expression and the stapedius muscle in the middle ear. The somatic sensory portion conducts sensation from a portion of the external ear canal and the mastoid region. The special sensory portion carries taste sensation from the anterior two-thirds of the tongue by way of the chorda tympani nerve. The parasympathetic portion permits lacrimation by way of the superficial petrosal nerve and salivation by way of the chorda tympani.

Motor function of the facial nerve is tested first by observation of the patient's facies at rest, with spontaneous emotional expression, and with commands to "close your eyes," "raise your eyebrows," "blow out your cheeks," and "purse your lips." Subtle asymmetries in the depth of nasolabial folds, palpebral fissures, and the position of the corners of the mouth are sought. The symmetry of the platysma should be observed as the patient attempts to growl. The strength of the orbicularis oculi and orbicularis ori may be tested by the examiner forcefully attempting to open the patient's eyes and mouth with the patient opposing these actions.

Taste sensation on the anterior two-thirds of the tongue can be tested with solutions of salt or sugar painted on the lateral aspects of the outstretched tongue. The patient shakes his head "yes" or "no" to indicate whether the solution can be tasted—before bringing the tongue back into the mouth. Somatic sensation is not ordinarily tested because of the facial sensory overlap of nerves V and IX and because of individual variation. Lacrimation can be tested with Schirmer's paper. Stapedius paralysis produces auditory hyperacusis, which can be determined by standard hearing tests, described under the discussion of cranial nerve VIII.

Facial hemiparesiscan be caused by a facial nerve lesion (lower motor neuron) such as in Bell's palsy, or by a supranuclear lesion (upper motor neuron) such as contralateral corticobulbar tract damage from hemispheric stroke. The upper half of the face receives bilateral supranuclear innervation to each facial nerve nucleus, whereas the lower half receives only unilateral supranuclear innervation. In an upper motor neuron lesion, there is only a lower-half paresis of the contralateral facial muscles, whereas in a facial nerve lesion, the entire ipsilateral half of the face is paretic. The strength of the orbicularis oculus muscle is the key to making the distinction. There is trace weakness of this muscle in an upper motor neuron facial hemiparesis, but profound weakness in a facial nerve lesion such as Bell's palsy.

Bell's palsy can impair other functions of the facial nerve in addition to causing facial muscular paresis, depending upon the location of the lesion. Consequently, the patient should be tested for taste, lacrimation, and auditory hyperacusis to survey whether these facial nerve functions are also affected.

Vestibuloacoustic Nerve (VIII)

The vestibuloacoustic nerve transmits the special sensations of hearing and balance from the inner ear to the brain stem. The vestibuloacoustic nerve has a division for each function: the cochlear division for hearing and the vestibular for balance.

Hearing is tested clinically by placing a sound stimulus of known loudness and pitch before each ear. A softly ticking watch is an adequate stimulus, but a 512 Hz tuning fork is better because it has a high pitch and can identify subtle hearing loss that especially affects high-frequency sounds. Furthermore, loudness can be regulated, and the patient's ability to hear can be compared with the examiner's ability. If unilateral hearing loss is detected, Weber's test can help classify the hearing loss as conductive or sensorineural. A 128 Hz tuning fork is sounded and placed in the center of the patient's forehead. If the unilateral hearing loss is conductive, the sound induced by the vibrating tuning fork will be heard louder in the affected ear. If the hearing loss is sensorineural, the sound will be louder in the normal ear.

The Rinne test measures the efficacy of air conduction of sound versus bone conduction. A 128 Hz tuning fork is sounded and placed on the mastoid process. The patient is instructed to indicate when he can no longer hear the sound. Then, the still vibrating tuning fork is placed next to the patient's ear and he is again asked to indicate when he no longer hears the sound. Because air conduction is greater than bone conduction, the time the patient can hear the tuning fork by air conduction should be twice the time it can be heard by bone conduction. If air conduction time is less than twice bone conduction time, a conductive etiology to the hearing loss is suspected.

The precise pattern and often the etiology of hearing loss can be determined by formal audiometry. Standard pure-tone audiograms can be supplemented with more sophisticated tests to differentiate cochlear versus retrocochlear lesions as well as types of conductive loss.

The vestibular division is not specifically tested in a general neurological examination, except when looking for nystagmus and for the extent to which the vestibular system contributes to coordination and gait. Vestibular imbalance produces vertigo or a sensation of movement. Nystagmus or positional nystagmus may be present in such cases.

Glossopharyngeal Nerve (IX), Vagus Nerve (X)

The glossopharyngeal and vagus nerves are usually tested together. The former carries motor fibers from the medulla to the stylopharyngeus muscle, conducts somatic sensory input from the middle ear and eustachian tube, provides special sensory taste input from the posterior one-third of the tongue, and regulates parasympathetic secretory activity of the parotid gland. The vagus nerve conducts somatic motor impulses from the medulla to the pharynx, soft palate, and larynx; autonomic impulses to the heart, esophagus, stomach, and small intestine; somatic sensation from the ear; and special visceral sensation from thoracic and abdominal viscera.

Ninth and tenth nerve testing begins with listening to the patient's voice. Pharyngeal paralysis increases the nasal quality of the voice. Unilateral vocal cord paralysis produces hoarseness. Bilateral vocal cord lesions produce a voice of reduced intensity, with an inability to make high-pitched sounds. Bilateral vocal cord paralysis in the abducted position produces cough, inspiratory stridor, and a brassy voice quality. Direct or indirect laryngoscopy can be performed by an otolaryngologist in cases of unexplained voice change to evaluate vocal cord movement.

The palate is examined as the patient says "Ahh." In unilateral pharyngeal weakness, the uvula and median raphe are deviated away from the paretic side to the normal side. Patients can be asked to repeat "ga-ga-ga" and "ka-ka-ka."

The swallowing of water is observed. Dysphagia is present with bilateral ninth and tenth nerve lesions (bulbar palsy) or with bilateral supranuclear corticobulbar lesions to these brain stem motor nuclei (pseudobulbar palsy). Swallowed fluids may be regurgitated through the nose in bilateral lesions of the ninth and tenth nerves.

The gag reflex is tested by touching each posterolateral pharyngeal wall sequentially with a wooden tongue blade. The normal response is contraction of the pharyngeal muscles, usually with gagging.

Lesions of both ninth and tenth nerves produce loss of the gag reflex. Supranuclear corticobulbar lesions often have an exaggerated gag reflex.

It is possible, but difficult, to test taste on the posterior one-third of the tongue, in a way that is analogous to taste testing for the facial nerve. Most clinicians omit this test because it is very difficult to place the gustatory stimulus solution on the outstretched posterior one-third of the tongue without the solution diffusing onto the taste buds inside the mouth.

The syndrome of pseudobulbar palsy results from bilateral corticobulbar tract lesions, most often caused by strokes, motor neuron disease, or multiple sclerosis. The patient with pseudobulbar palsy has dysphagia, dysarthria, dysphonia, hyperactive gag reflexes, hyperactive jaw jerk, and often exhibits pathological crying. Pseudobulbar palsy is an upper motor neuron paralysis of pharyngeal and laryngeal functions whose lower motor neurons are the ninth and tenth nerves.

This purely motor nerve, innervating the sternocleidomastoid and trapezius muscles, arises in the upper cervical spinal cord, ascends through the foramen magnum, and exits through the jugular foramen with the ninth and tenth nerves. Unilateral accessory nerve lesions produce paralysis, atrophy, and fasciculations of the ipsilateral sternocleidomastoid and trapezius muscles. Upper motor neuron lesions produce only mild weakness because of bilateral supranuclear innervation, analogous to the upper face.

The examiner notes the size, shape, and symmetry of the sternocleidomastoid and trapezius muscles; both muscles can be palpated easily. Trapezius power is tested by having the patient shrug the shoulders against the examiner's resistance. Sternocleidomastoid power is tested by having the patient turn his head in the direction opposite from the muscle tested, a useful point in the detection of factitious illness. However, many patients with acute hemispheric lesions lose ipsilateral function of the accessory nerve and have weakness in head turning in the direction opposite of the hemispheric lesion. Bilateral sternocleidomastoid muscle weakness, such as that seen in patients with myopathies, produces weakness in neck flexion with intact extension.

Hypoglossal Nerve (XII)

The hypoglossal nerve is a purely motor nerve that innervates the tongue. It arises in the medulla and passes through the hypoglossal foramen. It has primarily unilateral supranuclear control. Hypoglossal nerve lesions produce unilateral tongue weakness, atrophy, fasciculations, and dysarthria.

The examiner first observes the size and symmetry of the tongue as it rests on the floor of the mouth. Fasciculations should be sought in this position. The patient then protrudes the tongue. When there is weakness, the tongue deviates to the paretic side. Tongue deviation is usually more prominent in lower motor neuron lesions than in upper motor neuron lesions. The patient then pushes his tongue against the inside of his cheek while the examiner opposes this attempt with pressure on the outside of the cheek. The patient pronounces complicated phrases such as "Methodist-Episcopal," "Commonwealth of Massachusetts," and repetitive lingual syllables such as "la-la-la..." and "the-the-the..." while the examiner listens for dysarthria.

7. Motor

A complete motor examination includes tests and observations to assess muscle symmetry, size, shape, tone, and power; adventitious muscle movements; muscle coordination; mechanical muscle reactions; and muscle tendon reflexes. Examination of reflexes and coordination will be discussed in other sections of this chapter.

Size, Shape, and Symmetry

The motor exam begins with the inspection of the limb and trunk musculature for evidence of atrophy and hypertrophy. Subtle degrees of asymmetric limb atrophy may be established by measuring limb girths with a tape measure (at a constant distance proximal or distal to a joint) and comparing measurements. The patient's dominant arm may be 1 to 2 cm greater in circumference than his nondominant arm; asymmetries greater than 2 cm are significant.

Adventitious Movements

The limbs are inspected for evidence of involuntary, spontaneous, adventitious movements. Fasciculations are spontaneous synchronous contractions of the muscle fibers of a single motor unit as a result of denervation. They appear as minor muscle twitches not sufficiently strong to move a limb or to be obvious to the patient. They are seen in all denervating disease of the lower motor neuron, but particularly in diseases of spinal cord anterior horn cells. Myokymia is a continuous, regular, undulating, rippling fasciculation, usually of no pathologic significance. Fibrillations are contractions of individual muscle fibers, also the result of denervation. Because an individual muscle fiber is so small, fibrillations usually cannot be seen or felt, except in the tongue. They can be detected easily by electromyography, however. Tremor is a rhythmic, oscillatory dyskinesia, usually the result of sequential involuntary contractions of agonist and then antagonist muscles.

Chorea is a sudden, jerky, discrete, brief, irregular, purposeless, involuntary movement seen most often in the limbs and face. The amplitude of the dyskinesia is sufficient to move the part of the body affected. Choreiform movements occur in an unpredictable pattern and disappear with sleep. The affected patient will often attempt to incorporate the choreiform movement into an ostensibly voluntary movement. A sudden jerk of the patient's hand in the air may be followed by a voluntary smoothing down of the back of the hair, as if the entire movement was a volitional gesture. Chorea is seen most often in Huntington disease, Sydenham chorea, side effects of medication (oral contraceptives, levodopa), and unilaterally after strokes to the contralateral corpus striatum.

Athetosis is a distal, gross, slow, continuous, writhing movement in which there are varying degrees of tonic contraction of antagonistic muscles pulling the limb, face, or trunk in slow, contorted activity. It frequently coexists with chorea (choreoathetosis) in the disorders named above because both reflect damage to the corpus striatum. It is also seen as a type of cerebral palsy resulting from perinatal injury. Pseudoathetosis is a wavering, searching movement of the outstretched hands resulting from loss of proprioceptive input; it resembles true athetosis only superficially.

Ballismus is a sudden, rapid, violent, involuntary flailing or flinging of a limb that requires so much muscular exertion that it exhausts the patient. It is often seen unilaterally involving an arm and leg, contralateral to a stroke in the subthalamic nucleus. It is often associated with hemichorea.

Dystonia is a tonic, sustained involuntary muscular contraction of sufficient force to hold the affected body part in a "frozen," twisted, and contorted state. The basal ganglia is the site of dysfunction in the dystonias. Torticollis is a dystonia of the sternocleidomastoid muscles and sometimes other neck muscles. Dystonia musculorum deformans is a hereditary dystonia. Limb dystonias and the eye dystonia, oculogyric crisis, commonly are seen as an idiosyncratic reaction to the first dose of a neuroleptic drug. Intravenous diphenhydramine (Benadryl®) or benztropine mesylate (Cogentin®) will quickly reverse neuroleptic-induced dystonia. Blepharospasm, another focal dystonia, often is associated with oromandibular dystonia (Meige syndrome).

Myoclonus is a sudden, rapid muscle contraction of variable intensity. Multifocal myoclonus is an important sign of metabolic encephalopathy. It is commonly present in uremia and in hypoxic encephalopathies after cardiac arrest. Nocturnal myoclonus, especially of the legs, awakens affected patients many times nightly and disturbs sleep. The hypnic jerk is a single, synchronous myoclonic jerk that occurs normally as a person drifts off to sleep, particularly after an exhausting day. Palatal myoclonus is not true myoclonus, but a continuous tremor of the palate caused by brain stem-cerebellar disease of the pathways between the inferior olive, dentate nucleus and red nucleus. It is the only type of tremor that persists during sleep.

Asterixis or "flap," is an irregular, asynchronous movement of outstretched limbs in the patient with a metabolic encephalopathy. When asked to hold hands or feet outstretched, the muscle suddenly loses tone; this is followed by a compensatory movement to return the limb to its outstretched position. It is often seen with tremor and multifocal myoclonus. Electrophysiologically, asterixis is an intermittent, sudden, brief lapse of extensor tone during which there is electromyographic silence for less than 200 msec. The flap occurs just after the lapse of extensor tone.

Tics or habit spasms are learned, stereotyped, compulsive, complex movements, often of the face, that are under partial voluntary control. Patients asked to supress them become anxious and are relieved only when they can resume performing the tic. In Gilles de la Tourette syndrome, tics reach a magnitude where they become socially and physically debilitating. There is partial improvement in Tourette syndrome tics with haloperidol (Haldol®).

Muscle Tone

The examiner tests muscle tone by assessing resistance to passive muscle stretching. The patient is instructed to "relax" and "go loose" to try to induce a state of resting muscle tone. Many anxious patients are unable to fully relax in this situation; further admonishment only makes the situation worse. Such patients should be given mental tasks to distract them during the assessment, such as to spell "world" backwards, or to count backwards from 80 by sevens.

While testing tone, the examiner notes the range of motion of the joints, the presence of contractures, and the induction of pain upon movement of the extremity. Resting tone can be described as normal, flaccid, spastic, or rigid. Normal resting tone produces the slightest resistance to passive stretch. In flaccidity, the limb is moved as dead weight with no opposition to movement. Flaccidity characterizes lower motor neuron syndrome when a lesion is present in the anterior horn cell of the spinal cord, peripheral nerve, root, or plexus.

Spasticity is caused by an upper motor neuron (corticospinal tract) lesion in which inhibitory descending control on the spinal reflex arc is eliminated. Hyperreflexia and increased muscle tone are produced by the dysinhibition of the spinal reflex arc. Spasticity is a velocity-dependent increase in muscle tone, which is maximal at the onset of motion and decreases during motion. The "clasp-knife" quality is thus produced and a "giving way" is felt in the muscle during stretching. In very mild degrees of spasticity, only the spastic "catch" can be felt by the examiner when rapidly extending and flexing the patient's wrist or pronating and supinating the patient's arm. In severe spasticity, the arm tends to be held in a flexed posture at the elbow and wrist while the leg is held in extension at the knee and hip.

Rigidity is an extrapyramidal sign in which increased muscle tone is found throughout the range of passive movement. There is simultaneous contraction of agonist and antagonist muscles, often with tremor superimposed, producing "cogwheel" or "ratchety" rigidity. Limb rigidity has been called "lead pipe" rigidity because of the increased tone throughout the range of movement.

A similar type of rigidity is seen in acute and chronic states of bilateral hemispheric dysfunction. Known as paratonia, it is marked by the patient's resistance to passive movement with an involuntary, antagonistic movement that is identical in force but opposite in direction to that made by the examiner.

Muscle Power

Testing the strength of individual muscles is a vital part of the neurological examination. It is necessary to identify the pattern of weakness to localize the disorder in the nervous system. For example, if only those muscles innervated by the radial nerve below the mid-humerus are weak, the disorder is probably a radial mononeuropathy.

Muscle strength is tested by one of two techniques: 1) the patient is asked to hold a limb in a particular position and the examiner attempts to move it; or 2) the examiner begins to move a patient's limb and asks the patient to resist it. Experience dictates normal responses for age and sex. Women are usually weaker than men, particularly in triceps power. Muscle power usually declines with age. The nondominant upper extremity is weaker than the dominant.

Muscle power is customarily quantified on a 0-to-5 scale as follows:

0 No contraction

1 Flicker or trace of contraction

2 Active movement with gravity eliminated

3 Active movement against gravity

4 Active movement against gravity and resistance

5 Normal power

To these numbers may be appended with "+" or "-" to further quantify power. Alternatively, the terms "slight, mild, moderate, and severe" weakness may be applied.

Subtle degrees of muscle weakness may be appreciated by testing for "drift." The patient extends both arms with hands supinated and eyes closed. In mild states of unilateral weakness, particularly in pyramidal lesions, there is a slow descent of the involved arm and pronation of the hand. In cases of factitious weakness, drift without pronation may be seen. Patients with parietal lobe lesions affecting proprioceptive integration may elevate the affected hand when the eyes are closed.

Mechanical Muscle Reaction

Muscles should be palpated for consistency and tenderness. Increased consistency, with a feeling like hard rubber, is seen in muscular dystrophy and other primary myopathies. Muscle tenderness may be present in acute polymyositis, trichinosis, and viral myopathies. Denervating diseases and injuries produce muscles that are flabby and flaccid.

Muscle percussion normally induces the idiomuscular, or myotatic, response, a brief contraction that is akin to a deep-tendon reflex. This response is often absent in primary muscle diseases. If percussion of muscle induces a contraction that is sustained for several seconds or longer, percussion myotonia is said to be present. The muscles usually tested are the thenar eminence and the tongue. Contraction myotonia can be tested by having the patient sustain a contraction, then suddenly make a movement opposite to the contraction. For example, the patient squeezes his fingers tightly around the examiner's fingers for five seconds, then suddenly extends all his fingers. If myotonia is present, there is a delayed and difficult finger extension that can take five seconds or longer. Myotonia is seen in myotonic dystrophy, myotonia congenita, and other primary diseases of muscle.

Myoedema is an unusual response of muscle to percussion, in which localized swelling persists for several seconds at the site of percussion. This finding has been described in severe hypothyroidism and other chronic illness.

8. Sensory

The sensory examination is the most tedious, subjective, and variable part of the examination of the nervous system. Many examiners perform it at the end of an already lengthy exam when both the patient and examiner are tired. Because the examination is totally subjective—with the results depending entirely upon the patient's perception of the applied stimuli— patients who are suggestible, histrionic, or embellishing can mislead the examiner. An adequate sensory examination requires an attentive and cooperative patient.

Testable sensory modalities can be divided into two groups: 1) the "primary" sensations of pain, temperature, light touch, vibration, and position; and 2) the "secondary," or higher cortical, sensations of stereognosis, barognosis, graphesthesia, two-point discrimination, and double simultaneous stimulation. The primary group requires the nervous system to be intact from the periphery to the thalamus; the secondary group requires intact thalamocortical connections as well.

There is an important anatomic separation of the primary sensory modalities that becomes important in assessment. At the peripheral nerve level, vibration and position sensations are carried along the heavily myelinated A fibers, whereas pain is carried by the unmyelinated C fibers. At the level of the spinal cord, the pain and temperature fibers ascend crossed in the lateral spinothalamic tracts. The fibers for position and vibration ascend uncrossed in the posterior columns. At the brain stem level, the pain and temperature fibers ascend in the spinothalamic tracts of the lateral lemniscus, whereas the position and vibration fibers form the medical lemniscus.

There are several principles of sensory examination. A screening exam is performed first over the trunk and limbs. Specific areas are tested further in detail if the patient's complaint is from that area (eg, "my hands are numb"), or if the screening exam reveals an abnormality in that area. When a zone of decreased sensation is detected, the examiner should attempt to delineate the boundaries of the abnormality by marching repetitive sensory stimuli from the abnormal to the normal zones of sensation. Finally, if the primary modalities are markedly abnormal in an area, there is not much to be gained by testing the secondary modalities there.

Focal sensory abnormalities are discerned by comparison to zones of normal sensation on the patient. For lateralized abnormalities, comparison of sensation with homologous body regions is carried out. The patient is instructed to report only significant differences in perception of sensory stimuli.

Primary Sensory Modalities

Light Touch

Light touch is tested with a wisp of cotton applied to the skin in a nonrhythmic way. The patient closes his eyes and says "now" or "touch" when he perceives the light touch. The examiner should avoid stroking hairs because a stimulus of greater than intended magnitude is produced.

Pain

Pain sensation is best tested with an unused safety pin applied just to the point of being noxious but not to the point of piercing the skin or drawing blood. The clinician should never use the same safety pin between patients because it can carry transmissible diseases (eg, HIV, hepatitis B). Many neurologists avoid pins altogether and prefer to crisply break the stick of a cotton-tipped applicator and use the end as a sharp stimulus. The broken stick must be sharp to adequately test pain sensation. The patient is asked if the stimulus is felt to be sharp or painful.

Temperature

A simple and adequate test for temperature is to place one of the tines of an unstruck tuning fork against the patient's skin and ask if it feels hot or cold, then repeat the test with one end of a wooden tongue depressor. Because the metal conducts heat well, its room temperature will be felt as cool against the skin. Because the wood conducts heat poorly, it is perceived as a neutral thermal stimulus. Patients with normal temperature sensation can tell the "cold" from the "warm," and those with abnormal temperature sensation cannot.

Position

Joint position sensation is tested by the examiner moving the patient's distal finger or toe joint and asking him if the movement was up or down. The examiner must grasp the digit on the sides to minimize inadvertent cues provided to the patient. If the digit is grasped above and below, the patient might feel pressure on the bottom as the joint is moved up. Normally, the patient should feel a distal finger movement of 2 degrees and a toe movement of 5 degrees. If position sensation in a given joint cannot be reported accurately, the next most proximal joint should be tested until the patient can report movement correctly.

Vibration

Vibration sensation can be tested on bony prominences or on the skin. A 128 Hz or 64 Hz tuning fork should be used; the 256 Hz tuning fork does not impart a strong enough vibration to permit adequate testing. The examiner first applies the tuning fork to the patient's sternum to acquaint him with the feel of the stimulus. The tuning fork is then sounded and applied to the most distal bony prominences in the feet and hands. The patient reports when he can no longer feel the vibration stimulus. The examiner then applies the tuning fork to the same part of his own body to use himself as a normal control. Allowances should be made for the decrease in vibration sensation that occurs with normal aging. If distal impairment is present, the stimulus should be gradually moved proximally until the limit of normal sensation is identified.

Secondary Sensory Modalities

If the primary sensory modalities are grossly intact and the examiner wants to assess the component of sensation served by hemispheric thalamocortical pathways, the secondary sensory modalities may be tested. Patients with parietal lobe lesions may have normal primary modality sensation but impaired secondary modality sensation on the side of the body contralateral to the lesion. Usually performance on the two body sides is compared, using one side as a control for the other.

Secondary sensory modalities also can be used to further refine sensory testing in subtle lesions of the more peripheral sensory pathways. For example, some patients with minor symptoms of carpal tunnel syndrome may not have sensory loss over the median nerve distribution demonstrable by ordinary testing of pain, temperature, or touch. Two-point discrimination testing there, however, may be abnormal.

Two-point discrimination. The ability to discriminate between a single-point stimulus and two closely and simultaneously applied point stimuli is a parietal lobe function. The examiner may use a commercially available device specifically designed to test two-point discrimination. A handy alternative is to crisply break the stick of a cotton-tipped applicator into two sharp fragments and use the two resulting points. Normal two-point discrimination varies greatly over the skin surface. The lips and fingertips are most sensitive; the back is least sensitive. Whether a particular body part is adept at two-point discrimination depends not so much on the density or type of cutaneous receptors as it does on the amount of parietal cortex assigned to integrate the sensory input. Normal values for two-point discrimination over various body parts are:

Finger tips:	less than 4 mm
Palms:	less than 10 mm
Toes:	less than 10 mm
Hand dorsum:	less than 30 mm
Back:	less than 70 mm

It is crucial when testing two-point discrimination to apply the two stimuli simultaneously. An inadvertent, very slight time delay makes very simple the recognition of the stimuli as two, even in the presence of impaired two-point discrimination. The examiner alternates randomly between applying a single stimulus and two closely applied stimuli, each time asking the patient if he feels one or two points. The distance between the points is gradually increased until the threshold for accurate two-point discrimination is identified.

Double simultaneous stimulation. Thalamic and parietal lesions can produce extinction to double simultaneous stimulation on the side contralateral to the lesion. The patient is tested with his eyes closed. He responds verbally or by gesture to the exact location touched by the examiner. The examiner tests each hand and each side of the face separately.

Figure 7

Dermatomal sensory patterns

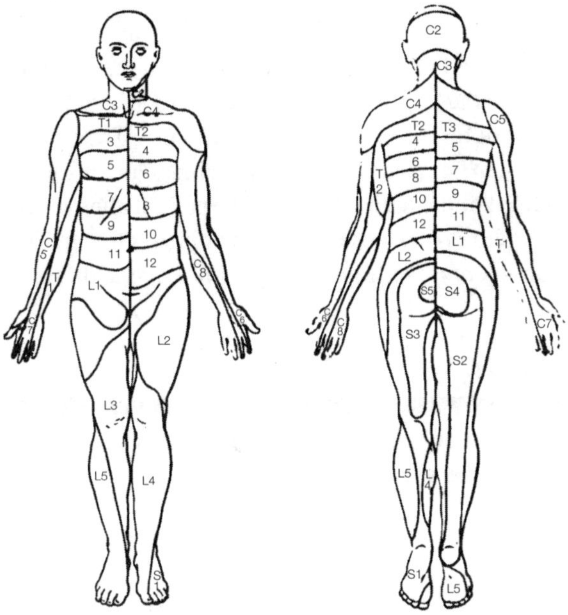

Ford FR. Diseases of the Nervous System in Infancy, Childhood and Adolescence. *3rd ed. Springfield, Ill: Charles C. Thomas; 1966.*

Then, without warning, the examiner touches homologous areas of both hands simultaneously and repeats the maneuver on other homologous body areas. Another type of extinction is "rostral dominance," the tendency to extinguish caudal stimuli in favor of rostral ones. Present in childhood, it may reappear in states of bilateral hemispheric dysfunction. Here, the patient may extinguish the hand stimulus when hand and face are touched simultaneously.

Graphesthesia is the ability to recognize letters or numbers sketched on the skin. Like two-point discrimination, there is great variation in the size of characters that can be felt in different areas of the skin. The examiner draws numbers or letters 0.5 to 1 cm in height on the fingertips. The process can be repeated on the palms with 4 cm characters.

Stereognosis is the ability to recognize common objects just by touching them. Examples of test objects include coins, a safety pin, a paper clip, a key, and a rubber band. Test objects are placed in each hand one at a time, and the patient names them. He is not allowed to transfer objects from one hand to the other. The test can be made more sensitive by double simultaneous presentation of test objects in both hands.

Barognosis is the ability to discriminate the weight of objects by holding them. With the patient's eyes closed, objects of similar shapes and sizes but different weights are placed in his hands. The patient tells which object is heavier. With parietal lobe damage, the contralateral hand usually feels the object as lighter, even if it is heavier.

Sensory Localization

If abnormalities are disclosed on the sensory exam, the clinician next must interpret their significance. The presence of normal primary modalities with abnormal secondary modalities suggests parietal lobe dysfunction. If the primary modalities are impaired, the clinician must first consider which modalities are affected. If the sensory loss is "dissociated" (abnormal pain and temperature with normal position and vibration) the lesion is probably in the spinal cord (eg, syringomyelia) or in the peripheral nerves (eg, amyloid neuropathy). Abnormal position and vibration sensation with intact pain and temperature sensation suggests a lesion of the posterior columns of the spinal cord, or of the peripheral nerves. The clinician must compare the pattern of sensory loss he detects with anatomic charts of known nerve root and peripheral nerve sensory distributions (Figures 7 through 9.)

9. Coordination

Coordination testing ordinarily is performed to examine the cerebellar contribution to motor function. But normal coordinated movements require the proper function of sensory input systems in addition to the motor and cerebellar system. Vision is necessary to precisely guide the intended movement; vestibular and proprioceptive inputs provide spatial orientation cues necessary for fine motor control. Because normal cerebellar function depends upon inputs from these sensory systems, impairments of coordination can arise from impaired visual, vestibular, or proprioceptive inputs as well as from intrinsic cerebellar dysfunction.

Coordination testing can be interpreted correctly only after examinations have clarified the patient's visual, vestibular, motor, and proprioceptive functions.

Coordination is tested by observing the accuracy, grace, and facility of fine movements of the extremities. In the finger-to-nose test, the patient extends his right forefinger and touches his nose. The examiner then holds his own right forefinger about 2 feet in front of the patient's nose. The patient alternately touches his own nose and the examiner's finger. The examiner moves his own finger into several differ-

Figure 8

Peripheral nerve sensory patterns (anterior view)

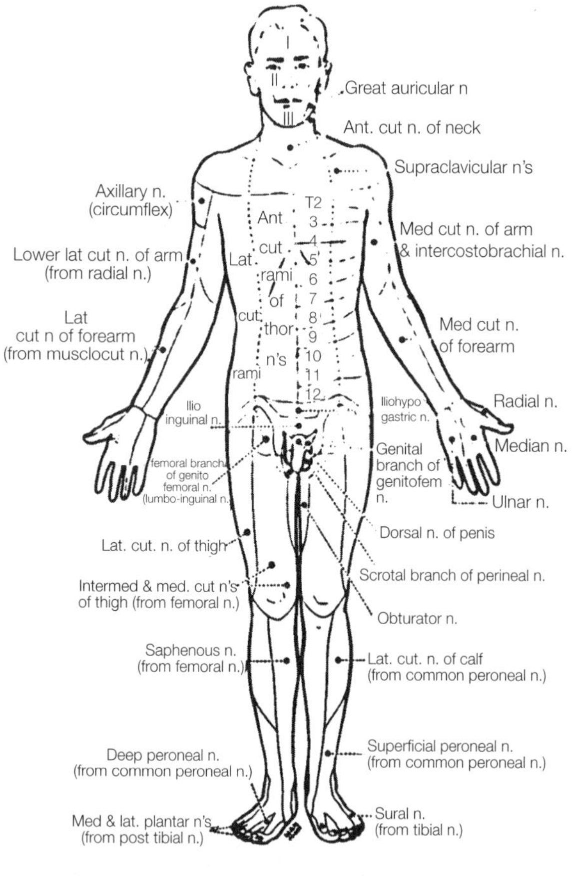

Haymaker W, Woodal B. Peripheral Nerve Injuries: Principles of Diagnosis. *Philadelphia, Pa: Saunders; 1945.*

Figure 9

Peripheral nerve sensory patterns (posterior view)

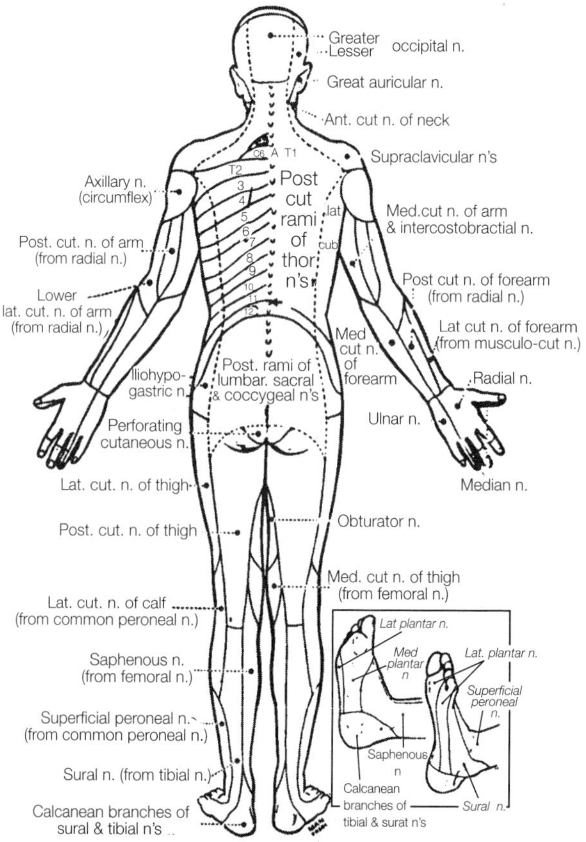

Haymaker W, Woodal B. Peripheral Nerve Injuries: Principles of Diagnosis. *Philadelphia, Pa: Saunders; 1945.*

ent positions for the patient to gauge and reach in successive attempts. The left side is tested similarly. The speed, accuracy, and finesse of each movement is assessed by the examiner.

The heel-to-shin test makes a similar assessment of leg coordination. While supine, the patient raises his right leg and lightly places his right heel on his left knee, then makes even hops with the heel about two inches apart, touching the shin and proceeding distally to the foot. Once at the foot, the process is performed in reverse back to the knee. It is then repeated for the left heel and right knee.

Rapid rhythmic alternating limb movements are assessed in both upper and lower extremities. The patient is asked to repetitively slap his right palm on his right knee as quickly and accurately as possible; then he alternately slaps the palm and the dorsum of his hand against his knee. A similar test is to touch the thumb and forefingers rapidly and repetitively, or the thumb and all fingertips in succession. Leg movements are tested by having the patient repetitively tap the floor with each foot.

In cerebellar ataxia, there is decomposition of movement, slowness, clumsiness, overshooting the mark, and action tremor. The more fine and rapid the movement, the worse the ataxia. Dysmetria, the inability to judge distances by limb movement, and dysdiadochokinesia, the inability to perform rapid, rhythmic movements, are classic cerebellar signs.

In cerebellar dysfunction, frequently there are hypotonia and also a loss of checking movements. Checking movements are assessed by having the patient contract the biceps muscle against resistance; the examiner then suddenly removes the resistance. Normal checking is present when the sudden release of the limb is recognized and stopped after only about 30 degrees of inadvertent elbow flexion. In loss of checking caused by cerebellar disease, the hand may continue flexion movement when released, to the extent of striking the patient in his face. The examiner must guard the patient's face with his forearm to prevent injury. The legs can be tested similarly.

Hypotonia is assessed by having the relaxed patient sit on the edge of a bed or table sufficiently high to prevent his feet from touching the floor. The examiner gently extends the patient's knees, one at a time, and allows them to swing like a pendulum. The hypotonic leg will swing more times than the normal leg before coming to rest.

Cerebellar ataxia also can be assessed by listening to phonation and by observing the movements of the patient's eyelids, tongue, and lips. The patient makes rapid repetitive movements and the examiner watches for irregularity and decomposition of movement. To test for labial and lingual ataxia, the patient alternately moves the tongue from side to side and says "la-la-la...," "pa-pa-pa...," "me-me-me...," etc. Phonation ataxia is tested by having the patient hold a note (eg, middle C) while saying "eeee..." for at least five seconds. With phonation ataxia, the pitch as well as the volume of the sustained note fluctuate, producing an exaggerated vibrato.

10. Gait and Station

Tradition has it that 19th-century clinicians needed only to watch a patient walk to make a correct neurologic diagnosis. Normal gait requires the proper functioning of nearly all the components of the nervous system: adequate consciousness, praxis, and spatial orientation; visual fields, acuity, and vestibular function; and motor, proprioceptive, and cerebellar functioning. Gait examination, therefore, supplements the examination of each subsystem and confirms the findings.

The patient is taken to a hallway or large room where objects do not encumber the path and there is at least a 30-foot space to walk. The patient is asked to walk normally. The examiner notes the balance, ease, grace, poise, presence of associated arm movements, symmetry, confidence, freedom and bounciness of gait. The patient is observed walking on his toes, then his heels. Tandem gait is tested by having the patient walk in a straight line with heel touching toe. Then, the patient walks on the lateral surfaces of his feet in a waddling fashion. Heel, toe, tandem, and lateral foot gait tests are designed to stress the nervous system to magnify minor asymmetries and amplify minor signs. For example, the patient with mild pyramidal dysfunction of the left arm may have normal, ordinary walking, but may exhibit dystonic posture and not swing the left arm normally during stressed gait testing.

Station is tested by observing the patient while sitting for evidence of "titubation," a swaying ataxia seen in advanced midline cerebellar disease. While the patient stands, the clinician observes the width of his base. Ataxic patients tend to adopt a wide base to maintain balance. The patient is asked to stand with his feet together, toes and heels touching. This position is very difficult for ataxic patients.

If the narrow-base position can be assumed, the patient is asked to close his eyes. The normal person may exhibit a trace of swaying, but he can usually stand with feet together and eyes closed for 30 seconds. In cases of sensory ataxia, there is absolute reliance on visual input to compensate for impaired proprioceptive input. Here, Romberg's sign is positive as the patient sways and falls when the eyes are closed but not when the eyes are open. In cerebellar ataxia, the patient has great difficulty standing with feet together with his eyes open or closed. Unilateral vestibular disease can also produce swaying and falling with eyes closed. The examiner must take care to guard the patient with his hands to prevent injury while testing for Romberg's sign.

In young patients with subtle forms of ataxia, the sharpened Romberg's test can be performed. The patient is asked to stand with his feet in the tandem position, with heel touching toe in a straight line. Normal young people should be able to stand in this position for 20 seconds with eyes closed.

A number of classic abnormal gait patterns have been described. More than one pattern can coexist; for example, the multiple sclerosis patient often has both spastic and ataxic components to his gait. Various degrees of severity may be present in all types.

Hemiplegic gait. Unilateral upper-extremity and lower-extremity pyramidal dysfunction produces hemiplegic or hemiparetic gait. The leg is extended at the knee and circumducted at the hip, with the toe scraping the floor. The arm is flexed at the elbow and wrist and associated swinging movement is decreased. Hemispheric stroke is the most common cause of hemiplegic gait.

Spastic gait. Bilateral leg pyramidal dysfunction produces the spastic "scissors" gait. The patient walks slowly and with difficulty with the knees extended and the hips moved in adduction movements with pelvic tilting movements. The thighs scraping each other in adduction produces a scissor-like movement. Cerebral palsy and multiple sclerosis are common causes of spastic gait.

Sensory ataxic gait. Impairment of proprioceptive input produces sensory ataxia. The patient may say he "does not know where the floor is" and slaps and stamps his feet as he walks. The gait is mildly wide-based and the feet are lifted high and uncertainly. The patient relies entirely upon visual cues and his eyes are fixed to the ground. Gait impairment is much worse in the dark. Normal people occasionally experience sensory ataxia when descending stairs. If a person is not looking and incorrectly expects one more step, he is surprised as his foot suddenly stamps the floor. This is what patients with sensory ataxia experience all the time. Disorders of peripheral nerves and posterior columns can produce sensory ataxia.

Cerebellar ataxic gait. This disorder is produced by dysfunction of the midline cerebellum (anterior superior vermis). The gait is erratic, irregular, reeling, imbalanced and very wide-based. Attempted compensatory movements often exacerbate the state of imbalance. This gait is seen in patients with cerebellar degeneration and midline cerebellar neoplasms.

Steppage gait. Patients with unilateral or bilateral foot drop must pick up their knee very high to avoid dragging the foot. There is a slapping quality as the foot is placed toe-first on the floor. There is inability to walk on the heels. The gait is often called "equine" because it is similar to that of a prancing horse. Foot drop may be the result of common peroneal mononeuropathy, hereditary motor-sensory neuropathy (Charcot-Marie-Tooth disease), or ruptured lumbar intervertebral disc with L5 root compression.

Waddling gait. In patients with primary muscle disease, proximal pelvic girdle muscle weakness produces characteristic walking called waddling or dystrophic gait. While walking, the patient's pelvis tilts inappropriately, producing swaying of the trunk that resembles a duck waddling. Myopathic diseases, including the muscular dystrophies and polymyositis, produce the waddling gait.

Parkinsonian gait. The patient with idiopathic or drug-induced parkinsonism walks with short steps (marche à petit pas), shuffling feet, stooped trunk, flexed head, arms flexed at the elbows and wrists, fingers adducted and flexed at the metacarpophalangeal joints, while extended at the interphalangeal joints. The patient also has decreased or absent arm swing, and acceleration (festination), as if the patient were trying to chase his own center of gravity that somehow got ahead of him. The patient often cannot initiate walking and exhibits retropulsion and rigid and clumsy en bloc turning.

Apraxic gait. Although perhaps a misnomer, patients with frontal lobe gait, particularly that resulting from bifrontal tumors or hydrocephalus, exhibit a distinct gait disorder. It has also been called Bruns' apraxia and "glue-footed gait." The patient cannot initiate walking—as if his shoes were stuck to the floor. Once walking, he shuffles and is clumsy. He cannot skip or hop. Disorders producing apraxic gait also produce urge urinary incontinence and subcortical dementia.

Senile gait. With advancing age, the gait begins to resemble mild parkinsonism with short steps, flexion, and some loss of associated movements.

Hysterical gait. A variety of bizarre, inconsistent, and exaggerated gait types are seen in conversion and malingering. Generally, the gait appearance does not fit a characteristic syndrome and is inconsistent with the findings on the rest of the exam. Often there is much lurching and exaggerated compensatory movements without falling. The clinician should exercise caution in assigning this diagnosis.

11. Reflexes

Reflex assessment is the most objective part of the examination of the nervous system. In addition to the cranial nerve reflexes already discussed, three types of reflex activity are commonly assessed: 1) deep-tendon (muscle stretch) reflexes; 2) cutaneous superficial reflexes; and 3) pathologic (regressive) reflexes.

Deep-Tendon Reflexes

Deep-tendon reflexes can be elicited from any muscle by suddenly stretching the muscle tendon. These monosynaptic reflexes receive descending inhibitory input from the corticospinal tract. Lesions of the lower motor neuron (anterior horn cell, nerve root, peripheral nerve) interrupt the reflex arc and cause hypoactivity or ablation of the reflex. Lesions of the corticospinal tract in the brain or spinal cord produce dysinhibition and hence hyperactivity of the reflex arc. The most severe form of deep-tendon reflex hyperactivity is clonus, wherein a persistently applied stretch to the tendon produces continuous rhythmic phasic muscle contraction. Deep-tendon reflexes increase with anxiety, hyperthyroidism, hypocalcemia, beta-adrenergic agonist drugs, and increases in muscle tone caused by injury and pain. There is a spectrum of normal reflex amplitude that each clinician must learn. Comparison between left and right sides is mandatory.

The clinician ordinarily assesses deep-tendon reflexes of the biceps (C5-C6), triceps (C7-C8), and brachioradialis (C5-C6) muscles in the arm, and of the quadriceps (L3-L4) and gastrocnemius (L5-S1) muscles in the leg. Other muscles easily tested include pectorals (C5-C6), finger flexors (C7-C8, T1), hamstrings (L5-S1), and leg adductors (L2-L4). The clinician usually taps the muscle tendon directly, but for biceps, pectorals, hamstrings, and leg adductors, it is easier for the examiner to tap his own fingertip placed over the muscle tendon.

Deep-tendon reflex activity is graded as follows:

0 absent

1 hypoactive

2 normal

3 hyperactive

4 hyperactive with sustained clonus

Subtle intermediate grades can be created by the addition of plus (+) and minus (-) quantifiers.

Complete relaxation and correct positioning are necessary for the proper assessment of reflexes. All arm reflexes can be tested with the arm flexed 90 degrees to 120 degrees. The gastrocnemius reflex (ankle jerk) requires the examiner to actively dorsiflex the foot to its maximum extent.

If a reflex cannot be obtained despite proper technique, positioning, and relaxation, methods of reinforcement should be attempted. These measures are designed to increase the general state of body tone and amplify the reflexes. Reinforcement of upper extremity reflexes is obtained by having the patient clench his teeth and close his eyes tightly just before and during the tendon tap. Reinforcement of lower extremity reflexes is obtained with Jendrassik's maneuver. The patient pronates one arm and supinates the other, locking the fingers of each hand together; just before and during the reflex, he pulls the left hand against the right. Only if no reflex can be obtained during reinforcement can the deep-tendon reflex in question be said to be absent.

Superficial Reflexes

In addition to corneal and gag reflexes, the superficial abdominal (T6-T12) and cremasteric (L1-L2) reflexes are ordinarily tested. The superficial abdominal reflexes are lost in pyramidal lesions, unlike the deep-tendon reflexes, which become hyperactive. (Superficial abdominal reflexes also are lost in lower motor neuron lesions of the thoracic spinal nerves.) They are tested with the patient supine, relaxed, and warm. Each quadrant of the abdomen is stroked briskly with a partially noxious stimulus. The ideal stimulus is a sewing pattern tracer, which is a device with a handle and a rotating circular head that contains radially oriented straight pins and that rolls across the skin as the device is moved. The clinician should take care to have the patient relax properly and should observe the abdomen carefully on the first stroke because the superficial abdominal reflexes often extinguish in normal people. The reflex is present when the umbilicus moves in the direction of the stimulated quadrant. In a young person, the absence of abdominal reflexes is an important sign of bilateral pyramidal dysfunction (usually of spinal cord origin) and is commonly seen in multiple sclerosis.

In men, the cremasteric reflex is tested by stroking the medial superior aspect of the thigh of the supine patient with a mildly noxious stimulus, such as the sewing pattern tracer, the edge of a broken tongue blade, or the edge of a cotton-tipped applicator. Normally, there is reflex contraction of the ipsilateral cremasteric muscle and elevation of the testicle. If the patient is cold, the testicle will already be elevated and the reflex cannot be appreciated.

The cutaneous anal reflex (S3-S5; anal wink) is occasionally tested in patients with presumed spinal cord lesions. The left, then right, perianal skin is once briskly stroked with the broken edge of a cotton-tipped applicator. Normally there is reflex contraction of the external anal sphincter, which can be seen or can be felt by the gloved finger.

Pathologic ("Regressive") Reflexes

A group of reflexes seen in normal neonates later become inhibited with maturation and pyramidal tract myelination. In disease of the pyramidal tracts, these reflexes become disinhibited and may reappear in their infantile form. The clinician should test for Babinski's sign and Wartenberg's sign in patients with suspected pyramidal tract lesions. Tests for suck, snout, glabellar, palmomental, and grasp reflexes (see below) are performed in any patient with suspected bilateral hemispheric dysfunction. These may be present in the normal elderly person.

Babinski's sign is a time-honored sign that nearly always indicates corticospinal tract dysfunction. The clinician strokes the most lateral portion of the supine patient's sole with a blunt object from the heel to the base of the fifth toe, then across the ball of the foot to the base of the great toe. A key, the broken edge of a wooden tongue blade, or two broken edges of a cotton-tipped applicator make good stimuli. The normal response to this plantar stimulation is flexion of the great toe. The pathologic response (positive Babinski's sign) is extension of the great toe and fanning of the remaining toes. It may be difficult to distinguish between an extension response and a voluntary withdrawal response. If voluntary withdrawal is suspected, the clinician should stroke more lightly or use other means to elicit the sign.

The clinician can test the same reflex with several alternative methods of stimulation. The lateral foot can be stroked (Chaddock's reflex) or both Babinski's and Chaddock's reflexes can be performed simultaneously with the tines of a tuning fork: one tine on the lateral foot, the other on the lateral sole. The anterior tibial surface can be stroked from proximally to distally (Oppenheim's reflex), the calf muscle can be squeezed (Gordon's reflex), or the toes 2 through 5 can be forcibly plantar flexed.

Wartenberg's pyramidal hand sign is the upper-extremity equivalent of Babinski's sign in the lower extremity. It is highly suggestive of corticospinal tract disease. The clinician bends his fingers 2 through 5 into partial flexion and places his fingertips against those of the patient, which are in the same position. The clinician and patient pull against each other and movements of the thumb are observed. Normally, there is no movement or slight flexion. The positive pathologic response is adduction of the thumb across the palm of the hand.

It has been incorrectly stated that Hoffman's sign necessarily has pathological significance. When the examiner briskly flicks the distal phalanx of the patient's middle finger, Hoffman's sign is said to be present if there is reflex flexion of the distal phalanx of the thumb and forefinger. This sign only represents hyperactivity of the finger flexor reflex (C7C8, T1). This hyperactivity may or may not be pathological.

Suck, snout, and grasp reflexes may indicate bilateral hemispheric dysfunction in the nonelderly patient. The suck response is tested by placing a tongue depressor in the patient's closed lips. Sucking or swallowing movements are the pathological response. Snouting is tested by lightly tapping the closed lips with a tongue depressor or the middle phalanx of the examiner's flexed index finger. Reflex pursing of the lips is the positive response.

Grasping is tested by stroking the patient's palm with the examiner's fingers. If the patient grasps the examiner's hand he should be asked to let go. Grasping itself is not necessarily abnormal, but forced grasping in which the patient cannot let go suggests bilateral hemispheric dysfunction.

The palmomental reflex is tested by firmly stroking the patient's thenar eminence with a tongue blade and observing the ipsilateral mentalis muscle for evidence of contraction. The sign is said to be positive if, after five consecutive stimuli, there is no extinction and each stimulus continues to provoke a response. This sign is seen in 10%-20% of normal people.

The glabellar reflex is tested by tapping the midline supraorbital ridge (glabella), approached from behind with the examiner's index or middle fingertip. A positive response is the absence of extinction of the blink response after the fifth stimulus. This sign is present in parkinsonism (Myerson's sign) and in some normal elderly patients.

The glabellar, palmomental, and snout reflexes may be seen normally, particularly in the elderly population. Their significance must be interpreted in the context of the entire examination.

12. Autonomic

The functions of the autonomic nervous system are not usually tested in a screening neurological examination but may be tested when symptoms suggest autonomic dysfunction. Symptoms of autonomic dysfunction may include bladder paralyis, orthostatic lightheadedness, anhidrosis, pupillary changes, sweating abnormalities, reduced tearing, and trophic or vasomotor skin changes. Pupillary abnormalities were discussed under "Cranial Nerves".

The skin can be examined for evidence of vasomotor skin changes such as acrocynaosis, pallor, mottling, flushing, coolness or anhidrosis. The skin also can be examined for trophic changes such as atrophy, shininess, nail thickening, and hypertrichosis.

Cardiovascular reflexes can be tested in cases of suspected orthostatic hypotension, syncope, and lightheadedness. The blood pressure and pulse should be measured lying, sitting, and standing. Orthostatic hypotension is confirmed when a drop in systolic blood pressure of 20 mm or greater occurs, or a drop in diastolic blood pressure of 10 mm or greater within three minutes of standing up. Normally, hypotension will induce reflex tachycardia. The absence of tachycardia in the face of a drop in blood pressure suggests autonomic insufficiency.

The integrity of the autonomic nervous system can be tested further using standardized tests. These test may be useful in several clinical circumstances: (1.) when generalized autonomic failure is suspected; (2.) to diagnose autonomic neuropathy; (3.) when a distal small-fiber neuropathy is suspected; (4.) to diagnose orthostatic intolerance; (5.) to detect a neuropathic basis for neurocardiogenic syncope; (6.) and to detect sympathetic dysfunction in pain syndromes (Low, 2003).

13. References

Brain M. *Guarantors of Brain: Aids to the Examination of thePeripheral Nervous System*. 4th ed. Philadelphia, Pa: Saunders; 2000.

Brazis PW, Masdeu JC, Biller J. *Localization in Clinical Neurology*. 5th ed. Philadelphia, Pa: Lippincott Williams & Wilkins; 2007.

(Contains practical advice on how to localize lesions in the nervous system by eliciting signs and symptoms.)

Campbell WW. DeJong's *The Neurologic Examination*. 6th ed. Philadephia, Pa: Lippincott Williams &Wilkins; 2005.

(An encyclopedic reference work to be consulted for detailed explanations, obscure signs, and alleponyms. Earlier editions have more detailed descriptions of signs and more interesting historical detail.)

Caplan LR, Hollander J. *The Effective Clinical Neurologist*. 2nd ed. Boston, Mass: Butterworth-Heinemann, 2001.

(Analytical account of neurological assessment by master clinicians. Shows how assessment is constructed by the iterations and revisions of successive hypotheses.)

Guarantors of Brain: Aids to the Examination of the Peripheral Nervous System. 4th ed. Philadelphia, PA: Saunders; 2000.

(Portable and indispensable reference for the examination of muscle weakness, particularly from peripheral nerve and nerve root lesions; very well illustrated.)

Low PA. Testing the autonomic nervous system. *Semin. Neurol*. 2003;23:407-421.

(Reviews autonomic testing and the evidence base for standardized tests of autonomic function.)

Mayo Clinic. Rochester, MN. *Mayo Clinic Examinations in Neurology*. 7th ed. Philadelphia, PA: Elsevier.

(The best short work devoted to the neurological examination; highly recommended.)

Rizzo M, Eslinger PJ. *Principles and Practice of Behavioral Neurology and Neuropsychology*. Philadelphia, Pa: Saunders; 2004.

(Contains good sections on the mental status exam, aphasia exam, and other aspects of examining patients with cognitive and language impairments.)

Strub RL, Black FW. *The Mental Status Examination in Neurology*. 4th ed. Philadelphia, Pa: FA Davis; 2000.

(Detailed discussion of performing and interpreting the bedside mental status examination.)

14. Questions

1. Which of the following is not a primary sensory modality?

   A. Vibration

   B. Temperature

   C. Graphesthesia

   D. Position

   E. Pain

2. Which feature is not part of the lower motor neuron syndrome?

   A. Spasticity

   B. Hyporeflexia

   C. Atrophy

   D. Weakness

   E. Fasciculations

3. What is the resting position of an eye with a pure oculomotor nerve palsy?

   A. Adducted and depressed

   B. Abducted and depressed

   C. Adducted and elevated

   D. Adducted and depressed

   E. Adducted

4. Which is the most prominent feature of conduction aphasia?

   A. Impairment of naming

   B. Impairment of repetition

   C. Impairment of written comprehension

   D. Impairment of auditory comprehension

   E. Paraphasias

5. Which of the following structures/functions are not innervated by the facial nerve?

   A. Muscles of facial expression

   B. Stapedius muscle

   C. Muscles of mastication

   D. Lacrimal glands

   E. Taste on the anterior two-thirds of the tongue

6. Why do many patients with hemispheric strokes have weakness of only the lower half of their face?

   A. Corticospinal fibers do not end on cranial nerve nuclei

   B. Corticobulbar fibers are the upper motor neuron of the hypoglossal nucleus

   C. The facial nerve nuclei are not affected in hemispheric strokes

   D. The patients are unaware of their upper facial weakness

   E. There is bilateral corticobulbar innervation of the upper facial nuclei

7. Which of the following is not a feature of the pupillary light reflex?

A. It may be affected by anticholinergic drugs

B. It may be affected by sympathomimetic drugs

C. It is normally direct and consensual

D. It may be affected by an optic neuritis

E. It may be abnormal in cortical blindness

8. Why is ptosis part of Horner syndrome?

A. Involvement of the levator palpebra muscle

B. Involvement of the oculomotor nerve

C. Involvement of the sympathetic Müller's muscle

D. Involvement of the Edinger-Westphal nucleus

E. Involvement of the optic nerve

9. What is the name given to gait imbalance resulting from a myelopathy or peripheral neuropathy impairing proprioception?

A. Astasia-abasia

B. Sensory ataxia

C. Charcot's gait

D. Cerebellar ataxia

E. Ataxic hemiparesis

10. Which is not an expected finding in a pure left afferent pupillary defect?

A. Impaired left pupilloconstriction shining light in the left eye

B. Impaired right pupilloconstriction shining light in the left eye

C. Impaired left pupilloconstriction shining light in the right eye

D. Intact right pupilloconstriction shining light in the right eye

E. Impaired vision in the left eye

F. A left Marcus Gunn pupil

Questions 11-15 concern the following case:

A 64-year-old man developed painless left-hand weakness that gradually spread over 8 months to produce right-hand weakness, leg stiffness and weakness, dysarthria, dysphagia for liquids, easy crying, and a 20-lb weight loss. His examination showed diffuse hyperreflexia, atrophy and fasciculations of his tongue and both hands, dysarthric-dysphonic speech, bilaterally increased leg tone, and normal sensation. Are the following statements true or false?

11. He has evidence of both upper and lower motor neuron dysfunction.

12. The findings could be explained by cervical spondylotic radiculomyelopathy.

13. The findings could be explained by peripheral neuropathy.

14. The easy crying suggests bilateral corticobulbar lesions.

15. Electromyography and electroneurography would be more useful to reach a diagnosis than MRI.

Questions 16-20 concern the following case:

A 68-year-old hypertensive man developed sudden vertigo with nausea and vomiting, numbness in his left face and right arm and leg, left Horner syndrome, dysphagia, and ataxia of his left arm and leg. Are the following statements true or false?

16. A single lesion of the central nervous system could account for all these findings.

17. His Horner syndrome suggests dysfunction of the pericarotid sympathetic chain.

18. His acute dysphagia requires bilateral central nervous system involvement.

19. An internal carotid artery dissection/occlusion could produce these findings.

20. Cardioembolism to the brain is a common cause for this symptom complex.

Answers

1. C. Graphesthesia is a cortical sensory function, not a primary sensory modality.

2. A. Spasticity is the result of corticospinal or corticobulbar tract dysfunction and therefore is an upper motor neuron sign.

3. B. The resting position of an eye with an oculomotor palsy is abducted and depressed because the vector of the remaining innervated muscles (superior oblique: IV nerve and lateral rectus: VI nerve) pulls the eye down and out.

4. B. Impairment of repetition is the most conspicuous feature of conduction aphasia because of involvement of the arcuate fasciculus connecting Broca's and Wernicke's areas.

5. C. Muscles of mastication are innervated by the trigeminal nerve.

6. E. Bilateral corticobulbar innervation of the upper facial nuclei prevents upper motor neuron weakness from a unilateral corticobulbar lesion.

7. E. Cortical blindness does not affect the pupillary light reflex.

8. C. The sympathetically-innervated Müller's muscle is responsible for a small portion of eyelid elevation, so mild ptosis is seen with sympathetic denervation.

9. B. Sensory ataxia refers to gait imbalance resulting from deafferentation of proprioception from the feet in myelopathies and peripheral neuropathies.

10. C. Shining a light in the unaffected right eye will produce direct and consensual pupilloconstriction in the presence of a left afferent pupillary defect.

11. True. The evidence of upper motor neuron dysfunction is spasticity and hyperreflexia. The evidence of lower motor neuron dysfunction is atrophy and fasciculations. Both can produce weakness.

12. False. Cervical spondylotic radiculomyelopathy may produce hand atrophy and weakness and leg spasticity and hyperreflexia but it cannot produce tongue atrophy and fasciculations.

13. False. A peripheral neuropathy cannot produce spasticity and hyperreflexia and very rarely produces tongue fasciculations.

14. True. Easy ("pathological") crying is a part of the syndrome of pseudobulbar palsy resulting from bilateral corticobulbar lesions.

15. True. Electromyography and electroneurography would be useful to prove the patient has ALS (the diagnosis here) by showing chronic partial denervation in limbs, face, and throat muscles with normal nerve conduction and muscle action potentials.

16. True. A single lesion in the left lateral medulla (the "lateral medullary syndrome") could account for all these findings.

17. False. Horner syndrome suggests sympathetic dysfunction but it could be first-, second-, or third-order sympathetic neuronal dysfunction.

18. False. Acute dysphagia is seen in unilateral infarctions of the lateral medulla because of involvement of the nucleus ambiguus.

19. False. Lateral medullary infarctions may occur from vertebral artery dissections but not from internal carotid artery dissections.

20. False. Cardioembolism to the brain is an uncommon cause of lateral medullary infarction. More common is vertebral artery occlusion resulting from atherothrombosis or vertebral artery dissection.

Chapter 3: The Neurological Examination: Pediatrics

Phillip L. Pearl, MD

Contents

1. Introduction

The pediatric adage that, "Children are not just small adults," rings true in neurology. While the foundation of pediatric neurology fits well within the framework of classical neurology, there are special considerations in the examination and evaluation of neonates, infants, and children. The clinician should endeavor to utilize the rostro-caudal organization of the neuraxis when presenting the examination, ie, an orderly presentation of mental status, cranial nerves, motor systems, and so forth. Yet the approach to the child must take into particular consideration a non-threatening, flexible style, requiring a patient demeanor and lighthearted affect. The pediatric neurologic examination relies on the time-honored discipline of neurologic localization, but also accounts for the process of normal development. This chapter will select aspects of the neurologic evaluation that supplement the adult examination and are of special emphasis in pediatrics. Particular key points will be made to aid in practical applications of common findings, although a comprehensive differential diagnosis of features on the examination is beyond the scope of this chapter. As the experienced clinician will often say that the lack of a diagnosis upon the completion of the history invariably means the lack of a diagnosis upon the completion of the physical, we will begin with some notes regarding the pediatric history.

2. Pediatric History

The breadth of pediatrics covers the fetal period to adolescence. Naturally, the history and examination will evolve over the individual's lifespan. The neonatal period includes the first 30 days post-term (called postconceptional age, although postmenstrual age is more accurate). The history of any neonate, infant, or child should include a thorough assessment of the pregnancy, labor, and delivery. The gestational history includes the mother's age, duration of pregnancy, and history of maternal illnesses or fetal exposures to teratogens such as drugs or radiation. The TORCH viral infections, causing fetal cerebral injury (and frequently deafness and ocular problems), refer to toxoplasmosis, syphilis, rubella, cytomegalovirus, herpes simplex, and HIV. The timing of an adverse exposure or illness during pregnancy is critical to the neurologic outcome. The nervous system begins with the process of neurulation, or formation of the neural tube, at 17 days post-conception, and this process continues until approximately 7 weeks post-conception. Ventral induction, or formation of the hemispheres, begins at 5 weeks post-conception; disruptions here may lead to holoprosencephaly, or a single, unilobar cerebrum, or to milder versions along this spectrum. Brain development proceeds with nerve cell proliferation between 2 and 4 months of gestation, then neuronal migration between 3 and 5 months, and then nerve cell organization and the formation of synaptic circuitry. Disorders of proliferation include macroencephaly and microcephaly vera. Migrational disorders include lissencephaly (smooth brain), pachygyria (thick gyri), polymicrogyria, and schizencephaly (congenital clefts). Myelination occurs, starting inferiorly and posteriorly, during the latter half of pregnancy and continues actively until two years post-term. Prenatal encephaloclastic lesions, whether from viral infections or vascular accidents during the fetal period, include porencephaly and hydranencephaly. Knowledge of the orderly process of congenital brain development lends perspective on congenital brain anomalies.

Certain patterns suggest prenatal problems. Maternal bleeding during pregnancy raises concerns regarding pre-existing placental or fetal abnormalities. Toxemia, with maternal edema, proteinuria, and hypertension, is associated with prematurity, placental insufficiency, *in utero* growth retardation (IUGR), and neonatal hypoglycemia. Infants of diabetic mothers have neonatal hypoglycemia and hypocalcemia, macrosomia, respiratory distress syndrome, and sometimes icterus. Mothers with hypothyroidism or phenylketonuria are at risk of producing offspring with cognitive deficiencies. Mothers with myasthenia gravis may produce infants with neonatal myasthenia, reflecting a transient condition due to passive transfer of acetylcholine-receptor antibody requiring supportive care until resolution. A history of maternal polyhydramnios suggests an infant with a neuromuscular problem who had decreased swallowing. A low maternal alpha-fetoprotein (AFP) suggests Down syndrome, versus high AFP incriminating a neural tube defect.

The perinatal history should include whether the amniotic fluid was clear or meconium stained, and whether the membranes ruptured spontaneously or with medical assistance. Rupture of membranes 24 hours prior to delivery increases the risk of fetal amnionitis, with common organisms being *Streptococcus* Group B, *E coli*, and *Listeria monocytogenes*. Either a prolonged, difficult or precipitous labor suggests problems with the newborn. A full-term infant is delivered between 37 and 42 weeks of gestation, and on average weighs 2500 grams. Infants small for gestational age are known as SGA or having IUGR, ie, *in utero* growth retardation. Infants born large for gestational age (LGA) should raise the question of maternal diabetes, which may have been limited to gestation and unrecognized.

The perinatal history should emphasize whether there was evidence for a newborn encephalopathy, ie, hypotonia, decreased motoric activity, apnea, seizures, temperature instability, or other problems referable to the nervous system. This is the best predictor of whether a neonate is at risk for neurodevelopmental sequelae related to the perinatal period.

The APGAR score is used to describe a newborn's transition from the *in utero* environment to normal breathing and activity during the first minutes after birth. It is a total of scores between 0 and 2 in five categories: Activity level (muscle tone), Pulse (heart rate), Grimace (reflex response to stimulation), Appearance (skin color), and Respirations [although this mnemonic belies that attribution for this scoring system belong to pediatrician Virginia Apgar (1909-1974)]. The APGAR scores, done on a scale of 0 to 10 (worst to best), indicate how well a newborn is doing at that time, but do not have long-term predictive value unless the very late APGAR scores (10 minutes and beyond, as opposed to the standard scores taken at 1 and 5 minutes) are very low. The primary risk factors for the development of cerebral palsy are prematurity and "multiples," ie, twins, triplets, etc., as opposed to birth asphyxia.

The pediatric neurological history also must concentrate on the developmental history. Each age has its own developmental norms, and premature infants are generally assessed for their "corrected" postconceptional age at least until 12 months. A newborn infant with normal vision should be able to briefly fixate with open eyes. A considerable amount of time, on average 16 hours out of 24, will be spent asleep, with a preponderance of "active" sleep (the forerunner of stage REM) in the first months of life. Screening tests such as the Denver Developmental Screening Test (Denver II) are available to assist with rapid identification of developmental norms and delays. Typical developmental milestones are noted in Table 1. It is important to recognize that there is a wide normative range, and multiple aspects of delay in a particular sphere (gross motor, fine motor, language, social) should be present, often in combination with multiple spheres, before diagnosing a child with a neurodevelopmental disorder.

Children often present with paroxysmal problems, whereupon only the history will provide clues unless the family can produce a videotape of the event. The differential diagnosis of seizures versus nonepileptic paroxysmal phenomena is wide, but special consideration is given to whether there are provocative features as expected in breath-holding spells, hypoglycemic events, conversion disorders, etc. The pediatric migraine spectrum includes many "equivalent" syndromes of variable prognoses, eg, benign paroxysmal vertigo, benign intermittent torticollis, periodic syndrome with vomiting, acute confusional migraine, alternating hemiparesis, and others.

The presenting problem must be defined not only by its special characteristics but also by the temporal course. In particular, one must emphasize whether

Table 1

Typical Developmental Milestones

1 month
- Spontaneous, symmetrical motor activity
- Lifts head when prone
- Regards surroundings
- Follows visually to midline

2 months
- Smiles spontaneously and reciprocally
- Coos
- Follows visually past midline

3 months
- Follows 180 degrees
- May wave at toy
- Turns head to sound
- In ventral suspension, head held above body

4 months
- Grasps rattle
- Good head control when placed in sitting position
- Laughs aloud
- Excites with feeding

6 months
- Reaches with either hand
- Rolls over, usually prone-to-supine first
- Sits briefly when placed
- Plays with examiner

7 months
- Transfers objects from hand-to-hand
- Imitates sounds
- Responds to name

8 months
- Sits independently
- Stands holding on
- Combines syllables
- Regards self in mirror

10 months
- Pulls to stand
- Thumb-finger opposition grasp
- Waves bye-bye
- May say "mama" or "dada" (specifically)

12 months
- Walks with support
- Stands alone
- Places cube in cup
- 2 words besides "mama" or "dada"

15 months
- Toddles
- Pats pictures
- Uses spoon
- Points or vocalizes to indicate wants
- 4 to 5 words

18 months
- Removes shoes/socks
- Climbs on furniture
- Stacks 3 to 4 cubes
- 10-word vocabulary
- Turns pages in groups

2 years
- Runs
- Walks up steps one at a time
- Begins to use pronouns, 3- word sentences
- Uses own name
- Toilet trained during day

2-1/2 years
- Partially undresses
- Attempts to put on socks
- Imitates horizontal or vertical line
- Helps put things away
- Knows name and sex

3 years
- Alternates feet upstairs
- Pedals tricycle
- Builds tower of cubes
- Copies a circle
- Speech at least 50% intelligible
- Buttons and unbuttons, puts on shoes

4 years
- Runs and climbs well
- Alternates feet downstairs
- Hops on one foot
- Throws ball overhand
- Copies a cross
- Asks questions
- Imaginative play

5 years
- Skips feet
- Copies a triangle
- Counts to 10 or higher
- Knows age
- Can tie shoelaces

6 years
- Draws person with hands and clothes
- Knows morning and afternoon
- Knows right from left

an encephalopathy appears static or nonprogressive versus progressive. The latter is taken to mean the presence of a deteriorating course, where there is regression, ie, loss of previously acquired skills, or a failure to properly acquire new skills. The presence of a progressive or intermittent pattern raises consideration of the inborn errors of metabolism. Such metabolic encephalopathies can be heuristically organized into several patterns. One scheme is to consider whether the disorder is typified by predominantly a leukodystrophy, with white matter involvement, or poliodystrophy, with gray matter involvement. The leukodystrophies typically present with the long tract signs of spasticity, hyperreflexia, and ataxia, as well as visual loss with optic atrophy and deafness. The poliodystrophies will present with more typical gray matter symptoms, such as dementia, seizures, or retinal pathology. As time proceeds, many of the metabolic encephalopathies will share features of both, and clarification of the findings at presentation may help to delineate which broad category is a better fit. Other taxonomic schemes will use classification by organelle, eg, mitochondrial versus peroxisomal. Newer information is permitting the definition of disorders by neurotransmitter metabolism, eg, Segawa DOPA-responsive dystonia with diurnal variation. Clues from the history, along with a knowledge base regarding these conditions, may lead to a well-honed diagnostic plan to verify a suspected diagnosis. Alternatively, less well-defined syndromes may be better evaluated through examinations that allow for screening of multiple potential disorders. The autism spectrum disorder, representing a syndrome that presents commonly to the child neurology clinic, has features of both a static and progressive course, oftentimes with periods of developmental plateau. Thus, the assessment of a temporal course to a child's neurodevelopmental disorder also requires a degree of flexibility that allows for vagaries attributable to the natural history of disease that do not follow the timelines of our diagnostic algorithms.

3. Family History

The family history is of particular importance and should not be dismissed or abrogated to a cursory review. The contributory value of the family history, while traditionally highly honored in child neurology, has become even more amplified with the information explosion in neurogenetics and mapping of the human genome. A family tree represents the optimal pictorial demonstration, and all first degree relatives (parents and siblings) should be represented at the very least, with inquiry into the medical status of grandparents and parents' siblings as well. Disorders of autosomal dominant (involving consecutive generations), autosomal recessive (skips generations), X-linked (maternal transfer of disorder to sons), or mitochondrial (maternal transfer to all her children) inheritance may be identified. Parental ancestry and assessment for consanguinity are key points.

4. Physical Examination

The examination is best used to confirm or refute the differential diagnosis as formulated following the history, and should emphasize apropos portions of particular relevance or interest. The pediatric neurology examination requires both the general and neurological examinations. Observing and playing with the child yield high impact information. The general examination in particular should assess for dysmorphic or cutaneous stigmata. Dysmorphic features may involve the cranium, facies, eyes, ears, mouth, skeleton, or extremities. The phenotype may immediately suggest a known syndrome, ranging from the upslanting palpebral fissures of Down syndrome to the shortened palpebral fissures with smooth philtrum and thin upper lip of fetal alcohol syndrome. Coarse facial features suggest the mucopolysaccharidoses.

Neuromuscular disorders may reveal themselves with their own physical signs. The presence of a high-arched palate or pectus excavatum suggests hypotonia of prenatal origin. In a hypotonic newborn, examination of the mother may reveal stigmata of myasthenia to support transient neonatal myasthenia, or myotonia manifest by a delayed handshake release to suggest neonatal myotonic dystrophy. In an older child or adolescent, pes cavus may be present along with chronic peripheral neuropathy as in Charcot-Marie-Tooth syndrome. Asymmetric movement of the upper extremities, with persistent forearm extension and pronation in an infant, is seen in Erb congenital brachial plexus palsy. The presence of a Horner syndrome, including heterochromic irides where the ipsilateral eye is lighter in color, indicates additional involvement of the lower plexus as in a complete (Klumpke) palsy.

The phakomatoses, or neurocutaneous disorders, provide a wealth of findings on the general physical examination. The cutaneous findings of tuberous sclerosis include the hypopigmented "ash leaf" maculae, typically lumbar shagreen patch, malar fibroadenomata (previously called adenoma sebaceum), and periungual fibromas around the nailbeds. Typically, the infant in whom the diagnosis is first considered, particularly in the setting of infantile spasms, will only demonstrate the ash leaf spots, which may be better visualized with the aid of a fluorescent (Wood's) lamp. A facial port-wine stain does not always mean there will be cerebrotrigeminal vascular angiomatosis of Sturge-Weber syndrome, but involvement of the eyelid and cranial nerve V-1 frontalis distribution is very suggestive. The prepubertal child with neurofibromatosis-1 will demonstrate at least six café au lait maculae greater than 5 mm, along with axillary or inguinal freckling. In incontinentia pigmenti, a female neonate will have transient vesicular lesions sometimes confused with neonatal acne, but which leave linear and whorled hyperpigmented patches seen in older infants and children.

The cranium deserves its own examination. All time-honored modalities of observation, palpation, auscultation, percussion, and transillumination are valuable. A newborn will commonly have some head molding, which resolves within the first weeks of life. Caput succedaneum is self-limited scalp edema. A cephalohematoma represents subperiosteal hemorrhage. Overriding sutures raise concern regarding microcephaly; split sutures and a bulging fontanelle suggest increased intracranial pressure. Anomalous cranial shapes may represent transient molding or a more significant craniosynostosis. The cranium will grow in the axis of the closed suture, so that sagittal synostosis leads to an abnormally elongated head (scaphocephaly), whereas coronal synostosis leads to a shortened, box-like shape (brachycephaly). As parents are now advised to place their children supine during sleep to decrease the risk of sudden infant death syndrome, more and more children present with simple molding, which can often be avoided by use of the prone position during waking hours and alternating the child's head position during sleep. Cranial bruits, while often normal in young children, may instead suggest the presence of a vein of Galen malformation, particularly in a young infant with macrocephaly and congestive heart failure.

The posterior fontanelle may be difficult to palpate, and is normally closed at birth, and no later than six weeks. Congenital hypothyroidism should be ruled out in a newborn with an open posterior fontanelle. The anterior fontanelle typically closes between 10 and 20 months of age. When palpated to assess for intracranial pressure, the infant should be sitting up and relaxed. It is normal to perceive the cardiac pulse while palpating the anterior fontanelle. The head circumference measurement should be taken as the largest consistent frontal-occipital measurement. While normative graphs should be used to calculate the percentile for a male versus female, the general rate of cranial growth is helpful to know at the bedside. A term infant has an average FOC (fronto-occipital circumference) of about 34 cm. The FOC grows rapidly, at a rate of 2 cm per month the first three months, reaching 40 cm at age three months. The rate slows to 1 cm per month the next three months, so that a six-month-old typically has an FOC of 43 cm. The growth is then on average 0.5 cm per month the next six months, or 46 cm at 12 months. Over the next two years, the rate is about 0.5 cm per six months, or 48 cm at 2 years and approximately 50 cm at 3 years. The FOC is about 52 cm at 8 years, and 54-55 cm in the adult. Macrocephaly is often a benign familial trait, but raises concern regarding a plethora of diagnoses, ranging from an intracranial tumor or posterior fossa cyst with hydrocephalus, eg, Dandy-Walker malformation, to subdural hematomata or hydrocephalus that may be related to child abuse.

The general examination may pick up many important findings that may not be manifest by an abnormal neurological examination early in life. A sacral dimple above the gluteal fold, possibly accompanied by a tuft of hair or sinus tract, may be the only clue to spinal dysraphism and a tethered spinal cord that will lead to later neurological deficits during growth. Involvement of other organ systems may provide important support of a potential neurological diagnosis, eg, hepatic or renal dysfunction in a neonate with suspected perinatal hypoxic-ischemic encephalopathy, or thrombocytopenia and hepatosplenomegaly in a neonate with a TORCH infection. A cardiac murmur may accompany the atrioventricular canal defect of Down syndrome, or a ventricular septal defect associated with fetal alcohol syndrome. An abdominal mass in an infant with proptosis is alarming for metastatic neuroblastoma. Clearly the distinction between benign variants and pathognomonic signs on the general examination is critical in pediatric neurology.

5. Neurological Examination

The classic mental status examination is obviously adjusted for the patient's age. A responsive and calm, or at least consolable, infant is more reassuring for normalcy than persistent irritability or unresponsiveness. A newborn with an excessive Moro response, or persistent jitteriness, raises concerns regarding neonatal drug withdrawal following maternal drug use, electrolyte disturbance including hypoglycemia or hypocalcemia, or other encephalopathy. An excessive startle reaction on the "nose tap" test is pathognomonic for hyperekplexia. Loss or lack of visual attentiveness is concerning in an infant, and sometimes is the first or only developmental change in infantile spasms. Auditory myoclonus to a startle is worrisome for various encephalopathies and is a well-known feature in Tay-Sachs disease.

The developmental milestones shown in Table 1 are helpful guideposts during the examination. In the preschool or school age child, age and grade relevant questions and even brief tests add considerable strength to the mental status examination. Screens such as the Beery Test of Visual Motor Integration (VMI), Draw A Person test, and WRAT-R (Wide Range Achievement Test—Reading) are readily available and allow for rapid acquisition and scoring. Referral for psychoeducational testing, whether through the school, clinical psychologist, or neuropsychologist, may be predicated upon the child's performance. A common presenting problem to the child neurologist is the question of a primary attention disorder, learning disability, or combination of these problems leading to academic or behavioral impairment.

The acquisition of language is of particular importance in the mental status examination. The early milestones are included in Table 1. The speech of a three-year-old should be at least 50% understandable. By this age, a child should also be using at least 2-3 word sentences. As the child becomes older, more correct use of pronouns, verb tense, and noun plurals emerges. The infant begins consonants with reduplicated babble, eg, dada-dada, then nonreduplicated babble, and then moves on to jabbering. The process of articulating the various combinations of consonant sounds occurs between the age of 3 and 7 years. Persistent difficulty with specific sounds may be secondary to misaligned dentition, or uncoordinated movements of the tongue and lips. Ongoing dysarticulation, or stuttering characterized by conscious tension and speech avoidance, should lead to referral for speech and language therapy.

Higher cortical functions can be screened during the neurological examination, and may be helpful in the evaluation of a child for the so-called soft or subtle neurologic signs that accompany ADHD and learning disabilities. Sequential complex movements, such as repeatedly tapping the palm to the thigh, then rotating 90-degrees to the ulnar hand surface, and then producing a fist, may demonstrate dyspraxia related to the contralateral prefrontal cortex of motor planning. Testing for finger gnosis may be done by having the child with closed eyes name the finger that is touched by the examiner. Right-left discrimination is learned at about age six years, and same-side commands can be accomplished, ie, "touch your right thumb to your right ear." Cross-sided commands are accomplished in the somewhat older child. Right-left discrimination may be impaired in normal individuals, but is also found in association with learning disabilities.

Cranial Nerves

The newborn infant should be able to show some visual fixation as well as reaction to olfactory, gustatory, and auditory stimuli. The facial grimace should be observed carefully. An asymmetric smile could represent congenital facial nerve palsy, although it may also manifest the asymmetric crying facies syndrome secondary to congenital absence of the depressor anguli oris muscle. This occurs in conjunction with a congenital heart defect in up to 20% of cases, and hence is known as the cardiofacial syndrome. The velocardiofacial syndrome may be detected by the combination of a palatal defect and a cardiac murmur; these infants have a telltale facial sign of a very wide nasal bridge. The cranial nerve functions are also examined by the rooting (CN V and VII) and sucking (CN V, VII, and XII) reflexes in the newborn.

Cranial nerve testing in young children often requires considerable adjustment in technique compared to the traditional neurological examination. Simple observation may be sufficient. Torticollis present from birth often reflects sternocleidomastoid muscle spasm of prenatal onset and responds to physical therapy with passive stretching. Acquired torticollis, however, suggests pathology involving the posterior fossa. Head tilt may be seen in the syndrome of spasmus nutans, with asymmetric ocular oscillations and head nodding. Alternatively, a head tilt could represent compensation for a contralateral CN IV palsy, or cerebellar tonsillar herniation through the foramen magnum, that may reflect a posterior fossa lesion. Amaurosis in combination with nonparalytic strabismus can be an unrecognized finding for a number of years. In the young child, visual acuity can be assessed indirectly by determining if the patient reaches for small objects. In a preschooler, one can use the direction of the "E" or three fingers, with the patient responding by showing the direction. If visual acuity appears to be deficient below the level of counting fingers or mimicking direction, a bright light in a dark room may be used to determine for light perception (LP). The ability to tell the direction from which the light is shining is called light perception with projection (LP with P). Opticokinetic nystagmus can be observed by using a large, commercially available drum, or tapes with bright figures or stripes in young children. The response may be deficient when targets are moved toward the involved hemisphere. The infant too young to follow the rotating drum will normally demonstrate so-called twirling nystagmus with a spinning movement. The oculocephalic, corneal and gag reflexes are present from birth. It is often best to delay the cranial nerve examination until the end of the session, due to its more threatening nature, although one risks the eventual fatigue and uncooperation of the patient.

Motor

Careful observation followed by gentle palpation and passive range of motion are first steps. At term, there is generally more flexor tone. There can be some persistence of clenched fists and internal thumbing until four months of age. In contrast, the premature infant will tend toward hypotonia. The degree of flexor tone predicts gestational age. Hypotonia in the term infant suggests neurological dysfunction, whether related to hemispheric, spinal cord, or lower motor neuron pathology. The most common causes will be central, and include a multitude of systemic problems as well as genetic syndromes and congenital brain malformations. Intracranial hemorrhage or spinal cord injury may produce persistent hypotonia, despite the upper motor neuron localization. A frogleg posture or reduced motoric activity in a young infant suggests a significant myelopathy or lower motor neuron disorder. Spinal muscular atrophy type I—Werdnig-Hoffman disease—presents within the first six months of life. This patient will typically have a very alert appearance but profound hypotonia and hyporeflexia.

Head and neck control develop over the first several months of life. The head lag as a child is pulled by the hands to a sitting position is resolved normally by 4 months of age. By this age, the child supports some weight with the legs. Sitting is achieved with confidence between 7-8 months, followed typically by creeping, crawling, and then cruising by 10 months. There is a wide normative range in development, especially in the gross motor realm. The significance of "late walking," or absence of crawling, should be judged in the context of associated motor findings. Associated hypotonia does raise the question of "benign congenital hypotonia" or "dysmaturation," which may have a benign outcome but raises the question of a motor system disorder. Motor activities become progressively more purposeful and complex throughout the first year of life, and any persistent asymmetry suggests a neurological problem, including prominent handedness before 9-12 months of age. During the second year, walking improves and becomes confident typically by 18 months, and running begins with reliance on the upper extremities for balance and protection.

Individualized muscle testing is often not evaluable, yet functional activity can be observed in a multitude of ways. The Gower's maneuver, a time-honored test for proximal weakness, is optimally done with the child beginning supine. The weak child will need to roll over to the side before arising, to be followed by climbing up one's own legs with sequential hand movements to reach the standing position.

Reflexes

The traditional reflexes, ie, deep tendon and superficial, are the parlance of traditional neurology and covered in the adult neurological examination. Other than a positive patellar tap, the deep tendon reflexes are difficult to elicit in the newborn. The ankle and triceps reflexes do not appear until several weeks of age, with the triceps being inconsistent until six months. Alternatively, hyperactive responses such as the crossed adductor are typical up to 7 months, and an extensor plantar response is common up to age one year and acceptable as normal until age 3 years. Sustained ankle clonus or reflex asymmetries, however, remain pathological signs.

The specific newborn and infantile reflexes, however, are the province of pediatric neurology and provide information on normal neurological development as well as pathological changes. Their age of appearance and disappearance are shown in Table 2. The Moro reflex is the startle response, and is provoked by gently dropping the head in the supine infant held supported with the neck slightly flexed. There should be symmetrical upper extremity abduction, extension, and circumduction, and lower extremity extension and then flexion. It is normally present at birth and involutes by 16-20 weeks. It is elicitable between 28 and 32 weeks in the premature, and serves as a clinical sign of neonatal encephalopathy when decreased. It is also a clue to a brachial plexus lesion, clavicle fracture, or hemiparesis when asymmetrical. The response should recede in time and should not be present beyond five months post-term.

The Galant is the truncal incurvation response. This is present between birth and three months of age. It appears by 24 weeks in the premature. The intact response is incurvation of the trunk ipsilateral to the side of stimulating the flank. The asymmetric tonic neck reflex (ATNR) describes the fencer's posture with ipsilateral arm extension and contralateral flexion upon rotation of the head to either side. A strong and long-lasting ATNR suggests pathology at any age, and the response is normally gone by six months. The sucking and rooting reflexes are present at birth. Sucking appears by 28 weeks and rooting, even more primitive, at 24 weeks of gestation.

A decrease in these responses suggests an encephalopathy. These responses disappear by the fourth month.

The palmar and plantar grasp responses are also present from birth. There is flexion of fingers and toes in response to gentle pressure to the palm and foot, respectively. The responses are clearly evoked in 32 week prematures. The so-called righting reflexes, present in the first four months, are responses by the infant to various movements and are part of the normal maturational response of developing protective responses. In the crossed leg extension reflex, the infant withdraws and flexes the stimulated leg and extends the other, as if pulling away from a threat and exerting antigravity resistance simultaneously. The neck-righting elicits an ipsiversive turning movement of the shoulders and trunk when the infant's head is turned. Similarly, there is a vertical righting response where the infant's lower extremities extend, followed by the trunk and head, when the infant is held flexed over the examiner's arm and the feet are stimulated.

In the parachute response, the infant extends the upper extremities toward the table as the examiner, supporting the prone infant, motions the head toward the examination table. This protective mechanism appears between 6 and 9 months of age and should be well-developed between 12 and 24

Table 2

Common Developmental Reflexes

Reflex	Age of Appearance	Age of Disappearance (post-term)
Moro	28-32 weeks GA	5-6 months
Rooting	24 weeks GA	4 months
Sucking	28 weeks GA	4 months
Grasp (palmar, plantar)	32 weeks GA	2 months
Galant (spinal incurvation)	24 weeks GA	3 months
ATNR	Birth	3-6 months
Crossed leg extensor	Birth	1 month
Placing	Birth	1-2 months
Stepping	10 days	1-2 months
Parachute	6-9 months	Persists
Landau (extends when supported prone)	10 months	24 months

GA = gestational age; ATNR = asymmetric tonic neck reflex

months. The Landau reflex, present by 10 months of age, evokes extension of the neck, trunk, and lower extremities when the infant is suspended by the examiner's hand in the prone position. Passive head extension results in further extension, and head flexion leads to flexion of the trunk and hips. Focal deficits such as hemiplegia or paraplegia, or exaggerated rigidity, may be detected by anomalous responses.

The antecedents to walking can be observed in the newborn reflexes. The steppage reflex is obtained by placing the infant's feet on a surface and alternating the shoulders forward to simulate walking. A heel take-off is reached by 40 weeks gestational age. In the placing reflex, the dorsum of the infant's foot is brought to the undersurface of a tabletop. The infant will raise the foot, placing it on the table in a stepping pattern. This reflex appears about ten days of age and its absence may indicate the presence of neurological deficits that are otherwise undetected by the examination.

Sensory

The sensory exam is particularly difficult in the child. Only major deficits will be detected in infants. In the young child, reliability of response is always a question, and the rhythm of testing should be altered to avoid automated answers. The preschooler can generally attend to double simultaneous stimulation and answer reliably enough to detect extinction of the stimulus on one side. Higher cortical modalities such as graphesthesia and stereoagnosia can be tested by seven to eight years of age.

Cerebellar Function

The cerebellar exam is traditionally directed toward this structure's role as a modulator of oscillatory activity, although functions related to frontal and striatal neural networks have greatly expanded our view of the cerebellum in clinical neurology. In the young child, offering toys will allow for evocation of cerebellar tremor or dysmetria. Asking the child to place a marble between the examiner's two fingers screens for incoordination. Other helpful maneuvers are having the child press the button on a tape measure, finger-to-nose testing, rapid alternating movements such as alternatively tapping the palm and dorsum of the hand on the thigh, or apposing the fingers to thumb as if playing the piano. The hands should be tested individually as the examiner assesses for the dysrhythmia of cerebellar disease, or the presence of extrapyramidal or adventitious movements suggestive of basal ganglia disease or dyspraxia. Excessive mirroring movements in the opposite limb represent so-called soft or subtle neurological signs, although extraneous movements may be normal until seven to eight years of age.

Gait is a screen of cerebellar function that signifies neurologic disease at all levels. Heel and toe gait can be reliably observed by four to five years of age. Impaired dorsiflexion as manifest by absent heel gait suggests a peripheral neuropathy. The waddling gait of pelvic girdle weakness is seen in muscle disorders, and coupled with oversized calves in a young boy suggests Duchenne muscular dystrophy. Excessive toe gait points to spasticity; absent toe gait may represent a lumbosacral spine lesion involving the conus medullaris or cauda equina. Impaired tandem gait implies problems with cerebellar pathways. A circumductive gait, coupled with decreased arm swing, suggests hemiparesis corresponding to a lesion of the contralateral cerebral hemisphere.

6. Conclusion

The history remains the cornerstone of the pediatric neurological examination. The chief complaint, more diplomatically referred to as the chief concern, is often best left in the family's own words. The history is best taken as a guided story provided by the family. The examination includes the general features, with emphasis on dysmorphic or cutaneous stigmata of a neurological disorder, and for the involvement of systemic organs. It is critical to account for the process of normal development, and its wide range of normalcy, during the enactment and interpretation of the pediatric neurological examination. As with the rest of clinical localization in the nervous system, the significance of the findings on examination depends upon the company that they keep. Are there supportive features in the history and examination to substantiate the finding under consideration? Are there related deficits in that developmental sphere to assign the presence of a neurological deficit? Are there deficits in other neurodevelopmental spheres to suggest the pattern of a syndrome? The examiner must continuously ask and reflect on these questions during the clinical evaluation. The neurological examination must emphasize simple observation and playful interaction with the child. While a successful examination requires both cleverness and originality, recruiting the child into challenging games invariably leads to an increased level of cooperation and rewarding physician-patient interaction.

7. References

1. V Gunn, C Nechyba, MA Barone, eds. *Johns Hopkins Hospital Children's Medical and Surgical Center. Harriett Lane Handbook: A Manual for Pediatric House Officers*. 16th ed. St. Louis, Mo: Mosby; 2002.

(This legendary manual is a must for pediatric residents and can ably assist the neurology house officer with practical synopses of all organ systems, including child neurology and development. There is an easily accessed formulary specifying pediatric (mg/kg) dosages.)

2. Jones KL. *Smith's Recognizable Patterns of Human Malformations*. 5th ed. Philadelphia, Pa: WB Saunders; 1997.

(The bible of dysmorphism. This features a fact-filled page and accompanying set of photographs on the recognizable patterns of human malformation, as well as normative data for multiple anthropometric measurements.)

3. DO Wiebers, AJ Dale, E Kokmen, JW Swanson, eds. *Mayo Clinic Examinations in Neurology*. 7th ed. St. Louis, Mo: Mosby; 1998.

(Both comprehensive and concise, this monograph covers the clinical neurologic examination and ancillary diagnostic procedures. A rich discussion of speech and language development and praxis is included in the chapter on the examination of infants and children.)

4. Volpe JJ. *Neurology of the Newborn*. 4th ed. Philadelphia, Pa: WB Saunders; 2001.

(The classic for neonatal neurology. This includes authoritative sections on the orderly process of fetal brain development and congenital malformations, as well as hypoxic-ischemic encephalopathy and other neurologic problems of the newborn.)

8. Questions

1. The findings of hepatosplenomegaly, petechiae, and microcephaly at birth are most consistent with:

   A. Perinatal hypoxic-ischemic encephalopathy

   B. Fetal alcohol syndrome

   C. Craniosynostosis

   D. TORCH infection

   E. Neonatal meningitis

2. Adrenoleukodystrophy is likely to present with which of the following patterns:

   A. Pigmentary retinopathy with seizures

   B. Cognitive decline

   C. Spasticity, ataxia, and visual loss

   D. Visual hallucinations

   E. Myoclonic epilepsy

3. In tuberous sclerosis, the initial cutaneous manifestation is likely to be:

   A. Adenoma sebaceum of the face

   B. Hypopigmented maculae of the skin

   C. Shagreen patch over the lumbosacral region

   D. Fibromata of the periungual nailbeds

   E. Pits of dental enamel

4. The hypotonic infant with hyperalert appearance is likely to have:

   A. Miller-Dieker syndrome

   B. Hyperekplexia

   C. Walker-Warburg syndrome

   D. Neonatal myasthenia

   E. Werdnig-Hoffman syndrome

5. Which of the following signs indicate an abnormality in a term newborn?

   A. Sustained ankle clonus

   B. Extensor plantar response

   C. Crossed adductor response

   D. Absent triceps reflex

   E. Closed posterior fontanelle

6. In the Landau reflex, there is extension of the neck, trunk, and lower extremities as the infant is held prone in the examiner's hand. This reflex normally appears by:

   A. Birth

   B. 1 month

   C. 6 months

   D. 10 months

   E. 12 months

7. The Moro or "startle response" is normally present during which of the following time intervals:

A. Perinatal period

B. Birth to 1 week

C. Birth to 1 month

D. Birth to 5 months

E. 1 week to 6 months

8. The head lag that appears as a child is brought from the supine to seated position should resolve by age:

A. 2 months

B. 4 months

C. 6 months

D. 8 months

E. 10 months

9. A healthy infant girl is able to pull herself up to stand and wave bye-bye. Her FOC measures 45 cm. What level of verbal language should be anticipated?

A. Cooing (long musical vowel sounds)

B. Reduplicated babbling (da-da-da)

C. Says mama and dada nonspecifically

D. Uses two words with meaning

E. Combines two words

10. By age three years, a child is expected to:

A. Copy a triangle

B. Hop on one foot

C. Distinguish left from right

D. Distinguish morning from afternoon

E. Pedal a tricycle

11. Ana is a 3-year-old girl. She sat independently at 12 months and walked initially at 23 months. She began using single words just after her 2nd birthday and only recently began stringing words together. She responds inconsistently to single-step commands and is starting to point to named body parts. She will remove shoes and socks and is otherwise dependent on her parents for dressing. She is showing some interest in toilet training. This child's condition is best summarized by which of the following:

A. Late walker

B. Global developmental delay

C. Autism spectrum disorder

D. Specific learning disability

E. Cerebral palsy

12. A newborn infant with imperforate anus is noted to have upslanting palpebral fissues and single palmar creases. A loud systolic cardiac murmur is demonstrated to indicate an atrioventricular canal cardiac defect on echocardiography. Which of the following is the most likely genotype on chromosome analysis?

A. 47 XXY

B. Trisomy 18

C. Trisomy 13

D. Translocation 14/21

E. 45 XO

C. PMP22

D. Spastin

E. MeCP2

13. Carlos presents at age 4 years with severe hyperactivity and stereotypical movements, eg, hand flapping, that occur with excitement or anxiety. Intellectual testing reveals mild intellectual disability (IQ 55-69). Family history reveals his mothers brother attended special education classes throughout high school. His mother is already monpausal at age 37. His mother's father has a form of parkinsonism associated with hand tremors, gait ataxia, and memory impairment. DNA testing on Carlos showed which of the following results:

A. 10 CGG repeats of the FMR1 gene

B. 100 CGG repeats of the FMR1 gene

C. 1000 CGG repeats of the FMR gene

D. 47 XYY karyotype

E. 47 XXY karyotype

14. Carla, age 2 years, had an uneventful gestational and perinatal history, but her head circumference growth revealed deceleration so that a measurement of 44 cm at nine months showed less than anticipated growth compared to a 50%-tile measurement of 43 cm at six months. More recently, she has lost purposeful hand movements, and instead brings her hands to her mouth or wrings them together. She has intermittent paroxysms of hard breathing and just had a first time convulsion. What gene mutation is most likely in this girl?

A. Fragile X

B. 45 XO

15. A six-month-old girl begins having flexor spasms shortly following arousal. Her MRI shows agenesis of the corpus callosum and choroid plexus cysts. You suspect Aicardi syndrome. What other examinations may help you confirm the diagnosis?

A. Karyotype

B. Vertebral radiographs

C. Echocardiogram

D. Opthalmological consultation

E. B and D

16. A 5-year-old boy has not developed kindergarten readiness skills. His examination reveals microcephaly and cognitive difficulties. His mother graduated high school with special assistance. She herself had been on a protein-restricted diet as a young girl, but she resisted this diet almost entirely in her adolescence. What is the mother's diagnosis?

A. Fragile X syndrome

B. Congenital hypothyroidism

C. Tay-Sachs disease

D. Adrenoleukodystrophy

E. Phenylketonuria

17. A one-week-old neonate has respiratory failure and hypotonia. The mother has a neuromuscular condition that has not been elucidated. Which of the following is the most likely diagnosis in the child?

A. Congenital myasthenia

B. Congenital Güillain-Barré syndrome

C. Infantile ALS

D. Congenital myotonic dystrophy

E. Spinal muscular atrophy

18. Charlie, age 3 years, was a content infant who smiled and babbled on time. By age 1 year, he was identifying most letters. Soon after, he was seemingly obsessed with naming and ordering letters and numbers, but had never used the words "momma" or "dada." He recited phrases from videotapes but rarely initiated any spontaneous speech. What is the most likely diagnosis?

A. Attention deficit hyperactivity disorder

B. Global developmental delay

C. Autism spectrum disorder

D. Asperger disorder

E. Rett syndrome

19. Devin, age 8 years, is unable to sit or complete his work in the classroom. He frequently gets out of his seat and answers questions without raising his hand. This year he has been involved in fights on the playground. His early history was notable for repeated pediatric visits for abdominal colic and a difficult temperament. His physical and neurological examinations were entirely normal other than possibly mild dysdiadochokinesia when testing rapid alternating and sequential movements of the hands and fingers, respectively. What is the most appropriate diagnosis?

A. Attention deficit hyperactivity disorder

B. Childhood depression

C. Autism spectrum disorder

D. Post-traumatic stress disorder

E. Adrenoleukodystrophy

20. Rose, age 5 years, was adopted from a Russian orphanage with a confirmed history of having been born at 30 weeks gestation and having had a Grade III intraventricular hemorrhage. She is excelling in kindergarten but runs stiffly. The examination reveals symmetrical spasticity, hyperflexia, and sustained clonus of the legs. The examination of the upper extremities and cranial nerves are normal. What type of cerebral palsy is indicated by this pattern?

A. Spastic hemiplegic

B. Spastic quadriplegic

C. Spastic diplegic

D. Choreoathetotic

E. Ataxic

21. A one-year-old girl is evaluated for rhythmic left arm muscle contractions lasting a few minutes several times a day. Her mother cannot say when these episodes began. Upon further examination, it is found that the child is unable to play pat-a-cake, put blocks in a cup, use two-word phrases or stand for two seconds. The child has one blue eye and one brown eye and a macular, light pink lesion across her right face encompassing her eyelids to cheeks. No other cutaneous lesions are found. The child's arms and legs are symmetrical. What is the most likely diagnosis?

A. Simple partial seizure

B. Systemic lupus erythematosus

C. Klippel-Trenaunay-Weber syndrome

D. Sturge-Weber syndrome

E. Von Hippel-Lindau syndrome

22. A 12-month-old girl presents with motor development regression. At 6 months, she was able to sit alone. Now at 12 months, she is not only unable to stand but has developed difficulty sitting without support. On physical exam, the patient is found to have tongue fasciculations and hypotonia. When her hands are held out, she has a fine tremor. No sensory deficits are noted. Her language development is beyond her age since half her speech is understandable, and she is able to name six body parts.

22A: What is her most likely diagnosis?

A. Spinal muscular atrophy

B. Duchenne muscular dystrophy

C. Becker muscular dystrophy

D. Botulism

E. Myasthenia gravis

22B: What is her most likely prognosis?

A. Death from complications of the disease by 18 months

B. Death due to respiratory complication between 2 year of life to third decade of life

C. Death during adolescence due to respiratory failure

D. Death during status epilepticus

E. Normal life expectancy

Answers

1. D.

The systemic findings of hepatosplenomegaly and petechiae in a newborn, associated with microcephaly, strongly suggest the presence of an *in utero* viral infection. The latter represents a group of viral infections summarized with the acronym TORCH, ie, toxoplasmosis, syphilis (O is for "other"), rubella, cytomegalovirus (CMV), Herpes simplex, and HIV. There are some classic distinguishing features, such as the patterns of intracranial calcifications. The calcifications in CMV are typically periventricular, and in toxoplasmosis are intraparenchymal. In perinatal hypoxic-ischemic encephalopathy, dysfunction of other organ systems, eg, hepatic and renal, should be present as well. Microcephaly may be found in children with a history of perinatal hypoxic-ischemic encephalopathy after some time, but not at birth.

2. C.

Adrenoleukodystrophy (ALD), also known as Lorenzo's disease (note the movie, *Lorenzo's Oil*), is a peroxisomal disease presenting with adrenal insufficiency and progressive dysmyelination which proceeds in a posterior to anterior distribution. Leukodystrophies such as ALD (as well as metachromatic leukodystrophy or MLD, or Krabbe disease) will present with long tract signs such as spasticity and ataxia, as well as visual loss due to optic atrophy. In contrast, gray matter degenerative diseases will present with primary neuronal symptoms, such as cognitive decline and seizures. Option A, pigmentary retinopathy with seizures, would be classic for neuronal ceroid lipofuscinosis (NCL), of which Batten disease is the type affecting school age children. Option E, myoclonic epilepsy, would be more representative of a gray matter than white matter disorder.

3. B.

The cutaneous findings of tuberous sclerosis complex include all of the listed items, although the earliest to appear are the hypopigmented maculae of the skin traditionally known as ash leaf spots. This descriptive term is somewhat amorphous, as ash leaves do not have a distinct shape. In any case, "hypopigmented maculae" is more descriptive and less confusing. Their detection is aided by the use of the fluorescent Wood's lamp in a dark room, particularly in individuals with light complexions. This is worthwhile in screening first degree relatives of patients, as this multisystem phakomatosis has wide phenotypic variation and asymptomatic parents are sometimes detected during the evaluation of their affected child.

4. E.

Hypotonia in an infant can be due to either an upper or lower motor neuron lesion. The association of profound hypotonia in an unusually alert appearing infant is classic for spinal muscular atrophy. Type I, with onset within the first six months of life, is known eponymically as Werdnig-Hoffman syndrome. These patients will have absent reflexes. The intermediate form, Type II, has onset after six months and features tongue fasciculations. The adolescent form is known as Kugelberg-Welander syndrome.

Miller-Dieker and Walker-Warburg syndromes are genetic forms of lissencephaly, a congenital brain anomaly of disordered neuronal migration leading to a smooth cerebral cortex. Hyperekplexia is a startle syndrome related to a mutation of the glycine inhibitory receptor. Neonatal myasthenia is a transient condition related to passive transfer of acetycholine receptor antibody from a myasthenic mother. This is in contrast to congenital myasthenia, which refers to a group of genetic disorders leading to abnormal formation of the neuromuscular junction.

5. A.

Sustained clonus would represent an abnormal neurological finding in a term newborn. An extensor plantar response is expected up to one year of age and acceptable up to three years of age. The triceps reflex may not be seen until six months of age in normal infants. An open posterior fontanelle at birth would raise concern about congenital hypothyroidism or increased intracranial pressure.

6. D.

The newborn and infant reflexes represent developmental patterns that presage later maturation. These appear and extinguish within normal time ranges, and late appearance or disappearance suggest abnormal development. The Landau reflex, manifest by extension as the infant is held prone, appears by ten months and disappears by two years of age.

7. D.

The newborn's startle response, known as the Moro, is present at birth. Absence may indicate a neurologically depressed infant; asymmetry suggests a hemiparesis, brachial plexopathy, or clavicle fracture. The response is typically gone by five or six months of age.

8. B.

By four months of age, an infant should have enough head support to maintain the cranium in line with the trunk while raised by the hands from supine to sitting. Persistent head lag suggests hypotonia, of either central or peripheral localization.

9. C.

This vignette depicts a normal nine month old. The cooing of long vowel sounds is heard at about three months of age. Reduplicated babbling, ie, ba-ba-ba, da-da-da, is present about six months of age, and combined syllables (nonreduplicated babbling) by eight months. Discriminate use of dada or mama is typical at 10 months. By one year, a child is expected to use two words with meaning (other than dada/mama). Two-word combinations typically appear at about 18 months.

10. E.

Three-year-olds ride three-wheel bikes! Of the "Gesell figures," a 15-month-old imitates a scribble; an 18-month-old scribbles spontaneously; a 2-year-old imitates a stroke; a 2-1/2-year-old differentiates a horizontal versus vertical line; a 3-year-old copies a circle; a 4-year-old a square; and a 5-year-old a triangle. A diamond is mastered at ages 6-7 years; cylinder while age 9; and a cube at age 11. A 4-year-old learns to hop. Left versus right and morning versus afternoon distinction are the province of the six-year-old.

11. B.

This child has global developmental delay involving multiple domains. This may represent an early manifestation of long-term intellectual disability, ie, mental retardation. This is distinguished from divergent development, where development may progress except in areas such as social communication. That pattern would be typical of autism spectrum disorder. Another aberrant pattern is known as dissociated development. An example of dissociated development would be academic problems with reading versus otherwise well-developed social and cognitive skills, ie, learning disability in reading (or dyslexia).

12. D.

This child has Down syndrome, clinically evident based on the general examination and endocardial cushion defect of the heart. Imperforate anus is seen in approximately 1% of newborns with Down syndrome. While 95% of Down syndrome individuals have trisomy 21, 4% will have a translocation, which commonly involves chromosome 21 with chromosomes 14, 21, or 22. The remaining 1% has mosaic trisomy 21, and typically show better cognitive development than those with trisomy 21 or translocation Down syndrome. Note that of the other options in the question, 47 XXY is Klinefelter syndrome, and 45 XO is Turner syndrome.

13. C.

Carlos has Fragile X syndrome, which is associated with at least hundreds of repeats of the trinucleotide sequence CGG of the Fragile X Mental Retardation 1 gene on the X chromosome. His mother has the premutation, associated with early ovarian failure and subsequently a common reason for infertility. His maternal grandfather has a more recently identified disorder of adulthood known as "FXTAS," ie, Fragile X-associated Tremor-Ataxia Syndrome.

14. E.

This girl, with deceleration of head growth, loss of purposeful hand skills, and onset of hand stereotypies, paroxysmal hyperpnea, and seizures, has Rett syndrome. The typical mutation involves the MeCP2 gene of the X chromosome. 45 XO is the karyotype of Turner syndrome. PMP22 is the gene for Charcot-Marie-Tooth disease (hereditary sensorimotor neuropathy), and spastin mutations are seen in familial spastic paraparesis, as well as Pelizaeus-Merzbacher disease.

15. E.

Aicardi syndrome is associated with chorioretinal lacunae and vertebral bony anomalies. These patients typically present with infantile spasms. While various mutations on the X chromosome have been incriminated in Aicardi syndrome, there is no standard genetic test for the disorder, and a karyotype will be normal.

16. E.

This mother has phenylketonuia (PKU), which is detected on newborn screens and treated with a phenylalanine-restricted diet. While historically the diet had been liberalized once patients entered adulthood, this is now considered inadvisable, especially during pregnancy. Although the proband in this vignette did not inherit the disease PKU, he sustained prenatal brain injury owing to untreated maternal PKU. Fragile X is incorrect in this scenario, although it should be recognized as the most common inherited cause of mental retardation (in males and females). Congenital hypothyroidism requires treatment with thyroid supplement beginning in the newborn period, although (as with PKU) it is silent in its clinical effects for a relatively long period (as opposed to other metabolic disorders presenting in acute metabolic crisis, eg, urea cycle disorders or organic acid disorders). Tay-Sachs disease is a relentlessly progressive disorder presenting with auditory hyperacusis and loss of developmental milestones in the first year of life. Adrenoleukodystrophy (ALD) is a peroxisomal disorder that is X-linked and predominantly affects boys with progressive dysmyelination beginning in the occipital lobes.

17. D.
Myotonic dystrophy is a trinucleotide repeat disorder that is autosomal dominant and maternally inherited when presenting in the newborn period. Congenital myasthenia and spinal muscular atrophy are autosomal recessive conditions and therefore much less likely even if one parent is affected. This is in contrast to neonatal myasthenia, which is a transient condition attributed to trans-placental transfer of acetylcholine receptor antibody from a mother with autoimmune myasthenia to her fetus. Güillain-Barré is an acquired inflammatory demyelinating polyneuropathy. ALS, or amyotrophic lateral sclerosis (Lou Gehrig disease), is not a congenital disorder.

18. C.
Charlie demonstrates autism spectrum disorder, ie, severe qualitative impairment in socialization, communication, and behavior. Dr. Hans Asperger described, in 1944, children with grossly normal early language development who had impaired socialization and language pragmatics. Attention deficit hyperactivity disorder does not present with the obsessiveness and script speech that is seen in autism. Rett syndrome almost exclusively affects girls and has associated motor impairment and loss of early developmental milestones, although girls with the disorder were initially classified as autistic before Dr. Andreas Rett from Vienna described the disorder.

19. A.
Devin has a typical history of attention deficit hyperactivity disorder (ADHD). The longstanding signs and symptoms of infantile colic and difficult temperament are characteristic, although more acute onset could suggest depression or an anxiety disorder. Post-traumatic stress disorder would be expected to follow a significant adverse event. ALD can present with similar manifestations but is rare and would be expected to have accompanying neurologic features of a leukodystrophy, which by this age would include spasticity, hyperreflexia, visual impairment, and loss of developmental skills.

20. C.
Rose was a premature newborn and sustained an intraventricular hemorrhage (IVH). The source of IVH in a premature is the germinal matrix, which normally involutes by term. IVH is rare in a fullterm baby, and emanates from the choroid plexus. In Rose's case, there is evidence for periventricular leukomalacia on MRI, which is related to having IVH in a premature. Prematurity is the leading cause of cerebral palsy, and is associated with the spastic diplegia form. A fullterm infant having had hypoxic-ischemic brain injury is more likely to exhibit spastic quadriparetic cerebral palsy. A child having had a prenatal infarction may present after six months of age with the first identifiable signs of a spastic hemiparesis. Choreoathetotic cerebral palsy is associated with injury to the basal ganglia, as seen with kernicterus from neonatal hyperbilirubinemia. Ataxic cerebral palsy refers to a syndrome of abnormal voluntary movements involving balance and position of the trunk and limbs, and may be associated with increased or decreased muscle tone.

21. D.
The patient presents with partial seizures, developmental delay, and port wine stain, which are all associated with Sturge-Weber syndrome, also known as encephalotrigeminal angiomatosis. Sturge-Weber syndrome is associated with angiomas involving the leptomeninges (arachnoid and pia mater) and skin of the face in the V1 and V2 distributions of cranial nerve V. Developmental delay correlates to the degree of neurological involvement, and thus is more likely to occur with bilateral involvement. Seizures are generally focal, but may become generalized. Possible physical exam findings include port wine stain (cutaneous angioma), macrocephaly, glaucoma, heterochromia of iris, tomato-catsup color of fundus (ipsilateral to nevus flammeus) with glaucoma, possibility of choroidal angioma, and soft tissue hypertrophy.

Although the patient described was suffering from simple partial seizures, this diagnosis alone does not best explain the findings.

Although the port wine stain may resemble the butterfly-shaped macular rash, and SLE can have neurological involvement in a minority of cases, SLE would be unusual in a child this age.

Klippel-Trenaunay-Weber syndrome is a rare disorder of blood vessels, skin and soft tissue characterized by port wine stain, varicose veins, and bony and soft tissue hypertrophy, typically involving one extremity and resulting in loss of symmetry of the extremities. Klippel-Trenaunay-Weber syndrome typically does not involve neurological symptoms.

Von Hippel-Lindau syndrome is an autosomal dominant disorder characterized by hemangioblastoma formation of the cerebellum, as well as involvement of the retina, kidney, and sometimes other organ systems.

22. A.
Spinal muscular atrophy.

22. B.
Death due to respiratory complications between 2 years of age to the third decade of life

Spinal muscular atrophy (SMA) is a group of genetic disorders characterized by progressive loss of lower motor neurons. There arc four subtypes: type I (Werdnig-Hoffman, aka acute infantile), type II (chronic infantile), type III (Kugelberg-Welander, aka chronic juvenile), and type IV (adult-onset). In general, patients present with weakness, and muscle wasting in the limbs, respiratory and bulbar muscles. Patients often have above-average IQ. Type I presents before 6 months of age and is characterized by severe, progressive muscle weakness and hypotonia, poor suck ability, poor swallowing ability, and respiratory failure, with life expectancy averaging 18 months. Type II, the most common subtype, presents between 6-18 months and is characterized by motor delay, postural tremor affecting fingers, and hyporeflexia. The lifespan for these patients is typically between 2 years to the third decade of life, and death is usually due to respiratory infections. Type III presents after 18 months of age and is characterized by slowly progressive proximal muscle weakness. The patients typically can stand and walk but have difficulty going upstairs. The disease is slowly progressive and patients have a normal lifespan. Type IV typically presents in the mid-30s and is characterized by mild progressive proximal muscle weakness. This form of disease is benign and patients have normal life expectancy.

Duchenne muscular dystrophy (DMD) is an X-linked recessive trait involving frame shift mutation resulting in deficient or dysfunctional dystrophin protein. Patients usually achieve early gross motor skills such as rolling over, sitting and standing, but begin to show signs of hip girdle weakness by age 3-6 years. Patients assume lordotic posture and manifest Gower's sign and Trendelenburg (hip waddle) gait. Eventually, patients become non-ambulatory and succumb to respiratory failure and death in late adolescence. Patients often manifest pseudohypertrophy of the calves, thigh muscle wasting, cardiomyopathy, and low intellect. Although girls may express the phenotype, their clinical manifestations are mild. DMD is not associated with fasciculations. Becker muscular dystrophy, an in-frame mutation of the dystrophin gene, is similar to DMD, but manifests at an older age with patients surviving longer.

Botulism is unlikely in this case because the patient's symptoms did not present acutely. Myasthenia gravis is unlikely in this patient since hypotonia and weakness would occur with muscle use. The patient is out of the window for both transient neonatal myasthenia (due to antibodies from the mother) and hereditary congenital myasthenia gravis. These conditions present very early birth with respiratory insufficiency, and difficulty sucking and swallowing.

Chapter 4: Review of Clinical and Functional Neuroscience

Rand Swenson, MD

Contents

1. Introduction

Most disorders of the nervous system either target particular brain structures or affect components of one or more functional systems of the brain. Therefore, an understanding of functional neuroanatomy is critical to localizing disease of the nervous system and to appreciating the origin of symptoms of nervous system damage. This chapter will consider the important elements of clinical neuroanatomy. There are several good texts that provide greater detail on these systems.[1-3] This chapter will discuss the cellular components of the nervous system first and then will consider the peripheral nervous system (PNS) before discussing the central nervous system (CNS). In the CNS we will first consider the sensory systems and then the motor systems before discussing limbic and higher cortical functions.

An atlas of brain structures is essential to the study of neuroanatomy. There are many good atlases,[4-6] and some can be found on the Web. One such atlas is located at www.dartmouth.edu/~rswenson/Atlas.

2. Cellular Constituents of the Brain

The brain consists of neurons and glia. While most of our discussion will focus on the functions of neurons, there is growing recognition of the important role of glial cells in maintaining critical functions of the brain. Therefore, glial biology will be considered at the end of the section.

The primary building block of the nervous system is the neuron. Each neuron has a cell body and processes, consisting of one or more dendrites, and axons. The cell body, also called the soma or perikarion, contains the metabolic machinery and the genetic material for the neuron. Dentrites are the main site of synapse with other neurons, often at knob-like projections called dendritic spines. The axon, beginning at the axon hillock, is the process that conveys the electrical signal from the neuron and it is often called the nerve fiber. Dendrites and axons usually have many collateral branches, and axo-dendritic synapses are the most common type of communication between neurons, though axosomatic and axoaxonic synapses are also frequent.

The neuron maintains a resting membrane potential. This potential is based on the concentration gradient of ions that is created by an energy-dependent sodium-potassium ATPase pump. This pump moves 2 potassium ions into the neuron in exchange for 3 sodium ions moving out of the cell. Therefore, this pump directly creates a slight electrical potential, with the outside of the cell being slightly positive. The pump is said to be electrogenic. However, most of the resting membrane potential does not derive directly from this effect of the pump but rather from the force of the concentration gradient created by the pump. Because potassium is in high concentration inside the neuron, there is a concentration gradient attempting to force potassium out of the cell. Similar forces will attempt to move sodium ions into the neuron.

The membrane of the neuron is a lipid bilayer with embedded proteins. Some of these proteins are pumps (like the sodium-potassium ATPase pump) but many are ion channels. These ion channels consist of transmembrane proteins with a complex configuration that includes a pore through which ions can pass. Some channels permit constant passage of ions (leak channels), while some are opened by voltage change (voltage-gated), or by chemical substances (ligand-gated). Most channels have selectivity, allowing only certain ions to pass when they are open. This selectivity is due to the particular conformation of the protein or the arrangement of charges in the ion pore.

The resting membrane is semipermeable, with much higher permeability to potassium than to sodium. This is due to potassium leak channels. Therefore, the potassium concentration gradient will force some positively charged potassium ions to escape from the cell. This is the primary generator of the voltage difference across the membrane, called the resting membrane potential. This potential is usually somewhere between -70 and -90 millivolts, with the inside of the cell negative because positive potassium ions have left the cell. The precise voltage depends on the force exerted by the concentration gradient. As potassium leaves the neuron, the inside of the cell will become progressively more negative, which will attract the positive potassium ions, preventing further exodus. If this electrical force is great enough, it will actually draw potassium ions from the outside of the cell back inside.

Potassium ions will escape from the neuron until the electrical attractive force of the developing negative charge inside the cell equals the force exerted by the concentration gradient that is forcing potassium out. Be aware that it doesn't take the movement of many positively charged potassium ions to create a significant electrical force, so the overall concentration gradient does not change very much by this movement. At the point where inward and outward forces balance, the neuron is in equilibrium, with one potassium ion moving into the neuron for every one that leaves. The transmembrane voltage at which this balance occurs is called the potassium equilibrium potential and can be calculated from the Nernst equation (Figure 1). This equation basically says that the equilibrium potential will be the product of a constant, multiplied by the natural logarithm of the ratios of concentration outside and inside the cell. A membrane potential can only be generated by ions that can actually cross the membrane. Since, in the case of neurons at rest, the membrane is much more permeable to potassium than to other ions, the potassium equilibrium potential nearly equals the measured resting membrane potential. However, it should be kept in mind that there is a very slight contribution to the membrane potential from movement of other ions. This contribution is proportional to their very low permeability. The Goldman-Hodgkin-Katz equation (Figure 1) takes these other ions into consideration, although, if the permeability to an ion is very small relative to potassium, the ion can be basically ignored when considering the resting membrane potential. It is important to understand the resting membrane potential, since this is necessary to understanding what happens when the neuron is excited.

Of course, all cells of the body have a resting membrane potential. This resting potential allows the cells to do work such as transporting molecules across their membranes. However, nerve and muscle cells are somewhat unique in that they have the property of being excitable. This excitability means that they can change their potential due to external chemical or mechanical factors.

Figure 1

A. Nernst equation

$$V = 58 \log \frac{[K^+]_{outside}}{[K^+]_{inside}}$$

At body temperature, the potassium equilibrium potential (which represents the great majority of resting membrane potential) is a constant times the logarithm of the ratio of concentrations of potassium outside and inside the cell.

B. Goldman-Hodgkins-Katz equation

$$V = 58 \log \frac{p_K[K^+]_o + p_{Na}[Na^+]_o + p_{Cl}[Cl^+]_i}{p_K[K^+]_i + p_{Na}[Na^+]_i + p_{Cl}[Cl^+]_o}$$

This is similar to the Nernst equation except that it adds a factor for permeability. If an ion is impermeable, its contribution to the membrane potential (V) is nil. The higher the relative permeability, the closer the membrane will be to the equilibrium potential for that ion.

When we discuss electrical changes in the neuronal membrane, this change is from the starting point of the resting membrane potential, where the cell is polarized, having an inside that is negative when compared to the outside. Depolarization makes the inside of the cell less negative and the outside less positive. Hyperpolarization is the opposite. Opening any ion channel will tend to bring the transmembrane voltage toward the equilibrium potential of whichever ions are permeable through that channel. For example, if a sodium channel were opened, the membrane potential would move toward the sodium equilibrium potential. Due to the concentration gradient of sodium, the sodium equilibrium potential occurs when the inside of the cell is slightly positive relative to the outside. Again, this does not require the movement of very many positively charged ions into the cell and can occur quite rapidly when the channel is opened. The term repolarization is applied to the process of reestablishing the resting membrane potential after an event that depolarizes the cell.

Certain ion channels in the neuronal membrane are opened rapidly when the membrane potential reaches a specific voltage. These are termed voltage-gated channels. The voltage at which the channel opens is called the threshold potential, and this corresponds with a sudden change in conformation of the transmembrane proteins comprising the ion channel. The channel then becomes permeable to all of the ions conducted by that particular voltage-gated channel. Since many of these voltage-gated channels are permeable to sodium, which is in high concentration outside the neuron, there is rapid movement of a few sodium ions into the neuron that reverses the normally negative potential of the inside of the cell to a slight positivity. This rapid depolarization is termed an action potential (Figure 2).

The open voltage-gated sodium channels rapidly close, a process called inactivation. This terminates the depolarization or rising phase of the action potential. Additionally, voltage-gated potassium channels open, which forces repolarization toward the potassium equilibrium potential by movement of potassium out of the cell. In fact, this produces slight hyperpolarization. During the brief period of

Figure 2

Action potential

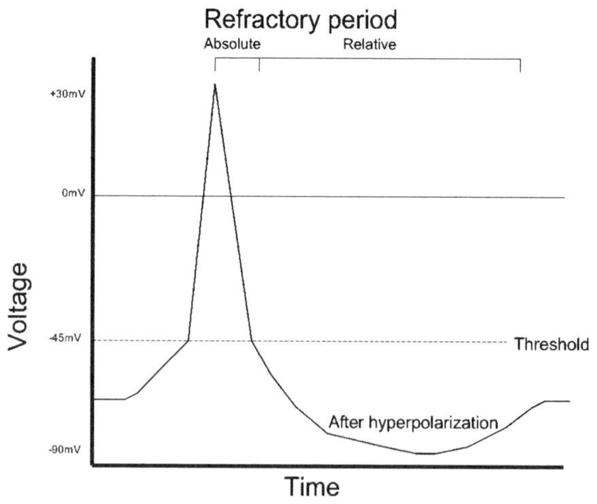

Depolarization is a graded phenomenon until threshold is reached. At that point, voltage-gated sodium channels are opened and the movement of sodium rapidly depolarizes the neuron. The voltage-gated sodium channels are then rapidly inactivated and voltage-gated potassium channels are opened, which drives the cell back toward the potassium equilibrium potential (near -90 μV). Until the cell repolarizes, the voltage-gated sodium channels are inactivated and another action potential cannot be generated (absolute refractory period). Until the voltage-gated potassium channels are inactivated it is harder (but not impossible) to generate an action potential (relative refractory period).

sodium channel inactivation, these channels cannot be opened again and the membrane cannot be depolarized. This is termed the absolute refractory period. During the period of hyperpolarization that follows the action potential, it takes a large stimulus to generate another action potential and this is termed the relative refractory period.

An action potential produces a large change in voltage of a portion of the neuron. Because ions spread through the cytoplasm and the extracellular fluid, the action potential also depolarizes adjacent areas of membrane. This depolarization opens voltage-gated ion channels in the adjacent membrane and the action potential is regenerated at these sites. This action potential then spreads over the nerve cell and is regenerated in all areas where there are voltage-gated ion channels. This includes spread down the axon. Because the potential is regenerated at each level of the neuron, the action potential can extend the length of the axon and into all branches without decreasing in amplitude. This is termed propagation of the action potential. Damage to an axon membrane or the presence of toxins that affect ion channels will affect the generation of the action potential or the conduction of the impulse.

The propagation of an action potential down an unmyelinated axon is quite slow due to the need for regeneration at each adjacent site. This usually restricts conduction to less than a meter per second. This speed can be increased by increasing the diameter of the axon, but is still quite slow. Myelination is a method for increasing the speed of conduction without making the axon too large. This process involves the wrapping of layers of cell membrane tightly around the axon. This has the function of preventing ions from moving through these insulated portions of the axonal membranes and also decreasing capacitance of the membrane by producing greater separation of the negative electrical charges inside from the positive charges outside the membrane.

In the central nervous system, the myelin sheath develops from oligodendroglial processes. In the peripheral nervous system, each segment of myelin is the result of wrapping of an individual cell, called a Schwann cell. There are recognition molecules in the membrane that initiate recognition between the axon and either the Schwann cell or the oligodendrocyte process. Other surface proteins are involved in causing the membrane to wrap around itself, and then to pack the external and internal parts of the membrane tightly. It is interesting that, although there are proteins performing each of these functions that are associated with the Schwann cell and the oligodendrocyte, the specific proteins are different in each case. This is part of the reason why the myelin is antigenically different in the CNS and the PNS.

There are gaps in between segments of myelin called the nodes of Ranvier. These are sites of high concentrations of voltage-gated ion channels. Because there is little movement of ions across the membrane where the myelin sheath is present, and because there is little charge concentration along the membrane in the internodal segment (due to low capacitance), ions can move relatively freely down the axon. This produces sufficient depolarization at the next node of Ranvier, which can be up to several millimeters away in heavily myelinated axons, without having to regenerate the action potential at each successive part of the axon. This markedly increases the speed of conduction of the axon, with the distance between nodes being directly proportional to the amount of the velocity increase. Damage to myelin significantly slows or can even block axonal conduction. The largest motor axons are those that connect the nervous system to skeletal muscle, and they conduct between 50 and 100-plus meters/second. Autonomic postganglionic motor axons to glands, organs and blood vessels are unmyelinated and conduct very slowly (usually less than 1 meter per second). Touch, pressure and muscle stretch sensation are conducted by large, myelinated fibers, and pain and temperature sensation is conducted by small myelinated or unmyelinated sensory fibers.

Most axons terminate in a "synapse" on the dendrites of other neurons, often on small dendritic spines. The synapse is the site of transmission between neurons. While there are rare gap junction-type synapses in which there is actual flow of ions between neurons, the vast majority of synapses are chemical synapses. These involve the release of neurotransmitter by the axon terminal when an action potential reaches it. The axon terminal contains vesicles or quanta of neurotransmitter, and release of transmitter from synaptic vesicles occurs by a multistep process. The action potential opens voltage-gated calcium channels on the nerve terminal, resulting in an inflow of calcium, because calcium is in higher concentration outside of cells. The calcium in the nerve terminal results in a series of chemical interactions between proteins in the nerve terminal that ultimately causes mobilization of vesicles of neurotransmitter, binding and then fusing them to the axonal presynaptic membrane. This fusion results in release of the content into the synaptic cleft. Some nerve terminals will release the contents of hundreds of vesicles every time an action potential reaches the nerve terminal. This is true of the neuromuscular junction. Some nerve terminals will release only one vesicle with a depolarization. This happens at many central nervous system axon terminals. In some synapses, only every second or third action potential actually results in the release of a vesicle of neurotransmitter.

The neurotransmitter diffuses across the synaptic cleft to the postsynaptic side (usually on a dendrite), where the transmitter binds with specific receptors. Many of these receptors are part of an ion channel called a ligand-gated ion channel. These ion channels have very specific permeability to particular ions. Depending on the particular ion permeability of the channels, the receptor may excite or inhibit the postsynaptic neuron. There are other receptors that are not ion channels. These receptors, termed metabotropic or second messenger receptors, are linked to internal processes within the postsynaptic neuron, such as enzymes that can change the function of the neuron. Many of these receptors are linked to g-proteins which can increase the intracellular concentration of compounds such as cyclic AMP, inositol triphosphate, or diacyl glycerol. Since these receptors frequently do not directly affect the membrane potential they are often described as being modulatory, and the transmitters that bind to these receptors are often termed neuromodulators. Because they can change many functions within the cell, their effects can be very long lasting.

The effect of the neurotransmitter is terminated by one of a few mechanisms. There may be enzymes that break down the neurotransmitter, such as the effect of acetylcholinesterase on acetylcholine. Blockade of acetylcholinesterase by drugs or toxins will prolong the effect of acetylcholine release. Another possibility is that the transmitter may diffuse away from the synaptic cleft, usually to be taken up by glial cells around the area. A third possibility is that the transmitter may be taken back up into the nerve terminal through specific transport mechanisms. In this case the transmitter may be repackaged for later release. Drugs such as the selective serotonin reuptake inhibitors affect this process.

In the case of ligand-gated ion channel-type receptor, the effect of opening the channel depends on the particular ions that can pass through it. In every case, opening these channels will tend to drive the membrane potential toward the equilibrium potential for the ions to which it is permeable. The voltage to which the membrane is driven has been termed the reversal potential for the receptor. If this reversal potential is at a level that would result in the membrane reaching threshold, it is termed an excitatory receptor since, if enough of these channels are opened, an action potential will be generated. For example, any ligand-gated receptor that is primarily permeable to sodium or calcium would be excitatory. If the reversal potential for a receptor is at a level that would not reach threshold, it would be an inhibitory receptor. Opening this type of channel would prevent the neuron from reaching threshold and therefore prevent it from generating an action potential. For example, opening a receptor that was permeable to potassium would be inhibitory.

The most common inhibitory receptor in the brain is the $GABA_A$ receptor that binds gamma aminobutyric acid and is permeable to chloride. This receptor is particularly important since many inhibitory drugs modulate the activity of this receptor, including alcohol, benzodiazepines and barbiturates. In the adult brain, since the reversal potential for an ion channel that is permeable to chloride is more negative than threshold, GABA is inhibitory when it binds to the $GABA_A$ receptor. Be aware, however, that at different chloride concentration (such as in the newborn brain), GABA may actually be excitatory.

If the cumulative activity of thousands of synapses brings the neuron to threshold through a process of summation, an action potential is generated and the process of transmission of the nerve impulse is begun once again. There are very few voltage-gated channels on the dendrites, and therefore, action potentials usually don't begin there. Voltage-gated channels are clustered in the axon hillock region at the beginning of the axon, which is the typical site of action potential generation. Depolarization of dendrites must spread to the axon hillock in order to summate into an action potential. Because the effect of this depolarization has to spread out over the neuron, it becomes smaller and smaller the further it has to travel. This is termed "electrotonic spread" of depolarization and means that a synapse located further out on a dendrite is going to produce less change at the axon hillock than would a similar synapse close to the soma.

Glial cells are important in the brain. We have already seen how oligodendrocytes comprise central nervous system myelin. Astrocytes surround neurons and blood vessels. These are responsible for the critical function of maintaining the normal ionic and nutritive environment around neurons. They remove ions and transmitters that accumulate due to neuronal activity and make sure the extracellular environment is ideal for the neuron. Recently, it has been recognized that glia can release growth factors and cytokines that are important for neuron health. Finally, they stimulate the brain capillaries to develop tight junctions and other specializations of endothelial cells that contribute to the blood-brain barrier (Section 12).

Ependymal cells are a type of glial cell that lines the ventricular system. These cells do not provide a barrier between the cerebrospinal fluid and the brain. Therefore, substances delivered to the CSF have direct access to the brain and spinal cord.

Table 1

Fiber Types and Functions (From Largest to Smallest)

Fiber Category	Size (microns)	Speed (meters/second)	Function
Aα Group IA and IB afferents	15	60-100	Large motor axons; muscle stretch and tension sensory axons
Aβ Group II afferents	12-14	30-60	Touch, pressure, vibration and joint position sensory axons
Aγ	8-10	15-30	Gamma efferent motor axons
Aδ Group III afferents	6-8	10-15	Sharp pain, very light touch and temperature sensation
B axons	2-5	3-10	Sympathetic preganglionic motor
C Group IV afferents	<1	<1.5	Dull, aching, burning pain and temperature sensation

3. Peripheral Nervous System

The peripheral nervous system is divided into somatic and autonomic components.

Somatic Nervous System

The somatic nervous system includes the sensory and motor nerves that innervate the limbs and body wall. These nerve fibers are classified as general somatic afferent (GSA) and general somatic efferent (GSE) fibers. GSA fibers in the peripheral nerves are the peripheral process of neurons in the dorsal root ganglion. The GSE fibers contained in peripheral nerves are the axons of anterior horn cells of the spinal cord.

Peripheral nerves have multiple layers of connective tissue surrounding axons, with the endoneurium surrounding individual axons, perineurium binding axons into fascicles, and epineurium binding the fascicles into a nerve. There are also blood vessels (vasa vasorum) and nerves (nervi nervorum) contained within the nerve. The axons that comprise the peripheral nerves are wavy, such that a length of peripheral nerve can be stretched to nearly half again its length before tension is directly transmitted to nerve fibers. Nerve roots have much less connective tissue, and individual nerve fibers within the roots are straight, leading to some vulnerability to damage, including by stretching.

Peripheral nerves receive collateral arterial branches from adjacent arteries. The arteries contribute to the vasa nervorum anastomose, with arterial branches entering the nerve above and below in order to provide an uninterrupted circulation along the course of the nerve. There is usually sufficient collateral circulation to survive damage to one of the feeding arteries. However, this is unpredictable.

Individual nerve fibers vary widely in diameter and also may be myelinated or unmyelinated. Myelin in the peripheral nervous system derives from Schwann cells, and the distance between nodes of Ranvier determines the conduction rate. Table 1 shows the functional categories of peripheral nerve fibers and their relative speeds of conduction. In this Table, please note that the function of an axon can be deduced from its diameter and from conduction velocity. Because certain conditions preferentially affect myelin, such conditions would be most likely to affect the functions mediated by the largest, fastest, most heavily myelinated axons (Table 1).

Figure 3

A myelomere of the spinal cord, and one of its two associated spinal nerves

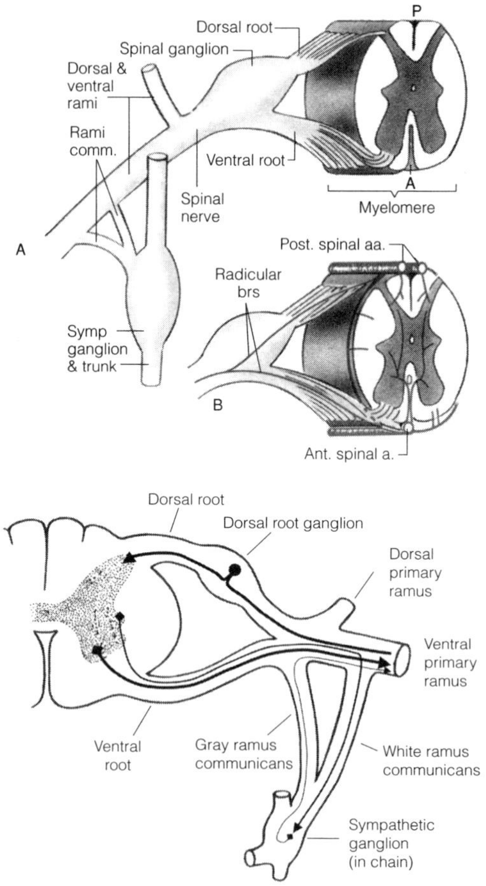

In A: A, anterior median fissure; P, posterior median sulcus. B shows the arterial supply to the cord. C depicts a sensory axon in the dorsal nerve root and a somatic motor axon in the ventral nerve root. Additionally, there is a sympathetic preganglionic axon arising from a neuron in the spinal cord lateral horn and this is traversing the white ramus communicans to the sympathetic gangliated chain, where it is synapsing on a small postganglionic neuron.

A and B from O'Rahilly R, Muller F. Basic Human Anatomy: A Regional Study of Human Structures. *Philadelphia, Pa: WB Saunders; 1982. By permission.*

Sensory neurons are somewhat unique, having an axon that extends to the periphery and another axon that extends into the central nervous system via the dorsal root (Figure 3). The cell body of this neuron is located in the dorsal root ganglion or one of the sensory ganglia of sensory cranial nerves. Both the peripheral and the central axon attach to the neuron at the same point, and these sensory neurons are called pseudounipolar neurons.

Before a sensory signal can be relayed to the nervous system it must be transduced into an electrical signal in a nerve fiber. This involves a process of opening ion channels in the membrane in response to mechanical deformation, temperature or, in the case of nociceptive fibers, various signals released from damaged tissue. Many receptors become less sensitive with continued stimulation, and this is termed adaptation. This adaptation may be rapid or slow, with rapidly adapting receptors being specialized for detecting changing signals.

There are several structural types of receptors in the skin. These fall into the category of encapsulated or nonencapsulated receptors. The nonencapsulated endings include free nerve endings, which are simply the peripheral end of the sensory axon. These mostly respond to noxious (pain) and thermal stimuli. There are some specialized free nerve endings around hairs that respond to very light touch, and also free nerve endings that contact special skin cells, called Merkel's cells. These Merkel's cells (discs) are specialized cells that release transmitter onto peripheral sensory nerve terminals. The encapsulated endings include Meissner's corpuscles, Pacinian corpuscles, and Ruffini endings. The capsules that surround encapsulated endings change the response characteristics of the nerves. Most encapsulated receptors are for touch, but the Pacinian corpuscles are very rapidly adapting and therefore are specialized to detect vibration. Ultimately, the intensity of the stimulus is encoded by the relative frequency of action potential generation in the sensory axon.

In addition to cutaneous receptors, there are muscle receptors that are involved in detecting muscle stretch (muscle spindle) and muscle tension (Golgi tendon organs). Muscle spindles are located in the muscle bellies and consist of intrafusal muscle fibers that are arranged in parallel with the majority of fibers comprising the muscle (ie, extrafusal fibers). The ends of the intrafusal fibers are contractile and are innervated by gamma motor neurons, while the central portion of the muscle spindle is relatively devoid of contractile elements and is wrapped by a sensory nerve ending, the annulospiral ending. This ending is activated by stretch of the muscle spindle or by contraction of the intrafusal fibers (Section 5). The Golgi tendon organs are located at the myotendinous junction and consist of nerve fibers intertwined with the collagen fibers at the myotendinous junctions. They are activated by contraction of the muscle (muscle tension).

The cutaneous distribution of sensory nerves is shown in Figure 4. There is a small area of overlap between sensory distributions of peripheral nerves. However, most named peripheral nerves have a distinct independent area of innervation, such that damage is likely to result in a well-defined region of anesthesia. It is important to note that there is significant variability in the precise borders of the peripheral distribution of nerves although the general pattern is quite consistent.

Spinal nerve roots supply dermatomes (Figure 5). With few exceptions, there is complete overlap between adjacent dermatomes. This means that the loss of a single nerve root rarely produces significant loss of skin sensitivity. The exception to this rule is found in small patches in the distal extremities, which have been termed autonomous zones. In these regions single nerve roots supply distinct and non-overlapping areas of skin. By their nature the autonomous zones represent only a small portion of any dermatome and only a few nerve roots have such autonomous zones. For example, the C5 nerve root may be the sole supply to an area of the lateral arm and proximal part of the lateral forearm. The C6 nerve root may distinctly supply some skin of the thumb and index finger. Injuries to the C7 nerve root may decrease sensation over the middle and sometimes the index finger along with a restricted area on the dorsum of the hand. C8 nerve root lesions can

Figure 4

The sensory distribution of peripheral nerves

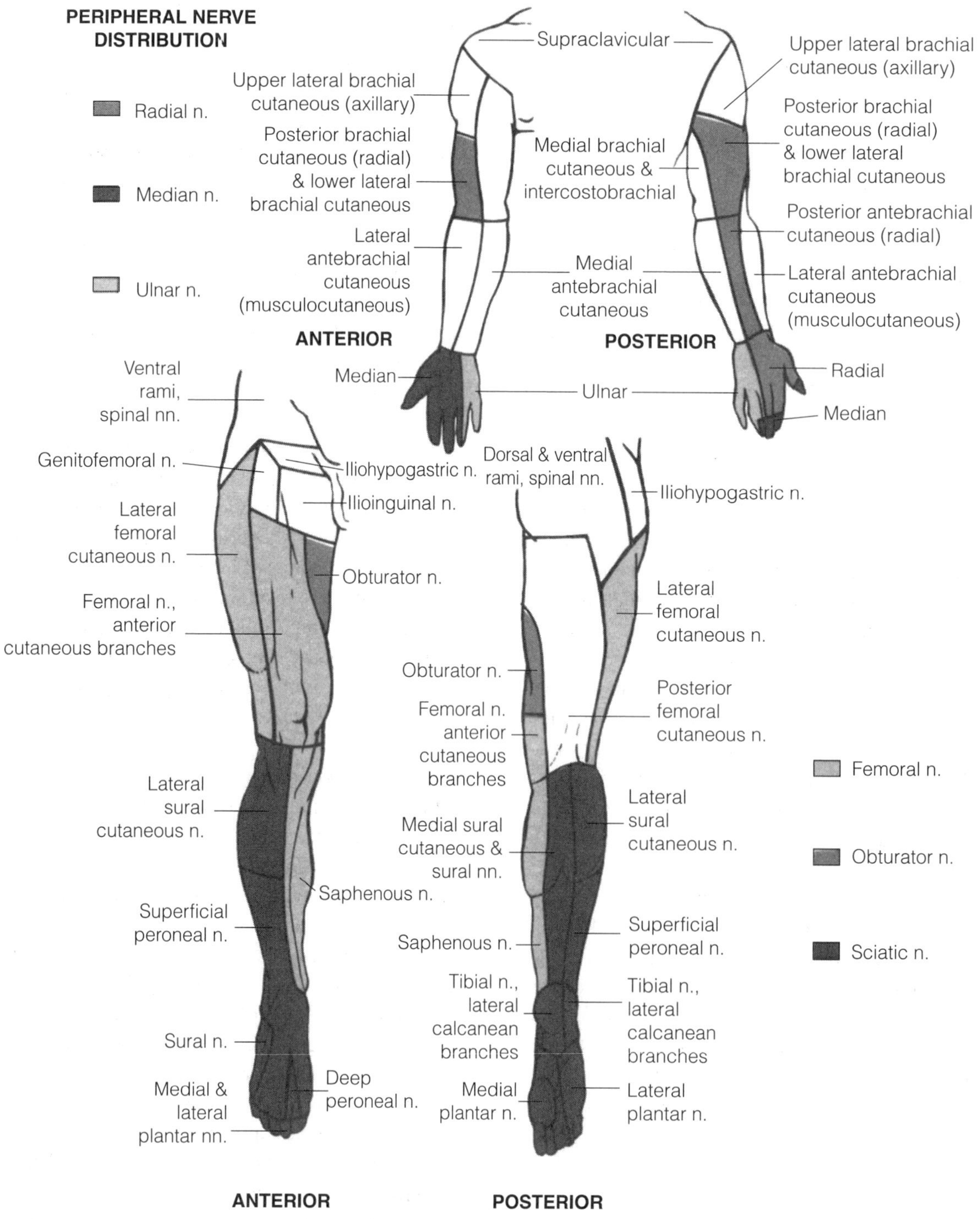

From O'Rahilly R, Muller F. Basic Human Anatomy: A Regional Study of Human Structures. *Philadelphia, Pa: WB Saunders; 1982. By permission.*

Figure 5

The approximate sensory distribution of dorsal roots (after Foerster)

Note that there is near complete overlap between adjacent nerve roots with the exception of a small distal portion of the distribution (so-called "autonomous zones").

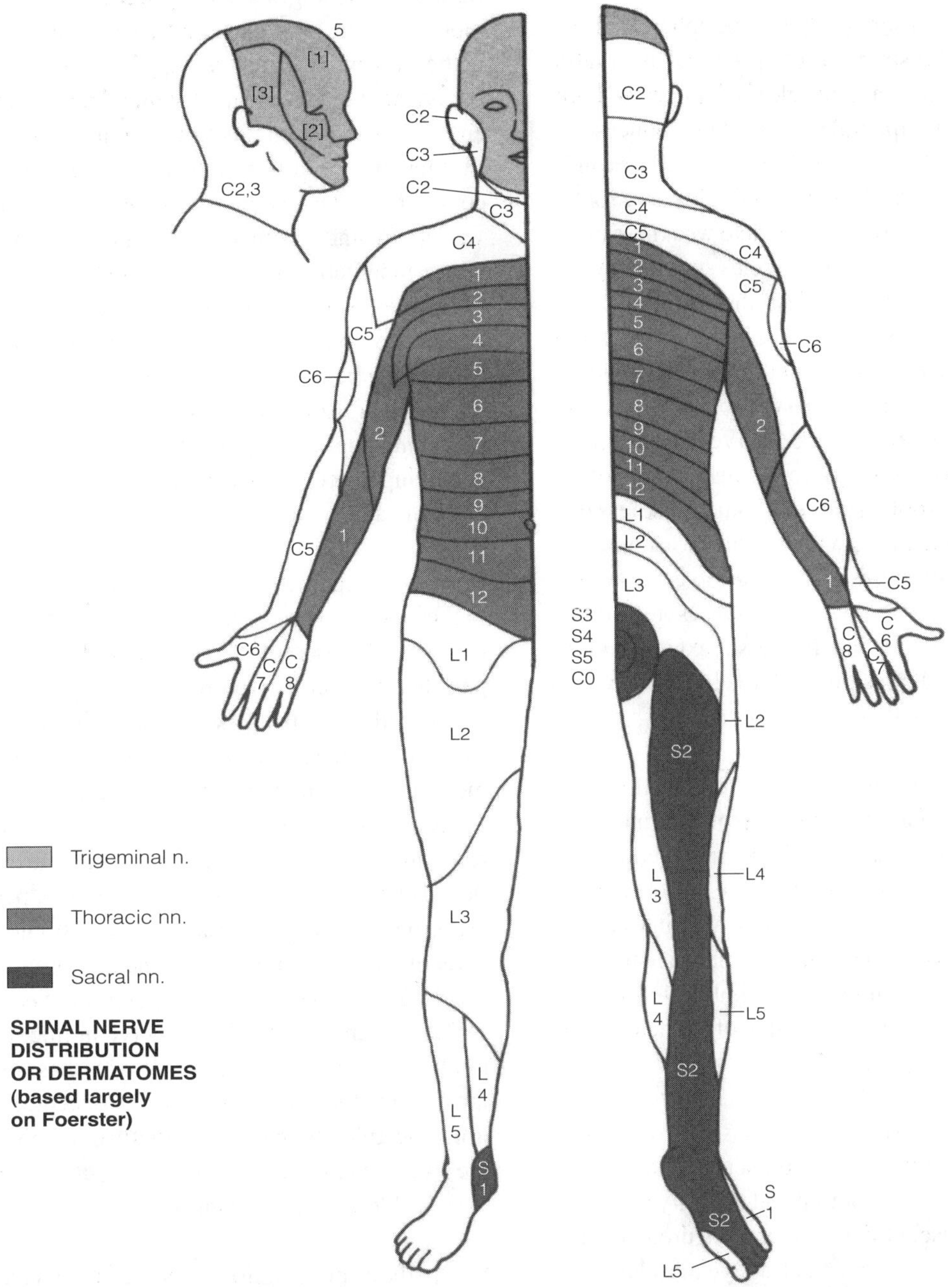

From O'Rahilly R, Muller F. Basic Human Anatomy: A Regional Study of Human Structures. *Philadelphia, Pa: WB Saunders; 1982. By permission.*

produce similar symptoms over the small digit, occasionally extending into the hypothenar area of the hand. In the lower limb, L4 nerve root damage may decrease sensation over the medial part of the leg, while L5 lesions affect sensation over part of the dorsum of the foot and great toe. S1 nerve root lesions typically decrease sensation on the lateral side of the foot.

In addition to sensory problems, peripheral nerve injury can affect strength. The principal innervation for the most important muscles is depicted in Table 2. Damage to peripheral nerves often produces a very recognizable pattern of severe weakness and (with time) atrophy. Damage to single nerve roots usually does not produce complete weakness of muscles since there are no muscles supplied by a single nerve root. Nonetheless, there is often detectible weakness. Examples in the upper extremity include weakness of shoulder abductors and external rotators with C5 nerve root lesions, weakness of elbow flexors with C6 nerve root lesions, possible weakness of wrist and finger extension with C7 nerve root lesions and some weakness of intrinsic hand muscles with C8 and T1 lesions. In the lower extremity, there may be some weakness of knee extension with L3 or L4 lesions, some difficulty with great toe (and, to a lesser extent, ankle) extension with L5 lesions and weakness of great toe plantar flexion with S1 nerve root damage.

Motor nerve fibers end in myoneural junctions. These consist of a single motor axon terminal on a skeletal muscle fiber. The myoneural junction includes a complex infolding of the muscle membrane, the ridges of which contain nicotinic acetylcholine receptors. There is also a matrix in the synaptic cleft containing acetylcholinesterase, involved in termination of action of the neurotransmitter.

One motor neuron has connections with many muscle fibers through collateral branches of the axon. This is called the motor unit and can vary from a handful of muscle fibers per motor neuron in muscles of very fine control (such as eye muscles) up to several thousands of fibers (as in the gluteal muscles).

Autonomic Nervous System

The autonomic nervous system consists of nerve fibers that have been classified as general visceral efferent (GVE), and appears in two main divisions, the sympathetic and the parasympathetic nervous systems. The sympathetic nerves are primarily involved in responses that would be associated with fighting or fleeing, such as increasing heart rate and blood pressure, as well as constricting blood vessels in the skin and dilating them in muscles. The parasympathetic nervous system is involved in energy conservation functions and increases gastrointestinal motility and secretion. It also increases contractility. There are some areas in which blood vessels are under competing sympathetic and parasympathetic control, such as in the nose or erectile tissues. There are some areas where there is a competitive balance between sympathetics and parasympathetics, such as the effects on heart rate or the pupil. For some functions, sympathetics and parasympathetics cooperate; an example being parasympathetic nerves, which are necessary for erection, and sympathetics for ejaculation.

Both the sympathetic and parasympathetic portions of the autonomic nervous system have a two-neuron pathway from the central nervous system to the peripheral organ. Therefore, there is a ganglion interposed in each of these pathways, with the exception of the sympathetic pathway to the adrenal medulla. The adrenal medulla basically functions as a sympathetic ganglion, with the ganglion cells releasing transmitter (epinephrine) into the circulation. The two nerve fibers in an autonomic pathway are termed preganglionic and postganglionic. At the level of the autonomic ganglia the neurotransmitter is typically acetylcholine. Postganglionic parasympathetic neurons also release acetylcholine, while norepinephrine is the postganglionic transmitter for most sympathetic nerve fibers. The exception is the use of acetylcholine in sympathetic transmission to the sweat glands and erector pili muscles, as well as to some blood vessels in muscle.

Sympathetic preganglionic neurons are located between T1 and L2 in the lateral horn of the spinal cord. Therefore, sympathetics have been termed the thoracolumbar outflow. These preganglionic visceral motor fibers leave the cord in the ventral nerve

Table 2

Strength Testing

Movements and the principal muscles, nerves and nerve roots involved in the movement. Parentheses indicate a smaller contribution.

Movement Tested	Main Muscles	Nerve Root Levels	Peripheral Nerve
Shoulder			
Shrug (elevation)	Trapizius	C2-5	Spinal accessory
Abduction	Deltoid/supraspinatus	C5 (6)	Axillary/suprascap.
External rotation	Infraspinatus/teres	C5 (6)	Suprascapular
Internal rotation	Pectoralis major	C5-7	Lateral pectoral
Adduction	Latissimus/pectoralis	C6-8	Subsapular/pectoral
Flexion	Deltoid/corachobr.	C5-6	Axillary/musculocut.
Elbow			
Flexion	Biceps/brachialis	C5-6	Musculocutaneous
	Brachioradialis	C5-6	Radial
Extension	Triceps	C6-7	Radial
Wrist			
Flexion	Flexor carpi mm.	C6-7	Median/ulnar
Extension	Extensor carpi radialis	C6-7	Radial
	Ext. carpi ulnaris	C7-8	Radial
Pronation	Pronator teres	C6-7	Median
Supination	Supinator	C5-6	Radial
Finger			
Flexion	Flexor digitorum mm.	C7-8	Median (ulnar)
Extension	Extensor digitorum	C7-8	Radial
Ab- & adduction	Interosseus muscles	C8-T1	Ulnar
Thumb abduction	Abductor pollicis	C8-T1	Median
Hip			
Flexion	Iliopsoas	L2-3 (L4)	Lumbar plexus
Extension	Gluteus	L5-S2	Inferior gluteal
Abduction	Gluteus medius	L5-S1	Superior gluteal
Adduction	Adductur mm.	L2-4	Obturator
Knee			
Flexion	Hamstring	L5-S1	Sciatic
Extension	Quadriceps	L2-4	Femoral
Ankle			
Dorsiflexion	Tibialis anterior	L4-5 (S1)	Peroneal
Plantar flexion	Gastroc/soleus	S1 (S2)	Tibial
Inversion	Posterior tibial	L5 (S1)	Tibial
Eversion	Proneal mm.	L5 (S1)	Peroneal
Great toe			
Dorsiflexion	Extensor hallucis	L5 (S1)	Peroneal
Plantar flexion	Flexor hallucis	(S1) S2	Tibial

Figure 6

Sympathetic pathway to the head

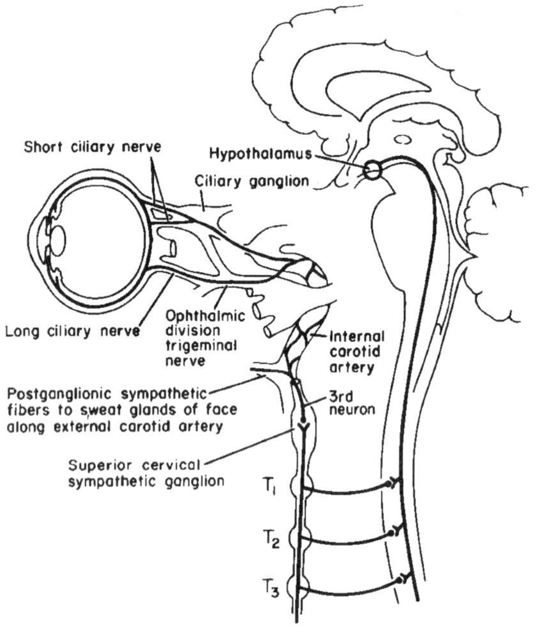

Note the descending connection from the hypothalamus through the brain stem and cervical spinal cord to the pregangilionic neuron in the upper thoracic cord. The axon from the preganglionic neuron exits the cord and joins the sympathetic gangliated chain. Those destined for the head ascend the cervical sympathetic chain to reach the superior cervical ganglion, where they synapse with postganglionic neurons. The axons from the postganglionic neurons join blood vessels to the head (those to the orbit are depicted in the figure as following the internal carotid to the ophthalmic artery).

From Reeves AG. Disorders of the Nervous System: A Primer. *Chicago, Ill: Yearbook Medical Publishing; 1981. With permission.*

root and then connect to the sympathetic gangliated chain through the white rami communicans (Figure 3). This chain of connected ganglia follows the sides of the vertebrae all the way from the head to the coccyx. These axons may synapse with postganglionic neurons in these paravertebral ganglia. Alternatively, preganglionic fibers can pass directly through the ganglionated chain to reach prevertebral ganglia along the aorta (via splanchnic nerves). Additionally, these preganglionics can pass rostrally or caudally through the ganglionated chain to reach the head or the lower lumbosacral regions. The sympathetic pathway to the head is shown in Figure 6. Sympathetic fibers can go to viscera by one of two pathways. Some postganglionics can leave the ganglionated chain and follow blood vessels to the organs. Alternatively, preganglionic fibers may pass directly through the ganglionated chain to enter the abdomen as splanchnic nerves. These synapse in ganglia located along the aorta (the celiac, renal, superior or inferior mesenteric ganglia) with postganglionic neurons. Again, the postganglionic nerve fibres follow the blood vessels to the organs.

Sympathetic postganglionic fibers from the ganglionated chain can go back to the spinal nerves (via gray rami communicans) to be distributed to somatic tissues of the limbs and body walls. For example, the somatic response to sympathetic activation will result in sweating, constriction of blood vessels in the skin, slight dilation of vessels in muscle, and in piloerection. Damage to sympathetic nerves to the head results in slight constriction of the pupil and loss of sweating on that side of the head (called Horner syndrome). This can happen anywhere along the course of the nerve pathway, including the upper thoracic spine and nerve roots, the apex of the lung, the neck, or the carotid plexus of postganglionics.

Parasympathetic preganglionic nerves arise with cranial nerves III, VII, IX and X, as well as from the sacral segments S2-4. Therefore, they have been termed the craniosacral outflow. Parasympathetics in cranial nerve III synapse in the ciliary ganglion and are involved in pupillary constriction and accommodation for near vision. Parasympathetics in cranial nerve VII synapse in the pterygopalatine ganglion (lacrimation) or the submandibular ganglion (salivation), while those in cranial nerve IX synapse in the otic ganglion (salivation from parotid gland). The vagus nerve follows a long course to supply the thoracic and abdominal organs up to the level of the distal transverse colon, synapsing in ganglia very close to (or within) the organ walls. The pelvic parasympathetic nerves, which appear as pelvic splanchnic nerves, activate bladder contraction and also supply lower abdominal and pelvic organs.

4. Development

The brain begins as an infolding of ectoderm on the dorsal aspect of the embryo around 18 days from conception (Figure 7). The ectoderm has a default program to develop the neural tube, but produces a protein–bone morphogenic protein (BMP) that blocks development of neural tube. This is one of the transforming growth factor beta (TGF-beta) family of proteins. The notochord secretes several factors (noggin, chordin and folistatin) that inhibit BMP, triggering formation of the neural epithelium over the notochord. This produces a dorsal longitudinal fold, the neural groove, that begins closing into a tube in the cervical area at around day 20. It "zips up" rostrally and caudally to close the tube around 28 days. The hollow of the tube becomes the ventricular system and the walls become the brain and spinal cord.

The cells comprising the walls of the neural tube undergo massive proliferation. Some of these cells become neural precursors (neuroblasts) and some become glial precursors (glioblasts) under the influence of proteins called notch and delta, which are expressed on these cells. This prevents all cells from developing into neurons or all into glia.

Cells proliferate in the region of the tube adjacent to the cavity (the ventricular zone). There are long, thin glia (radial glia) that maintain contact between the inner and outer edges of the wall of the tube. There are contact factors on the surface of the radial glia and on the developing neurons that guide radial migration of cells from the ventricular zone of the tube into the mantle zone of the neural tube, a layer that adds to the outside of the neural tube. This mantle zone becomes most of the substance of the spinal cord and brain. As axons begin to move out from the cells, they enter the periphery of the tube, comprising the marginal zone. The spinal cord maintains this general organization into adulthood, with the ependymal cells being the only remnant of the ventricular zone, the gray matter representing the marginal zone and the white matter the mantle zone.

Migration is a little more complex in the rostral part of the brain, the portion that becomes the cerebral cortex. Radial glia maintain connections to the very surface of the cerebral cortex for a long time (this surface layer becomes cortical layer I). Then there are 5 waves of neuronal migration into the cerebral cortex (representing cortical layers II-VI). Each wave migrates though the prior set of neurons until they bump up against cortical layer I. This means that the oldest layer of the cortex is layer I, but the next oldest (developmentally) is layer VI. Migration continues for quite some time and is subject to being disrupted.

The head end of the neural tube folds ventrally at the cervical flexure and cephalic (mesencephalic) flexure and then expands into primary brain vesicles. These primary vesicles are, from caudal to rostral, the rhombencephalic, mesencephalic and prosencephalic vesicles. The primary vesicles become secondary vesicles. A dorsal fold develops in the rhombencephalon (pontine flexure) that divides the rhombencephalic vesicle into the myencephalic vesicle (the myelencephalon becomes the caudal

Figure 7

Progressive stages of development of the neural tube

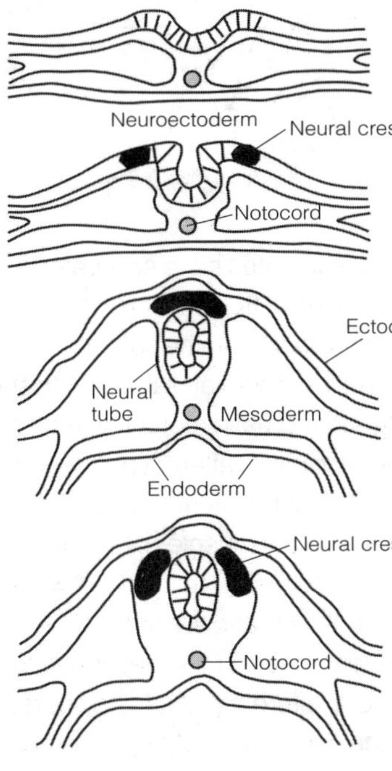

The black represents the location of neural crest cells. The light gray circle (directly below the neural tube) is the notocord.

part of the 4th ventricle, ie, the medulla) and the metencephalic vesicle (the metencephalon becomes the rostral part of the 4th ventricle, ie, the pons).

Rostrally, the prosencephalic vesicle develops a midline vesicle (the diencephalic vesicle, that becomes the third ventricle) and lateral outpouchings (that become the telencephalic vesicles, which develop into the lateral ventricles).

The neural tube has a ventral portion (the basal plate) and a dorsal portion (the alar plate). The main signal that triggers the development of the ventral part of the neural tube is a gene product called Sonic Hedgehog (Shh), which is produced by the notochord and the floorplate of the neural tube. Absence of Sonic Hedgehog will result in holoprosencephaly. There are other signals that are responsible for the development of the dorsal aspect of the neural tube. These derive from overlying skin and include many of the TGF-beta family (including BMP, vitamin A and dorsalin). Ventral-dorsal gradients of these various molecules pattern the development of the spinal cord and brain stem.

The basal plate in the spinal cord and brain stem is destined to contain most of the motor neurons while the alar plate contains sensory neurons. Additionally, cells in the developing cervical region accumulate retinoic acid that diffuses rostally into the developing head. The expression of different patterns of Hox genes is dependent on the specific concentration of retinoic acid to which a developing neuron is exposed. The set of Hox genes expressed will determine the rostral-caudal organization of the brain stem from the developing neural tube. This is why vitamin A (or lack of this vitamin) or administration of analogues of vitamin A can be so teratogenic.

Throughout the brain stem, the general organization of the spinal cord is maintained. However, with the expansion of the fourth ventricles on the dorsal side, the alar plates are displaced laterally (Figure 8). As a result, the cranial nerve nuclei that are located ventrally and medially (in the basal plate) are motor, and those that are in the dorsal and lateral part of the brain stem are sensory. There is a shallow groove on the floor of the fourth ventricle (the sulcus limitans)

Figure 8

A. A view of the dorsal aspect of the embryo showing the location of the neural epithelium and the successive stages of closure of the neural tube

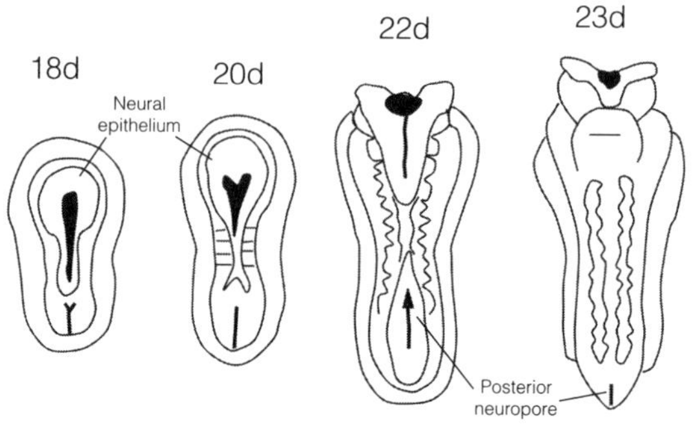

Note that the anterior and posterior neuropore are open at each end in the lower figure.

B. The neural tube in the region that will be the spinal cord (left) and brain stem (right)

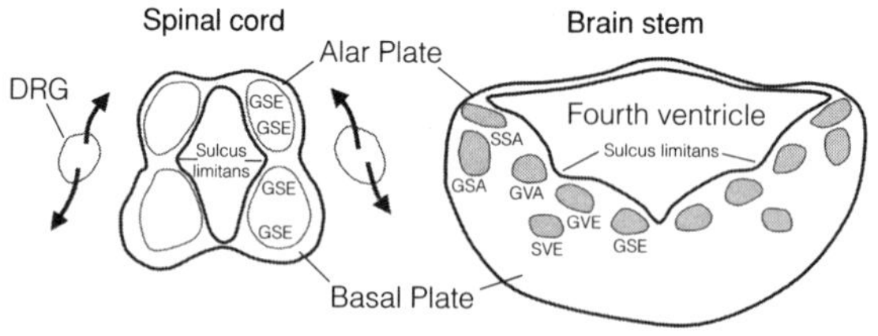

Note how the alar plates have separated from one another in the view at the left. The motor cranial nerve nuclei are ventromedial to the sulcus limitans and the sensory nuclei are dorsolateral. GSE = general somatic efferent (somatic motor to eyes and tongue); GVE = general visceral efferent (parasympathetic); SVE = special visceral efferent (branchial motor to larynx, pharynx and jaw muscles); GVA = general visceral afferent (visceral sensory); GSA = general somatic afferent (somatic sensory); SSA = special somatic afferent (hearing and vestibular function). Special visceral afferent (SVA; taste fibers) terminate in nuclei in the same general region as GVA.

that defines the separation between alar and basal plates, and cranial nerve nuclei located near this sulcus are associated with visceral functions.

The retina develops directly from the neural tube as an outpouching from the diencephalic vesicle, while inner ear formation is induced in the overlying ectoderm by the presence of the rhombencephalon.

The cerebellum undergoes very late development from the dorsal lips of the metencephalon (rhombic lips). This region continues to develop even postpartum. The frontal lobes of the cerebral cortex are also rather late to develop, particularly in terms of myelination of the white matter connections.

Much of the peripheral nervous system develops from neural crest cells (Figure 7). All of the sensory neurons and postganglionic sympathetic neurons develop from these cells, as do the supporting cells of the ganglia and the Schwann cells. Neural crest cells also become all of the chromaffin cells, the melanocytes and, in addition, contribute to development of the outer layers of the eye and many of the skull bones.

It appears that the ultimate fate of the developing neurons depend on several factors. First of all, neurons respond to the environment through which they migrate, changing their character depending on environmental signals. Additionally, it is critical that neurons make appropriate connections since, if they do not, they undergo apoptosis (a noninflammatory, non-necrotic form of cell death). This appears to be dependent on appropriate and complex trophic interaction between neurons and targets.

A large amount of study has been devoted to the topic of axonal guidance. All growing axons (neuritis) develop a broad lamellipodium at their tip (the "growth cone"), which extends filopodia through assembly of globular actin into fibrillar actin. If there are factors in the environment of the filopodium that stabilize the fibrillar actin, that filopodium will stabilize, with the assembly of tubulin into microtubules. This will become the platform for further axonal outgrowth and the axon will extend in that direction. There are apparently soluble factors as well as contact factors that can result in stabilization (or destabilization) of the growth cone, attracting or repelling the growth cone. Some of these factors include interaction with an already successful "pioneer" fiber through cell adhesion molecules on the growth cone and the pioneer fiber. There are a couple of classical model systems that are known in some detail. One of these is the optic chiasm, where retinal ganglion cells from the temporal retina, which express a specific Eph receptor, are repelled by the specific type of ephrin that is expressed by the glia of the optic chiasm. This allows only the axons from the nasal retinal ganglion cells to cross. Another model system is the spinal decussation of spinothalamic tract fibers. This appears to occur via a different mechanism in which the developing growth cones express netrin receptors that result in attraction of the growth cone to the region of high concentration of netrin located in the floorplate of the developing neural tube. Exposure of the nerve process to this high concentration of netrin, however, results in downregulation of the expression of netrin receptors and an upregulation of expression of the gene for Robo. Neuritis expressing Robo are repelled by another diffusible protein, "slit" that is present in the floorplate. This repels the growth cone and prevents it from recrossing the midline. While it is safe to say that only the broadest outlines are known about how the nervous system is wired, it is clear that gradients of diffusible attractant and repulsive molecules, coupled with contact interaction between adjacent fibers, represent the prime mechanisms of axonal guidance. There are also known molecular mechanisms for target recognition and stabilization of appropriate synapses; however, these signals are only known for a limited number of systems, including the neuromuscular junction. Neurons that do not make appropriate connection undergo apoptosis in a process of self-selection that continues through most of early development.

5. Spinal Cord

Anatomy

The spinal cord is composed of a core of gray matter surrounded by white matter (Figure 3). The white matter appears in three locations: lateral, anterior, and posterior to the gray matter (the lateral, ventral and dorsal funiculi, respectively). The white matter consists of tracts that interconnect segments of the spinal cord or connect the spinal cord with the brain. The gray matter appears in a butterfly shape, with ventral and dorsal horns, an intermediate gray matter and, in the thoracic cord, a lateral horn (sympathetic neurons). The dorsal horn contains neurons that represent some of the processing mechanisms for sensory signals, and the ventral horn contains motor neurons.

The gray mater of the spinal cord consists of layers (Rexed's lamina), which basically progress from posterior to anterior (lamina I-IX). Laminae I-III are usually included in the "substantia gelatinosa". This is where many sensory fibers terminate and are initially processed. Laminae IV and V includes the neurons that give rise to the spinothalamic tract. Lamina IX is the location of the alpha motor neurons. There is a topographic organization of motor neurons in the ventral horn, with motor neurons to extensor muscles placed more anteriorly and flexor motor neurons more posteriorly in Lamina IX of the anterior horn.

Laminae VII and VIII are often included in the "intermediate gray matter" of the spinal cord. This is the location of most of the interneurons that are part of reflex pathways. These interneurons often interconnect with one another and receive processed signals from sensory systems and eventually (often through some chain of interneurons) connect with motor neurons. Interneurons mostly use glutamate as excitatory transmitter or glycine for inhibition. There are interneurons that have axons that cross the spinal cord, synapsing on the contralateral side of the cord, and others that travel for many segments, contributing to intersegmental reflexes and motor patterns (such as normal locomotor patterns or reciprocal arm and leg swing). Most of the axons that travel between segments travel in the white matter immediately adjacent to the gray matter (so-called propriospinal fibers). Interneurons of the intermediate gray are under descending control. Most of the tonic descending control is inhibitory, primarily mediated through medullary reticulospinal tract fibers.

The cervical and lumbar enlargements of the spinal cord result form enlargement of the gray matter that contains the neural machinery necessary to operate the limbs. The cord ends in the upper lumbar region (L1-2) at the conus medullaris. Of course there are nerves to the lower extremities that exit the spine all the way down to the sacrum. Therefore, the lower lumbar and sacral nerve roots must leave the spinal cord in the lower thoracic/upper lumbar regions and course within the canal made by the vertebrae down to their point of exit. This bundle of nerve roots is called the cauda equina and can be injured in the low back with catastrophic consequences (including loss of bladder and bowel control). The filum terminale interna is a continuation of pia matter that continues to the lower end of the thecal sac (around S2). It then continues, along with a contribution from the dura matter, the filum terminale externa, to attach to the coccyx, anchoring the lower end of the spinal cord.

Reflexes

Reflexes, at a minimum, require a sensory signal and a motor response of some type. There are often interneurons present that pattern the reflex response. In the case of spinal reflexes, the intermediate gray (Rexed's lamina VII) contains interneurons that pattern reflex responses.

Muscle stretch (myotatic) reflexes are mediated purely at the spinal cord level, with monosynaptic connections between muscle spindle afferents and motor neurons to the muscle that was stretched. There is polysynaptic facilitation of agonist muscles and polysynaptic inhibition of antagonist muscles. The sensitivity of this reflex can be adjusted by activation of small gamma motor neurons in the ventral horn. These small motor neurons contract the intrafusal fibers of the muscle spindle and increase the sensitivity to stretch. This reflex is under a constant degree of inhibition via descending tracts (particularly medullary reticulospinal tracts).

There is an inverse myotatic reflex that involves inhibition of muscles as a result of very forceful stretching of the muscle. This involves massive activation of Golgi tendon organs and is apparently protective (preventing the muscle from tearing). It is only normally seen when a muscle is stretched to the breaking point, although it is seen as the "give-way" portion of the clasp-knife response observed in patients with spasticity.

There is a third type of reflex, the withdrawal reflex to noxious stimuli. These reflex responses are mediated via polysynaptic pathways that actually involve both sides and many levels of the cord. This reflex response, which results from activation of nociceptive nerve fibers (particularly the Aδ fibers), includes withdrawal (physiologic flexion) of the limb, along with extension of the contralateral limb. In fact, there is some effect on all four limbs when this reflex is activated, making this a very complicated reflex. Spinal reflexes are normally kept in check by descending pathways. Damage to the spinal cord usually results in exaggerated reflexes below the level of the lesion after a brief period of "shock." This may be overactivity of muscle stretch reflexes (hyper-reflexia; clonus), inverse myotatic reflexes ("clasp-knife") or withdrawal reflexes (Babinski response).

6. Brain Stem Organization

The brain stem contains the origin of motor cranial nerves and the termination for all of the sensory cranial nerves except for vision and olfaction. Due to the fact that the dorsolateral brainstem develops from the alar plate of the neural tube (see Section 4), it is the locus of most of the sensory cranial nerve nuclei. Therefore, damage to the lateral brain stem often affects sensory cranial nerve nuclei such as the vestibular nuclei (where vertigo would be the primary complaint and nystagmus would be the main exam finding) or the trigeminal nuclei (affecting facial sensations, particularly pain and temperature sense as well as the corneal reflex). The corneal (blink) reflex, which is a brain stem mediated reflex, requires intact corneal sensation, and also intact facial nerves since this consensual reflex is mediated via bilateral connections between the spinal nucleus of the trigeminal and the facial nuclei. Motor cranial nerve nuclei are located ventromedially in the brain stem due to their embryonic origin in the basal plate.

Patients with cranial nerve damage often have problems with their voice or with swallowing. The nucleus ambiguus is the location of the majority of the motor neurons to the larynx, pharynx and soft palate. These fibers travel with the vagus and, to a lesser extent, the glossopharyngeal nerve. The gag reflex has a sensory limb that involves sensations from the back of the pharynx via the glossopharyngeal nerve to the medulla, with subsequent activation of vagal nerve fibers that should cause the pharynx to contract bilaterally and the soft palate to elevate. The larynx is innervated by the vagus nerve, via the recurrent laryngeal branch. This nerve enters the chest and ascends to the neck, passing posterior to the thyroid gland to reach the larynx.

Visceral sensations arriving at the brain stem with the vagus and glossopharyngeal nerves traverse the solitary tract to the solitary nucleus. These visceral sensory fibers include chemoreceptor inputs from the carotid and aortic body, baroreceptor inputs and inputs from pulmonary stretch receptors. These sensory fibers participate in a variety of visceral reflexes including the baroreceptor reflex as well as respiratory reflexes.

Cranial parasympathetic nuclei include the salivatory nuclei (that send fibers into the facial and glossopharyngeal nerves), the dorsal motor nuclei of the vagus (that are the origin for most of the vagal parasympathetics), and the Edinger-Wesphal nucleus (that is the origin for oculomotor parasympathetic nerves to pupillary constrictors and the cilary muscle for the lens).

Eye movement is controlled by somatic efferent neurons in the oculomotor (midbrain), trochlear (midbrain) and abducens (pons) nuclei (Section 8).

Much of the core of the brain stem consists of reticular formation (RF). While there are some well-localized nuclei within the RF, most of the RF is involved in integrative functions. There are some regions that are more focused on particular functions (for example, most of the respiratory centers and some centers for cardiovascular control are portions of the RF). Additionally, there are regions in the rostral pons that play a role in patterning gait in many species (probably including humans) and also the RF is involved in modulating muscle tone. Descending projections from the medullary reticular formation have a strong inhibitory effect over spinal cord interneurons (and therefore over reflexes). Despite what have been termed physiologic "centers," it is better to think of the RF as collections of neurons serving a variety of important functions, with some regional differences in the primary functions that are influenced.

One special case includes the midbrain reticular formation, which is the foundation for the reticular activating system. This system involves diffuse projections through the intralaminar and midline thalamic nuclei to the cerebral cortex. Damage to midbrain reticular formation interferes with normal arousal and produces coma by interfering with this mechanism.

There are very specific neurotransmitter systems in the brain. Most of these systems are modulatory. For example, most of the serotonin in the brain arises from raphe nuclei and most of the norepinephrine arises from the locus ceruleus. These nuclei have terminations in virtually all areas of the central nervous system (Figure 9) and are involved in such diffuse processes as sleep/wake, pain modulation, and regulation of mood.

Figure 9

Efferent connections from the raphe nuclei (serotonin; A) and from the locus ceruleus and medullary reticular formation (norepinephrine; B)

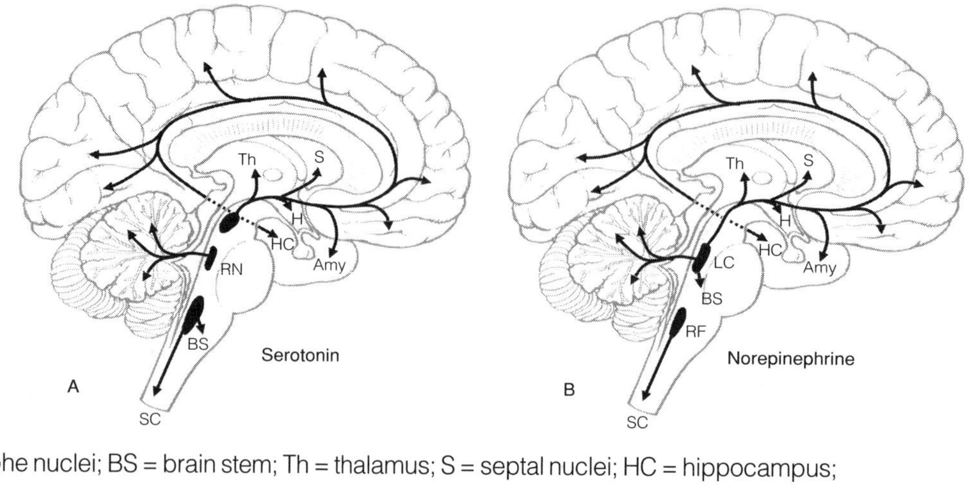

RN = raphe nuclei; BS = brain stem; Th = thalamus; S = septal nuclei; HC = hippocampus; Amy = amygdala; H = hypothalamus; LC = locus ceruleus; RF = reticular formation

7. Sensory Systems

The sensory pathways begin with sensory receptors that transduce the signal (light, sound, touch, etc.) and follow the peripheral nerves (as described in Section IIIa) or cranial nerves. There are several pathways that convey this information through the central nervous system. Some of these pathways terminate in the cerebral cortex, providing the basis for conscious sensation. Other sensations are unconscious, particularly those from muscle spindles and muscle stretch receptors. These pathways terminate in the cerebellum, where they participate in control of movement; or in the brain stem, where they participate in many reflex responses.

Somatosensory Systems

The nervous system has many more sensory fibers and sensory pathways than motor fibers. This stems from the importance of properly understanding the environment prior to responding. These ascending tracts provide the bridge between the inputs from the environment and the organizing centers of the brain that generate the complexity of our responses. Collectively, somatosensory systems are termed "general somatic afferents" (GSA). The somatosensory systems include the receptors as well as the pathways for transmission of sensory information from the soma to the portions of the brain that need to integrate it and act upon it. While much of this is conscious, there are also ascending systems that convey unconscious information involved in coordination (proprioception) and brain stem reflexes.

There are several different modalities that fall under the broad topic of exteroception. These sensations include well-localized touch (2-point discrimination), light touch, pain, temperature and vibration sense. These sensations can all be tested clinically. Proprioception is the ability to detect the position of the body in space. This may be consciously perceived, such as with joint position sense, or it may be a sensation that is not perceived consciously, such as from muscles and ligaments.

Most of the receptors are sensitive to mechanical deformation. There are ion channels in the membranes of these mechanically sensitive fibers that open with deformation of the membrane, resulting in a "generator potential". If this is sufficient to reach threshold potential, an action potential is generated. The intensity of the stimulus is encoded by the frequency of firing of action potentials. Receptors can be divided into rapidly adapting and slowly adapting. This property describes what happens to the frequency of firing when the stimulus continues to be applied. Rapidly adapting fibers will cease to fire after a short period, therefore being specialized to signal change. Slowly adapting fibers continue to fire as long as the stimulus is present and are involved more in signaling intensity. Another property that describes sensory fibers is whether they are low- or high-threshold. High-threshold receptors, for example, require an intense stimulus and are often associated with pain.

Often the somatosensory receptor simply consists of the peripheral terminal of the sensory nerve fiber. The simplest of these receptors consist of free nerve endings, which are often high threshold and slowly adapting. Many of these free nerve endings are also sensitive to chemical activation by products of tissue breakdown and of inflammation, and serve as pain fibers. Hair receptors consist of nerve fibers wrapped around the follicle and can detect the slightest movement. Other receptors are associated with a connective tissue encapsulation that modifies the stimulus. Meissner and Pacinian corpuscles are the best-known examples. These are for well-localized touch and, in the case of Pacinian corpuscle, vibration. There are other receptors that consist of specialized skin cells (Merkle cells) that release transmitter on the sensory axon, activating it. Receptors for muscle stretch (muscle spindle) and for muscle tension (Golgi tendon organ) have been described above.

We will first discuss the pathways for conscious perception before considering unconscious sensation. These pathways for conscious somatic sensation, at their simplest, require three neurons (and two relay sites) from the periphery all the way to termination of the cerebral cortex. These steps are often described as first, second and third order neurons in the sensory pathway. The signal can be modified by control mechanisms at each of the relay points (nuclei).

The pathways for detection of pain, temperature and very light (poorly localized) touch are distinct from those conveying well-localized touch, pressure,

Figure 10

Spinothalamic tract

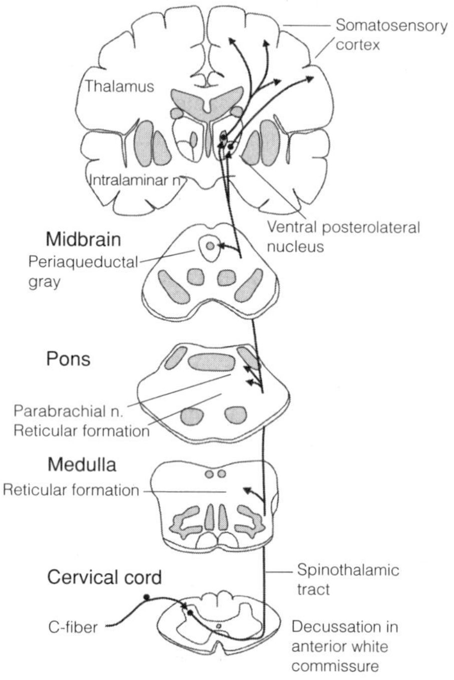

Spinal cord at the bottom and cerebral cortex at the top. Note that the sections are not to scale.

vibration and conscious proprioception. We will first consider the pathways for pain, temperature and light touch (Figure 10). Thinly myelinated and unmyelinated nerve fibers (first order nerve fibers) convey these modalities from the periphery. As with all sensations from the body, the neuronal perikarya for these sensory axons are located in the dorsal root ganglion. The central processes from these small neurons enter the spinal cord in the lateral part of the dorsal root. As these lightly myelinated and unmyelinated nerve fibers enter the spinal cord, they give rise to collateral branches that ascend and descend several segments in a region near the cap of the dorsal horn of the spinal cord, called the tract (or zone) of Lissauer. These collateral branches enter the dorsal horn and synapse in the substantia gelatinosa, located in the dorsal part of the dorsal horn. This synapse occurs within several segments of entering the spinal cord.

Pain, temperature and light touch nerve fibers synapse on several cell types in the dorsal horn. Some of these neurons are involved in local circuitry, including interneurons involved in local reflexes, particularly the withdrawal (flexor) reflex. They also synapse on neurons involved in sensory transmission. There are two groups of transmission neurons in the dorsal horn. There are marginal neurons that are located in the most dorsal part of the dorsal horn. Since these neurons respond almost exclusively to noxious inputs, they have been termed nociceptive specific neurons and appear to be most involved in signaling the presence and location of pain. There is a population of transmission neurons located more deeply in the dorsal horn, termed wide dynamic range neurons (WDR) because they respond with increasing frequency of discharge to more intense stimuli. These neurons have been studied intensively since they are involved in signaling the intensity of pain and also because their response characteristics can be altered by certain inputs in a process similar to "memory."

The substantia gelatinosa of the dorsal horn contains enkephalinergic interneurons and other inhibitory neurons that are involved in modulating pain. Descending pathways containing serotonin and norepinephrine are capable of activating inhibitory local circuits, as can certain direct somatosensory inputs to the spinal cord (Figure 11).

The axons from the transmission neurons (ie, the second order neurons in the pathway) comprise the spinothalamic tract or anterolateral system that conveys pain and temperature sensation (Figure 10). These axons decussate in the anterior white commissure of the spinal cord within several segments of their origin, although about 10% of sensory fibers remain ipsilateral. The decussating axons enter the anterolateral portion of the white matter of the spinal cord where they ascend the spinal cord as the spinothalamic tract. Historically, this tract has been divided into a lateral and ventral spinothalmic tract, with the lateral being more for pain and the ventral for thermoreception. However, the distinction is not as clear as would be suggested by this nomenclature and most authors consider them together. The fibers that arise from the sacral spinal cord are closest to the surface of the cord, with sensory fibers from the upper portion of the spinal cord

Figure 11

Descending pathways modifying pain perception

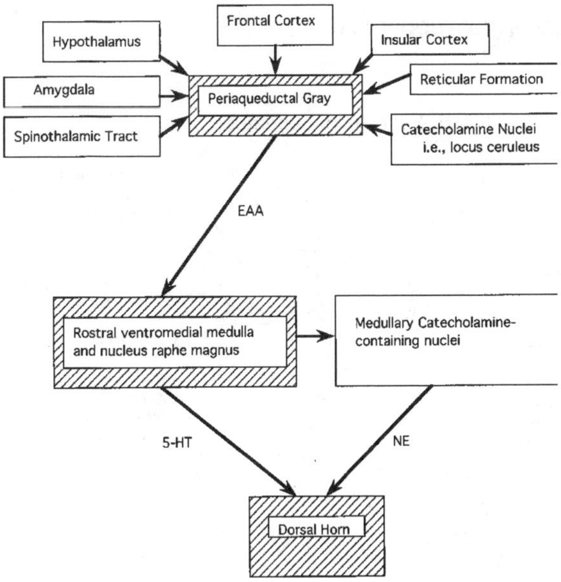

Regions that are cross-hatched contain enkephalinergic interneurons. EAA = excitatory amino acids; NE = norepinephrine; 5-HT = serotonin

layered more towards the center of the cord. These fibers comprise the spinothalamic tract, which extends through the ventrolateral part of the tegmentum of the brain stem to terminate mainly in the ventral posterolateral nucleus of the thalamus. There are additional terminations in intralaminar and posterior thalamic nuclei.

While there is some evidence for crude pain perception in the thalamus, most pain perception and discrimination occurs at the level of the cerebral cortex. The third order neuron for transmission of pain, temperature and light touch to the cerebral cortex begins in the VPL of the thalamus. Axons from these thalamic neurons follow the thalamic radiations to terminate in the primary somatosensory cortex (Brodman's areas 3, 1, 2 of the postcentral gyrus) in a topographic manner (See Section 11).

Somatosensory information regarding well-localized touch, pressure, vibration and joint position follows a different pathway to the cerebral cortex (Figure 12). Large, myelinated sensory nerve fibers that conduct these modalities are located in the medial aspect of the dorsal root as they enter the spinal cord. Some of these sensory fibers terminate directly at the level of entry to the cord, where they participate in reflex responses to touch and also are involved in inhibiting pain transmission through the substantia gelatinosa. However, the great majority of large-diameter sensory fibers enter the dorsal column of the spinal cord. These sensory axons ascend the length of the spinal cord to the level of the brain stem. Collectively, these fibers are called the dorsal columns since they comprise the entire region of the dorsal funiculus of the spinal cord. The afferent fibers from the lower half of the body (the fasciculus gracilis) are medial to those from the upper body (the fasciculus cuneatus) since fibers add to the dorsal columns from the lateral side at progressively higher levels of the cord. Note that the sensory fibers in the dorsal columns have not synapsed and therefore are still the primary or "first order" sensory fibers.

The first order sensory fibers in the dorsal column tracts ascend to the level of the medulla. Here they synapse in the dorsal column nuclei, which include the nucleus gracilis and nucleus cuneatus located within the dorsal aspect of the caudal medulla. Projection neurons of the gracile and cuneate nuclei, that is, the second order neurons for the pathway, give rise to axons that arch ventrally within the medulla (internal arcuate fibers). These axons decussate and reach the medial lemniscus. The medial lemniscus is a tract consisting of axons that connect the dorsal column nuclei with the ventral posterolateral nucleus of the thalamus.

The medial lemniscus has a topographic organization. The axons that arise from neurons in the nucleus gracilis, that is, axons that convey information from the legs, enter the ventral part of the medial lemniscus in the medulla with fibers from the nucleus cuneatus traversing more dorsal portions of the tract. As the medial lemniscus reaches the pons, it changes its orientation, such that the

Figure 12

Dorsal columns pathways, medial lemniscus pathway

A. Fasciculus gracilis (from lower limb). B. Fasciculus cuneatus (from upper limb)

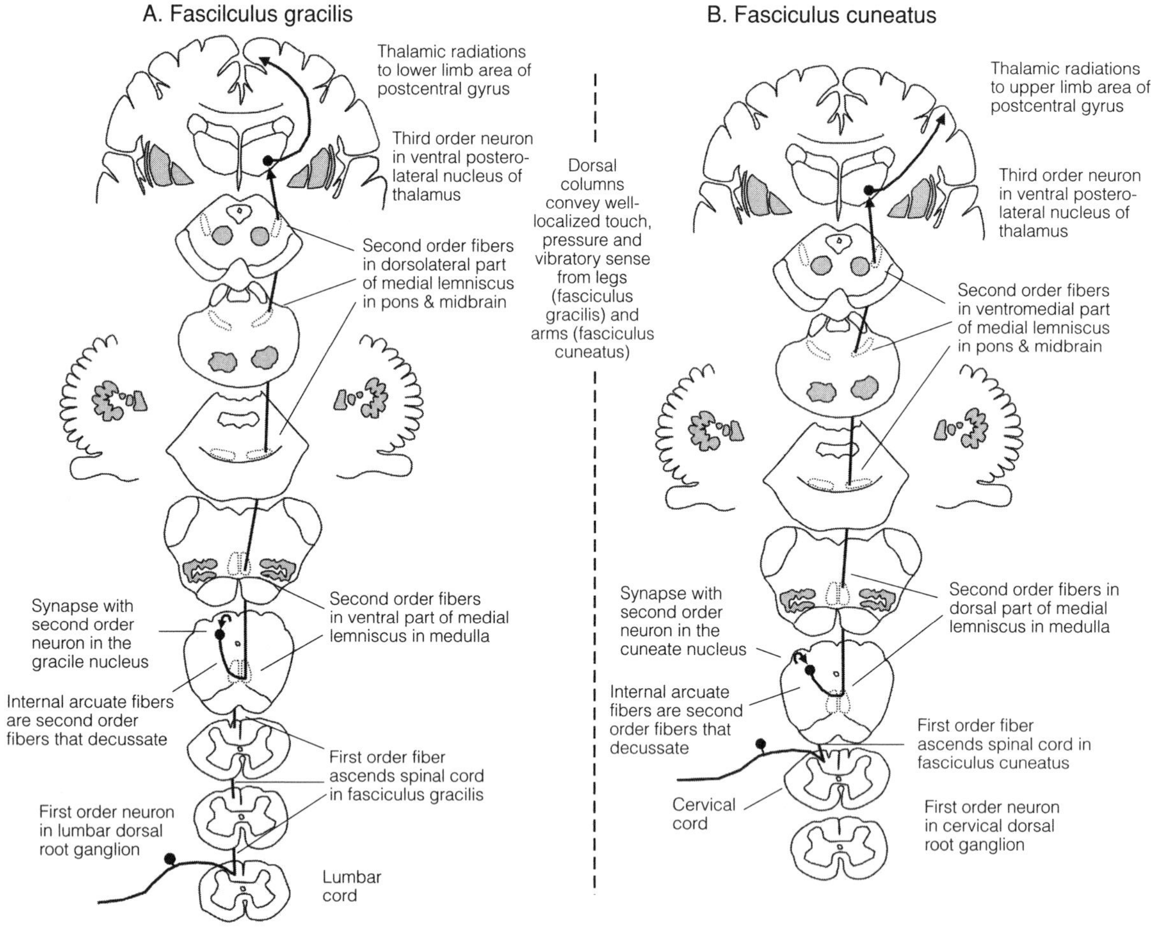

fibers from the legs are in the lateral portion of the tract. This shift in orientation is depicted in Figure 12.

The medial lemniscus terminates in the VPL of the thalamus. The third order neuron, located in the VPL, relays to the primary somatosensory cortex (postcentral gurus; cortical areas 3, 1, 2) in the topographic manner discussed above. The primary somatosensory cortex is connected to other parietal lobe regions immediately adjacent, which are responsible for synthesizing this somatosensory information into a recognizable pattern. Damage to this somatosensory association cortex produces an inability to interpret a sensory signal, even though it can be detected (somatosensory agnosia).

Figure 13

Spinocerebellar pathways

A. Dorsal (posterior) spinocerebellar tract. B. Cuneocerebellar tract.

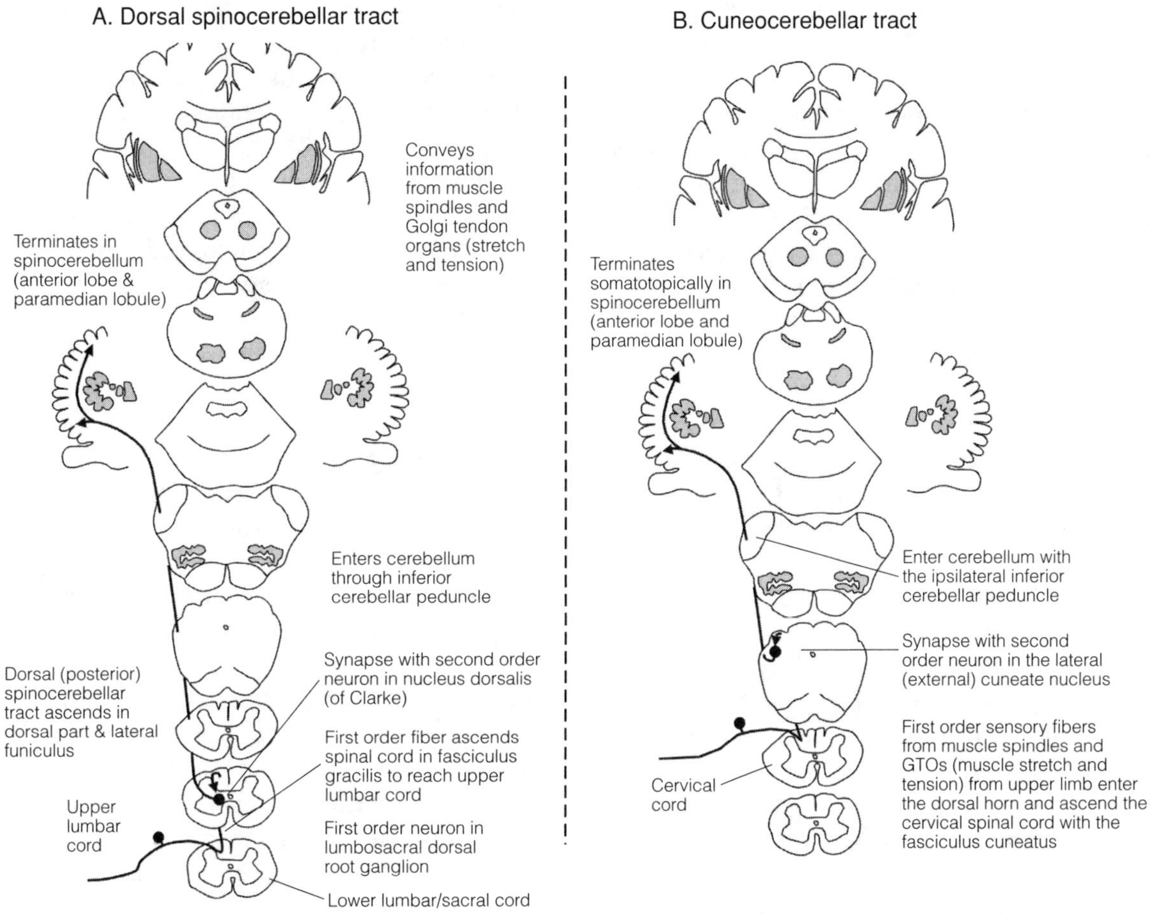

There are other ascending somatosensory pathways. Spinoreticular fibers are mostly collateral branches of the spinothalamic tract. These fibers terminate in the reticular formation and participate in various reflex reactions to pain, as well as alerting reactions. For example, these responses can include autonomic reflex responses and some behavioral reactions to pain. Additionally, relay from the reticular formation to more rostral aspects of the nervous system is an alternate route for pain to reach the cerebral cortex. The spinotectal tract that terminates in the superior colliculus contributes to reflex orientation of the head and eyes toward a somatic stimulus. Spinal projections to the periaqueductal gray can activate descending pain-suppression pathways.

In addition to these long ascending pathways, there are fibers that connect one segment of the spinal cord to neighboring portions of the cord. These fibers are located in the deepest part of the white matter, immediately adjacent to the gray matter. Therefore, they are named propriospinal fibers. These fibers participate in patterning intersegmental reflexes but also provide an alternate route whereby crude sensory information can reach the higher centers of the brain.

There are several pathways for unconscious proprioception. These transmit information necessary for the maintenance of normal muscle tone and posture as well as for coordination. Much of this information arises from muscle stretch and tension receptors and also from spinal interneurons that participate in reflexes and regulate motor output. While this is important information if movements are to be performed smoothly, there is very little conscious awareness of these sensations. The pathways for unconscious proprioception primarily terminate in the ipsilateral cerebellum, in two topographic maps in the spinocerebellum (anterior lobe and paramedian lobule). Some of these pathways, such as the dorsal spinocerebellar tract and the cuneocerebellar tract, require only 2 neurons, while some pathways are polysynaptic. Many of the polysynaptic pathways synapse on neurons of brain stem nuclei that, in turn, project to the cerebellum (the so-called precerebellar nuclei).

The dorsal spinocerebellar tract is the best studied of these tracts (Figure 13). Sensory information conveying muscle stretch and tension (ie, afferent fibers from muscle spindles and Golgi tendon organs), terminate in the nucleus dorsalis (of Clarke). This is a collection of neurons located in the central gray matter of the spinal cord between the C8 and L3 levels. Muscle proprioceptive fibers from all muscles that are innervated below the level of the neck terminate within this nucleus. Since the nucleus dorsalis does not exist below the L3 level, fibers conveying muscle stretch and tension information that enter the cord with the sacral and lower lumbar nerve roots joins the fibers of the dorsal columns and ascends the spinal cord to reach the upper lumbar region before synapsing. Therefore, damage to the lower portions of the dorsal columns, or to the large muscle stretch and tension afferent nerve fibers, can produce loss of coordination of the legs that has the appearance of cerebellar damage.

Projection neurons within the nucleus dorsalis give rise to second order sensory fibers that ascend the ipsilateral dorsal part of the lateral funiculus of the spinal cord. At the level of the medulla these fibers enter the cerebellum through the inferior peduncle. They terminate in a topographic fashion within the spinocerebellum and provide the cerebellum with muscle stretch and tension information.

Since the nucleus dorsalis does not extend into the cervical spinal cord above C8, the dorsal spinocerebellar tract does not convey information from the upper limb. Therefore, there is another pathway for muscle stretch and tension information from the arms, the cuneocerebellar tract (Figure 13). Afferent nerve fibers arising from muscle spindles and Golgi tendon organs in the upper limb join the fasciculus cuneatus and ascend the cervical spinal cord to reach the medulla. These fibers terminate in the lateral (external) cuneate nucleus. The second order neurons in this pathway enter the ipsilateral inferior cerebellar peduncle, terminating topographically in the spinocerebellum (Section 8).

The ventral spinocerebellar tract arises from neurons in the intermediate gray matter of the thoracic and lumbar spinal cord. These spinal interneurons participate in reflexes and regulate activity of the motor neurons in the cord. Axon collateral branches from these interneurons decussate in the anterior white commissure and ascend in the ventral part of the lateral funiculus as the ventral spinocerebellar tract. This tract is adjacent to the spinothalamic tract. These axons can be followed through the brain stem to the level of the rostral pons, where they turn dorsally and join the superior cerebellar peduncle. They enter the cerebellum and, for the most part, recross to terminate ipsilaterally. These fibers are important since they convey the level of activity in spinal cord interneurons. Since these interneurons are part of the control mechanism for most voluntary movements, it is important that the cerebellum have access to this information in order to participate in coordination of activity.

There are several other direct and indirect spinocerebellar pathways. These pathways provide necessary information regarding the current status of reflex pathways, as well as muscle tone, length and tension. This is all critical information to permit the cerebellum to coordinate motor activity.

There are several additional ascending spinal pathways with which you should have some passing familiarity. The spinocervical tract is an important pain pathway in some species, although its role in humans is less well understood. This tract relays in the lateral cervical nucleus and projects to the VPL of the thalamus. The spinohypothalamic and spinoamygdalar tract provides sensory input to areas of the nervous system involved in controlling autonomic, endocrine and emotional responses. It is important to know the location of the principal sensory pathways in the spinal cord. These are depicted in Figure 14.

Trigeminal Sensory System

The trigeminal nerve is the principal sensory nerve of the head. It supplies most of the face (to near the vertex of the skull), but does not extend to the angle of the jaw and only slightly onto the auricle. The trigeminal nerve also is the somatic afferent innervation of the nose, mouth and eyes. It provides sensory innervation of the dura and most of the cranial

Figure 14

Location of ascending and descending tracts of the spinal cord

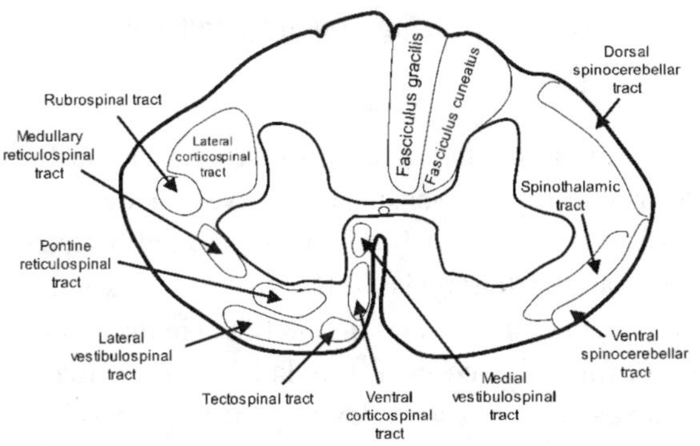

Ascending tracts on the right and descending on the left.

blood vessels, where its peripheral terminals can release a variety of vasoactive compounds that may be involved in the generation of headaches.

Most sensory fibers in the trigeminal nerve have their cell bodies in the trigeminal (semilunar, Gasserian) ganglion. This is located in the lateral wall of the cavernous sinus, immediately lateral to the pituitary gland. There is one very unusual exception to this rule. Sensory cell bodies of trigeminal proprioceptive nerve fibers are located inside the CNS, in the mesencephalic nucleus of the trigeminal.

The trigeminal nerve enters the brain stem through the middle cerebellar peduncle of the pons (Figure 15). There is a large sensory and a small motor root for this nerve.

Once inside the pons, sensory fibers segregate into three bands. The largest, most heavily myelinated fibers (proprioceptive fibers) extend into the mesencephalon to reach their sensory ganglion cells, located in the mesencephalic nucleus of the trigemi-

Figure 15

Ventral view of the brain stem including the locations of the cranial nerves

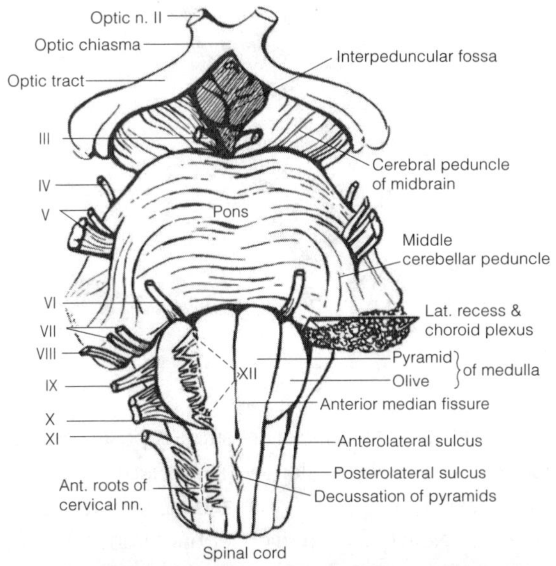

From O'Rahilly R, Muller F. Basic Human Anatomy: A Regional Study of Human Structures. *Philadelphia, Pa: WB Saunders; 1982. By permission.*

nal. Sensory axons conveying touch, pressure and vibration terminate in the chief or principal sensory nucleus of the trigeminal, located in the pons immediately lateral to the entry site of the nerve.

The small diameter sensory nerve fibers conveying temperature and pain sensation run caudally along the lateral side of the brain stem through the pons and medulla (Figure 16). They comprise a tract of fibers called the spinal tract of the trigeminal, and they terminate in a long nucleus called the spinal nucleus of the trigeminal. This nucleus extends into the upper cervical spinal cord. The spinal nucleus of the trigeminal has a similar cytoarchitecture and neurochemistry to that found in the substantia gelatinosa of the spinal cord, which is also a site of processing of pain and temperature information. From the spinal nucleus of the trigeminal, second order sensory axons decussate in the brain stem to

Figure 16

Trigeminal sensory systems

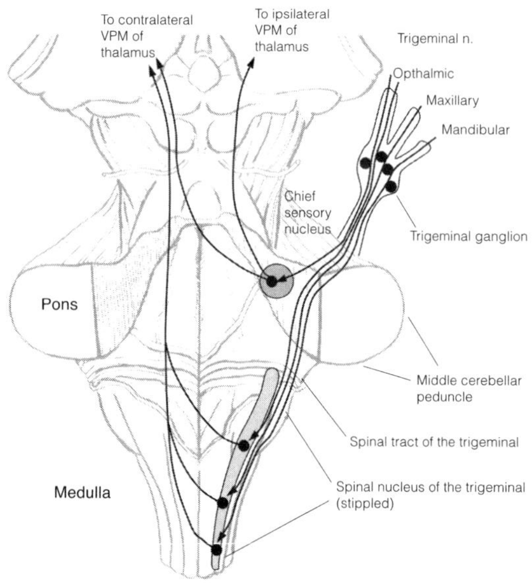

Trigeminal tracts and nuclei are superimposed over a dorsal view of the brain stem with the caudal medulla at the lower aspect of the figure and the midbrain at the upper. Note that the mesencephalic tract and nucleus are not shown.

lie in close proximity to the spinothalamic tract. These nerve fibers have been called the trigeminal lemniscus or the ventral trigeminothalamic tract. This tract terminates in the contralateral ventral posteromedial nucleus (VPM) of the thalamus.

Second order sensory fibers from the chief sensory nucleus of the trigeminal (conveying touch and pressure sensation) also decussate to follow the ventral trigeminothalmic tract (Figure 16). However, some fibers from this nucleus also follow the dorsal trigeminal thalamic tract to the ipsilateral VPM of the thalamus. Therefore, touch, pressure and vibration sensory fibers terminate bilaterally in the VPM. For this reason, it is very unusual to lose all sensations on one side of the face from unilateral lesions of the brain.

The third order neuron from the VPM of the thalamus projects to the face area of the somatosensory cortex on the inferior portion of the postcentral gyrus, where initial cortical processing takes place.

Many cranial nerves contain some GSA axons and these nerve fibers will terminate in the spinal nucleus of the trigeminal regardless of the nerve that they follow in the head. For example, there are GSA nerve fibers in the facial, glossopharyngeal and vagus nerves (from the ear, pharynx and tongue and larynx, respectively). Additionally, the spinal trigeminal nucleus extends well into the neck. Upper cervical nerve roots terminate on trigeminal sensory cells, providing an important substrate for referred pain in the head and neck. The spinal trigeminal nucleus is also important on the sensory side of many cranial reflex pathways, such as the corneal reflex, sneezing, coughing and gag responses.

Some of these reflexes are easily tested, such as the corneal reflex (consensual reflex eye closure to corneal stimulation). Some are not as readily tested. For example, tearing is a reflex that involves activation of general visceral efferent fibers in the facial nerve following corneal stimulation. Also, some reflexes have very complex responses, such as coughing and sneezing in response to irritation of the larynx and nose, respectively. The oculo-cardiac reflex involves a slowing of the heart following pressure on the eyeball, with a reflex loop involving the trigeminal nerve (input) and the vagus nerve (output).

The trigeminal motor root is relatively small. It distributes only with the mandibular division of the trigeminal and goes to muscles of mastication. When the patient attempts to forcibly open their mouth, the jaw will deviate towards the weak side if there is unilateral weakness. This is due to imbalance in strength in the lateral pterygoid muscles. The jaw jerk (pontine) reflex is a monosynaptic muscle stretch reflex which is mediated by the muscle stretch (afferent) fibers associated with the mesencephalic nucleus of the trigeminal, while the motor response is mediated via activation of neurons in the motor nucleus of the trigeminal, located in the pons.

Taste and Smell

Taste and smell are considered to be "special visceral" sensations (SVA). These are chemical sensations with receptors being activated by odorants and tastants that interact with specific membrane molecules. Olfaction is highly complex due to the number of molecules that are detected and, to this point, there are no recognized number of "primary olfactory" stimulants from which all odors are created. This has limited the ability to analyze odors mechanically. The primary olfactory epithelium is in the upper part of the nasal cavity. Olfactory epithelial cells have processes containing membrane receptors for a specific molecular structure. These epithelial cells are neural structures that have axons traversing the cribriform plate of the ethmoid bone to reach the olfactory bulb. In the olfactory bulb, olfactory epithelial cells synapse with processes of mitral cells in glomeruli. Each glomerulus includes only axons from olfactory epithelial cells that detect the same odorant. The mitral cells give rise to axons comprising the olfactory tract, which are located immediately ventral to the frontal lobes. The olfactory tract trifurcates, with some fibers terminating directly in the anterior perforated substance of the ventral forebrain, and other fibers splitting into lateral and medial olfactory stria. These stria terminate on the ipsilateral and contralateral olfactory regions of the temporal lobes, respectively. In the temporal lobes, there are terminations in the olfactory cortex (prepiriform part of the parahippocampal gyrus covering the uncus) and the amygdala. This latter structure, especially, participates in visceral and behavioral responses to odorants.

Taste—representing the primary sensations of sweet, salty, sour and bitter—results from activation of specific molecular receptor mechanisms in the cells of the taste buds. Of course, olfaction is a major component of what patients recognize as taste. Taste itself is conveyed along fibers of the facial, glossopharyngeal and vagus nerves (the latter is minimal) from anterior to posterior on the tongue. These fibers terminate in the gustatory nucleus of the brain stem. Relay from taste is through the parabrachial nucleus and part of the VPM of the thalamus to the inferior part of the postcentral gyrus.

Auditory System

There are three components of the ear subserving hearing function: outer ear, middle ear, inner ear. The outer ear consists of the pinna, which collects sound waves, and the external auditory meatus, ending at the tympanic membrane. Internal to this tympanic membrane is the middle ear containing three bones—the malleus, incus and stapes. Air pressure in the middle ear is equilibrated with the external environment via the auditory (Eustachian) tube. The ossicular chain ends at the oval window on the medial wall of the middle ear. The footplate of the stapes and its ligaments seal the opening into the inner ear that contains the cochlea and the vestibular apparatus (the semicircular canals and organs of the vestibule, discussed in the next section). The chief functions of the outer and middle ear are to transmit sound waves from air into fluid of the inner ear via the tympanic membrane and ossicular chain. Since it takes almost 13 times more energy to vibrate fluid than it does air, sound waves from a large amount of air have to be focused on a small area, a process called impedance matching. This is why the tympanic membrane is about 13 times larger than the footplate of the stapes. Anything that impedes vibration of the tympanic membrane or ossicular chain would produce conductive deafness in which a vibrating tuning fork placed on the head would actually seem to be louder in the deaf ear (vibrations of the skull bypass the ossicles).

There are two muscles that can modulate the movement of the bones of the inner ear. The tensor tympani muscle, innervated by the trigeminal nerve, is attached to the handle of the malleus. The stapedius muscle, innervated by the facial nerve, is attached to the stapes. Contraction of these muscles attenuates the movement of the bones, and therefore diminishes sound before it reaches the inner ear.

The frequency of vibration in the air indicates the pitch, while the amplitude of the vibrations equates to the loudness of the sound. Human hearing is in the range of 20 to 20,000 Hz. The upper limit of this frequency greatly exceeds the maximum frequency at which a nerve can conduct action potentials. Therefore, these frequencies of sound cannot be translated by the auditory system directly into frequency of action potentials.

The inner ear consists of a bony cavity (the bony labyrinth), which is filled with perilymph, and a watertight membrane-lined sac (membranous labyrinth) containing endolymph inside. The membranous labyrinth is much like a fluid-filled balloon inflated in a bottle containing a different fluid (Figure 17). The receptive cells for hearing are contained within the cochlea. This cochlea, which is coiled for 2.5 turns, contains three fluid-filled compartments. The oval window, noted above, displaces perilymph in the vestibule of the inner ear. The vestibule is continuous with the scala vestibuli.

At the tip of the cochlea (the helicotrema), the perilymph of the scala vestibuli communicates with the perilymph of the scala tympani, which ends blindly at the round window. The round window appears on the medial wall of the middle ear and is closed by a membrane. Displacement of the oval window by movement of the stapes produces a pressure wave that is transmitted along the scala vestibuli and tympani, ultimately vibrating the membrane closing the round window. The perilymph that fills the scala vestibuli and tympani has a composition very similar to that of extracellular fluid and may represent an

Figure 17

Structure of the ear

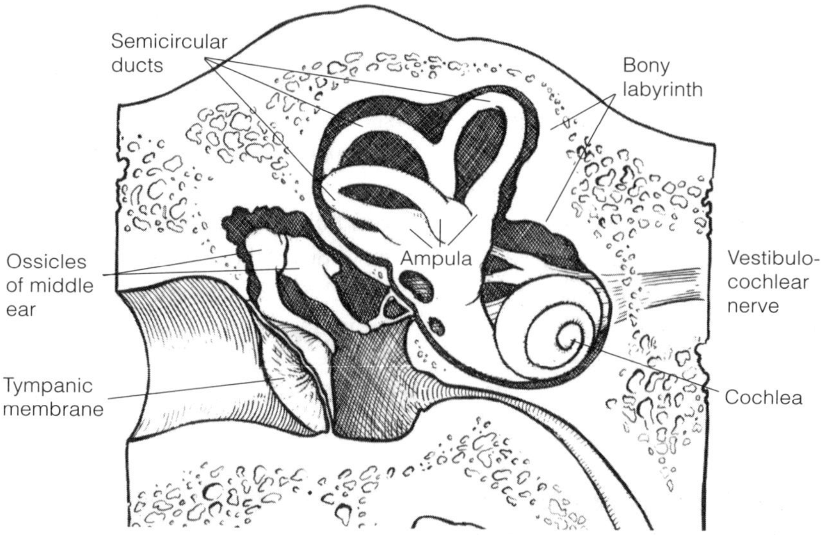

Note that the inner ear consists of a cavity in the bone (bony labyrinth) containing a sac. This sac consists of the coiled cochlear duct (hearing) and vestibular elements that include three semicircular ducts that are oriented at right angles to one another.

ultrafiltrate of plasma. This fluid communicates with cerebrospinal fluid through the perilymphatic duct. This connection represents a potential route of spread of infection from the meninges to the inner ear.

Separating the scala vestibuli from the scala tympani is a duct that is part of the membranous labyrinth called the scala media or cochlear duct. The cochlear duct is triangular, with the vestibular (Reisner's) membrane separating it from the scala vestibuli and the basilar membrane separating it from the scala tympani. The third side of the triangle is comprised of the spiral ligament that contains the blood vessels of the stria vascularis, which are responsible for production of endolymph. The cochlear duct is a blind sac, filled with endolymph, which differs in composition from the perilymph in that the potassium concentration is much higher. This endolymph more closely resembles intracellular fluid. Due to this ion gradient, there is a potential difference of +80 mV between the endolymph and perilymph. Hair cells are the receptive cells of the inner ear. These cells maintain a potential of -45mV compared to the perilymph and -125mV compared to endolymph. This potential difference is critical to the function of the inner ear.

These hair cells are stretched along the cochlear duct in two rows (the inner and outer hair cells) positioned on a thickened ridge of the basilar membrane. Upon each segment of the basilar membrane are three outer hair cells and one inner hair cell. In humans, outer hair cells are more numerous (approx. 12,000) than inner hair cells (approx. 3,500). The "hairs" on these cells project toward the

Figure 18

Location of the semicircular ducts in the head

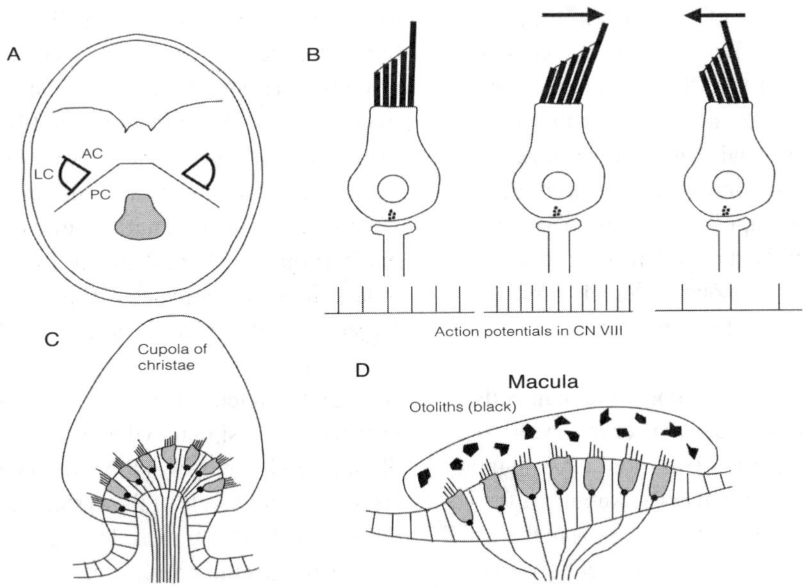

A. Note that the anterior semicircular duct of one ear is in the same plane as the posterior canal from the other ear. AC = anterior semicircular canal; PC = posterior semicircular canal; LC = lateral semicircular canal.
B. The structure of hair cells. Note that the kinocilium is longer and is attached to the tip of the other cilia by a filament. Tension on this filament will open ion channels and result in an increase in action potentials in the nerve (below). C. Structure of a christae. Note that all of the hair cells are polarized in the same direction.
D. Structure of a macula. Note that the hair cells have different polarization.

inside of the cochlear duct and are embedded in a covering membrane (the tectorial membrane). Collectively, these structures are termed the organ of Corti and this is the location of sound transduction. The "hairs" consist of a series of cilia and one longer steriocilia (called the kinocilium), which is located off to one side of the hair cell (Figure 18B). At the apex of the cilia there are protein filaments that attach to adjacent cilia. These filaments are anchored to proteins that comprise an ion channel that is opened when tension is placed on the filament. Deformation of the cilia towards the kinocilium places tension on the filaments. This results in a rapid influx of potassium due to the high concentration of this ion in the endolymph and the fact that the potassium equilibrium potential is less negative than -125mV. This results in a rapid depolarization of the hair cell, which increases release of neurotransmitter from the base of the hair cells. When the hair cell is depolarized, calcium enters the cell, and neurotransmitter (probably glutamate) is released onto peripheral terminals of afferent fibers in the vestibulocochlear nerve. Potassium can be rapidly cleared from the hair cell simply by opening potassium channels in the base of the hair cell (the part that is exposed to the perilymph). This is a passive process since the potential difference with the perilymph is significantly less negative than the potassium equilibrium potential. This rapid passive movement of potassium into and then out of the hair cell occurs extremely rapidly and does not require energy on the part of the hair cell. It is part of the capacity of this cell to respond extremely rapidly and for sustained periods to sound stimuli.

Despite the fact that there are more outer hair cells, the inner hair cells have much denser innervation and the auditory system receives more afferent input from the inner than outer hair cells. Another difference between inner and outer hair cells is in their efferent innervation. Both receive projections from the brain stem, mostly the superior olivary nucleus (olivocochlear bundle). When activated, these fibers release neurotransmitter, probably acetylcholine, which hyperpolarizes the inner and outer hair cells. Such inhibition is more effective for the outer hair cells since efferents end directly on the cell body (as opposed to ending on the afferent axons of the inner hair cells). This olivocochlear efferent innervation can "fine-tune" auditory perceptions.

Different frequencies of vibration in the perilymph will produce specific patterns of maximal vibration in the basilar membrane due to varying length, and stiffness of the membrane at different parts of the cochlea. For example, low frequencies produce a maximal displacement of the apical end of the cochlea whereas high frequencies produce a maximal displacement of the base. This mapping of frequency of vibration (ie, pitch) onto location in the cochlea is the reason that the brain is able to detect different frequencies of sound. These frequencies are transmitted to the central nervous system via the central process of the neurons of the spiral ganglia. These axons comprise the vestibulocochlear nerve.

The hallmark of the central auditory pathways is divergence. Such divergence commences immediately upon the afferent fiber entering the brainstem, with a bifurcation to terminate in the dorsal and ventral cochlear nucleus. The cochlear nuclei have a tonotopic organization, with cells of progressively higher frequency characteristics being arrayed in a progression along the axis of the nuclei. Neurons of the ventral cochlear nucleus send fibers to the medial and lateral superior olivary nuclei on the ipsilateral and contralateral sides of the brain. Divergence continues with neurons of the olivary nuclei projecting to both the ipsilateral and contralateral lateral lemniscus. The lateral lemniscus projects to neurons of the inferior colliculus of the midbrain, which relay the signal to the medial geniculate nucleus of the thalamus; this nucleus, in turn, relays the signal to the primary auditory cortex of the superior temporal lobe (transverse gyri of Heshel). At all levels of the system, a tonotopic representation is maintained. The auditory association area surrounds the primary auditory cortex and is necessary for recognition of the significance of sounds. In the dominant hemisphere, this is particularly important for recognition of language (Wernicke's area) and includes much of the angular and supramarginal gyrus.

This divergence of auditory information from the cochlea is evidenced by the finding that many neurons along the "auditory pathway" receive information from both ears. There is a difference in arrival time from each ear (the binaural beat) that the brain uses to lateralize sounds. Also, progressively more complicated stimuli are necessary in order to activate neurons at progressively higher centers of the auditory pathway. Thus, despite the general tonotopic representation, many neurons in the brainstem do not respond to a pure tone, but only to more complicated frequency patterns.

The divergence within the auditory system also makes it exceedingly improbable that any single lesion involving the brainstem or cerebral cortex will cause deafness in both ears or even total deafness in one ear.

Vestibular System

The vestibular system is important for normal function in several ways. It is a critical system for detecting the position and motion of the head, particularly angular motions such as rotation. It is through this system that the eyes are stabilized when the head is moving and also for adjusting neck and body muscle tone during movements.

General principles of the inner ear anatomy are introduced in the preceding section on hearing (Figure 17). The vestibular organs are located in portions of the membranous labyrinth contained in the vestibule (the saccule and utricle) and in the semicircular ducts that fill the semicircular canals. There are receptive organs within the membranous labyrinth, the macula in the saccule and utricle and christae in the semicircular canals. Each of these receptive organs contains hair cells that were described in the section on hearing. These cells are polarized by the presence of the kinocilium, such that bending the cilia toward the kinocilium results in increased neurotransmitter release from hair cells and increased activity in the vestibulocochlear nerve. Deflection away from the kinocilium results in the opposite. There is a constant background release of transmitter, meaning there is a tonic activity in the vestibular nerve (Figure 18). Therefore, each nerve fiber can signal movement of the cilia toward or away from the kinocilium by increasing or decreasing its firing rate, respectively.

Maculae and christae have some structural similarities and some differences (Figure 18C, D). Both types of organs include a thickened epithelium with the cilia of their hair cells being embedded in a gelatinous covering. In the case of the maculae, which are located in the utricle and saccule, this gelatinous covering is studded with calcium carbonate crystals (otoliths). These crystals are heavy and will distort the hairs by the effect of gravity. Additionally, they will lag behind if the head is accelerated in a linear direction. There are hair cells that are polarized in many different directions in each macula. Therefore, the macula can detect the orientation of the head in relation to gravity and the direction of linear acceleration.

In the case of the semicircular ducts, a dilated ampula is associated with each duct. The ampula contains a flame-shaped christae (Figure 18C). In the christae, the gelatinous cap (the cupula) protrudes into the canal. Movement of the endolymph through the canal results in a deflection of the christae, thereby deflecting the hairs. Each christae contains hair cells that are polarized in a single direction. So fluid movement in one direction will excite all of the hair cells and movement in the opposite direction will inhibit all of them. Each ear has three semicircular canals (containing semicircular ducts) that are at right angles to one another. These canals are not purely horizontal, coronal and sagittal. The horizontal canals are oriented at approximately 20 degrees, with the anterior side elevated. The posterior and anterior canals are oriented in a manner such that the anterior canal of one ear is basically in the same plane as the posterior canal of the other ear. This allows each ear to function as a backup for the other.

Angular acceleration of the head (ie, rotation, lateral flexion or nodding) will cause fluid to tend to lag behind the movement of the head in relation to the canal that moves with the head, so there will be relative movement of the fluid. This relative movement will be greatest if the head movement is directly in the plane of the semicircular duct. Therefore, the christae signal angular acceleration.

Of course, vestibular receptors would not be of much use if they were not connected to the brain. The vestibular part of the vestibulocochlear nerve consists of nerve fibers that have contacted hair cells in the macula and christae. These sensory fibers have bipolar cell bodies located in the vestibular ganglion. The central processes of these bipolar neurons enter the brain stem in the rostral medulla, where they synapse in the vestibular complex. Additionally, many vestibular nerve fibers terminate in the flocculonodular lobe of the cerebellum (the vestibulocerebellum) (Figure 19).

The vestibular complex of the brain stem is so-called because it actually consists of several nuclei. For the purposes of this discussion, we will not consider them separately. The vestibular complex is located in the dorsolateral portion of the rostral medulla and caudal pons and receives several types of input in addition to primary vestibular afferent information. For example, input from the spinal cord allows proprioception (particularly of the neck) to influence vestibular functions. The vestibular complex has a very important reciprocal connection with the flocculonodular lobe of the cerebellum (the vestibulocerebellum).

One of the most important roles of the vestibular complex is to keep the eyes focused on target when the head moves. This is termed the vestibulo-ocular reflex (VOR) (Figure 20). When the head jerks in one direction the eyes move in an equal and opposite direction. The reflex is mediated via connections from the vestibular complex to the extraocular nuclei (ie, those nuclei that control eye muscles). Many of these connections traverse the medial longitudinal fasciculus. The VOR must be adjusted from time to time in order to keep it accurate over the course of one's life, especially as the inner ear becomes less sensitive with age and disease. This "fine-tuning" of the reflex is dependent on activity of the vestibulocerebellum, which is critical in order to assure that the reflex continues to produce accurate eye movements.

Figure 19

Central connection of the vestibular nerve

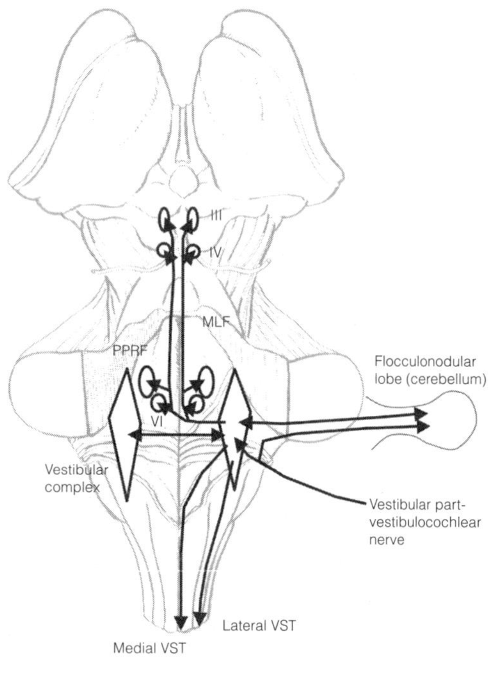

PPRF = paramedian pontine reticular formation (para-abducens nucleus; pontine lateral gaze center). Cranial nerve nuclei noted in Roman numerals; MLF = medial longitudinal fasciculus; VST = vestibulospinal tract.

Figure 20

Schematic of connections of vestibulo-ocular reflex (VOR)

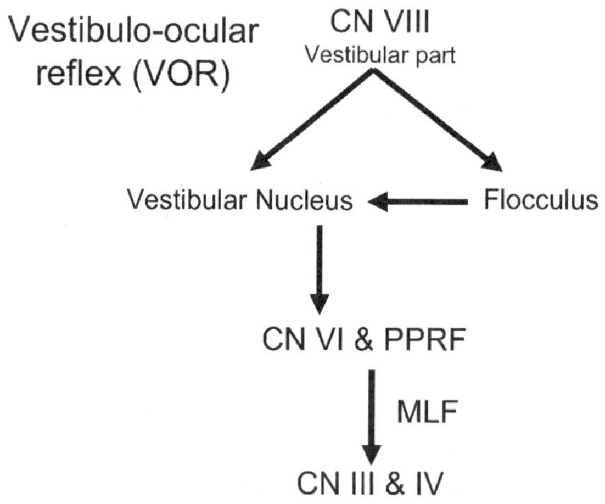

See legend of Figure 18 for key to abbreviations

The vestibular complex projects to other portions of the nervous system. The lateral vestibulospinal tract arises from neurons in the lateral vestibular nucleus (Deiter) and projects through the ventral part of the lateral funiculus to activate extensor motor neurons at all levels of the cord. The medial vestibulospinal tract arises from the medial vestibular nucleus and projects through the descending medial longitudinal fasciculus (MLF) to enter the anterior funiculus of the spinal cord and affect neck muscle activity bilaterally. These vestibulospinal tracts adjust the muscle tone and position of the body in response to vestibular stimulation and are the physiological basis for vestibular righting reflexes and tonic neck reflexes.

In addition to projections to the spinal cord, there are projections from the vestibular complex to the reticular formation. Intense vestibular stimuli can produce vomiting and even influence blood pressure. Additionally, there are projections to the thalamus that relay to poorly defined portions of the inferior parietal lobe that permit the conscious perception of movement.

Visual System

Visual pathways are interesting and clinically important. The retina is a complex structure that consists of three main cellular layers, with interspersed layers of connections containing other cells that modify the signals. The deepest layer contains the rods and cones, which themselves have an inner and outer segment. The receptive element of the rods and cones are contained on lamella of membranes in the outer segment, meaning that light has to pass through all retinal layers to produce its physiologic effects. Rods are very sensitive to a small number of photons of light; they are used in low-light situations but do not convey color information. There are three types of cones representing the three primary colors, distinguished by their photoreceptive pigment. The rods and cones are constantly depolarizing and releasing neurotransmitter (called the dark current). Stimulation by light closes the ion channels that produce the dark current and results in hyperpolarization with a decrease in neurotransmitter release onto bipolar cells. Bipolar cells do not generate action potentials. However they do release transmitter onto ganglion cells, which are the first site of action potential generation in the visual system. Ganglion cells receive input from many bipolar cells, some of which are excitatory and some inhibitory. Uniform lighting of the receptive field of a bipolar cell will produce no response. Some ganglion cells respond to a pinpoint of light illuminating the center of the receptive field (on-center) and some are inhibited by light falling on the center (off-center). This makes the ganglion cell signals very good at discriminating edges and points.

Figure 21

Optic pathways

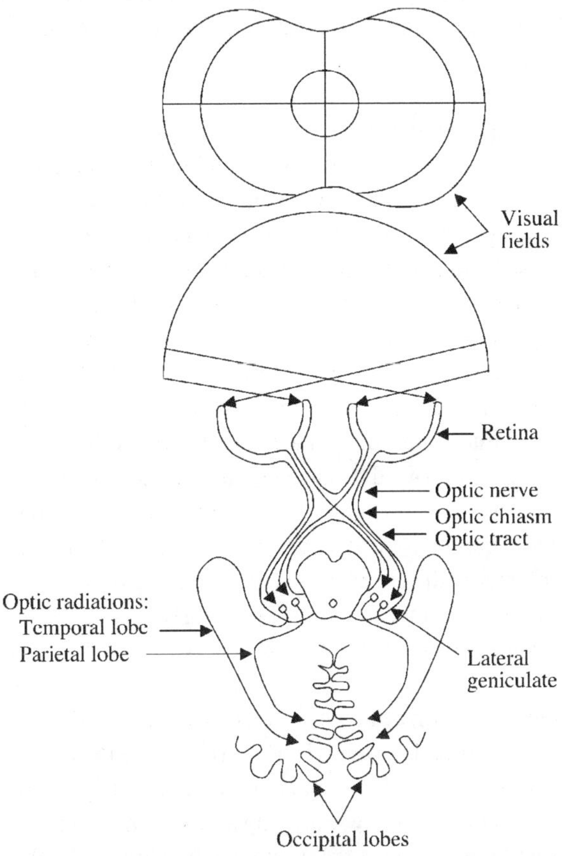

The optic nerve consists of the myelinated processes of ganglion cells (Figure 21), which leave the retina at the optic disc (a physiologic blind spot because there are no photoreceptors). The nerve leaves the orbit through the optic canal to reach the optic chiasm located just superior to the pituitary gland. The ophthalmic artery has a branch that enters the optic nerve (central retinal artery) and supplies the inner part of the retina. In the optic chiasm, the nerve fibers from the nasal side of the retina cross to the contralateral side. These crossing fibers convey signals from the lateral (temporal) visual fields. As the retinal axons progress posteriorly from the optic chiasm, those from the nasal part of the retina that have just crossed the midline join those from the opposite temporal part of the retina in the optic tract. Note that the nasal part of the retina of one eye and the temporal part of the retina of the other eye detect light from an overlapping part of the visual field. Therefore, the left optic tract contains all of the signals from the right side of the visual world. All portions of the visual system posterior to the optic chiasm convey information from overlapping (homonomous) portions of the visual world.

The optic tract terminates in the lateral geniculate nucleus of the thalamus. This nucleus has 6 layers, each one receiving input from one or the other eye. The optic radiations are a broad band of fibers that arise from neurons in the lateral geniculate and terminate in the primary visual cortex located in the medial occipital lobe adjacent to the calcarine sulcus. Information from the lower contralateral visual world passes through optic radiations that traverse the white matter of the parietal lobe to terminate on the gyrus above the calcarine sulcus (the cuneus) and that from the upper visual world passes through the temporal lobe (Meyer's loop) to reach the gyrus inferior to the calcarine sulcus (the lingula). Central vision is represented most posteriorly, right at the occipital pole of the cerebral cortex.

Geniculo-cortical connections terminate in adjacent, vertically oriented stripes (therefore the name "striate cortex" for visual cortex). These stripes represent input from overlapping areas of each eye (ocular dominance columns). Each column of cells receives input from one eye and the column adjacent to it receives input from portions of the retina of the other eye that detect light from the same portion of the world. It is at this level that inputs from the two eyes begin to be integrated.

The visual cortex does not function as a camera conveying point-to-point information. Instead, neurons are arranged to be responsive to progressively more complex functions (lines, edges, or particular orientations or directions of movement of edges). The visual association areas surrounding the primary visual cortex are responsible for synthesizing the information into recognizable and useful representation of the world. There are certain specific areas of critical importance, such as the posterior part of the middle temporal gyrus (MT) that are necessary for processing information about movement, and part of the inferior temporal gyrus that is necessary for facial recognition.

8. Motor Systems

Pyramidal System

Many corticofugal axons terminate in the brain stem (corticobulbar) and others continue through the brain stem and into the spinal cord where they are called the corticospinal or "pyramidal" tract.

Corticospinal

The corticospinal tract (Figure 22) represents the highest order of motor function in humans and is most directly involved in control of fine, digital movements. This tract arises in pyramidal neurons of layer V of the precentral gyrus, the primary motor cortex. Betz cells are the largest of these pyramidal neurons. There is a motor homunculus in this gyrus, with the feet represented near the superomedial part of the motor cortex and the leg, trunk, arm, hand and head represented progressively further inferior on the lateral side of the brain. Axons arising from neurons in the precentral gyrus exit through the white matter and pass through the internal capsule where they are topographically arranged in the posterior limb. The fibers controlling the lower extremity are posterior to those of the upper limb. Corticospinal fibers traverse the middle portion of the cerebral peduncle of the midbrain and then the basal pons. They enter the pyramids of the medulla (from whence they get their name). Over 90% of the axons in the pyramids decussate just before reaching the upper cervical spinal cord (the pyramidal decussation) and they enter the lateral funiculus of the spinal cord to become the (lateral) corticospinal tract (Figure 22). Most of these axons terminate in the intermediate gray matter of the cord, although some enter the dorsal horn (where they can have an effect on sensory transmission) and a few terminate directly on alpha motor neurons, contributing to rapid voluntary movement. Most of these fibers terminate on interneurons of the spinal cord. These interneurons are responsible for reflexes and, therefore, most motor activity actually occurs by the regulation of reflex excitability in the spinal cord.

A few corticospinal axons descend the anterior funiculus of the spinal cord as the anterior (ventral) corticospinal tract. This is more involved in axial (trunk and neck) movements and terminates bilaterally.

Corticobulbar

Many projections from the cerebral cortex terminate in the brain stem (generically called corticobulbar projections). These projections have several functions including voluntary control over cranial nerves, relay to the cerebellum, activation of other descending pathways (ie, indirect corticospinal projections) and modulation of sensory processing.

Many cranial nerve nuclei receive direct and indirect (through the reticular formation) cortical input via nerve fibers arising from the motor cortex and traversing the genu of the internal capsule. Most corticobulbar connections are bilateral, meaning that unless both sides of the nervous system are affected, there is no loss of motor control. However, the facial nucleus to the lower face receives only input from the contralateral motor cortex and, therefore, there will be weakness of voluntary movement of the lower face on the side opposite damage to corticobulbar neurons (with sparing of movements of the upper face).

The majority of corticobulbar projections terminate in the ipsilateral basal pontine nuclei. These nuclei relay to the cerebellar cortex via projections that decussate in the pons and enter the cerebellum through the middle cerebellar peduncle (see below). These represent, by far, the largest input to the cerebellum.

There are several brain stem nuclei that project to the spinal cord. The cerebral cortex projects to most of these and, therefore, may affect them as indirect corticospinal projections. These areas include the red nucleus, which gives rise to the rubrospinal tract that decussates in the midbrain and descends the lateral funiculus near to the location of the lateral corticospinal tract (Figure 14). The reticular formation gives rise to several descending pathways, one from the rostral pons that helps pattern locomotion, one from the caudal pons that can affect head movement to coincide with eye movement, and one from the medulla that mostly inhibits reflex activity in the spinal cord. This latter tract is excited by cortical input and, therefore, cerebral motor cortical output is mostly inhibitory to spinal cord reflexes via this

Figure 22

Corticospinal and corticobulbar pathways

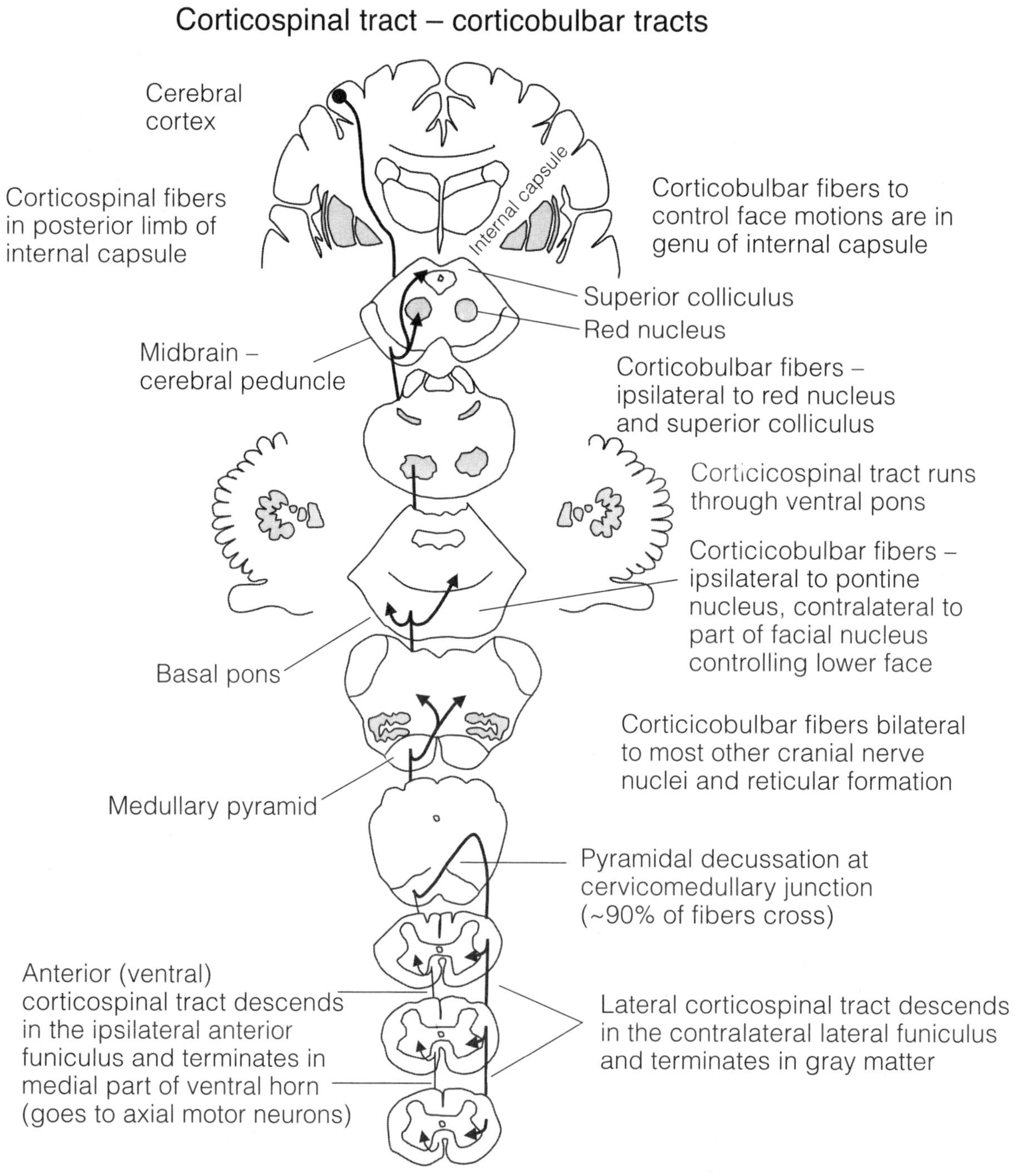

indirect pathway. For this reason, interruption of corticobulbar projections typically increases reflexes.

Cerebral cortical projections also go to the superior colliculus, a region that gives rise to a tectospinal tract as well as projections to eye movement centers. The superior colliculus is mostly responsible for reflex head and eye movement toward novel stimuli. The cerebral cortical projections to the superior colliculus may affect movement via these projections.

Cerebellum

The cerebellum is a region of the brain that functions largely outside of the realm of conscious awareness. Its best known functions are involved in coordinating motor activities and learning new motor skills. It is particularly involved in adjusting activities to meet new conditions. However, in addition to these well-known functions, there is a growing awareness that cerebellar systems may be involved in other types of learning and also in emotional reactivity.

The cerebellum, located dorsal to brain stem, is partially hidden by the large occipital lobes of the cortex. The cerebellar cortex is deeply grooved and appears as thin, transverse leaves called folia. There is a deeper transverse fold on the superior aspect of the cerebellum termed the primary fissure. This fissure defines the posterior end of the anterior lobe. The posterolateral fissure divides the small flocculonodular lobe from the remainder of the cerebellum. The portion of the cerebellum in the midline is not as prominent as the lateral hemispheres and is termed the vermis. It is important to note that the cerebellum is connected to ipsilateral body functions. Therefore, whenever the cerebellum connects to portions of the brain that have crossed functions (such as the cerebral cortex), the connection must cross.

There are three functional subdivisions of the cerebellum. The flocculonodular lobe is called the vestibulocerebellum or archicerebellum. The spinocerebellum (paleocerebellum) includes the anterior lobe and paramedian lobules. The neocerebellum (pontocerebellum) makes up the lateral hemispheres.

The cerebellum is connected to the brain stem by three peduncles. The middle peduncle is, by far, the largest of the peduncles, connecting the pons to the cerebellum. The inferior peduncle connects the medulla to the cerebellum, while the superior peduncle connects the cerebellum to the midbrain. Most input to the cerebellum is through the middle and inferior peduncles and most of the output from the cerebellum is via the superior peduncle.

The deep cerebellar nuclei are within the cerebellum, with the fastigial nucleus being the most medial, the interposed nuclei, comprised of the small globose and emboliform nuclei, located immediately lateral to the fastigial nucleus, and the massive dentate nucleus being the most lateral. The cerebellar cortex is connected to the deep nuclei. The vermal zone of cortex connects to the fastigial nucleus, the paravermal zone connects to the interposed nuclei, and the lateral hemispheres connect to the dentate nucleus.

The cerebellar cortex only connects to the deep cerebellar nuclei and to the vestibular nuclei. Neurons in the deep cerebellar nuclei represent virtually all of the output from the cerebellum. The fastigial nuclei are connected to the reticular formation by two pathways. The interposed nuclei are connected through the superior cerebellar peduncle primarily to the red nucleus. The dentate nucleus has a massive connection through the superior peduncle to the ventral lateral nucleus of the thalamus, which relays to the cerebral motor cortex.

Before proceeding with a discussion of the connections of the various regions of the cerebellum, it is appropriate to describe the cerebellar cortex (Figure 23). The cellular structure of the cerebellar cortex is completely monotonous, with every region of the cortex, regardless of its functions or connections, appearing identical. Therefore, the differences in function from one area to another are based entirely on difference in inputs and output from the cortex. It is interesting to note that there are more neurons in the cerebellar cortex than the rest of the brain combined. Furthermore, there are only five different

Figure 23

Wiring of the cerebellar cortex

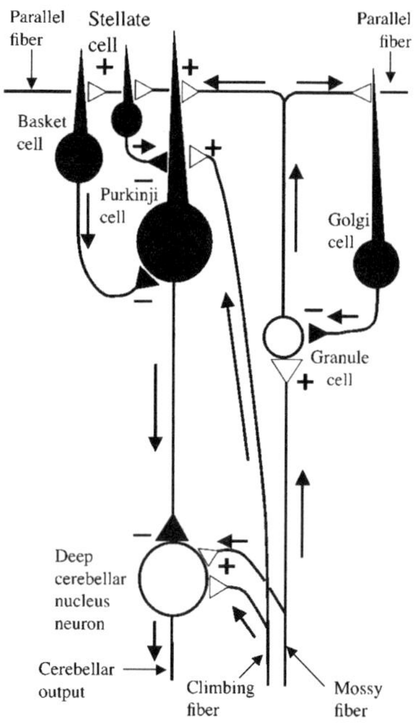

Neurons represented by circles
(filled = inhibitory neurons; open = excitatory)
Synapses represented by triangles
(filled = inhibitory neurons; open = excitatory)

types of neurons in the cortex. These appear in three layers—the granule cell layer is deepest, the Purkinje cell layer is in the middle, and a superficial layer is termed the molecular layer. Not surprisingly, granule cells (the most numerous cell type in the human brain) are in the granule cell layer along with Golgi cells. The Purkinje cells appear in a single layer. Finally, the molecular layer contains basket and stellate cells. All of these cell types, with the exception of the granule cells, use the inhibitory neurotransmitter, GABA. It is also important to note that the Purkinje cell is the only neuronal type that has an axon that leaves the cerebellar cortex. The remaining cell types make connections only within this thin layer of the cerebellar cortex.

The circuitry of the cerebellar cortex is also quite well understood, and was largely established by Sir John Eccles and colleagues. There are only two types of axons that enter the cerebellum, mossy fibers and climbing fibers. Climbing fibers arise only from the inferior olivary nucleus, while mossy fibers comprise all of the other cerebellar inputs. Both of these fiber types release excitatory neurotransmitter, glutamate in the case of the mossy fibers, and aspartate in the case of climbing fibers. As they enter the cerebellum, both the mossy and climbing fibers have collateral branches that synapse on (and excite) the deep cerebellar nucleus neurons. However, these two fiber types have quite different terminations and effects in the cerebellar cortex.

Mossy fibers branch extensively as they enter the cortex. Each mossy fiber terminal synapses on a group of granule cell dendrites, exciting the granule cell. The granule cell axon runs toward the cortical surface, into the molecular layer where it divides in a "T." These granule cell axons run along the axis of the cerebellar folia, crossing the dendritic arbors of many Purkinje cells, with which they make excitatory en passant synapses. There are millions of granule cell axons packed into each folia and they are called parallel fibers. Several hundred thousand parallel fibers synapse with (and excite) each Purkinje cell. Parallel fiber axons are also the main excitatory input to the Golgi, stellate and basket cells. Each parallel fiber input makes a minute input, but they can summate to activate the Purkinje cell.

The Purkinje cell axons are the only nerve fibers to actually leave the cerebellar cortex, and they synapse on deep cerebellar nucleus neurons and on some vestibular neurons, inhibiting them powerfully. Therefore, the excitatory input that entered the cerebellum with the mossy fiber was responsible for exciting the deep nucleus neuron and then for exciting granule cells that stimulate Purkinje cells that "turn off" the deep nucleus neuron. It is critical that the correct amount of inhibition arrive at the deep cerebellar nucleus in order to produce an appropriate output, inhibiting unwanted activity in the deep nuclei. This is a process akin to sculpture, where the unwanted parts of the stone are removed to create a pattern.

The cerebellar climbing fibers synapse directly on the Purkinje cells and powerfully excite them. There is only one climbing fiber per Purkinje cell and each climbing fiber only goes to one to three Purkinje cells. Therefore, there is an intimate connection between the neurons of the inferior olivary nucleus and the Purkinje cells. Current concepts of inferior olivary function place it as an "error detector." When a particular action goes off target, inferior olivary nucleus neurons are activated. This results in powerful activation of the target Purkinje cells through the climbing fibers. This powerful activation of Purkinje cells inhibits the deep cerebellar nucleus neurons, hopefully terminating the unwanted component of the action.

If this is how the cerebellum works, then how does the cerebellum contribute to motor learning, so that the next time the movement is performed, it is more accurate from the beginning? This appears to be the result of plasticity of the synapse between the parallel fiber and the Purkinje cell. At the moment of activation of the Purkinje cell by the climbing fiber, all of the parallel fiber synapses that were recently active will undergo a process of long-term depression. This long-term depression occurs by a complicated molecular mechanism that has been well studied and depends on the near simultaneous activation of parallel fibers and climbing fibers to the Purkinje cell. This mechanism warrants some discussion because it represents a fundamental example of the plasticity of neuronal response and of a type of "learning" in the nervous system. Parallel fibers release glutamate at their synapse on the Purkinje cell dendrite. This input activates metabotropic glutamate receptors at the same time that it activates the inotropic AMPA receptors. This is how parallel fibers normally excite Purkinje cells. The metabotropic glutamate receptors activate phospholipase C, which results in creation of IP3 and DAG. These molecules contribute directly and indirectly to formation of protein kinase C (PKC). This PKC will phosphorylate proteins associated with the AMPA (inotropic glutamate) receptors. Under most circumstances this phosphorylation is quite minor. However, the activation of PKC is massively increased in the setting of high levels of calcium in the dendrite, a situation that results from Purkinje cell activation via climbing fibers (aspartate, the neurotransmitter at the climbing fiber to Purkinje cell synapse, opens calcium channels). This high level of PKC results in internalization of phosphorylated AMPA glutamate channels. This produces a long-term depression of subsequent responses to input along the particular parallel fiber that was active immediately before the parallel fiber input. In other words, the synapses that were active around the time of climbing fiber input will be weakened, so that the next time the specific parallel fiber is active, it will have less of an excitatory effect on the Purkinje cell. Since our current concept of the climbing fiber function is that they convey an error signal, the granule cell to Purkinje cell synapses that were active at the time of the error will be inhibited. This is appropriate since these synapses were probably at fault in the unwanted activity in the first place. Therefore, each synapse can be adjusted during a process of learning to produce the correct cerebellar output. In the case of motor patterns, this allows for procedural learning, where each time an action is performed, it becomes somewhat more accurate since the "right synapses" are contributing to the response.

Less is known about the activity of the other neurons of the cerebellar cortex. It is noteworthy that all of the other three cell types (Golgi, stellate and basket cells) are inhibitory. Each of these cell types is excited by the parallel fibers and each feeds onto a certain part of the circuit. Golgi cells feed back inhibition to the granule cells. Parallel fiber activation of the stellate cells will feed forward and inhibit Purkinje cells shortly after they themselves are excited by the parallel fibers. This inhibition may be necessary to "clear" the activity of the Purkinje cells shortly after they have been excited, allowing the Purkinje cell to respond to only the immediate activity in granule cells and parallel fibers. The basket cells are a special case, since their axons usually go to surrounding Purkinje cells, not the ones to which they are adjacent. This may "turn off" activity in Purkinje cells at a certain distance surrounding the focus of activity. While there are concepts of how these inhibitory neurons of the cerebellar cortex work, suffice it to say that all of the details are not understood and, despite its rather simple architecture, we do not have a working computer model of cerebellar control of any of the complex activities that it so ably regulates. This is mostly being investigated in control of vestibulo-ocular reflex functions, where the inputs and outputs can be more precisely measured. It is clear, however, that damage to the deep cerebellar nuclei or the Purkinje cells have severe and potentially devastating effects, which are most obvious in the area of motor control.

If the cerebellar cortex is a sea of monotonous circuitry, what distinguishes the different parts of the cerebellum? In a word, these areas are distinguished by their specific inputs, most dramatically by the particular origins of the mossy fibers that terminate in the cortex. Also, although all of the climbing fibers arise from the inferior olive, there is a very precise topography of origin of climbing fibers within the olive. We will discuss three basic parts of the cerebellum: the vestibulocerebellum, the spinocerebellum, and the neocerebellum.

The vestibulocerebellum, or flocculonodular lobe of the cerebellum, receives a substantial amount of its input from the vestibular nerve. This is unique since no other portion of the cerebellum receives direct input from a sensory nerve. Additionally, there are connections from the vestibular nuclei to the vestibulocerebellum. Another unique feature of this portion of the cerebellum is that Purkinje cells in this region actually have axons that leave the cerebellum to synapse in portions of the vestibular nuclear complex in the dorsolateral brain stem. This is the only portion of the cerebellar cortex to have any direct connections other than to deep cerebellar nucleus neurons, and suggests that the vestibular complex may have some similarity with deep cerebellar nuclei.

The vestibulocerebellum is an important regulator of the vestibular system. Damage to this region will result in vertigo and nystagmus. However, the most important function of this part of the cerebellum is to allow adaptation to vestibular damage. The effects of damage to the vestibular system—for example, by damaging the inner ear—are severe. However, with time, these injuries will be well compensated. This compensation does not happen if the vestibulocerebellum is also injured. The vestibulo-ocular reflex has been the basis for much of the research into cerebellar plasticity, since this reflex is precise in stabilizing the eyes during movement and adjusts to vestibular damage.

The spinocerebellum is important in regulating muscle tone and in adapting the body to changing circumstances. This portion of the cerebellum includes vermal and paravermal zones of the anterior lobe and part of the posterior lobe. Therefore, it receives extensive input from the spinal cord. As described in Section VIIa, several direct and indirect spinocerebellar pathways terminate in the spinocerebellum in a topographic manner in two somatotopic maps (one in the anterior lobe and one in the paramedian lobule). The input from muscles and the spinal cord reflex pathways are necessary for proper regulation of muscle tone and movement.

Since the spinocerebellum includes both vermal and paravermal zones of the cerebellum, there are connections with both the fastigial nuclei and the interposed nuclei. The fastigial nuclei, in turn, connect to the reticular formation (Figure 24), which can affect muscle tone and crude movements via the reticulospinal tracts. The interposed nuclei connect predominantly to the contralateral red nucleus through the superior cerebellar peduncle (Figure 24). This nucleus is the origin for the rubrospinal tract that mainly influences limb flexor muscles. Therefore, the spinocerebellum can influence both muscle tone and coordination of the extremities. Additionally, the cerebellum is important in determining the appropriate response to changing situations. For example, when attempting to resist a force on the extremities, a sudden release of force would result in a rebound of the limb. The ability to rapidly check this motion requires feedback from muscle stretch and tension receptors.

The neocerebellum receives the vast majority of its input from the pontine nuclei. The pontine nuclei receive input from the majority of the cerebral cortex via corticopontine fibers. The pontine nuclei project exclusively through the middle cerebellar peduncles to the cerebellum, where these axons terminate as mossy fibers. It is the largest input to the cerebellum and almost exclusive input to the neocerebellum (which comprises most of the lateral hemispheres of the cerebellum). The neocerebellum connects to the dentate nuclei via its Purkinje cell axons, and the dentate nucleus, in turn, projects to the ventral lateral nucleus of the thalamus, which relays back to the cerebral cortex (Figure 24). Therefore, the lateral hemispheres of the cerebellum are involved in regulating the cerebral cortical motor output. The best-known effect of this is in procedural learning. Activities such as riding a bike or learning to ski involve activity of the cerebellar hemispheres. Damage to the lateral hemispheres results in lack of coordination of limb movement, with overshoot and undershoot (intention tremor).

The discussion to this point has largely focused on control of balance and of skilled voluntary movements. In addition to these functions, the cerebellar vermis receives visual input from the superior colliculus and is involved in coordinating eye movements. It also coordinates speech. Drunken speech, for example, derives from the effect of alcohol on the vermal portions of the cerebellum.

Finally, there has been increasing recognition of the role of the cerebellum in learning and regulating many behaviors at the level of the cerebral cortex. For example, there are abnormalities in the cerebellum in such diverse conditions as schizophrenia and autism, indicating a much broader range of effects than previously appreciated. Of course, the anatomy of the cerebellum does provide a substrate for this interaction, with afferent input to the cerebellar cortex via corticopontine, pontocerebellar fibers from diverse areas of the cerebral cortex. Also, the dentato-thalamo-cortical connection distributes to many regions of the cerebral cortex beyond the clas-

Figure 24

Cerebellar efferent connections

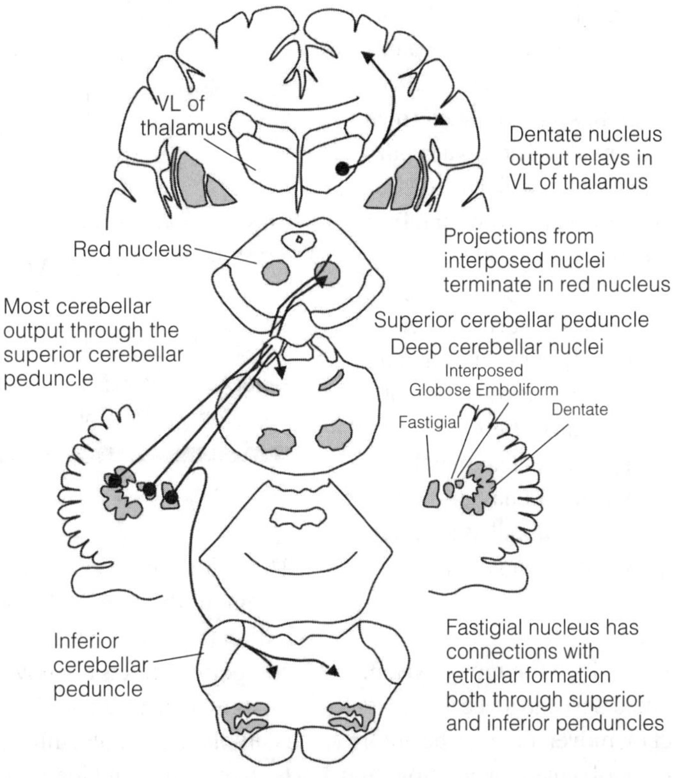

sic projections to the ventrolateral thalamic nucleus and motor cortex. However, a full appreciation for these aspects of cerebellar function represents the frontier of research into cerebellar functions.

Basal Ganglia

The extrapyramidal system consists of a series of functionally related nuclei in the telencephalon, diencephalon and midbrain. The basal ganglia represent the largest component, and include the caudate, putamen and globus pallidus. The pars reticulata and pars compacta of the substantia nigra of the midbrain, as well as the subthalamic nucleus, which is located in the caudal diencephalon, are functionally connected to this system.

The caudate and putamen are functionally and histologically similar nuclei located on either side of the internal capsule. Collectively, they are called the striate nuclei, the neostriatum, or the striatum. The caudate nucleus is on the ventrolateral side of the lateral ventricle. The caudate has a very large head with a body that follows most of the sweep of the lateral ventricle. The tail enters the temporal lobe with the temporal horn of the lateral ventricle. The globus pallidus is immediately medial to the putamen and has a medial and lateral segment. Collectively, the putamen and globus pallidus are termed the lenticular or lentiform nuclei. There's a small rind of cells called the claustrum, which is separated from the putamen by the external capsule and from the insular cortex by the extreme capsule.

The extrapyramidal system has historically been viewed as a part of the motor system, since damage to these areas affect muscle tone, posture, voluntary movements, and can also produce abnormal movements. It has become increasingly clear that this system is also used for control of behavioral "tone" and emotional "posture" of the animal as a whole. This will be discussed toward the end of this section.

Most of our discussion will focus on motor systems, since that has been studied best and since the lessons learned from the effect on movement may be applicable to understanding involvement in emotions and behaviors.

Fundamentally, the principal connections made by the extrapyramidal system are via closed circuits that receive input from the cerebral cortex and project reciprocally back to the cerebral cortex (Figure 25). When considering the motor functions of the extrapyramidal system, the greatest input arises from the premotor cortex. This portion of the cortex is most involved in planning, patterning and initiating movements. The circuit passes through several nuclei in the system, each of which is involved in processing.

Figure 25

Fundamental wiring of basal gangliar circuitry

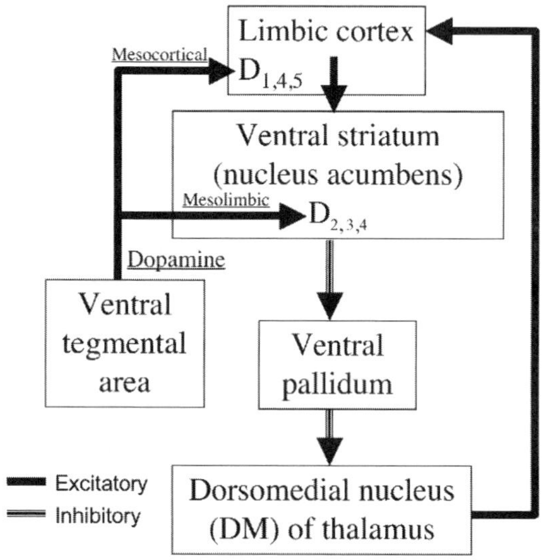

D1 and D2 refer to the principal types of dopamine receptors located on striatal neurons participating in the direct and the indirect pathways, respectively.

There are two described pathways for transmission of signals through the basal ganglia, a direct and an indirect pathway (Figure 25). These pathways have competing effects on movement and there is often thought to be a balance between these systems that is involved in establishing and regulating tone. In both the direct and indirect pathways, the caudate and putamen represent the first synapse in the system. These nuclei receive afferent nerve fibers from virtually all portions of the cerebral cortex, but especially from the premotor areas. The caudate and putamen also receive input from the intralaminar nuclei of the thalamus as well as from several neurotransmitter systems that modulate the activity of the neurons. For example, the substantia nigra pars compacta provides critically important dopaminergic innervation, and several raphe nuclei give rise to serotonin input to the basal ganglia. Therefore, drugs that affect these transmitter systems can have major effects on movement.

Output from the striatum is all via GABAergic, inhibitory neurons. The striatum projects to the medial and lateral segments of the globus pallidus as well as to the substantia nigra, pars reticulata. This latter nucleus is best thought of as a functional part of the globus pallidus since its neurons have similar inputs and response characteristics to those of the globus pallidus.

The globus pallidus itself has two components, a medial (internal) and lateral (external) segment. The globus pallidus has an interesting physiology since its output is solely via inhibitory GABAergic neurons that are tonically active. Therefore, in the absence of any input, there would be a tonic inhibitory signal arising from these neurons. The lateral or external segment of the globus pallidus is a part of the indirect pathway, while the medial segment is a component in both the direct and indirect pathways. We will first discuss the direct pathway and then the indirect.

In the direct pathway (Figure 25), cerebral cortical input to the striatum activates the inhibitory projection neurons in the striatum. This increases the inhibitory output to the tonically active medial globus pallidus. The output of the medial globus pallidus is to the ventral anterior and ventrolateral nucleus of the thalamus via two pathways. The lenticular fasciculus cuts through the internal capsule while the ansa lenticularis courses ventral to the internal capsule. These two pathways meet at the thalamic fasciculus and terminate in the thalamus in two adjacent regions, the ventral anterior nucleus (VA) and the rostral part of the ventral lateral nucleus (VL). The VA and VL of the thalamus project via excitatory pathways primarily to the premotor cerebral cortex. This feedback is involved in regulating the tonic level of excitation in the premotor cortex, an area involved in planning and initiating of movement.

In considering the physiology of the direct pathway, note that the cortical input to the striatum would excite the inhibitory projection neurons to the medial globus pallidus. This would decrease activity in the tonically active projection neurons in the medial globus pallidus and, in turn, would decrease the tonic inhibitory pressure on the VA and VL of the thalamus. Ultimately, there would be disinhibition of thalamic excitation of the cerebral cortex. In other words, this pathway results in a net facilitation of the cerebral cortex. In the case of the motor cortex, activation of the direct pathway would increase the ease of movement and of initiating movement.

The indirect pathway (Figure 25) is inhibitory to movement. Excitatory projections from the cerebral cortex facilitates inhibitory projection neurons in the striatum. These project to the lateral (external) globus pallidus where they inhibit the tonic inhibitory output neurons. This decreases tonic inhibition of the subthalamic nucleus, resulting in increased excitatory output to the medial globus pallidus. The subthalamic nucleus is a small collection of excitatory neurons located at the junction between the midbrain and diencephalons. This excitatory input to the medial globus pallidus increases the inhibitory output from the medial globus pallidus to the thalamus, ultimately decreasing the excitatory feedback to the cerebral cortex. Note that the indirect pathway has opposite effects on the medial segment of the globus pallidus than does the direct pathway. Ultimately, the indirect pathway is inhibitory to motor cortical activity.

Dopamine projections from the substantia nigra, pars compacta to the striatum have complex, and ultimately opposing effects on activity in the direct and indirect pathways (Figure 25). For example, dopamine acts primarily through dopamine D1 receptors on the neurons that participate in the direct pathway, exciting these neurons. It acts on dopamine D2 receptors on the striatal neurons that are involved in the indirect pathway. The D2 receptors are inhibitory. Therefore, dopamine excites the direct pathway and inhibits the indirect pathway, with a net effect to increase facilitatory inputs to the motor regions.

Most of the output from the basal ganglia goes through the thalamus to the cerebral cortex, affecting movement by influencing motor cortex activity. However, there are some other outputs from the basal ganglia. The striatum projects to the substantia nigra pars reticulata. Just like the globus pallidus, the substantia nigra reticulata contains tonically active GABAergic output neurons. Efferent projections from the reticulata project to several places. These include the dorsomedial thalamic nucleus that feeds back on several cerebral cortical sites, particularly those affecting motivation and mood. Also, the reticulata projects directly to the brain stem reticular formation (affecting muscle tone) and to the superior colliculus (affecting eye movements). Altered activity in this system can be seen as the slow and irregular eye movements seen in patients with Parkinson disease.

The extrapyramidal system is involved in setting the level of external responsiveness to stimuli and also in establishing tones and postures of the body. Many neurons in the basal ganglia begin to show activity before movement actually takes place. These have been termed "getting set cells." Additionally, damage to the basal ganglia can result in abnormal involuntary movements, termed dyskinesias. These movements can take several forms that may give clues as to the cause of the abnormality.

It has become increasingly apparent that the basal ganglia are involved in more than motor control. Recent attention has been directed to the mesolimbic dopamine reward system, an important system for the control and reinforcement of behavior (Figure 26). There is a system that has many similarities to the direct pathway that we have previously described. It is primarily involved in controlling emotional tones and responsiveness to the world. This system has also been termed the ventral striatal system and begins with projections from emotional portions of the cerebral cortex, often termed the limbic cortex, to the ventral striatum. This is located where the head of the caudate and the putamen meet, called the nucleus accumbens. The nucleus accumbens projects to the ventral pallidum, a region

Figure 26

Organization of the "ventral striatal system"

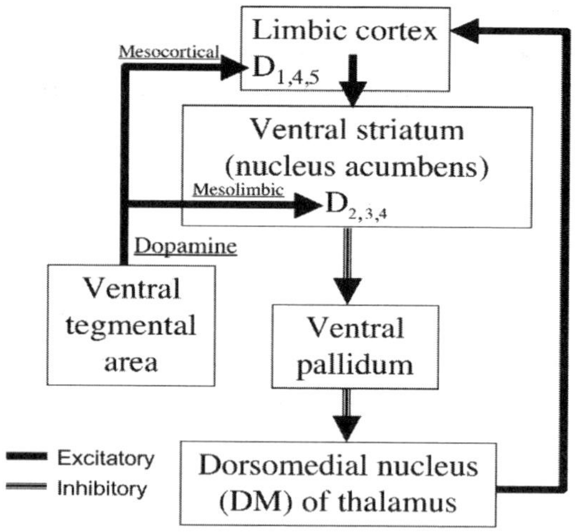

This system is similar in organization to the other portions of the extrapyramidal system and includes a feedback loop involving a striatal element (the nucleus accumbens), a palidal element (the ventral palidum), a thalamic relay nucleus (the dorsomedial nucleus), and a source of dopamine (the ventral tegmental area). Note that dopamine acts on different types of receptors depending on the location.

that is immediately ventral to the anterior commissure in the basal forebrain. Note that it is close to the globus pallidus. The ventral pallidum projects to the dorsomedial nucleus of the thalamus, which, in turn, projects to the limbic areas of the cerebral cortex. These areas are important for maintaining behavioral tone and motivation. In most respects this pathway is similar to the direct pathway, which results in increased thalamic feedback to the cerebral cortex. Just like the direct pathway, dopamine is important in increasing activity in striatal neurons. In this case, the dopamine input derives from the ventral tegmental area, which is located in the ventromedial aspect of the midbrain. It appears to act primarily on the D3 subtype of dopamine receptor.

This dopamine system appears to be stimulated by most drugs of abuse and may be overactive in schizophrenia.

Control of Eye Movements

Although the eyes can be moved voluntarily, most eye movements are through reflexes. The principal types of movement include voluntary motion (both vertical and horizontal), tracking (both voluntary and involuntary), and convergence. Additionally, there are pupillary reactions and control of the lens.

Eye position and motion is controlled by six muscles in each eye. All muscles are tonically active to maintain stability of the eyes. Each eye can be adducted, abducted, elevated, depressed, intorted or extorted. Additionally, this motion must be conjugate in order to prevent diplopia. Horizontal eye movements are controlled by the medial and lateral rectus muscles (adduct and abduct the eyes, respectively). Every movement that elevates the eye above or depresses below the horizontal plane requires the participation of at least two muscles because the axis of the orbit and the muscles of the eye are not directly in line with the visual axis. Accordingly, isolated contraction of the superior or inferior rectus muscles or the superior or inferior oblique muscles results in torsion and deviation of the eye during the process of elevation and depression. For this reason, at least two muscles are primarily active whenever the eyes are elevated or depressed. When looking straight up, the superior rectus and inferior oblique act together. Looking straight down employs the inferior rectus and superior oblique. The six positions of gaze are used to simplify analysis of eye muscle weakness (Figure 27).

There are three cranial nerves innervating eye muscles. The oculomotor nerve, CNIII, innervates all of the extraocular muscles with the exception of the lateral rectus and superior oblique. It also innervates the elevator of the upper lid. These motor nerve fibers arise from the oculomotor nucleus, located within the midbrain just ventral to the periaqueductal gray. In addition to motor nerve fibers, the oculomotor nerve contains parasympathetic preganglionic nerve fibers. These nerve fibers synapse in the ciliary ganglion with postganglionic fibers going to the constrictor of the pupil and to the ciliary muscle. Contraction of the ciliary muscle results in the lens becoming rounder, to allow for close focus. The parasympathetic nerve fibers in the oculomotor nerve arise from the Edinger-Westphal nucleus, which is located in the midline between the left and right oculomotor nuclei.

The oculomotor nerve leaves the midbrain in the interpeduncular fossa (Figure 15), passes between the superior cerebellar artery and the posterior cerebral artery, and enters the dura. It passes through the wall of the cavernous sinus to reach the superior orbital fissure of the skull, which is how it enters the

Figure 27

Six positions of gaze

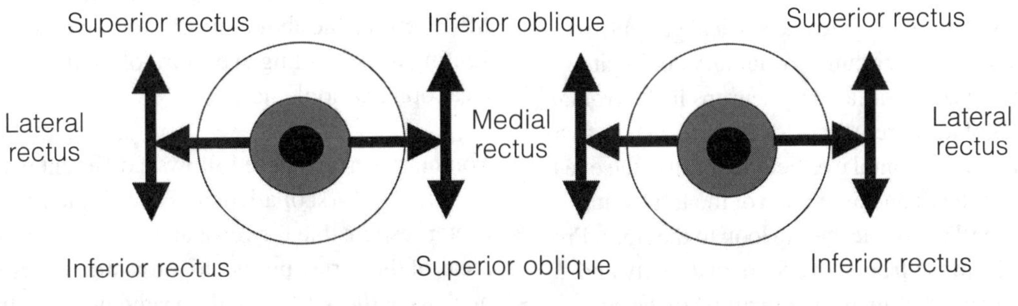

Note that vertical movements of an adducted or abducted eye are the responsibility of a single muscle and that there are always at least 2 muscles that are active when the eyes are moved vertically.

orbit. The cavernous sinus is immediately adjacent to the sella turcica at the skull base, which contains the pituitary gland.

The trochlear nerve, CNIV, arises from the trochlear nucleus (Figure 15), crosses within the brain stem, and exits from the dorsal side of the brain stem at the ponto-mesencephalic junction. As with the oculomotor nerve, the trochlear nerve passes through the superior orbital fissure after traveling within the wall of the cavernous sinus and innervates the superior oblique muscle.

The abducens nerve, CNVI, innervates the lateral rectus muscle. This nerve arises from motor neurons in the abducens nucleus, which is located at the facial colliculus in the floor of the fourth ventricle in the caudal pons. This nerve exits from the pontomedullary junction and follows a long course through the dura (Figure 15). The abducens nerve courses through the cavernous sinus in contact with the internal carotid artery and passes into the orbit through the superior orbital fissure. Neurons in extraocular nuclei have tonic activity.

When the nerve or nucleus is damaged, the eye will drift in the direction of pull of the remaining, intact muscles. Abducens palsy (lateral rectus weakness) will result in medial drift of the eye, while damage to the trochelar nerve (superior oblique weakness) results in extorsion of the eye.

Voluntary eye movements occur in small jumps called saccades. These rapid movements occur so fast that the eye cannot see during the movement. Frequent small jumps (microsaccades) occur even when the eye is still.

Voluntary horizontal gaze and vertical gaze utilize different neuronal circuitry. Voluntary conjugate horizontal gaze is initiated by neurons in the frontal eye fields of the cerebral cortex (Figure 28). Activation of the right frontal eye field will cause the eyes to look to the left and activation of the left frontal eye field will cause the eyes to look to the right. Projections from the frontal eye field go directly and indirectly (via the superior colliculus) to the contralateral paramedian pontine reticular formation (the PPRF). The PPRF, the region of reticular formation immediately ventral to the abducens nucleus, contains neurons that are critical for generating horizontal saccades. Damage to the left PPRF, for example, will completely prevent the movement of either eye to the left. Projections from the PPRF go to the ipsilateral abducens nucleus and through the medial longitudinal fasciculus to the contralateral oculomotor nucleus. This results in conjugate eye movement away from the frontal eye field that started the process and towards the side of the PPRF that was involved in the movement. The medial longitudinal fasciculus (MLF) is the link that yokes the medial movement of one eye to lateral movement of the other eye during lateral gaze. Damage to the MLF permits the abducting eye to move, while preventing the adducting eye from following (internuclear ophthalmoplegia).

Voluntary vertical gaze follows a different pathway (Figure 29). First of all, there is no single cortical center responsible for vertical gaze. Instead, diffuse areas of the cortex project to the rostral interstitial nucleus of the MLF (Cajal; located in the rostral midbrain). This nucleus projects bilaterally to the oculomotor and trochlear nuclei, with many of these fibers passing through the posterior commissure.

Figure 28

Circuitry for voluntary conjugate horizontal gaze to the left

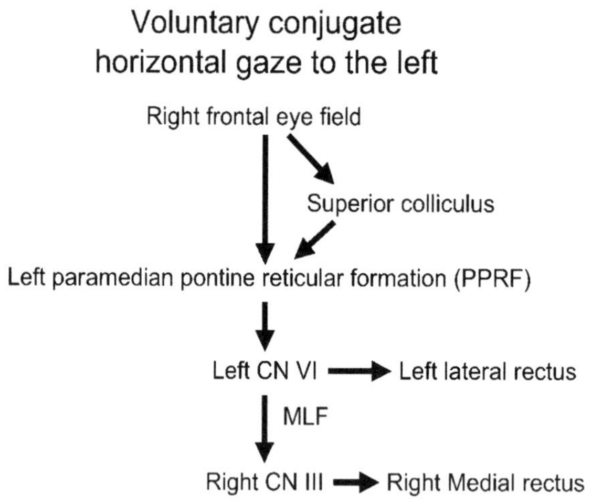

Roman numerals indicate cranial nerve nuclei

Figure 29

Circuitry for voluntary vertical eye movements

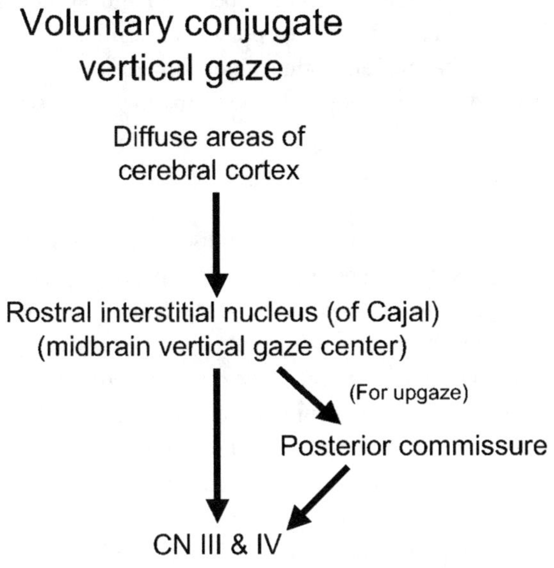

Note that there is no single cerebral cortical vertical gaze center.

Damage to the rostral interstitial nucleus or the posterior commissure can impair voluntary vertical gaze while still permitting reflex vertical movement. This can be seen with pathology of the rostral, dorsal midbrain.

The vestibulo-ocular reflex (VOR) (Figure 20) produces eye movement in response to changes in head position. This is an extraordinarily accurate reflex that allows the eyes to remain focused on a target when the head moves. This is reflected in a 1:1 "gain" of this reflex (ie, 3 degrees of head motion should cause an opposing 3 degrees of eye movement). Projections from the vestibular nerve terminate in the vestibular nucleus and cerebellar flocculus. Many neurons in the vestibular nucleus project to the extraocular nuclei and paramedian pontine reticular formation. The medial longitudinal fasciculus carries many of these connections. With abnormal vestibular input, the eyes will drift away from the direction of perceived motion (vertigo). However, if the person is awake, there will be saccades to reacquire the visual image as it begins to drift. This is the substrate for jerk nystagmus.

The VOR is a reflex response that must be adjusted over time. For example, if there is damage to the vestibular apparatus of an ear, there will be diminished input on that side. Nonetheless, the reflex must still maintain a "gain" of 1:1, causing the eyes to move contrary to head movement if vision is to be stabilized.

Most of our normal voluntary eye movements are not smooth, but rather occur in saccades. However, we are able to move our eyes smoothly when tracking a moving object (Figure 30). Smooth pursuit eye movements utilize some of the vestibulo-ocular reflex pathways and require a visual input to the occipital cortex in order to permit locking of the eyes onto the target. The occipital eye fields are not as well defined as the frontal eye field. They are located in the region near the junction of the occipi-

Figure 30

Circuitry for smooth pursuit eye movements

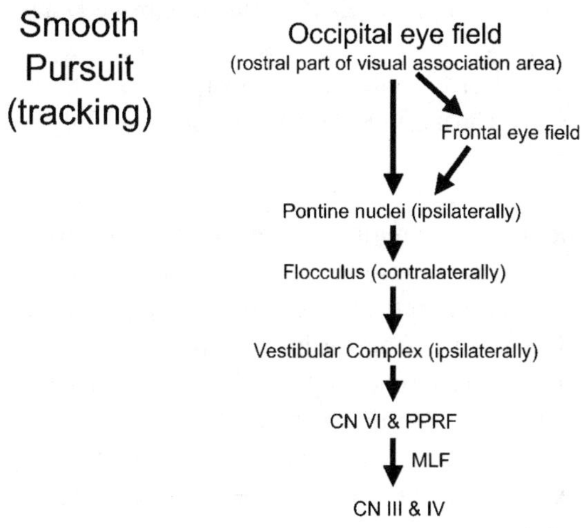

Note that this uses much of the same circuitry as the vestibulo-ocular reflex (see Figure 19). Ipsilateral and contralateral are in relation to the preceding element in the system.

tal lobes with the posterior parietal and temporal lobes (including visual association areas that are involved in detecting motion).

The occipital eye fields project directly and indirectly to the pontine nuclei. Pontocerebellar fibers carry these signals to the flocculus of the cerebellum. As described above, the flocculus is part of the vestibulo-ocular circuitry. The flocculus, in turn, is connected to the vestibular complex and, as described above, the vestibular complex is capable of generating smooth eye movements in all directions via connections to the extraocular nuclei.

There are two reflexes that use the same wiring as smooth pursuit movements (Figure 30). These are the fixation reflexes and the optokinetic reflexes. Fixation reflex refers to the ability to fixate on a target that is moving. When the head is moving, this reflex complements the VOR to stabilize the eyes. The optokinetic reflex (nystagmus; OKN) is an involuntary fixation on objects that are moving in relationship to the head. This is classically observed when looking out of the side of a moving vehicle, and has been termed railway nystagmus. The eyes will have the tendency to track moving objects, especially if they have very starkly contrasting features. They will track for a distance and then subsequently saccade in the opposite direction to reacquire a target. If one visual cortex is damaged, optokinetic nystagmus will be lost when objects move toward the side of the cortex lesion (that is, if they approach an individual from the side of vision impairment).

Another type of normal movement is called vergence. This refers to convergence or divergence of the eyes in order to focus on objects that are closer or further away from the individual. Vergence requires that the occipital lobes be intact and the pathway involves the rostral midbrain reticular formation (adjacent to the oculomotor nuclei) where there are neurons that are active during vergence activities. The details of this pathway are less well understood than for some of the other eye movement pathways, although it is wired in parallel with accommodation (contraction of the ciliary muscle and pupillary constrictor muscle). This linkage appears to be due to interconnections between midbrain neurons projecting to the Edinger-Wesphal nucleus (for accommodation) and neurons projecting to the oculomotor nucleus to adduct (converge) the eyes.

The pupillary light reflex is consensual (bilateral) constriction of the pupil in response to light stimuli. Collateral axons from the optic nerve terminate in the pretectal nuclei. Light triggers bilateral projections from the pretectum to the Edinger-Westfall nucleus to produce pupillary constriction via the parasympathetic division of CNIII.

The superior colliculus is less important in humans than many other species (where it may be the primary generator of eye movements). Nonetheless it is a center for certain head and neck reflex movements. The superior colliculus receives retinotopic visual input, auditory input (from the inferior colliculus), somatic sensation from the spinal cord, as well as input from the cerebral cortex and substantia nigra, pars reticulata. It projects to areas controlling eye movements, such as the PPRF and midbrain reticular formation, as well as to the cervical spinal cord. These latter projections are through the tectospinal tract. It is likely that the superior colliculus triggers reflex head and eye movements towards stimuli of interest, such as flashes of light or loud noises.

In summary, there are several types of eye movements that have distinct anatomy and physiology. Pathways for voluntary horizontal gaze and for voluntary vertical gaze are distinct from one another and can be damaged separately. The vestibulo-ocular reflex is critical for stabilizing the eyes when the head is moving and utilizes many of the same neuronal pathways used by smooth pursuit or tracking eye movements. Vergence and the responses of accommodation for near vision are triggered simultaneously when examining objects nearer than a few meters from the eyes.

Initiation of Movement

Simple motor responses, particularly ones that are repetitive or well rehearsed, often require only activity of motor cortex itself. On the other hand, somewhat more complex movements requiring some decision typically activate the premotor and supplementary motor as well as the motor region.

The premotor cortex is active in the planning stages of a motion, even when no movement ultimately takes place. Therefore, one could conclude that areas such as the premotor cortex are involved in planning movements, while the motor cortex is more involved in its execution. For example, lesions of the supplementary motor area can produce a condition called abulia in which initiation of movement is nearly impossible even though all other elements of the motor system are intact. More complex movements, particularly those where significant planning is required, typically begin with activity in the parietal lobes. For example, there is an area in the lower posterior parietal lobe that is necessary for initiating accurate finger grasp.

9. Limbic System

The limbic system is a convenient way of describing several functionally and anatomically interconnected nuclei and cortical structures that are located in the telencephalon and diencephalon. These nuclei serve several functions; however, most have to do with control of functions necessary for self-preservation and species preservation. They regulate autonomic and endocrine function, particularly in response to emotional stimuli. They set the level of arousal and are involved in motivation and reinforcing behaviors. Additionally, many of these areas are critical to particular types of memory. Some of these regions are closely connected to the olfactory system, since this system is critical to survival of many species.

Areas that are typically included in the limbic system fall into two categories. Some of these are subcortical structures, while many are portions of the cerebral cortex. Cortical regions that are involved in the limbic system include the hippocampus as well as areas of the neocortex, including the insular cortex, orbital frontal cortex, subcallosal gyrus, cingulate gyrus and parahippocampal gyrus. This cortex has been termed the limbic lobe because it makes a rim surrounding the corpus callosum, following the lateral ventricle. Subcortical portions of the limbic system include the olfactory bulb, hypothalamus,

Figure 31

Pathways interconnecting elements of the limbic system

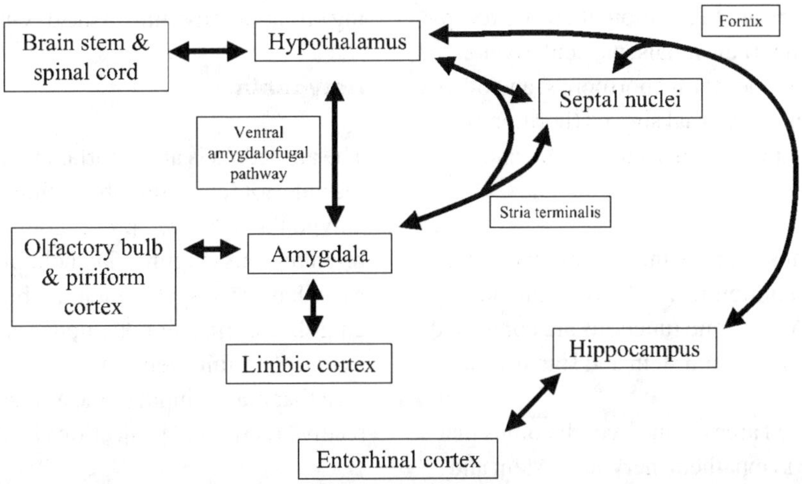

amygdala, septal nuclei and some thalamic nuclei, including the anterior nucleus, and possibly the dorsomedial nucleus.

One way in which the limbic system has been conceptualized is as the "feeling and reacting brain" that is interposed between the "thinking brain" and the output mechanisms of the nervous system. In this construct, the limbic system is usually under control of the "thinking brain" but obviously can react on its own. Additionally, the limbic system has its input and processing side (the limbic cortex, amygdala and hippocampus) and an output side (the septal nuclei and hypothalamus). Most of these regions are connected by pathways that are shown in Figure 31.

Hypothalamus

The hypothalamus, the primary output node for the limbic system, has many important connections. It is connected with the frontal lobes, septal nuclei and the brain stem reticular formation via the medial forebrain bundle. It also receives input from the hippocampus via the fornix and the amygdala via two pathways (ventral amygdalofugal pathway and stria terminalis). The hypothalamus has centers involved in sexual function, endocrine function, behavioral function, and autonomic control.

In order to perform its essential functions, the hypothalamus requires several types of inputs. There are inputs from most of the body as well as from olfaction, the viscera, and the retina. It also has internal sensors for temperature, osmolarity, glucose and sodium concentration. In addition, there are receptors for various internal signals, particularly hormones. These include steroid hormones, and other hormones as well as internal signals (hormones involved in appetite control such as leptin and orexin).

The hypothalamus strongly influences many functions including autonomics, endocrine functions and behaviors. Autonomic functions are controlled via projections to the brain stem and spinal cord.

There are localized areas in the hypothalamus that will activate the sympathetic nervous system and some that will increase parasympathetic activity. Endocrine functions are controlled either by direct axonal connections to the posterior pituitary gland (vasopressin and oxytocin control) or via infusion of releasing factors into the hypothalamic-hypophyseal portal system (to influence anterior pituitary function). There are also projections to the reticular formation that are involved in certain behaviors, particularly emotional reactions. Some functions are intrinsic to the hypothalamus.

These are functions that require a direct input to the hypothalamus and where the response is generated directly via hypothalamic outputs. Included are such things as temperature and osmolarity regulation. There are many functions where the hypothalamus monitors the internal milieu and produces a regulatory response. These include the regulation of endocrine functions and appetite. For example, the ventromedial nucleus of the hypothalamus is considered a satiety area, while the lateral hypothalamic area is a feeding center.

Additionally, there are many complex behaviors that are patterned by the hypothalamus, including sexual responses. The preoptic area is one of the areas of greatest sexual dimorphism (ie, difference in structure between the sexes) and, along with the septal nuclei, is an area of gonadotropin-releasing hormone projections to the median eminence region of the hypothalamus. These sexual responses involve autonomic, endocrine and behavioral responses.

Finally, the suprachiasmatic nucleus receives direct retinal input. This nucleus is responsible for entraining circadian rhythms to the day-night cycle.

Amygdala

The amygdala is an important structure located in the anterior temporal lobe within the uncus. The amygdala makes reciprocal connections with many brain regions (Figure 32), including the thalamus, hypothalamus, septal nuclei, orbital frontal cortex, cingulate gyrus, hippocampus, parahippocampal gyrus, and brain stem. The olfactory bulb is the only area that makes input to the amygdala and does not receive reciprocal projections from the amygdala.

Figure 32

Connections of the amygdala

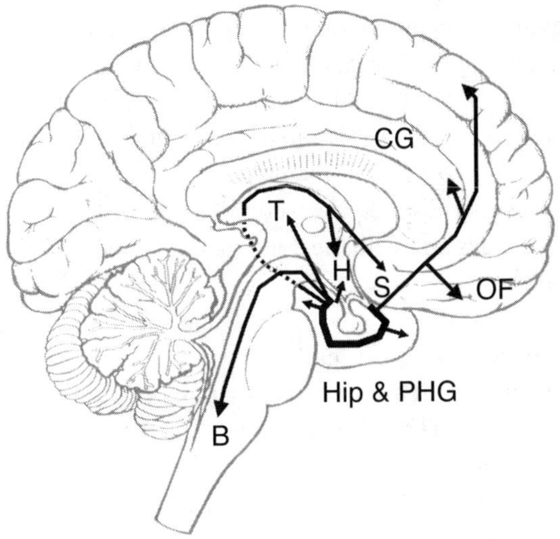

B = brain stem; T = thalamus; S = septal nuclei;
Hip = hippocampus; PHG = parahippocampal gyrus;
H = hypothalamus; OF = orbital frontal cortex;
CG = cingulate gyrus.

The amygdala is a critical center for coordinating behavioral, autonomic and endocrine responses to environmental stimuli, especially those with emotional content. It is important to the coordinated responses to stress, and integrates many behavioral reactions involved in the survival of the individual or of the species (particularly to stress and anxiety). Lesions of the amygdala reduce responses to stress, particularly conditioned emotional responses. Stimulation of the amygdala produces behavioral arousal and can produce directed rage reactions.

Various stimuli produce responses mediated by the amygdala. The convergence of inputs is important since it allows the generation of learned emotional responses to a variety of situations. The amygdala responds to a variety of emotional stimuli, but mostly those related to fear and anxiety.

Hippocampus

The hippocampus is an ancient area of cerebral cortex that has three layers. This is located in the medial aspect of the temporal lobe, forming the medial wall of the lateral ventricle in this area. The hippocampus has several parts. The dentate gyrus contains densely-packed granule cells. There is a curved area of cortex called the cornu ammonis (CA) that is divided into four regions called the CA fields. These are designated as CA1 to CA4. These contain prominent pyramidal cells. The CA fields blend into the adjacent subiculum, which, in turn, is connected to the entorhinal cortex on the parahippocampal gyrus of the temporal lobe.

There are several sources of hippocampal afferents. These are primarily from the septum and hypothalamus via the fornix and from the adjacent entorhinal cortex. This cortical region receives input from diffuse areas of the neocortex, especially the limbic cortex, and from the amygdala. The entorhinal cortex projects to the dentate gyrus of the hippocampus via the perforant pathway, synapsing on granule cells. These granule cells connect to pyramidal neurons in the CA3 region, which, in turn, project by Schaeffer collaterals to CA1 pyramidal cells. It is these latter cells that give rise primarily to the fornix. The physiology of these pathways has been studied extensively, particularly in terms of long-term physiological changes associated with memory. Hippocampal neurons have been studied extensively in terms of long-term potentiation. This requires activation of glutamate receptors and results in long-term changes in neural excitability by way of calcium mediated physiological effects.

Outputs from the hippocampus pass primarily via two pathways. The first of these outputs is through the fornix. These fibers project to the mamillary bodies via the postcommissural fornix, to the septal nuclei, to the preoptic nucleus of the hypothalamus, to the ventral striatum and to portions of the frontal lobe through the precommisural fornix. There are large numbers of projections from the hippocampus back to the entorhinal cortex.

Figure 31 demonstrates many of the important pathways within the limbic system. Note that the hippocampus has reciprocal connections with the cortex as well as outputs along the fornix. Historically, the loop starting with the hippocampus projecting to the mamillary bodies, with relay to the anterior thalamic nucleus—then the cingulate gyrus, entorhinal cortex and back to the hippocampus—was thought to be an important circuit (the Papez circuit). The circular nature of this connection, however, does not appear to be of functional significance.

The hippocampus has several functions. It helps control corticosteroid production. It also contributes significantly to understanding spatial relations within the environment. Additionally, the hippocampus is critically involved in many declarative memory functions.

There are several types of memory. Explicit or declarative memory refers to the memory of facts and events. Any memory that can be completely explained in words is of this type. Implicit or nondeclarative memory, however, is also very important. The learning of skills as well as associative learning, such as conditioned and emotional responses, are common examples of nondeclarative or implicit memory. Explicit memory depends on the medial temporal lobe and the relationship between the hippocampus and entorhinal region of the parahippocampal gyrus.

There are several areas involved in explicit memory. The hippocampus plays a critical role in short-term memory, which is absolutely necessary if long-term memory patterns are to be established. Lesions of the hippocampus do not affect old, established memories. These lesions affect new declarative learning. Ultimately, memory storage is transferred to other areas of the cerebral cortex, and the location of encoding of these memories may be a function of the type of memory. Established memories involve association areas in the frontal lobe and parietotemporo-occipital association cortex.

The hippocampus is not only active in encoding memories but also in retrieval of them. Activation of the hippocampus can be seen in this case of learning about new surroundings and of retrieving directions.

Limbic Cortex

The prefrontal cortex is anterior to the premotor cortex. The orbital frontal cortex is the portion over the orbits. This part of the cortex is extremely well developed in humans and is critical to judgment, insight, motivation and mood. It is also important for conditioned emotional reactions. The prefrontal cortex receives input from the other areas of the limbic cortex, from the amygdala and from septal nuclei, and has reciprocal connections with each of these areas and with the dorsomedial nucleus of the thalamus.

Damage to the prefrontal area produces difficulties with abstract reasoning, judgment moods, and puzzle solving. The effect of frontal lobe damage on mood depends on the specific part of the prefrontal cortex damaged. The patient's behavior is often described as tactless. Also, this part of the cortex can be strongly affected by alcohol.

Prefrontal cortex function is abnormal in mood disorders. Depression is most often associated with increased activity in portions of the frontal lobe, especially the medial regions, including the subgenual portion of the anterior cingulate cortex, and decreased activity in the posterior cingulate gyrus.

Olfaction makes strong connections with the anterior portions of the temporal lobe and the amygdala. The olfactory cortex is structurally simpler than other portions of the cerebral cortex and is termed the allocortex (Section 11). It includes the prepiriform and periamygdaloid cortex that comprises the anterior part of the parahippocampal gyrus covering the uncus. In some species, of course, olfaction is more important than in others. Olfactory filaments cross the cribiform plate and synapse with mitral cells in the olfactory bulbs. Axons from these cells make up the olfactory tract, which extends to anterior temporal structures bilaterally, as well as the basal forebrain.

Olfactory signals are relayed to several other brain regions after their initial termination in the olfactory cortex. The olfactory cortex affects the frontal lobe through connections with the dorsomedial nucleus of the thalamus. Olfactory cortex projections to the

Figure 33

Structure and connections of the thalamus

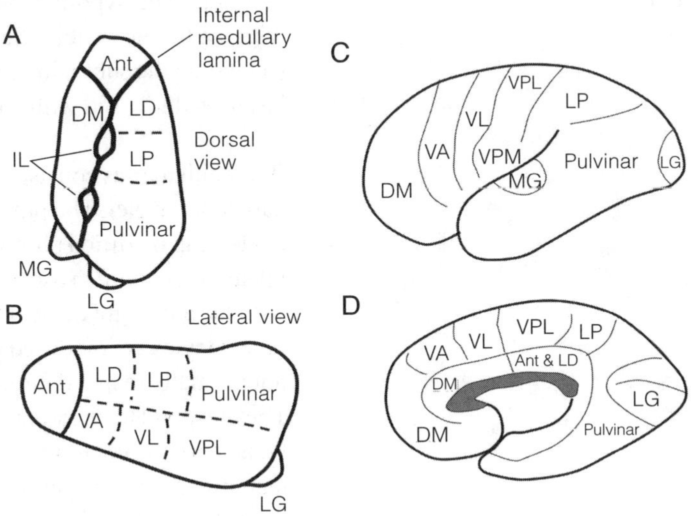

A. View of the right thalamus from the dorsal aspect (anterior toward the top of the page). The internal medullary lamina divides the thalamus into lateral, medial and anterior regions. B. View of the thalamus from the lateral aspect. C & D. Shows the cerebral cortical regions that are reciprocally connected with the labeled thalamic regions. C is a lateral view of the hemisphere while D is a view of the hemisphere from the medial aspect. See Figure 34 for details on cerebral cortical organization. DM = dorsomedial; VA = ventral anterior; VL = ventral lateral; VPL = ventral posterolateral; Ant = anterior; LD = lateral dorsal; MG = medial geniculate; LG = lateral geniculate; LP = lateral posterior; IL = intralaminar.

amygdala can influence emotional and endocrine reactions, particularly via connections with the hypothalamus.

There are several interesting syndromes that elucidate aspects of limbic functions. The Kluver-Bucy syndrome occurs with bilateral lesions of the temporal lobes. It blocks emotional responses in animals, which become quite docile. They are unafraid of things that their species should react to, for example, in the case of an ape, a length of rope. Animals become hypersexual and engage in compulsive exploration behavior, especially with the mouth.

As previously described, there are pathways through the forebrain that are involved in reinforcement of behaviors and in "reward." Electrical stimulation of these sites is highly reinforcing for behavior. Many of these pathways involve dopamine and are commonly affected by drugs of addiction. Habituation in these pathways with chronic administration of addicting drugs is one of the most important targets of addiction research. Figure 26 shows the ventral striatal projections to the ventral pallidum which, in turn, projects through the dorsomedial nucleus of the thalamus to limbic areas of cortex. The ventral striatum mostly consists of the nucleus accumbens, which is an important target of dopaminergic projections from the ventral tegmental area.

Various addictive compounds affect activity of the dopamine transmission in the nucleus accumbens (mesolimbic) and frontal cortical (mesocortical) systems. Additionally, these pathways appear to be functionally unbalanced in patients with schizophrenia. It appears that patients with schizophrenia have diminished dopamine effects through mesocortical systems to the prefrontal cortex. This could produce symptoms such as social withdrawal and diminished emotional responsiveness. Concurrently, there is a relative increase in dopamine effects via the mesolimbic system to the ventral striatal system, resulting in positive symptoms of delusions and hallucinations.

10. Thalamic Organization

The diencephalon consists of the hypothalamus, subthalamus, dorsal thalamus and epithalmus. These structures basically surround the third ventricle, and comprise the lateral wall and floor of this ventricle. The hypothalamus has been discussed with the limbic system (Section 9). The subthalmus (including the subthalmic nucleus and zona incerta) has been discussed with the basal ganglia.

The epithalamus consists of the pineal gland and habenular nuclei. The pineal is an interesting area containing modified photoreceptor cells. These release melatonin in a circadian rhythm associated with the day/night cycle. Despite the fact that pinealocytes are modified photoreceptors, they do not normally respond directly to light in humans. They respond to circadian differences in sympathetic nervous system activity. This may be important in sleep-wake cycles and, in many species, it is the critical trigger for hibernation and sexual maturation.

The habenular nuclei receive input from several limbic structures (including the ventral forebrain and septal nuclei) via the stria medullaris thalami. This tract can be seen on the third ventricular surface of the thalamus. The habenular nuclei project to the interpeduncular nucleus of the midbrain via the fasciculus retroflexus. This is a pathway by which limbic structures may influence brain stem (reticular formation) function.

The remainder of this discussion will deal with the dorsal thalamus, usually just called the thalamus.

Some of the functions of the thalamus have been discussed in prior sections. This section will put thalamic functions in a more integrated construct. The thalamus is the largest component of the diencephalon. It is the primary site of relay for all of the sensory pathways, except olfaction, on their way to the cerebral cortex. Even olfactory signals reach the thalamus via indirect connections with the cortical regions initially receiving the olfactory signal.

The thalamus is a site where sensory inputs can be modulated. It is also a site of relay for cerebellar and basal ganglia inputs to the cerebral cortex. Remember, these are feedback pathways, since the cerebellum and basal ganglia respond to outputs from the cerebral cortex (Section 8). Limbic pathways also make input to the dorsal thalamus.

All thalamic nuclei, with the exception of the reticular thalamic nucleus, project primarily to the cerebral cortex. Additionally, each portion of the thalamus receives a reciprocal connection from the same portions of the cerebral cortex, whereby the cortex can modify thalamic functions. This may provide a mechanism for filtering thalamic inputs to the cerebral cortex.

All thalamic nuclei contain many inhibitory interneurons (GABAergic and peptidergic) that can modulate the transmission of signals through the thalamus. Additionally, many neuromodulatory neurotransmitter systems (such as serotonin and norepinephrine systems) have terminations within thalamic nuclei. Therefore, it appears that the ability to filter signals is important to thalamic function and plastic changes in this filtering function may be physiologically important. There are two basic types of inputs to the thalamus. The first of these is input that is being relayed to the cortex. The second is modulatory input, which primarily arises from the cerebral cortex, as well as from the reticular thalamic nucleus and various brain stem areas. These modulatory pathways affect transmission.

Each thalamic projection neuron can exist in one of two basic physiological states, tonic mode and burst mode. Burst mode has also been called oscillatory mode, since neurons in this state have an intrinsic rhythmicity. In tonic mode, the neurons respond like other neurons to depolarization and hyperpolarization. Burst mode is found when neurons are tonically hyperpolarized. When they are in this mode, a special class of calcium channels are opened, which result in rhythmic depolarization, producing a rhythmic burst of action potentials in the thalamic projection neurons.

During sleep, most thalamic neurons are in burst mode. During waking, many thalamic neurons remain in burst mode. In burst mode, neurons cannot communicate specific information. However, if a novel stimulus is presented, the sudden change from burst to tonic mode may be a major factor in alerting the cortex. Additionally, this intrinsic rhythmicity probably contributes to the generation of cortical electroencephalographic rhythms.

The thalamus is divided into three regions that are anatomically defined by a "Y"-shaped bundle of nerve fibers termed the internal medullary lamina (Figure 32A). Broadly, there is an anterior, lateral and medial subdivision of the thalamus. Within each of these divisions there may be subnuclei with distinct connections. The anterior thalamic nucleus has a single nucleus, the anterior nucleus. This is between the arms of the rostral parts of the internal medullary lamina. The medial portion of the thalamus contains the medial dorsal nucleus (MD; also called the dorsal medial nucleus – DM), as well as smaller midline nuclei (located right beneath the wall of the third ventricle). The lateral region is subdivided into ventral and dorsal tiers, each of which contain subnuclei.

The ventral tier of the lateral division contains the ventral posterior, the ventral lateral (VL) and ventral anterior (VA) nuclei. The ventral posterior is further divided into the ventral posteromedial (VPM) and ventral posterolateral nuclei (VPL). The dorsal tier contains, from caudal to rostral, the pulvinar, the lateral posterior (LP), and the lateral dorsal (LD) nuclei.

The intralaminar nuclei are found within the internal medullary lamina and include the central median and parafascicular nuclei. The reticular thalamic nucleus is a thin shell of neurons covering the entire lateral aspect of the thalamus. This is separated from the thalamus by the external medullary lamina.

The metathalamus includes nuclei that protrude from the posterior aspect of the pulvinar of the thalamus. These include the medial geniculate body (an auditory relay nucleus) and the lateral geniculate body (the principal visual relay).

There are three basic types of thalamic nuclei: 1) relay nuclei; 2) association nuclei; and 3) nonspecific nuclei. Relay nuclei receive very well-defined inputs and project this signal to functionally distinct areas of the cerebral cortex. These include the nuclei that relay primary sensations (the ventral posterolateral – VPL, ventral posteromedial – VPM, medial geniculate and lateral geniculate nuclei) and also the nuclei involved in feedback of cerebellar signals (ventral lateral – VL) and in feedback of basal gangliar output (part of the VL and the ventral anterior nucleus – VA). The association nuclei are the second type of thalamic nuclei and receive most of their input from the cerebral cortex and project back to the cerebral cortex in the association areas where they appear to regulate activity. The third type of thalamic nuclei are the nonspecific nuclei, including many of the intralaminar and midline thalamic nuclei that project quite broadly through the cerebral cortex, and may be involved in general functions such as alerting.

Given the various functions of the thalamus, it is not surprising that each of the thalamic nuclei has distinct connections to the cerebral cortex (Figure 32B). We will first discuss connections of specific nuclei before discussing the association and nonspecific nuclei. The VPL and VPM nuclei are part of the somatosensory system. The VPL relays medial lemniscal and spinothalamic connections to the cerebral cortex. The VPM receives trigeminothalamic input and relays to the inferior portion of the postcentral gyrus.

The lateral and medial geniculate nuclei are specific nuclei that relay vision and hearing, respectively. The lateral geniculate receives retinotopic input via the optic tract from the contralateral homonomous visual world. This projects in a topographic manner to the primary visual cortex via the optic radiations. The optic radiations from the upper visual world loop through the temporal lobe white matter on the way to the visual cortex (Meyer's loop), while optic radiations from the lower visual world pass just deep to the parietal lobe.

The medial geniculate receives tonotopically organized auditory afferents from the inferior colliculus via the brachium of the inferior colliculus. This projects to the primary auditory cortex on the superior temporal gyrus (transverse gyrus of Heschel).

The VL receives input from the cerebellum, mainly from the dentate nucleus. There is a small input from the basal ganglia to the rostral part of the VL as well. The VL projects to the primary motor area, area 4, of the precentral gyrus and also has a smaller projection to premotor areas. The VL is thus involved in motor feedback from the cerebellum and basal ganglia to the cerebral cortex.

The VA nucleus receives most of its input from the basal ganglia, especially the medial globus pallidus and substantia nigra, parts reticulata. This projects to premotor cortex, including the supplementary motor area of the frontal lobes, and is involved in planning and initiating movements. The centromedian nucleus (one of the intralaminar nuclei) has reciprocal connections with the globus pallidus and with the premotor cortex. It appears to function as part of the basal gangliar feedback system.

There are a substantial number of association nuclei. Remember, these nuclei receive the largest input directly from the cerebral cortex. The pulvinar is the largest of these association nuclei, occupying the posterior part of the dorsal tier of the thalamus. This receives afferent projections from the superior colliculus as well as from the association cortex. It projects to secondary visual areas and to association areas in the parietotemporal region. This contributes to visual perception and eye movements, probably relating to attention to these stimuli. The LP has very similar connections and function to the pulvinar.

The dorsomedial nucleus (DM; also known as the mediodorsal nucleus—MD) is an association nucleus that has a medial and lateral subdivision. The lateral part receives projections from the superior colliculus, olfactory cortex and the ventral pallidum. It has efferent projections to the frontal eye fields and to the anterior cingulate cortex of the frontal lobes. This is involved in controlling eye movements and attending to visual stimuli, but it also plays a role in emotional "tone."

The medial portion of the MD, along with the midline nuclei, receives inputs from several brain areas including the solitary nucleus, substantia nigra reticulata, amygdala and ventral pallidum. It projects to limbic areas of the cortex, including insular cortex, orbital frontal cortex and subcallosal region. These cortical areas are involved in autonomic regulation and emotions. Damage to this area can also impair memory, as may happen with the amnestic syndrome due to alcoholism.

The anterior nucleus of the thalamus has connections similar to the LD nucleus. It receives input from the hippocampus via the mamillary bodies and projects to the posterior cingulate cortex. The functions are not entirely clear, although it appears to have some role in emotional learning.

The reticular thalamic nucleus receives afferents from the brain stem reticular formation as well as from the cerebral cortex and thalamus. This makes a strongly inhibitory input to thalamic nuclei. This nucleus may be important in sleep-wake cycles and may be an important regulator of signals relaying through the thalamus.

Many of the intralaminar nuclei and midline nuclei have diffuse projections to the cortex and have been termed "nonspecific." These nuclei are probably mostly involved in arousal and alertness.

11. Cerebral Cortical Organization

The cerebral cortex is the outer covering of gray matter over the hemispheres. This is typically 2-3 mm thick, covering the gyri and sulci. Certain cortical regions have somewhat simpler functions, termed the primary cortices. These include areas directly receiving sensory input (vision, hearing, somatic sensation) or directly involved in production of limb or eye movements. The association cortices subserve more complex functions. Regions of association cortex are adjacent to the primary cortices and include much of the rostral part of the frontal lobes, and also regions encompassing areas of the posterior parietal lobe, the temporal lobe and the anterior part of the occipital lobes. These areas are important in more complex cortical functions including memory, language, abstraction, creativity, judgment, emotion and attention. They are also involved in the synthesis of movements.

Most of the cerebral cortex is neocortex. However, there are phylogenetically older areas of cortex termed the allocortex. These more primitive areas are located in the medial temporal lobes and are involved with olfaction and survival functions such as visceral and emotional reactions. In turn, the allocortex has two components: the paleocortex and archicortex. The paleocortex includes the piriform lobe, specialized for olfaction, and the entorhinal cortex. The archicortex consists of the hippocampus, which is a three-layered cortex dealing with encoding declarative memory and spatial functions.

The neocortex represents the great majority of the cerebral cortex. It has six layers and contains between 10 and 14 billion neurons. The six layers of this part of the cortex are numbered with Roman numerals from superficial to deep. Layer I is the molecular layer, which contains very few neurons; layer II is the external granular layer; layer III the external pyramidal layer; layer IV the internal granular layer; layer V the internal pyramidal layer; and layer VI the multiform, or fusiform layer. Each cortical layer contains different neuronal shapes, sizes and density, as well as different organizations of nerve fibers.

Functionally, the layers of the cerebral cortex can be divided into three parts. The supragranular layers consist of layers I to III. The supragranular layers are the primary origin and termination of intracortical connections, which are either associational (ie, with other areas of the same hemisphere), or commissural (ie, connections to the opposite hemisphere, primarily through the corpus callosum). The supragranular portion of the cortex is highly developed in humans and permits communication between one portion of the cortex and other regions.

The internal granular layer, layer IV, receives thalamocortical connections, especially from the specific thalamic nuclei. This is most prominent in the primary sensory cortices.

The infragranular layers, layers V and VI, primarily connect the cerebral cortex with subcortical regions. These layers are most developed in motor cortical areas. The motor areas have extremely small or nonexistent granular layers and are often called agranular cortex. Layer V gives rise to all of the principal cortical efferent projections to basal ganglia, brain stem and spinal cord. Layer VI, the multiform or fusiform layer, projects primarily to the thalamus.

There are several identifiable cell types in the cerebral cortex. The pyramidal cells are the main cell type within layers III and V. These cells can be extremely large in layer V of the motor cortex, giving rise to most corticobulbar and corticospinal fibers. The largest of these neurons are called Betz cells.

These cells are pyramidal in shape, with an apical dendrite that extends all the way to layer I of the cortex. There are also several basal dendrites projecting laterally from the base of these neurons. Dendrites of cortical neurons have many spines that are sites of synapse. The thin axon that arises from the base of the pyramidal cell has collaterals and a long process that leaves the cortex. This is the process that connects with other brain regions by extending through the white matter deep to the cortex.

Stellate or granule cells are most prominent in layer IV. Their axons remain in the cortex. There are several less common cell types, including horizontal cells, fusiform cells, and the cells of Martinotti. It's not important that you know about these minor cell types; however, it is important to note that pyramidal and granule cells are not the only cell types in the cortex.

Figure 34

Map of the cerebral cortex (Korbinian Brodmann, 1909)

The numbers refer to his numbering scheme for cytoarchitectural subdivisions (see text)

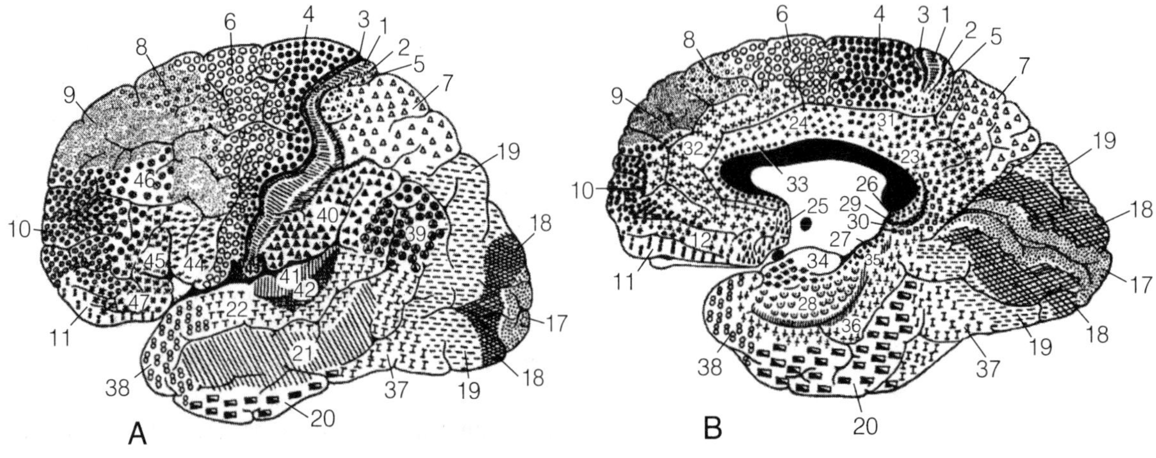

Cerebral cortical cytoarchitecture was described by Brodmann in 1908 and 1909 (Figure 34). While this study was done purely on the basis of cellular composition of the cortex (and the cortical layers), the map that he created corresponds very well with functional mapping of the cortex. We will employ this numbering scheme in the following discussion.

Primary somatosensory cortex (SI; areas 3, 1, 2) is located in the postcentral gyrus. This receives somatotopic input from the VPL and VPM of the thalamus. Histologically, this area would consist of granular cortex. The sensory homunculus includes cortical representation of the body based on the degree of sensory innervation. There are actually four submaps, one each in area 3a, 3b, 1 and 2. Very sensitive areas such as the lips and the fingertips have a huge representation. Neurons within each cortical site (particularly layer IV) are arranged in columns representing specific body regions. If a region is amputated (such as a finger) there is reorganization with neurons responding to stimulation of adjacent body parts. This can also happen as the result of increased use of a body part. Damage to the sensory cortex results in decreased sensory thresholds, an inability to discriminate the properties of tactile stimuli, or to identify objects by touch.

The secondary somatosensory cortex (SII; area 40) is in the lower parietal lobe. This receives connections from the primary sensory cortex and also less specific thalamic nuclei. This responds to sensory stimuli bilaterally, although with much less precision than the primary cortex. Nonetheless, lesions to this area may impair some elements of sensory discrimination.

The somatosensory association cortex (areas 5 and 7) is directly posterior to the sensory cortex in the superior parietal lobes. This receives synthesized connections from the primary and secondary sensory cortices. These neurons respond to several types of inputs and are involved in complex associations. Damage can affect the ability to recognize objects even though the objects can be felt (tactile agnosia). Damage also can cause neglect of the contralateral side of the world, especially with nondominant hemisphere lesions.

The primary visual cortex (VI; area 17), also called the striate cortex, surrounds the calcarine sulcus. This area has a large granular layer with dense columns of neurons, called ocular dominance columns. Adjacent columns come from the same homonomous portions of the left and right eyes (ie, portions that detect images from corresponding portions of the visual world). The macula, the most sensitive portion of the center of the retina, is represented at the posterior tip of the occipital lobe. The upper part of the world projects to the lower part of the striate cortex. Lesions of the occipital lobe would cause cortical blindness and difficulty tracking objects.

The primary visual cortex projects to cortical areas surrounding it, called the visual association areas (V2,V3; areas 18 and 19), where signals are interpreted and form is recognized. In addition to connections from the visual cortex, there are also inputs to visual association areas directly from the lateral geniculate. Selective lesions of these association areas will produce an inability to recognize objects even when they may be seen. There are additional aspects of visual function that are represented in other regions of adjacent cortex. V4 is necessary for color recognition, and V5 (which resides in the posterior part of the middle temporal gyrus – also called MT) is responsible for recognizing movement.

The primary auditory cortices (AI; area 41) are on the transverse temporal gyri, extending into the lateral fissures. These gyri are situated on the upper part of the superior temporal gyri. There are tonotopic maps for different tones. Unilateral cortical lesions do not affect hearing because of completely bilateral sound representation.

There are auditory association areas surrounding the primary auditory cortex (AII; area 42). These areas are involved in the interpretation of sound. In the dominant hemisphere, the cortex surrounding the auditory cortex (area 22) is required for understanding language. This is called Wernicke's area. Damage to this area can produce inability to understand language, including written language. In the nondominant hemisphere, this may be involved in understanding the tone of voice.

Taste is detected in the inferior part of the postcentral gyrus, bilaterally extending into the lateral fissure, including the insula. Vestibular afferent sensations are processed in the superior temporal or inferior parietal gyri. The primary motor cortex (MI; area 4) is in the precentral gyrus. This is the origin of most of the corticospinal tract and a large number of cortical bulbar fibers, particularly those controlling motor cranial nerves. This also has projections to the thalamus and basal ganglion. The VL of the thalamus makes significant input to this nucleus, and the precentral gyrus also receives significant input from sensory cortical areas, as well as from the premotor portions of the cerebral cortex. There is a very well-defined somatotopic organization of the motor cortex and this is the region of cortex from which movements can be generated by the lowest intensity of electrical stimulation. Specific movements tend to be represented (such as elbow flexion) rather than specific muscles. Lesions produce spastic contralateral weakness, which is most prominent in the distal extremities.

The premotor cortex (area 6) is immediately anterior to the motor cortex and has many of the same connections as the motor cortex. However, most of its output is to the motor cortex, with a smaller output to the brain stem and the spinal cord. This region receives input from the sensory association cortex as well as feedback from the basal ganglia via the VA and VL of the thalamus. Electrical stimulation of this area tends to produce more complex movements and at a higher stimulus intensity than the simple movements from MI. Lesions produce less severe weakness but greater spasticity than patients with isolated precentral gyrus lesions.

The supplementary motor area (MII, superiomedial part of area 6) is a part of the premotor cortex that extends onto the medial side of the hemisphere. This projects to the primary motor cortex, basal ganglia, thalamus and brain stem, and also has connections with the contralateral supplementary motor area. This area becomes active before movement and is felt to be involved in initiation of motion. Lesions of this area can cause inability to initiate motions, called abulia.

The frontal eye fields (inferior area 8) are located just inferior and rostral to the premotor cortex. Activity in this region results in conjugate horizontal eye movement away from the stimulus. This receives input from the medial dorsal nucleus of the thalamus as well as other areas of the cerebral cortex. It makes output to the superior colliculus and the PPRF. Lesions of this area initially block voluntary movement away from the side of lesions, although patients will slowly compensate for this deficit.

The occipital eye fields are located in the visual association cortex. This projects to the frontal eye fields as well as to the pontine nuclei to generate smooth pursuit eye movements. Lesions will produce difficulty in fixing on a target and also will produce abnormalities in optokinetic responses. There are areas of the cerebral cortex of particular importance. The receptive language area (Wernicke's—area 22) is in the upper temporal lobe, extending back to the supramarginal (area 40) and angular (area 39) gyri. Lesions produce receptive aphasia with problems understanding spoken and written language.

Lesions of the opercular and triangular portions of the inferior frontal gyrus (areas 44 and 45), called Broca's area in the dominant hemisphere, produce expressive or motor aphasia. These patients have difficulty in generating spoken or written language.

In the nondominant hemisphere, lesions of the regions of the brain that are analogous to Wernicke's and Broca's areas affect the ability to understand or to generate inflections of voice, respectively.

The prefrontal cortex is extremely well-developed in humans. It also undergoes the greatest amount of postnatal development. There are two main portions of this cortex, the dorsolateral prefrontal cortex (DLPC; mostly areas 9 and 10) and the orbitomedial prefrontal cortex (especially areas 11 and 12). The DLPC is primarily involved in executive functions.

These include working memory, judgment, planning, sequencing of activity, abstract reasoning, and dividing attention. The orbitomedial prefrontal cortex is involved in impulse control, personality, reactivity to the surroundings, and mood. A particular area, the anterior cingulate gyrus (areas 24 and 25; subcallosal and subgenual regions) appears to be most associated with mood (particularly depression and mania). While laterality is not as well recognized in the prefrontal cortex as it is in language, there does appear to be some laterality, with lesions of the dominant cortex tending to produce depression, and of the nondominant hemisphere tending to produce mania.

The first and most striking example of frontal lobe functions came from the description of the results of lesions of the orbital and medial prefrontal cortex in a railway construction supervisor, Phineas Gage, whose frontal lobes were destroyed by a tamping rod that passed vertically through his skull, primarily damaging the orbitomedial frontal regions bilaterally. The description of his subsequent behavior by Harlow in 1868 remains a classic:

"The equilibrium or balance, so to speak, between his intellectual faculties and animal propensities, seems to have been destroyed. He is fitful, irreverent, indulging at times in the grossest profanity (which was not previously his custom), manifesting but little deference for his fellows, impatient of restraint or advice when it conflicts with his desires, at times pertinaciously obstinate, yet capricious and vacillating, devising many plans of future operation, which no sooner arranged than they are abandoned... in this regard his mind was radically changed, so decidedly that his friends and acquaintances said that he was 'no longer Gage.'"

The frontal lobes connect to all other cortical regions through association fibers. It receives particularly strong input from limbic cortex, amygdala and septal nuclei, areas involved in emotional responses. Patients with lesions in this area are often referred to as having a changed personality.

Finally, regions of the cerebral cortex are tied together by bundles of white matter fibers. There are association bundles that connect one part of the cortex to another. These association fibers typically arise from layer III and terminate in layers I and II. These may be short and connect adjacent gyri or may connect one lobe to another. Common pathways include the superior longitudinal (arcuate) fasciculus, the superior occipital frontal fasciculus, the inferior occipital frontal fasciculus, the uncinate fasciculus, and the cingulum.

Commissural fibers connect one hemisphere with the other. The largest commissural connection is the corpus callosum, which consists of about 300,000 fibers. Damage to this pathway can produce a "split brain" in some individuals, where an individual may literally appear to have two minds. The anterior commissure represents a smaller connection between the hemispheres that links anterior temporal lobe structures, including the amygdala and other olfactory lobe structures.

Figure 35

Arteries of the brain

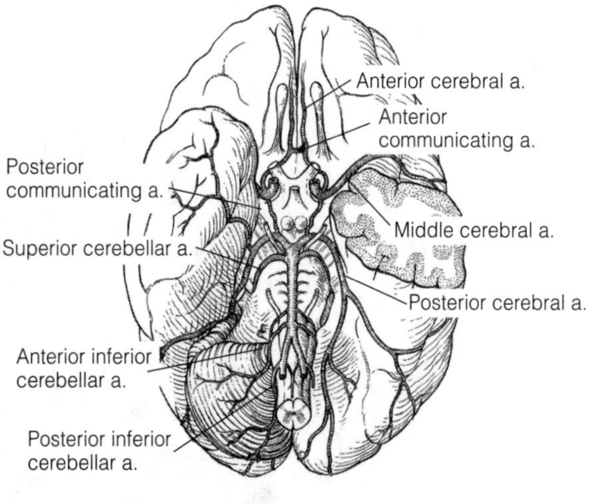

12. Nutrition of the Brain

Circulation of the Brain

There are four arteries supplying the brain (Figure 35). The two carotid arteries and their branches comprise the anterior circulation and the two vertebral arteries comprise the posterior circulation. There are small penetrating blood vessels that come off the larger vessels. These nourish deep areas of brain, while the larger branches remain on the surface. Figure 36 shows the distribution of superficial vessels on the top and deeper vessels in the lower figure. The internal carotid arteries pass through the cavernous sinus (carotid siphon) and give rise to ophthalmic arteries immediately after exiting from the anterosuperior part of the sinus. They give rise to anterior choroidal branches that follow the optic tract posteriorly and then divide into anterior cerebral and middle cerebral branches. The anterior cerebral arteries enter the fissure separating the left and right hemispheres, supplying the medial and superior surface of the cortex. The middle cerebral artery traverses the Sylvian fissure, sending branches onto the lateral part of the cerebral cortex.

The posterior circulation begins with the vertebral arteries that typically join one another just ventral to the rostral medulla. There they form the basilar artery. There are several cerebellar branches off the vertebrobasilar system, as well as penetrating branches into the brain stem and thalamus. The basilar artery ends as the posterior cerebral arteries that supply the medial temporal lobes and most of the occipital lobe.

Figure 36

Distribution of penetrating arteries

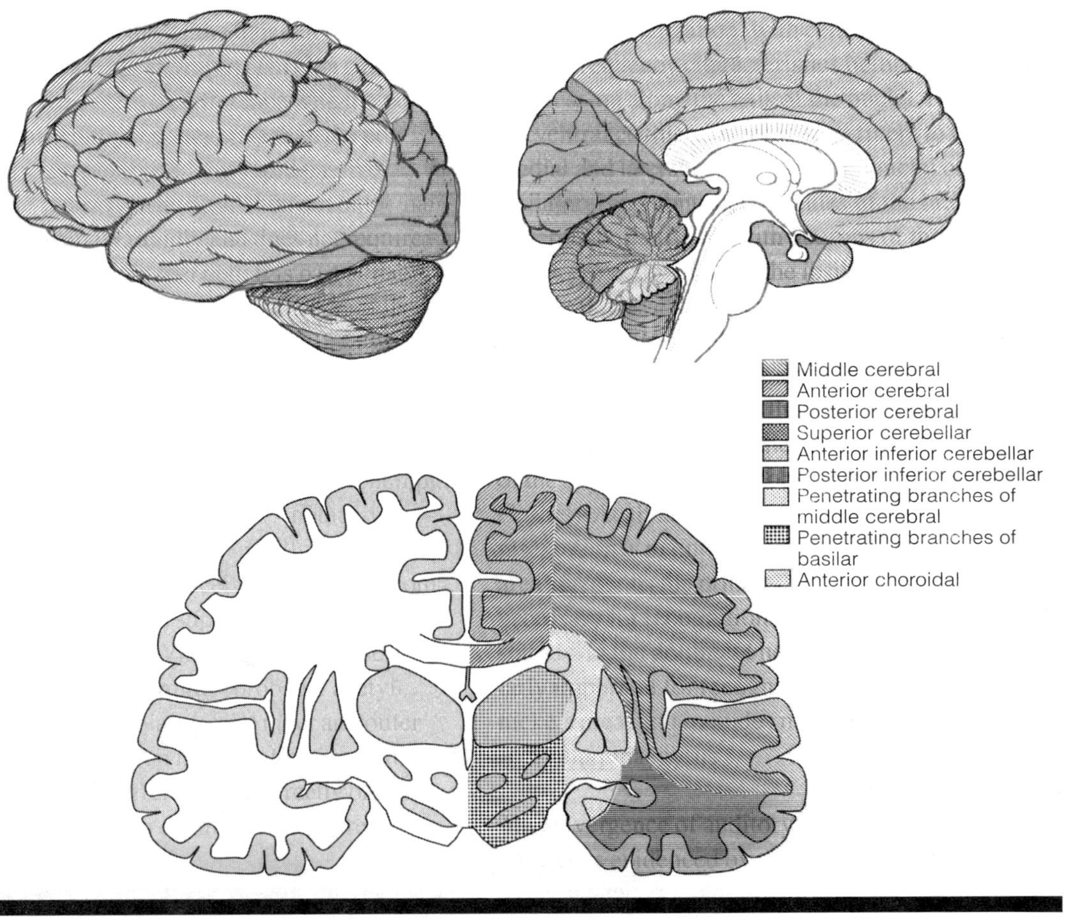

Figure 37

Venous dural sinuses

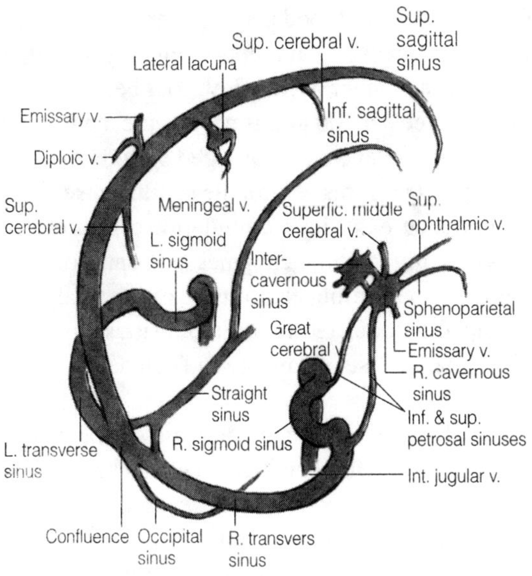

From O'Rahilly R, Muller F. Basic Human Anatomy: A Regional Study of Human Structures. *Philadelphia, Pa: WB Saunders; 1982. By permission.*

Neurons obtain virtually all of their nutrition via aerobic metabolism of glucose. Since this process requires large amounts of oxygen, the nervous system requires a high blood flow, typically around 50 cc/100 grams of tissue/minute. If this value falls below around 15 cc/100 grams of tissue/minute, neurons will begin to malfunction and lower levels result in death quite rapidly.

Most of the venous drainage of the brain is into "sinuses" that are tunnels in the dural coverings of the brain (Figure 37 and 38). The largest, the superior sagittal sinus, is located where the falx cerebri attaches to the dura over the skull. There are bridging veins that cross from the brain to the sinuses and there is one particularly important vein that drains the deep structures of the brain (the great cerebral vein of Galen).

Figure 38

Cerebrospinal fluid pathways

A, cerebral artery; C, cerebral vein; D, diploic vein; E, emissary vein; M, meningeal vein; 3 and 4, third and fourth ventricles. The lowermost part of the figure shows the caudal end of the spinal cord. Lumbar puncture (LP) is performed in the lumbar cistern (below the termination of the spinal cord).

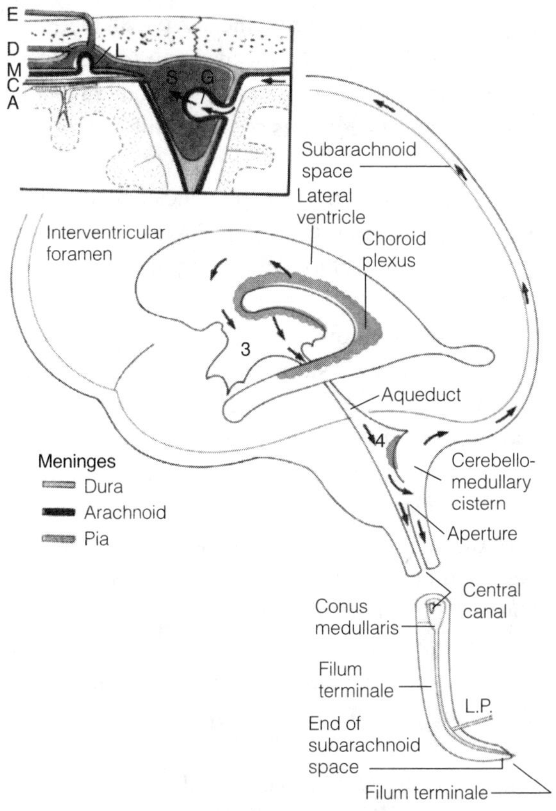

From O'Rahilly R, Muller F. Basic Human Anatomy: A Regional Study of Human Structures. *Philadelphia, Pa: WB Saunders; 1982. By permission.*

Blood-Brain Barrier

The blood-brain barrier is represented by the specialized endothelium that is present in brain capillaries. These specializations (by comparison with most somatic capillaries) include: tight junctions between endothelial cells; few pinocytotic vesicles; no fenestra; and high amounts of metabolic activity involved in active transport. These specializations develop under the influence of footplates of astrocytes, which basically cover the abluminal aspect of the endothelium.

The blood-brain barrier permits selective entry of substances into the brain. Highly lipophilic substances enter the brain by directly crossing the membrane. Water will also cross by simple diffusion. Very small molecules are also somewhat more likely to cross, although even these are usually tightly regulated and transport of ions is via active pumps. Most nutrients cross the barrier via facilitated diffusion, usually by mechanisms that couple the movement of the nutrient with movement of an ion that is moving down its concentration gradient.

There are regions of the brain that lack a blood-brain barrier. These are in brain regions that are responsible for sensing the internal milieu of the body (such as serum osmolarity) or in areas that are involved in either sensing hormone levels or releasing hormonal factors into the blood stream. In the former category are areas such as the subfornical organ or the area postrema of the brain stem. The infundibulum of the hypothalamus and the pituitary gland are examples of the latter category. Releasing factors enter the capillaries of the infundibulum and travel to the anterior pituitary gland where they influence the release of the trophic hormones. This circulation from the hypothalamus to the pituitary gland is called the hypothalamo-hypophyseal portal system and contains fenestrated capillaries.

There are specialized glial cells called tanycytes that separate those areas of the brain with and without blood-brain barriers. This is necessary in order to prevent substances from moving between these brain regions, circumventing the blood-brain barrier.

There is no barrier between the cerebrospinal fluid and the brain. Therefore, there must be a barrier between the blood and CSF. This barrier is formed by the epithelium of the choroids plexus, which has very well-defined, tight junctions between cells, as well as a high metabolic rate, and specific transport mechanisms for nutrient passage and electrolyte regulation.

Control of Regional Blood Flow

Cerebral blood flow is highly regulated and is activity dependent. At baseline, the flow in gray matter is about 50-70 cc of blood per 100 grams of tissue per minute. White matter has approximately half of the flow of gray matter. When flow goes below approximately 15 cc per 100 grams per minute, neurons begin to suffer and any prolonged period below 10 cc per 100 grams per minute results in ischemic injury to neurons with accumulation of free radicals, release of intracellular enzymes, and entry of calcium into the neuron. Neurons do not normally have the capacity for anaerobic metabolism, so hypoxia is a primary cause of damage and cell death.

Cerebral blood flow is regulated by several mechanisms. There are myoepithelial cells in brain precapillaries that contract when stretched. This is an intrinsic property of these cells and does not require innervation. Therefore, when blood pressure rises, the precapillaries constrict, preventing much rise in blood flow. Blood flow will remain constant through all normal ranges of mean arterial blood pressure. This autoregulation can be exceeded by malignant hypertension and can result in damage to the endothelium and the blood-brain barrier. Long-standing hypertension results in a shifting of this autoregulatory curve such that low-normal pressures can result in tissue ischemia.

There are a variety of substances present in the circulation or released from brain cells that dilate cerebral blood vessels. These include CO_2, low pH (which can occur because of increased CO_2), adenosine, and nitric oxide. These latter compounds are often released in regions of increased neuronal activity and result in increased blood flow (beyond that needed for the increased metabolism) in active areas of the brain.

Cerebrospinal Fluid

Cerebrospinal fluid (CSF) is created in the choroid plexi via an active process. These highly vascular structures are located within the ventricles (Figure 38). This fluid, amounting to about 75 cc, has few cells and a low concentration of protein. It does contain 1/2 to 3/4 the concentration of blood glucose. CSF circulates, and turns over several times per day (depending on the level of hydration). The fluid in the lateral ventricles enters the third ventricle via the foramen of Monroe. The third ventricle connects to the fourth ventricle via the narrow cerebral aqueduct, which is located in the core of the midbrain. The fourth ventricle, which lies dorsal to the tegmentum of the pons and rostral medulla, connects with the tiny central canal of the caudal medulla at the obex. This canal continues through the caudal medulla and spinal cord to end blindly in the sacral spinal cord. The fourth ventricle also connects with the subarachnoid space via the midline foramen of Magendie and the two lateral foramina of Lushka.

The subarachnoid space surrounds the brain and spinal cord and provides buoyancy for the brain. It also provides some nourishment for the brain. There are several subarachnoid collections of CSF called cisterns. The largest is the lumbar cistern located between the end of the spinal cord (around the L1 disc) and the end of the thecal sac, around S2 (Figure 38). Other cisterns include the cisterna magna, located between the dorsal medulla and the posterior part of the cerebellum, the quadrigeminal cistern, located dorsal to the midbrain and containing the pineal gland, and the basal cistern, located ventral to the hypothalamus and containing the beginning of the great vessels.

Cerebrospinal spinal fluid is resorbed into the venous system at the arachnoid granulations that are associated with the venous dural sinuses, especially the superior sagittal sinus. Any condition that impairs this circulation of CSF is likely to result in increase in pressure inside the head and may result in herniation or other neurologic catastrophes.

13. Conclusion

An understanding of normal structure and function is critical to appreciating the many ramifications of neoplasms affecting the nervous system and to understanding their treatment. This review of the structures and functions of the nervous system provides a foundation for understanding the pathophysiological processes to be discussed in the subsequent chapters.

14. References

1. Purves D, et al, eds. *Neuroscience*. 4th ed. Sunderland, Mass: Sinauer; 2007.

(Excellent text of basic neuroscience. It is somewhat deficient in neuroanatomy, but it is very clear and easy to follow. There are interesting digressions that are provided as separate short articles that are set off in boxes from the rest of the text.)

2. Nolte J. *The Human Brain: An Introduction to Its Functional Anatomy*. 5th ed. St. Louis, Mo: Mosby; 2002.

(Standard text of neuroscience utilized in many medical schools. It is comprehensive but not overly detailed.)

3. Kandel ER, Schwartz JH, Jessell TM. *Principles of Neural Science*. New York, NY: McGraw-Hill; 2000.

(This is the "bible" of neuroscience texts. Well organized, but quite heavy in sections. It extensively references primary sources and introduces methodology. This is a wonderful text for the graduate or the advanced student of neuroscience. Each section can be studied on its own by the student with a background in neuroscience.)

4. Haines DE. Neuroanatomy: *An Atlas of Structures, Sections, and Systems* (book with CD-ROM). 5th ed. Philadelphia, Pa: Lippincott Williams & Wilkins; 2002.

(Comprehensive atlas: includes a large number of schematic drawings of functional systems of the brain.)

5. Nolte J, Angevine JB. *The Human Brain: In Photographs and Diagrams*. 2nd ed. St. Louis, Mo: Mosby; 2000.

(This atlas includes many illustrations that provide a 3-dimensional feel for brain structures.)

6. Martin JH, Leonard ME, Radzyner HJ. *Neuroanatomy: Text and Atlas*. 3rd ed. New York, NY: McGraw-Hill; 2002.

(Atlas is incorporated in a text with more description than is found in most atlases.)

15. Questions

1. The neural tube undergoes many structural changes over the course of development. Which of the following is true regarding brain flexures in the developing embryo?

   A. The cephalic flexure bends the brain dorsally

   B. The pontine flexure separates the metencephalon (developing pons) from the mesencephalon

   C. The cervical flexure bends the developing nervous system dorsally

   D. The cephalic flexure separates the diencephalon from the telencephalon

   E. The pontine flexure bends the brain dorsally

2. Which of the following is true concerning the sodium-potassium ATPase pump?

   A. This is necessary in order to generate every action potential

   B. This is an essential step in repolarization of neurons

   C. Blocking it will initially have no effect on nerve conduction

   D. This is necessary for release of neurotransmitter from the nerve terminal

3. You are asked to see a 58-year-old man with sudden onset of "numbness" over the left side of the face. On examination, you determine that this involves diminished pain and temperature sensation with preserved touch and pressure sense. You correctly deduce that this is due to damage to the spinal tract of the trigeminal. Which of the following statements regarding this nucleus is CORRECT?

   A. It is confined to the medulla

   B. It is so-called because its neurons send fibers to the spinal cord nuclei

   C. Axons from neurons of the spinal trigeminal nucleus are distributed to the thalamus as fibers in the spinal tract of the trigeminal nerve

   D. It has characteristics shared with the dorsal horn gray matter of the spinal cord, especially with the substantia gelatinosa

   E. It receives stretch receptors from the muscles of mastication

4. Your patient presents with spastic paraparesis. In the process of evaluating her you consider the course and function of the descending motor tracts. Regarding the lateral corticospinal tract, which statement is INCORRECT?

   A. Decussates in the caudal medulla

   B. Proceeds down the spinal cord in the lateral funiculus

   C. Is primarily concerned with proper function of the axial musculature

   D. Contains axons of neurons located in both motor and sensory areas of the cortex

   E. Occupies a small portion of the posterior limb of the internal capsule

5. Cerebrovascular disease is a frequent cause of focal damage of the cerebral cortex. Localization of the lesion depends on an appreciation of the localized functions of the cortex. Which of the following statements is INCORRECT regarding the cerebral cortex?

   A. The association cortex of the human brain is far more extensive than the primary sensory and motor cortices combined

B. Association cortices are anatomically situated adjacent to their related primary cortices

C. Broca's speech area (areas 44-45 Brodmann) occupies the opercular and triangular portion of the inferior frontal gyrus

D. Wernicke's area is located in the posterior superior part of the dominant temporal lobe

E. The auditory association area lies in the orbital portion of the frontal lobe

6. A 65-year-old man presents with gradually increasing rigidity, resting tremor in the right hand and difficulty initiating movements. You correctly consider Parkinson disease, which is characterized by degeneration of dopaminergic neurons of the substantia nigra, pars compacta, which are involved in regulating the function of the basal ganglia. In considering the structure and function of the basal ganglia, which of the following is FALSE?

A. The caudate nucleus and the putamen are termed the striatum or neostriatum

B. The lateral segment of the globus pallidus is connected to the subthalamic nucleus by fibers that cross the internal capsule

C. The thalamic fasciculus from the globus pallidus to the thalamus terminates primarily to the anterior nucleus of the thalamus

D. The globus pallidus is called the pallidum, or paleostriatum

E. There are neurons having spontaneous activity in the globus pallidus

7. The thalamus is an important area that is comprised of subnuclei with extensive reciprocal connects to the cerebral cortex. These subnuclei also receive input from other brain regions that they process and relay to the cerebral cortex. Which of the following nuclei projects to the ventral posterolateral nucleus (VPL) of the thalamus?

A. Nucleus gracilis

B. Pontine nucleus

C. Inferior olivary nucleus

D. Substantia nigra

E. Spinal nucleus of the trigeminal

8. Your 34-year-old patient with multiple sclerosis has an apparent exacerbation characterized by the development of intention tremor and severe ataxia of the right upper extremity. An MRI scan shows a new lesion in the right brachium conjunctivum (superior cerebellar peduncle). Concerning this structure:

A. It is comprised of axons of Purkinje cells

B. It decussates in the pons

C. It projects to the red nucleus and the ventrolateral nucleus (VL) of the thalamus

D. It plays an important role in visceral reactions to sensory stimuli

E. It forms the medial portion of the cerebral peduncle in the midbrain

9. Afferent input to the cerebellar cortex terminates as either climbing or mossy fibers. Cerebellar climbing fibers arise from neurons located in the:

A. Inferior olivary nuclei

B. Lateral reticular nuclei

C. Pontine nuclei

D. Inferior colliculus

E. Red nuclei

10. A number of reflexes occur purely at the spinal level and do not require participation of supraspinal components of the central nervous system. In which of the following spinal reflexes would the time be shortest between activation of the receptor and the response?

A. Excitation of motoneuronal activity to flexor muscles of the knee in the ipsilateral leg following activation of pain receptors (withdrawal reflex)

B. Excitation of motoneuronal activity to extensor muscles of the knee following stretching of the patella tendon (myotatic reflex)

C. Inhibition of motoneuronal activity to flexor muscles of the knee following elicitation of myotatic reflex

D. Inhibition of motoneuronal activity to extensor muscles of the knee following stimulation of Golgi tendon organs (inverse myotatic reflex)

E. Excitation of motoneuronal activity to extensor muscles of contralateral knee following activation of pain receptors (crossed extensor reflex)

11. The motor system use both alpha and gamma motoneurons. Which of the following distinguishes these two types of motoneurons?

A. Only alpha motoneurons have cell bodies in the spinal cord

B. Only alpha motoneurons have axons that exit the spinal cord via the ventral roots

C. Only gamma motoneurons have axons that are myelinated

D. Only gamma motoneurons innervate intrafusal muscle fibers

E. Only gamma motoneurons are directly activated by Ia afferents from muscle spindles

12. Sound stimuli are transduced by the cochlear membrane and hair cells of the cochlea. Which is a CORRECT statement concerning this transduction?

A. High frequency sound causes a greater displacement of the apex than the base of the cochlea

B. With a doubling of the frequency of a sound, the frequency of action potentials in all fibers of the auditory nerve doubles

C. The hair cells of the cochlea have no electrical potential gradient, compared to the perilymph

D. Depolarization of the hair cells can cause the release of neurotransmitter without an action potential

E. Efferents from the central nervous system end only on the inner hair cells

13. One test for the integrity of the semicircular canals is the "caloric" test in which warm and cold solutions are introduced into the auditory canal with the patient supine. Introduction of these solutions induces nystagmus. Which of the following is CORRECT for this test?

A. The rapid phase of nystagmus is toward the same side regardless of whether warm water or cold water is introduced to the same ear

B. The solutions induce the nystagmus by activation of free nerve endings in the external meatus

C. Warm solutions cause the endolymph to rise and flow around the semicircular canals producing a rapid phase of nystagmus toward the side of fluid introduction

D. Nystagmus will still be induced following sectioning of the VIII cranial nerve on the side of water introduction

E. The movements of the eyes to the left and right during the test occur at the same speed

14. The sympathetic and parasympathetic nervous systems have many similarities and some important differences. Which of the following is unique to the parasympathetic nervous system?

A. Acetylcholine is used as a neurotransmitter from preganglionic neurons

B. Release of transmitter from postganglionic neurons always decreases activity of the organ innervated

C. The preganglionic parasympathetic neuron has axons that are always shorter than preganglionic neurons of the sympathetic nervous system

D. The preganglionic neuron can have cell bodies of origin in the brainstem

E. The postganglionic neuron releases norepinephrine

15. The extracellular fluid (ECF) of the brain and cerebrospinal fluid (CSF) are derived from arterial blood. Which of the following is a CORRECT statement concerning these fluids?

A. The concentrations of protein in the ECF and CSF are the same as arterial blood

B. The cerebral capillaries, through which substances are transported from blood to the extracellular fluid, are identical to the capillaries in the systemic circulation

C. Carbon dioxide and oxygen pass readily through cerebral capillaries

D. Transport of substances from arterial blood to the cerebral spinal fluid is entirely passive, ie, no active transport is involved

E. A change in ionic composition of arterial blood results in an essential instantaneous change in the composition of the extracellular fluid of the brain

16. A 62-year-old man with a long history of poorly controlled hypertension was brought to the ED with symptoms of sudden onset of headache associated with nausea/vomiting and right-sided weakness. He was able to be aroused only to intense stimulation. A CT scan showed extensive left-sided basal gangliar hemorrhage in the region of the putamen. Which of the following is true regarding this patient?

A. This condition probably resulted from rupture of an aneurysm of the distal anterior cerebral artery

B. The posterior cerebral artery is the main supply of blood to the putamen

C. This condition probably resulted from rupture of a vessel passing through the anterior perforated substance

D. The anterior choroidal artery is probably the vessel that has ruptured

E. An arteriovenous malformation affecting a branch of the basilar artery is probably at fault for the condition

17. Lesions of the nervous system can damage the ability to perceive certain sensations. These sensory signals follow complex pathways through the central nervous system. Of the following, what is the TERMINATION of the SECOND order neuron in the pathway conveying vibration sensation from the index finger to the somatosensory cortex?

A. The ventral posterolateral nucleus of the thalamus

B. The cuneate nucleus

C. The substantia gelatinosa

D. The cerebellum

E. The ventral anterior nucleus of the thalamus

18. The cerebellum has several functions and its connections to other regions of the brain and spinal cord allow it to serve these functions. Which portion of the cerebellum is most directly connected with the vestibular nuclei?

A. Lingula

B. Anterior lobe

C. Lateral hemispheres

D. Flocculus

E. Posterior lobe

19. The basal ganglia are areas of the brain that are important to the regulation of muscle tone and posture as well as to the initiation of movement and regulation of stereotyped movements. The neostriatum (caudate and putamen) is a large portion of the basal ganglia. Which of the following is FALSE regarding the neostriatum?

A. Cerebral cortical inputs excite neostriatal neurons

B. Neostriatal projections to the medial globus pallidus (paleostriatum) are inhibitory

C. The lenticular fasciculus is comprised of neostriatal projections to the thalamus

D. The substantia nigra projects to the striatum

E. The components of the neostriatum (caudate and putamen) are separated by the anterior limb of the internal capsule

20. Your 78-year-old patient with severe cerebrovascular disease presents with a stroke due to occlusion of a paramedian branch of the basilar artery in the pons on the left. The patient has right-sided weakness of an upper motor neuron type. In addition to this, eye movements are affected. In considering the effects of this, you remember that the left paramedian pontine reticular formation (PPRF):

A. Will make the eyes deviate conjugately to the right when stimulated

B. Receives strong input from the right frontal eye field

C. Receives most of its input from the temporal cerebral cortex

D. Is NOT involved in vestibulo-ocular reflexes

E. Is critically important to upgaze

21. The cerebral cortex has a well-defined organization, with each layer subserving particular functions and making specific connections. Which layer of the cerebral cortex contains the majority of pyramidal neurons that project into the corticospinal tract?

A. Layer II

B. Layer III

C. Layer IV

D. Layer V

E. Layer VI

22. One important function of the hypothalamus is regulation of endocrine function. Which hypothalamic nucleus has the greatest concentration of neurons containing the hormonal releasing and inhibiting factors?

A. Suprachiasmatic nucleus

B. Mamillary body

C. Arcuate nucleus

D. Supraoptic nucleus

E. Preoptic area

23. Your 75-year-old patient with Alzheimer disease is showing progressive loss of short-term memory. You understand that the hippocampus is important for short-term memory and is also heavily affected in Alzheimer disease. You further learn that the majority of input to the hippocampus comes from the:

A. Amygdala

B. Entorhinal cortex

C. Hypothalamus

D. Angular gyrus

E. Prefrontal cerebral cortex

24. A 62-year-old patient is brought to you because of change in personality accompanied by socially inappropriate behavior. The portion of the cerebral cortex that is most involved in inhibiting socially inappropriate behavior is the:

A. Parietal association cortex

B. Cingulate cortex

C. Parahippocampal gyrus

D. Prefrontal cortex

E. Angular gyrus

25. You are asked to evaluate a right-handed patient with some vision disturbance that is characterized by an inability to read. As part of your examination, you determine that she is able to write, to speak and to follow commands normally. This can happen with damage to the:

A. Left occipital cortex and splenium of the corpus callosum

B. Left superior parietal cortex and body of the corpus callosum

C. Left frontal cortex and body of the corpus callosum

D. Wernicke's area and the angular gyrus

E. Wernicke's area and the superior longitudinal fasciculus

26. The hair cells of the semicircular canals have a specific arrangement. Due to this arrangement, which of the following is correct for hair cells of ampulla of the horizontal semicircular duct during a turning of the head to the left?

A. All of the hair cells on both sides of the body will be depolarized

B. The hair cells in the ampulla on one side will be depolarized whereas those on the other side will be hyperpolarized

C. Hair cells will remain depolarized at the same level during entire motion and the vestibular nerve will have the same frequency of action potentials throughout the movement

D. Hair cells have a resting membrane potential of +90 mV that increases to +100 mV with any movement

E. Hair cells on one side will be depolarized as the stereocilia are deflected towards the kinocilium, whereas on the other side, a deflection of stereocilia towards the kinocilium will result in hyperpolarization

27. You are asked to evaluate a 57-year-old woman with some visual difficulty. On examination you identify a loss of vision in the upper left quadrant of the visual field in both eyes (left homonomous superior quadrantanopia). Which of the following lesions could produce this symptom?

A. Lesion of the optic tract in the left-hand side of the brain

B. Lesion just above the calcarine sulcus of the primary visual cortex in the right occipital lobe

C. Lesion just below the calcarine sulcus of the primary visual cortex in the left occipital lobe

D. Lesion of the fibers in Meyer's loop in the right temporal lobe

E. A pituitary tumor that compresses the optic chiasm

28. You are called to the ED to see a patient in status epilepticus. As an initial measure you want to use a benzodiazepine. You know that this drug potentiates the action of gamma-aminobutyric acid (GABA), which increases chloride conductance, resulting in inhibition. This occurs through:

A. Activation of $GABA_A$ receptors

B. Activation of $GABA_B$ receptors

C. Activation of second messenger-mediated ion channels

D. Inhibition of NMDA receptors

E. Allosteric modulation of voltage-gated chloride channels

29. The amygdala is an almond-shaped nucleus located in the region of the uncus of the temporal lobe that is frequently involved in seizures affecting the medial portion of the temporal lobe. Which of the following is NOT true regarding the amygdala?

A. It is a site of generation of integrated autonomic, endocrine and behavioral response

B. Destruction of this nucleus results in exaggerated autonomic responses

C. It receives input from the olfactory system

D. It has connections with the piriform part of the cerebral cortex over the uncus

E. It has extensive connections with the hypothalamus

30. The thalamus (dorsal thalamus) consists of many subnuclei subserving different functions. Injury to the ventrolateral (VL) nucleus of the thalamus would likely result in which of the following?

A. Distortion of cognitive activity

B. Contralateral anesthesia

C. Ataxia—motor incoordination

D. Sham rage

E. Personality deterioration

Answers

1. E.

There are several flexures that develop at the rostral end of the embryo. Most of these flexures fold the neural tube ventrally. The cervical flexure is a ventral bend between the cervical cord and rhombencephalon (the developing caudal brain stem). The cephalic flexure is another one of the primary bends, and it is a ventral flexure at the level of the midbrain, separating the rhombencephalon from the prosencephalon. The pontine flexure is a secondary bend that is dorsally directed and which separates the rhombencephalon into the mylencephalon and metencephalon (the developing medulla and pons).

2. C.

The sodium potassium ATPase pump is necessary to establish a concentration gradient of ions between the inside and outside of cells. This concentration gradient is the primary generator of the resting membrane potential. Blocking this pump will initially have no effect on neural function, since only a few ions need to move in order to conduct impulses or release transmitter. However, after a prolonged period, the ion gradient will run down and function will cease.

3. D.

The spinal nucleus of the trigeminal is located in the dorsolateral part of the brain stem and it extends down into the cervical spinal cord. This nucleus receives general somatic afferent information predominantly from the trigeminal nerve, but also from other cranial nerves and even upper cervical nerve roots. The spinal tract of the trigeminal nerve consists of primary sensory fibers of the trigeminal. This tract consists of the small diameter fibers of the trigeminal nerve as they descend the ipsilateral side of the brainstem to reach the more caudal levels of the nucleus. The spinal nucleus of the trigeminal is the terminal nucleus for pain and temperature sensory nerve fibers, and it has the characteristics of the substantia gelatinosa in the spinal cord. This includes various modulatory mechanisms for pain transmission. It does not receive other types of trigeminal sensory information, such as well-localized touch, pressure or vibration sense. Information is transmitted to the thalamus through the ventral trigeminothalamic tract.

4. C.

The lateral corticospinal tract is the principal tract controlling skilled movements of the distal extremity. It does not affect axial movements. This tract begins in the primary motor and primary sensory cortices and descends through a restricted portion of the posterior limb internal capsule, the cerebral peduncle, and medullary pyramids until its decussation at the caudal-most end of the medulla. After decussating, it descends in the lateral funiculus and it is mainly involved in controlling distal axial muscles.

5. E.

The auditory association area is adjacent to the primary auditory cortex on the superior-most portion of the lateral temporal lobe. The primary auditory cortex extends into the lateral fissure as the transverse gyri (of Heshel). Cortical association areas are typically adjacent to the primary sensory cortices. The association areas are substantially larger than the primary sensory cortices. Wernicke's area is a portion of the auditory association cortex in the dominant hemisphere and Broca's area is on the inferior frontal lobe immediately anterior and inferior to the primary motor cortex.

6. C.

The basal ganglia consist of several interconnected areas in the forebrain along with certain functionally related brain stem nuclei. The primary components of the system include the striatum (caudate and putamen), the globus pallidus, the subthalamic nucleus, the substantia nigra and associated thalamic regions. These thalamic regions include the ventral anterior nucleus and the rostral part of the ventral lateral nucleus. Several portions of the system include spontaneously active neurons, most notably the globus pallidus. Parkinson disease, which results from degeneration of the substantia nigra, produces symptoms by loss of dopamine modulation of striatal neuronal activity.

7. A.

The ventral posterolateral nucleus (VPL) of the thalamus is a somatosensory nucleus associated with relaying somatosensory information from the body. The nucleus gracilis is a somatosensory nucleus in the dorsal column pathway for transmission of touch, pressure and joint position sense from the lower extremity. Therefore, this nucleus will send fibers to the VPL. The spinal nucleus of the trigeminal, which is a somatosensory nucleus for the head, relays to the cortex through the ventral posteromedial nucleus. The other nuclei listed are more involved in motor systems. The substantia nigra connects with the basal ganglia and the inferior olivary and pontine nuclei connect to the cerebellum.

8. C.

The superior cerebellar peduncle is comprised of axons arising from neurons in deep cerebellar nuclei (specifically, the dentate and interposed nuclei). These axons traverse the superior cerebellar peduncle in their course toward termination in the red nucleus and ventral lateral nucleus of the thalamus. These fibers decussate in the midbrain and are generally involved in cerebellar feedback, controlling and regulating movement. With regard to other potential responses, axons from Purkinje cells do not leave the cerebellum (with the modest exception of those going to the vestibular nuclei). The cerebral peduncle is a structure located in the ventral midbrain that contains cortical efferent fibers.

9. A.

Cerebellar climbing fibers only arise from the inferior olivary nucleus. Inputs to the cerebellar cortex from all other sources terminate as mossy fibers. That would include spinal cord inputs as well as inputs from various precerebellar nuclei as well as the prominent pontine nuclei (that relay cortical information to the cerebellum).

10. B.

Spinal reflexes consist of muscle stretch (myotatic) reflex, the inverse myotatic (clasp-knife) reflex, as well as withdrawal reflexes. Of these three spinal reflexes, the muscle stretch reflex is a monosynaptic reflex elicited by muscle stretch. Large, fast-conducting sensory fibers from the muscle spindle terminate directly on alpha motor neurons that return to the muscle, resulting in contraction. Therefore, this is the fastest of all the reflexes since it utilizes the fastest sensory and motor fibers and since it only has one synapse. The other reflexes are polysynaptic and use somewhat slower afferent nerve fibers.

11. D.

Alpha and gamma motor neurons have many similarities and some important differences. They are both located in the ventral horn of the spinal cord, and have myelinated axons that extend out in peripheral nerves. Gamma motor neurons are significantly smaller, however, and conduct more slowly. They also innervate intrafusal muscle fibers of the muscle spindle, which do not actually result in any visible muscle contraction of the extrafusal muscle fibers, but rather regulate muscle spindle sensitivity. Muscle stretch afferent fibers from the muscle spindle can activate both alpha and gamma motor neurons.

12. D.

The process of sound transduction involves hair cells of the inner ear. These cells do not generate action potentials, though they release neurotransmitter when depolarized. The other responses are wrong. There is an electrochemical gradient (membrane potential) that is very important both with the perilymph as well as the endolymph. This is critical to normal ion movement when ion channels are opened. High-frequency sound causes a greater displacement of the basilar membrane at the cochlear BASE and the frequency of a sound wave is not transmitted directly to frequency of firing of auditory afferent nerve fibers, but rather is related to the specific location of greatest movement of the basilar membrane. Efferent projections from the central nervous system end predominantly on outer hair cells and can "fine tune" the inner ear.

13. C.

Convection currents in the endolymph of the inner ear are capable of activating hair cells. Slow movement of the eyes will occur in the direction opposite to perceived motion. In the awake individual, rapid corrective eye movement will occur in the opposite direction (jerk nystagmus). With the patient lying on her back, the infusion of warm solutions into the ear canal will warm fluid in the lateral aspect of the lateral semicircular canal. This will cause the endolymph in the lateral part of the canal to rise and the patient will perceive that they are spinning towards the warm ear. There will be relatively slow drift of the eyes away from that ear, with rapid corrective jerks toward the side of fluid introduction. Damage to the eighth cranial nerve or inner ear will limit or completely prevent this eye movement.

14. D.

The parasympathetic nervous system has occasionally been called the "craniosacral outflow" because parasympathetic preganglionic neurons have origins in the brainstem and sacral spinal cord. Sympathetic preganglionic neurons are only located in the thoracic and upper lumbar spinal cord. The synapse between preganglionic and postganglionic neurons take place in autonomic ganglia and use acetylcholine both in sympathetic and parasympathetic ganglia. Postganglionic neurons in the parasympathetic nervous system typically release acetylcholine, which can have several effects depending on the specific type of receptor upon which this acts. Usually, parasympathetic nerves have rather short postganglionic courses and the ganglia are generally located very close to or within the wall of the innervated organ. This is somewhat different from the sympathetic nervous system, where postganglionic axons can be quite long and highly branched. Therefore there is quite a bit of divergence in these fibers resulting in more widespread sympathetic responses.

15. C.

Extracellular fluid of the brain and cerebrospinal fluid are quite similar since there is no barrier between them. Both of these fluids have very low protein levels, and the specific ion concentration within ECF of the brain and the CSF is tightly regulated by the blood-brain barrier and blood cerebrospinal fluid barrier. Both of these barriers can be crossed easily by gases such as carbon dioxide and oxygen, though many things are excluded and many nutrients are actively transported. These barriers also protect the brain from rapid changes in ion concentrations in the peripheral blood.

16. C.

The arterial branches to the basal ganglia are damaged by systemic hypertension and diabetes mellitus. Hemorrhages into the area of the putamen typically result from rupture of branches of the lenticulostriate arteries. These arteries are branches of the proximal middle cerebral artery that traverse the anterior perforated substance. The distal anterior cerebral artery supplies portions of the cerebral cortex superficially, while the posterior cerebral artery supplies the occipital lobe, and much of the medial temporal lobes. The anterior choroidal artery follows the optic tract and often supplies part of the thalamus, but does not supply basal ganglia. The basilar artery gives rise to most of the perforating branches that traverse the posterior perforated substance to supply much of the midbrain and caudal diencephalon. However, these branches do not reach the basal ganglia.

17. A.

Most somatic sensory pathways to the cerebral cortex follow three neuron pathways. The third neuron in the pathway is a thalamocortical projection neuron, and therefore the second order neuron must terminate in the thalamus. Since somatic sensation relays in the ventral posterolateral nucleus of the thalamus, that is the correct answer in this case. The cuneate nucleus would be the origin of the second order fiber (or the termination of the first) relaying the sensation, while the substantially gelatinosa of the spinal cord is the termination of the first order fiber transmitting pain and temperature sense from the body.

18. D.

The flocculonodular lobe of the cerebellum is extremely important for vestibular function. This part of the cerebellum receives primary vestibular afferent nerve fibers and is interconnected with vestibular nuclei. Damage to the flocculonodular lobe results in vestibular symptoms and will also limit the ability to recover from vestibular damage.

19. C.

The neostriatum (caudate and putamen) is one of the principal components of the basal ganglia. Excitatory input arises from the cerebral cortex, while inhibitory output neurons project to the globus pallidus and the subthalamic nucleus depending on whether these neurons are part of the "direct" or "indirect" pathway through the basal ganglia, respectively. Modulatory, dopaminergic input to the striatum arises from the substantia nigra, pars compacta. The anterior limb of the internal capsule separates the two components of the neostratum, the caudate and putamen, from one another. These nuclei do not connect directly to the thalamus, as suggested by choice "C", but instead connect to the globus pallidus, which in turn connects to the ventral anterior and part of the ventral lateral nucleus of the thalamus via the ansa lenticularis and the lenticular fasciculus.

20. B.

The paramedian pontine reticular formation (PPRF) is also known as the para-abducens nucleus or the pontine lateral gaze center. This region receives input from the contralateral frontal eye fields and connects to the adjacent abducens nucleus. Therefore, activation of the left PPRF will result in leftward eye deviation. The left abducens nucleus connects to the right ocular motor nucleus through fibers traversing the medial longitudinal fasciculus (MLF) to activate the right medial rectus muscle. While the PPRF is a critical location for controlling lateral gaze (including that induced by the vestibulo-ocular reflex), it is not necessary for upgaze, the centers for which are in the rostral midbrain and caudal diencephalon.

21. D.

Each layer of the cerebral cortex subserves a different function. Layer V of the cerebral cortex contains large pyramidal neurons that project through the corticospinal tract. The granular layer, layer IV, receives thalamic input, while the supragranular layers, layers II and III, are the primary layers receiving and giving rise to (respectively) cortical interconnections. Layer VI gives rise to many projections to the thalamus that are important regulators of thalamic function.

22. C.

The arcuate nuclei, located in the region of the median eminence of the infundibulum of the hypothalamus, are a primary site of release of the several compounds that regulate the release of hormones by the anterior pituitary gland. This region does not have a blood-brain barrier in order to allow these compounds to reach the hypothalamo-hypophyseal portal system. Other hypothalamic regions subserve different functions. For example, the suprachiasmatic nucleus is associated with circadian rhythms, the mammary body is associated with limbic circuitry, the supraoptic nuclei are associated with the posterior pituitary gland, and the preoptic area is associated with sexual differentiation and some elements of behavior. The latter is a sexually dimorphic nucleus.

23. B.

This region has strong interconnections with other regions of association cortex in the brain. The hippocampus has a prominent connection with the hypothalamus and septal area through the fornix. However, this is not as functionally important.

24. D.

The prefrontal cortex is the region most associated with regulation of socially inappropriate behaviors. The other areas that are listed do not have this as a major function. For example, the parietal association cortex is most involved in integrating and interpreting sensory inputs, and distributing attention appropriately. The cingulated cortex appears to have its strongest effects over emotional experiences, while the parahippocampal gyrus is most associated with short-term memory and other hippocampal functions. The angular gyrus includes part of Wernicke's area in the dominant hemisphere, and is part of the auditory association cortex.

25. A.

Alexia without agraphia is an unusual syndrome in which patients are able to write despite their inability to read. This typically occurs with damage to the dominant visual cortex such that there is a homonymous vision loss on the dominant side of the body. This also must include damage to the posterior part of the corpus callosum (splenium) in order to prevent visual information from the non-dominant hemisphere from being transferred to Wernicke's area where interpretation of written (as well as spoken) language takes place. This syndrome that is described cannot be due to direct damage to Wernicke's area, since that will also affect the ability to comprehend spoken language (a receptive aphasia). Damage to Wernicke's area would also affect the ability to write a complex phrase that was dictated to the patient.

26. B.

The horizontal semicircular canals function in concert when the head is rotated. The hair cells in the semicircular canal on one side of the head will be depolarized, resulting in increased release of neurotransmitter, while on the other side they will be hyperpolarized, with a decrease in transmitter release. This will result in increased frequency of action potentials in one vestibulocochlear nerve, and a decrease on the other side. The hair cells are all polarized by the specific orientation of placement of the kinocilium. Deflection of stereocilia towards the kinocilium will result in depolarization, and deflection away will result in hyperpolarization of the hair cell.

27. D.

A superior quadrantic visual field defect is a classic manifestation of damage in Meyer's loop. This loop consists of fibers in the inferior part of the optic radiations from the lateral geniculate to the visual cortex. These fibers, which "loop" laterally into the temporal lobe, convey visual signals arising from the contralateral upper visual world. These fibers will terminate in the lower bank of the calcarine sulcus. The fact that the visual field deficit was on the left side indicates a right-sided lesion. This makes response "C" wrong. A lesion in the right occipital lobe, just below the calcarine sulcus, while unusual, could produce a similar picture. Lesions of the optic chiasm affect temporal vision in both eyes, while optic tract lesions (even if they were on the correct side) would not produce such specific symptoms.

28. A.

Gamma aminobutyric acid acts at several receptors in the nervous system. The most clinically important of these is the $GABA_A$ receptor, which is a chloride channel that can be allosterically modulated by many drugs, chemicals and toxins. This is the primary site of action of benzodiazepines, for example. These channels are ligand-gated and are not responsive to voltage change. GABAS, acting at these receptors, is the most important inhibitory receptor system in the adult nervous system.

29. B.

The amygdala is an important nucleus involved in integrating stress responses. Bilateral damage to this nucleus has been described as part of the Kluver-Bucy syndrome, which blunts autonomic responses to stressors. Stimulation of the nucleus may result in rage-type reactions. Seizures affecting this nucleus often result in unpleasant odors, and the amygdala is a site of primary olfactory termination. The amygdala is connected directly with the hypothalamus by two pathways, and is important in producing integrated responses to stress.

30. C.

The ventral lateral nucleus of the thalamus is part of the feedback system from the cerebellum to the cerebral cortex, though it also receives some basal gangliar import. The primary effects of damage to this nucleus would include difficulties with movement, with contralateral ataxia being a prominent feature.

Chapter 5: Practical Neurochemistry

Russell H. Swerdlow, MD

Contents

Energy Metabolism and Energy Metabolism Diseases

Overview

You learned a number of biochemical pathways relevant to energy production in the first year of medical school and then (most likely) promptly and gratefully forgot about them. While at this point it is not critical to memorize pathway details, it is nevertheless worthwhile to recognize the overall scheme and how pathways relate to each other. Moreover, particular pathways or parts of them occur within defined compartments (for example, within the mitochondria or cytoplasm). Figure 1 provides an overview of pathway links and compartmentalization.

Energy is ultimately produced via catabolism of carbohydrates, fatty acids, and (if necessary) amino acids. Breakdown products in each case converge on acetyl CoA, in which the acetyl group flows into the Krebs cycle. The Krebs cycle occurs within mitochondria. Primary Krebs cycle disorders (such as fumarase deficiency) are rare, conceivably because it is the nexus of several different catabolic pathways. Other factors, though, may lead to acquired Krebs cycle dysfunction. For instance, one of the key regulatory Krebs cycle enzymes is the thiamine-dependent α ketoglutarate dehydrogenase complex (KDHC). Thiamine deficiency can impair KDHC, as can valproic acid.

Carbon movement through the Krebs cycle generates NADH and $FADH_2$, which can then provide reducing equivalents (electrons) for the electron transport chain (ETC). The ETC resides on the mitochondrial inner membrane and consists of four enzyme complexes. The full name of complex I is NADH:ubiquinone oxidoreductase, as it accepts electrons from NADH and transfers them to coenzyme Q_{10} (ubiquinone). Complex II is also the succinate dehydrogenase of the Krebs cycle, and is alternatively called succinate:ubiquinone oxidoreductase. It passes electrons from $FADH_2$ to ubiquinone. In either case, ubiquinone carries its acquired electrons to complex III, which hands them off to cytochrome c. Complex III is thus called

Figure 1

Overview of Energy Production

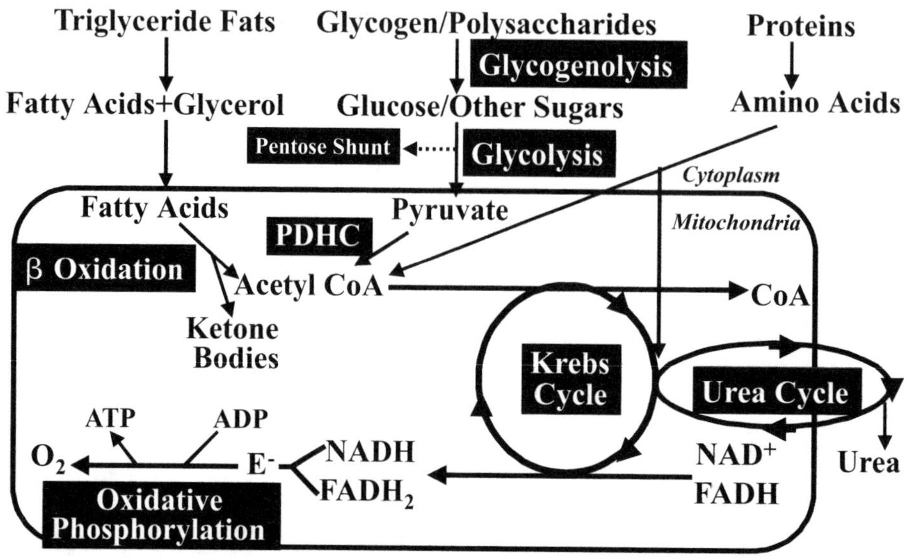

Figure 2

The mitochondrion

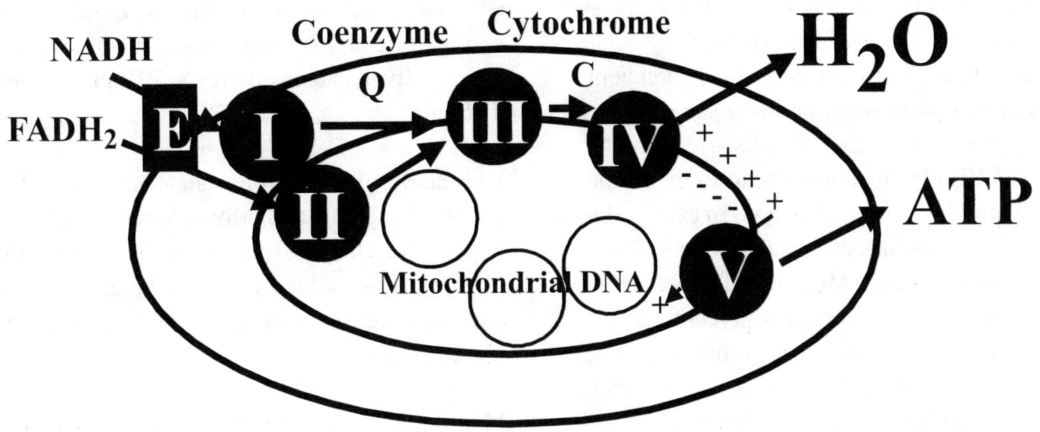

cytochrome c reductase. Complex IV, also called cytochrome c oxidase, takes the electrons from cytochrome c and transfers them to molecular oxygen (O_2), forming H_2O. This "aerobic" metabolism is the primary site of body oxygen consumption. The brain accounts for about 20% of the body's total O_2 consumption.

The ETC apparatus passes electrons from high to low energy states, and this expended energy is used to pump protons across the inner mitochondrial membrane, from the mitochondrial matrix to the intermembrane space. In this way, the original electron energy is used to generate a proton gradient, with the intermembrane space becoming positively charged and the matrix side of the inner membrane becoming negatively charged. Naturally, the exuded protons want to reaccess the matrix according to the electrochemical gradient, but the nonporous inner membrane won't permit this. A fifth enzyme complex found in the inner membrane, complex V, does permit protons to reenter the matrix, and has evolved to harvest energy from this proton flux to phosphorylate ADP into ATP. Complex V is also called ATP synthase. Together, these five enzyme complexes enable the process of oxidative phosphorylation, which is depicted in Figure 2.

All but complex II of the five oxidative phosphorylation enzyme complexes are partly encoded by mitochondrial genes and partly by nuclear genes (complex II is solely nuclear encoded). Some diseases are either caused by or associated with defects of these enzymes. Mitochondrial encephalopathy, lactic acidosis, and stroke-like symptoms (MELAS), Leber hereditary optic neuropathy, Alper disease, and Parkinson disease are some disorders in which complex I dysfunction occurs. Complex III dysfunction is seen in some mitochondrial myopathies. Complex IV defects are noted in MELAS, myoclonic epilepsy with ragged red fibers (MERRF), Kearns-Sayre syndrome, Alper disease, Menke kinky hair disease, Leigh disease, and Alzheimer disease. Leigh disease and the neuropathy, ataxia, retinitis pigmentosa syndrome (NARP) are associated with mutations in a mitochondrial DNA gene that encodes a complex V subunit. Oxidative phosphorylation enzyme inhibitors include MPTP, rotenone, haloperidol (complex I); malonate (complex II); antimycin A (complex III); cyanide, sodium azide, carbon monoxide (complex IV); and oligomycin (complex V).

Carbohydrates

Glycolysis occurs in the cytoplasm, although largely in cytoplasm adjacent to mitochondria. Indeed, hexokinase, the first enzyme of the pathway, often functions tethered to mitochondria. Deficiencies of particular glycolytic enzymes are associated with myopathies. Tarui disease is due to deficient activity of phosphofructokinase, the second enzyme of the glycolytic pathway. Tarui disease is also called type VII glycogenosis, because despite the fact it is a problem of the glycolysis, it causes abnormal muscle glycogen accumulation. Clinically, Tarui disease resembles McCardle disease. Phosphoglycerate kinase and phosphoglyceromutase deficiences are also rarely seen glycolysis disorders. Under conditions of aerobic metabolism, the end product of glycolysis is pyruvate. When anaerobic metabolism is required, lactate dehydrogenase (LDH) can reduce pyruvate to form lactate. LDH deficiency diseases exist. Of note, mannose is the only sugar other than glucose that crosses the blood-brain barrier, and it can also feed into energy metabolism.

Pyruvate is then transported into the mitochondrial matrix, where pyruvate dehydrogenase complex (PDHC) converts it to acetyl CoA, which then enters the Krebs cycle. PDHC is thiamine dependent, and thiamine deficiency will cause secondary PDHC deficiency. One of its components is coded for on the X chromosome, and mutation of this component (E1) causes X-linked Leigh disease (25% of Leigh disease), as well as an X-linked intermittent ataxia. In general, PDHC deficiency will cause myopathy and lactic acidosis.

Liver and muscle are capable of storing glucose as glycogen. This process is called glycogenesis. Glycogen consists of glucose chains (connected by 1,4 linkages) that intermittently form branches that arise from α 1,6 linkages. Glycogenolysis refers to the process via which glucose molecules are retrieved from glycogen. A number of glycogenolysis biochemical defects (in conjunction with other disorders with abnormal glycogen storage) comprise the glycogenosis disorders, or the glycogenoses.

When glucose is needed, glycogen phosphorylase (called myophosphorylase in muscle) starts breaking α 1,4 linkages to yield glucose 1-phosphate. Enzymatic failure at this point in muscle yields McCardle disease (glycogenosis type V). An enzyme called phosphorylase B kinase is needed to activate a glycogen phosphorylase initiation pathway; failure of this kinase has been observed to occur in liver, causing the Type VIII glycogenosis disorder.

Ultimately, glucose 1-phosphate is converted to glucose 6-phosphate, and prior to leaving the liver is dephosphorylated to glucose by the enzyme glucose 6-phosphatase. Glucose 6-phosphatase deficiency clinically is called von Gierke disease, or Type Ia glycogenosis.

Myophosphorylase will not work within 4 glucose residues of an α 1,6 branch. Degradation of glycogen near branches requires a set of debranching enzymes. Debranching enzyme deficiency is called Cori disease (glycogenosis type III). Lysosomes contain a special enzyme called acid maltase, which can break α 1,4 linkages to directly yield glucose (instead of stopping at glucose 1phosphate). Deficiency of this lysosomal enzyme causes Pompe disease (type II glycogenosis).

Lipids

Fatty acid catabolism occurs inside mitochondria. The enzyme carnitine palmitoyl transferase (CPT) is needed to transport fatty acids across mitochondrial membranes. CPT deficiency diseases can occur as a consequence of either dysfunction of CPT I, which transfers the fatty acid acyl group across the mitochondrial outer membrane as a carnitine ester; or of CPT II, which transfers the acyl group across the mitochondrial inner membrane before handing it over to a CoA moiety in the mitochondrial matrix.

Next, in the process of β oxidation, acetyl groups are successively removed from the parent acyl CoA, and conjugated to another CoA to form acetyl CoA. Acetyl CoA molecules generated in this way can enter the Krebs cycle. Depending on the length of the acyl CoA at a given point, β oxidation is performed by either long, medium, or short chain acyl CoA dehydrogenases. The most common clinical disease to arise at this step relates to failure of the medium chain acyl CoA dehydrogenase (MCAD

Figure 3

Fatty acid beta oxidation

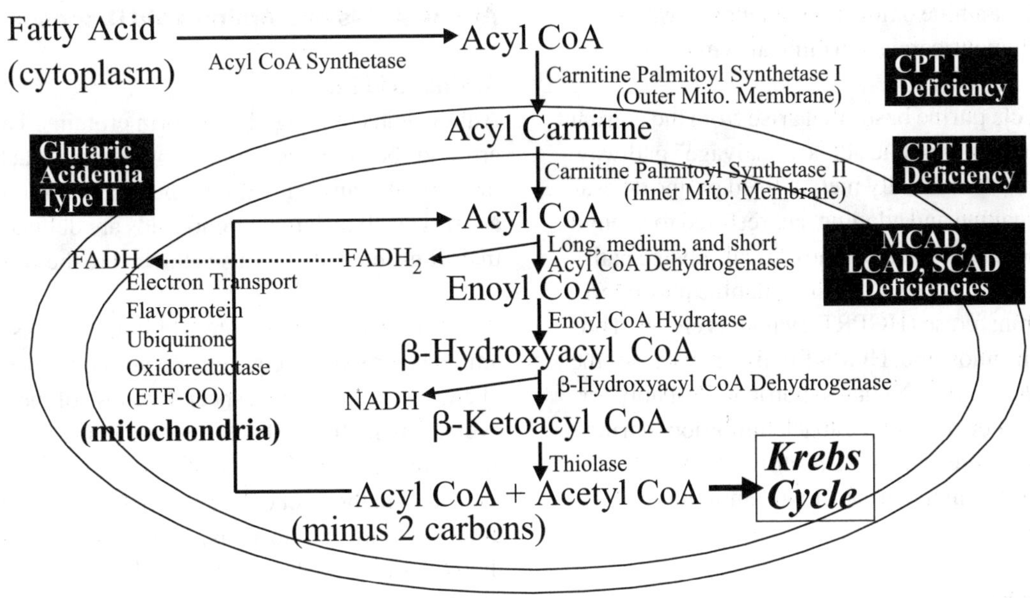

deficiency). Long chain acyl CoA dehydrogenase (LCAD) and short chain acyl CoA dehydrogenase (SCAD) deficiencies are less common. $FADH_2$ is also generated during β oxidation, and this reducing equivalent can donate electrons to the ETC by way of the enzyme electron transport flavoprotein:ubiquinone oxidoreductase (ETF-QO). Type II glutaric acidemia arises when ETF-QO is unable to oxidize β-oxidation-generated $FADH_2$.

The liver plays an important role in assuring the brain gets adequate fuel. When insulin levels drop low enough, the liver diverts oxaloacetate (a Krebs cycle intermediate) to gluconeogenesis. The subsequently formed glucose is secreted. A secondary consequence of this is that acetyl CoA produced by liver fatty acid β-oxidation cannot enter the Krebs cycle, because Krebs intermediates have been seized for gluconeogenesis. Two acetyl CoA molecules can alternatively condense to form the ketone bodies acetoacetate and α-hydroxybutyrate. Both species enter the blood, cross the blood brain barrier, and split into two acetyl CoA molecules in the mitochondria. These acetyl CoAs then serve as a brain energy source.

Keep in mind it is low insulin levels rather than low glucose levels that actually turn on liver ketone body production. Limiting glucose intake so insulin drops is the rationale behind ketogenic diets.

Nucleic Acid Metabolism and Nucleic Acid Metabolism Diseases

Purines

The pentose phosphate pathway converts 6 carbon sugars to 5 carbon sugars. These ribose sugars are used to synthesize the purine nucleotides adenylic acid and guanylic acid. A *de novo* purine synthesis pathway requires glutamine, glycine, and aspartate. Folate coenzymes are also required at several steps.

Phosphoribosyl pyrophosphate (PRPP) levels help regulate synthesis rates.

Purines are degraded to uric acid, which is excreted in the urine. Uric acid formation requires the enzyme xanthine oxidase, deficiency of which causes hypouricemia and clinical symptoms.

To recycle purine bases that arise from the constant breakdown of nucleic acids, a "salvage" pathway exists in which mildly metabolized purine derivatives, guanine and adenine, are restored to adenylic acid and guanylic acid. One critical salvage pathway enzyme is hypoxanthine:guanine phosphoribosyl transferase (HGPRT), which is encoded on the X chromosome. HGPRT deficiency causes the sex-linked Lesch-Nyhan syndrome. Probably for reasons of decreased feedback inhibition, purine salvage failure causes the *de novo* pathway to rev up, resulting in hyperuricemia, xanthinuria, and hypoxanthinuria.

Pyrimidines

The pyrimidine bases uridylic acid, thymidylic acid, and cytidylic acid are produced in the cytoplasm by a process that requires ATP, glutamine, aspartate, and PRPP. As with purine synthesis, PRPP levels control pathway activity. The enzyme that initiates pyrimidine synthesis is a cytoplasmic form of carbamoyl phosphate synthetase (CPS II). Orotic acid is an intermediate of pyrimidine synthesis, and failure of the pathway beyond its formation results in a clinical syndrome that is characterized by orotic aciduria. Also, some drugs increase pyrimidine synthesis rates and therefore increase orotic acid levels. As orotic acid is secreted and reabsorbed in the kidney by a saturable transporter, such overproduction can also cause an orotic aciduria. It is worth noting that orotic acid and uric acid both use the same transporter, so orotic aciduria may also cause uric aciduria.

At the biochemical level, xeroderma pigmentosa and Cockayne syndrome involve problems with pyrimidines. These problems result from defects of pyrimidine repair systems. For example, xeroderma pigmentosa results from an inability to repair UV light-induced pyrimidine dimerization.

Pyrimidines are catabolized to alanine and aminoisobutyrate. This generates NH3, which is excreted in the urea cycle (to be discussed later in this chapter).

Amino Acids and Amino Acid Diseases

Amino Acid Basics

Amino acids link together to form proteins. They are acids because they are carboxylated. Attached to the carbon is an amino group (hence, an amino acid). The 20 different amino acids are defined by their R group, which is also attached to the carbon.

Aside from serving as protein building blocks, amino acids exist in equilibrium with intermediates of energy metabolism, especially those of the Krebs cycle. When glucose levels are low many amino acids enter into the Krebs cycle, convert to oxaloacetate, and in the liver enter gluconeogenesis (the gluconeogenic amino acids). Some amino acids, though, are not in direct flux with Krebs cycle intermediates and can only access the Krebs cycle via formation of acetyl CoA. As discussed above, two acetyl CoA molecules can condense under gluconeogenic conditions to form ketone bodies. Such amino acids are called the ketogenic amino acids.

Amino Acid Metabolism and Transport Disorders

As the different amino acids basically represent variants of a common plan, it is not surprising that one amino acid may serve as the building block or precursor of another. Failure of these synthetic pathways result in a number of metabolic diseases:

1. Tyrosine is produced from phenylalanine. When the enzymes that mediate this are dysfunctional, phenylalanine cannot undergo conversion to tyrosine, and it gets diverted to phenylketones. The key enzyme in this conversion, phenylalanine hydroxylase, is biopterin dependent. Biopterin deficiency can also cause phenylketones to appear in urine.

2. Tyrosine is metabolized to fumarate, a Krebs cycle intermediate. Failure of the enzymes that mediate this results in tyrosinemia.

3. Cysteine, a sulfur-containing amino acid, is produced from methionine, the other sulfur-contain-

ing amino acid. In this synthesis, methionine is first converted to S-adenosyl methionine and then to the homocysteine intermediate. The enzyme that catalyzes the next step, conversion of homocysteine to the cysteine precursor, cystathionine, is called cystathionine synthase. Deficiency of cystathionine synthase causes homocysteine accumulation. Homocysteine can convert to homocystine, a related molecule. Homocysteine/homocystine elevation due to cystathionine synthase deficiency is known as Type I Homocystinuria. It is also important to know that the enzyme methionine synthase can reverse-metabolize homocysteine back to methionine. This reaction is cobalamin and folate dependent. Cobalamin and folate deficiencies respectively cause Homocystinuria Types II and III, since this results in homocysteine/homocystine elevation.

4. Serine is produced from glycine via an enzyme called the glycine cleavage system. The glycine cleavage system is localized within mitochondria, and is pyridoxine, folate, and lipoic acid-dependent. Failure of the enzyme causes a "nonketotic hyperglycinemia". Alternatively, this enzyme may lose function when exposed to ketoacids, causing a "ketotic hyperglycinemia". Valproate can also induce hyperglycinemia.

5. Tryptophan is an amino acid that undergoes renal filtration and reabsorption via a specific reuptake transporter. Failure of the tryptophan renal reuptake transporter causes Hartnup aminoaciduria. Tryptophan itself is a ketogenic amino acid that ultimately gets converted to acetoacetate. Failure to metabolize tryptophan per se can cause tryptophanaemia. One intermediary of the tryptophan metabolic pathway is glutaryl CoA. Failure of the enzyme glutaryl CoA dehydrogenase causes type I glutaric acidemia. Improper tryptophan renal reabsorption or metabolism to acetoacetate can reduce nicotinamide synthesis and mimic niacin deficiency.

6. Lysine, along with the other dibasic amino acids arginine and ornithine, is also renally excreted

Figure 4

Tryptophan and lysine disorders

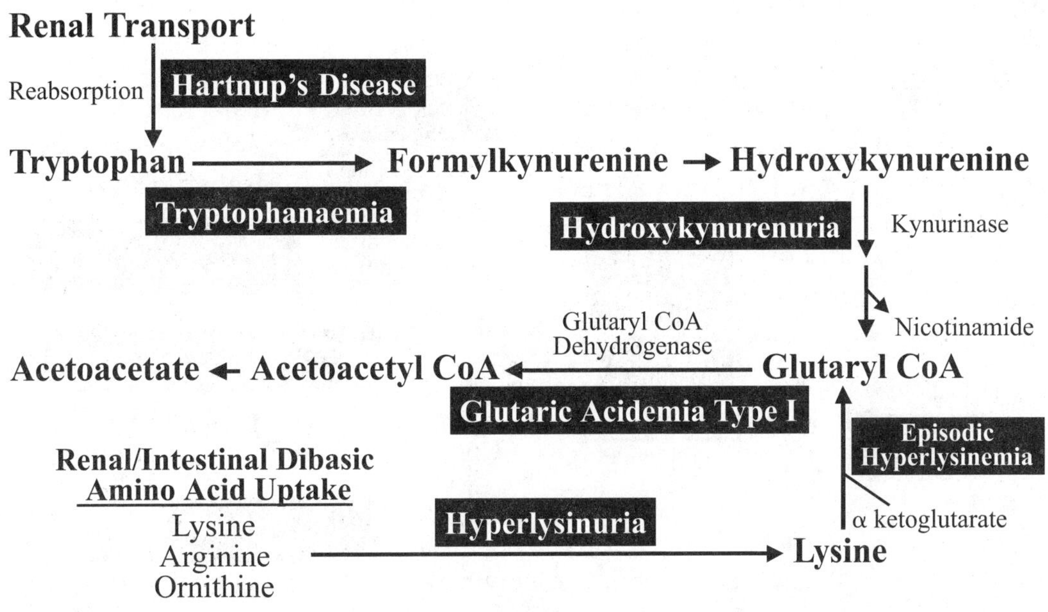

and reabsorbed. Failure to reabsorb causes hyperlysinuria. Like tryptophan, lysine is also a ketogenic amino acid that gets metabolized to acetoacetate. Inability to metabolize lysine per se can cause episodic hyperlysinemia. As is the case with tryptophan, glutaryl CoA is an intermediary metabolite of lysine metabolism, so lysine loading can exacerbate type I glutaric acidemia.

Organic Acids

The branched chain amino acids (leucine, isoleucine, and valine) are deaminated within mitochondria to branched chain ketoacids, which are then converted by branched chain ketoacid dehydrogenase (a thiamine-dependent enzyme) to particular organic acids. Deficiency of this enzyme causes the branched chain ketoaciduria of maple syrup urine disease. Thiamine deficiency can also result in branched chain ketoaciduria. Organic acids (such as isovaleric acid, methylbutyric acid, and isobutyric acid) are further metabolized to a Krebs cycle intermediate, succinyl CoA. A key enzyme in this conversion is proprionyl CoA carboxylase, deficiency of which causes proprionic acidemia. Proprionyl CoA carboxylase is biotin-dependent, and biotin deficiency can cause proprionic acidemia as well. In some cases, biotin deficiency arises from a deficiency of a synthetic enzyme, biotinidase. As many carboxylase enzymes require biotin, this can lead to a state called multiple carboxylase deficiency, of which organic aciduria is a feature.

The final step of organic acid detoxification involves conversion of L-methylmalonyl CoA to succinyl CoA. The enzyme that does this, methylmalonyl CoA, is cobalamin dependent. Cobalamin deficiency causes L-methylmalonyl CoA to accumulate and back-metabolize to methylmalonic acid.

It is believed that organic acids are toxic to mitochondria. Mitochondrial excretion of organic acids across mitochondrial membranes cannot happen spontaneously since they are not lipid soluble. Fortunately, organic acid esterification can occur with carnitine, which can then remove the organic acid moieties as carnitine esters. Over time, this can lead to a secondary carnitine deficiency. As valproate is itself an organic acid, it is partly excreted as a carni-

Figure 5

Organic acids

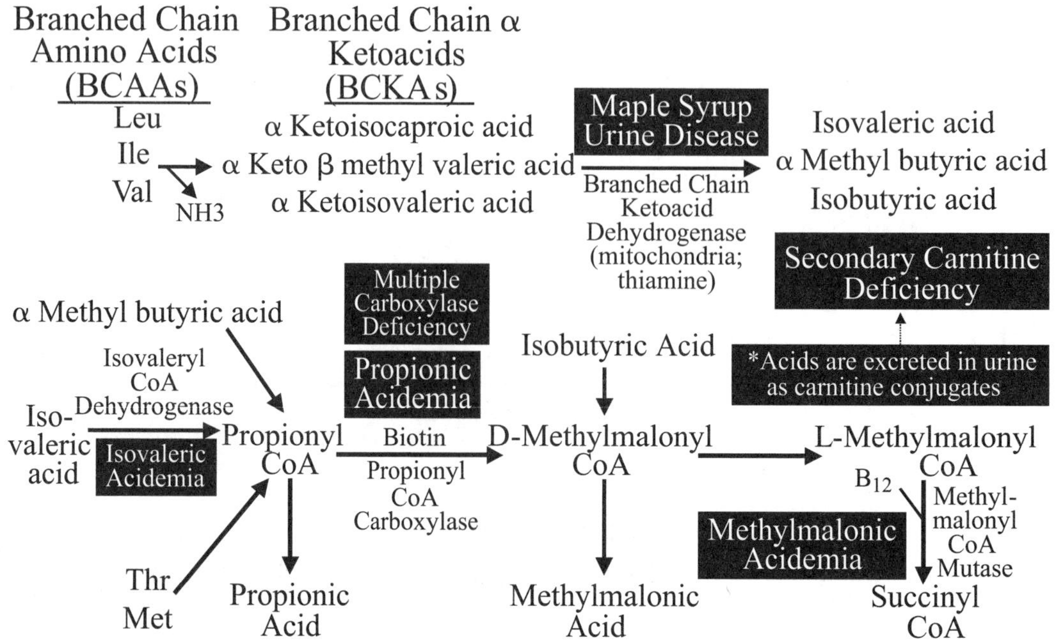

tine ester. Valproate can therefore also cause a secondary carnitine deficiency.

Vitamins and Coenzymes

Vitamins are organic molecules required for certain metabolic functions, and must be supplied in very small amounts (less than 50 mg/day). The water soluble vitamins (B and C) act as coenzymes (nonprotein organic molecules that bind to an enzyme to aid in the transfer of specific functional groups) or coenzyme precursors. Vitamin C is an antioxidant and its deficiency causes scurvy. Deficiencies of various vitamin B derivatives can cause a number of neurologic diseases and symptoms.

The role of certain vitamin coenzymes in a variety of enzymatic reactions was previously discussed. For example, cobalamin (B_{12}) serves in the conversion of homocysteine to methionine by methionine synthase, and in the conversion of methylmalonic acid to succinyl CoA by methylmalonyl CoA mutase. B_{12} deficiency will therefore cause elevations of serum homocysteine and methylmalonic acid. Thiamine (B_1) is used by pyruvate dehydrogenase complex, α ketoglutarate dehydrogenase complex, branched chain ketoacid dehydrogenase, and transketolase (an enzyme of the pentose shunt pathway). Deficiency can cause, among other problems, Wernicke's encephalopathy. Pyridoxine (B_6) mediates decarboxylation reactions. Deficiency can cause neonatal seizures and excess can cause sensory neuronopathy. Biotin is required for various carboxyl group transfers, and its deficiency can cause organic acidosis. Pantothenate and lipoamide participate in acyl group transfers.

The fat soluble vitamins are A, D, E, and K. They don't serve as coenzymes. Vitamins A and E are antioxidants. Vitamin E deficiency is associated with opthalmoplegia and ataxia.

It is important to recognize the role carnitine plays in metabolism. It is necessary for the carnitine palmitoyl transferase-mediated mitochondrial

Figure 6

The urea cycle

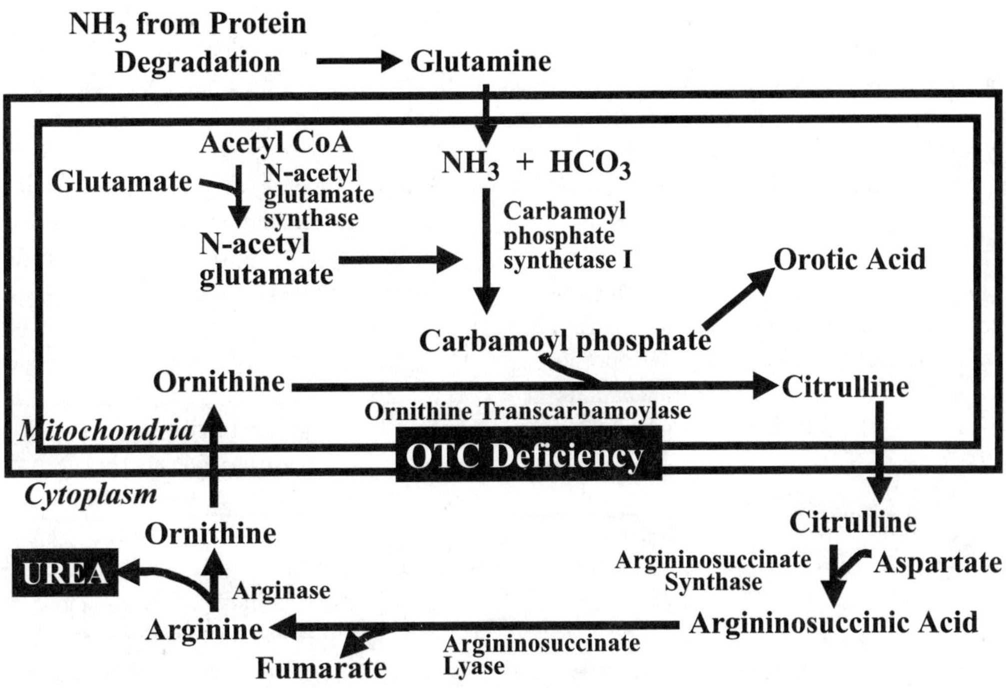

import of fatty acids. It contributes to organic acid detoxification. It lowers mitochondrial acyl CoA levels, which is important given that acyl CoA elevations are likely also toxic to mitochondria. Increased acyl carnitine:free carnitine ratios in urine are associated with Reye-type syndromes.

Special Cases

Urea Cycle

The urea cycle is designed to dispose of NH3, which is largely generated by protein and pyrimidine metabolism. This NH3 is used to generate carbamoyl phosphate in the mitochondria by the mitochondrial form of carbamoyl phosphate synthetase (CPS I). Ornithine transcarbamoylase takes this carbamoyl phosphate and uses it to generate citrulline, which exits the mitochondria for the cytoplasmic portion of the cycle. The cytoplasmic reactions require aspartate and generate fumarate. In the final step, NH3 is removed from the cycle in the form of urea, which is excreted in the urine.

Urea cycle defects cause hyperammonemia. In urea cycle failure, backed up carbamoyl phosphate can be shunted into pyrimidine synthesis, with a resultant orotic acidemia. Deficiency diseases are recognized for virtually all of the urea cycle enzymes. The most common is the X-linked ornithine transcarbamoylase (OTC) deficiency.

Poryphyrin Cycle

Heme is produced from glycine and succinyl CoA via a series of porphyrin intermediates. The pathway begins with the creation within mitochondria of delta amino levulinic acid (ALA). ALA then moves out of the mitochondria, where it goes through a number of enzymatic modifications. The coproporphyrin form returns to the mitochondria where it is eventually converted to heme.

A number of autosomal dominant porphyrin metabolism disorders are recognized (the porphyrias), three of which are associated with neurologic symptoms:

Acute antermittent porphyria is the most common form. It is due to deficiency of the porphobilinogen deaminase complex (usually the uroporphyrin-1 synthetase portion). It manifests as an elevation of urine ALA and porphobilinogen with no increase in stool coproporphyrins.

Hereditary coproporphyria is due to coproporphyrinogen oxidase deficiency. Urine ALA and porphobilinogen are elevated, as are stool and urine coproporphyrins.

Variegate porphyria is seen primarily in South African Caucasians. It is due to protoporphyrinogen oxidase (ferrochelatase) deficiency. Urine ALA, porphobilinogen, and coproporphyrin are elevated, as are stool coproporphyrins and protoporphyrins.

Peroxisomes

Peroxisomes are organelles that contain a large number of metabolic enzymes. A number of different peroxisomal disorders are recognized, and are classified into three groups:

1. Group I disorders are characterized by peroxisomes that are absent or empty. They arise from an inability to transport peroxisomal enzymes into the peroxisome itself. The quintessential group I disorder is Zellweger syndrome.

2. Group II disorders arise from the defect of a single enzyme within the peroxisome. Examples include X-linked adrenoleukodystrophy, Refsum disease of phytanic acid metabolism, and pipecolic acidemia.

3. Group III disorders occur when there are multiple biochemical defects within the peroxisome. The quintessential group III disorder is rhizomelic chondrodysplasia punctata.

As a related aside, peroxisomes can also catabolize fatty acids, including very long chain fatty acids. One particular peroxisomal enzyme (the ATP-binding transport protein, ALDP, also called ABCD1) is encoded on the X-chromosome. ALDP plays a role in the peroxisomal activity of an enzyme called very long chain acyl CoA synthetase. Mutation of ALDP ultimately lead to failure of hexacosanoic acid (C26) very long chain fatty acid metabolism, the characteristic biochemical lesion of X-linked adrenoleukodystrophy.

Figure 7

Poryphyrin pathway

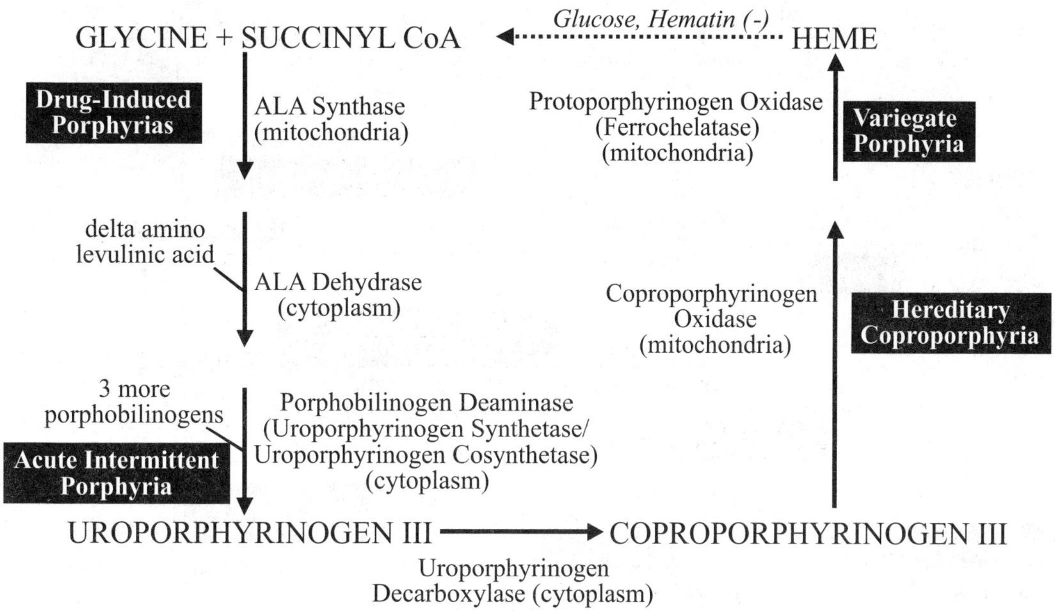

Sphingolipids

The simplest sphingolipid consists of a sphingosine fatty acid linkage (a ceramide sphingolipid). Ceramides can be further linked to a hexose sugar (a cerebroside), sugar chains or modified sugar derivatives (a ganglioside), phosphorylcholine (sphingomyelin), or a sulfated galactose (a sulfatide).

The enzymes that catabolize sphingolipids are housed in lysosomes. Deficiencies of most of these enzymes result in aberrant lysosomal sphingolipid storage, and are recognized clinically as the sphingolipidoses:

1. Hexosaminidase A deficiency: Tay-Sachs

2. Hexosaminidase A+B deficiency: Sandhoff

3. α Galactosidase deficiency: Fabry. Treatment for Fabry disease is now available in the form of recombinant galactosidase beta (agalsidase), which replaces the missing enzyme. This approach is quite expensive, costing about $183,000 per year to treat an adult.

4. Beta glucosidase deficiency: Gaucher

5. Sphingomyelinase deficiency: Niemann-Pick

6. Arylsulfatase A deficiency: metachromatic leukodystrophy

7. Galactosyl ceramide β galactosidase deficiency: Krabbe globoid cell leukodystrophy. Umbilical cord blood cell grafts from unrelated donors may offer a potential therapy for this disorder.

8. Ceramidase: Farber

Mucopolysaccharides

Mucopolysaccharides (glycosaminoglycans) consist of proteins conjugated to repeating sulfated disaccharide units. Four main sulfated disaccharide units exist. They are dermatan sulfate, heparan sulfate, keratan sulfate, and chondroitin sulfate. Enzymes that perform mucopolysaccharide catabolism are lysosomally stored.

Figure 8

The sphingolipidoses

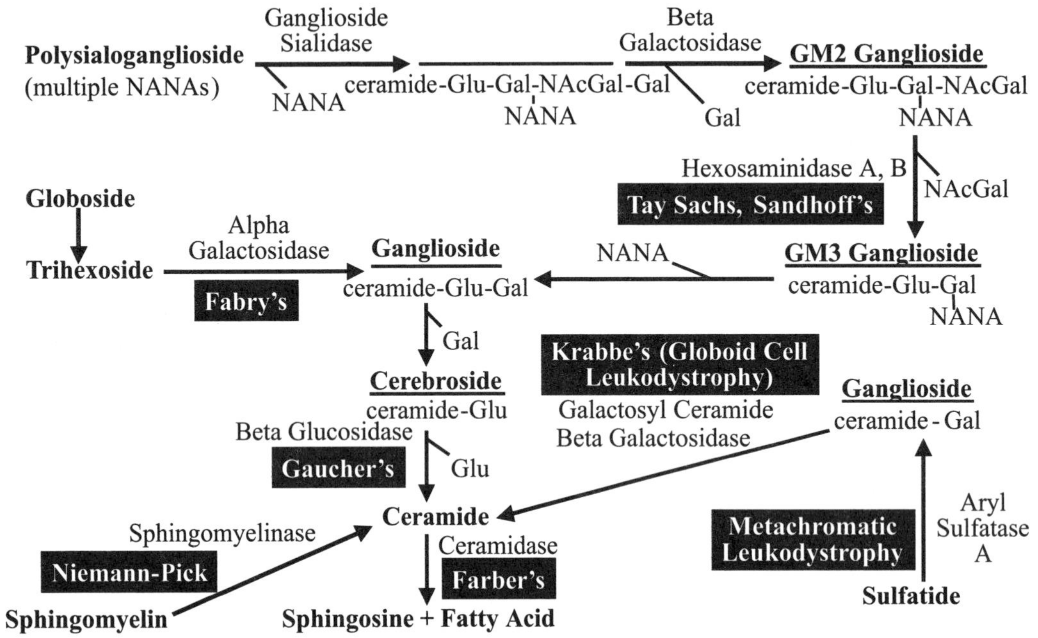

First, sulfated disaccharide repeats are removed from the mucopolysaccharide so that they can undergo degradation to monosaccharides. Abnormalities of specific lysosomal enzymes that degrade these sulfated sugars cause the mucopolysaccharidoses family of lysosomal storage diseases. Buildup of a particular polysaccharide is associated with its increased urinary excretion. These diseases are defined by which type of saccharide chain cannot be metabolized, and are diagnosable by urinalysis:

1. Dermatan and heparan sulfate:
   Hurler (Type I-H)
   Scheie (Type I-S)
   Hurler-Scheie (Type I-H/S)
   Hunter (Type II)
   Sly (Type VII).
   Treatment is available for Type I (Hurler types) who are α-L-iduronidase deficient; replacement with recombinant enzyme costs approximately $176,000 per year.

2. Heparan sulfate only: Sanfilippo A, B, C, D (Type III).

3. Dermatan sulfate only: Maroteaux-Lamy (Type VI).

4. Keratan sulfate (+ heparan sulfate): Morquio A, B (Type IV).

Cholesterol

Systemically produced cholesterol does not appear to easily enter the brain. The brain therefore synthesizes its own cholesterol. Cholesterol plays an important role in lipid membrane formation, and also serves as an antioxidant. Brain cholesterol is metabolized to the 24 hydroxycholesterol metabolite, which is transported across the blood-brain barrier into the blood. It is carried to the liver where it is further metabolized. Most plasma 24 hydroxycholesterol is brain-derived.

Abetalipoproteinemia (Bassen-Kornzweig) is an autosomal recessive disorder caused by impaired gastrointestinal fat absorption. Lipoproteins, which consist of fat conjugated to protein, therefore cannot be made. Without lipoproteins, cholesterol transport is impaired. Bassen-Kornzweig presents biochemically with a combination of low cholesterol, low triglycerides, and low vitamin E.

Cholesterol is also used to synthesize the bile acid chenodeoxycholic acid. Rarely, a defect of the enzyme sterol 27 hydroxylase precludes this synthesis, with accumulation of an intermediate metabolite, cholestanol. Cholestanol accumulation is the key biochemical feature of a lipid storage disease, cerebrotendinous xanthomatosis.

Cholesterol is delivered to individual cells as cholesterol esters. Cholesterol esters are in turn internalized by lysosomes, where the lysosomal enzyme acid lipase (cholesterol ester hydrolase) deesterifies the cholesterol. Failure of this enzymatic de-esterification leads to abnormal cell accumulation of unesterified cholesterol. Clinical variants of this biochemical defect include Wolman disease and cholesterol ester storage disease.

2. Membrane Potentials and Ion Channels

Overview

Cells are demarcated by their plasma membranes. These lipid bilayers are impermeable to charged ions. The only way ions can pass between the cell intracellular space (cytoplasm) and the extracellular space is via ion channels (ionophores). Ion channels can exist in open or shut states. This open or closed state is determined either by ligand binding to an associated receptor, or by the local membrane potential (voltage gating). Specific ion channels permit passage of Na^+, K^+, Cl^-, or Ca^{++}.

Na^+ channels are impermeable when the cell is at rest. Therefore, Na^+ cannot enter the cell easily, and its concentration is substantially higher in the extracellular space. This renders the outside of the plasma membrane positive and the inside negative. Several types of K^+ channels exist. One type is the "leak channel", which lets K^+ into the cytoplasm. Because the cytoplasm is negatively charged, K^+ concentrates within the cell. Cl^- channels are relatively permeable at rest, but the positive charge outside the cell keeps Cl^- levels relatively high in the extracellular space. The overall balance of these ions on either side of the membrane defines the membrane potential (usually around -70 μV), and is mathematically predictable by the Nernst Equation, or its practical derivative, the Goldman-Hodgkin-Katz equation.

Mutations of ion channel genes are clinically relevant and constitute a category of disease called channelopathies. Cl^- channel mutations cause myotonia congenita, and Na^+ channel mutations can cause both hyperkalemic periodic paralysis and paramyotonia congenita (of von Eulenberg).

Na^+ nevertheless does trickle across the membrane. To prevent this from causing dissipation of the membrane potential, an ATP-dependent sodium-potassium pump is employed. This pump exchanges 3 intracellular Na^+ ions for 2 extracellular K^+ ions. It is inhibited by dinitrophenol and ouabain.

Voltage gated Na^+ channels open (activate) with mild cell depolarizations and close (inactivate) with larger cell depolarizations. They permit Na^+ influx, and are blocked by tetrodotoxin (puffer fish) and saxitoxin (from dinoflagellates that parasitize shellfish). Batrachotoxin (arrow poison), grayanotoxin,

Figure 9

Determinants of the resting membrane potential

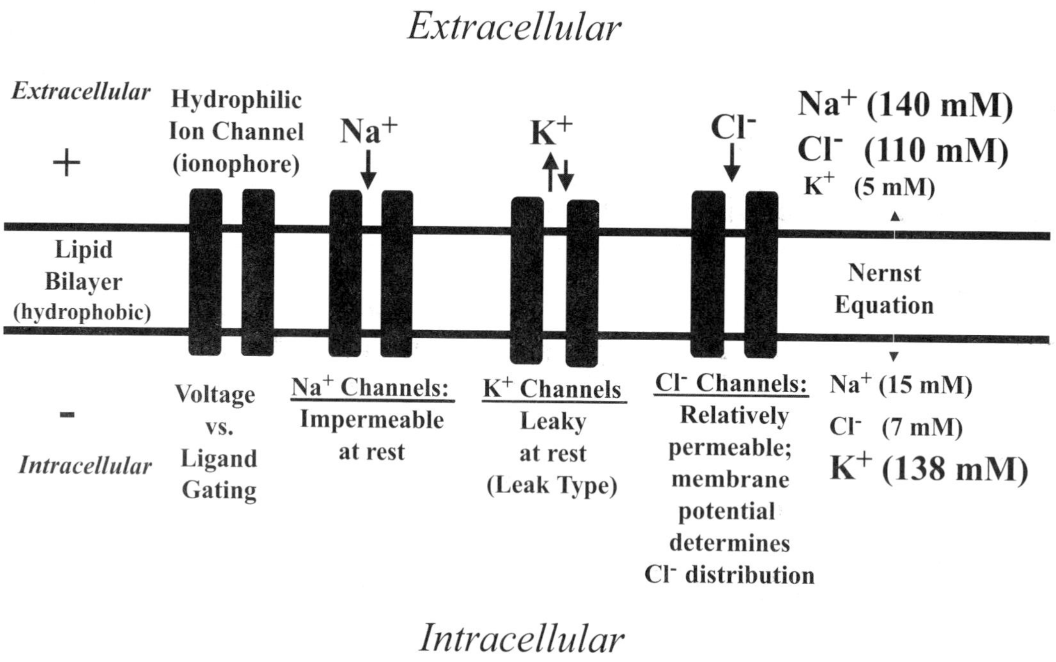

and veratridine open Na^{++} channels. Scorpion and sea anemone toxin block Na^{++} channel inactivation.

The nonleak type voltage-gated K^+ channels activate with cell depolarization and inactivate with repolarization. They permit K^+ efflux. The two types of nonleak K^+ channels are the Hodgkin-Huxley Delayed Type (blocked by tetraethyl-ammonium chloride, TEA), and the Fast A (Maxi) Type (blocked by 4-aminopyridine, which facilitates AP propagation). Some K^+ channels are activated by calcium (ie, when calcium is present, they require less depolarization to open).

Action Potentials

Ligand-gated Na^+ channels are concentrated around the axon hillock. When these channels are stimulated to open, Na^+ enters the cell to cause depolarizing excitatory postsynaptic potentials (EPSPs). Hyperpolarizing inhibitory postsynaptic potentials from the opening of nearby ligand-gated K^+ and Cl^- channels may counter this. If enough EPSPs summate to depolarize the axon hillock area to about -55 μV, voltage-gated Na^+ channels will begin opening down the axon. This permits a rapid all-or-nothing depolarization spike to about +40 μV (the action potential). As this depolarization shift proceeds, it becomes large enough to inactivate voltage-gated Na^+ channels and the action potential terminates. Meanwhile, voltage gated K^+ channels remain open, and K^+ efflux helps repolarize the cell. This period, in which voltage-gated Na^+ channels are utterly inactivated, is called the absolute refractory period. Eventually, the K^+ efflux tends to overshoot, and the cell briefly becomes hyperpolarized relative to its resting state. During this period of hyperpolarization, voltage-gated Na^+ channels are able to open if the action potential threshold is reached, but reaching the action potential threshold is unlikely because of the state of cell hyperpolarization. This period is known as the relative refractory period.

In myelinated neurons, Na^+ channels are concentrated at nodes of Ranvier. This allows for saltatory conduction, which greatly increases the rate at which an action potential is conducted.

Excitation-Secretion Coupling

When the action potential reaches the axon terminal, it opens voltage-gated Ca^{++} channels. Ca^{++} entry into the cell can proceed via three types of Ca^{++} channels. The N Type open briefly. Some Ca^{++} entry can activate a protein kinase that phosphorylates the L Type channel, which is slow to inactivate. L Type channels are also found linked to inhibitory G proteins. Calcium channel blocker drugs act at L Type channels. T Type channels are responsible for oscillatory behavior in places like the inferior olive. In any case, Ca^{++} influx triggers exocytosis of transmitter-containing secretory granules, a process called excitation-secretion coupling. Ca^{++} channel mutations are a cause of hypokalemic periodic paralysis.

Neurotransmitter Binding and Receptor Activation

Although some glial cells and rare brainstem nuclei neurons have direct electrical synapses (gap junctions), most intercellular communication in the nervous system occurs via chemical synapses. When excitation-secretion coupling occurs, neurotransmitter(s) are delivered into the synaptic cleft. Dale's Principle emphasizes that axon terminals arising from a single neuron utilize the same chemical message, be it a single transmitter or a combination of transmitters. Synaptic connections can be axospinous, axodendritic, axosomatic, and axoaxonal. Dendrodendritic synapses also exist.

To convert the chemical signal back to an electrical signal at the postsynaptic neuron, postsynaptic receptors are in place to bind the released neurotransmitter. Two main classes of neurotransmitter exist: 1) ion channel-coupled ionotropic receptors (class I receptors, fast receptors) that are directly linked to ion channels; and 2) second messenger coupled metabotropic receptors (class II receptors, slow receptors).

Metabotropic receptors contain transmitter receptor sites that consist of seven membrane-spanning segments. This receptor portion is often linked to a

Figure 10

The action potential

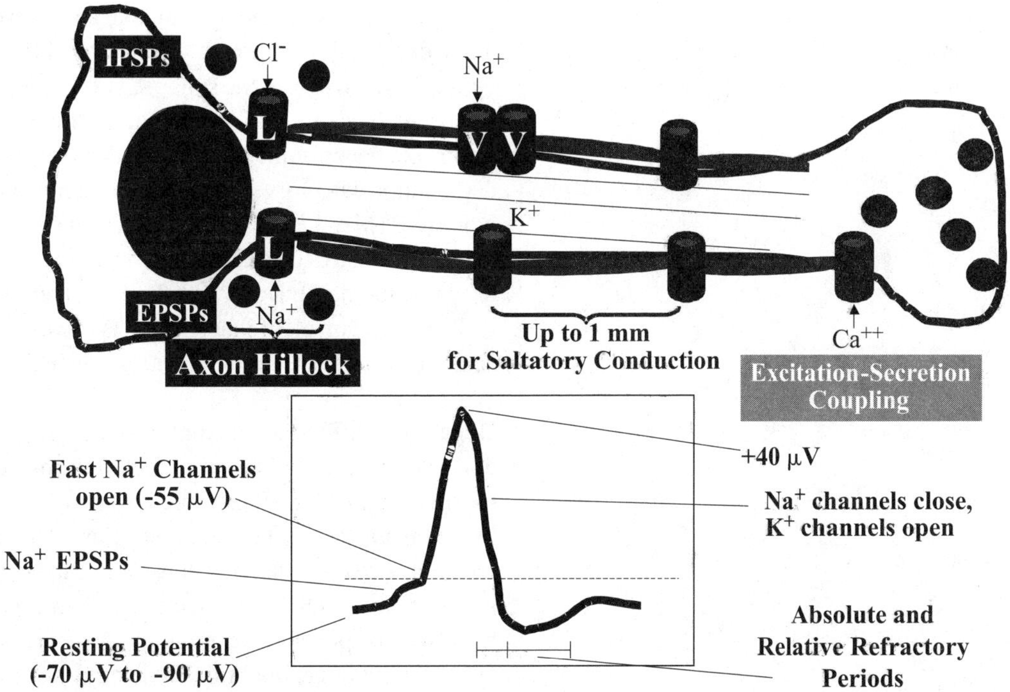

three-part G protein heterotrimer (because it binds GTP/GDP). When transmitter binds the receptor, the previously resting G protein exchanges a GDP for a GTP. One of the G protein subunits (the α subunit) detaches from the others, taking the GTP with it, and activates a second messenger. Eventually, the GTP hydrolyzes to GDP, the α subunit inactivates, and the G protein trimer reforms.

Second messenger signaling can proceed via different pathways. These pathways are stimulated or inhibited by the activated G protein (this depends on whether the G protein is stimulatory (Gs) or inhibitory (Gi)). These pathways include: 1) an adenylate cyclase-modulated cAMP cascade; 2) a guanylate cyclase cGMP cascade; and a 3) phospholipase C-mediated hydrolysis of phosphoinositides (to arachidonic acid, diacylglycerol, and inositol triphosphate). The end result of the second messenger cascade is to influence a biological response, which can include opening or closing of a channel. Presynaptically and at axoaxonic synapses, the final result is to alter transmitter release. Postsynaptically, it is to alter cell firing patterns.

3. Pharmacology

Overview

Neurotransmitters are compounds that are: 1) synthesized and released presynaptically; 2) have an effect; and 3) are inactivated. This is in contrast to neuromodulators, which are compounds that are only active in the face of ongoing synaptic activity, and neurohormones, which are compounds that pass through the circulation.

Catecholamines

Catechols are monoamines that contain a catechol group. The catecholamine dopamine is synthesized from tyrosine. The key enzyme in dopamine synthesis is tyrosine hydroxylase (TH), which converts tyrosine to DOPA. Aromatic amino acid decarboxylase converts DOPA to dopamine. Alternatively, DOPA can be converted to 3-O-methyldopa by catechol O-methyl transferase (COMT).

Dopamine acts to inhibit its own synthesis by competing with the tetrahydrobiopterin cofactor used by TH. Autoreceptor binding also downregulates TH. Conversely, high action potential "impulse flow" rates and sometimes interruption of impulse flow upregulate TH via phosphorylation of the enzyme.

Dopamine is inactivated by reuptake and then enzymatic degradation, although some dopamine inactivation likely occurs at the synapse before reuptake can occur. Cocaine, amphetamine, mazindol, buproprion, and benztropine block reuptake. Enzymatic degradation can proceed either through monamine oxidase B (MAO B) and then COMT, or COMT and then MAO B. MAO itself is localized to mitochondrial membranes, but may also be extraneuronal as well. The end result of inactivation is homovanillic acid (HVA). HVA levels are measurable in the CSF.

Dopamine's effects are mediated, of course, via dopamine receptors. These are metabotropic receptors that are primarily classified into two families based on how they affect adenyl cyclase. D_1 type receptors activate adenyl cyclase, and can be further subclassified as D_1 and D_5 subtypes. D_2 receptors, which can be presynaptic as well as postsynaptic, either inhibit or are not linked to adenyl cyclase. They can be further subclassified as D_2, D_3, and D_4 receptors.

D_1 and D_2 subtypes are important in the nigrostriatal dopaminergic pathway, and so help regulate movement. D_3 and D_4 subtypes probably figure more prominently in the mesocortical and mesolimbic dopaminergic pathways, and are targeted by atypical antipsychotics.

Dopaminergic neurons arise from the midbrain, in the ventral tegmentum and the substantia nigra. In addition to nigrostriatal, mesocortical, and mesolimbic pathways, a tuberoinfundibular pathway exists that arises from the arcuate and periventricular nuclei of the hypothalamus. In this pathway, which uses D_2 receptors, dopamine appears to act as a prolactin inhibitory factor.

The catecholamine norepinephrine (NE) is structurally similar to dopamine. In fact, it is synthesized from dopamine by the enzyme dopamine β-hydroxylase. The adrenal medulla contains an additional enzyme, phenylethanolamine N-methyl transferase, which can methylate NE to form epinephrine. Epinephrine levels are low in brain.

NE inactivation is initially by reuptake, which is an energy and Na^+ dependent process. Some NE inactivation nevertheless likely occurs at the synapse before reuptake occurs. Cocaine, tricyclics, and amphetamines block NE reuptake. Like dopamine, it is enzymatically degraded by COMT and MAO (A or B forms). MAO A is inhibited by clorgyline, and MAO B is inhibited by deprenyl (selegiline). Both types are inhibed by pargyline. MAO degradation yields an aldehyde derivative that is dehydrogenated in the peripheral nervous system (PNS) to vanilyl-mandelic acid (VMA), and reduced in the CNS to 3-methoxy-4-hydroxy phenyl glycol (MHPG). Determining serum VMA and CSF MHPG levels is occasionally of clinical use.

NE receptors are metabotropic. The two classes of NE receptors are the α and β types. β receptors are the main type in the CNS, and are further subclassified as β1 and β2 receptors. Binding to these receptors activates adenyl cyclase. Propranolol is a nonselective β receptor antagonist, and isoproterenal is an agonist. α Receptors are further subclassified as α1 and α2 receptors. α2 Receptors inhibit adenyl cyclase. α1 Receptors likely trigger phospholipase C-related pathways, and may end up opening Ca^{++} channels as their effect. Prazosin is an α1 antagonist, clonidine is an α2 agonist, yohimbine is an α2 antagonist, and phentolamine is a nonselective α antagonist.

NE is largely produced in the locus ceruleus of the caudal pontine central grey area. Neurons from here project to the diencephalon and telencephalon, and also to the cerebellum (via the superior cerebellar peduncle) and spinal cord (ventrolateral column thoracolumbar levels). Except for the sudomotor system, NE is the transmitter that is used at postganglionic PNS sympathetic synapses.

Rauwolfia alkaloids (reserpine, tetrabenazine) block NE storage. In addition to blocking reuptake, amphetamines may activate release. α Methyltyrosine inhibits tyrosine hydroxylase, and can be used to treat inoperable pheochromocytomas.

Indolamines

Like dopamine and NE, serotonin (5-hydroxytryptamine; 5-HT) is a monoamine. However, it is an indolamine rather than a catecholamine. It tends to be an inhibitory neurotransmitter. Serotonin is synthesized from tryptophan by the enzymes tryptophan hydroxylase and amino acid decarboxylase. These enzymes are not easily saturated, and therefore tryptophan availability determines synthesis rates. In the pineal gland, enzymes are present that can further convert it to melatonin.

Serotonin is first inactivated by an energy-dependent reuptake system. Reuptake is blocked by tricyclics (amitriptyline and imipramine tend to nonselectively block biogenic amine reuptake in general). Some drugs are more selective blockers of serotonin reuptake (the tricyclic clomipramine, trazodone, selective serotonin reuptake inhibitors). Reuptake is followed by enzymatic degradation. Typically, degradation occurs via MAO-A and aldehyde dehydrogenase, yielding 5 hydroxyindole acetic acid (5-HIAA).

Seven serotonin receptor types are currently recognized:

1. $5HT_{1B}$ and $5HT_{1D}$ receptors are metabotropic presynaptic autoreceptors that inhibit adenyl cyclase. Their activation decreases serotonin release. $5HT_{1D}$ receptors are found in the basal ganglia, and sumaptriptan is an agonist. $5HT_{1B}$ receptors are found in the globus pallidus and substantia nigra.

2. $5HT_{1C}$ and $5HT_2$ receptors are metabotropic postsynaptic receptors that activate phospholipase C. $5HT_{1C}$ receptors are found in the choroid plexus, and bind LSD and methysergide. $5HT_2$ receptors are found cortically, and are antagonized by risperidone and clozapine. $5HT_2$ receptors also play a role in facial motor nucleus activation.

3. $5HT_3$ receptors are unique in that they are ionotropic channels that permit Ca^{++} influx. They exist in entorhinal cortex and the area postrema. Ondansetron and metaclopramide are $5HT_3$ antagonists.

4. $5HT_{1A}$ is a metabotropic postsynaptic receptor that inhibits adenyl cyclase. It seems to open a K^+ channel. Buspirone is a $5HT_{1A}$ agonist. An adenyl-cyclase stimulating population of $5HT_{1A}$ receptors may reside in the hippocampus.

5. $5HT_4$ receptors are metabotropic postsynaptic receptors that stimulate adenyl cyclase. They are also called $5HT_{1P}$ receptors, and are found in the gut.

Serotonin is largely synthesized in the brainstem raphe nuclei. The dorsal and median raphe nuclei of the midbrain and pons project to the pineal gland, cerebral hemispheres, and cerebellum. The pontomedullary raphe nuclei (nucleus raphe magnus and nucleus gigantocellularis) project to the area postrema of the medulla and also the spinal cord dorsal horn substantia gelatinosa.

Serotonin supplies are also depleted by reserpine. Serotonin levels can be increased by tryptophan loading (in the past this was occasionally used to treat myoclonus). Lysergic acid diethylamide (LSD) is a partial agonist, and methysergide is an agonist.

Acetylcholine

Acetylcholine is produced by the choline acetyl transferase-mediated condensation of acetyl CoA and choline. Acetyl CoA is produced in mitochondria. As choline acetyl transferase (CAT) is hard to saturate, choline availability tends to serve as the rate-limiting factor in its synthesis. CAT activity is decreased in Alzheimer disease.

Acetylcholine inactivation differs from that of the biogenic amines in that it is first enzymatically degraded, with reuptake occurring only after this degradation takes place. Acetylcholine is degraded primarily in the CNS/PNS by acetylcholinesterase, and in some areas by related butyrylcholinesterase enzymes. The degradation products are acetic acid and choline. Choline undergoes presynaptic reuptake via a sodium dependent transporter. Hemicholinium blocks choline reuptake.

In the CNS, acetylcholinesterase is inhibited by physostigmine, tacrine, donepezil, rivastigmine, and galantamine. In the PNS, acetylcholinesterase is inhibited by pyridostigmine, neostigmine, and edrophonium (tensilon). Organophosphate pesticides and carbamate nerve gas also irreversibly inhibit acetylcholinesterase. With pesticide or nerve gas exposure, 2-pyridine aldoxime methiodide (PAM) or HI-6 can dislodge the inhibitor and restore enzyme activity.

Acetylcholine receptors fall into two families, nicotinic and muscarinic. Nicotinic receptors are agonized by nicotine and are ionotropic. They consist of four subunits $[\alpha, \beta, \gamma, \Delta]$ in varying combinations. Although N1-N4 types are known, they can be grossly subdivided into N1 and N2 subtypes. In the CNS, nicotinic receptors are found pre- and postsynaptically, and are concentrated in the superior colliculus. In the PNS, N1 receptors are found at neuromuscular junctions and N2 receptors are found at preganglionic synapses. Muscarinic receptors that are agonized by muscarine are metabotropic, and are linked to G proteins that open or close K+, Ca++, or Cl- channels. They can be subdivided into those muscarinic receptors that activate phospholipase C (M1, M3, M5), and those that inhibit adenyl cyclase (M2, M4). In the PNS, muscarinic receptors are found at autonomic target organs in the parasympathetic system, as well as at sweat glands in the sympathetic autonomic nervous system (ANS). M1, M3, and M5 receptors seem to be the most used type in the CNS. M2 receptors are presynaptic. The following facts pertain to acetylcholine pharmacology:

1. N1 agonist: phenyltetramethylammonium

2. N1 antagonists: tubocurarine (reversible), α bungarotoxin (irreversible)

3. N2 agonist: tetramethylammonium

4. N2 antagonists: trimethaphan, hexamethonium

5. Decrease nicotinic tone by nondepolarizing blockade: curare, procainamide, aminoglycosides

6. Decrease nicotinic tone by depolarizing blockade: succinylcholine

7. Decrease nicotinic tone by blocking acetylcholine release: botulinum toxin, Lambert-Easton myasthenic syndrome, tick paralysis

8. Increase nicotinic tone by increasing release: latrotoxin (the black widow spider toxin)

9. Block muscarinic receptors: atropine, scopalamine, artane

10. Agonize muscarinic receptors: amanita mushrooms, pilocarpine, and carbachol.

Hyponicotinic states are characterized by weakness. Hypomuscarinic states are characterized by decreased autonomic activity ("dry as a stone, red as a beet, mad as a hatter"). Hypermuscarinic states present as increased sweating, salivation, miosis, GI hypermotility, and airway constriction/secretion. Dizziness, confusion, weakness, and coma can also occur.

Spinal cord Renshaw neurons are cholinergic. In the PNS, motor neurons that synapse on muscle are cholinergic. In the ANS, pre- and postganglionic parasympathetic neurons are cholinergic, as are sympathetic preganglioinic neurons. It is worth noting postganglionic sudomotor sympathetic neurons are also cholinergic, which is unusual since postganglionic sympathetic neurons typically use NE.

Figure 11

Autonomic and peripheral nervous system acetylcholine

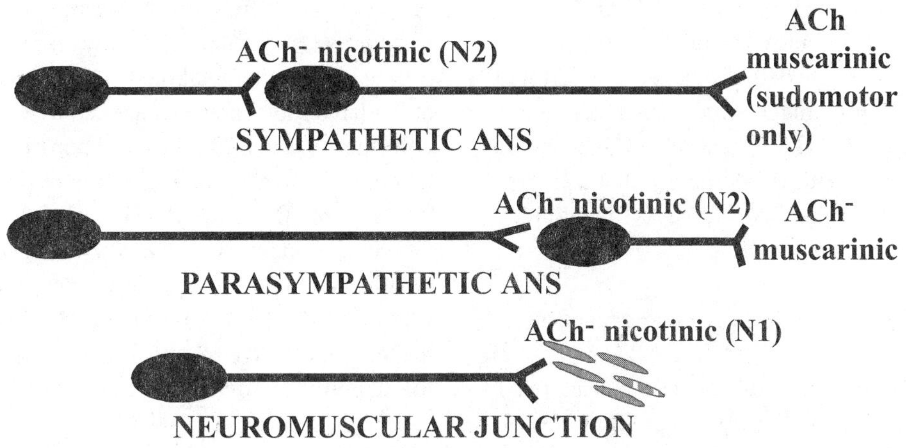

In the CNS, acetylcholine is used at cranial nerve nuclei. It is the transmitter of local circuit neurons in the striatum, nucleus accumbens, and olfactory tubercle interneurons. Two cholinergic projection systems are known. One arises from the pontomesencephalotegmental complex. The main one, though, arises from the basal forebrain cholinergic complex. The basal forebrain cholinergic complex consists of several components. The largest part is the substantia innominata, and much of the substantia innominata consists of the nucleus basalis of Meynert. The other cholinergic nuclei of the basal forebrain complex include the nuclei of the diagonal band of Broca and the medial septal nuclei. Together, these three nuclei (Meynert, diagonal band, medial septal) project throughout the cortex by way of the fornix, internal capsule, and other tracts.

Amino Acid Neurotransmitters

GABA (γ-aminobutyric acid) is the main CNS inhibitory neurotransmitter. It does not cross the blood-brain barrier, so it must be synthesized in the CNS itself. It is synthesized from glutamate by glutamic acid decarboxylase (GAD), which is a pyridoxine-dependent enzyme. Pyridoxine deficiencies can therefore be associated with seizures.

GABA is enzymatically degraded in a way that it primes its own resynthesis. This degradation-resynthesis pathway is called the "GABA shunt". In the GABA shunt, GABA is deaminated by GABA-ketoglutarate transaminase (GABA-T) in mitochondria. The removed amino group is attached by glutamate dehydrogenase to α ketoglutarate, creating glutamate (which can then regenerate GABA). The GABA-T generated GABA degradation product is further modified so that it enters the Krebs cycle as succinate. GABA-T is inhibited by vigabatrin and valproate.

GABA is also removed from synaptic spaces by glial uptake. As glia also contain GABA-T, they can convert GABA to glutamate. Further, glia are rich in the enzyme glutamine synthase. This facilitates conversion of glial glutamate to glutamine, which is released from glial cells and taken up by neighboring neurons. Once in the neuron, glutamine can be converted to glutamate by glutaminase, and then on to GABA. This cycle by which glia help replenish/maintain neuronal GABA levels is called the "glutamine loop."

GABA receptors consist of two types, $GABA_A$ and $GABA_B$ receptors. $GABA_A$ receptors are ionotropic, and facilitate Cl^- entry into cells (hence their inhibitory effect). They are found in the hippocampus, striatum, spinal cord, and cerebellar granular layers. $GABA_A$ receptors are activated by muscimol and inhibited by both bicuculline and picrotoxin, which clinically can induce seizures. These are allosteric receptors, whose activation thresholds are modified by other molecules that can also bind them (benzodiazepines, barbiturates, and steroids). Benzodiazepines increase GABA binding affinity, and thus increase the frequency of channel opening that follows GABA binding. Barbiturates potentiate GABA by prolonging GABA-induced channel opening.

$GABA_B$ receptors are metabotropic. They are found presynaptically and postsynaptically at axoaxonal synapses. Baclofen is a $GABA_B$ receptor agonist. When it binds at its receptor at axoaxonal synapses, it acts to diminish excitation-secretion coupling by diminishing action potential-mediated Ca^{++} channel opening. The end result is less neurotransmitter release by the targeted neuron. $GABA_B$ receptors are not bound by benzodiazepines or barbiturates.

Glycine is an inhibitory neurotransmitter found mostly in spinal cord and brainstem interneurons. It is synthesized from serine by serine hydroxymethyltransferase, and is inactivated by reuptake. It is removed through metabolism to other amino acids and related molecules. As with GABA, it increases chloride conductance via activation of an ionotropic receptor. This receptor also activates (less efficiently) with β-alanine, taurine, alanine, and serine. Glycine receptors are selectively antagonized by strychnine. In the CNS, an important role of glycine is to prevent desensitization of NMDA receptors during prolonged exposure to glutamate. Tetanus toxin inhibits glycine release (and also blocks GABA release as well).

Glutamate is the main CNS excitatory neurotransmitter. It can be synthesized from α ketoglutarate (by glutamate dehydrogenase), glutamine (by glutaminase), and aspartate (by aspartate aminotransferase). It is metabolized to related molecules, such as GABA, and is one of the amino acids in glutathione.

Glutamate receptors are named after their specific agonists. NMDA, AMPA, and kainate receptors are ionotropic. Early glutamate receptor studies recognizing only NMDA, AMPA, and kainate receptors collectively referred to AMPA and kainate receptors as "non-NMDA receptors". Subsequently, metabotropic receptors that are agonized by L-AP4 and APCD were also described.

AMPA receptors are the major source of EPSPs in the CNS, and likely play a role in convulsions. When agonized by beta-N-oxalylamino-L-alanine (BOAA) they can cause lathryrism. Meta-N-methyl-amino-L-alanine (BMAA) from cycads may also mediate neurotoxicity via AMPA receptor agonism. Kainate receptors are in the limbic system and hippocampus, may be presynaptic, and may play a role in seizure disorders. L-AP4 receptors are inhibitory autoreceptors and activate adenylate cyclase. ACPD metabotropic channels operate through phospholipase C-mediated pathways.

NMDA receptors are found in particularly high amounts in the hippocampus and forebrain, and appear to play a role in long-term potentiation (and therefore learning). They are interesting for a number of reasons. Unlike other ionotropic glutamate receptors, in addition to Na^+ passage they permit Ca^{++} passage. Also, in addition to ligand gating there is also an element of voltage gating. This is possible because under resting cell conditions, Mg^{++} occupies the channel and impedes calcium's ability to enter the cell. When cells depolarize, however, the Mg^{++} ion block is removed and Ca^{++} can more rapidly access the cytosol. Other sites on the NMDA receptor can bind glycine (which prevents desensitization in the face of repetitive glutamate activation), PCP (which inhibits activation), and zinc (which inhibits activation). Ketamine, memantidine, and amantadine are NMDA receptor antagonists.

Aspartate is also a CNS excitatory neurotransmitter. It is largely synthesized by the transamination of oxaloacetate, but can also be synthesized from asparagine and glutamine.

Histamine is synthesized from the amino acid derivative histidine. The enzyme that catalyzes this, histidine decarboxylase, is pyridoxine-dependent. Neuronal reuptake of histamine is not recognized. In the CNS glial cells, histamine is metabolized by MAO and an aldehyde dehyrodenase to an imidazole derivative, tele-methyl imidazole acetic acid. In the PNS, it is metabolized to a related but distinct imidazole, imidazole acetic acid.

Three metabotropic types of histamine receptor are recognized. H_3 receptors are presynaptic autoreceptors. H_3 activation blocks further histamine release. H_1 receptors are found in the cortex, and inhibit phospholipase C-mediated phosphoinositide hydrolysis. They are antagonized by diphenydramine. H_2 receptors are found in the striatum, and stimulate adenyl cyclase. They are antagonized by cimetidine.

Histamine is produced in large amounts at the hypothalamus. It is utilized in the hypothalamic median eminence, where it may alter food/water intake and thermoregulation. Histaminergic neurons also project to the midbrain reticular formation and cortex, and appear to play a role in arousal. Hypothalamic histaminergic neurons also project to the spinal cord.

Neuroactive Peptides

Many different neuroactive peptide molecules are produced from a relatively restricted set of genes. Neuroactive peptide proliferation is made possible from differential splicing of mRNA transcripts and variable endopeptidase modifications that produce distinct prohormones in the cell soma. These prohormones, following axonal transport to the cell terminal, are further posttranslationally modified to form actual neuroactive peptide molecules. They are inactivated by peptidases.

Neuroactive peptides can diffuse over large areas. They largely serve as neuromodulators and neurohormones, although in some instances they can also act as neurotransmitters. When neuroactive peptides act as neuromodulators, they are concomitantly stored and released with the neurotransmitters they influence. Neuroactive peptides are grouped into two main families, the nonopioid and opioid peptides.

Nonopioid neuropeptides include the hypothalamus-produced releasing hormones, such as corticotropin releasing factor (CRH). CRH may play a role in seizures, such as infantile spasms, and can induce anxiety. Somatostatin inhibits growth hormone release. Vasopressin (from the hypothalamic supraoptic nuclei) and oxytocin (from the hypothalamic paraventricular nuclei) are considered neurohormones. Substance P is a tachykinin peptide, and is found in the substantia gelatinosa of the spinal cord. Vasoactive intestinal polypeptide is a glucagon-related peptide. Neurotensin may potentially affect the circulatory sytem, analgesia, and thermoregulation. Neuropeptide Y is a pancreatic polypeptide-related peptide that is a potent vasoconstrictor. Cholecystokinin (CCK) may antagonize opioids. Angiotensin II is active in circumventricular areas.

Opioid peptide synthesis appears dependent on cAMP pathways. There are three basic opioid prohormones: prodynorphin, propiomelanocortin, and proenkephalin. The proenkephalin prohormone gets modified into a series of smaller enkephalins, including two five amino acid pieces (met enkephalin and leu enkephalin). These two five amino acid pieces form the amino ends of all the other opioid peptide derivatives, no matter which prohormone they derive from. Prodynorphin gives rise to neodynorphin, dynorphin A, and dynorphin B. Propriomelanocortin gives rise to three neuroactive peptides, including ACTH, melanocyte stimulating hormone, and β-lipotropin. α-Lipotropin is further modified to form the endorphins (α, β, and γ endorphin).

Opiate receptors are metabotropic and uniformly inhibitory. There are currently three known types, and each modifies adenyl cyclase activity. Mu receptors are utilized by endorphin molecules, and are found in the pituitary and hypothalamus. β-Endorphin binding at mu receptors produces long-lasting analgesia. Delta receptors are utilized by enkephalins, and are present in the spinal cord. Enkephalin binding inhibits the release of substance P in the cord. Kappa receptors are utilized by dynorphins. Previously, an additional opioid receptor titled the sigma receptor was postulated, but it now appears sigma receptors are not actually opioid receptors. All opioid receptors are antagonized by naloxone, although mu and delta receptors are inhibited more avidly than kappa receptors. Opiate transmitter postsynaptic activity it terminated by extracellular proteases or diffusion.

Nitric Oxide

Nitric oxide (NO) can act as a second messenger that activates guanylate cyclase, raising cGMP levels. It also can diffuse across membranes and act as a neurotransmitter. It is synthesized from arginine by the enzyme nitric oxide synthase (NOS), which exists in tissue-specific isoforms (neuronal NOS, endothelial NOS, and inducible NOS). Neuronal NOS is activated by Ca^{++} when it accesses cell cytoplasm via NMDA receptor channels. It was previously postulated that via its role as a glutamate-activated second messenger, NO may potentially play a role in long-term potentiation/synaptic memory.

When an oxidative balance is present in the cytoplasm, NO acts as a free radical that can diffuse over distances, a characteristic not typical of most free radicals. NO acting as a free radical can react with the superoxide radical to form a more toxic free radical intermediate, peroxynitrite, via the "peroxynitrite reaction". Peroxynitrite can further degrade to hydroxyl radical, which is perhaps the most toxic radical of all. NO under appropriate conditions may therefore play a role in neurodegeneration.

4. Neurodegeneration

Oxidative Stress

Oxidative stress is observed in a variety of neurodegenerative disease states and may play a physiologically important role in such. A state of oxidative stress is said to exist when cell free radical production is elevated to the point that cell free radical scavenging systems cannot keep up. Oxidative stress can also develop under conditions of normal free radical production when free radical scavenging capacity is reduced.

Free radicals are molecules that contain an unpaired electron in their outer orbital shell and are thus inherently unstable. In essence, they would like to either unload their unpaired electron or else acquire an electron from somewhere else in order to alleviate the unpairing. When oxygen carries the unpaired electron, the free radical molecule can be designated as a "reactive oxygen species" (ROS). Reactive nitrogen species (RNS) arise when nitrogen carries an unpaired electron. Free radicals will react with DNA, protein, and lipid molecules within cells. Byproducts of such abnormal oxidation reactions are evident as hydroxyguanosine (DNA); hydroperoxides, hydroxynonenal, malondialdehyde, isoprostanes, thiobarbituric acid reactive substances (lipids); and carbonyls, aromatic hydroxylation, nitration, and nitrosylation (proteins).

The most active site of cell free radical production tends to be the mitochondrial ETC. They are also produced as a byproduct of arachidonic acid metabolism (both lipoxygenase and cyclooxygenase pathways), oxidase catalyzed reactions (NADPH oxidases, xanthine oxidase, MAO), tyrosine hydroxylase, and activated macrophages/phagocytes.

The most common ROS is superoxide anion, which is molecular oxygen that has accepted an extra (unpaired) electron. Superoxide can be dismuted by superoxide dismutase (SOD) to form H_2O_2. There are two main types of SOD, a mitochondrial form that contains manganese (MnSOD), and a predominantly cytoplasmic form that contains copper and zinc (CuZn SOD). It is important to subsequently eliminate H_2O_2, since upon exposure to iron H_2O_2 it can give rise to the extremely toxic hydroxyl radical via a chemical process called the Fenton reaction. Also, H_2O_2 can react with superoxide to produce hydroxyl radical. This process is called the Haber-Weiss reaction. Fortunately, catalase (in the cytoplasm) and glutathione peroxidase (in mitochondria) can convert H_2O_2 to H_2O. As mentioned above, nitric oxide and superoxide react to form peroxynitrite, which can also form hydroxyl radical via the peroxynitirite reaction.

Excitotoxicity

Glutamate, the main brain excitatory neurotransmitter, activates NMDA receptors. This activation allows calcium to access neuronal cytoplasm, where it activates intracellular signaling cascades. Under some conditions, such as stroke, glial cells release glutamate into the extracellular space and this glutamate is believed to cause excessive NMDA receptor activation and excessive cell calcium entry. Of course, cells will attempt to restore cytoplasmic calcium homeostasis by pocketing it into other compartments, such as the endoplasmic reticulum. Mitochondria, which contain negatively charged matrices, are also an avid site of calcium cation storage. In this form of excitotoxicity, mitochondria take on excessive calcium to the point that mitochondrial dysfunction occurs. When mitochondria fail to the point that ATP is no longer produced, cells die via a process called necrosis, a form of cell death that is not energy dependent. When ATP supplies are adequate, but mitochondria depolarize beyond a critical threshold, apoptotic programmed cell death may ensue.

Mitochondrial dysfunction is observed in various neurodegenerative disease states, and this may limit the ability of mitochondria to buffer even normal levels of NMDA channel-derived calcium. In this case, cytoplasmic calcium levels rise pathologically and may act in a neurotoxic fashion. This situation represents a distinctly different form of glutamate excitotoxicity from that which is proposed for conditions of acute hypoxia.

Apoptosis

Apoptosis is an energy dependent form of programmed cell death. In neurodegenerative disease states, data implicate activation of an intrinsic apoptosis pathway that initiates in mitochondria. Either as a result of mitochondrial bioenergetic failure (low energy), oxidative stress, or depolarization,

Figure 12

Mitochondrial role in oxidative stress, excitotoxicity, and apoptosis

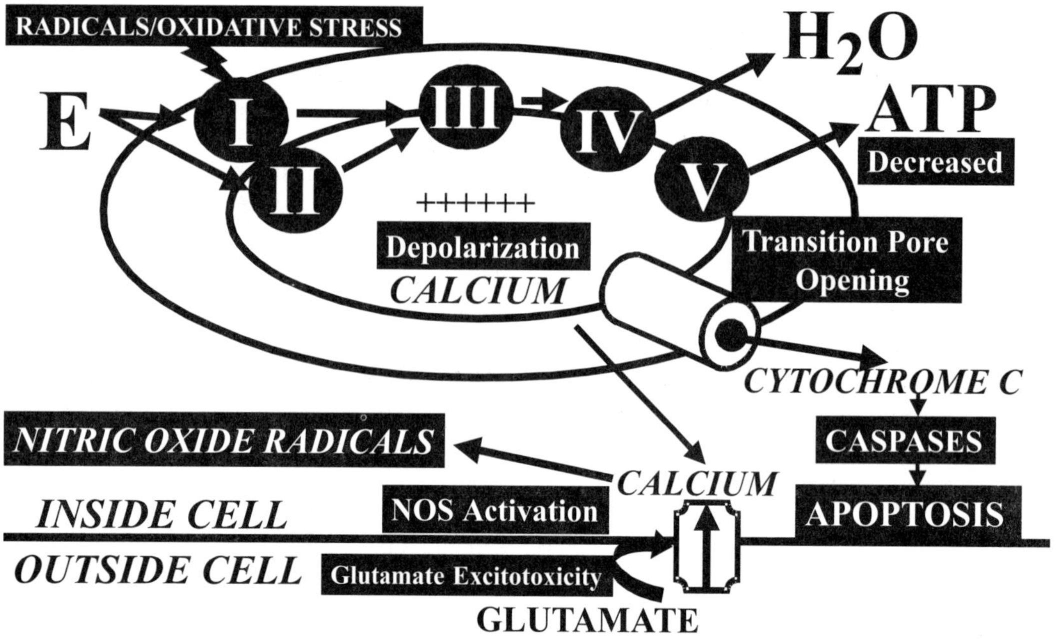

molecules that are typically sequestered within mitochondria (cytochrome c, apoptosis initiating factor) are released into the cytoplasm. In the case of cytochrome c, binding with other cytoplasmic molecules (APAF 1, procaspase 9, ATP) leads to activation of a caspase enzyme cascade that ultimately results in cell elimination.

5. Other Topics

Axonal Transport

Anterograde transport from the cell soma to the cell terminal can occur via slow (0.5-4 mm/day), intermediate (15-50 mm/day), and fast (200-400 mm/day) modes. Retrograde transport in the opposite direction is only designed to occur in the fast mode (200-300 mm/day).

Slow transport is basically due to cytoplasmic flow down the axon (axoplasmic flow). It facilitates movements of cytoskeletal elements. Fast transport is an active, ATP-dependent process that requires microtubules. It is inhibited by the microtubule disrupting drugs colchicine and vinblastine. Organelles and neurotransmitters use fast transport. Tetanus toxin and viruses can undergo retrograde transport.

When axonal transport down the axon is disrupted, retrograde messages return from the site of disruption. This message triggers activation of the cell body with dissolution of the cell's Nissl substance (rough endoplasmic reticulum), with migration of the nucleus to an eccentric location. This process is called chromatolysis.

Blood-Brain Barrier

Three main features characterize the blood-brain barrier. First, endothelial capillary cells contain tight junctions and no fenestrations. Second, a thick basement membrane surrounds the endothelial cells. Third, astrocytes provide perivascular capillary cuffing (the glia limitans). Transport across the BBB requires carrier-mediated mechanisms for most molecules. Highly lipophilic molecules can diffuse across.

There are six areas in the brain where the blood-brain barrier is not present. These areas are called the circumventricular organs. They allow for CNS monitoring of the somatic environment.

In addition to the blood-brain barrier, a blood-cerebrospinal fluid (CSF) barrier exists. This barrier exists to prevent contents of choroid plexus capillaries from freely mixing with the ventricular CSF. The choroid plexus capillaries themselves are fenestrated, and permit egress of plasma contents, but lining the choroid plexus is a tight-junctioned epithilium. It is this choroid plexus epithilium that actually creates the blood-CSF barrier. Finally, there

Figure 13

The blood-brain barrier and circumventricular organs

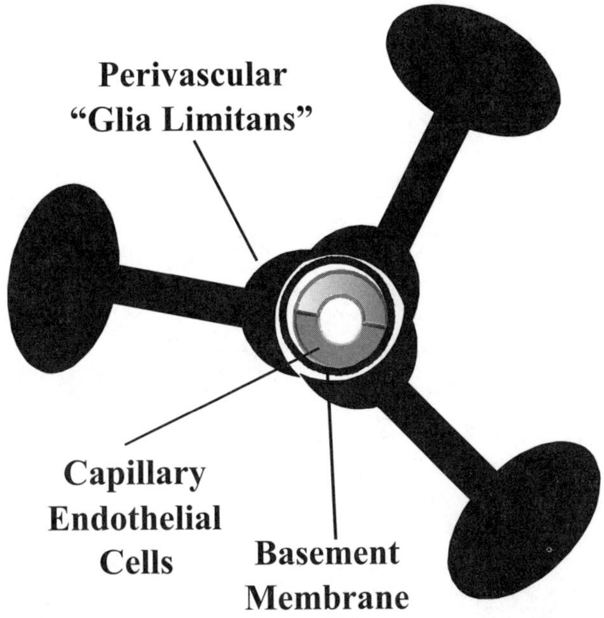

Exceptions:
The "Circumventricular Organs"
Pineal gland
Neurophypophysis
Area postrema
Subfornical organ
Organum vasculosum of the lamina terminalis
Median eminence of the hypothalamus

is "CSF-brain barrier", which is defined by the ventricular ependymal lining. Cells of the ependymal lining, however, do not contain tight junctions. Mixing of ventricular fluid and extracellular fluid can therefore occur.

Neurotoxins

Clinically relevant neurotoxins are typically divided into metal and organic types. Toxin related symptoms tend to overlap, and affect cognition, behavior, movement, and the peripheral nervous system. Toxicity is often due to interference with metabolic pathways. Some toxins, though, can be associated with very particular clinical symptoms and signs. Arsenic-induced neuropathy is more sensory than motor. In adults, lead poisoning can result in motor neuropathy. Trichloroethylene can cause trigeminal nerve damage, as well as other cranial neuropathies.

6. References

1. Cooper JR, Bloom FE, Roth RH. *Biochemical Basis of Neuropharmacology*. 8th ed. Oxford: Oxford University Press; 2002.

2. Griggs RC, Mendell JR, Miller RG. *Evaluation and Treatment of Myopathies*. Contemporary Neurology Series. Philadelphia, Pa: FA Davis; 1994.

3. Nestler ER, Hyman SE, Malenka RC. *Molecular Neuropharmacology: A Foundation for Clinical Neuroscience*. New York: McGraw Hill; 2001.

4. OMIM-Online. Mendelian inheritance in man. Link: www.ncbi.nlm.nih.gov.

5. Siegel GJ, Agranoff BW, Albers RW, Fisher SK, Uhler SD, eds. *Basic Neurochemistry: Molecular, Cellular, and Medical Aspects*. 6th ed. Philadelphia, Pa: Lippincott Williams & Wilkins; 1999.

6. Gene clinics. Link: www.geneclinics.org.

7. Questions

1. Which of these is not a disorder of glycogen catabolism?

   A. Cori disease

   B. Pompe disease

   C. McCardle disease

   D. Scheie disease

2. Which of the following diseases results from a problem with the second step of glycolysis?

   A. Von Gierke disease

   B. Tarui disease

   C. Andersen disease

   D. Hers disease

3. Which statement about pyruvate dehydrogenase complex is not true?

   A. Thiamine is a cofactor

   B. Dysfunction can cause Leigh syndrome

   C. Dysfunction can cause lactic acidosis

   D. Catabolizes products of the Krebs cycle

4. Which of these peroxisomal disorders is associated with a single enzyme defect?

   A. X-linked adrenoleukodystrophy

   B. Neonatal adrenoleukodystrophy

   C. Zellweger syndrome

   D. Infantile Refsum disease

5. Which statement about ketone bodies is true?

   A. Acetoacetate and malonate are major species

   B. Are produced in the starving brain

   C. Feed into the Krebs cycle

   D. Are neurotoxic

6. Leucine, isoleucine, valine, and ketoacids in urine are typical of what disorder?

   A. Maple syrup urine disease

   B. Multiple carboxylase deficiency

   C. Isovaleric acidemia

   D. Hartnup disease

7. All of the following may alleviate an organic aciduria except:

   A. Biotin

   B. Carnitine

   C. Protein restriction

   D. Pyridoxine

8. Which of these is not part of the mitochondrial electron transport chain?

   A. Malonate reductase

   B. Succinate dehydrogenase

   C. NADH dehydrogenase

   D. Cytochrome c oxidase

9. Mitochondrial depolarization is not associated with which of the following events:

A. Loss of permeability transition

B. Glutamate excitotoxicity

C. Increased cytoplasmic calcium

D. Apoptosis

10. Which is correct about axonal transport?

A. Fast transport is not energy dependent

B. Chromatolysis is due to anterograde transport

C. Colchicine and vinblastine interfere with fast transport

D. Microtubules don't participate in fast transport

11. Which of these statements about membrane potentials is incorrect?

A. The Na-K pump is blocked by dinitrophenol

B. The Na-K pump is blocked by oubain

C. The resting membrane potential is -55 mV

D. During action potentials the cell depolarizes to 40 mV

12. Which of the following channelopathy associations is incorrect?

A. Sodium channels – hyperkalemic periodic paralysis

B. Calcium channels – hypokalemic periodic paralysis

C. Chloride channels – myotonia congenita

D. Potassium channels – paramyotonia congenita

13. Which of the following channel-inhibitor pairings is incorrect?

A. Potassium channels – tetramethylammonium chloride

B. Potassium channels – 4 aminopyridine

C. Sodium channels – saxitoxin

D. Calcium channels – tetrodotoxin

14. Which of these receptors is not coupled to a G-protein?

A. $GABA_A$

B. M_1 acetylcholine

C. M_2 acetylcholine

D. Dopamine

15. Binding at which of these dopamine receptor types activates adenyl cyclase?

A. D_1

B. D_2

C. D3

D. D_4

16. Which statement about norepinephrine metabolism is true?

A. It is formed by dopamine methylation

B. Epinephrine is made by norepinephrine demethylation

C. Reuptake is its major mode of inactivation

D. It is degraded in the CNS to vanilyl mandelic acid

17. Which statement about acetylcholine is true?

A. Synthesis occurs in mitochondria

B. Choline acetyltransferase activity is rate limiting in acetylcholine synthesis

C. Is primarily inactivated by reuptake mechanisms

D. Choline reuptake is sodium dependent

18. All of the following are inhibitory amino acid neurotransmitters except:

A. GABA

B. Glycine

C. Homocysteic acid

D. Taurine

19. Which of the following statements about GABA is incorrect?

A. It is directly synthesized from glutamate

B. Cobalamin is required for its synthesis

C. It can be metabolized to enter the Krebs cycle

D. It undergoes glial reuptake

20. Which sphingolipidosis – enzyme defect pairing is incorrect?

A. Tay-Sachs – hexosaminidase A

B. Metachromatic leukodystrophy – arylsulfatase A

C. Krabbe – beta glucosidase

D. Niemann Pick – shingomyelinase

Answers

1. D.

2. B.

3. D.

4. A.

5. C.

6. A.

7. D.

8. A.

9. A.

10. B.

11. C.

12. D.

13. D.

14. A.

15. A.

16. C.

17. D.

18. C.

19. B.

20. C.

Chapter 6: Practical Neuroradiology

John J. McIntyre, MD
Margaret Montana, MD

Contents

1. Introduction

Neuroimaging is arguably the most exciting and rapidly progressing area in imaging. In the span of approximately four decades, the arsenal of the neuroimaging specialist has evolved from 4-view skull series and spine radiographs to now include molecular level imaging and therapeutic interventions in the small vessel vascular bed. The depiction of the neuroanatomy is to submillimeter resolution. The anatomical assessment is complemented by tissue characterization, which can often aid non-invasive diagnosis. Connections among the components of the central nervous system are being defined and mapped to allow assessment of functional relationships and their disruption in maldevelopment of and injury to the neural tissues. Neuroimaging is a frontier that is on the move.

It is a somewhat daunting task to attempt to summarize and present some basic principles of neuroimaging. It's like chasing a moving target as the technology evolves so quickly. However, an attempt will be made to introduce the reader to some common principles of neuroimaging, the relative strengths and weaknesses of the imaging repertoire, and some of the generally accepted algorithms for patient management in several, more common neurological clinical scenarios. Additionally, some concepts of "what to watch for" in the near future of neuroimaging will be presented.

2. Technologies of Neuroimaging

The technologies of neuroimaging represent a wide spectrum of choice. Each modality offers strengths and weaknesses that must be understood to fully realize their respective potential. The optimum use of these modalities represents a partnership among the varying modalities to best define the anatomy, the functional consequences, and the therapeutic options of treating neurological disease.

The work engines of neuroimaging are MRI and CT. Their use has expanded to now represent a majority of all imaging done in the United States. What was once a "simple" CT has now evolved to include multi-detector CT with CT angiography and perfusion study capability. MRI now encompasses MR spectroscopy, diffusion-weighted imaging, and perfusion studies. In some centers, functional MRI is requested daily. The choice of imaging sequences for a MRI exam is expanding and allows the imager to tailor the exam to best assess the clinical concerns.

Computed tomography takes advantage of the different x-ray attenuation of tissues to generate an image. The contrast among bone, air, fluid and soft tissue is great. The contrast between grey matter and white matter is less evident. The multi-detector capability now common in CT equipment can generate images that are submillimeter thick that retain high signal-to-noise ratio and allow reformation in multiple planes. The near instantaneous post-processing capability in CT angiography allows display of intracranial vessels similiar to digital subtraction angiography or display with the background of the environs of the vessels included. 3D reformations are generated within seconds of data acquisition. The advantages and weaknesses of CT are noted in Table 1.

Magnetic resonance imaging uses the different responses of nuclei in varying chemical environments to radiofrequency pulses and gradient coils to generate an image. The basic sequences in MRI are the T1- and T2-weighted sequences. With hardware development, these sequences can now be obtained within seconds to minutes with "turbo" or "fast" imaging. Basically, the T1-weighted images offer high contrast between gray and white matter. Anatomy is very well depicted with T1-weighted images. Water and CSF are rendered black on T1-weighted images. The T2-weighted images offer

Table 1

CT Overview

Strengths	Weaknesses
Wide availability	Radiation exposure
Quick	Less soft tissue contrast Less motion artifact (with respect to MRI)
Relatively less expensive	May need iodinated contrast (contraindicated in renal insufficiency, allergic patients)
Excellent bone detail	
High spatial resolution	
Acute trauma evaluation	
Multiplanar reconstruction capability	

tissue characterization and detection of abnormalities because of the conspicuity of water in this pulse sequence.

Cerebrospinal fluid and water are of high signal (white) on T2-weighted images, as are most pathologic abnormalities. Contrast enhancement with gadolinium is often used—not so much for the detection of abnormality, as is typical with iodinated contrast enhancement in CT, but with the goal of further characterization of an already detected abnormality.

FLAIR (fluid attenuated inversion recovery) images are T2-weighted images that suppress the high signal of CSF in the ventricles and sulci but retain high signal in water containing lesions adjacent to these areas. This allows improved contrast between the abnormal tissue and the CSF and therefore, improved detection. The basic "screening" brain MRI will generally include T1-weighted images, often in a sagittal projection, and axial T2 and FLAIR images.

Diffusion-weighted images assess the movement or restriction of movement of water among cells. With unrestricted movement or Brownian motion, the diffusion coefficient of water is high and the DWI image signal is low (dark), and the apparent diffusion coefficient (ADC) is high (white). This is because the protons which were acted on by the gradient pulse and then rephased have moved to another location before they can be measured. With water motion restriction as seen in acute ischemia, the diffusion is low, the signal on DWI is high (white), and the ADC is low (black). This is because the rephased protons in water in the damaged swollen cells have not moved and will be present when it is time to be measured. Much work has been done to assess the DWI appearance of several pathologies in the brain and spine including the differentiation of abscess and neoplasm, acute vs. chronic spinal fracture, ongoing demyelination in normal-appearing white matter, etc., to aid the non-invasive diagnosis of neural pathology.

Gradient recall echo (GRE) images are modifications of the basic T1- and T2-weighted images that can be obtained very fast and offer a high sensitivity to blood products. These sequences will often be added to the routine sequences in patients with a history of trauma, vascular malformations, etc. They do, however, suffer from a heightened sensitivity to motion and artifact at bone-air interfaces; eg, temporal bone region. Susceptibility-weighted imaging (SWI) consists of using both magnitude and phase images from a high-resolution gradient-echo sequence. SWI is currently being used as an emerging technique to improve diagnosis of neurological trauma, brain neoplasms, and neurovascular diseases such as vascular malformations and amyloid angiopathy because of its sensitivity in revealing microhemorrhage (Figure 1a, 1b).[24,25,26]

Spectroscopy in MRI offers an analysis of the molecular composition of the neural tissues. No images are generated— only spectra that highlight the molecular composition of tissues. The most common cellular entities assessed in neuroradiology include N-acetyl aspartate (NAA), choline (Cho), creatine (Cr), lactate, myo-inositol (myo), and lipids. The most frequent uses currently are as an adjunct to anatomic imaging in the further characterization of masses suspect for malignancy, confirming abscess in the setting of a rim enhancing mass with a differential of necrotic neoplasm, and the differentiation of radiation necrosis and tumor recurrence in the setting of recurrent enhancement after radiation therapy (Figure 2a, 2b). One rare lesion where spectroscopy can be helpful is Lhermitte Duclos. Lactate peaks are seen without elevation in the choline and a relatively blunted Na peak.[27]

CT perfusion is a relatively new qualitative and quantitative technique that generates perfusion maps using the central volume principle (CBF = CBV/MTT) to generate maps of Cerebral Blood Flow (CBF), Cerebral Blood Volume (CFV), and Mean Transit Time (MTT). Most currently available CT vendors offer software applications to create perfusion maps. CT perfusion has been useful in the evaluation of ischemia, infarction, and vasospasm. Used in conjunction with an acetazolamide challenge, CT perfusion is used in the evaluation of cerebrovascular reserve in the setting of

Figure 1a

SWI Images

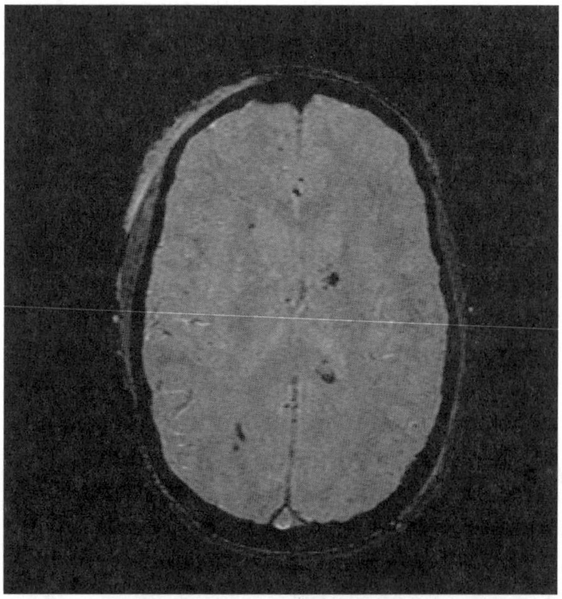

Figure 1b

Demonstrates blood products in left splenium of the corpus callosum, left deep white matter of the basal ganglia and the grey white junction over the convexity in the left frontal lobe.

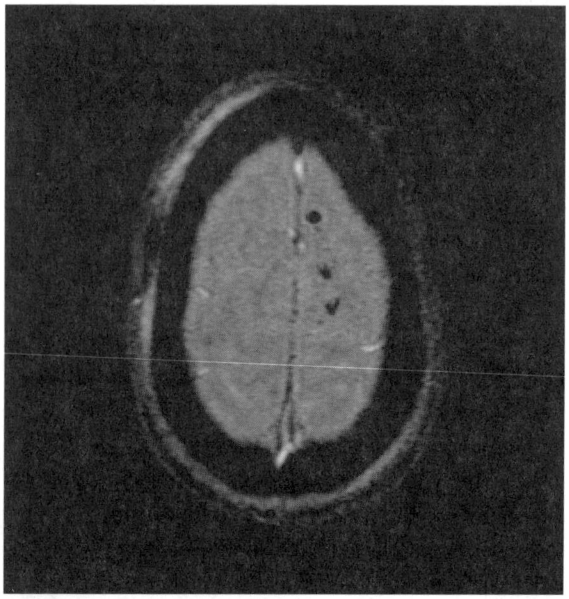

Figure 2a and 2b

Post-gadolinium T1 image and spectroscopy in patient with recurrent GBM

Demonstrating a rim-enhancing lesion with malignant Spectra. There is an elevated choline peak at 3 ppm (parts per million) and a blunted NAA peak at 2 ppm.

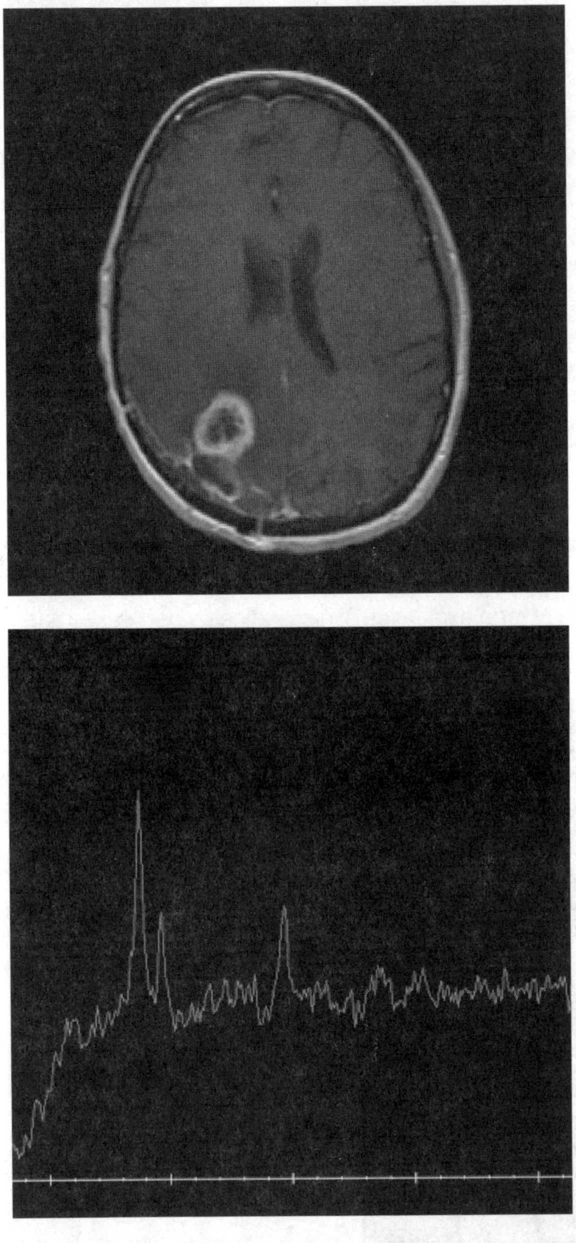

vascular stenosis. MRI perfusion images combined with DWI images have the added advantage of being able to assess jeopardized but potentially viable brain tissue, ischemic penumbra. These techniques can be helpful to vascular neurologists evaluating stroke symptoms, neurosurgeons considering revascularization, or doctors contemplating surgery that may alter cardiac output such as cardiac bypass surgery (Figure 3a, 3b).[28]

Technological advances in MR imaging offer the possibility of producing a diagnostic image in a moving subject or an unsedated patient. MR imaging now offers an alternative to CT in the evaluation of hydrocephalus, without the inherent risks of ionizing radiation for either the child or an adult immobilizing the child. An added benefit of MR is the additional information resulting from improved contrast in the brain parenchyma and multiplanar capabilities.

Propellar Imaging

Periodically rotated overlapping parallel lines with enhanced reconstruction (PROPELLER) is a technique of data collection and reconstruction used to compensate for head motion during MR imaging in adults and the unsedated pediatric patient. This correction is made possible with the acquisition of data with a series of concentric blades, each of which rotates through the center of k-space.[29]

The "art" of MRI is to utilize a variety of imaging parameters to selectively assess these different responses of molecules to help characterize the tissue. For instance, the evolving blood products of a hematoma generate different signal intensities on T1-weighted images as compared to T2-weighted images, as compared to gradient echo images during the course of radiographic follow-up. This pattern of evolution may allow an estimate of radiographic "dating" of the acuity of the hemorrhage, as well as assess for underlying pathology that might be related causally to the hematoma. The expected pattern of the evolution of brain parenchymal hemorrhage is presented in Table form (Table 2). This pattern should be used as a guide only and cannot be extrapolated to extra parenchymal hemorrhages. Though the changing appearance of parenchymal hemorrhage on MRI has been described, this

Figure 3a

CT perfusion images demonstrate diminished Cerebral Blood Flow, diminished Cerebral Blood Volume, and an increase in the Mean Transit Time consistent with an acute infarction in the left MCA territory.

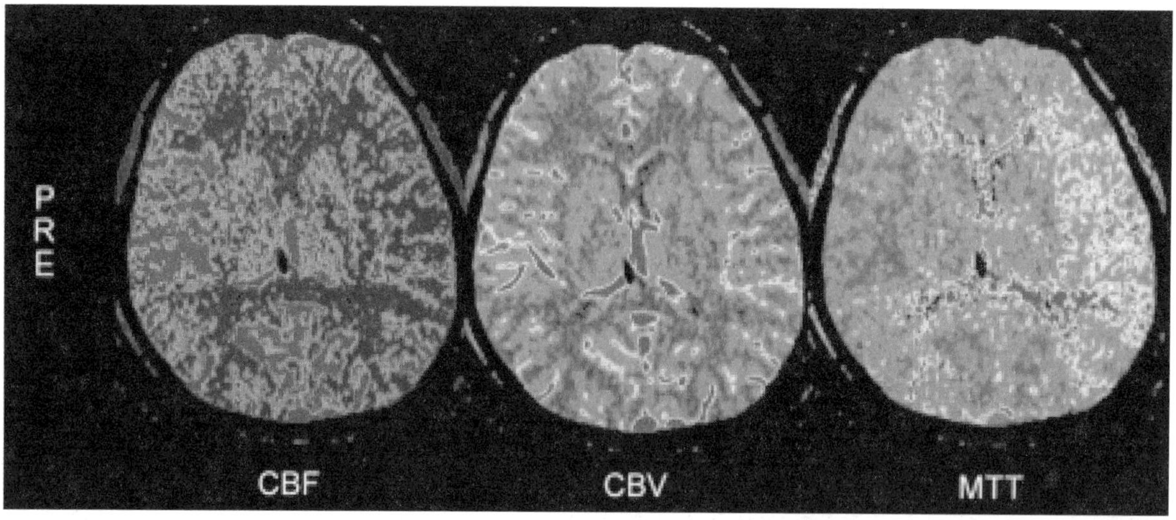

Figure 3b

MRI perfusion images pre- and post-diamox demonstrate areas of perfused viable brain tissue which show decreased perfusion after the administration of the vasodilator, acetazolamide, which indicates decreased vascular reserve in the affected areas relative to the normal brain parenchyma.

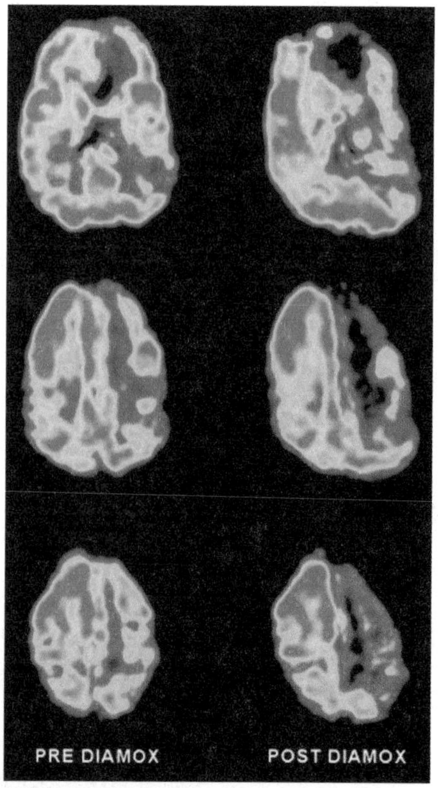

Image courtesy of Cliff Eskey, M.D.

information is controversial, with some evidence pointing to the relatively nonspecific appearance of parenchymal hemorrhage with time.[30]

The paradigm shift in imaging represented by MRI is that no longer are imagers relegated only to assessment of the anatomy of the neural tissues—although the anatomy is portrayed in exquisite detail. Now, with MRI and its partner technologies, cellular-level imaging is available. The membrane turnover in multiple sclerosis can be reflected in an elevated choline spike in MR spectroscopy (MRS) in areas of normal-appearing white matter. A subtle gyral bulge anatomically associated with an elevated choline and decreased N-acetyl-asparate (NAA) on MRS is very worrisome for a low-grade tumor. A hyperacute stroke, within hours of ictus, may only be depicted by increased signal on diffusion-weighted imaging, representing the cytotoxic edema resulting from breakdown of the ATPase cellular energy machinery.

Not all patients can undergo MRI imaging, however. Several relative and absolute contraindications exist, as noted in Table 3. With the growing indications for MR imaging, however, work is advancing on the development of surgical materials and clips that are safe for MRI. Some centers now are reporting MRI examinations performed safely on patients with cardiac pacemakers—albeit with a cardiologist in attendance during and after the exam. A good source to remain abreast of the changes in MRI safety is *MRISafety.com*.

MRI will remain a mainstay for neuroimaging and grow in its application, speed, and availability. The strengths and weakness of MRI are detailed in Table 4.

With CT and MRI as the mainstays of neuroimaging, conventional angiography, ultrasound, and PET serve as complementary modalities in patient assessment. Guide catheter and microcatheter technology allows cannulation of small vessels of the CNS for treatment of vascular malformations, delivery of chemotherapy, preoperative embolization, and embolization of life-threatening epistaxis. These microcatheters and the development of mechanical thrombolytic devices have changed the management of acute vascular occlusion through both directed delivery of intraarterial thrombolytic agents as well as the mechanical removal or ablation

Table 2

Evolution of Hematoma

	T1WI	T2WI	GRE
Hyperacute (4-6 hours)	Isointense	Hyperintense	Very hypointense
Acute (7-72 hours)	Isointense	Hypointense	Very hypointense with "blooming"
Early subacute (3-7 days)	Hyperintense	Hypointense	Very hypointense with "blooming"
Late subacute (1 week – months)	Hyperintense	Hyperintense with hypointense rim	Very hypointense with "blooming"
Chronic (months – years)	Hypointense to isointense	Hypointense	Very hypointense with "blooming"

Table 3

MRI Contraindications

Absolute
Cardiac pacemaker
Cochlear implant
Electronic stimulator implant
Orbital metal
Relative
Claustrophobia
Body habitus precludes positioning (Consider open magnet)
Recent surgery (usually wait 6-8 weeks to image) (More relevant re abdominal and general surgery where clips have been used)
Pregnancy (Especially first trimester) (Gadolinium has not been approved for use)

of thrombus. Vascular stenting of both extracranial and intracranial vessels and nonoperative treatment of cerebral aneurysms with coils delivered by microcatheter are rapidly expanding areas of neuroradiology and have replaced or become adjuncts to surgical treatments in many cases.[31]

Ultrasound is somewhat more limited in application in neuroimaging, but has an undeniable role in the assessment of the carotid bifurcation and neonatal brain. Ultrasound screening for the high-risk, asymptomatic patient for carotid stenosis is an easily obtained, relatively inexpensive triage study. Transcranial Doppler can be used in the post-operative patient for assessment of vascular compromise and spasm.

Table 4

MRI Overview

Strengths	**Weaknesses**
Soft tissue contrast	Relatively longer exam
Multiplanar capability	Contraindications (Table 3)
Tissue characterization	Relatively expensive
Cellular function	
High sensitivity to abnormality	
Improved specificity	

PET scanning offers a new tool in the assessment of dementia, epilepsy, and movement disorders. Depending on the isotope used, neurotransmitter function can be assessed. The hope is that different patterns of isotope uptake will help diagnosis different dementias prior to the destruction of neural tissue that is apparent on the anatomical studies. Malignant lesions demonstrate increased uptake of FDG when compared with surrounding brain parenchyma. Because of relatively low spacial resolution and the relatively high glucose avidity of normal gray matter, PET imaging is not used as a routine element of the imaging workup for patients presenting with a symptom or sign of a brain parenchymal mass lesion.

Uses of FDG PET in the evaluation of patients diagnosed with or suspected of having a brain tumor include grading, localization for biopsy, differentiation of radiation necrosis from tumor recurrence, therapeutic monitoring, and assessment for malignant transformation of what were originally low-grade gliomas. More specific radiopharmaceuticals are on the horizon that may enable specific targeting of tumor cells, improving the tissue contrast between normal brain and tumor.[32]

The caveat to these choices in neuroimaging is that communication between the neurological clinician and imager must be enhanced and maintained. Contrary to a rose, a brain MRI is not a brain MRI is not a brain MRI. Choices abound regarding the modality, sequences, and protocols to consider in neuroimaging, and a complete history and expression of the clinical concern and question are necessary to optimize patient care and management.

Figure 4

Right MCA infarct

Note the hyperdense right MCA with loss of the grey-matter delineation of the lentiform nuclei and edema and loss of sulci of the right cerebral hemisphere.

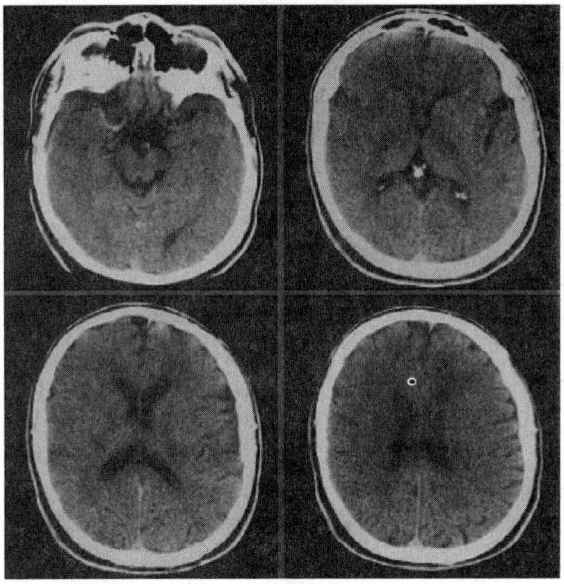

3. Ischemia and Infarction

Stroke remains the third leading cause of death in the United States and the leading cause of disability. Some 750,000 people a year suffer a first or recurrent stroke. For many people, the spectre of a stroke-induced disability, loss of speech and/or motor skills, or the inability to care for oneself is a haunting prospect indeed.

The role of imaging in the acute setting of a possible stroke is to assess for possible stroke mimics, the extent of the ischemia, evaluate for complicating hemorrhage and/or brain swelling and edema, and to triage patients for rapid therapeutic intervention. While MRI is becoming a more valuable and utilized imaging modality in the acute setting, CT often remains the initial examination. It is widely available, rapid, relatively easy to interpret, and very sensitive to the presence of hemorrhage.

The signs of acute ischemia on CT are as follows (Figure 4):

1. Swelling and edema;

2. Loss and obscuration of the grey-white matter delineation;

3. Hyperdense MCA (neither a sensitive nor specific finding);

4. Hemorrhage may or may not be present (occurs in 15% of acute embolic strokes).

Swelling and edema are represented by effacement of the sulci in the distribution of the ischemia and low density in the ischemic area. In major arterial ischemia, the edema and swelling are in the vascular territory of the vessel. Comparison of right and left sides is very helpful in detecting subtle sulcal loss. The sylvian fissures may be asymmetrical. If severe, the ipsilateral ventricle may be compressed and the midline falx shifted away from the side of ischemia. The basal cisterns may be small or non-visualized, reflecting herniation.

The grey-white matter delineation should be sharp throughout the brain. A typical pattern in ischemia in the MCA distribution is poor delineation of the lentiform nuclei and/or insular ribbon, secondary to the swelling of ischemia. This can be very subtle in the acute stage, and follow-up CT in 24 hours may well define the ischemic change more precisely. It is helpful, though, to view the CT images at a variety of level and window settings: a narrower window offers greater soft tissue contrast and the loss of the grey-white matter delineation may be better defined.

Detecting hemorrhage is a strength of CT. In the acute stage, the hyperdensity of hemorrhage is easily visualized. Patients who have suffered a stroke involving a third or more of the MCA territory are at greater risk for hemorrhagic transformation and thrombolytic intervention is contraindicated.

As the stroke evolves, the hypodensity of edema resolves. The brain parenchyma may appear normal, but if extensive enough, with time, the infarcted tissue will become of low density and demonstrate volume loss. This is the pattern of lacunar infarcts of the basal ganglia and cerebellum. Encephalomalacia becomes evident in the cerebral hemispheres as the infarction evolves.

The limitation of CT in the detection of acute stroke without hemorrhage is that within the first 6 hours of ictus only about 38%-45% of acute strokes are appreciated on CT. In many cases, this does not affect patient management in that in the appropriate clinical situation and with no evidence of hemorrhage or other intracranial process causing the patient's symptomatology, treatment can proceed. The touted advantage of MRI is that there can be earlier detection and definition of the ischemic insult in as short as 2-3 hours after ictus. No prospective studies have yet been completed to assess improved patient outcome with MRI as compared to CT, but this is a very active area of clinical research.

The findings of ischemia on MRI are similar to those of CT: edema and swelling are seen as decreased signal intensity on T1-weighted images and increased signal on T2-weighted and FLAIR images. The grey-white matter signal differences are blunted and there may be mass effect and shift. The hyperdense MCA seen on CT is depicted as increased signal within the vessel lumen, implying clot. Normally, vessels of high flow such as the arteries of the circle of Willis and the dural venous sinuses demonstrate a lack of signal ("flow void phenomenon") because of the signal loss of the red blood cells leaving the image plane with vascular flow.

Diffusion imaging is the added jewel of imaging ischemia with MRI. DWI depicts the early consequence of disruption of the ATPase energy generating system of cellular metabolism. With ischemia, the ATPase system can no longer function. The cells lose their control of the influx of sodium and water and there is a swelling of the cells (cytotoxic edema). This occurrence is imaged as increased signal on DWI with a decrease in apparent diffusion coefficient (ADC). This pattern can be detected within hours of the vascular compromise and peaks over 3 days. Reported sensitivities range from 80%-100%. After 3-7 days, the DWI images may appear normal as the brain begins its repair process.

This cytotoxic edema of ischemia should be differentiated from vasogenic edema, which represents a breakdown of the blood-brain barrier. In contradistinction to cytotoxic edema, vasogenic edema demonstrates an increased signal on DWI but with a normal or elevated ADC. This results in the so-called "T2 shine-through" phenomenon where the vasogenic edema is visualized as increased signal on both T2WI and DWI. Vasogenic edema is generally reversible. Cytotoxic edema is not, and cell loss is expected in the area of cytotoxic edema. Vasogenic edema develops later in the course and evolution of the ischemia and infarct. The vasogenic edema of infarction will generally peak within the first 3-5 days of an infarct and often begins to resolve by the first week. It may take weeks for all the edema to resolve, however. The diagnosis of posterior reversible encephalopathy syndrome, seen in hypertensive encephalopathy, eclampsia, and preeclampsia, is characterized by the reversible pattern of vasogenic edema on DWI.

The role of contrast enhancement in the acute setting of ischemia has evolved to CT angiography and CT and/or MRI perfusion studies. MR angiography is performed without gadolinium enhancement required. MR perfusion does require gadolinium injection. There are typical patterns of enhancement of an evolving stroke on both CT and MRI, which can aid confirmation of the diagnosis if some uncertainty exists. However, more importantly for the immediate management of the patient, the angiographic studies are performed to assess the extent of the vascular occlusion that has led to the ischemia. This serves not only for diagnosis, but if intra-arterial therapy is indicated, can aid the neurointerventionalist as a "roadmap" to expedite the therapeutic procedure. The perfusion patterns of the brain are studied for asymmetry and extent of the insult. Parameters depicted with perfusion studies include cerebral blood volume (CBV), mean transit time (MTT), and cerebral blood flow (CBF).

In MR perfusion studies, correlation with diffusion-weighted images is being used to assess for the penumbra of "at-risk" but not yet infarcted neural tissue. Areas with diminished perfusion, but normal diffusion appearance represent the target tissue for intervention and attempted protection. These areas represent tissues with some compromise of blood flow, depicted on the perfusion images, but cell damage and malfunction has not yet occurred, as indicated by the normal appearance on diffusion-weighted images. These concepts continue to be areas of active clinical investigation.

Imaging of white matter disease has blossomed with the advent of MRI. Lesions can be depicted on CT as low-density foci, but their depiction can be quite subtle and the extent of disease is often underestimated on CT. However, MRI has a high sensitivity for white matter lesions, particularly with the development of FLAIR sequences. In fact, when MRI was first introduced, many reports noted "UBOs," the unidentified bright objects in the brain—of unknown etiology and significance. Understanding of these lesions has increased, and there now is an appreciation that the pattern and distribution of white matter lesions can offer a more specific diagnosis and guidance for patient management.

The prototypical white matter disease evaluated with imaging is multiple sclerosis. In the United States, 0.1%-0.2% of the population is affected, and the disease typically strikes young adults. The prerequisite change of lesions over time and locale are reflected both clinically and on imaging.

Imaging sequences best utilized for detection and characterization of lesions include proton-density weighted images and FLAIR images. Gadolinium is often used as a marker for determination of lesion activity and acuity. Enhancement implies an active lesion and the enhancement would be expected to lessen and /or resolve within 3-6 months. T1-weighted images are useful for the detection of "black holes," purportedly the end-stage of axonal degeneration or demyelination.

Follow-up studies are used to assess for new lesions, enlarging lesions, resolving lesions, and change in contrast enhancement. An attempt has been made by the Consortium of Multiple Sclerosis Centers to standardize the imaging parameters of multiple sclerosis patients to aid in this longitudinal followup. The criteria for the diagnosis of MS using MRI are detailed in Table 5.

The lesions are typically ovoid in shape and oriented perpendicular to the ventricles (Dawson's fingers). Lesions can be ring-shaped and demonstrate solid, ring, or no enhancement. Callosal volume loss and diffuse cerebral volume loss should also be assessed. A single lesion may also be noted, the so-called tumefactive MS, and can mimic tumor or abscess (Figure 5).

Figure 5

Multiple sclerosis

The FLAIR images (lower left image) best demonstrates the ovoid white matter lesions with a perpendicular orientation to the lateral ventricles.

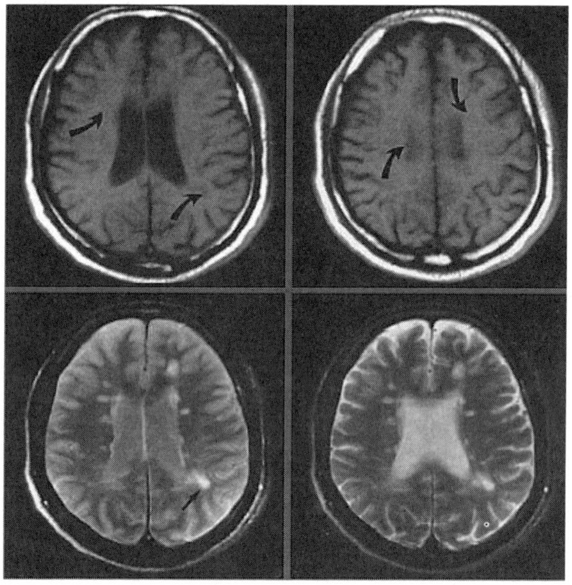

Several etiologies of white matter disease may present with similar imaging findings as multiple sclerosis. Those most often seen clinically include Lyme disease, vasculitis of several causes, and complex migraine. Most often, the clinical presentation allows differentiation among them. A more difficult differentiation can be between MS and microvascular ischemic change and microangiopathy. Both conditions can result in periventricular lesions. However, the lesions of MS are typically ovoid in contradistinction to the usually round morphology of microangiopathy. The corpus callosum, cerebellar peduncles, juxtacortical white matter, and the spine are more typically involved in MS. Pons involvement and gray matter lacunae are more typical of microangiopathy. At some point in the temporal evolution, at least some of the lesions of MS will demonstrate contrast enhancement. No contrast enhancement is seen in microangiopathy and microvascular ischemic change.

Dilated perivascular spaces (Virchow-Robin spaces) must be differentiated from white matter

Table 5

MRI Criteria for the Diagnosis of Multiple Sclerosis

Paty et al 1988	4 lesions >3 lesions, including 1 periventricular lesion
Fazekas et al 1988	3 lesions with 2 of the following: Infratentorial Periventricular >5 mm in diameter
Barkhof et al 1997	Cumulative based on 4 lesion characteristics: >1 juxtacortical >1 enhancing or >9 nonenhancing >1 infratentorial >3 periventricular

lesions. The dilated spaces are generally considered of no clinical significance, but can be dilated in fungal infections, especially *Cryptococcus neoformans*. Rarely, the perivascular spaces may enlarge to exert mass effect, but even then, the relationship of the large giant perivascular space to neurological complaints is uncertain. The imaging sine qua non of the dilated perivascular spaces is isointensity to CSF on all imaging sequences. This is particularly well depicted on FLAIR sequences. No contrast enhancement is seen. Additionally, the dilated spaces are typically seen in the basal ganglia, thalamus, and along the course of penetrating arteries of the midbrain.

5. Intracranial Infections

Intracranial infection can have manifold presentations, and most often, a specific etiology is not determined by the imaging findings. However, the pattern of imaging findings often allows an educated determination of the category of disease whether viral, bacterial, fungal, parasitic, etc. Biopsy is often needed, but the imaging findings can help direct the biopsy to the most efficacious area of a lesion to make a diagnosis. The strength of imaging in infection is the determination of the compartment(s) of the brain involved (parenchyma, leptomeninges, ventricles, extra-axial spaces, osseous structures), the evolution of lesions, response to therapy, and associated complications.

Cerebritis is most often a result of hematogenous seeding from an extracranial infection. More directly, sinus and/or mastoid infections can locally extend intracranially, often via a retrograde thrombophlebitis. These situations can be complicated by abscess formation, empyema and/or meningitis.

The imaging findings of a cerebritis reflect its stage of maturation. Early cerebritis, seen in the first 3 to 5 days of infection, can result in an ill-defined area of low density on unenhanced CT, often with an illudane, mottled pattern of enhancement in the infected area. On MRI, the cerebritis demonstrates a subtle decrease signal on T1-weighted images and increased signal on T2-weighted images. The diffusion-weighted images will demonstrate a vasogenic edema pattern of increased signal intensity with normal ADC. Some "T2 shine-through" may also be evident. Contrast enhancement is mottled and low-grade. The cerebritis typically is at the gray-white matter junctional area and the frontal and parietal brain are the areas most affected. Occasionally, especially in the immunocompromised patient, multiple lesions may occur.

With ongoing evolution, the late cerebritis stage is characterized by a more focal, somewhat better defined lesion. This stage occurs from about 4-5 days after insult and continues for about 10-14 days. The center of the lesion becomes more liquefied and thus of less density on CT. An ill-defined rim is seen with contrast enhancement, surrounded by progressive edema. On MRI, the central necrotic area demonstrates increased signal on T2-weighted images and the developing rim exhibits prominent contrast enhancement. Peripheral edema is readily apparent on T2 and diffusion images with low intensity of the edema apparent on T1-weighted images. Satellite lesions of rim enhancement may now be seen on both CT and MRI, a helpful characteristic to suggest infection.

With further evolution, the rim of the developing abscess becomes better defined and organized. At about 2 weeks, the early capsule stage is typified by a strongly-enhancing rim, often thin but well-delineated and continuous. A common finding is that the rim is thinner on its border nearest the ependyma and thickest on the border nearest the cortex—a propensity of evolution often cited as to the etiology for ventricular rupture and the development of ventriculitis and ependymitis. Vasogenic edema is yet prominent at this stage (Figure 6). As the late capsule stage begins, which may last for weeks to months, the abscess cavity begins to shrink and the vasogenic edema resolves. The rim often persists and can become of decreased signal intensity on T2-weighted images. This loss of signal within the rim reflects the collagen that has been deposited in the rim during its evolution.

The rim-enhancement is not unique to bacterial infection and developing abscess. The differential for rim-enhancing masses include primary and metastatic tumor, subacute hematoma, tuberculoma, granuloma, fungal and parasitic infection, multiple sclerosis, infarct, thrombosed vascular malformation, and thrombosed aneurysm. Clinical presentation and assessment are obviously crucial to the differentiation among these lesions, but often biopsy is required. Diffusion weighted images are very often diagnostic as brain abscess will demonstrate increased signal on trace diffusion images with decreased signal on ADC maps, with a similar pattern to infarction. In contrast, a necrotic tumor will most often demonstrate increased signal on diffusion imaging with a normal to increased ADC, primarily due to T2 shine through. On MR spectroscopy, the central necrotic area of an abscess will have increased lactate in its spectrum. Fungal infections are more likely to be associated with perivascular infiltration and resulting vascular compromise than are bacterial infections. Fungal infections may

Figure 6

Bacterial cerebral abscess with vasogenic edema, rim enhancement, and mass effect

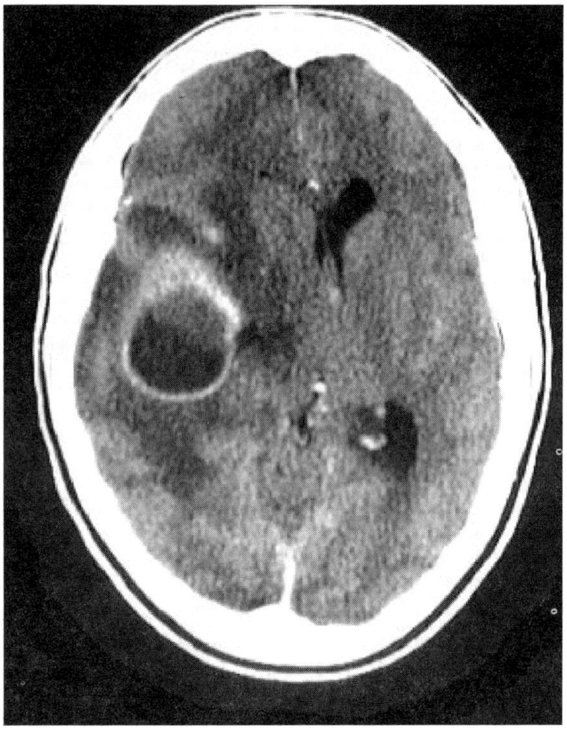

be complicated by infarcts, hemorrhage and or vascular thrombosis (Figure 7a and 7b)

Viral infections do not typically develop into abscesses. Viral meningitis is not usually imaged unless there is clinical uncertainty. If imaged, there may be mild meningeal enhancement and/or increased signal in the sulcal CSF spaces on FLAIR images.

The viral encephalitides are most often of herpetic origin and include Herpes simplex virus 1 and 2, Epstein-Barr, CMV, and varicella-zoster. Cases of Western equine, Eastern equine, and St. Louis encephalitis have been reported.

The herpes simplex 1 virus accounts for over 90% of adult encephalitis with a mortality rate of 50%-70%. The imaging findings can be suggestive

Figures 7a and 7b

A rim-enhancing lesion on post Gd T1-weighted image with central high signal on DWI trace image

The ADC map was lower in signal centrally. This finding of restricted diffusion is highly specific for pyogenic abscess where the initial post Gd T1 image is relatively nonspecific for other entities including hemorrhage and necrotic neoplasm.

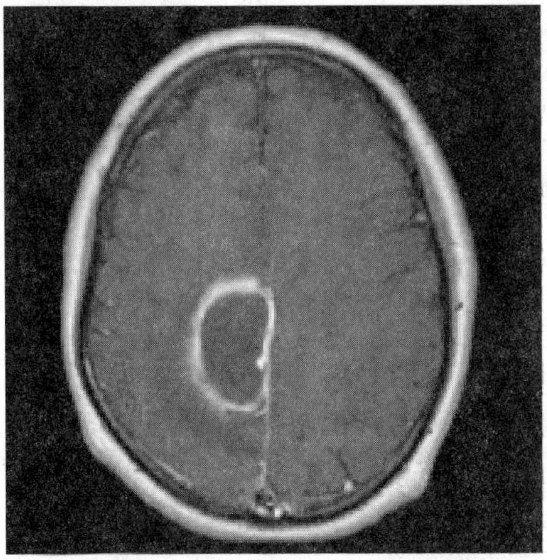

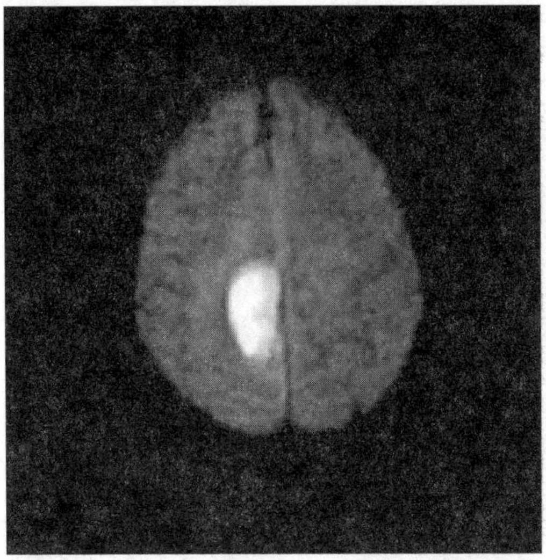

of the pathogen and may support the earlier institution of appropriate therapy. Typical findings on CT include edema and low density in the temporal lobe(s).

Some medial frontal lobe involvement may also be evident and petechial hemorrhage may occur. On MRI, these findings are reflected earlier than on CT and with improved sensitivity. The MRI findings include swelling of the gyri and high signal in the temporal and frontal lobes on T2-weighted and FLAIR images with low signal on T1-weighted images. Gradient-echo images are very sensitive to the detection of the petechial hemorrhages. Some indistinct enhancement in the areas of involvement may be seen on both CT and MRI. In the late stages of the disease, atrophy and calcifications develop.

The imaging of the neurotropic effects of the HIV virus are nonspecifiic. Imaging may be normal even in the presence of clinical ramifications. The most common finding is volume loss. Multiple scattered subcortical white matter lesions may also be seen, most commonly in the frontal lobes. These lesions eventually coalesce, but do not exert mass effect and no contrast enhancement is evident. The grey matter is typically spared. These imaging findings reflect the demyelination that occurs with the viral infection.

More vivid imaging is present with the superimposition of the opportunistic infections and/or tumors associated with the HIV infection and resulting AIDS. Fungal infections, parasitic infections, particularly toxoplasmosis, and TB can result in contrast-enhancing masses, mass effect, prominent vasogenic edema, and hydrocephalus. The superimposition of infection with the group B human papovaviruses can result in progressive multifocal leukoencephalopathy. Demyelination is the predominant insult of PML and is reflected in the imaging findings of confluent white matter increased signal, typically in the parietoccipital regions, most often bilateral but possibly asymmetric, and without contrast enhancement (Figure 8).

Acute disseminated encephalomyelitis represents an immune-mediated neural injury initiated by viral exposure, including vaccination. Symptoms typically begin 4-21 days after the exposure and include headache, fever, meningeal irritation, and change in consciousness. The proposed mechanism is an immune reaction to the myelin of white matter, and on imaging, areas of increased signal are seen on T2-weighted images and FLAIR. Typically, the subcortical white matter is involved, but grey matter and spinal cord can be affected as well. Both supratentorial and infratentorial involvement may develop. Enhancement is common. The imaging differential is primarily multiple sclerosis and sometimes only time will tell: ADEM occurs once; MS is multiphasic.

6. Intracranial Tumors

The spectrum of imaging appearance of brain tumors is very wide and variable, and generally, biopsy is necessary to define the tumor type and classification. However, imaging is a necessary partner in the delineation of tumors at the time of diagnosis, aiding therapy and surgical planning, and monitoring response and/or complications to therapy. The goals of imaging include depiction of the location and extent of the tumor; any associated complications of the tumor such as hydrocephalus, herniation, mass effect, and/or hemorrhage; providing an assessment of probable tumor grade; and offering a differential diagnosis for tumor mimics.

The patient's age offers a first-line distinction of tumor types, followed by location. In the adult population, the most common posterior fossa tumor is a metastatic tumor. Multiplicity of lesions also suggest metastatic disease (Figure 9) although a multicentric glioblastoma can occur and intracranial lymphoma is often multifocal. Glial tumors are the most common primary tumor in the adult.

Figure 8

PML in a HIV+ patient with AIDS

Note the confluent white matter lesions with a parietal occipital predominance.

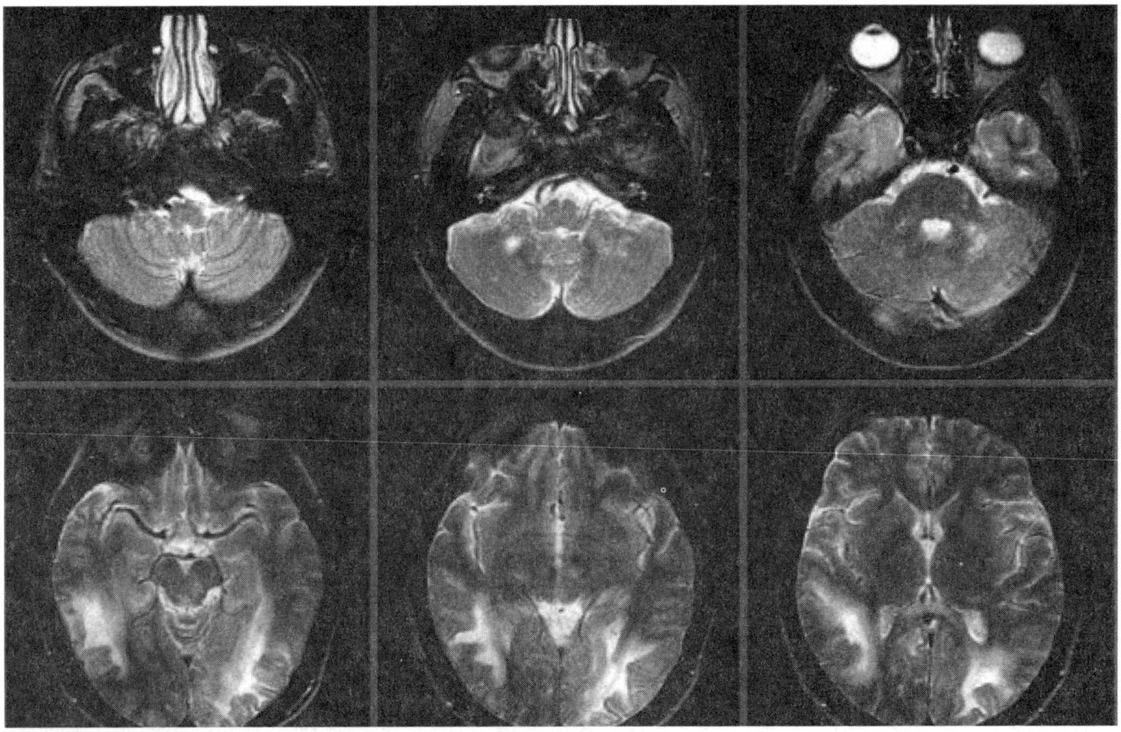

Figure 9

Intracranial metastatic lesions

Note multiplicity of enhancing lesions with propensity to be at the grey-white matter junctional region. Multifocal infection could result in this appearance as well.

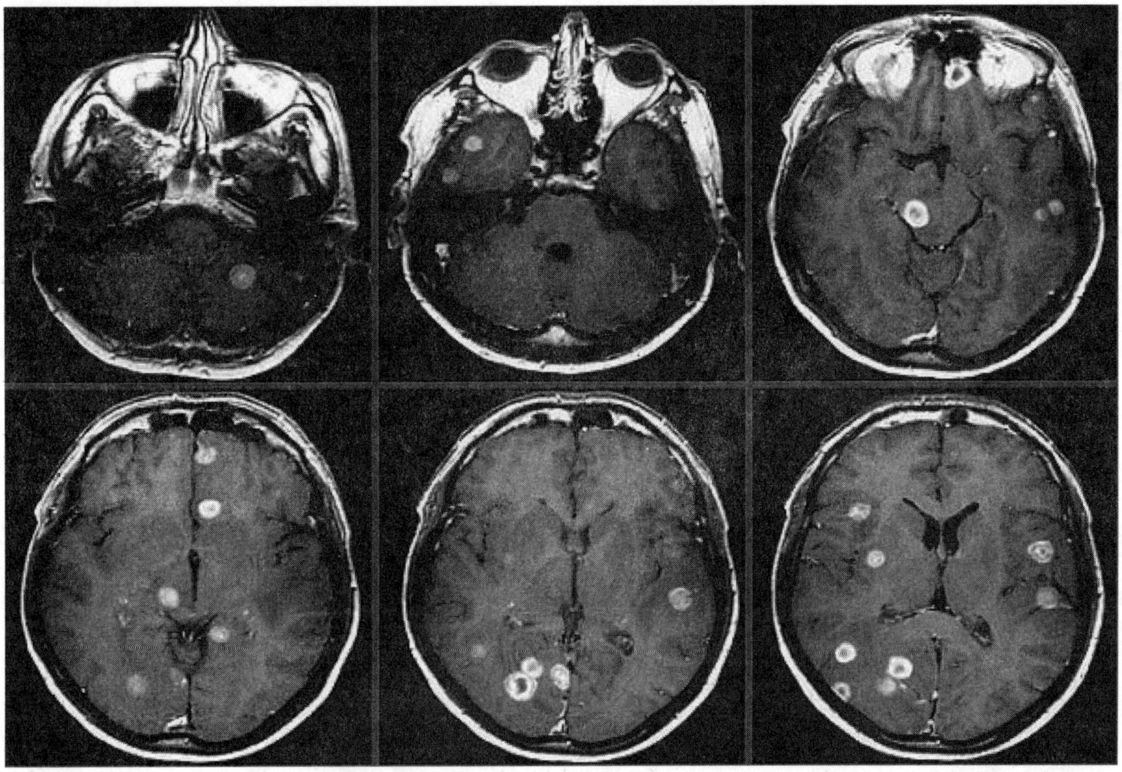

A primary distinction to be made on imaging is whether the tumor is intra-axial or extra-axial. Criteria for this assessment are noted in Table 6.

Tumors that bleed can suggest a more limited differential. The high-grade primary tumors, typically glioblastoma multiforma and anaplastic astrocytoma, can present with hemorrhage. The metastatic tumors that are associated with hemorrhage include melanoma, renal cell, choriocarcinoma, thyroid, lung and breast cancer.

Calcification within a tumor can be helpful as well, as noted in Table 7.

Attempts to preoperatively grade a tumor with imaging have classically been based on the presence and degree of contrast enhancement. The greater the enhancement, the higher the pathological grade, in general, reflecting a greater disruption of the blood-. brain barrier. The presence of necrosis also suggests a high-grade tumor (WHO III-IV). In addition, the areas of contrast-enhancement within the tumor are also usually targeted for image-guided biopsy as most probably representing the areas of most prominent tumor aggressiveness (Figure 10).

More recently, attempts to preoperatively grade tumors are being developed using PET. On PET studies, the higher-grade tumors will typically demonstrate a higher metabolic rate with 2-(18F)

Table 6

Intra-axial versus Extra-axial Masses

Gray-white junction	Displaced outwardly	Displaced inwardly
Gyral pattern	Enlarged	Compressed
Pial vessels	Peripheral displacement	Central displacement
Extra-axial CSF rim	Effaced	Widened at margin of lesion
Dural displacement	Outward	Centrally
Bony changes	Unusual	Common

Figure 10

Glioblastoma multiforme

Note the irregular, prominent contrast enhancement, associated edema, and mass effect upon the falx and ventricles.

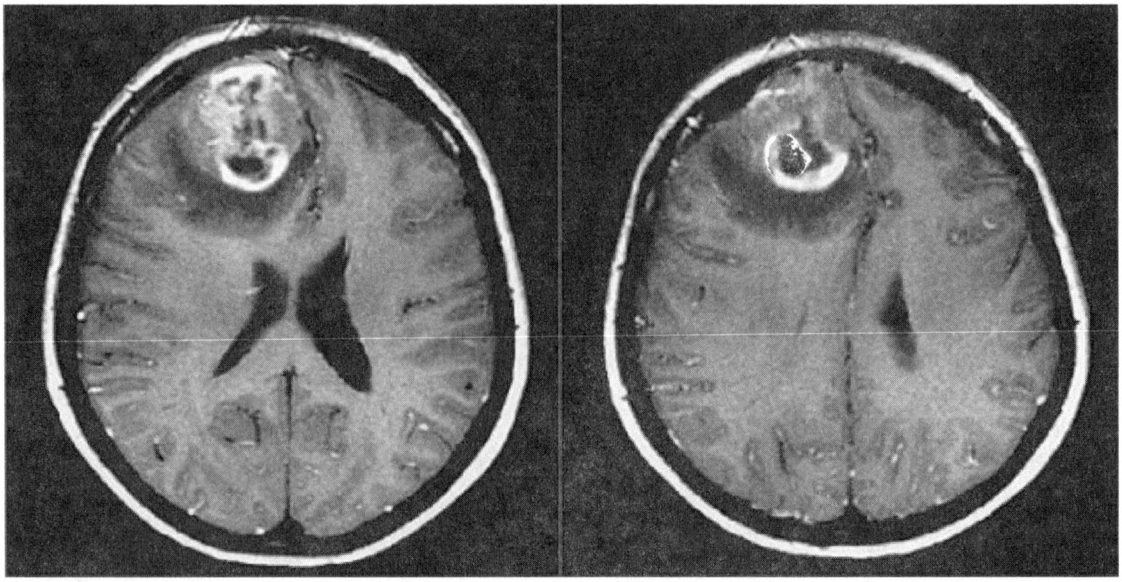

Table 7

Tumors with Calcification

Metastatic Tumors	Primary CNS Tumors	Tumors After Radiotherapy
Mucinous adenocarcinoma		
Colon	Oligodendroglioma	
Stomach		
Ovary		
Breast		
Osteosarcoma	Ependymoma	

fluoro-2-deoxy-D-glucose (FDG) than normal white matter, and a rate that approximates the metabolic rate of gray matter. A lower grade tumor (WHO I-II) will generally demonstrate a metabolic rate similar to white matter. One study noted a 94% sensitivity and a 77% specificity in preoperative tumor grading using PET. MRI perfusion offers another opportunity to further characterize the tumor's neovascularization. This shows some promise in tumor grading and the evaluation of tumor mimics. Angiogenesis, a process necessary for tumor growth can be evaluated with relative Tumor Blood Volume (rTBV). Several studies have shown that tumor grade correlates with tumor blood volume as measured relative to white matter. The absence of angiogenesis may be seen in tumor mimics such as tumefactive demyelinating disease, infarction, radiation necrosis, and cerebral abscess (Figure 11a, b, c).[33,34]

As with PET imaging of other body tumors, research is continuing on the patterns of PET imaging in tumors and the relationship to prognosis and response to therapy. Radiation necrosis often presents as a ring-enhancing mass, often with mass effect, in the initial and adjacent tumor bed, and the differentiation from recurrent tumor can be impossible with anatomical imaging modalities. PET scanning can help make this differentiation. The recurrent tumor will usually demonstrate high metabolic activity and increased FDG uptake whereas radiation necrosis will not be associated with increased metabolic activity (Figure 12a, b, c).

While most tumors are readily imaged and confirmed on CT and/or MRI, occasionally a low-grade tumor may be difficult to confirm. Such a tumor may present as a subtle enlargement of a few gyri, but with no mass effect discerned. No contrast enhancement is apparent, and it can be difficult to be confident in the diagnosis. In such cases, MR spectroscopy offers a helpful alternative. With tumors, the normal N-acetyl aspartate (NAA) peak may be diminished, reflecting destruction of neural tissue. Additionally, the choline (Cho) peak is elevated, reflecting the metabolic turnover of cellular membranes and hypercellularity. Creatine (Cr) is often diminished in tumors. Works-in-progress include attempts to grade various tumors using differences in the metabolic spectrum of tumors, including NAA, Cho, Cr, alanine, lactate, and lipids.

Figures 11a, 11b and 11c

Post-Gd T1 image in patient with treated GBM

Shows recurrent rim enhancement with differential of recurrent tumor or post-radiation necrosis. There is increased perfusion relative to the adjacent white matter consistent with recurrent tumor.

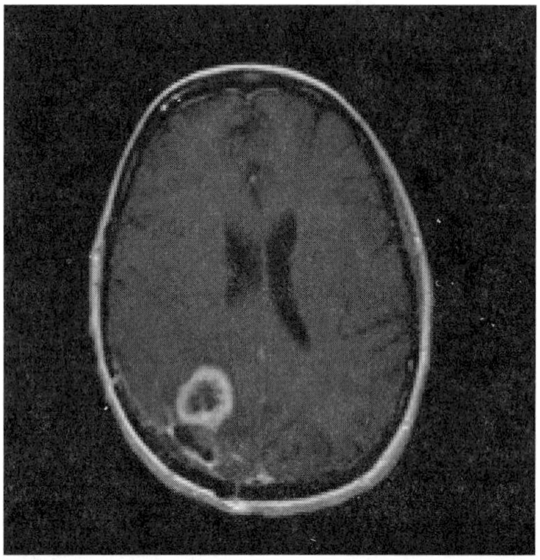

A.

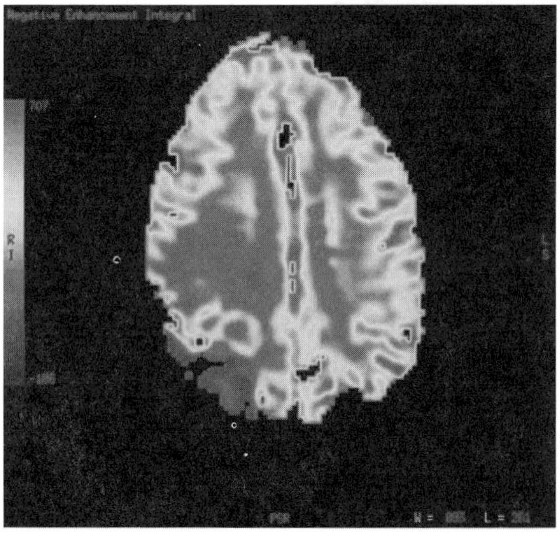

B.

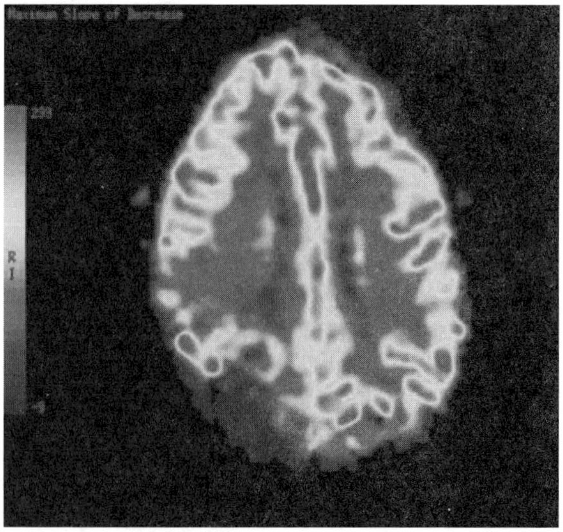

C.

Figure 12a

Patient with known GBM status post-surgery, chemotherapy and radiation therapy

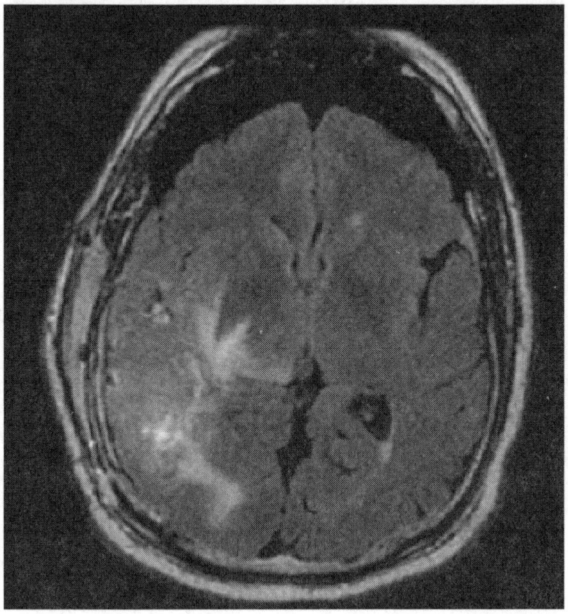

Figure 12b

Post-gadolinium image

Shows peripheral enhancement adjacent to the surgical bed, which is nonspecific for tumor recurrence and radiation necrosis.

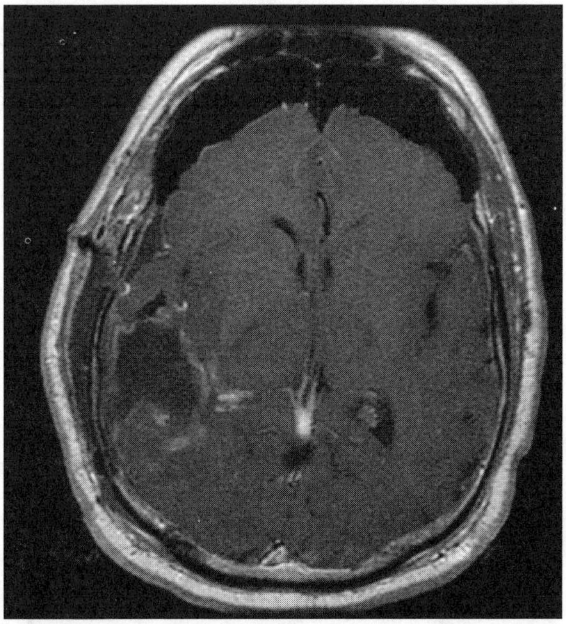

Figure 12c

FDG PET image

Demonstrates increased metabolic activity compared to the adjacent white matter in the anterior aspect of the surgical bed consistent with tumor recurrence.

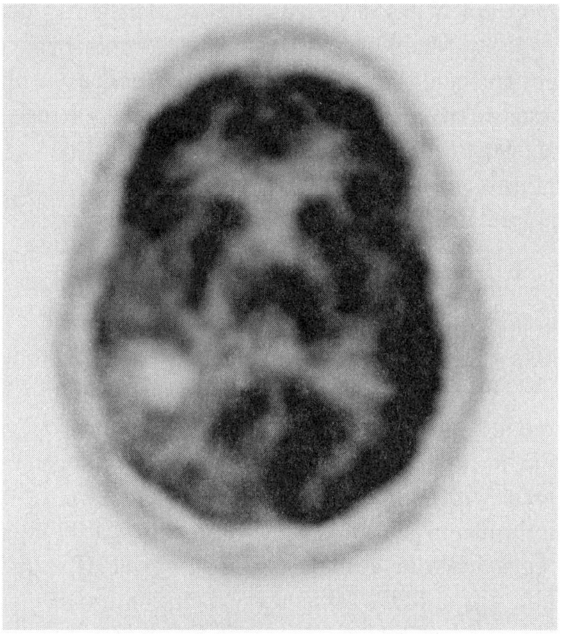

Image courtesy of Mark Seltzer, M.D., Dartmouth Hitchcock Medical Center.

7. Epilepsy and Seizures

In the not too distant past, EEG and electrophysiological studies were the mainstay for the diagnosis and localization of epileptogenic lesions. With the advent of high-field strength magnets, high-resolution phased array coils, and functional and metabolic imaging, neuroimaging has become a more potent ally in the management of patients with epilepsy. Neuroimaging can aid the detection of an epileptogenic focus in complex partial epilepsy with a sensitivity of 75%-95% for hippocampal sclerosis and 90% for other focal lesions, such as tumors, gliosis, and infarct. MRI and neuroimaging are less helpful in the patient with generalized epilepsy.

In addition to defining a lesion as the focus of epileptic activity, the role of imaging includes an assessment as to whether the surgical excision of the lesion is possible, what functional, normal brain might be at risk, and to allow some assessment of the functional interconnections of the epileptogenic focus with normal brain areas. The anatomical information generated with MR imaging can be co-registered with the metabolic imaging of PET scanning and/or SPECT scanning to help confirm the abnormal neural function. On PET scanning, typically performed interictally, the abnormal focus is typically hypometabolic. On SPECT imaging, which can be performed during the seizure ictus, the abnormal focus is hyperperfused.

The imaging evaluation of epilepsy requires attention to detail with thin images and high contrast between grey and white matter. Contrast enhancement is not often helpful in the epileptic patient without tumor, infarct, or infection. Image sequences typically include T1, T2, and FLAIR sequences of the entire brain. Thin, oblique coronal images perpendicular to the axis of the temporal lobes and hippocampus are necessary for optimal evaluation of the hippocampus and parahippocampal regions in the assessment for mesial temporal sclerosis. High-resolution 3D IR-SPGR images offer excellent grey-white matter contrast and are invaluable in the assessment of developmental dysmorphic brain changes.

The assessment of the images requires concentration and a directed, patterned approach. Several of the possible findings in epilepsy are subtle and difficult to detect. Several lesions represent abnormal patterns of morphology without abnormal signal intensity (eg, heterotopia). Some authors suggest the use of the HIPPO SAGE mnemonic to guide the analysis of the images (Table 8).

Table 8

HIPPO SAGE Mnemonic

H:	Hypothalamic hamartoma; hippocampal size and signal abnormality
I:	Internal auditory canal and atrial asymmetry
P:	Periventricular heterotopia
P:	Peripheral abnormalities
S:	Sulcal morphologic abnormalities
A:	Atrophy
G:	Gray matter thickening
E:	Encephalocele of anterior temporal lobe
O:	Obvious lesion

The positioning of the patient can be crucial in epilepsy evaluations. Some tilting or rotation of the patient's head can make it very difficult to assess for and confirm gyral asymmetry, heterotopia, or lissencephaly. Some volumetric evaluation is being done in academic centers, research centers, and progressive communities. The programs are cumbersome to use and require establishment of unique normative values for a given institution, however, which hampers widespread use. An appreciation of normal variations is also required in the assessment of the epileptic patient. Virchow-Robin spaces (dilated perivascular spaces), arachnoid cysts, choroidal fissure cyst, venous angiomas, etc., are common findings on MR imaging, but have not been implicated as epileptogenic foci.

The detection of mesial temporal sclerosis is a success story for MRI with a sensitivity of over 75% reported. In patients with refractory temporal lobe seizures, the depiction of the abnormal focus may determine surgical excision and possible cure and if not, decreased refractoriness to medical therapy.

The predominant findings of mesial temporal sclerosis are depicted on the coronal thin T2 and/or FLAIR images and the high-contrast SPGR images. The normal hippocampus is isointense to gray matter. A mild increase of signal can be seen in the hippocampus on FLAIR images, which is felt to be secondary to some partial volume artifact from adjacent CSF signal. The typical findings of mesial temporal sclerosis are volume loss of the involved hippocampus and abnormal increased signal intensity. These imaging findings reflect the neuronal loss of Ammon's horn and dentate nucleus of the hippocampus with associated gliosis (Figure 13).

Additionally, ancillary findings of mesial temporal sclerosis can be seen and include atrophy of the ipsilateral fornix and mammillary body, temporal lobe volume loss, dilation of the ipsilateral temporal horn reflecting the temporal lobe volume loss, and white matter loss and/or signal abnormality in the anterior temporal lobe.

Developments in epilepsy imaging will undoubtedly include higher resolution with 3T machines, improved volumetrics, diffusion-weighted imaging with tractography to delineate abnormal white matter connections, and more widespread functional MRI to assess the connections of the epileptogenic focus throughout the brain. MR spectroscopy has begun to be used as well. A decrease in the NAA/creatine or NAA/creatine + choline ratio has been helpful in localization of the side of the epileptogenic focus in 65%-95% of patients with bilateral abnormal MRI studies and in 20% of patients with normal MRI studies. As spectroscopy is expanded to include neurotransmitters, some assessment of the metabolic derangements in epilepsy may be better assessed. A role for such assessment in monitoring response to therapy may develop.

Figure 13

Mesial temporal sclerosis

Note the volume loss of the hippocampus bilaterally.

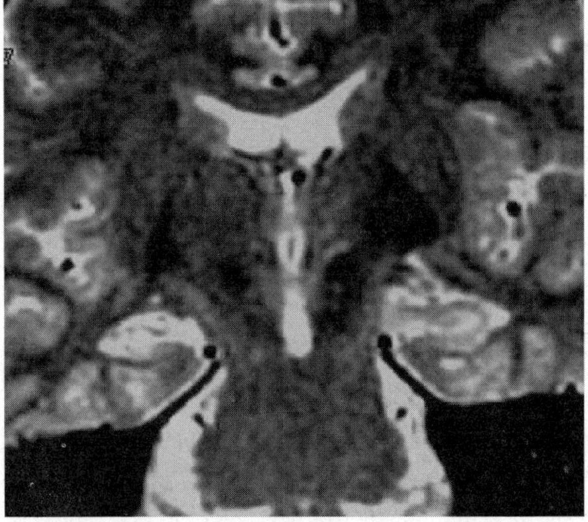

8. Dementia and Degenerative Diseases

With the aging of the population, the dementias and degenerative diseases of the brain represent a growing societal burden reflected in rising health care costs and increased need for nursing home care. The dementias also offer an exciting area of active research into the natural history of the diseases, their pathophysiology, and the clinical and imaging markers that might help predict and thus treat early the dementia and/or degenerative processes. Previously, imaging was used only to exclude other, treatable causes of dementia. More recently, patterns of abnormality are being defined to aid in the actual diagnosis of the dementia or degenerative process.

The developmental degenerative processes such as the inherited mucopolysaccharidoses, mitochondrial diseases, and other metabolic storage diseases are beyond the scope of this chapter. Typically, these patients will present in infancy or young childhood, and the diseases represent a destruction of previously developed, normal white matter and neurons.

The most pervasive imaging finding in dementias is volume loss. The pattern and location of the volume loss may be helpful in defining a particular type of dementia. Volume loss typically is associated with ventricular enlargement, and it may be a difficult assessment to distinguish between cerebral volume loss and hydrocephalus. A summary of helpful criteria are presented in Table 9.

The most prevalent dementia is Alzheimer disease. Estimates suggest that over 10% of persons over 65 years of age and 50% of those over 85 years of age are affected by AD. The defining imaging pattern of AD is hippocampal and medial temporal lobe volume loss. Often a more generalized atrophy is also apparent. White matter lesions in themselves are not a prominent feature of AD imaging. Compare Figure 14 of hydrocephalus with Figure 15 of volume loss of Alzheimer disease. Pick disease, in contrast, demonstrates a predominant frontal lobe volume loss with some temporal lobe atrophy as well.

Normal-pressure hydrocephalus can be a difficult diagnosis radiographically, and a challenge to distinguish from volume loss. A disproportionate ventriculomegaly with the degree of sulcal prominence can suggest NPH. A smooth pattern of signal increase in the periventricular white matter, typical of transependymal migration of CSF, is also suggestive of NPH. Radionuclide cisternography with 111In-DTPA can be helpful. In NPH, there is no flow of the isotope over the convexities and ventricular reflux persists at 24-48 hours. The normal cisternography can demonstrate transient ventricular reflux of the isotope on early images, but the ventricular reflux does not persist to 24 hours. Additionally, there will be flow of isotope over the convexities in the normal patient. In some cases, a trial of high-volume CSF removal will be necessary.

Table 9

Hydrocephalus versus Volume Loss

Criteria	**Hydrocephalus**	**Volume Loss**
Sulci	Effaced, small	Large
Ventricles	Enlarged with bulging contours	Enlarged with more normal contours
Fourth ventricle	Enlarged	Normal
Corpus callosum	Stretched	More lax in contour
Transependymal migration of CSF	Present acutely	Not evident
Mammillopontine distance	Decreased	Increased

Figure 14

Hydrocephalus

Note normal to small size of sulci with ventriculomegaly. Increased signal about the ventricles suggests transependymal migration of CSF.

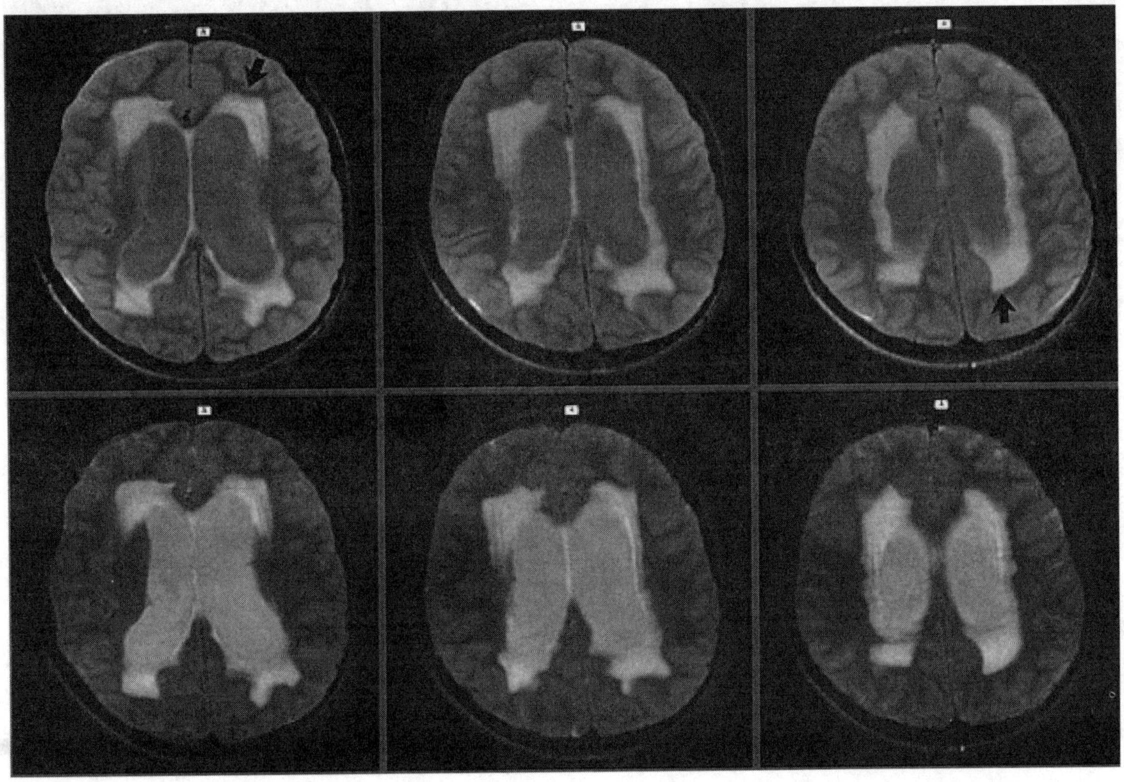

The multi-infarct dementia, sometimes called Binswanger disease, is a microvascular ischemic dementia, often caused by hypertension and related risk factors. In contrast to AD, images demonstrate a predominance of white matter changes, particularly in the peritrigone regions and periventricular white matter frontally. The white matter lesions are "lumpy-bumpy" in the periventricular regions and distributed throughout the corona radiata. Gray matter lacunar infarcts are a common feature and pontine involvement is not uncommon. Volume loss is typical as well.

The prion dementia of Creutzfeldt-Jakob disease, also termed spongiform encephalopathy, typically demonstrates increased signal in the basal ganglia on T2 images with volume loss. This increase in signal probably represents the increased water content of the spongy, vacuolized cells seen pathologically. Recent reports indicate that diffusion weighted images may detect these changes earlier than the T2 and/or FLAIR images.

Parkinson disease can be associated with dementia in 30% of the affected patients. The clinical symptoms are related to the depletion of pigmented cells that produce dopamine in the substantia nigra. This depletion is reflected as a thinning of the pars compacta of the substantia nigra on T2-weighted images. In the Parkinson-plus syndromes, increased iron deposition is noted in the basal ganglia, which results in

Figure 15

Alzheimer disease with predominant temporal parietal volume loss, prominent sulci and no evidence of transependymal migration of CSF

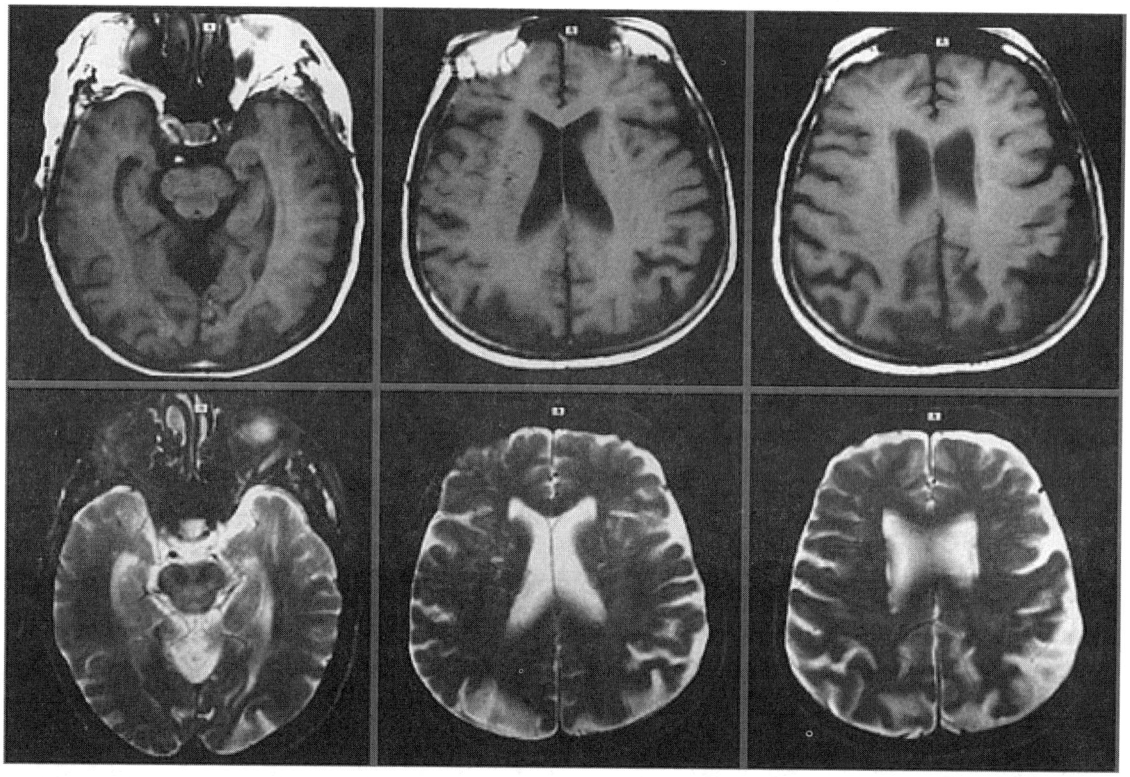

decreased signal intensity in the putamen as compared to the globus pallidus on T2-weighted sequences. In the normal person, the globus pallidus demonstrates decreased signal intensity as compared to the putamen. In striatonigral degeneration, the iron deposition is predominantly in the caudate nuclei, which then demonstrate decreased signal intensity. Volume loss is also a prominent imaging finding in the Parkinson-plus syndromes.

Metabolic diseases and inherited disorders can be associated with gray matter degenerative disease processes. Increased signal intensity on T1-weighted images in the basal ganglia should raise the concern for hepatocellular disease (Figure 16), total parenteral nutrition, manganese toxicity, hyperparathyroidism, hypoparathyroidism and pseudohypoparathyroidism, hemorrhage, and neurofibromatosis type 1. Normal calcifications in the basal ganglia can also cause increased signal on T1 images.

The abnormal copper accumulation of Wilson disease (hepatolenticular degeneration) can result in typical imaging findings as well. On CT, the basal ganglia and thalami are hypodense. On T2-weighted images, the basal ganglia (especially the putamen) and thalami are hyperintense and may be atrophic.

Huntington's chorea will result in caudate atrophy. Increased signal intensity may also be apparent. Some frontal volume loss may also occur (Figure 17).

PET imaging is on the frontier for imaging of the early, preclinical metabolic derangements of dementia detectable prior to the anatomic changes of the disease. The characterization of "typical" patterns of altered metabolic function in the various types of dementia may lend more specificity to the imaging

Figure 16

Increased signal of the basal ganglia in a patient with cirrhosis

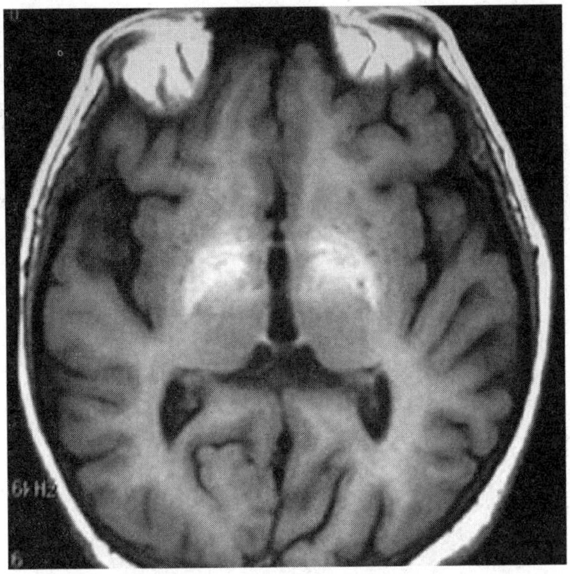

Figure 17

Huntington's chorea

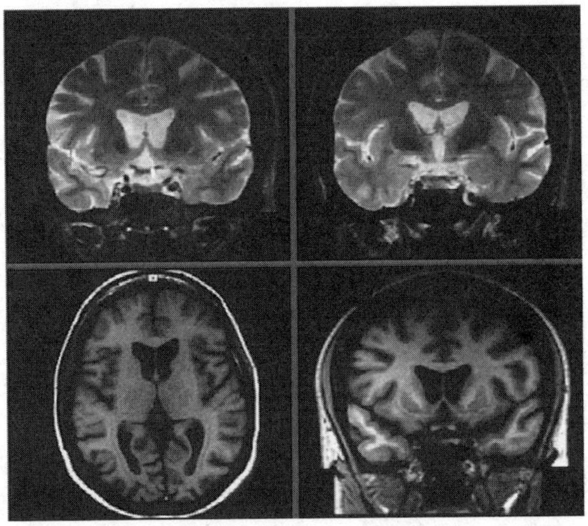

and clinical diagnosis of a particular dementia and may help identify patients at risk for the development of full-blown AD or other dementia. This assessment may help the development of therapy and monitoring of interventions. Patterns are developing which suggest that an early decrease in FDG uptake in the cingulate gyrus and parietal temporal brain is suggestive of AD. A frontal lobe dementia such as Pick demonstrates decreased FDG uptake in the frontal regions. Parkinson disease demonstrates the findings of AD with more occipital lobe involvement as well. This research is ongoing and only recently has the federal government added PET imaging for dementia to its roster of reimbursable indications for PET scanning.

9. Spine Imaging

Briefly, spine imaging is well served by either CT or MRI, with MRI taking precedence. The depiction of disc herniations, stenosis, and vertebral compressions is a daily bread-and-butter role of imaging. The detection of cord abnormalities such as myelitis, infarct, hemorrhage, demyelination, and tumor optimally requires MRI and gadolinium contrast agents. The detection of bone marrow abnormalities is most sensitive with MRI. For instance, inversion recovery imaging (STIR) is assuming a preeminent role in the determination of the acuity of spinal fractures. An acute fracture will demonstrate increased signal intensity on STIR images as a result of the bone marrow edema. Some differentiation between an uncomplicated osteoporotic compression fracture from a pathological compression fracture can also be assessed with MRI.

10. Summary

This chapter has introduced some of the current concepts of neuroimaging with comment on the areas of ongoing research and imaging development. The modalities of neuroimaging offer a variety of strengths, often complementary to each other, and need to be utilized in a cost-effective, efficacious partnership—a goal best served by continued and precise communication between the referring clinician and/or neurologist and the neuroradiologist.

11. References

1. Lester K. Localized MR Spectroscopy: basic principles. *Neuroimaging Clinics of North America*. 1998;8(4):713-731.

2. Castillo M, Kwock L. Proton MR spectroscopy of common brain tumors. *Neuroimaging Clinics of North America*. 1998;8(4):733-752.

3. Frank Shelleck. *MRISafety.com*

4. Romero J, Schaefer P, Grant PE, Becerra L, Gonzalez RG. Diffusion MR imaging of acute ischemic stroke. *Neuroimaging Clinics of North America*. 2002;12(1):35-53.

5. Osborn, AG. *Diagnostic Neuroradiology*. St. Louis, Mo: Mosby; 1994.

6. Grossman R, Yousem DM. *Neuroradiology: The Requisites*. St. Louis, Mo: Mosby; 1994.

7. Latchaw RE, Kucharczyk J, Moseley ME. *Imaging of the Nervous System: Diagnostic and Therapeutic Applications*. Philadelphia, Pa: Elsevier Mosby; 2005.

8. Gonzalez RG, Schaefer PW, Buonanno FS, et al. Diffusion-weighted MR imaging: Diagnostic accuracy in patients imaged within 6 hours of stroke symptom onset. *Radiology*. 1999;210:155-162.

9. Lovblad K, Laubach H, Baird A, et al. Clinical experience with diffusion-weighted MR in patients with acute stroke. *Am J Neuroradiology*. 1998;19:1061-1066.

10. Gaskill-Shipley, MF. Routine CT evaluation of acute stroke. *Neuroimaging Clinics of North America*. 1999;9(3):411-422.

11. Marks MP. CT in ischemic stroke. *Neuroimaging Clinics of North America*. 1998;8(3):515-523.

12. Yoshiura TW and Sorensen AG. Advanced MR techniques: diffusion MR imaging, perfusion MR imaging, and spectroscopy. *Neuroimaging Clinics of North America*. 1999;9(3):439-453.

13. Consortium of Multiple Sclerosis Centers, *mscare.org*

14. Butma, JA, Frank JA. Overview of imaging in multiple sclerosis and white matter disease. *Neuroimaging Clinics of North America*. 2000;10(4):669-688.

15. Salzman K, Osborne, AG, House P, Jinkins JR, Ditchfield A, Cooper JA, Weller RO. Giant tumefactive perivascular spaces. *American Journal of Neuroradiology*. 2005;26:298-305.

16. Inglese M, Salvi F, Iannucci G, Mancardi G, Luigi MM, and Filipi M. Magnetization transfer and diffusion tensor MR imaging of acute disseminated encephalomyelitis. *American Journal of Neuroradiology*. 2002;23:267-272.

17. Honkaniemi J, Dastidar P, Kahara V, Haapasalo H. Delayed MR imaging changes in acute disseminated encephalomyelitis. *American Journal of Neuroradiology*. 2001;22: 1117-1124.

18. Donovan Post M J, Yiannoutsos C, Simpson D, Booss J, Clifford DB, Cohen B, McArthur J, Hall CD. Progressive multifocal leukoencephalopathy in AIDS: are there MR findings useful to patient management and predictive of patient survival? *American Journal of Neuroradiology*. 1999;20:1896-1906.

19. Wong T Z, van der Westhuizen GJ, Coleman RE. Positron emission tomography imaging of brain tumors. *Neuroimaging Clinics of North America*. 2002;12:615-626.

20. Castillo M, Kwock L. Proton MR spectroscopy of common brain tumors. *Neuroimaging Clinics of North America*. 1998;8(4):733-752.

21. Bronen RA. Is there any role for gadopentetate dimeglumine administration when searching for mesial temporal sclerosis in patients with seizures? *Am J Roentgenology*. 1995;164:503.

22. Vattipally V, Bronen RA. MR Imaging of epilepsy: strategies for successful interpretation. *Neuroimaging Clinics of North America*. 2004;14:349-372.

23. Minoshima S. Imaging Alzheimer's disease: clinical applications. *Neuroimaging Clinics of North America*. 2003;13:769-780.

Technologies of Neuroimaging

24. Haackea EM, DelPropastob ZS, Chaturvedic S, Sehgalb V, Tenzere M, Neelavallid J, Kidof D. Imaging Cerebral Amyloid Angiopathy with Susceptibility-Weighted Imaging. *Ameri Jour Neuro*. 2007;28:316-317.

25. Sehgal V, DelProposto ZS, Haacke EM, et al. Clinical applications of neuroimaging with susceptibility-weighted imaging. *J Magn Reson Imaging*. 22; 2005:439–50.

26. Tong KA, Ashwal S, Holshouser S, et al. Improved detection of hemorrhagic shearing lesions in children with post-traumatic diffuse axonal injury: initial results. *Radiology*. 227; 2003:332–39.

27. Nagaraja S, Powell T, Griffiths PD, Wilkinson ID, MR imaging and spectroscopy in Lhermitte-Duclos disease. *Neuroradiology*. 2004; 46(5):355-358.

28. Hoeffner ED, Case I, Jain R, Gujar SK, Shah GV, Deveikis JP, Carlos RC, Thompson BG, Harrigan MR, Mukerji SK. Cerebral Perfusion CT: Technique and Clinical Applications. *Radiology*. 2004; 231:632-644.

29. Forbes KP, Pipe JG, Karis JP, Farthing V, Heiserman JE. Brain imaging in the unsedated pediatric patient: Comparison of periodically rotated overlapping parallel lines with enhanced reconstruction and single-shot fast spin-echo sequences. *AJNR AM J Neuroradiol*. 2003; 24(5):794-798.

30. Alemany Ripoll M, Stenborg A, Sonninen P, Terent A, Raininki R. Detection and appearance of intraparenchymal haematomas of the brain at 1.5 T with spin-echo, FLAIR and GE sequences: poor relationships to the age of the haematoma. *Neuroradiology*. 2004; 24(5): 435-43.

31. Safety of Mechanical Thrombectomy and Intravenous Tissue Plasminogen Activator in Acute Ischemic Stroke. Results of the Multi Mechanical Embolus Removal in Cerebral Ischemia (MERCI) Trial, Part I. *Amer Jour of Neuroradio*. 2006; 27:1177-1182.

32. Hammoud DA, Hoffman JM, Pomper MG. Molecular Neuroimaging: From Conventional to Emerging Techniques. *Radiology*. 2007; 245:21-42.

Intracranial Tumors

33. Cha S, Knopp EA, Johnson G, Wetzel SG, Litt AW, Zagzag D. Intracranial Mass Lesions: Dynamic Contrast-Enhanced Susceptibility-Weighted Echo-Planar Perfusion MR Imaging. *Radiology*. 2002;223:11-29.

34. Al-Okaili RN, Krejza J, Wang S, Woo JH, Melhem ER. Advanced MR Imaging Techniques in the Diagnosis of Intraaxial Brain Tumors in Adults. *RadioGraphics*. 2006; 26:S173-S189.

12. Questions

1. Complications of intracranial infection that can be imaged include:

   A. Abscess

   B. Ventriculitis

   C. Venous thrombosis

   D. Empyema

   E. All of the above

2. A decrease in metabolic function demonstrated in the cingulate region of the parietal brain would be most suggestive of:

   A. Pick disease

   B. Creutzfeldt-Jakob

   C. Parkinsonism

   D. Alzheimer disease

   E. Infarct

3. A focus of increased signal intensity on DWI with a normal ADC signal is consistent with:

   A. T2 shine-through

   B. Infarct

   C. Cytotoxic edema

   D. Vasogenic edema

   E. A & D

4. Cytotoxic edema is characterized by:

   A. Increased signal on T2 images, increased signal on DWI, and decreased signal on ADC maps

   B. Increased signal on T2 images, decreased signal on DWI, and decreased signal on ADC maps

   C. Increased signal on T2 images, increased signal on DWI, and increased signal on ADC maps

   D. Decreased signal on T2 images, increased signal on DWI, and decreased signal on ADC maps

5. An intracranial hemorrhage that is of increased signal on T1-weighted images and decreased signal on T2-weighted images would be expected to be:

   A. Older than 2 weeks

   B. About 3-7 days

   C. Chronic and older than one month

   D. Less than one day in acuity

6. A rim-enhancing mass could be:

   A. Hematoma

   B. Tumor

   C. Abscess

   D. Multiple sclerosis plaque

   E. Any of the above

7. The "H's" of the search pattern for a seizure focus include all of the following except:

   A. Hippocampus

   B. Hydrocephalus

C. Heterotopia

D. Hypothalamus

8. A corpus callosum that is normal in volume, lax in contour, and associated with an increased distance between the mammillary bodies and the pons would typically be seen in all of the following except:

A. Alzheimer disease

B. AIDS

C. Aqueductal stenosis

D. Parkinson disease

E. Multiple sclerosis

9. Abnormal signal intensity on MRI or abnormal density on CT in the basal ganglia are common findings. Match the following pattern of abnormality with the most likely etiology.

A. Infarct	I. Increased density on CT
B. Hepatocellular disease	II. Decreased signal on T1 and T2 images
C. Acute hemorrhage	III. Increased signal on T2, FLAIR, & DWI
D. Perivascular space	IV. Increased signal on T1
E. Chronic hemorrhage	V. Decreased signal on T1; increased T2

10. The following CT image is best explained as:

A. Early cerebritis

B. Herpes encephalitis

C. Early MCA infarct

D. Normal variant

E. Low-grade tumor

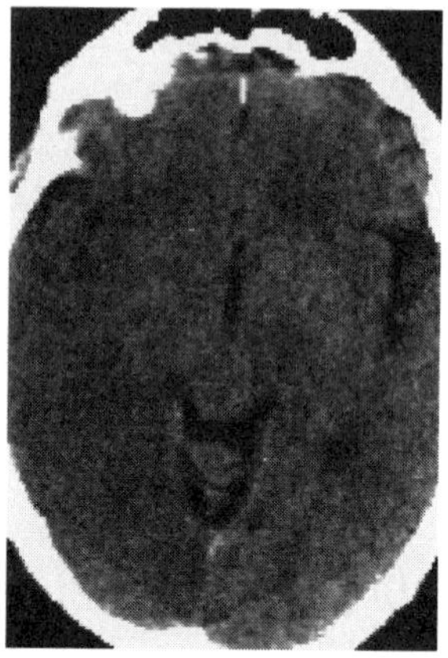

11. The following MRI image is most characteristic of:

A. Metabolic defect

B. CO poisoning

C. CJD sporadic variety

D. Perinatal ischemia

E. Total parenteral nutrition

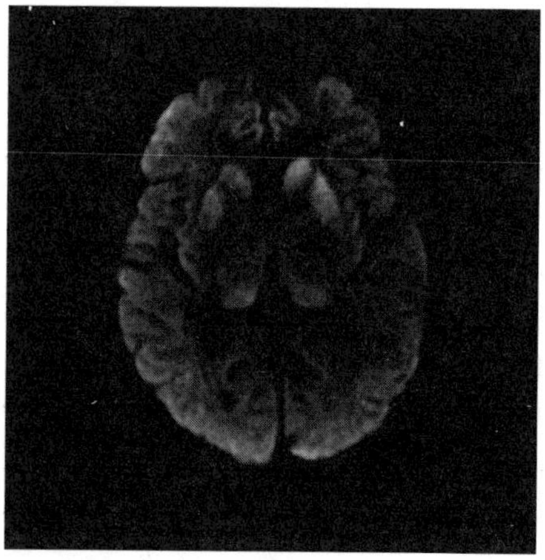

12. This patient presented with what problem?

A. Developmental delay

B. Seizures

C. Papilledema

D. Hemiparesis

E. Meningeal signs followed by obtundation

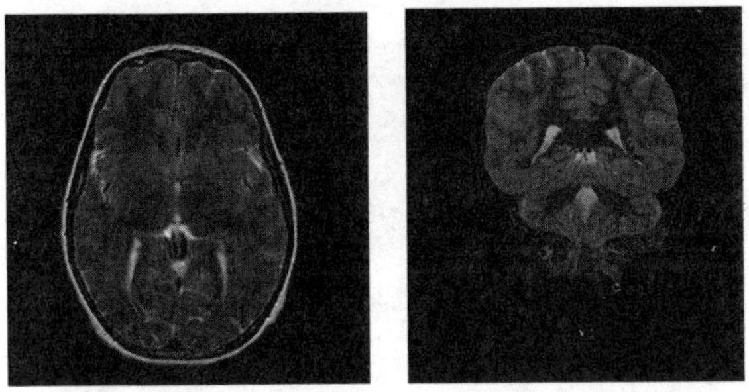

13. What is the diagnosis?

A. Bacterial meningitis

B. Lymphoma

C. Carcinomatous meningitis

D. Venous infarction

E. Intracranial hypotension

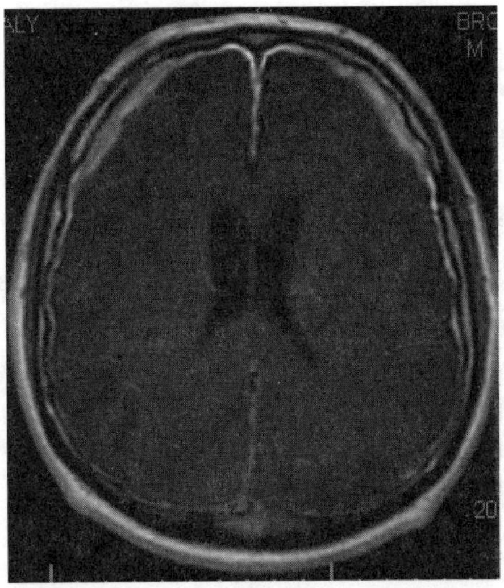

14. What is the most likely diagnosis?

A. Vestibular schwannoma

B. Meningioma

C. Epidermoid tumor

D. 5th nerve schwannoma

E. Aneurysm

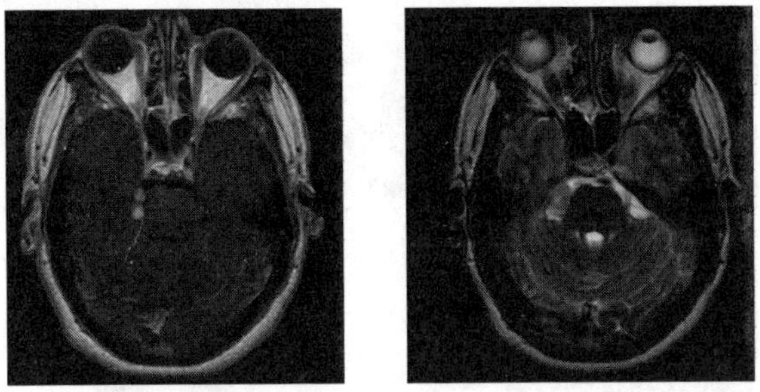

15. What is the most likely diagnosis?

A. Embolic infarction

B. Posterior reversible encephalopathy syndrome

C. Acute disseminating encephalomyelitis

D. Glial neoplasm

E. Venous infarction

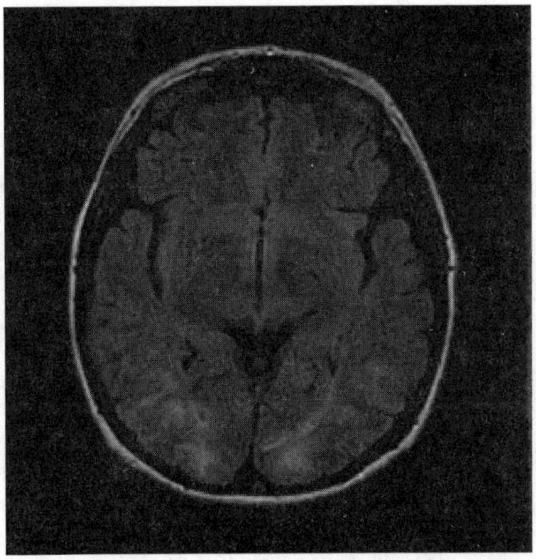

16. The differential diagnosis includes all of the following except:

A. Total parenteral nutrition

B. Liver failure

C. Lymphoma

D. Wilson disease

E. NF1

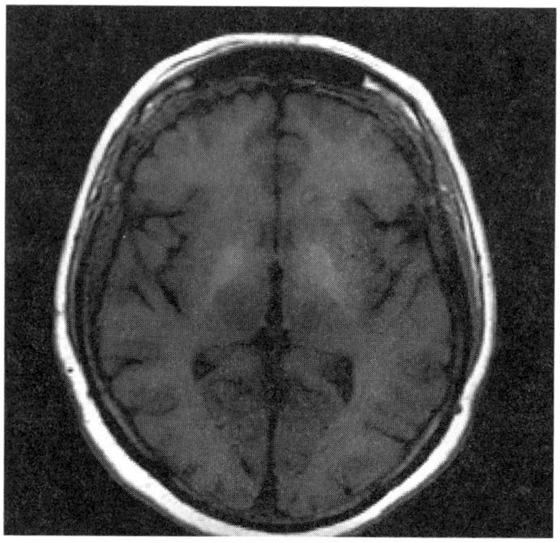

17. What is the most likely diagnosis?

A. Tuberous sclerosis

B. Acute hemorrhage

C. Metastatic disease

D. Heterotopia

E. Developmental venous anomaly

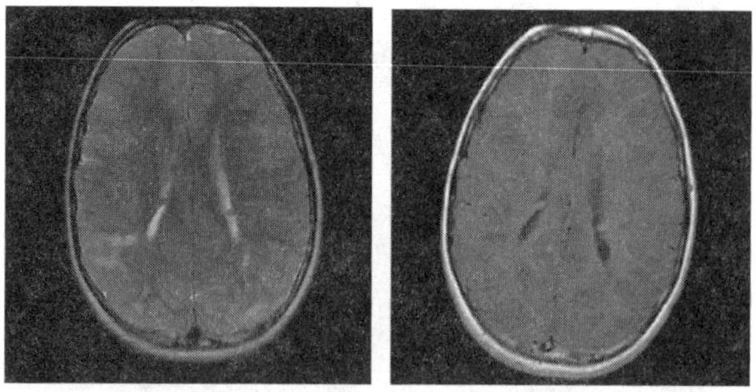

18. All are possible as a diagnosis except:

A. Subarachnoid hemorrhage

B. Carcinomatous meningitis

C. Tuberculosis

D. Intracranial hypotension

E. Sarcoid

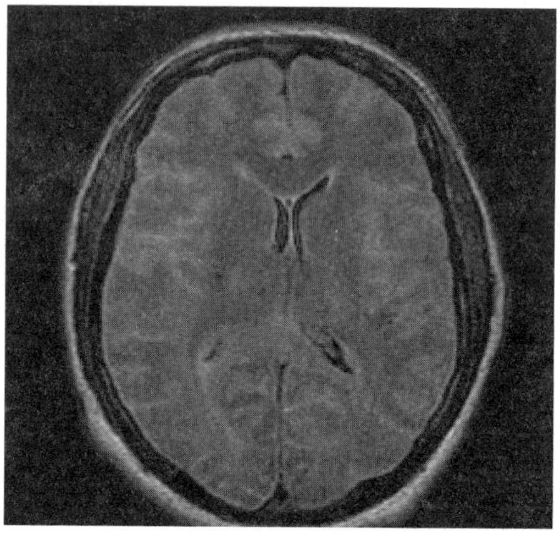

19. What is the most likely diagnosis?

A. NF1, schwannoma

B. Resolving hemorrhage

C. Hemangioblastoma

D. Metastatic disease

E. Medulloblastoma

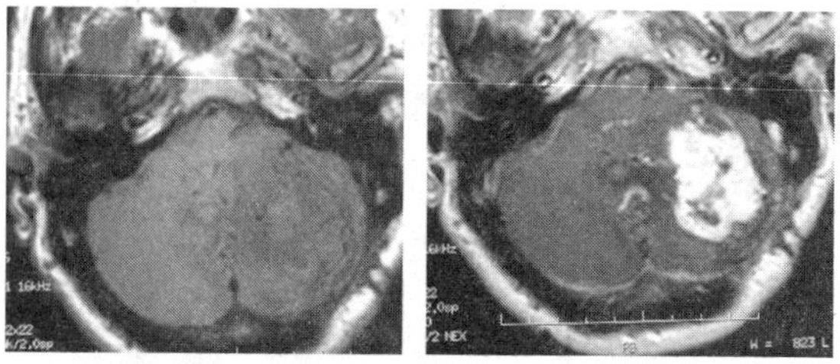

20. What is the most likely diagnosis given the imaging appearance of this recurrent mass?

A. Metastatic disease

B. Infarction

C. Glial neoplasm

D. Lymphoma

E. Lhermitte-Duclos

21. What is the spectroscopy finding that adds relative specificity to the diagnosis of the entity in question 20?

A. Elevated choline

B. Elevated creatine

C. Elevated lactate

D. Elevated NAA

E. Elevated myoinositol

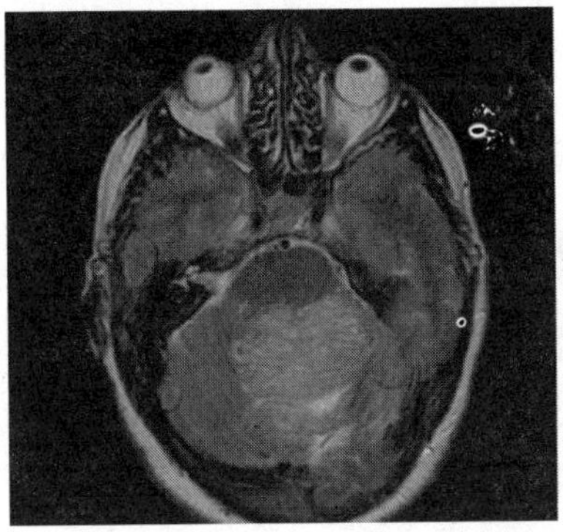

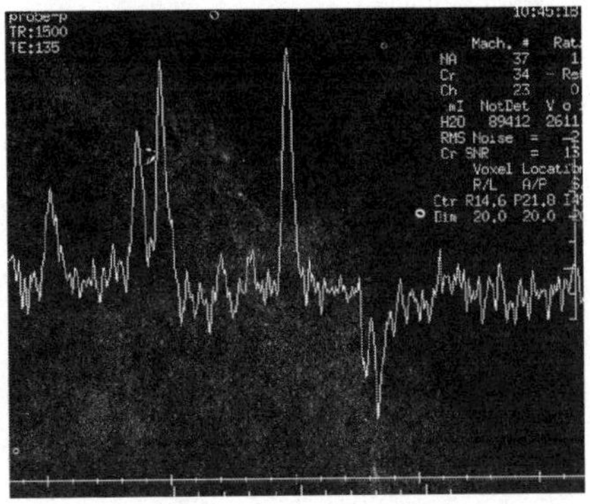

Answers

1. E.

2. D.

3. E.

4. A.

5. B.

6. E.

7. B.

8. C.

9. A. III; B. IV; C. I; D. V; E. II

10. C.

11. C.

12. B. The diagnosis is band heterotopia.

13. E.

14. D.

15. B.

16. C.

17. A.

18. D.

19. C.

20. E.

21. C. At 1.3 ppm, this is an inverted doublet.

Chapter 7: Topics in Neuropathology

Brent T. Harris, MD, PhD

Contents

1. Introduction

The field of neuropathology is a vast and varied landscape which every neurologist must traverse throughout their career. During training, neurology house officers work closely with neuropathologists, reviewing surgical specimens, participating in brain cutting sessions, and attending didactic lectures. In most programs residents often spend time learning about the neuropathology service. When in practice, the neurologist will need to maintain their relationship with neuropathologists either at their own hospital or as consultants from academic medical centers. For example, neuropathologists will need from the neurologist a clear clinical picture prior to nerve or muscle biopsy, to help decide how to properly process tissues and interpret results or may need to discuss the clinical progression of a patient who had dementia prior to performing an autopsy. Clinical-pathological correlation and good communication are essential between neurologist and neuropathologist. Most importantly, an understanding of neuropathological processes is essential for all practicing neurologists as they care for patients, provide prognoses and treatment, and search for cures to neurological disease.

The goal of this short chapter is not to provide a comprehensive discourse on all aspects of neuropathology–a challenge even for most textbooks. Subjects such as muscle/nerve, perinatal/developmental, epilepsy, dysmyelinating, infectious, and toxic/metabolic disorders cannot be covered in this short chapter but are discussed in other portions of this manual. Instead, highlighted here are a sampling of some important and better understood examples of neuropathological processes with a focus on gross and microscopic findings. Combined with these "classic" neuropathologies are discussions of some of the current findings regarding pathogenesis and methods that pathologists use to make a pathological diagnosis. Readers should only use this information as a quick starting point in their search for knowledge about particular diseases that can be found in the periodical literature, advanced texts, and in the ever-expanding electronic literature.

The study of neuropathology is a complex endeavor requiring a basic familiarity with both neuroanatomy and neurophysiology. Many of the disease entities encountered in the central nervous system (CNS) and peripheral nervous system (PNS) have no parallels in other organs. This is a reflection of the features that set the nervous system apart from all other bodily components. These features include:

a.) Complex but highly integrated anatomic structure;

b.) Grouping of many disparate functions (such as endocrine, homeostatic, memory, movement, personality, etc.) in one organ;

c.) Limited capacity for many neural components to regenerate;

d.) Glial rather than a fibroblastic infrastructure;

e.) Presence of blood-brain barrier: a functional boundary at the level of the blood vessel wall, which restricts free passage of most serum components into the nervous system;

f.) Absence of typical lymphoid drainage;

g.) Encasement within rigid, nonexpanding bony structures;

h.) Markedly different levels of tolerance for variations in oxygen, glucose and pH relative to that encountered in other organs.

Each of these features when damaged/altered alone or as a group will result in specific neuropathological conditions. Nevertheless, in dissecting and understanding neuropathological disorders, the basic principles of general pathology still apply.

2. Cellular Pathology of the Nervous System

A quick review of the cellular changes in response to injury that occurs in the central and peripheral nervous system sets the stage for the more complex multicellular processes that underlie virtually all neurological diseases. All cells respond to changes in their environment as well as to an internally programmed set of instructions dictated by the regulation of their genes. This interplay of cellular "nature and nurture" guides a cell through its relatively long life in the case of neural cells.

The following discussion is to familiarize you with the common pathological reactions in the CNS. We will return to each of these reactions at times later in the chapter when specific diseases are discussed. Note that cells in the nervous system, like those in other organs, have a limited number of ways of reacting to pathological stimuli.

Changes in Neuronal Cell Body (Perikaryon)

Ischemic/hypoxic change. Contracted neuron with hyper-eosinophilia of cytoplasm ("red-dead neuron") and pyknosis of nuclei. Severely damaged neurons will eventually disappear (Figure 1, color plates).

Neuronal atrophy. Gradual shrinkage of cell body and withering of its dendritic tree (eg, neurodegenerative diseases, disuse atrophy, trans-synaptic atrophy).

Neuronal loss. Can only be appreciated microscopically when there is approximately 30% cell loss; to determine fewer losses, computerized counting machines are now being used.

Chromatolysis. In Nissl preparations, Nissl granules disappear; sign of retrograde degeneration following injury or transection of axons. It can also be seen in some toxic-metabolic disorders without axonal damage, as in pellagra for instance (Figure 2).

Ferrugination (mineralization, incrustations). Mineral (Ca and Fe) deposits in damaged neurons.

Neuronophagia. Phagocytosis of a degenerated neuron by macrophages/microglia (Figure 3).

Apoptosis. Genetically controlled programmed cell death as a normal part of development or as a part of neurodegenerative diseases. Apoptosis mechanisms may be circumvented in neoplasia.

Accumulation of Abnormal Material

Lipofuscin – "wear-and-tear" pigment. Insoluble mixture of lipids and proteins that accumulate during the course of aging. Some cells such as in the inferior olivary nuclei will exhibit lipofuscin earlier than in Purkinje cells, which are relatively resistant to such an accumulation. If a lipofuscin-like material (ceroid) is seen in neurons in early life, it indicates a form of storage disease, ceroid-lipofuscinosis.

Lipid storage material. According to the site of catabolic enzymatic block, various sphingolipids or gangliosides accumulate in perikaryon, causing the cells to distend, enlarge, and assume a globular shape.

Neurofibrillary tangles are bundles of abnormal filaments seen in such disorders as Alzheimer disease.

Inclusions may be nuclear and/or cytoplasmic; seen in degenerative diseases such as idiopathic parkinsonism—Lewy bodies, Pick disease—Pick bodies, or ALS—Bunina bodies. Also in certain viral infections, such as in herpes encephalitis—Cowdry type A inclusions (Figure 4, color plates).

Changes in Neuronal Processes

Wallerian degeneration. Degeneration of an axon distal to injury. If the axon is myelinated, the myelin sheath will fragment as a secondary effect.

"Dying-back." Degeneration of the most distal segments of an axon due to inability of the cell body to maintain adequate axoplasmic flow or produce needed nutrients seen in some toxic neuropathies and certain neurodegenerative diseases (system degeneration).

Axonal spheroids. Focal bulbous swellings of axons, usually the result of sublethal injury.

Demyelination. a) Primary insult to myelin sheath or myelin forming cell (oligodendroglia in CNS and Schwann cell in PNS), or b) secondary to degeneration of axons as in Wallerian or dying-back.

Figure 2

Neurons with chromatolytic change

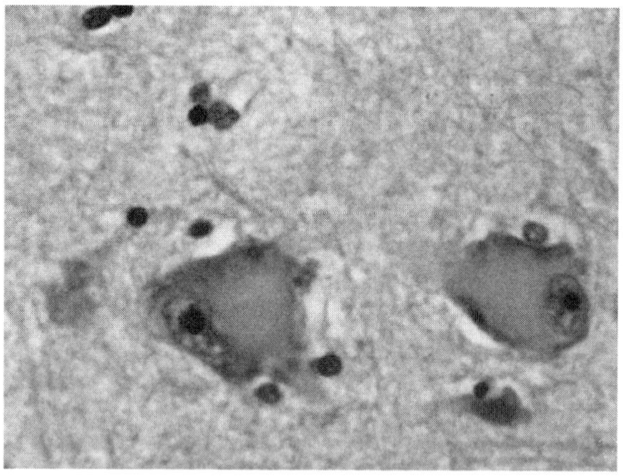

Figure 3

Neuronophagia by macrophage/microglia

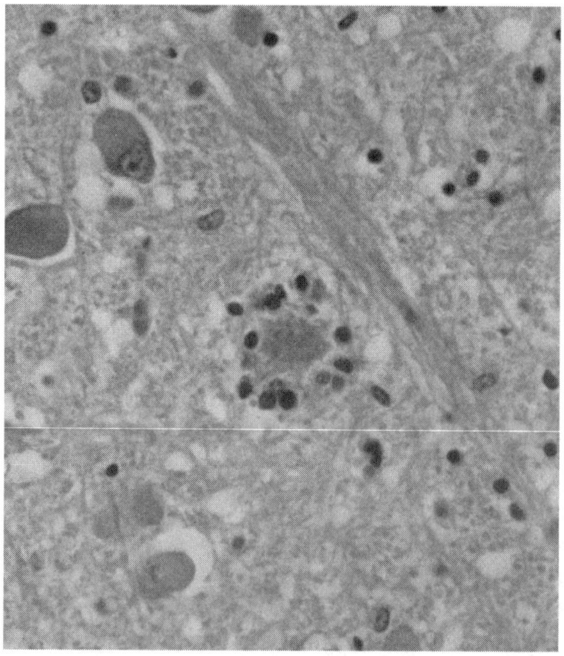

Dendrites. Abnormal spine configuration or loss. Loss of dendritic branches is often seen in developmental disorders, both congenital and acquired.

Changes in Neuroglia

Neuroglia are neuroectodermal in origin and far outnumber their neuronal counterparts, though their roles in the nervous system are largely not as well understood as those of neurons. Glia of the CNS comprise astrocytes which can be protoplasmic (gray matter) or fibrillar (white and gray matter), oligodendrocytes, ependymal cells and epithelium of choroid plexuses. Their function is to maintain a constant internal environment and to ensure optimal conditions for neuronal function. In addition, each cell type has its own specialized functions.

Astrocytes respond to almost any stimulus, first by enlarging (reactive astrocytes, Figure 5) and then retracting fibrous astrocytes when the injurious process subsides. The cell processes of fibrous astrocytes form a network (glial scar or gliosis) that mends an injured area. Most scars in the CNS are glial; fibrous scars formed of fibroblasts only occur in abscess walls or are post-traumatic when meninges (mesodermal tissue) are driven into brain tissue. Sometimes, protoplasmic astrocytes may proliferate and undergo a peculiar alteration known as Alzheimer's type II glia in conditions with electrolyte abnormalities or where the blood and CSF ammonia levels are elevated, such as in hepatic encephalopathy. The nuclei of Alzheimer type II glia are large, often bi-lobed, with clear karyoplasm and chromatin distributed under nuclear membrane.

Oligodendrocytes form and maintain central myelin; their destruction will lead to demyelination as in progressive multifocal leukoencephalopathy (PML), a viral condition that selectively "colonizes" oligodendrocytes, or multiple sclerosis. Inclusions within oligodendroglial cells can be seen in multiple system atrophy, progressive supranuclear palsy, and corticobasal degeneration.

Ependymal and choroid plexus cells are of glial derivation arising from the neuroectoderm. Ependymal cells line ventricles and maintain equilibrium between cerebrospinal and interstitial fluids of the brain. They are tall columnar ciliated cells, but show

Figure 5

Reactive astrocytes immunostained for GFAP

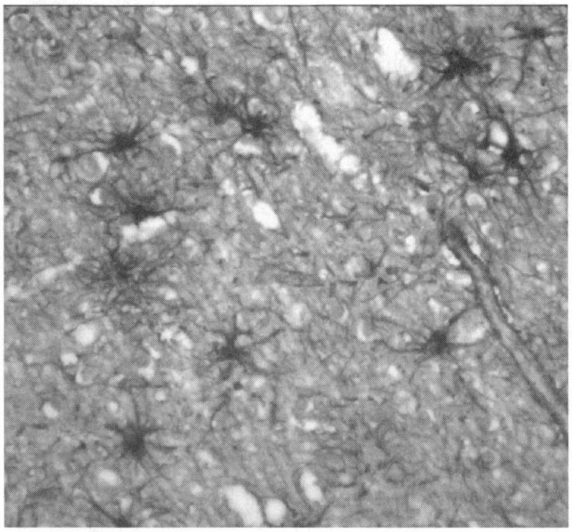

regional variations in cell configuration reflecting modified function, eg, over the choroid plexuses they acquire a more cuboidal appearance, have prominent microvilli, and develop the ability to secrete CSF.

Microglial cells may not actually be glial cells at all, but a specialized monocyte/macrophage which arises in the bone marrow and populates the CNS before birth. They are believed to assist in the extensive remodeling of the fetal CNS by phagocytizing cells that expire by apoptotic cell death. In postnatal life they are small, dense, elongated nuclei without identifiable cytoplasm. Special stains to reveal their cytoplasm show it to be arranged as thin branches radiating from the nuclear zone. Microglia establish individual, nonoverlapping territories. They comprise about 8%-10% of all CNS cells, and are inconspicuous until reaction is required in the neural parenchyma. They respond to myriad challenges including: neuronal death, trauma, inflammation/infection, tumor infiltration, and infarction. In conditions where neuronal death occurs by viral infection microglial stars/nodules form in the parenchyma or at the sight of the dead neuron. The term neuronophagia (neuron eating) refers to these microglial nodules around a degenerating neuron (Figure 6). In some conditions like AIDS encephalopathy, or in some enzymatic deficiency diseases, these cells can form multinucleate giant cells.

Schwann cells carry out similar functions to astrocytes, oligodendrocytes, and microglia in the peripheral nervous system. They ensheathe motor and sensory axons to improve conduction velocities. They are also important components of the synapse at the neuromuscular junction (NMJ) and have the capacity to ingest tissue debris and promote regeneration after injury. They also can proliferate as neoplasms (Schwannomas) or after injury in a hyperplastic fashion (traumatic neuroma).

Figure 6

Metastatic lung cancer

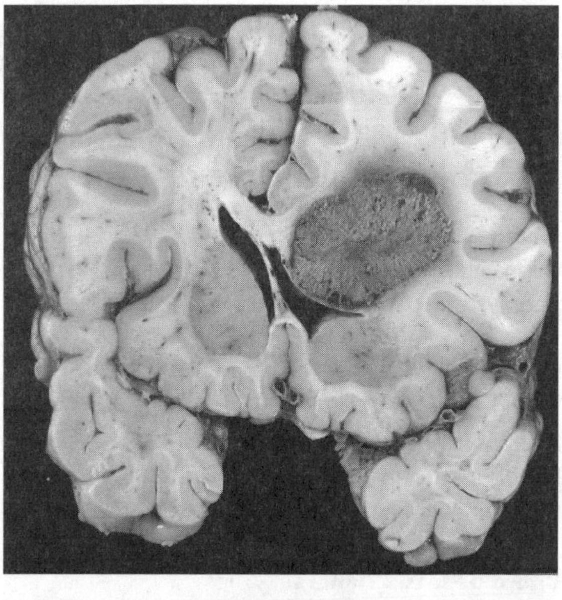

3. Neural Tumors

As with other areas of oncology, the explosion of knowledge about the molecular pathways of neoplastic transformation has brought about better understanding and therapeutic advances for CNS tumors. Molecular diagnostics that embrace such techniques as PCR, immunohistochemistry, and FISH (fluorescence *in situ* hybridization) analyses all serve to better define unique molecular signatures within a patient's resected or biopsied tumor. In fact, molecular diagnostics are being developed in combination with radiological techniques such as positron emission tomography (PET) and nuclear magnetic resonance (NMR), and serum or CSF proteomics to define tumor markers even before the surgeon takes scalpel in hand. The advanced techniques of diagnosis now go hand in hand with traditional histological evaluation of tumors, which will be focused on in this section. Despite these promising advances, malignant brain tumors are encountered in virtually all age groups with high morbidity and mortality.

The World Health Organization (WHO) classification is a comprehensive and established working list for CNS neoplasms that gets updated on a periodic basis. The most current classification was defined in 2007, and an abridged list is shown in Table 1. Most types of tumors are generally categorized based on the proposed cellular origin for the inciting tumor. There is a range of low-grade, sometimes "benign" to intermediate, and high-grade "malignant" tumors. Unlike neoplasms in the rest of the body,

Table 1

WHO Classification of Tumors of Neuroepithelial Tissue (abridged)

Astrocytic Tumors
Diffuse astrocytoma (variants)
Anaplastic astrocytoma
Glioblastoma
Pilocytic astrocytoma
Pleomorphic xanthoastrocytoma
Subependymal giant cell astrocytoma

Oligodendroglial Tumors
Oligodendroglioma
Anaplastic oligodendroglioma

Mixed Gliomas
Oligoastrocytoma
Anaplastic oligoastrocytoma

Ependymal Tumors
Ependymoma
Anaplastic ependymoma
Myxopapillary ependymoma
Subependymoma

Choroid Plexus Tumors
Choroid plexus papilloma, carcinoma

Glial Tumors of Uncertain Origin
(eg, chordoid glioma of the 3rd ventricle)

Neuronal and Mixed Neuronal-glial Tumors
(eg, dysembryoplastic neuroepithelial tumor; ganglioglioma; central neurocytoma)

Neuroblastic Tumors
Pineal Parenchymal Tumors
(eg, pineocytoma; pineoblastoma)

Embryonal Tumors
(eg, medulloblastoma; atypical teratoid/rhabdoid tumor)

Tumors of the Meninges
Tumors of Meningothelial Cells
Meningioma variants
Atypical meningioma
Anaplastic meningioma

CNS tumors usually do not have a propensity to metastasize to other organs but instead injure with local spread and develop mass effect. Even so-called "benign" tumors like low-grade meningiomas can have devastating mass effect, suggesting that benign and malignant are not necessarily the best descriptors for CNS neoplasms. As with most other peripheral cancers, CNS/PNS neoplasms are thought to often arise from progenitor stem cells that are still residing in these structures, and somehow signaled through intrinsic genetic means and/or by extrinsic signals such as radiation or chemical carcinogens to begin abnormal proliferation. Metastases from non-CNS tumors represent about 40% of intracranial tumors, with the most common sites being lung, breast, melanoma, renal, and colon (Figure 6). Knowing the age of the patient and the neuroanatomical site where the tumor arises helps tremendously in the differential diagnosis of tumors.

Gliomas make up a broad group on CNS neoplasms that are derived from glial cell origin, with the most common being astrocytomas, oligodendrogliomas, and ependymomas.

1. Astrocytomas are of astrocytic lineage and found in virtually all areas of the brain and spinal cord, as one would expect with the ubiquitous astrocytes. WHO grade I pilocytic astrocytomas are usually encountered in infants and children or, rarely, adults. They are often cystic with solid tumor nodules, and found more commonly in the posterior fossa. Microscopically, their hallmark is the fine fibrillar "hair-like" processes that can be seen best on smear preparation of fresh tumor (Figure 7). Other features are a biphasic growth pattern with loose areas and denser tumor cell accumulates around blood vessels. Proteinacious eosinophilic structures called eosinophilic granular bodies and Rosenthal fibers are often seen in these tumors (Figure 8, color plates).

   Diffuse and anaplastic astrocytomas make up the Grade II and III astrocytomas, respectfully. They are characterized by tumor cells with angulated and hyperchromatic nuclei and increasingly pleomorphic (variably shaped) nuclei and mitotic figures. Grade II astrocytomas are also called fibrillar or diffuse astrocytoma, and do not have as

Figure 7

Smear preparation of a pilocytic astrocytoma

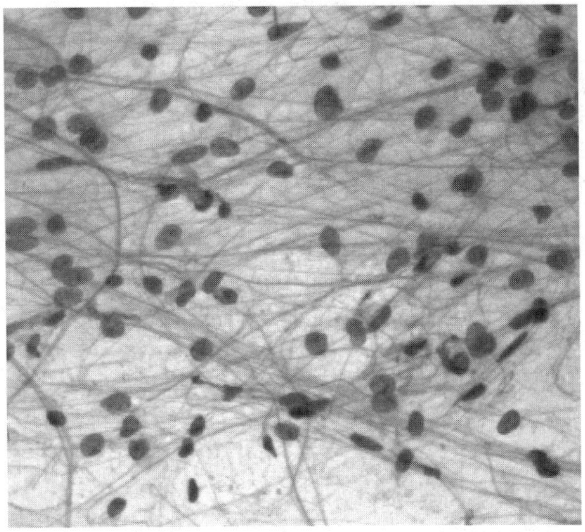

high a density of tumor cells in a given area as the anaplastic astrocytomas. In addition, the higher-grade astrocytomas elicit interesting vascular responses to small and larger vessels by secreting vascular proliferating substances. This results in endothelial proliferation and larger vessel neovascularization in many instances. Astrocytomas overexpress glial fibrillary acidic protein (GFAP), which is an important target for immunohistochemistry, an ancillary laboratory technique often used in diagnosing these tumors. This overexpression of GFAP is particularly seen in gemistocytic astrocytomas, a variant showing tumor cells with large, eosinophilic cell bodies and with a propensity to progress to higher-grade astrocytomas.

The highest-grade astrocytomas (WHO Grade IV) are called glioblastoma or glioblastoma multiforme (GBM) because of the many forms that the tumor cells can take. Unfortunately, these tumors are the most common, the most malignant, and the least effectively treatable of the astrocytomas. These tumors have high tumor cell density, often markedly pleomorphic nuclei (though a more uniform "small cell GBM" variant is observed), numerous mitotic figures, extensive endothelial proliferation, and often necrosis with surrounding tumor cells (called pseudo-palisading necrosis) (Figure 9). It has been suggested for some time that pathogenesis of glioblastomas follows one of two pathways: primary glioblastomas that occur *de novo*, often in older individuals, and secondary glioblastomas that progress, like many tumors, from lower-grade astrocytomas. Molecular characterization has further aided in this distinction with primary GBMs often showing amplification of the epidermal growth factor receptor (EGFR), MDM2 overexpression, p16 deletion, and PTEN mutations, while secondary GBMs often have inactivation of the tumor suppressor p53 and overexpression of platelet-derived growth factor A.

2. Oligodendrogliomas are less common than astrocytomas but also encountered throughout the CNS. The clinical presentation is often a middle-aged individual with new onset of seizures. WHO Grade II oligodendroglioma and Grade III anaplastic oligodendroglioma are comprised of transformed oligodendroglial cells in low density with little cytological atypia or mitotic activity to more densely packed tumor cells, with more pleomorphic nuclei and greater mitotic activity, respectively. These tumors are usually not GFAP immunoreactive like astrocytomas except for a small subset of tumors with mini-gemistocytic forms. The tumor cells are also different from astrocytomas in that the nuclei are often round and in some cases there is an artifactual peri-nuclear clearing giving the tumor cells a "fried-egg" appearance (Figure 10). Molecular diagnostics has had a direct clinical impact in the case of oligodendrogliomas. Findings of chromosome 1P and 19Q deletions within oligodendroglial tumor cells (especially in anaplastic oligodendroglioma) has been found to correlate with a better response to therapy (chemotherapy and radiation therapy) as opposed to those tumors that do not show these deletions and are usually refractory to these therapies. Mixed glial tumors exist and are called (anaplastic) mixed oligoastrocytomas.

Figure 9

Glioblastoma multiforme

A) MRI displaying gadolinium enhancing GBM
B) Malignant growth of GBM across the midline
C) Pseudo-palisading necrosis of GBM tumor cells

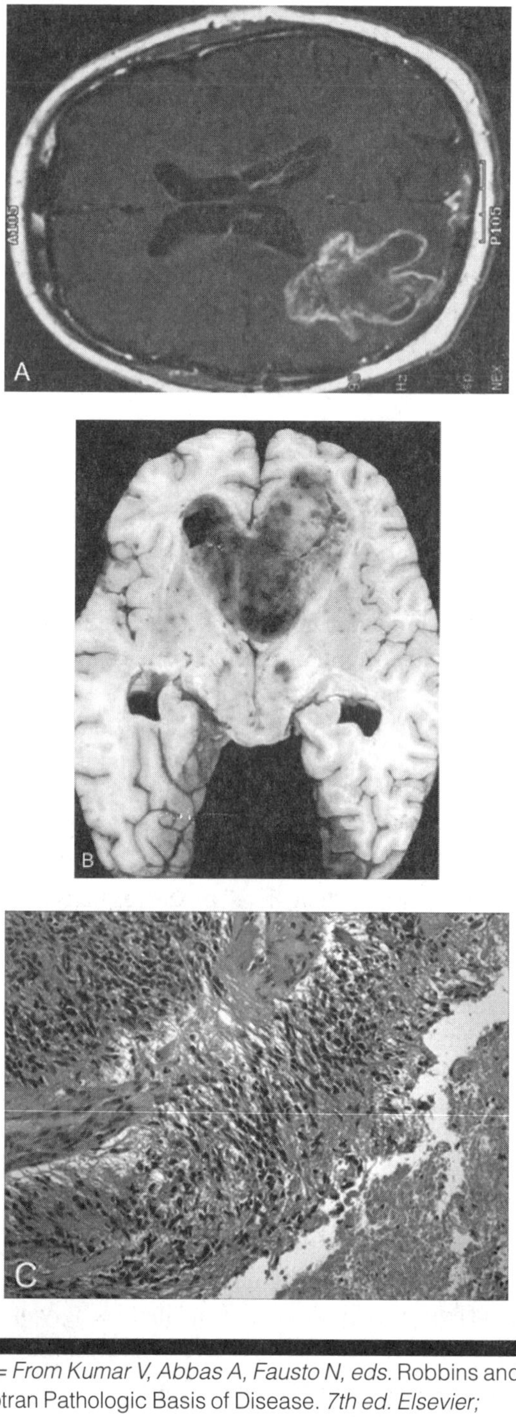

B = From Kumar V, Abbas A, Fausto N, eds. Robbins and Cotran Pathologic Basis of Disease. *7th ed. Elsevier; 2005. With permission.*

3. Ependymomas occur in the cerebrum, brainstem, and spinal cord, generally around the ventricular system or spinal central canal, respectively. However, they can also be encountered away from the ventricles where ependymal remnants still exist long after development. Ependymomas exist as WHO Grades I (subependymoma, myxopapillary ependymoma), II (ependymoma), and III (anaplastic ependymoma) tumors. Very slow-growing subependymomas are commonly found around the wall of the fourth ventricle, sometimes projecting into lumen and causing obstruction and symptoms of increased intracranial pressure. Myxopapillary ependymomas, so named because of the microcystic myxoid material they produce and papillary growth pattern, are nearly exclusively found in the conus medullaris/cauda equina area of the spinal cord most often in young adults. Ependymomas account for nearly 60% of the gliomas in the spinal cord. Microscopically they are usually easily recognized with their uniform nuclei often arranged around vessels (perivascular pseudorosettes) or around tubular lumen that recapitulate the lining of ventricles or central canals (ependymal rosettes) (Figure 11). GFAP immunostaining is usually present and helps to highlight the resetting features of this tumor. Anaplastic ependymomas have increased cell density, pleomorphic nuclei, increased mitotic activity, and occasionally necrosis.

Figure 10

Oligodendroglioma (WHO Grade II)

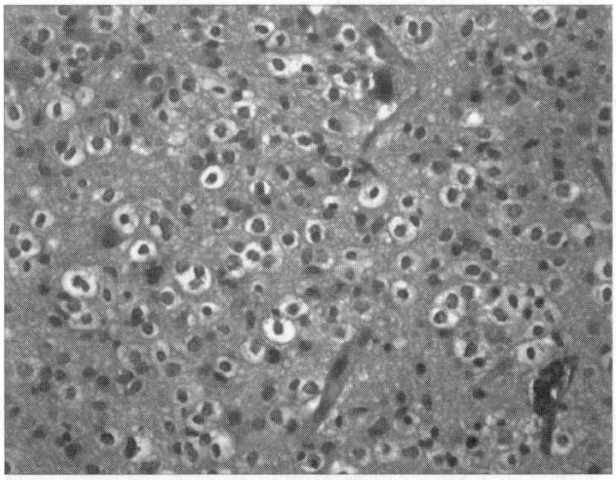

Figure 11

Ependymoma displaying vascular pseudorosettes

Insert shows gross tumor growing from filum terminale

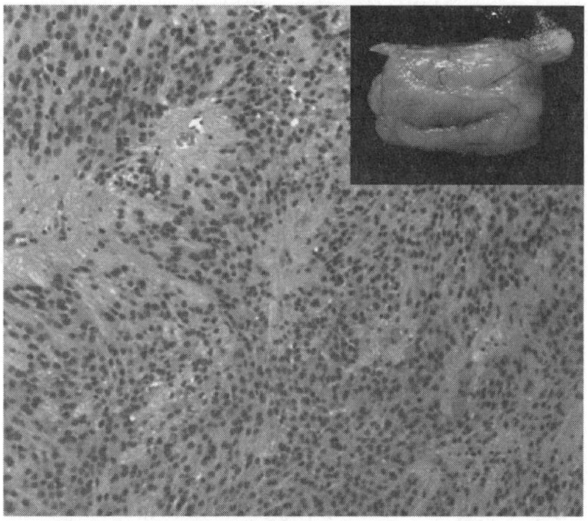

Meningiomas arise from the arachnoid cells of the meninges and with growth often into or onto the dura mater and occasionally into the brain or spinal cord parenchyma. They are usually slow-growing tumors that begin to elicit symptoms as they compress local structures. Multiple meningiomas are encountered in patients with type 2 neurofibromatosis (NF2), though in most cases they occur sporadically. Alterations in NF2 gene expression are seen in both familial NF2 and sporadic tumors.

A number of microscopic variants of meningioma are known, providing a challenge at times even to experienced neuropathologists. These are listed in Table 2. More common histological features of low-grade meningiomas include a syncytial appearance with indistinct cell borders, whorling patterns of tumor cell growth, and findings of psammoma bodies (mineralized concretions often within the whorls) (Figure 12). The tumor cells usually have abundant cytoplasm and round-to-oval nuclei, occasionally with pseudo-nuclear inclusions. Higher-grade atypical meningiomas can show increased cellularity, large nucleoli, patternless sheet-like growth, and increased proliferative activity. Malignant (anaplastic) meningiomas show frankly malignant cytological features, high mitotic activity, and often, invasive growth pattern into brain parenchyma. This latter feature, though not alone sufficient to diagnose a Grade III malignant meningioma, can sometimes be seen in lower-grade meningiomas.

Neuronal and neuronal-glial tumors occur in several forms within the nervous system. Gangliocytomas are composed entirely of tumor cells with mature-appearing neurons, often with the appearance of large ganglion cells, whereas gangliogliomas have an admixture of ganglion type cells and glioma tumor cells (Figure 13). Both are generally slow-growing tumors, but gangliogliomas do have the capacity for malignant transformation. Surgical resection often cures these patients that usually present with seizure disorders. Neurocytomas are tumors of neuronal lineage that occur in or around the ventricular system, and are composed of slowly proliferating tumor cells with small, round neuronal type cells which express synaptic apparatus proteins like synaptophysin. Dysembryoplastic neuroepithelial tumors (DNT) are generally found in superficial cortical locations of children or teens, and are also usually cured with surgical resection. They are made up of small, oligodendroglioma-type cells and microcystic collections with mature neuronal-type cells "floating" in these cleared cystic areas (Figure 14).

Table 2

Meningiomas

WHO Grade I	WHO Grade II
Meningothelial	Atypical
Psammomatous	Chordoid
Fibrous	Clear Cell
Transitional	
Angiomatous	**WHO Grade III**
Microcystic	Malignant (anaplastic)
Secretory	Papillary
Lymphoplasmacyte-rich	Rhabdoid

Figure 12

Gross and microscopic appearance of typical low grade meningioma with whorls and a large calcified psammoma body

Insert shows meningioma growth on fragment of dura

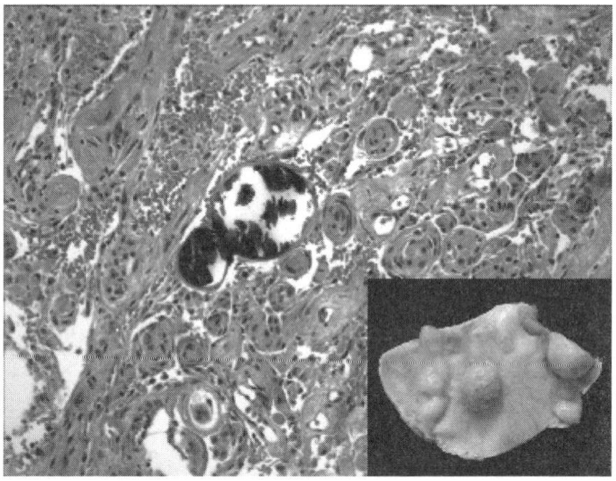

Medulloblastomas are poorly differentiated, highly malignant neoplasms of childhood usually located within the midline of the cerebellum. While a number of genetic alterations have been identified in these tumors, the most common is a deletion from the chromosome 17p thought to harbor an as yet unidentified tumor suppressor gene. Alteration in the Sonic Hedgehog®/patched and WNT pathways have also been identified in some medulloblastomas, and the tumors are found as part of Gorlin and Turot syndromes. Aggressive surgical resections and full cranio-spinal radiotherapy because of frequent drop metastases has increased 5-year survival rates to about 75%. Microscopically, these tumors show highly proliferating cells with small, angulated, and hyperchromatic nuclei arranged in sheets or distinctive Homer-Wright rosettes (Figure 15). One of the variants, termed desmoplastic medulloblastoma, has more of a nodular growth pattern, with the nodules separated by dense, collagenous septa.

Neurofibromas and Shwannomas comprise the

majority of peripheral (including cranial) nerve-related tumors. Most occur sporadically and are benign. Perhaps they are best known, though, because of their associations with NF1 and NF2, and in these genetic settings they can be either benign or malignant. Schwannomas can occur on any cranial nerve but are most commonly found in the cerebellar-pontine angle on the eighth nerve sporadically, or often bilaterally, in NF2. Whether on a peripheral or cranial nerve, they have similar histological findings of biphasic growth patterns with cellular areas (Antoni A areas) and looser areas (Antoni B). Characteristic Verocay bodies often assist with diagnosis (Figure 16). The tumor cells have elongated cigar-shaped nuclei which can show some pleomorphism.

Neurofibromas are encountered in the skin or in larger nerves as solitary lesions or as multiple lesions associated with NF1. In both locations, the tumor is formed of a loose, myxoid collection of spindle-shaped cells with fine nerve twigs coursing through the mass. A variant of neurofibroma found nearly exclusively in NF1 is called the plexiform neurofibroma. It is encountered densely enmeshed within larger nerves making surgical removal difficult. These latter tumors have the potential to transform into malignant peripheral nerve sheath tumors that are highly invasive sarcomas with metastatic potential.

Figure 13

Ganglioglioma with occasional binucleate neuronal forms

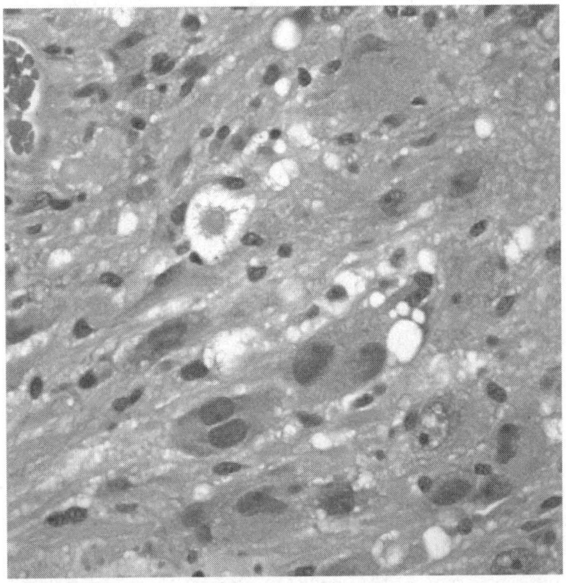

Figure 14

Microscopic appearance of a dysembryoplastic neuroepithelial tumor (DNT)

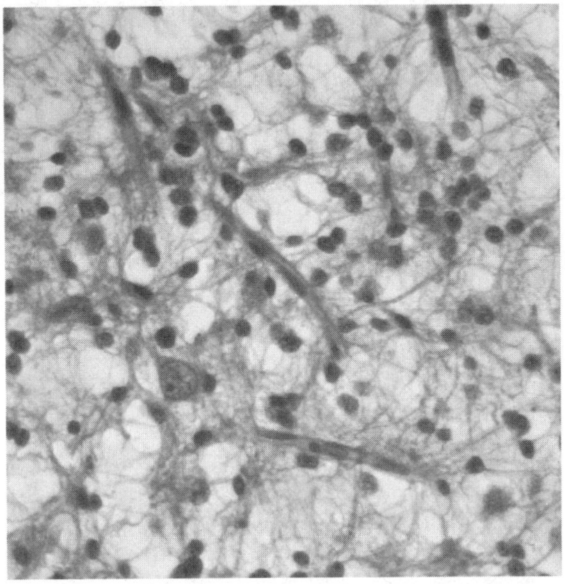

Figure 15

Medulloblastoma with Homer-Wright rosettes

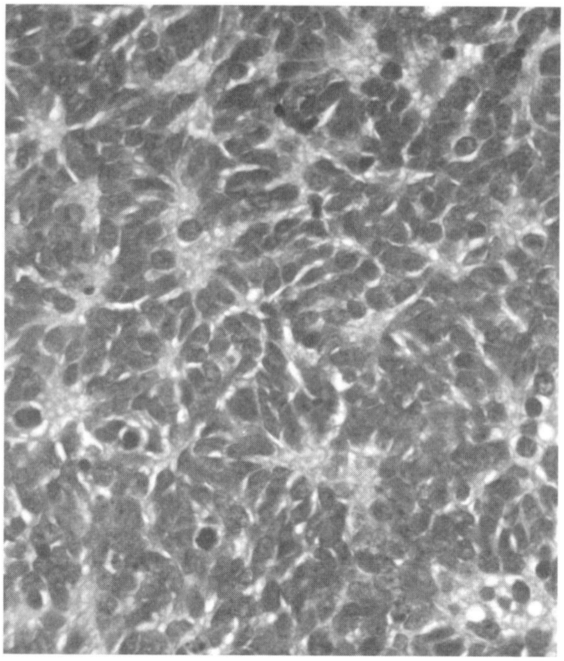

Figure 16

Verocay bodies within a schwannoma

Insert shows gross tumor attached to peripheral nerve

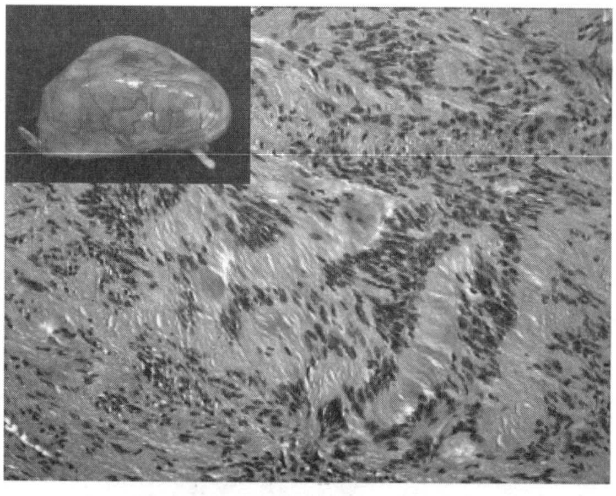

4. CNS Trauma and Hemorrhages

In industrialized societies, head injuries have become one of the leading causes of death, especially for individuals below 40 years of age. Vehicular accidents are by far the most important cause of head and spinal injuries of adults and older children. Deaths due to head injury account for 1%-2% of all deaths, and are the leading cause of death among young people. Many factors can contribute to the pathogenesis of brain damage in a patient who suffers a head injury. Reconstruction of the events of an accident that have led to the head injury, especially in fatalities from car crashes, is very important. During such accidents, the brain is subjected to all kinds of physical forces, such as acceleration, deceleration movements, linear or rotational impacts, fractures of the skull, etc., making it difficult to single out a special mechanism as having caused the most damage to the brain.

For practical purposes, head injuries have been classified into open and closed. Open injury is one in which the intracranial contents come in contact with the external environment, such as in compound fractures of the skull or following penetrating wounds such as caused by missiles. Closed injury results from a blow to the head (impact injury) or acceleration/deceleration motions (non-impact injury); the type of brain injury then largely depends on whether the head was restrained or in motion.

Closed Injuries

Focal Injuries Include Fractures of Skull, Contusions and Lacerations of Brain and Intracranial Hemorrhages

Fractures of skull attest to the severity of the impact, but are by no means an invariable finding in fatal head injuries; 20% of fatal cases have no fractures. Depressed fractures are important because of the extensive damage that they may cause to the underlying brain (Figure 17).

Contusions and lacerations are surface bruises of the brain, occurring primarily at the crests of gyri. Their locations contrast with those of ischemic lesions, which tend to preferentially involve the depths of sulci. Histologically, contusions show hemorrhages with variable degrees of necrosis and edema. A sequence of tissue reactions occurs, which

Figure 17

CT displaying depressed cranial fracture

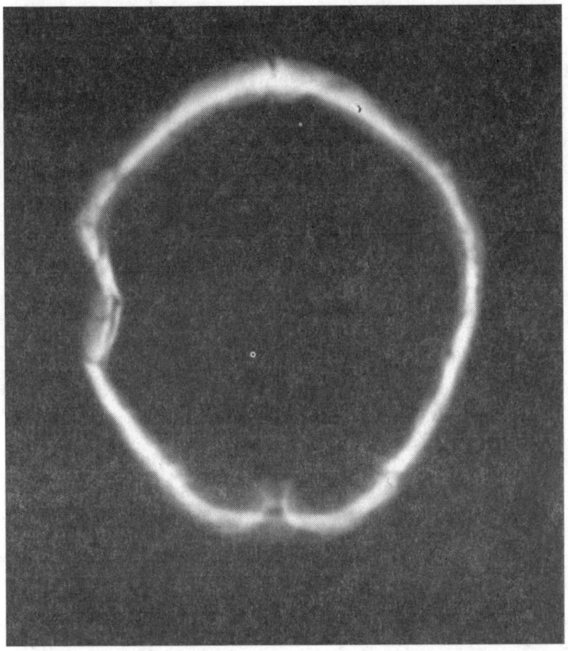

allows dating of recent contusions, and which eventually over months to years leaves a depressed scar, often yellow stained, at the gyral crests—plaques jaunes. If the blow is severe, as with depressed fractures, pia-arachnoid (mesenchymal tissue) is driven into brain parenchyma. During the subsequent tissue reactions, arachnoid and glia proliferate to form gliomesenchymal scars, which in turn account for some cases of post-traumatic epilepsy. In a laceration, there is more disruption of tissue and more hemorrhage than in a contusion.

Several mechanisms determine the locations of contusions and lacerations. A direct blow to a restrained head or a resting but moveable head will produce maximal lesions at the site of maximal impact (coup lesions), while injuries in which the head is accelerating or decelerating at impact, as in vehicular accidents, for instance, result not only in contusions at the site of impact, but also in more serious contusions in other areas (contrecoup lesions) (Figure 18). The contrecoup lesions may be found directly opposite the site of impact, but more often they have a propensity to occur in the orbital surfaces of the frontal lobes or tips of the temporal lobes after impacts at a variety of other sites. This singular involvement of basal areas is determined by the anatomy of the skull, and the fact that the largely incompressible brain is only allowed to undergo a "swirling" movement when the head sustains a rotational acceleration force. As a result, the base of the brain, especially rostrally, is rubbed against the bony ridges of the floor of the anterior cranial fossa and lesser wing of the sphenoid bones (Figure 19).

The brain stem may also be contused during impact (closed) injuries. The lesions in brain stem contusion are characteristically located along the lateral tegmental areas of the mid-brain and pons. They can usually be distinguished from the secondary brain stem hemorrhages (Duret hemorrhages) which tend to occupy mid-line zones in both the tegmentum and base of the mid-brain and pons (Figure 20). Brain stem contusions are almost invariably associated

Figure 18

Diagram representing coup (A) and contracoup (B-E) injuries

Arrows indicate point of impact and direction of force; black areas indicate areas of contusion

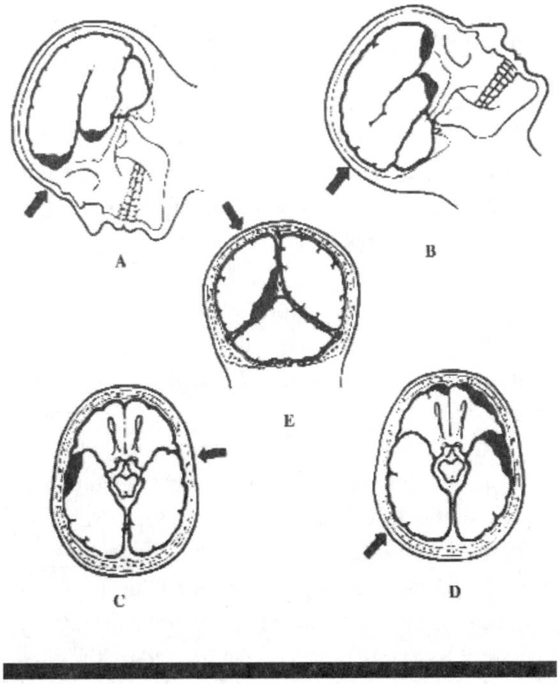

Figure 19

Base of frontal lobes show old contusion injury

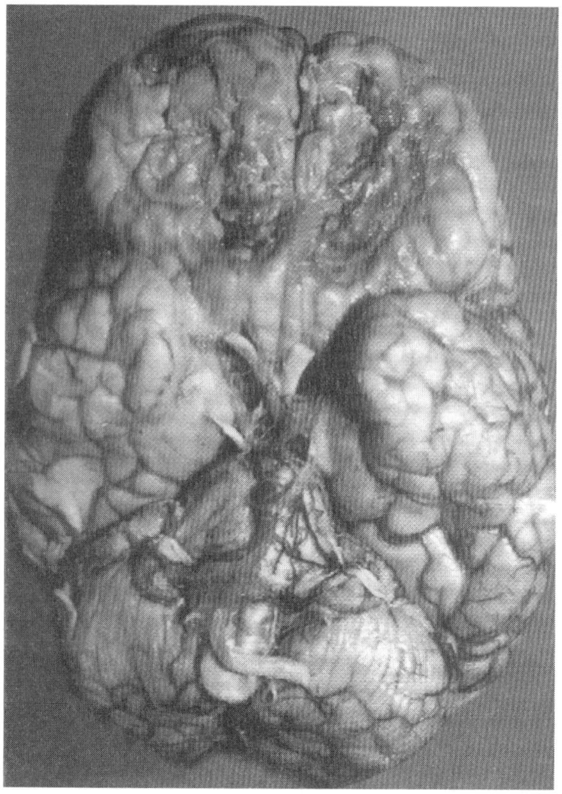

From Gray F, De Girolami U, Poirier J, eds. Escourolle and Poirier Manual of Basic Neuropathology. *4th ed. London: Elsevier; 2004. With permission.*

with diffuse axonal injury (DAI, see below).

Hemorrhages. Blood may collect in the following spaces: epidural, subdural and arachnoid, or may occur in the brain parenchyma itself.

Epidural hematoma. Blood accumulates between dura and skull and is almost always associated with skull fractures—except sometimes in children the vessels may tear without actual fractures. The most common site is the temporoparietal region where the bone is thin and flexible and where the anterior branch of the middle meningeal artery courses in a bony tunnel in the inner table. A fracture, usually linear, lacerates this artery and causes the hematoma, which expands rapidly under arterial pressure. Its extent is somewhat limited by the close apposition of dura to skull. Nevertheless, a rapidly enlarging mass may cause fatal tentorial herniation or brain stem compression by the time it has reached 75-100 cc in volume (Figure 21). Subtentorial epidural hematomas are usually caused by basilar skull fractures which lacerate a dural sinus. Being venous in origin, they may cause a clinical course that is less acute than those in the supratentorial compartment. A posterior fossa expanding mass, however, results in cerebellar and brain stem compression as well as cerebellar herniation.

Subdural hematoma. The blood accumulates between dura and arachnoid in what is normally a potential space and two types are to be distinguished: acute and chronic. The source of subdural bleeding in chronic subdural hemorrhage is caused by a tear of one of the "bridging" veins which drain the cortex as they cross the subdural space to enter the dural sinuses. The bridging veins, which are tethered in the subarachnoid spaces, are not well supported in this potential space and are therefore susceptible to acceleration/deceleration forces. As a result of brain atrophy in the elderly, the space enlarges further, increasing the risk of tears to the vessels. Indeed, most chronic subdural hematomas are largely seen in elderly patients in whom sometimes the head injury may have been no more than a jolt. As the venous blood oozes, it separates the dura from the arachnoid and spreads over a large area of

Figure 20

Duret hemorrhage in pons

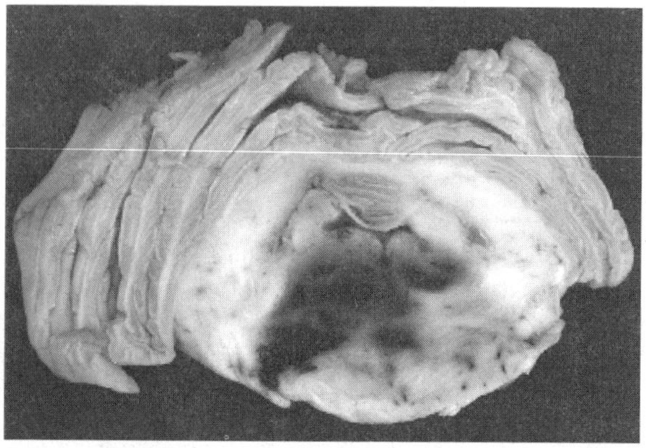

Figure 21

Epidural and subdural hematomas after motor vehicle accident

Insert CT showing typical lentiform shape of a rapid expanding epidural hemorrhage

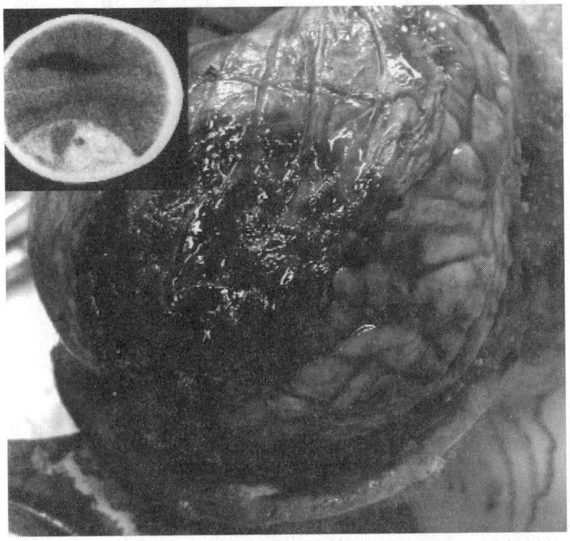

the hemisphere. Several hundred ccs of blood can thus accumulate in this space without causing any symptoms, at least initially (Figure 22). Acute subdural hematomas, on the other hand, are associated with severe head injuries that cause brain contusions. Accumulation of blood is often rapid. Like epidural hemorrhages, acute subdural hematomas are regarded as neurosurgical emergencies. Subdural hematomas evoke a peculiar reaction of the overlying dura, resulting in loculation of the blood by granulation tissue, which resolves by forming outer and inner membranes—chronic subdural hematoma. The blood in the center gradually liquefies and is resorbed. Re-bleeding within chronic hematomas, however, can occur and accounts for progressive enlargement of this "space-occupying lesion" with a wide variety of slowly-worsening clinical signs and symptoms ranging from focal compression signs to dementia due to hydrocephalus. The kinetics of tissue reactions in the outer and inner membranes can be used to date a subdural clot histologically.

Diffuse Brain Injury

Diffuse axonal injury (DAI). This term refers to widespread tearing of axons, primarily in white matter, and has been known by several terms over the past 25 years (diffuse degeneration of white matter, diffuse white matter shearing injury, etc.). This type of injury is usually produced during angular acceleration or deceleration of the head and impact is not necessary to produce it. The usual setting is a motor vehicle accident. Injury patterns in primate studies comparable to those of man have underscored that rapid acceleration of the head without impact can produce a spectrum of injuries ranging from immediate coma due to DAI to less severe forms of brain injuries such as mild to moderate concussions. The severity of the lesions largely depends on the acceleration force and posi-

Figure 22

CT scan of chronic subdural hematoma depressing underlying brain without causing midline shift

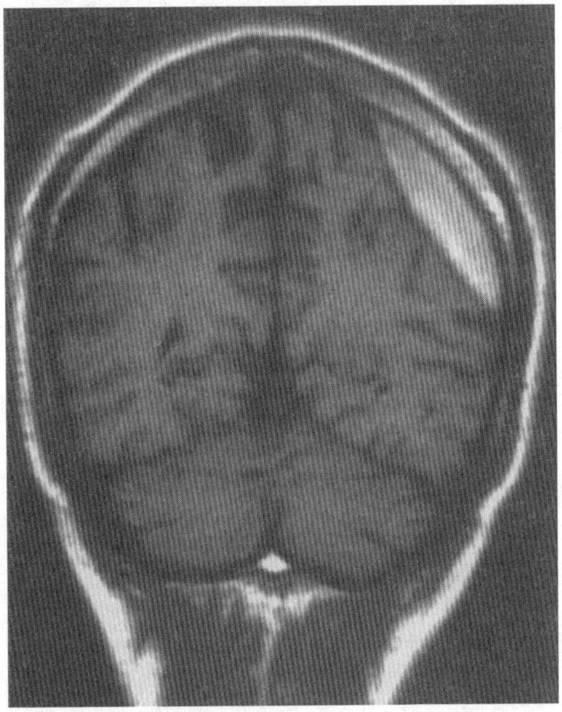

From Gray F, De Girolami U, Poirier J, eds. Escourolle and Poirier Manual of Basic Neuropathology. *4th ed. London: Elsevier; 2004. With permission.*

Figure 24

Diffuse cerebral edema

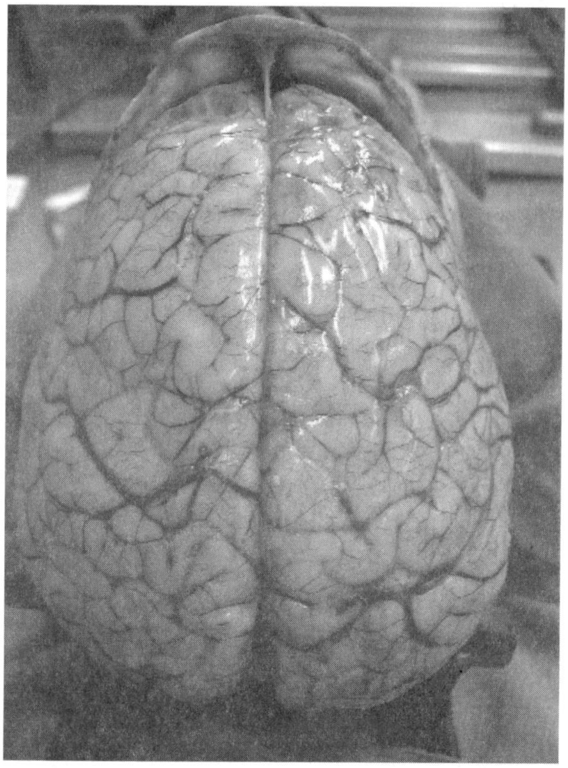

tion of the head–same-acceleration force causing more DAI when the head is in coronal motion than when jolted in sagittal plane. During the rapid angular acceleration, shearing forces generated within the brain can be great enough to tear blood vessels (leading to focal hemorrhages) and axons as well. In addition to being diffusely present in white matter of the cerebral hemisphere, DAI can be found in the corpus callosum, walls of the third ventricle, dorsolateral surface of rostral brain stem, and periaqueductal grey matter. Microscopically, axonal "retraction bulbs" or "spheroids" are apparent within hours of injury. An early marker of these spheroids is upregulation of beta-amyloid protein that can be visualized with immunohistochemistry (Figure 23, color plates).

Microglial "nodules" develop at these damaged sites and persist for a few weeks to disappear later, leaving behind an attenuated corpus callosum and white matter, the result of Wallerian degeneration of the affected axons. The typical patient with DAI is comatose immediately after injury and does not exhibit a lucid interval, as is often the case with epidural hematomas. Should the patient survive, many may become severely cognitively impaired or live in apallic or vegetative state with variable degrees of brain stem activity but little cortical function.

Diffuse edema is a complication of several forms of head injury. For as yet unknown reasons, swelling of one hemisphere may accompany an acute subdural hematoma on the same side. Bi-hemispheric swelling after head trauma appears in young children and is thought to result from loss of normal vasoregulation which then leads to an increased cerebral blood flow (Figure 24). The increased intracranial pressure seen in this setting is due to increased intracranial blood volume.

Diffuse hypoxic brain damage is also common in patients dying as a result of nonimpact head injury. A proportion of this damage is clearly related to a combination of one or more of the following, namely: brain shifts, raised intracranial pressure, systemic hypoxia and arterial spasm. Ischemic changes are often seen in the arterial boundary zones, so-called "watershed infarcts". Patients who have survived following prolonged hypoxia/ischemia are often left in a coma or persistent vegetative state. At autopsy, they often will show marked cortical thinning with tremendous neuronal loss (Figure 25).

Diffuse vascular injury. Multiple small hemorrhages throughout the brain, associated with rapid death.

Open Injuries

The majority of open craniocerebral wounds are caused by gunshot injuries. The extent of damage along the trajectory of a bullet largely depends on the speed and weight of the bullet. Usually, a low velocity bullet causes much greater damage at the site of entry. If it enters the cranial cavity with little remaining energy, it becomes arrested in its course

Figure 25

Prolonged cortical ischemia/hypoxia

Note the thinned cortex on the left compared to normal on right

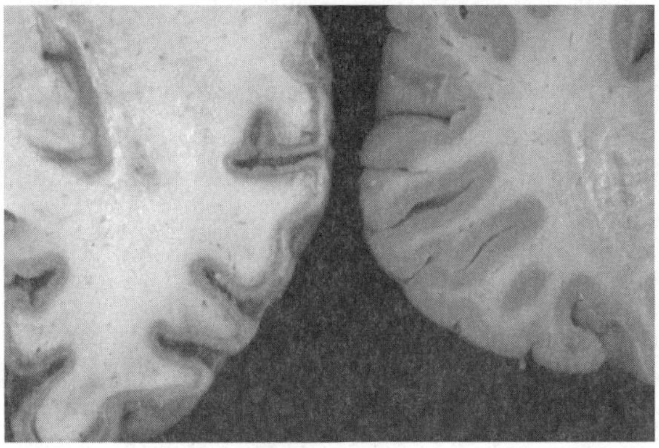

before reaching the opposite side. With a slightly higher velocity it may reach the opposite side and may even ricochet once or twice. This kind of gunshot wound is called "penetrating" in contrast to "perforating" in which the bullet traverses the head, as with high-velocity bullets. A bullet passing through the brain with very high velocity pushes the tissues radially aside, producing a momentary expansion or "cavitation" of the bullet track and displacing the surrounding brain structures. A caudal shift of the cerebellar tonsils and their jamming into the foramen magnum accounts for the fatal outcome of some cases of gunshot injuries. In more severe cases, the built-up pressure may be so forceful as to cause an explosive outward bursting of the skull. The exit wound in the skull is characteristically larger than the entry site. Severe lacerations of the brain may also result when fragments of skull bones, scalp or cloth are driven into the brain tissues, especially with low-velocity bullets.

Shaken Infant Syndrome

This is a controversial area in forensic neuropathology. The approximate incidence of child abuse in the United States is 1%, but exact numbers are difficult to determine. After SIDS, child abuse is the second leading cause of death among infants under one year old. The syndrome includes: retinal hemorrhage, subdural and/or subarachnoid hemorrhages, damage to the brainstem or high spinal cord, and sometimes little or no external injury. Many subdural hematomas in infants are the result of abuse. Pathologic findings may also include white matter tears and DAI. The above findings in and of themselves, though, are not entirely diagnostic of abusive injury, and other objective findings in the autopsy and circumstances of the injury are necessary to indicate abuse versus accidental injury. Severe brain swelling can lead to clinical sequelae including seizures, vomiting, lethargy, coma, mental retardation, motor dysfunction, and death.

Nontraumatic Intracranial Hemorrhages

The commonest cause of spontaneous cerebral hemorrhage is hypertensive vascular disease. Berry aneurysms and vascular malformations are next in frequency. Blood neoplasms and infections make up the remaining.

Hypertensive CNS Complications and Hemorrhage

The wall of a normal cerebral artery, unlike muscular arteries, lacks an external elastica and its media and adventitia are thinner. In long-standing "benign" hypertension, the arteries respond by muscular hypertrophy, which is often overshadowed by degenerative changes in the media and excess deposition of collagen in the adventitia. As these degenerative changes set in, the arteries lose their elasticity, elongate and acquire a tortuous course, becoming prone to focal thrombosis. Lacunar infarcts can result from hypertensive vascular change. They show an area of cavitary necrosis around an affected vessel often containing hemosiderin-laden macrophages (Figure 26). In accelerated or "malignant" hypertension, on the other hand, the characteristic change is fibrinoid necrosis of arterioles.

The pathogenesis of hypertensive cerebral hemorrhage is intimately related to microaneurysms, first described by Charcot and Bouchard in 1868. These are found in 46 out of 100 hypertensive patients and in only 7 out of 100 normotensives. These microaneurysms are numerous (average 20 in number) and are found in basal ganglia along the smaller branches of the lenticulostriate arteries, subcortical white matter, pons and cerebellum, in that order of

Figure 26

Lacunar infarct due to hypertensive vasculopathy

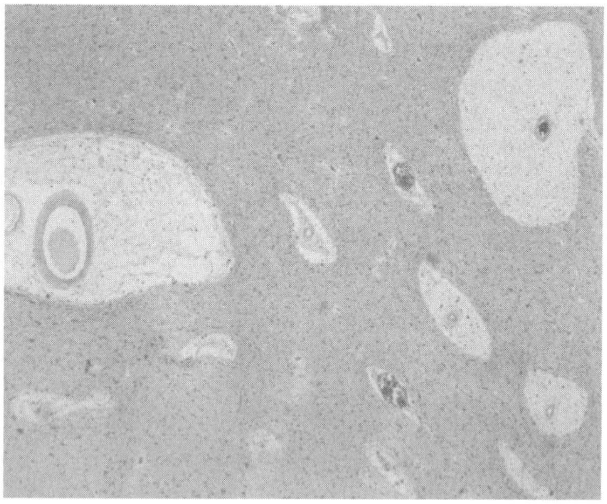

rapidly fatal, but early diagnosis and evacuation of the clot may save the patient's life. Hemorrhage in the pons is almost always in the basis pontis, while in the cerebellum the region of the dentate nucleus is a favorite site. It is not infrequent for a cerebellar hemorrhage to find its way into the cavity of the IVth ventricle, or sometimes extend to the surface with associated subarachnoid hemorrhage.

The CNS consequences of systemic hypertension are: 1) vascular changes (loss of elasticity), 2) microaneurysms, 3) hypertensive hemorrhages, and 4) lacunes.

Aneurysms

Berry aneurysm is the second most common cause of intracranial hemorrhage. The hemorrhage is usually in the subarachnoid space. The pathogenesis of "berry, saccular" or "congenital" (probably a misnomer, as not all are formed during development) aneurysms remains controversial. Failure of the muscle coat to fuse at the point of bifurcation during angiogenesis is considered responsible for their fre-

frequency. The diameter is usually about 500 μm and only rarely do they reach 2 mm. The wall of the aneurysm is formed by variable amounts of collagen and the rest is made up of hyaline amorphous material and blood clot in various stages of organization (Figure 27). The surrounding brain tissue usually contains a few hemosiderin-containing macrophages, variable amounts of gliosis, and occasionally frank interstitial hemorrhages. Interestingly, microaneurysms and occurrence of large cerebral hemorrhages are both uncommon in young hypertensives. It appears that aging is essential for their development.

Massive hypertensive hemorrhages occur first in putamen, globus pallidus, thalamus, pons and deep cerebellum. Those in the putamen and pallidum may involve the internal capsule. It is often difficult to ascertain the source because of the extensive destruction these bleeds cause. Sometimes, the hematoma ruptures into the ventricle (ie, hemoventricle), usually a fatal condition. Thalamic hemorrhages extend into the mesencephalon. Pontine hemorrhages are almost invariably and rapidly fatal. Cerebellar hemorrhages, on the other hand, are also

Figure 27

Small vessel microaneurysm secondary to hypertension

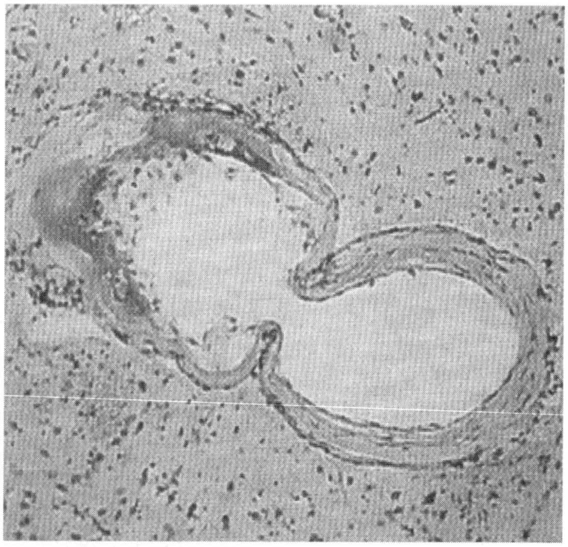

From Gray F, De Girolami U, Poirier J, eds. Escourolle and Poirier Manual of Basic Neuropathology. *4th ed. London: Elsevier; 2004. With permission.*

quency. The diameter is usually about 500 μm and only rarely do they reach 2 mm. The wall of the aneurysm is formed by variable amounts of collagen and the rest is made up of hyaline amorphous material and blood clot in various stages of organization (Figure 27). The surrounding brain tissue usually contains a few hemosiderin-containing macrophages, variable amounts of gliosis, and occasionally frank interstitial hemorrhages. Interestingly, microaneurysms and occurrence of large cerebral hemorrhages are both uncommon in young hypertensives. It appears that aging is essential for their development.

The incidence of berry aneurysm is said to be about 0.7% in some series, but higher figures are reported in other series depending on the interest of the pathologists and the criteria used to define what constitutes an aneurysm. The incidence of multiple aneurysms is about 10%. Eighty percent to 90% of all aneurysms in the circle of Willis are related to the anterior circulation and about 12% occur in the posterior circulation. The size ranges from a few mm up to several cm; the commonest size is about 1 cm. An aneurysm has a neck, body and a fundus and lies in the subarachnoid space (Figure 28).

Rupture usually takes place at the fundus, causing massive extravasation of blood into the subarachnoid space. The event is often acute and catastrophic, with patients presenting with complaints of having "the worst headache of my life." However, in some cases, minor episodes of leakage may occur, leading to fibrosis. The aneurysm in these cases becomes firmly bound to the surface of the brain, and should a forceful bleeding occur at a future date, blood tears its way through brain tissue and forms a cerebral hematoma. Cerebral infarction is another dangerous complication. This cerebral infarct may be caused by compression or stretching of the blood vessel by the subarachnoid hematoma. Spasm of the artery due to vasoactive substances released from platelets and a drop in perfusion pressure due to shunting of blood into the subarachnoid space have all been widely discussed as possible causes for the infarctions which follow the rupture.

Cerebral arteries, like any other arteries, are also prone to develop atheromatous, or fusiform aneurysms. Fusiform aneurysms occur frequently in the basilar artery, rarely rupture, and usually are asymptomatic. However, they may act as a space occupying mass and cause compression of brain stem structures.

Figure 28

Berry aneurysm

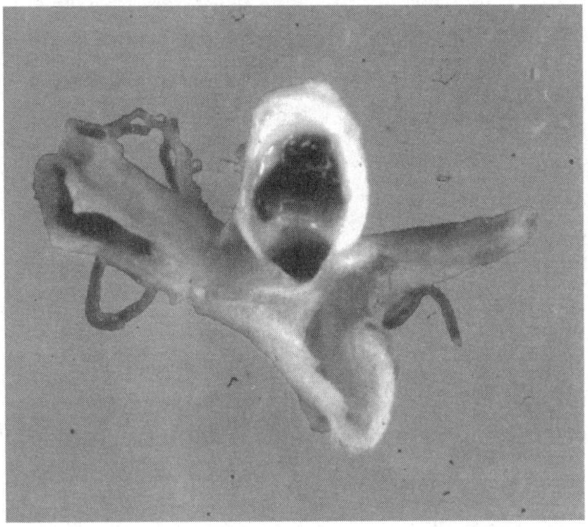

Vascular Malformations

The third cause of intracranial hemorrhage is rupture of vascular malformation. Three types of vascular malformations are distinguished pathologically: telangiectasias, cavernous hemangiomas and arteriovenous malformations.

Telangiectasias are for the most part of no clinical importance. They consist of multiple widened capillaries separated by normal neural tissue, an arbitrary point of distinction between telangiectasia, and cavernous hemangioma. Telangiectasia is often seen in the pons.

Cavernous hemangiomas. These often cause recurrent hemorrhages (subarachnoid or intraparenchymatous) and focal seizures. They consist of large, closely-packed channels with no intervening neural tissue. Thick collagen bands lined with a single layer endothelium form the wall of these abnormal channels. The subcortical tissue in the region of the Rolandic fissure is frequently involved.

Arteriovenous malformations (AVM). These are tortuous vascular masses usually in the leptomeninges, though the brain itself may also be affected (Figure 29). Unlike cavernous hemangiomas, the main arteries and veins leading to and from the mass are also enlarged. The abnormal channels consist of variable sized arteries and "arterialized" veins. Ischemic neurological manifestations may be associated with the vascular anomalies because degenerative changes within the vessels cause narrowing and predispose to thrombosis. Also in cases of AVM, blood may be shunted, creating some kind of an "internal steal" phenomenon. Some of the distended vessels may rupture and destroy the parenchyma. Pure venous varicosities (varices) are rare and more frequent in the spinal cord than in the brain.

Figure 29

Large arteriovenous malformation (AVM)

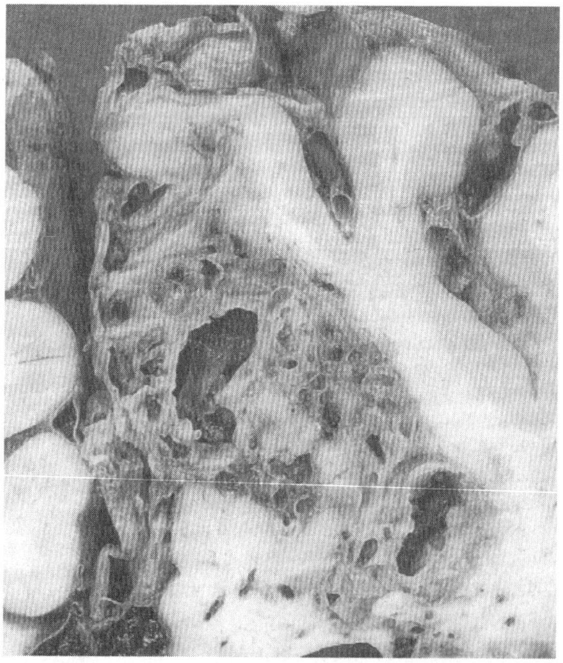

From Gray F, De Girolami U, Poirier J, eds. Escourolle and Poirier Manual of Basic Neuropathology. *4th ed. London: Elsevier; 2004. With permission.*

5. Neurodegenerative Diseases

The ravages of advanced age affect both mind and body, and perhaps nowhere do we recognize this more so than with the degenerative diseases of the nervous system. Combined now with the gross and microscopic changes that have been known for more than 100 years for many of the neurodegenerative ailments are an armamentarium of genetic and molecular data that have transformed how we look at and classify these diseases. Many of these disorders have both sporadic and familial forms, providing clues to the pathogenetic basis of these diseases. Described in this section are some of the more prevalent and better studied, though unfortunately, still not fully understood disorders with an emphasis on pathological findings.

Misfolding and aggregation of proteins is a hallmark of many neurodegenerative diseases, though it is still not known in many cases whether these phenomena are central to the pathogenesis, secondary injury, or perhaps even protective to the cell. Aggregates that form are multimeric but often have a predominant protein and tend to affect certain neuronal or glial cells in different diseases (Table 3). Aggregates can form intracellularly in cytosol, nucleus, or neuritic processes, or extracellularly with diverse cellular pathological consequences, often including cell death.

Alzheimer Disease

Alzheimer disease (AD) is the most common of the neurodegenerative diseases, with an increasing incidence in every decade of life. The prevalence roughly doubles every five years, starting from a level of 1% for the 60- to 64-year-old population and reaching 40% or more for the 85- to 89-year-old cohort. Brains from afflicted individuals grossly show variable cerebral atrophy with hippocampi and adjacent medial temporal cortices showing consistent diminution in size. Frontal and parietal lobes also often show diffuse atrophy with narrowed gyri and widened sulci, and occipital lobes are often unaffected. Coronal slices invariably show thinned cortical gray strips and enlarged ventricular system underscoring the widespread neuronal loss.

The microscopic hallmarks of this disease are plaques, neurofibrillary tangles, neuronal loss and reactive glial changes. Many aging brains have

Table 3

Neurodegenerative Diseases and their Associated Protein Aggregate Pathology

Neurological Disease	Primary Cell Type Affected	Anatomical Region Affected	Protein Aggregation
Alzheimer disease	*Neurons*	*neocortex, hippocampus, entorrhinal cortex*	*Neurofibrillary tangles and amyloid plaques*
Parkinson disease	*Neurons*	*substantia nigra, nucleus basalis, locus ceruleus*	*Lewy bodies*
Lewy body disease	*Neurons*	*substantia nigra, neocortex*	*Cortical Lewy bodies*
Amyotrophic lateral sclerosis	*Upper and lower motor neurons*	*motor cortex, lower motor neurons anterior horn of spinal cord*	*Bunina bodies, skein-like aggregates*
Corticobasal degeneration	*Neurons and glia*	*basal ganglia and cerebral cortex*	*Tau inclusions cytoplasmic and processes*
Multisystem atrophy	*Glia and neurons (less)*	*brainstem, midbrain, cerebellum, striatum*	*Synuclein/ubiquitin inclusions*
Prion diseases	*Neurons*	*variable and diffuse depending on subtype*	*Amyloid and prion plaques*
Frontotemporal dementias	*Neurons*	*hippocampus, frontal and temporal cortices*	*Tau tangles/pretangles (Pick bodies in Pick disease)*
Huntington disease	*Neurons*	*caudate, putamen, and cerebral cortex*	*Polyglutamine tract inclusions in neurites and nuclei*
Progressive Supranuclear Palsy	*Neurons and glia*	*globus pallidus, midbrain, pons, subthalamic nucleus*	*Globose neurofibrillary tangles (neurons), Coiled bodies (oligos), Tufted and thorn (astrocytes)*

Figure 32

Spinal cord in ALS with pallor of the corticospinal tracts (Loyez stain)

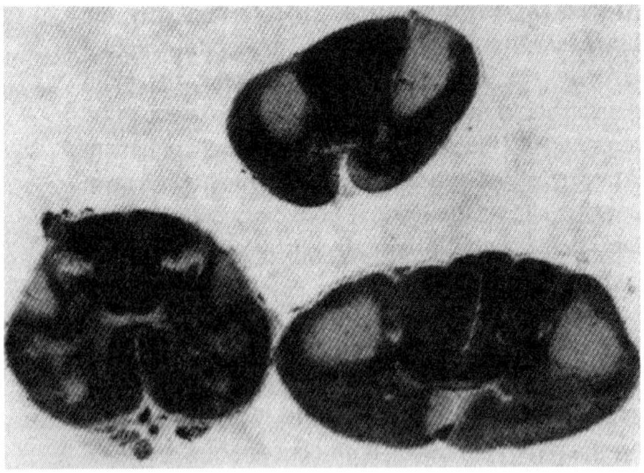

From Gray F, De Girolami U, Poirier J, eds. Escourolle and Poirier Manual of Basic Neuropathology. *4th ed. London: Elsevier; 2004. With permission.*

diffuse type plaques composed of collections of atypical neurites seen best with special silver stains, but AD plaques (also called mature, senile or neuritic plaques) are somewhat different. AD plaques are composed of Abeta protein deposits forming amyloid surrounded by degenerating neuritic processes. The amyloid can be visualized with a stain called Congo red which imparts an orange-red color by standard brightfield microscopy and an apple-green birefringence with polarized light. A vast majority of AD brains also show amyloid angiopathy to some degree. Activated microglia and astrocytes can also be found in and around these plaques.

Neurofibrillary tangles are intracellular inclusions of a variety of shapes composed of several proteins, with tau being the predominant. The tangles can be seen well with silver stains such as Bodian or Bielschowsky or by immunohistochemistry to tau (Figure 30, color plates). An increased number of plaques and tangles combined with the appropriate clinical course are used to make the diagnosis of AD, and most pathologists will generally follow diagnostic guidelines of the NIA-Reagan and CERAD (Consortium to Establish a Registry for AD) criteria.

While there is intense research being performed on uncovering the pathogenesis of AD, there is still some controversy as to the relative importance of the plaques and tangles in the disease process.

Approximately 75% of AD cases are thought to be sporadic, and 25% hereditary, with the latter group showing either early or late onsets. Mutations in presenilin ([PSEN], *PSEN1, PSEN2*), or amyloid precursor protein (*APP*) genes account for the majority of early onset familial AD, but there exists a wide spectrum of mutations in these genes as well as variable clinical and pathologic presentations. Individuals with trisomy 21 who survive beyond 45 years of age nearly all develop AD genes. A genetic susceptibility gene for the apolipoprotein E (ApoE) protein has been identified in sporadic AD. ApoE has 3 alleles: ApoE ε2, ApoE ε3, and ApoE ε4. Individuals that produce the ε4 form are a greater risk for developing AD, while those that have the ε2 have decreased risk. Polymorphisms in the APOE isoforms may also confer variable susceptibility. Genetic testing for the ApoE alleles is not generally done outside of the research setting, as the beneficial/detrimental effects are not absolute.

Figure 34

Pick's brain with severe cortical atrophy

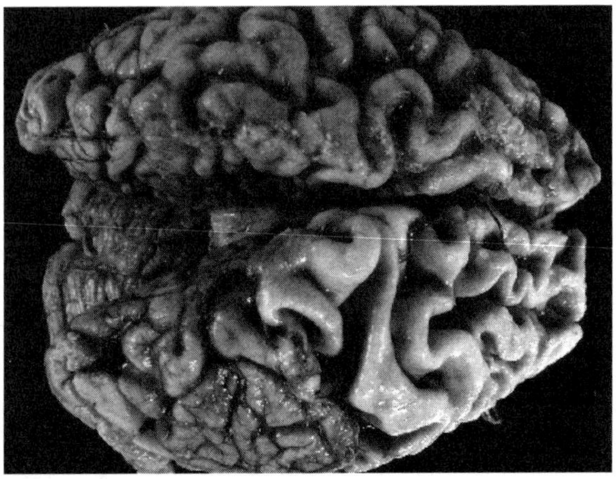

Parkinson Disease

The nonspecific clinical features of bradykinesia, rigidity, and tremor are typically found in Parkinson disease (PD), though other neurodegerative or even vascular diseases can manifest these symptoms as well. The pathological findings of (PD) are well known to all neurologists. These include the gross finding of pallor within the substantia nigra of the midbrain and locus ceruleus of the pons due to loss of dopaminergic and noradrenergic neurons of these nuclei, respectively (Figure 31, color plates). Lewy bodies are the eosinophilic cytoplasmic inclusions found within neurons of the substantia nigra, locus ceruleus, and nucleus basalis of Meynert of PD patients. These inclusions are composed of and can be immunostained for alpha-synuclein, ubiquitin, parkin, and neurofilaments. Lewy bodies are also found in cortical neurons in another disease that presents with more profound dementia with or without parkinsonism, called either diffuse Lewy body disease or dementia with Lewy bodies.

Multiple System Atrophy

This disorder actually encompasses three distinct clinical diseases: sporadic olivopontocerebellar atrophy (characterized by cerebellar ataxia); Shy-Drager syndrome (primary autonomic failure); and striatonigral degeneration (parkinsonism). What they share in common are unique inclusion bodies found within glial cells (usually oligodendroglial) and less commonly neurons concentrated within their respective areas but often widespread. Neuronal loss and gliosis is found within these areas as well. Silver staining is used to highlight the inclusions. The inclusions also contain alpha-synuclein, and so MSA disorders can be considered as an alpha-synucleinopathy like PD.

Amyotrophic Lateral Sclerosis (ALS)

ALS is a disease of upper and lower motor neurons, with an unknown cause in the majority of cases, that occurs sporadically in older individuals (50-70 years). However, less than 10% of cases are familial (usually autosomal dominant) and mutations have been identified in genes encoding the ubiquitous superoxide dismutase (SOD1) protein or neurofilaments proteins. The altered SOD1 or neurofilament proteins are thought to cause a toxic "gain of function" that somehow leads to motor neuron death by some as yet unknown mechanism. Other genetic loci have also been identified in familial cases. Some of the cellular pathological mechanisms that have been proposed in ALS include glutamate excitotoxicity, altered axonal transport, deficient growth factors and/or receptors, mitochondrial toxicity and apoptosis, oxidative damage, and damage from inclusions. Whatever the mechanisms involved, the end result is depletion of upper and lower motor neurons as well as cranial nerve motor neurons. When examined microscopically, peripheral motor nerves and corticospinal tracts are depleted of large myelinated fibers (Figure 32). Remaining cranial nerve and spinal motor neurons can show cytoplasmic inclusions called Bunina bodies. Reactive astrocytes and microglia are found in the anterior horns of the cord and motor cortex, especially in layer V where the Betz corticospinal neurons are depleted.

Prion Diseases

These familial and sporadic diseases are unique disorders caused by abnormally conformed prion proteins that are adherently expressed in patients (Creutzfeldt-Jakob disease ((CJD)); fatal familial insomnia, (Gerstmann-Staussler-Scheinker ((GSS)) disease), transmitted by ingesting tainted beef (new variant nvCJD) or other affected human tissues (Kuru), or iatrogenically introduced by tainted

Figure 36

Spinal cord in Friedreich's ataxia (Loyez stain)

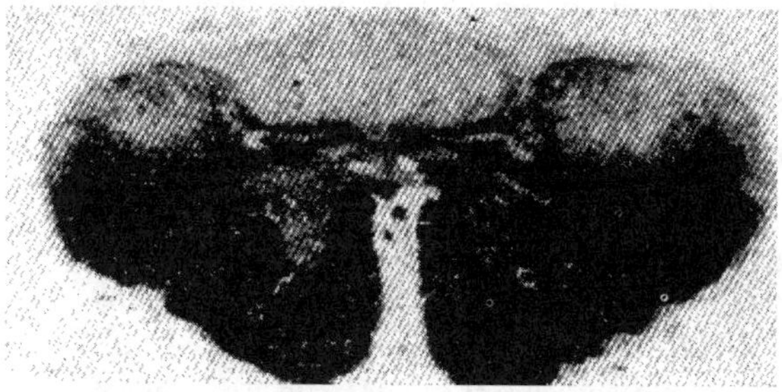

From Gray F, De Girolami U, Poirier J, eds. Escourolle and Poirier Manual of Basic Neuropathology. *4th ed. London: Elsevier; 2004. With permission.*

transplants or improperly cleaned surgical/dental equipment. They all cause some degree of spongiform encephalopathy, though the areas involved and clinical pictures are somewhat different. The spongiform change is accompanied by neuronal loss, gliosis, and distinctive plaque in the case of nvCJD and Kuru (Figure 33, color plates). These findings can be somewhat focal, are not obvious from gross examination of the brain, and may require extensive sampling. Immunohistochemistry or Western blot analysis to recognize the abnormal prion protein is generally performed to confirm the diagnosis. In the United States, tissues are generally submitted to the National Prion Disease Pathology Surveillance Center established by the American Association of Neuropathologists for these studies. Regular close physical contact by family members or by health care workers caring for these patients does not result in transmission of the disease.

Frontotemporal Dementias (FTD)

This group of disorders is characterized by degenerative changes of the frontal and temporal lobes and clinical findings of language dysfunction and behavioral changes. Pick disease, among the first described but likely only one subtype of the emerging field of frontotemporal dementias or frontotemporal lobar dementias (FTLD), is usually a sporadic but occasionally familial disorder. Brains display often pronounced, sometimes asymmetric "knife-edge" atrophy (Figure 34) of frontal and temporal lobes with conspicuous sparing of the anterior two-thirds of the superior temporal gyrus. On cut surface the caudate and putamen nuclei may be atrophied. The hallmark histological findings are Pick cells with their cytoplasmic inclusions that stain with silver stains, ubiquitin, and sometimes tau, placing the disease among the "tauopathies" (see discussion in the chapter on dementia). These cells are usually found in the dentate granule neurons (Figure 35, color plates) of the hippocampus but also in deep gray nuclei and cortex in some cases. Frontotemporal dementia associated with parkinsonism linked to chromosome 17 (FTD(P)-17) often shows little-to-moderate gross atrophy and tau positive neurofibrillary tangles in neurons, and sometimes glial cells in frontal and temporal lobes. Variable nigral degeneration is observed in such cases.

Spinocerebellar Ataxias (SCA)

Genetic characterization of these diverse diseases has aided helping to define distinct subsets of the cerebellar ataxias (as well as frustrating the neuropathology and neurology candidates studying for their boards!). One way of genetically defining these diseases is by autosomal dominant (SCA1-17) or recessive (Friedreich's ataxia, ataxia-telangiectasia ((AT)) inheritance pattern. Many of the dominant forms are related to trinucleotide repeats (often CAG) that encode for a polyglutamine tract within some known and other unknown proteins that accumulate within inclusions in affected cells. The greater the number of repeats, the earlier the age of onset. Another method of distinguishing them is by considering them as primary (inherited and sporadic forms) or secondary (neurometabolic, prion disease, toxic, infective, vascular, paraneoplastic). Morphological/neuropathological classification, at one time the gold standard, is now used in close conjunction with genetic/molecular characterization and, of course, clinical history to best define the distinct disease process. Clinically, these disorders are defined by signs and symptoms referable to the cerebellar system (progressive ataxia), brainstem, spinal cord, and peripheral nerves.

Pathologically, three main patterns of degeneration are recognized: cerebellar cortical atrophy, cerebellopetal atrophy, and cerebellofugal atrophy. In the cortical atrophy disorders, Purkinje cell loss is the hallmark finding, with associated Bergman gliosis. Secondary loss of inferior olivary neurons in the medulla is a result of transynaptic degeneration. Gliosis is also seen in both structures and is called Bergman gliosis in the cerebellum. Olivopontocerebellar atrophy is the classic form of the cerebellopetal atrophies with selective degeneration of basis pontis nuclei and pontocerebellar fibers. The cerebellum shows loss of white matter tracts, gliosis with less pronounced Purkinje or granular cell loss. Olivary nuclei show neuronal loss as well. Cerebellofugal atrophies are characterized by dentate nucleus atrophy, loss of their efferent fibers through the cerebellar peduncles, and red nucleus atrophy. Globus pallidus atrophy accompanies in the polyglutamine disorder dentato-rubro-pallido-luysian atrophy (DRPLA).

Friedreich's ataxia is an autosomal recessive disorder that has been mapped to chromosome 9 and involves a trinucleotide repeat in a protein called frataxin. This altered protein has been shown to involve dysregulation of iron levels and mitochondrial dysfunction. Morphologically, there is loss of corticospinal and spinocerebellar tracts (Figure 36), as well as neuronal loss of Betz cells, Clark's column, dorsal root ganglia, some cranial nerve, and dentate and Purkinje cell neurons. Myocardial fibrosis leading to cardiac failure is present in many patients.

Ataxia telangiectasia (AT) is caused by mutations in a gene designated as the AT-mutated (ATM) gene on chromosome 11, and is associated with telangiectasias, immune deficiencies, increased risk of cancers, and cerebellar signs and symptoms. There is marked loss of Purkinje and granule neurons in the cerebellum, degeneration of inferior olives and posterior columns in the brainstem, and sometimes loss of anterior horn and dorsal root ganglion cells with peripheral neuropathy.

Huntington Disease

This autosomal dominant transmitted disease is clinically characterized by chorea and progressive dementia. Genetically it is caused by mutations in the huntingtin gene located on chromosome 4 that confers variable polyglutamine copies to the protein. Patients with Huntington disease have expanded repeats that cause an accumulation of the abnormal protein and formation of nuclear inclusions within cells of the striatum and cortex. How these inclusions lead to cellular dysfunction and degeneration is not known. The classic gross appearance of the brain on coronal section is widened lateral ventricles and atrophied, flattened caudate and putamen nuclei (Figure 37).

Figure 37

Huntington disease brain with flattened atrophic caudate (Loyez stain)

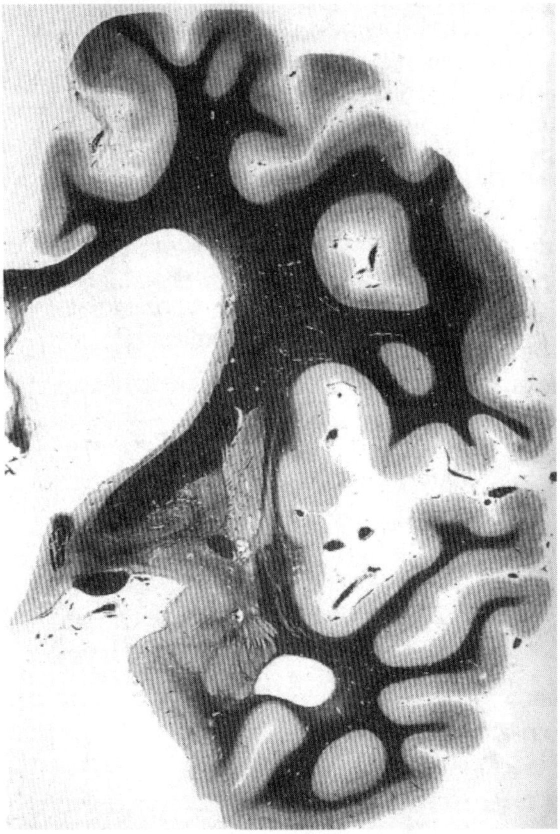

From Gray F, De Girolami U, Poirier J, eds. Escourolle and Poirier Manual of Basic Neuropathology. *4th ed. London: Elsevier; 2004. With permission.*

6. References

1. Bruijn LI, Miller TM, Cleveland DW. Unraveling the mechanisms involved in motor neuron degeneration in ALS. *Annu Rev Neurosci*. 2004;27:723-749.

2. Dickson D. *Neurodegeneration: The Molecular Pathology of Dementia and Movement Disorders*. Basel: ISN Neuropath Press; 2003.

3. Graham D, Lantos P. *Greenfield's Neuropathology*. 7th ed. London: Arnold; 2002.

4. Gray F, De Girolami U, Poirier J, eds. *Escourolle and Poirier Manual of Basic Neuropathology*. 4th ed. Philadelphia, Pa: Butterworth and Heinemann; 2004.

5. Kumar V, Abbas A, Fausto N, eds. *Robbins and Cotran Pathologic Basis of Disease*. 7th ed. London: Elsevier; 2004.

6. Louis, D.N., Ohgaki, H., Wiestler, O.D., Cavenee, W.K. *WHO Classification of Tumours of the Central Nervous System*. 4th ed. Lyon: IARC Press; 2000.

7. Questions

1. Which of the following is the INCORRECT statement about prion diseases?

A. The majority of prion diseases are sporadic and called Creutzfeldt-Jakob disease.

B. Kuru and new variant CJD are similar in that they both show unique speculated plaques that are not seen in sporadic CJD.

C. The common histological findings of prion diseases are vacuolation (spongiform change), neuronal loss, and gliosis.

D. Prion diseases have been shown to be transferred from person to person by close physical contact.

2. Which of the following cells become "reactive" with increased cytoplasmic GFAP and altered physiology in the CNS in response to ischemic/hypoxic, infectious, neoplastic, and traumatic insults?

A. Neurons

B. Oligodendroglia

C. Astrocytes

D. Fibroblasts

3. A relatively common type of bleed in the elderly patients, often due to tearing of the meningeal "bridging" veins is:

A. Epidural hemorrhage

B. Subdural hemorrhage

C. Subarachnoid hemorrhage

D. Intraparenchymal hemorrhage

4. All of the following are common sites for diffuse axonal injury (DAI) except:

A. Cerebellar cortex

B. Corpus callosum

C. Periaqueductal gray matter

D. Walls of the third ventrical

5. A woman has been found lying on the floor in a pool of blood apparently emanating from a large scalp laceration on her forehead. Closer examination reveals a large, depressed skull fracture to her occiput. Professor Plum has been accused of the heinous act of murdering Miss Scarlet with a lead pipe in the ballroom. Which of the following pathologic findings on brain examination at autopsy is least likely to relate to her acute demise?

A. Subarachnoid hemorrhage

B. Coup-contacoup contusions

C. Subdural and/or subarachnoid hemorrhages

D. Plaques jaunes degenerative changes

E. Skull fracture

6. Often presents as a "space occupying lesion" and neurosurgical emergency after skull fracture and laceration of the middle meningeal artery.

A. Epidural hematoma

B. Subdural hematoma

C. Both of the above

D. Neither of the above

7. Sometimes occurs during even minor head trauma, with rebleeding forming inner and outer membranes:

A. Acute subdural hematoma

B. Chronic subdural hematoma

C. Acute epidural hematoma

D. Chronic epidural hematoma

E. Subarachnoid hemorrhage

8. A nine-month-old infant presents to you in the ER comatose with the report of "falling out of the crib and hitting her head." On exam she doesn't seem to have any head surface contusions. After investigating a little further, you find out that she has had several hospital visits for "accidental" trauma, and you suspect child abuse and possibly shaken infant syndrome. Which of the following is least likely to be present in this case if your diagnosis is correct?

A. Diffuse axonal injury

B. Retinal hemorrhages

C. Subdural and/or subarachnoid hemorrhages

D. Skull fracture

E. Contusional tear in the white matter

9. A large intraparenchymal hemorrhage is found on autopsy in the region of the basal ganglia. The most common clinical setting for this to occur would be in:

A. A person in shock with a "borderzone" infarction

B. An elderly person after a recent fall with trauma to the brain

C. A young patient with atrial fibrillation who is "throwing off" cardiac thromboemboli

D. An elderly hypertensive patient with history of TIAs (transient ischemic attacks)

10. All of the following are true of berry aneurysms except:

A. They most commonly occur at bifurcation points around the circle of Willis.

B. Hypertension has been documented in about half the cases.

C. Rupture of even small berry aneurysms (<1 cm) is inevitable; so they must all be surgically treated.

D. Rupture can cause a large subarachnoid hemorrhage and patients presenting with complaints of "the worst headache of my life."

E. They have been associated with syndromes like: Marfan, Ehlers-Danlos, and autosomal dominant polycystic kidney disease.

11. True or False:

A sudden drop in perfusion pressure to the brain can cause a bilateral "watershed" or "borderzone" infarction.

12. All of the histological changes are considered in determining the grade of an astrocytoma, EXCEPT:

A. Necrosis

B. Metastatic implants found outside the CNS

C. Endothelial proliferation

D. Mitotic activity

E. Nuclear pleomorphism

13. Which of the following subtypes of meningioma has been found to have a more aggressive clinical behavior?

A. Papillary

B. Meningothelial

C. Psammomatous

D. Lymphoplasmacytic

E. Transitional

14. The following tumor found predominantly in the pediatric population often has a benign clinical course once resected:

A. Fibrillary astrocytoma

B. Pilocytic astrocytoma

C. Medulloblastoma

D. Ependymoma

15. Parkinson disease and multiple system atrophy have the following in common:

A. They both present with disturbances of the autonomic nervous system

B. Both display neurofibrillary tangles

C. Both show inclusions containing alpha-synuclein

D. Lewy bodies are present in both

16. Which of the following in NOT true of ALS?

A. ALS is a disease affecting both corticospinal neurons and spinal motor neurons

B. Many patients with the sporadic form of ALS have mutations in the SOD1 gene

C. The number of sporadic cases of ALS far outnumbers the familial cases

D. Bunina bodies are the characteristic inclusions found in ALS

E. A muscle biopsy is generally not necessary in making the diagnosis of ALS

17. Which of the following neurodegenerative diseases is characterized by gross "knife-edge atrophy of the frontal cortex?"

A. Alzheimer disease

B. Multiple system atrophy

C. Pick disease

D. Prion disease

E. Huntington disease

Answers

1. D.
Prion diseases can be transferred via tainted surgical instruments or tissues iatrogenically, ingesting tainted food (nvCJD), or genetically (FFI, GSS disease).

2. C.
Astrocytes change structurally and functionally in response to many neuropathological insults.

3. B.
Subdural hemorrhages can be chronic or acute and may represent a neurosurgical emergency when they expand precipitously as space occupying lesions.

4. A.
DAI is widespread tearing of axons, primarily in white matter, usually produced during angular acceleration or deceleration of the head. It tends to occur where bundles of tracts are exposed to rotational forces.

5. D.
Plaques jaunes degenerative changes would have occurred over months to years from contusion injuries and aren't related to this acute and heinous crime.

6. A.
Epidural (also called extradural) hemorrhages are often arterial and represent a neurosurgical emergency.

7. B.
Chronic subdural hematomas, if small, sometimes go unnoticed by patients. They can re-bleed multiple times and form membranes composed of fibrovascular connective tissues and inflammatory infiltrates.

8. D.
All of the answers are often found to varying degrees with inflicted, traumatic infant head injury. A skull fracture would be unlikely in this particular case, as no external head contusions were observed.

9. D.
Hemorrhagic basal ganglia infarcts are nearly always seen in the setting of acute severe hypertension or, more commonly, chronic poorly controlled hypertension patients. Brain stem and cerebellar hemorrhagic infarcts are other common locations.

10. C.
Many small berry aneurysms do not rupture, are clinically silent, and are uncovered as incidental findings at autopsy.

11. True
because this watershed area is a borderzone between major arterial distributions, and is the most susceptible to infarction in low perfusion settings.

12. B.
Glial tumors very rarely metastasize outside of the CNS.

13. A.
Of these subtypes listed only papillary meningiomas, a rare subtype, are considered WHO Grade III based on architectural subtype alone.

14. B.
Pilocytic astrocytomas are considered WHO Grade I because resection often cures the patient with usually no need for radiation or chemotherapy as opposed to other glial tumors that often recur even in the face of a good resection, radiation and/or chemotherapy.

15. C.
These diseases are considered among the synucleinopathies.

16. B.
Sporadic ALS patients do not show mutations in the SOD1 gene. Some familial patients show SOD1 mutations, though other genes have also been implicated in familial ALS.

17. C.
Pick disease, one of the more common fronto-temporal dementias shows the gross finding of "knife-edge" atrophy of the gyri in these regions.

Color Figures

Figure 1

Acute hypoxic-ischemic changes in "red-dead" neurons

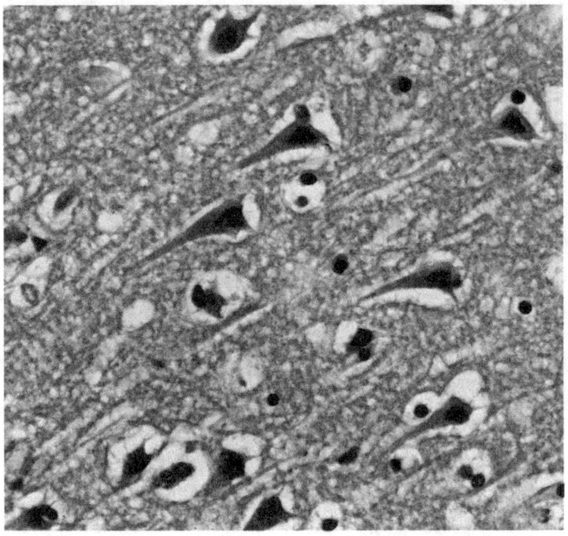

Figure 4

Cowdry type A inclusion in neuron

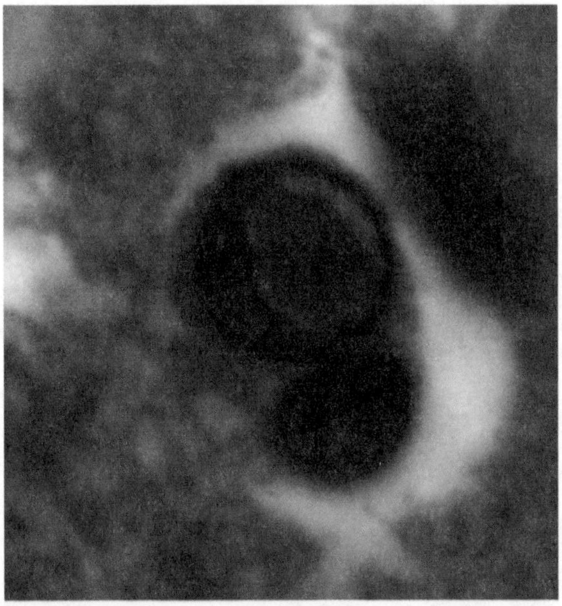

Figure 8

Eosinophilic granular bodies (A) and Rosenthal fibers (B) in a pilocytic astrocytoma

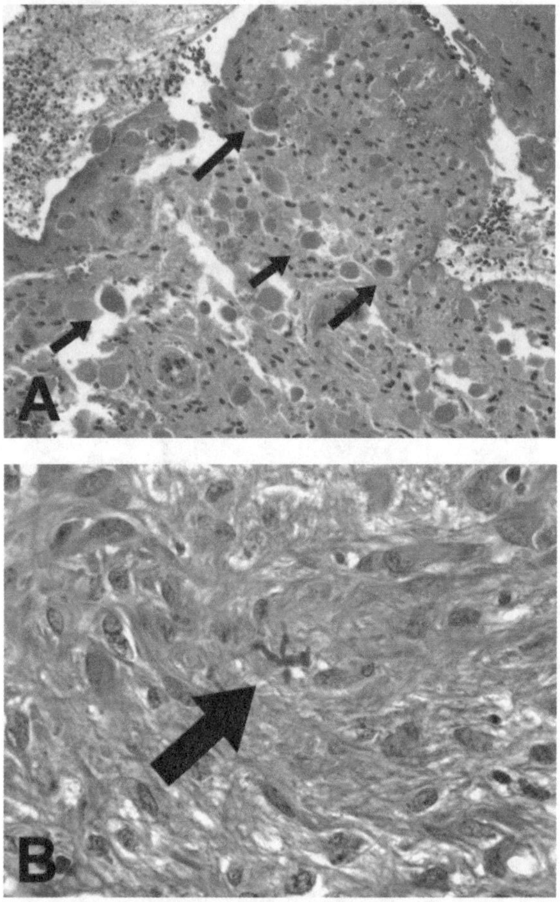

Figure 23

A) Axonal spheroids seen after diffuse axonal injury, B) Beta-amyloid staining of spheroids and injured axons

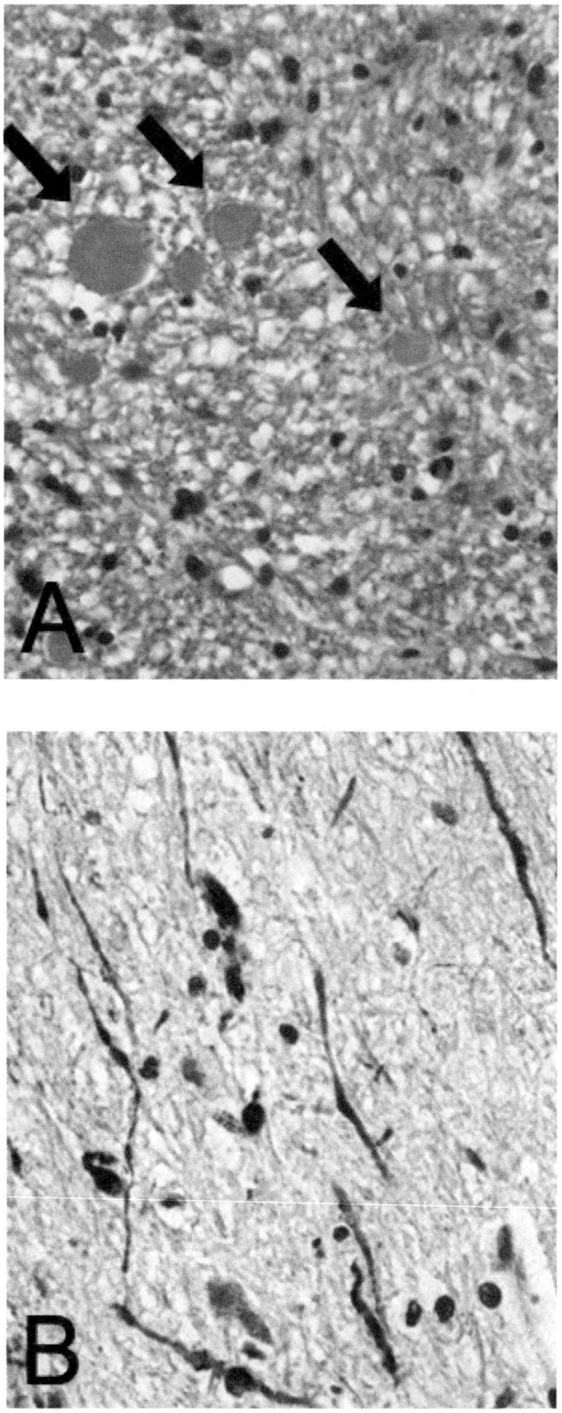

From Gray F, De Girolami U, Poirier J, eds. Escourolle and Poirier Manual of Basic Neuropathology. *4th ed. London: Elsevier; 2004. With permission.*

Figure 30

Neurofibrillary tangles (arrows) and Alzheimer-type plaques in patient with AD (tau immunostain)

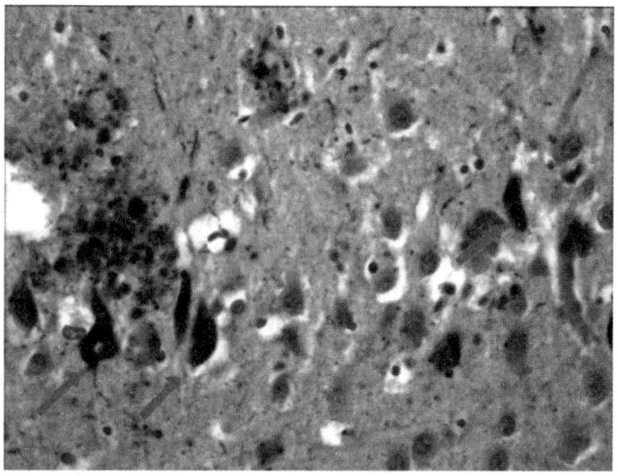

Figure 31

A) Normal midbrain with well-pigmented substantia nigra,
B) Parkinson's patient midbrain, C) SN neuron with Lewy body

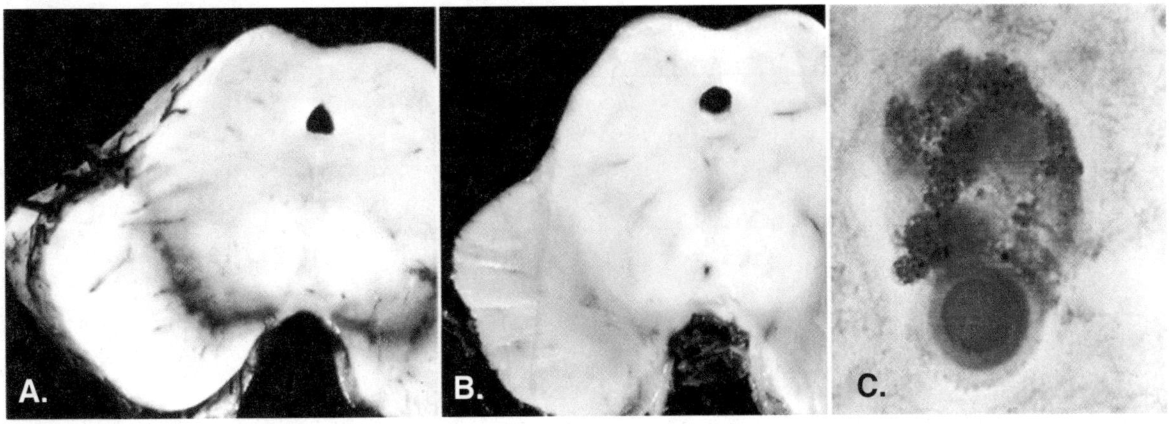

From Kumar V, Abbas A, Fausto N, eds. Robbins and Cotran Pathologic Basis of Disease. *7th ed. Elsevier; 2005. With permission.*

Figure 33

New variant CJD with vacuolations and spiculated plaques (arrows)

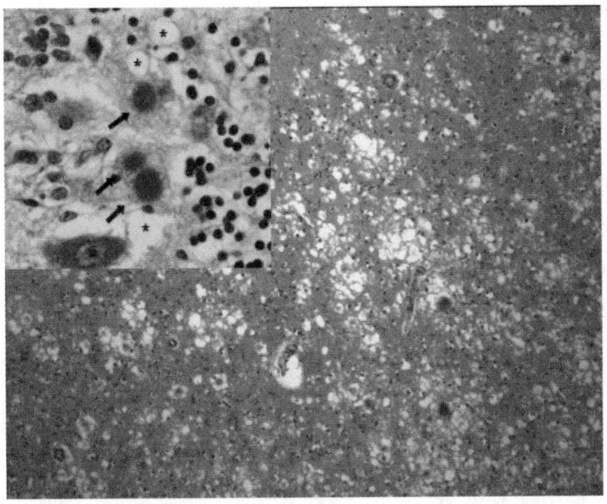

Figure 35

Ubiquitin immunostaining of hippocampal dentate nucleus in Pick disease

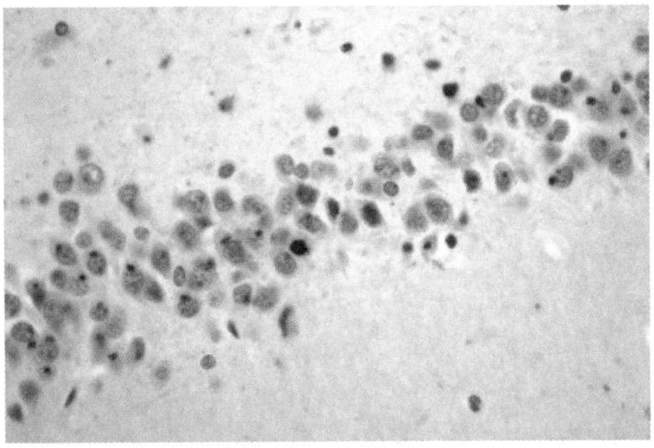

Chapter 8: Coma and Confusion

Morris Levin, MD

Contents

Introduction

The comatose patient requires rapid evaluation and often rapid treatment. Unfortunately, diagnosis can be challenging due to the limited information available. There are a wide variety of conditions which can either cause coma or a syndrome resembling coma. Medical status can dramatically worsen during coma, and few signs may indicate this. Hence accurate assessment of causes and progression of pathophysiology are crucial goals.

Confusion, often described as the rather vague "altered mental state," in many instances may herald depression of consciousness, and eventually coma. The differential diagnosis of the confusional state thus overlaps with that of coma. This chapter will deal first with the pathophysiology, diagnosis, treatment and prognosis of patients with a depressed level of consciousness, followed by a similar discussion of the confusional state.

1. Coma and Altered Level of Consciousness

Terms

There is a long list of terms used to describe different altered states of consciousness, and definitions are difficult to agree upon. Consciousness is probably best used to describe the normal state of awareness with full responsiveness. However, attention, cognitive dysfunction, and emotional states can alter the appearance of consciousness dramatically. Additionally, the normal state of consciousness may fluctuate throughout the awake period. Coma should be reserved for patients who are not conscious and that cannot be aroused. This differentiates it from sleep, from which one can be aroused. (There are other physiological differences between sleep and coma which can be measured, including EEG patterns and cerebral utilization of oxygen.) Stupor is used to refer to patients who are unconscious but who can be aroused to some degree of responsiveness. Somnolence refers to patients who tend to drift into stupor without constant stimulation. Terms like obtundation, lethargy, and organic brain syndrome are best avoided.

Anatomy

In order to maintain consciousness, the reticular activating system (RAS) in the brainstem (upper pons through midbrain), diencephalon (thalamus), and cerebral hemispheres must be functional. Due to redundancy of function, only one side is required for consciousness, thus bilateral pathology is required in this system for an alteration in consciousness. The brainstem portions of the RAS are located in paramedian regions and the thalamic structures involved in the RAS include the paramedian, parafascicular, centromedian, and intralaminar nuclei. The RAS receives input from multiple ascending sensory systems and projects to widespread areas of the cortex.

Localization of Lesions and Differential Diagnosis of Coma

There are three broad categories of lesions or illnesses which produce coma (see Table 1):

1) *Supratentorial mass lesions* which are either large enough (or under enough pressure) to cause dysfunction in the upper portions of the RAS bilaterally, or produce downward herniation of the brain causing compression of the brainstem RAS.

2) *Infratentorial mass lesions* with compression, or insult to the brainstem.

3) *Diffuse or multifocal* brain disease.

Supratentorial mass lesions, eg, hemorrhage, tumor, or abscess, may be of such magnitude as to put pressure on the cerebral portions of the RAS. This is rarely missed on neuroimaging and often subfalcial herniation is seen, along with dramatic effacement of ventricles and cortical sulci. Alternatively, supratentorial masses may produce downward herniation of brain structures, either in a symmetric or asymmetric fashion.

With symmetric (central) transtentorial herniation, for example due to thalamic hemorrhage, the force is exerted in a rostral caudal direction and leads to

Table 1

Differential Diagnosis of Coma

Supratentorial Mass

Intracerebral hemorrhage
Cerebral abscess(es)
Neoplasm: primary or metastatic
Cerebral contusions
Subdural hematoma
Epidural hematoma

Infratentorial Mass or Other Lesions

Cerebellar hemorrhage
Cerebellar abscess
Cerebellar or brainstem neoplasm
Posterior fossa subdural hematoma

Diffuse or Multifocal Causes

Multiple CVA
Cerebral venous thrombosis
Vasculitis
Subarachnoid hemorrhage
Diffuse hypoxia/ischemia (cardiac, pulmonary)
Infections: meningitis, encephalitis
Concussion
Drug intoxication: alcohol, barbiturates, neuroleptics, anticonvulsants

Diffuse or Multifocal Causes

Drug withdrawal
Neuroleptic malignant syndrome
Toxins: Sedatives, narcotics, industrial toxins, cyanide, heavy metals
Hypoglycemia, diabetic ketoacidosis, nonketotic hyperglycemic coma
Wernicke-Korsakoff
Reye syndrome
Hepatic or renal encephalopathy
Thyrotoxicosis or myxedema
Hypo- or hyperadrenal state
Hypertensive encephalopathy
Electrolyte derangement: Na, acidosis, alkalosis, Mg, Ca, Phosph
Central pontine myelinolysis
Hypothermia, heat stroke
Seizure: nonconvulsive status epilepticus, postictal state

Psychogenic Coma

Catatonia
Conversion disorder
Malingering

ventral movement of the diencephalon with early brainstem dysfunction. Coma is an early result as the RAS is affected at the onset. Small but reactive pupils are seen as a result of hypothalamic (sympathetic) dysfunction but extraocular movements tend to be preserved initially. Decerebrate and decorticate posturing occur, although some authors emphasize the early decorticate stage followed by a (supposedly irreversible) later decerebrate stage. Respiration is affected, often producing hyperventilation and then more ataxic patterns. Later, brainstem function is lost, pupils become fixed, and death ensues.

Asymmetric downward brain herniation is the result of a unilateral lesion becoming so massive as to produce downward movement of the inferior portions of the temporal lobe (including the uncus) toward the lateral aspect of the brainstem (Figure 1). Typical causes include subdural hematoma or temporal lobe neoplasm. This uncal transtentorial herniation tends to produce a sequence of observable events. First the medial-inferior temporal lobe compresses the exiting oculomotor nerve against the brainstem, which leads to ipsilateral pupillary dilation, followed by dysconjugate eye movements. A paradoxical ipsilateral hemiparesis occurs next due to compression of the midbrain peduncle against the contralateral Kernohan's notch of the tentorium. Respiration often deteriorates, but the pattern can vary including Cheyne-Stokes or hyperventilation. Decorticate and/or decerebrate posturing may occur and eventually bilateral paresis and posturing are seen. If the process is not arrested, bilateral fixed pupils, and then death, occur.

Table 2 summarizes the presentations of central and uncal transtentorial herniation.

Table 2

Signs of Central and Uncal Transtentorial Herniation

Central transtentorial herniation

1. Early coma
2. Small pupils
3. Normal EOMs
4. Posturing
5. Later – Bilateral fixed pupils, respiratory arrest, death (similar to late stage of uncal herniation)

Uncal transtentorial herniation

1. Medial temp lobe (compresses III → ipsilateral pupil) dilation then poor EOM
2. Ipsilateral hemiparesis due to compression of midbrain peduncle by Kernohan's notch of tentorium
3. Cheyne-Stokes or hyperventilation
4. Posturing
5. Bilateral fixed pupils, death

Infratentorial mass lesions such as hemorrhage, tumor, or abscess produce altered consciousness including coma as a result of brainstem compression. Focal brainstem lesions of other types, such as brainstem stroke or central pontine myelinolysis (CPM) are also possible causes. Tracts and cranial nerve nuclei are subject to damage which is apparent on examination (eg, hemiparesis, hemisensory loss, pupillary changes, dysconjugate gaze, absent corneal reflex, facial paresis). In the more alert patient, diplopia, vertigo, and dysarthria can be observed. Clinical clues suggestive of brainstem lesions include:

1. Bilateral motor or sensory loss

2. Crossed syndromes – eg, facial weakness and body weakness on opposite sides

3. Miosis

4. Loss of lateral gaze with preserved vertical gaze, or dysconjugate gaze

5. Abnormal respiratory pattern early in the course, including Cheyne-Stokes pattern.

Coma resulting from metabolic derangement, or diffuse or multifocal brain disease is due to bilateral damage to the RAS, diffuse cerebral insult or to increased intracranial pressure (ICP). A myriad of illnesses can lead to coma on this basis including multifocal strokes; cerebral venous thrombosis; subarachnoid hemorrhage; diffuse hypoxia/ischemia (eg, due to cardiac or pulmonary disease); infections such as meningitis or encephalitis; medications and toxins such as sedatives, narcotics, anticonvulsants, industrial toxins, cyanide, heavy metals; cerebral vasculitis; metabolic derangements such as hypoglycemia, hypo- or hypernatremia, acidosis, alkalosis, magnesium or calcium abnormalities; hepatic, renal, or thyroid dysfunction; Wernicke encephalopathy; Reye syndrome; hypothermia; heat stroke; non-convulsive status epilepticus; and postictal state. Respiratory depression may occur early and myoclonus or posturing may be seen. A telling feature in some metabolic causes of coma is the preservation of pupillary reactivity. Non-penetrating brain injury can also lead to transient coma as part of the concussion syndrome (see below).

Conditions which Mimic Coma

Locked-In Syndrome

The "locked-in syndrome" implies total paralysis of limbs and most cranial nerves, with preserved mentation and presumably some afferent input. Patients with brainstem stroke, CPM, Güillain-Barré syndrome, and amyotrophic lateral sclerosis (ALS) have been described with locked-in syndrome. Often, when midbrain or other anatomical structures are left intact, some extraocular movements can be spared. This can be the sole avenue for patients to interact with the environment. Jean Dominique Bauby, a brainstem stroke survivor, who became "locked-in," wrote an entire book, now a film, *The Diving Bell and the Butterfly*, painstakingly indicating to a stenographer one letter at a time via a system of left eyelid signals (the only motor function he retained). Fortunately, most patients are only partially locked in. It is crucial to realize in these cases that while central nervous system function may appear to be severely impaired, it is mainly efferent activity that is dysfunctional, and they may perceive things such as conversations at the bedside. Often patients appear comatose or stuporous due to their inability to respond to the examiner, particularly if eyes are closed. With aggressive supportive care, significant improvement may occur, particularly in the first days after injury.

Persistent Vegetative State (PVS) and Brain Death

In this condition, destruction of most of the cerebrum has occurred, sparing much of the brainstem and diencephalon (thalamus/hypothalamus). As a result, thought processes are essentially absent but neural activity sufficient to sustain basic metabolism (respiration, cardiovascular function, and even sleep wake cycling to some extent) remains. Patients are unconscious but can appear conscious (especially to medically unsophisticated observers), and it is difficult for families of patients to accept the reality of what is, essentially, death of the individual. Some patients can, for example, display reflex reactivity to pain stimuli, moan and seem to open or close their eyes following stimulation. The most common cause of PVS is diffuse brain anoxia, but multifocal strokes or other lesions can also produce a similar state. There is no treatment with any hope of improving the patient's status.

Some extremely rare reports of patients "waking up" from PVS have led some to question the permanence of this condition. However, these cases were almost certainly misdiagnosed, and rather than PVS, may have been in the so-called "minimally conscious state," the definition of which is still being debated.

Drawing the conclusion of "brain death" is a delicate process, but important because it can: 1) give loved ones closure, and avoid depletion of financial resources, and 2) make organ donation possible. However, in most institutions, brain death is defined as the absence of both cerebral and brainstem function (including respiratory drive), so chronic vegetative state does not meet criteria.

Akinetic Mutism (AK)

This is not generally mistaken for coma as patients with AK are generally awake appearing. However, the extreme unresponsiveness they display may seem deeply stuporous, particularly if eyes are partially or completely closed. This condition is generally the result of bilateral anterior frontal lobe lesions (sparing motor and sensory functions) resulting in extreme abulia (loss of impulse to perform action). Interestingly, these patients are able to perceive events around them and can form memories.

Psychiatric Causes of Coma and Altered Consciousness

Catatonic stupor is characterized by either acute or subacute development of stupor with waxy flexibility of limbs and sometimes echolalia and echopraxia and/or periods of greater activity. Catatonia is an uncommon manifestation of schizophrenia, but a similar state can be seen in severe depression. Intravenous sodium amytal can improve responsiveness temporarily and so may help to confirm the diagnosis. EEG shows normal background alpha activity, unlike other comatose conditions.

Conversion disorder may manifest as a state of unresponsiveness and apparent unconsciousness. Like catatonia, EEG looks relatively normal and sodium amytal can normalize behavior to some extent. According to the *DSM-IV-TR*, this psychogenic coma is considered a dissociative disorder.

Figure 1

Uncal herniation

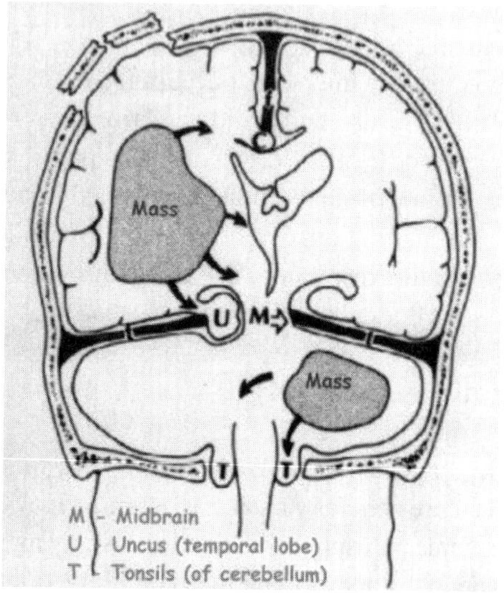

Lesion exerting downward pressure on the inferior portion of the temporal lobe, producing downward and medial shift toward the brainstem

Source: http://rad.usuhs.mil/rad/herniation/herniation.html

Coma due to malingering is not difficult to diagnose with general and neurological examination and simple provocative testing.

Examination of the Comatose Patient

Level of Consciousness

As mentioned earlier, the terms awake, somnolent, stupor, and coma are useful when describing a patient's level of consciousness. Differentiating deep sleep from coma can be challenging at the bedside. Fluctuating level of consciousness, for example from somnolence to deeper stupor, can be confounding as well. Experienced nurses are often best at characterizing this assessment as they make more sustained observations. Stimulation is essential to assess responsiveness, and can be done progressively, beginning with verbal stimuli, then louder noises, tactile stimulation, and finally pain. Stimulatory tests must be done carefully.

Respiratory Pattern

Breathing is entirely under neurological control. The three known paired respiratory "centers" in the brainstem lie in the tegmentum of the medulla and pons, and send descending axons to the anterior horn cells controlling the right and left diaphragm (C3-5). When these centers or tracts are damaged, the patient's automatic respiratory pattern becomes altered. Older literature postulated a number of specific centers (eg, the "apneustic center"), which when damaged, were supposed to produce a specific breathing pattern. This is usually not accurate as the interconnections between these areas are not straightforward.

Voluntary respiration is controlled by frontal cortical centers, which probably interconnect with the brainstem centers, but which also directly stimulate phrenic nerve motor neurons in the anterior horn at the first three cervical levels.

The *Cheyne-Stokes respiratory pattern* (CSR) consists of hyperventilation alternating with apnea in a crescendo-decrescendo fashion. It can be seen in a number of conditions including metabolic encephalopathy, increased ICP, bilateral cerebral insults, and upper brainstem lesions. *Cluster breathing* is similar but consists of apneic spells separated by shallow hyperventilation without

Figure 2

Respiratory patterns

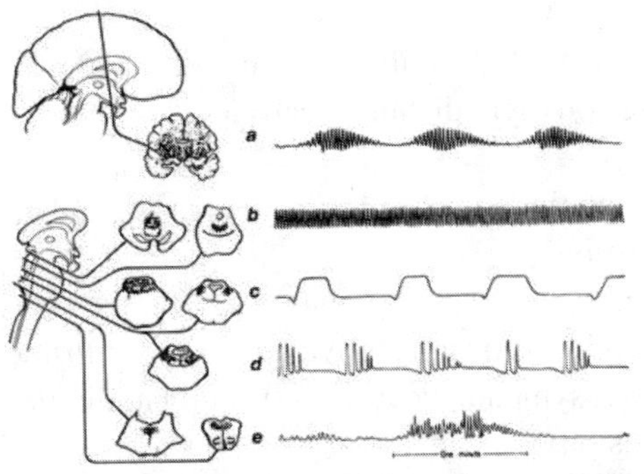

Figure 6a, c, e (p. 34) From 'Diagnosis of Stupor and Coma 3E' by Plume, Fred & Posner (1980). By permission of Oxford University Press, Inc.

crescendo-decrescendo pattern of CSR. This is supposedly seen with cerebellar or pontine damage. *Hyperventilation* is seen in metabolic acidosis and rostral brainstem lesions. *Apneustic breathing*, which consists of inspiratory pauses, is rare but can be seen in pontine lesions. *Ataxic breathing* is disorganized and ineffectual; it is usually seen in cases of medullary damage (see Figure 2).

Pupils

Pupillary size is controlled by muscles under sympathetic and parasympathetic control. Sympathetic innervation consists of a 3-neuron chain beginning in the hypothalamus, where neurons send axons caudally in the ipsilateral lateral brainstem tegmentum. 2nd order neurons in the intermediolateral column in spinal segments C8-T2 send axons via the T2 ventral root, through the stellate ganglion to synapse at the 3rd order neuron in the superior cervical ganglion. From there, fibers are found along the internal carotid through the cavernous sinus where they join the ophthalmic division of the trigeminal nerve (V1), then the long ciliary nerve to the pupillodilator muscle. Branches also innervate Mueller's muscle of eyelid, and facial sweat glands.

Parasympathetic nerves emanate from ganglia in viscera, which in the case of papillary function, is the Edinger-Westphal (EW) nucleus in the upper midbrain. Axons accompany the oculomotor nerve to synapse in the ciliary ganglion in orbit. Short ciliary nerves to sphincter pupillae constrict the pupil.

Pupillary reflexes thus involve a number of structures. The pathway of the direct and consensual light reflex proceeds as follows:

Retina

- >optic tract
- >synapse in pretectal nucleus in the high midbrain
- >intercalated neurons
- >synapse in ipsilateral and contralateral EW nucleus
- >parasympathetic pathway via the oculomotor nerves
- >synapse in ciliary ganglion
- >constrictor muscle of iris

The accommodation/convergence reflex, which can only be tested in cooperative patients, is not useful in coma and stupor.

The ciliospinal reflex is tested by delivering a painful stimulus to the upper neck (C1-3), which elicits pupillary dilation via reflexive stimulation of sympathetic pathways. This is usually not impaired in central sympathetic lesions, so if lost in a patient with miosis and ptosis, one should suspect a peripheral sympathetic lesion.

Normal pupil size is between 2 and 6 mm. It is important to remember that an asymmetry of .5 mm is normal in 20% of people. A blind eye leads to an unreactive pupil but consensual response in that eye should be normal. This is the Marcus Gunn pupil or

"Gunn pupil," which can be tested with the "swinging flashlight test" (flashlight shined at the normal eye produces constriction in both eyes; when "swung" to the deafferented eye, the pupil returns to normal size (appearing to dilate in response to light). Lack of direct and consensual responses in an eye suggests efferent parasympathetic paralysis.

Horner syndrome (miosis, ptosis, anhydrosis) can occur with ipsilateral hypothalamic, brainstem, or peripheral sympathetic lesions. Enophthalmos can occur as an illusion due to the palpebral fissure narrowing due to ptosis.

A "blown pupil" (unilateral mydriasis) can result from parasympathetic interruption at the level of the midbrain (EW nucleus) or oculomotor nerve dysfunction (eg, compression by tumor or aneurysm). Adrenergic or anticholinergic eye drops, or even aerosolized adrenergic medication, can produce ipsilateral or bilateral mydriasis, so these possibilities must be excluded.

Loss of both parasympathetic and sympathetic innervation leads to midposition fixed pupils at 4-7 mm. This generally requires a midbrain lesion.

Pinpoint reactive pupils requires bilateral sympathetic dysfunction, typically a pontine lesion.

With anisocoria, it is sometimes a challenge to decide which is the "bad" eye. A useful line of reasoning is as follows:

— if large pupil is abnormal, it should fail to constrict to light

— if small pupil is abnormal, it should fail to dilate in dark

In other words, light exaggerates a parasympathetic (usually 3rd nerve) lesion, and darkness accentuates a sympathetic lesion (Horner syndrome).

A quick approach to analyzing pupillary clues in comatose patients might be as follows:

- Enlarged pupil on one side → parasympathetic dysfunction (often III lesion)
- Enlarged pupils bilaterally → bilateral 3rd nerve lesions, anti-parasympathetic (anticholinergic) medications, barbiturate intoxication, postictal state
- Constricted pupils → sympathetic pathway lesion (hypothalamic, carotid)
- Pinpoint pupils → lesion in pons, opioid intoxication
- Midposition unreactive pupils → sympathetic + parasympathetic lesions (usually midbrain lesion)

Extraoccular Movements

Conjugate gaze depends on intact cranial nerves III, IV, and VI, their nuclei and interconnections. The frontal gaze center is responsible for eye deviation to the opposite side. The pontine gaze center is responsible for conjugate eye movement toward the ipsilateral side.

Testing extraocular movement is usually possible with oculocephalic maneuvers, but care must be taken so as not to displace endotracheal tubes, central lines, and other instrumentation. Oculocephalics cannot be done unless the cervical spine is known to be stable. The vestibulocaloric maneuver is an alternative which relies on the ability of cold water irrigation of the tympanic membrane (TM) to induce currents in the endolymph of the semicircular canals. This in turn leads to a particular pattern of tonic eye movements: If cold water is infused into one external auditory canal and makes good contact with the TM, eyes should deviate in a conjugate fashion toward the side of the stimulus.

If there is conjugate deviation at rest, an ipsilateral cerebral lesion or contralateral brainstem lesion is suggested. If dysconjugate eye movements are seen at rest or with maneuvers, a brainstem lesion is likely (skew deviation suggests a pontine lesion). Roving conjugate eye movements suggest that the brainstem is intact. Downward deviation indicates thalamic or upper brainstem dysfunction. Ocular bobbing is sometimes seen in lesions of the pons or cerebellum.

The corneal reflex (blink of the eye after cornea is stimulated with a wisp of cotton) involves the ophthalmic nerve, which carries afferent activity from the cornea and the facial nerve, which stimulates the orbicularis oculi muscle.

Motor Activity

Spontaneous movement is a sign of corticospinal tract integrity. When spontaneous limb movements are not seen, response to tactile or painful stimulation should be carefully observed.

Postures are generally a sign of motor system interruption. Decorticate posturing (arm adducted, elbow and wrist flexed, fist clenched; hip and knee extended) is seen in lesions involving the corticospinal tract in the deep hemisphere or upper midbrain. Decerebrate posturing (arm adducted, elbow extended and wrist flexed; hip and knee extended; toes pointed) suggests a lesion of the low midbrain or below.

Convulsive activity can be obvious, or, at times, very subtle. Eye flutter, brief clonic movements of a limb, or tonic postures may be the only clues. EEG is essential when this is suspected. Alternatively, presumptive treatment with an antiepileptic medication such as intravenous lorazepam can be diagnostic, although results may be difficult to interpret.

Myoclonus can be focal or generalized and may also be the result of seizure activity. It may alternatively be the sign of anoxic injury, infection or other CNS insult.

Initial Treatment of Coma

Initial steps

Early intervention in comatose patients must include assessment and stabilization of the cervical spine and search for body trauma, assurance of adequate airway, support of respiration if necessary, support of circulation if necessary, monitoring for arrhythmias, and searching for sites of hemorrhage and means of stopping it. Immediate labs should include blood levels of glucose, electrolytes, BUN, creatinine, and liver enzymes, complete blood count, ESR, blood gases, clotting parameters, and toxicology screen. Treatment with thiamine (100 mg IM) should be done in case Wernicke's encephalopathy is present. Naloxone .4-.8 mg IV should be given if there is any possibility of opioid overdose since respiratory arrest can be sudden. .2 to 1 mg of flumazenil should be given intravenously if benzodiazepine intoxication is possible. It should not be used if there is a suspicion of seizure, as it may precipitate seizures. 50% dextrose (D50) should be administered in 50 cc doses.

If at all possible (eg, from family, friends) a history should be obtained including past medical history (seizures, trauma, cerebrovascular disease) and

Table 3

Initial Management of Coma and Stupor

1.	Stop hemorrhage, maintain airway, support respiration if necessary, support circulation
2.	If trauma, assess for organ damage and cervical spine fracture
3.	Get quick history – seizure, medications, trauma
4.	ECG to monitor for arrhythmias
5.	Blood for glucose, electrolytes, BUN, creatinine, liver enzymes, CBC, ESR
6.	Arterial blood gases
7.	Urine or blood toxicology
8.	If fever or stiff neck — LP (after CT), consider starting antibiotic coverage
9.	CT, MRI
10.	EEG
11.	If elevated intracranial pressure – intubation and hyperventilation, osmotic diuretics, and dexamethasone, neurosurgical assistance
12.	Treat with thiamine and naloxone

medications. If fever or stiff neck is present, lumbar puncture should be done, preferably after CT or MRI of the head. ECG is important in evaluating for arrhythmia. EEG may not only help in the diagnosis of epilepsy, but can also help to explore the possibility of encephalitis, and provide information about cerebral function. (See Table 3 for summary of initial treatment of coma.)

Table 4

Glasgow Coma Scale

Eye Opening	
Spontaneous	4
To sound	3
To pain	2
None	1
Best Motor	
Obeys	6
Localizes	5
Withdraws	4
ABN flexion	3
ABN extension	2
None	1
Verbal	
Oriented	5
Confused	4
Inappropriate	3
Incomprehensible	2
None	1

Respiratory Support and Sedation

These two needs go hand in hand since agitation can impair respiratory efficiency, supported or unsupported. Early intubation is sensible for any stuporous or comatose patient having respiratory distress, hypoxemia, and/or hypercarbia or who appears to be at risk of aspiration. Intubation generally requires some sedation to avoid an increase in intracranial pressure, and often analgesic and paralytic agents as well. One good option is fentanyl 3 mcg/kg, but lidocaine and etomidate can also be used. Succinylcholine may be necessary for paralysis.

During mechanical ventilation, a number of sedative agents may be used, but most commonly in our institution propofol is chosen for its good efficacy and short action (it can be held for a short time allowing for more useful neurological examina-

Table 5

Management of Increased ICP

Elevate head of bed
Intubate
Hyperventilation (temporary) aimed at keeping pCO_2 between 25-30 mmHg
Mannitol 100-200 mL of 20%: effects in 20 min then 100 mL q4 to maintain ICP <15-20 mm
Furosemide: 20-40 mg IV
Barbiturates: 50-100 mg pentobarbital q1h
Corticosteroids: Decadron® 10 mg IV, 4-6 mg q 6 h

tion). Fentanyl at 2-3 mcg/kg/hr is also useful and other options include the benzodiazepines midazolam and lorazepam. The goals of mechanical ventilation include: 1) maximizing oxygenation, and 2) maintaining normal intracranial pressure. Typical initial respirator settings might include: 100% FiO_2, rate or 10-12, positive end expiratory pressure of 5 cc H_2O and tidal volume of 5-10 cc/kg (generally 5-7.5 cc/kg in adults).

Evaluation and Treatment of Increased Intracranial Pressure (ICP)

When intracranial pressure is elevated for more than brief periods, cerebral blood flow (CBF) becomes reduced. When increased ICP occurs, due to trauma or other causes, signs may be lacking in comatose or stuporous patients, particularly when the GCS score is below 8 (see Table 4). Even when evidence of neurological compromise is present, it is often too late to be useful. "Cushing's response" — hypertension, bradycardia and slow, irregular breathing — is an unreliable clue.

In these situations ICP monitoring is worth considering. Imaging evidence of compartment shifts and/or expanding lesions also warrant monitoring. Neurosurgical placement of a "bolt" allows insertion of pressure sensing devices extradurally, subdurally and intraparenchymally. Parenchymal monitoring of pressure is considered the most accurate but it does carry some morbidity. Intraventricular monitoring via ventriculostomy is also accurate, and is particularly useful in cases with ventricular outflow obstruction, to drain CSF. When pressure remains above 18 cm H_2O, intervention is reasonable.

Management of increased ICP includes hyperventilation, diuretic agents, and sedatives (see Table 5). Corticosteroids may be of benefit in some disease states, particularly with expanding edematous parenchymal lesions. When increased ICP persists and is intractable, consideration of craniotomy is reasonable.

Long-Term Treatment of the Patient in Coma

Numerous complications occur after the acute stage of coma if unresponsiveness persists, including seizures, infections, thrombosis, arrhythmias, metabolic derangement, and temperature dysregulation. Seizures should be treated acutely and prophylactically, with monitoring of anti-epileptic medication levels since clinical assessment of adverse effects is difficult. Aspiration pneumonia is a significant risk and measures must be taken to prevent it (ie, endotracheal intubation, clearing of secretions, positioning). Lower extremity venous thrombosis with embolization must be prevented with subcutaneous heparin and compression stockings. Cardiac and metabolic function must be monitored extremely carefully as bodily control of fluid and electrolyte levels may be poor. Temperature regulation may be dysfunctional so hyperthermia or hypothermia may ensue and must be controlled. Decubitus ulceration must be prevented, and careful monitoring for infection (urinary, respiratory) should be done.

Several Conditions Presenting With Coma

Concussion

Concussion, from the Latin "concussus," which means "a shaking," is best defined as a closed head injury of sufficient force to cause either a loss or alteration of consciousness followed by some period (even brief) of altered mentation. The mechanism of concussion symptoms is not clear, but must involve temporary paralysis of some central nervous system functions, due to the transmission of acceleration and/or deceleration forces. The range of sequelae following concussion is large. Some patients pass through a brief period of disorientation and memory dysfunction, or even temporary delirium, and return to normal completely. At the other extreme there are patients who remain comatose or stuporous for some time. A number of patients develop a long-standing syndrome including an array of symptoms including headache, cognitive dysfunction, depression and sleep dysregulation. This "post-concussion syndrome" is felt by many researchers to be due to diffuse axonal injury, presumably related to stretching injury to white matter tracts.

Prolonged coma is rare after concussion, so when it occurs, more serious traumatic injury, such as cerebral contusion, subdural hematoma and epidural hematoma must be ruled out. CT or MRI is indicated in all cases of concussion, although these will usually prove to be normal.

Sedative Intoxication

This is a life-threatening state, which may be untreatable in some cases. Barbiturates have a generally depressing effect on CNS function including respiratory centers. Presentation often offers few clues although, when available, appropriate drug and medication history as well as psychiatric history is valuable. On exam, lateralizing signs may be lacking and signs of cerebral and brainstem activity may be absent save pupillary reactivity. (However, sometimes even pupils are affected as well.) Hypothermia and hypotension may occur. EEG usually shows increased fast activity. Spinal fluid analysis, CT and MRI are normal. Barbiturates in urine or blood yield the answer.

Figure 3

Post-anoxic pattern of cerebral ischemia, with border zone infarctions

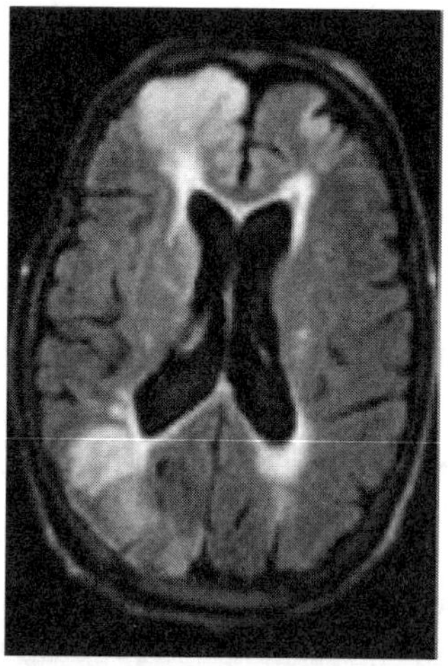

Reprinted with permission from Postoperative Stupor and Coma, Mayo Clinic Proc. 2005; 80:350-354 Dowden Health Media.

Diffuse Anoxic Injury

An often encountered neurology consultation involves the patient in coma following a hypoxic or presumed hypoxic injury to the CNS, generally after cardiac or pulmonary arrest. Neurological examination findings in the patient depend on the extent of CNS damage, which in turn depends on many factors, including the length of time the brain was deprived of oxygen. Myoclonus can be a relatively poor prognostic sign, but some patients with the persistent form recover neurological function. The longer the post-arrest patient is in coma the less likely he/she is to awaken from it (and length of coma also correlates with degree of permanent neurological deficit). Most patients who awaken from post-arrest coma will do so within the first 3 days. Motor response in particular tends to predict ultimate neurological outcome as does GCS score, but examination features in coma can depend on several factors including medications, systemic cardiovascular status, metabolic factors and seizure activity. Certain EEG findings such as burst suppression,

Figure 4

Central pontine myelinolysis – MRI showing hyperintense T2 lesions in pons

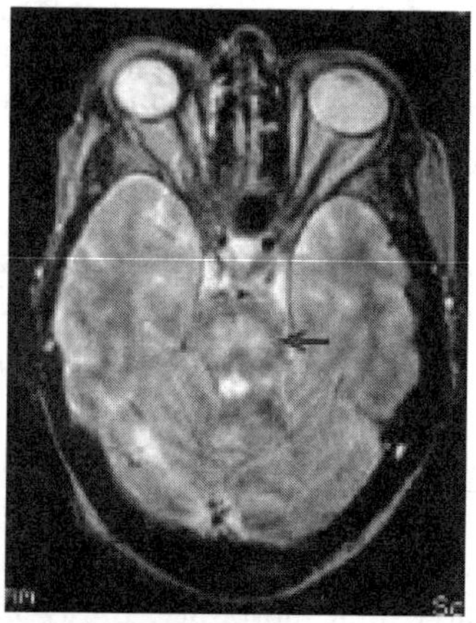

Reprinted with permission from eMedicine.com, 2007. Available at: http://www.emedicine.com/neuro/topic50.htm

periodic epileptiform activity, electrographic status epiliepticus, and alpha coma carry a poor prognosis for neurological recovery.

MRI findings after anoxic injury tend to include evidence of infarction in border zone areas, posterior cerebral artery territories, hippocampus, parahippocampal gyrus, basal ganglia and cerebellar hemispheres (Figure 3). The degree of brain imaging abnormalities, particularly the degree of edema, is of prognostic value.

Central Pontine Myelinolysis

The pathophysiological changes seen in the pons in this disease are due to demyelination of the central portions of the pons, thought to result from cellular derangement accompanying the too-rapid correction of hyponatremia. There is some doubt about this since animal trials of induced hyponatremia with rapid correction have not consistently led to CPM. Nutritional issues may contribute since CPM is frequently seen in patients with nutritional deficiencies. It is not known why the white matter of the central pons is uniquely affected. In some cases, there is "extra-pontine myelinolysis" (eg, thalamus, basal ganglia, internal capsule and cerebellar white matter).

The clinical presentation can range from minor long-tract signs to quadriplegia, locked-in syndrome and coma. Delirium is common. There is usually a lag period of 1-2 days between the rapid shift in sodium and the presentation of CPM symptoms. In many cases there is an association with another life-threatening illness such as severe liver disease, renal disease, carcinoma, and infection.

MRI shows hypointense T1 lesions, or hyperintense T2 lesions in the pons in a "bat-wing" pattern (Figure 4). CSF in CPM is generally unremarkable. Differential diagnosis includes acute demyelinating disease of the brain stem and basilar artery occlusion.

2. Confusional State and Delirium

Definitions

Confusion might be defined as "the inability to think clearly." It is a state most, if not all, people have experienced. A number of illnesses can lead to or present with confusion. Several states can mimic confusion. For example, inattentive states can simulate confusion and, if severe (such as in the neglect syndrome), the distinction is not meaningful. Patients with psychiatric conditions from dissociation to disordered thoughts or even affective disorders can appear quite confused. Language derangement, particularly receptive aphasia, may also appear as confusion in many cases.

Delirium is a term seen throughout medical literature and essentially implies a confusional state with any of a number of other symptoms including clouding of consciousness (which may fluctuate), inattentiveness, hallucinosis, tachycardia, diaphoresis, tremor and agitation. The classic delirium is that seen in alcohol withdrawal (delirium tremens). The term "organic mental state" is essentially useless.

Confusion can occur as part of several broad categories of cortical dysfunction: 1) an altered state of consciousness (eg, somnolence), 2) a general derangement of CNS function (as in intoxications), 3) dysfunction in a specific region of the brain – particularly in language areas, occipital lobe or bifrontally, or 4) as part of an ongoing dementia with acute exacerbation due to any cause.

Differential Diagnosis of the Acute Confusional State

The differential diagnosis of confusional state is large and essentially includes any process that either caused diffuse cortical dysfunction, dysfunction in the reticular activating system (without producing stupor or coma), or focal dysfunction in a part of the brain which is essential for the maintenance of lucidity (Table 6).

Vascular causes include stroke, intracerebral hemorrhage, subarachnoid hemorrhage, hypertensive encephalopathy, and cerebral venous thrombosis.

Table 6

Differential Diagnosis of Acute Confusional State

Vascular

Stroke
Intracerebral hemorrhage
Subarachnoid hemorrhage
Hypertensive encephalopathy
Cerebral venous thrombosis

Infectious

Brain abscess
(bacterial or parasitic: toxo, cysticercus)
Bacterial, fungal or TB meningitis
Encephalitis (HSV, et al)
Neurosyphilis
Lyme disease
HIV encephalitis
Septicemia or systemic infection

Trauma

Postconcussive state
Cerebral contusions
Subdural hematoma
Epidural hematoma

Autoimmune

SLE
MS

Metabolic / Toxic

Hepatic stupor
Uremia
Dialysis
Hyponatremia
Hypoxia
Hypercapnia
Hypoglycemia

Metabolic / Toxic

Hyperglycemia
Porphyria
Thyrotoxicosis
Hypothyroidism
Drug or alcohol intoxication
Drug or alcohol withdrawal
Carbon monoxide

Iatrogenic

Drug toxicity
Medication effects: Psychotropics, steroids, digoxin, cimetidine, anticonvulsants, antihistamines, anticholinergics, dopaminergics, indomethacin, lithium, opiates, benzodiazepines
Postoperative, ICU psychosis

Neoplasm

Primary or metastatic brain tumor
Paraneoplastic encephalopathy
("limbic encephalitis" with small-cell lung carcinoma)

Seizure, etc.

Postictal state
Nonconvulsive status epilepticus
Transient Global Amnesia
Migraine

Psychiatric

Mania
Psychosis
Depression
Beclouded dementia

Infectious causes include brain abscess (bacterial or parasitic); bacterial, fungal or tuberculous meningitis; encephalitis (Herpes simplex, et al); neurosyphilis; Lyme disease; HIV encephalitis; and systemic infection.

Post-traumatic causes include prolonged post-concussive state, cerebral contusions, subdural hematoma, and epidural hematoma.

Autoimmune causes include SLE and multiple sclerosis. Abnormal metabolic states which produce confusion include hepatic stupor, uremia, hyponatremia, hypoxia, hypercapnia, hypoglycemia, hyperglycemia, porphyria, and thyrotoxicosis. Toxic states which may produce confusion include intoxication or withdrawal from all drugs of abuse, including alcohol, carbon monoxide and a number of industrial solvents.

The most common iatrogenic causes of confusion involve prescription drug toxicity or idiopathic reactions to medications. This is an especially common problem with elderly patients. Drugs which commonly cause confusion include: psychotropics, steroids, digoxin, cimetidine, anticonvulsants, antihistamines, anticholinergics, dopaminergics, indomethicin, lithium, opiates, and benzodiazepines.

Primary or metastatic brain tumors may cause confusion, particularly if ICP is elevated due to tumor size or surrounding edema. Paraneoplastic encephalopathy ("limbic encephalitis") can be seen with small-cell carcinoma of the lung and has also been reported with other primary neoplasms.

Non-convulsive status epilepticus, as well as postictal confusion, may produce confusion. Transient Global Amnesia (see below) and migraine can cause a confusional state, which gradually clears spontaneously.

A myriad of psychiatric conditions may produce a syndrome which appears to be a confusional state, including mania, psychosis or depression. Patients with dementing illness typically become acutely confused following any number of possible triggers. This "beclouded dementia" is discussed further below.

Clinical Approach to the Patient With Confusional State

History from patient and witnesses can often supply the answers needed for rapid diagnosis. Things to focus on include: when mental status changes began and if there is a history of similar spells; history of head trauma; the presence of any other new symptoms or behaviors; history of any underlying medical conditions, such as diabetes mellitus, seizure disorder, or psychiatric history; and medication, drug and alcohol history. Checking medication bottles is worth the effort.

General examination must include vital signs. Searching for signs of head trauma (raccoon eyes, Battle's sign, CSF leaks) is essential since history of trauma may be lacking due to the confusion.

Fundoscopy is essential. Meningeal signs — nuchal rigidity, Kernig's sign (elevated leg with knee bent; attempts to straighten leg meet with resistance), and Brudzinski's sign (passively flexing the neck lead to knee and hip flexion) — are also crucial. Pulmonary examination should be done carefully, assessing for distress, tachypnea, and rales. Cardiac exam, looking for tachycardia, irregular rhythm, and murmurs should be included as well as abdominal exam, to rule out hepatomegaly. Skin examination may reveal bruising, splinter hemorrhages, diaphoresis, or signs of trauma. Extremities may reveal edema.

Neurological examination should begin with assessment of level of consciousness, searching for signs of somnolence. Attentiveness must be assessed, since the remainder of the mental status exam will depend on it. Orientation is checked by asking the patient to name him/herself, and to describe people in the room. Perseveration and impersistence are assessed. Language is tested including repetition, fluency, comprehension, and naming. Memory functions can be difficult to assess in the confused patient. Immediate recall of 3 words and short-term memory of these items at 5 minutes may be possible. Long-term memory is assessed in conversation generally but this can be done more specifically, asking the patient about recent and remote significant events. Calculation can be assessed with serial 7 subtractions, and construction is usually testable with copying simple figures. These higher cortical functions are important to assess to rule out focal cortical dysfunction as opposed to a more generalized process.

Affect, thought processes, and thought content should be assessed to explore the possibility of psychiatric illness. Affect, the observed manifestations of mood, may give a clue to depression. Thought processes can be quickly assessed by analyzing the linkages between thoughts, and thought content assessment should focus on delusions, illusions and hallucinations.

Cranial nerve exam should include pupil exam and visual acuity as well as facial sensation, facial movement, hearing, articulation, and swallowing. Assessment of motor power and tone is important as well as observation for tremor, asterixis, and myoclonus. Reflexes, including plantar reflexes, are important. Gait and tandem gait should be assessed, as well as Romberg testing.

Laboratory testing in the confused patient should include complete blood count and differential, erythrocyte sedimentation rate, electrolytes, glucose, calcium, phosphate, renal and liver function testing. Urine and/or blood toxicology, and urine and blood cultures might be warranted. Pulse oximetry is usually sufficient to assess oxygenation but arterial blood gas is worth checking in patients with possible respiratory disease.

Chest radiograph and electrocardiogram may reveal pulmonary or cardiac issues which require immediate management. CT or MRI of the brain is essential if the cause of confusion is not readily determined. EEG is the ideal way to rule out status epilepticus, but a trial of lorazepam IV may be diagnostic if necessary. Lumbar puncture should be done in any patient suspected of having subarachnoid hemorrhage, encephalitis or meningitis.

Initial Management of Confusional State

After assuring a good airway, normal respiration, and adequate circulation, history (including gathering of information from family and friends) and exam can be done. If the patient is agitated or combative, haloperidol can be given 2-10 mg IM. An alternative sedative is a benzodiazepine which can be given intravenously as well. (Caution should be exercised in elderly patients.) This is particularly useful in alcohol or benzodiazepine withdrawal and hepatic encephalopathy. A good choice is lorazepam 1-2 mg IM or IV, although much higher doses may be needed (see discussion of delirium tremens below).

Naloxone (Narcan®) should be given in any case of possible opioid intoxication, as 1-2 ampules (.4-.8 mg) IV, but more may be required (up to 5 or more mg). .2 to 1 mg of flumazenil should be given if benzodiazepine intoxication is possible. It should not be used if there is a suspicion of seizure, as it may precipitate seizures. 50% dextrose (D5O) should be administered in 50 cc doses. Thiamine (100 mg IM) should always be administered with D50 to prevent exhaustion of supply, which might induce Wernicke disease. If the patient has headache, fever or meningismus LP should be done. If there are any neurological deficits or signs of increased intracranial pressure, CT is done prior to LP. In cases suspicious for CNS infection where there is any delay in performing LP – for example, suspicion of mass lesion, and CT must be done first – antibiotic coverage for meningitis and encephalitis should be started.

Some Specific Syndromes Causing Confusional State

Transient Global Amnesia (TGA)

This syndrome consists of relatively sudden anterograde amnesia (inability to form new memories) with essentially no other cognitive dysfunction. In some cases there is some difficulty with retrograde memory over the past several days or weeks. Immediate recall is good. There is often a great deal of anxiety and the prevailing feeling seems to be one of bewilderment, with patients typically asking "Where am I"? and "What is happening?" repeatedly.

The pathophysiology has been debated for many years and it is still not clear. The possibilities proposed include TIA (involving the thalamus or temporal lobes), migraine (of the confusional type), or non-convulsive seizure activity, also presumably involving bitemporal cortical regions. EEG evidence for seizure activity is lacking and no clear cerebrovascular pathophysiology has been proven in any case. MRI is usually normal, although diffusion weighted image changes have been seen in several cases. The absence of headache in these patients speaks against migraine, although acephalic migraine is possible.

TGA typically occurs in middle aged or elderly patients. The syndrome resolves by the next day and in many cases is better within hours. Examination, other than memory testing, is normal. As noted, EEG and MRI are generally normal. Complete recovery is the rule. Recurrence, while unusual, can occur.

Systemic Lupus Erythematosus
SLE produces mental status changes in a number of patients, sometimes acutely. (There is some cerebral involvement in 25% of patients.) SLE does not produce vascular inflammation (hence the term "lupus cerebritis" is a poor one). Rather, symptoms are due to diffuse deposition of immune complexes in small vessels resulting in microinfarctions (or larger areas of ischemia).

The CNS lupus syndrome consists of seizures, psychosis, cognitive disturbances, chorea, and cranial nerve dysfunction, some or all of which may occur in a given patient. Other CNS vasculitides can cause confusional state including poloyarteritis nodosa, Wegener's granulomatosis, lymphomatous angiitis, and primary CNS angiitis. These are generally associated with headache and with focal neurological deficits. CNS lupus rarely causes abnormal CSF, and brain MRI is often entirely normal. EEG is likewise unhelpful. As a result, diagnosis rests upon the clinical picture and serology.

Non-convulsive status epilepticus (NCSE, a.k.a. Temporal Lobe Status Epilepticus)
This is usually found in patients with focal cortical injury (neoplasm, anoxia, inflammatory/infectious process), but it can be seen in metabolic disorders. Cortical irritation is required, so strictly subcortical lesions are unlikely to produce this state.

Patients seem distracted, slow to respond, and "disconnected." Their level of arousal and attentiveness may seem to fluctuate. Occasionally, minimal clonic movements or automatisms may be seen. A history of epilepsy is a significant clue.

Electroencephalography is diagnostic, but there have been cases where even EEG is unhelpful. When EEG is not available or is equivocal, a trial of intravenous lorazepam (1-4 mg) may provide the answer, while at the same time improving the patient's status. Still, this is most helpful when done with simultaneous EEG monitoring.

Delirium Tremens

This component of alcohol withdrawal usually occurs approximately 48 hours after cessation of drinking. Autonomic irritability leads to fever, tachycardia, and fluctuation in blood pressure. Hallucinosis is classic but may be minor or absent, with only confusional state noted.

Treatment is reasonably effective when begun in a timely manner and continued throughout the withdrawal period, which may last for many days. A commonly effective approach is to administer diazepam (Valium®) 5-10 mg IV to load, then 2-5 mg IV every 30-60 min. Dose should be titrated with effects on tremulousness and agitation. An alternative is chlordiazepoxide (Librium®) 25-100 mg every 6 hrs orally. Oxazepam is another useful alternative. Beta blockers and clonidine can help control the hypermetabolic state symptoms of tachycardia, hypertension, and tremor. Steroids are useless in DT. Thiamine 100 mg daily (IV, IM, or orally) is reasonable since deficiency is common. (Again, it is particularly important to give thiamine when using glucose solutions, as the last reserves of B vitamins might be mobilized and precipitate Wernicke disease).

Neuroleptic Malignant Syndrome (NMS)

NMS presents with rigidity or dystonia and some or all of the following: fever, tachycardia, diaphoresis, hypo- or hypertension, and tachypnea. Patients have a depressed level of consciousness and can become comatose. White blood cell count may be

Figure 5

EEG in Herpes encephalitis showing 1 Hz lateralized epileptiform discharges

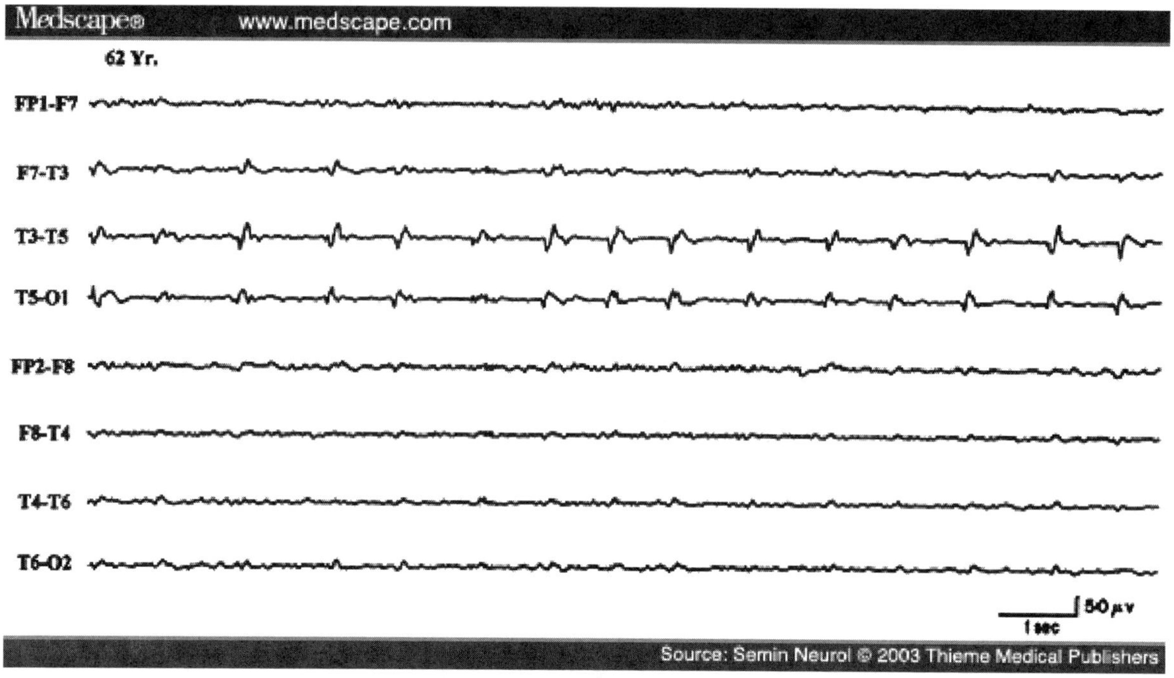

Markand O. Pearls, Perils, and Pitfalls in the Use of the Eletroencephalogram. Semin Neurol. *23(1):7-96,2003. Reprinted by permission.*

high, and CPK levels are almost always elevated. Liver enzyme levels may also be elevated. CSF is normal and neuroimaging is unremarkable.

While neuroleptic dopamine antagonist medications of all types (as well as dopamine depleters like reserpine) have led to this syndrome, the pathophysiology is not clear. It can occur soon after the first dose or after an increase in dosage. Dehydration or hyperthermia may lead to the syndrome.

Life threatening consequences include renal failure due to myoglobinuria, and respiratory failure due to the rigidity.

Neuroleptic medication should be discontinued. Treatment consists of dantrolene sodium or bromocriptine, although these have not been proven to be effective in controlled trials. Prognosis is generally good if supportive treatment is instituted. Neuroleptic medication can usually be restarted after all symptoms and signs of NMS are gone.

Herpes Encephalitis

This is the most common non-epidemic encephalitis. It is caused by Herpes simplex virus type 1 (HSV-1). Infection seems to predominantly affect temporal and frontal hemispheres, which explains why confusion is the typical presenting feature.

Other than alterations in mental state, most patients complain of some degree of headache. Fever may occur. Seizures may occur early. CSF shows mild lymphocytic pleocytosis, red blood cells (sometimes in the hundreds per hpf), and increased protein (although it may be normal). PCR testing of CSF is sensitive and specific.

Brain MRI can show focal inferior temporal and frontal lesions. EEG often shows focal epileptiform discharges, particularly periodic lateralized epileptiform discharges (Figure 5). Brain biopsy is definitive, showing eosinophilic intracellular (Cowdry type) inclusions, but it is rarely indicated.

Treatment should be instituted as soon as the diagnosis is entertained since early treatment can be lifesaving. Acyclovir 10-12.5 mg/kg IV every 8 hours for 14 days is generally effective if begun early. Some advocate the prophylactic use of anticonvulsants. Prognosis depends on diagnosis and prompt treatment. Herpes encephalitis is fatal in 40% of untreated patients.

Hepatic Encephalopathy

The mechanism for CNS compromise in hepatic failure involves the following process: Increased or continued protein load leads to toxic ammonia accumulation in brain, which induces neuronal dysfunction and damage and resulting encephalopathy. Liver cirrhosis, chronic hepatitis, or malignancy involving the liver (primary or metastatic) are the usual causes, and the pathophysiology probably involves some degree of brain edema. Moreover, ammonia is probably not the only brain toxin involved, with other candidates including manganese.

Examination reveals any or all of the following: ascites, hepatomegaly, asterixis, inattention, disorientation, and varying degrees of somnolence and/or agitation. In later stages, focal signs such as dysconjugate gaze, hemiparesis, and sensory deficits may occur.

Treatment is aimed at reducing the protein load with dietary restriction, reduction of ammonia-producing flora with neomycin 2-4mg daily by mouth, and lactulose 15-45 mL 2-4x daily to reduce gut flora further. Lactulose can lead to adverse effects including severe diarrhea, electrolyte disturbances, and hypovolemia, which can further exacerbate the encephalopathy, so caution is essential. Valium 5-10 mg every 8 hours is effective for agitation.

Wernicke Encephalopathy

The mechanism for the production of this syndrome is felt to be related to thiamine deficiency. Mamillary body lesions are consistently seen in Wernicke encephalopathy, but lesions in hypothalamus, thalamus, midbrain and cerebellar vermis (primarily affecting Purkinje cells) are also seen in some cases.

The clinical syndrome consists of a tetrad:

1. lethargy or confusional state

2. truncal ataxia

3. ophthalmoplegia (VI, III, IV)

4. nystagmus

Treatment is repeated intramuscular injections of thiamine 100 mg daily for at least 3 days.

Post-op and ICU "Psychosis"

This is a syndrome which, rather than representing a particular diagnostic entity, is probably a group of disorders. In fact, in most cases the causes are multiple, and sometimes determining the specific mechanism(s) is not possible.

In evaluating altered mental status in the intensive care setting it is essential to rule out the following potentially reversible causes: electrolyte imbalance, endocrinological dysfunction, medication effects, drug withdrawal, hypoxic brain injury, stroke, intracranial hemorrhage, seizures, and neurological or systemic infections.

In some cases the confusional state is related to fear, sensory overload, immobilization, sleep deprivation, or depression. An often overlooked cause is underlying dementia with acute worsening in the setting of stress and reduced environmental cueing.

Dialysis Dysequilibrium Syndrome

Somnolence, delirium or even coma may appear toward the end of a renal dialysis treatment. Headache and nausea may herald the development of the encephalopathy, which may even occur after a lag time of up to 24 hours, and may persist for several days.

The etiology is believed to be brain edema resulting from hydrostatic forces set up by changes in blood osmotic conditions. Increased intracranial pressure ensues. Papilledema may be appreciated on fundoscopy, and brain enlargement may even be seen on MRI or CT scan.

DDS must be distinguished from other causes of confusion or altered consciousness. It is usually self-limited.

3. Conclusion

Coma and confusional state in a sense represent two ends of a spectrum, since many disease states may in fact begin as a "change in mental status" and eventually lead to coma. Hence the overlap in the differential diagnosis of these two syndromes. A common challenge in these two presentations is that history and examination data may be frustratingly sparse. Still, a careful assessment of available data generally yields enough clues to allow meaningful decision making about diagnostic testing and initial treatment.

4. References

1. Bateman DE. Neurological assessment of coma. *Jourl Neurol, Neurosurg & Psy*. 2001, 71(1).

2. Bernat, JL. Brain Death. In *Ethical Issues in Neurology*. Boston, Butterworth Heinemann, 2002, pp. 243-282.

3. Bernat, JL. The persistent vegetative state and other related states. In *Ethical Issues in Neurology*. Boston, Butterworth Heinemann, 2002, pp. 283-306.

4. Booth CM, Boone RH, Tomlinson G, Detsky AS. Is this patient dead, vegetative, or severely neurologically impaired? Assessing outcome for comatose survivors of cardiac arrest. *JAMA*. 2004, 291(7):870-879.

5. Carolei A, Sacco S. Central nervous system vasculitis. *Neurol Sci*. 2003, 24(1):S8-S10.

6. Cartlidge N. States related to or confused with coma. *Jour Neurol, Neurosurg & Psy*. 2001, 71(1).

7. Claassen J, Mayer SA, Kowalski RG, Emerson RG, Hirsch LJ. Detection of electrographic seizures with continuous EEG monitoring in critically ill patients. *Neurology*. 2001, 62(10):1743-1748.

8. Devinsky O, Bear D, Volpe BT. Confusional states following posterior cerebral artery infarction. *Arch Neurol*. 45:160-163, 1988.

9. Felix MM, Castro LH, Maia AC, Jr., da Rocha AJ. Evidence of acute ischemic tissue change in transient global amnesia in magnetic resonance imaging: case report and literature review. *Jour Neuroimag*. 2005, 15(2):203-205.

10. Henderson, GV. Coma, Head Trauma, and Spinal Cord Injury. In: *Manual of Neurologic Therapeutics*. Samuels, MA, ed. Philadelphia, Lippincott Williams & Wilkins, 2004, pp. 1-8.

11. Koontz DW, Fernandes Filho JA, Sagar SM, Rucker JC. Wernicke encephalopathy. *Neurology*. 2004, 63(2):27.

12. Laureys S, Owen AM, Schiff ND. Brain function in coma, vegetative state, and related disorders. *Lancet Neurol*. 2004, 3(9):537-546.

13. Malik K, Hess DC. Evaluating the comatose patient. Rapid neurologic assessment is key to appropriate management. *Postgraduate Medicine*. 2002, 111(2):38-40.

14. McLean SA. Permanent vegetative state and the law. *Journal Neurol, Neurosurg & Psy*. 2001, 71(1).

15. Morcos Z, Kerns SC, Shapiro BE. Wernicke encephalopathy. *Arch Neurol*. 2004, 61(5):775-776.

16. Ronthal, M. Confusional States and Metabolic Encephalopathy. In: *Office Practice of Neurology*. Samuels, MA, and Feske, SK, eds. Philadelphia, Churchill Livingstone, 2003, pp. 886-890.

17. Siva A. Vasculitis of the nervous system. *Jour Neurol*. 2001, 248(6):451-468.

18. Smith E, Delargy M. Locked-in syndrome. *BMJ*. 2005, 330(7488):406-409.

19. Tirschwell, DL. Coma in the intensive care unit: Predicting awakening following cardiac and respiratory arrest. *Continuum*. 12,1: 46-69.

20. Tong DC, Grossman M. What causes transient global amnesia? New insights from DWI. *Neurology*. 2004, 62(12):2154-2155.

5. Questions

1. Which of the following differentiate coma and sleep?

    a. Motor function

    b. Sensory function

    c. Arousal response to stimuli

    d. Language

    e. Hearing

2. A 63-year-old man was found on the floor of his bedroom "unresponsive," and was brought to the ER. His level of consciousness is reported to fluctuate. He appears asleep, but when aroused can converse briefly, but without much depth. Without verbal stimulation he quickly becomes unconscious again. The best description for this patient's state of consciousness is:

    a. Somnolence

    b. Stupor

    c. Obtundation

    d. Light coma

    e. Delirium

3. Lesions in which of the following areas would be likely to cause coma?

    a. Pons

    b. Hypothalamus

    c. R thalamus

    d. L temporal lobe

    e. Frontal white matter

4. A 23-year-old with a history of depression was found in coma with an empty bottle of barbiturate sedative medications nearby. Which feature of her examination is inconsistent with transtentorial herniation?

    a. Preserved pupillary reflexes

    b. Bilateral Babinski reflexes

    c. Decerebrate posturing

    d. Reactivity to painful stimulation

    e. Cheyne-Stokes respiratory pattern

5. A 39-year-old patient on the neurology service has the following examination: Complete paralysis of all four extremities and the face; preserved corneal reflexes and some vertical eye movements; need for mechanical ventilation with no triggering breaths; and preserved hearing. Which are possible causes of this condition?

    a. Pontine stroke

    b. Multiple sclerosis

    c. Acute demyelinating polyradiculopathy

    d. Central pontine myelinolysis

    e. All of the above

6. A comatose patient exhibits a respiratory pattern of shallow breathing at 24 breaths per minute with intermittent apneic spells. This respiratory pattern is most consistent with:

    a. Cheyne-Stokes respiration

    b. Central hyperventilation

    c. Apneustic breathing

d. Cluster breathing

e. Ataxic breathing

7. Of the following, which is the most likely lesion site in the preceding case?

a. Bilateral cerebral hemispheres

b. Cerebellum

c. Thalamus

d. Hypothalamus

e. Upper cervical spinal cord

8. A stuporous 85-year-old man is found to have a small but apparently reactive R pupil. He has a normal brain CT scan. The pupillary abnormality could be due to which of the following:

a. L sympathetic dysfunction

b. R sympathetic dysfunction

c. L parasympathetic dysfunction

d. R parasympathetic dysfunction

e. R parasympathetic and sympathetic dysfunction

9. The lesion in the preceding case could involve any of the following EXCEPT:

a. Hypothalamus

b. R carotid artery

c. R III nerve

d. R cavernous sinus

e. R cervical intermediolateral column

10. A comatose patient has no reaction to oculocephalic maneuvers or vestibulocaloric stimulation on the right, but intact vestibulocaloric response with left ear cold irrigation. Which of the following might explain this?

a. R internuclear ophthalmoplegia

b. L frontal gaze center damage

c. R frontal gaze center damage

d. L pontine gaze center damage

e. R pontine gaze center damage

11. With painful stimulus, a comatose patient extends his right upper and lower extremities.

Which of the following is the most likely site of lesion:

a. L pons

b. L upper midbrain

c. R cerebellum

d. L thalamus

e. L frontal lobe

12. Concussion must include:

a. Some permanent cognitive change

b. Loss of consciousness

c. Memory loss

d. Altered mentation

e. Headache

13. Confusion can occur as the result of all of the following except:

a. A medullary lesion

b. An altered state of alertness

c. A general derangement of CNS function

d. A L occipital lobe lesion

e. As part of an ongoing dementia

14. A 26-year-old known poly-drug abuser is in an agitated delirium. Good choices for initial therapy include all but which of the following:

a. Glucose and thiamine

b. Naloxone

c. Flumazenil

d. Sedation with haloperidol

e. Sedation with lorazepam

15. A 55-year-old man is brought to the ER confused and agitated. On exam he is uncooperative and seems to have pronounced gait difficulty. Likely diagnoses include all of the following except:

a. Wernicke encephalopathy

b. Non-convulsive generalized status epilepticus

c. Alcohol intoxication

d. Amphetamine intoxication

e. Alcohol withdrawal

16. The patient in the preceding case is later, when calmer, found to have nystagmus and dysconjugate gaze. Best treatment for him at that point is to administer:

a. Diazepam

b. Glucose

c. Glucose and thiamine

d. Haloperidol

e. Naloxone

17. A 58-year-old man is brought to the ER by his wife who says he is "mixed up." He continually asks "Where am I?" and "What's going on?" but appears calm, and other than being apparently unable to form new memory, is non-focal on examination. Which is NOT typical of his most likely diagnosis?

a. Long-term memory loss is noted

b. Short-term memory loss is noted

c. Duration is generally only several hours

d. Recurrences are rare

e. Etiology is unclear but may represent cerebrovascular compromise

18. CNS involvement in SLE is generally due to:

a. Vasculitis

b. Secondary infection of the CNS

c. Psychiatric disease

d. Metabolic encephalopathy

e. Multifocal ischemia

19. Patients with akinetic mutism usually have:

a. Bifrontal lesions

b. L temporal lesions

c. Amnesia

d. Agitation

e. Stupor

20. A 26-year-old motor vehicle accident victim has no evidence of cortical activity on neurological examination 1 week later. Which of the following would argue against the diagnosis of persistent vegetative state?

a. Occasional smiling and moaning

b. Regular respirations

c. Rudimentary but purposeful withdrawal to painful stimulus

d. Apparent sleep/wake cycles

e. Good pupillary response to light both direct and consensually

Answers

1. C.
Sleep, as opposed to coma, carries the implication that one can be aroused. Language, hearing, motor function and response to sensation will vary with sleep stage or cause of coma.

2. B.
Stupor is exemplified by this patient who is basically unresponsive unless stimulated, at which time he can be aroused even to the level of rudimentary conversation. Terms like "light coma" and "obtundation," may be useful to some, but their definitions are not universally agreed upon. Somnolence is really akin to sleepiness, with consciousness tending to drift into sleep without stimulation. Delirium is a confusional state with additional features.

3. A.
A pontine lesion could easily affect both right and left RAS pathways. None of the other sites would be as likely to do so.

4. A.
Barbiturate coma can be extremely deep, with pathological reflexes, posturing, and dysfunctional respiration, as can also be seen in herniation syndromes. However, pupillary function is often preserved as opposed to cases with transtentorial herniation.

5. E.
This patient is in a locked-in state, ie, generally lacking efferent function. This can occur with brainstem lesions such as stroke, MS, and CPM. AIDP can also lead to the same clinical picture.

6. D.
Cluster breathing is defined as bursts of rapid breathing separated by apneic spells. Refer to Figure 2 to compare the types of abnormal respiratory patterns seen with CNS insults.

7. B.
Cluster breathing seems to occur with lesions in the pons or cerebellum.

8. B.
A small but reactive pupil (often difficult to assess) is generally due to ipsilateral sympathetic dysfunction.

9. C.
Sympathetic interruption could occur at a number of sites from the hypothalamus to descending sympathetic tracts in the brainstem, to the intermediolateral column in the thoracic spinal cord, to the carotid artery, and then via the cavernous sinus region to the eye. The oculomotor nerve carries parasympathetic nerves, and lesions of it do not generally affect sympathetic function.

10. E.
Failure to respond to vestibulocalorics on the R implies either a R pontine horizontal gaze center lesion or some mechanical reason for this provocative measure to have failed, such as blockage of the auditory canal with cerumen. Frontal gaze centers do not have to be functional for the vestibulocaloric reflex to operate. Left pontine horizontal gaze center seems intact.

11. A.
Decerebrate posturing as displayed by this patient is thought to arise after corticospinal tract lesions below the level of the red nucleus in the midbrain.

12. D.
While at one time the term "concussion" implied a loss of consciousness following closed head trauma, it has now been expanded to include any patient who has experienced a closed head injury of any type, followed by any change in mentation. While there is almost always some memory loss, this is not required.

13. A.
Medullary lesions should not cause confusion unless there is some depression of respiration and ensuing hypoxia, etc. The other choices are much more common causes of confusion, including simply being somnolent or inattentive.

14. E.
Lorazepam is not considered the best choice in cases of possible drug overdose since it can be a respiratory depressant, and therefore a possible additional suppressant of respiratory drive along with whatever other sedatives the patient has taken. Glucose, thiamine, naloxone and flumazenil are all reasonable treatment. If sedation is important, haloperidol should be effective.

15. B.
Agitated delirium can result from a number of drug intoxications but amphetamine intoxication is classic. Alcohol intoxication of course can produce the same picture, and the alcohol withdrawal state (delirium tremens) is entirely consistent with this presentation. Wernicke's encephalopathy can present with delirium but NCSE generally presents with a dazed, abulic sensorium, closer in appearance to akinetic mutism.

16. C.
This case now begins to resemble the triad of Wernicke's encephalopathy: confusion, ataxia, and diplopia/nystagmus. Hence, treatment with thiamine should begin immediately.

17. A.
This patient seems to have a classic Transient Global Amnesia, a mysterious condition that seems to produce short-term memory dysfunction in isolation. Long-term memories (name, address, knowledge base, etc.), are spared. The phenomenon is self-limited, and usually does not recur.

18. E.
While the term "lupus cerebritis" still circulates, CNS involvement in SLE is not really an inflammatory phenomenon at all, but rather a multifocal ischemic syndrome probably related to numerous sites of immune complex mediated vascular occlusion. The psychiatric and neurological presentations are varied and may be related to several as yet unspecified mechanisms.

19. A.
Akinetic mutism is generally the result of bilateral anterior frontal disease or injury. They are aware of their surroundings and can form memory. They are generally not agitated and while they appear stuporous, testing reveals that they are conscious.

20. C.
PVS requires the complete lack of meaningful response to stimuli, so even rudimentary but purposeful withdrawal behavior suggests some cerebral function. Smiling, moaning, respiration, and pupillary responses can all occur at the brainstem level and sleep/wake cycling can even occur in PVS.

Chapter 9: Infections of the Central Nervous System

Barbara Jobst, MD

Contents

1. Introduction

Central nervous system infections are frequent and can present with a variety of symptoms depending on the underlying organism. The incidence of bacterial meningitis varies between 3 and 5 per 100,000 per year, and more than 2000 deaths are annually recorded due to bacterial meningitis. Opportunistic CNS infections like toxoplasmosis, tuberculosis and syphilis have significantly increased due to AIDS and the increased use of immunosuppressants. New variants of Creutzfeldt-Jakob disease, which are related to bovine spongiform encephalitis (BSE), have caused worldwide public health concerns. It is crucial for the neurologist to readily diagnose, treat and understand the implications of CNS infections.

2. Diagnosis of CNS Infections

Most central nervous system infections present with fever and headache. Focal neurological signs, mental status changes, coma, seizures or hemiparesis can occur depending on the underlying organism. Meningismus (nuchal rigidity) suggests meningeal irritation, also suggested by Brudzinski's and Kernig's signs. Brudzinski's sign is spontaneous knee flexion with passive neck flexion. Kernig's sign is resistance to passive extension of the leg at the knee. Other CNS infections such as fungal, parasitic, myobacterial and spirochetal are more insidious in onset and present with intermittent headaches and cognitive changes. These infections are frequently referred to as "chronic" meningitis.

Most central nervous system infections are diagnosed with CSF analysis. Imaging may be required to assess for a possible mass lesion, such as abscess, before lumbar puncture for CSF analysis is performed. Although imaging is usually readily available, the patient should be assessed for papilledema with a careful fundoscopic examination. CSF analysis can usually clarify whether an infection is viral, bacterial or chronic (Tables 1 and 2). Specific cultures are needed to identify the organism.

Table 1

Normal CSF Analysis

Routine CSF Analysis	Normal Values
White blood count	<5 cells/mm^3
Red blood count	<5 cells/mm^3
Protein	< 45 mg/dL
Glucose	2/3 of serum glucose
Opening pressure	<200 mmH_2O
Gram stain	negative
Oligoclonal bands	negative

An increase of white blood cells in the CSF over 7-10 cells/mm^3 is considered meningitis. Meningitis is an inflammatory response or infectious process of the meninges. If there is invasion of the brain parenchyma with subsequent focal neurological signs—seizures, aphasia or motor weakness—this process is considered encephalitis. An abscess is a mass caused by infection. An empyema is a space-occupying infectious process in the subarachnoid or subdural space. Imaging studies (CT and MRI) are essential to diagnose infectious mass lesions. Meningeal enhancement on MRI suggests meningitis. This needs to be distinguished from meningeal enhancement that is noted after a previous lumbar puncture.

Table 2

Differential Diagnosis and CSF Findings in CNS Infections

	Bacterial Meningitis	**Viral Meningoencephalitis**	**Chronic Meningitis**
Clinical manifestations	Fever, headaches, coma, septic shock	Viral aseptic meningitis: fever, headache, normal mentation Viral encephalitis: fever, headache, seizures, coma	Chronic headaches, dementia
Time course	Acute	Acute	Protracted
Most common organism	*Streptococcus pneumoniae, Neisseria meningitidis*	Viral menigitis: unknown Viral encephalitis: Herpes simplex	*Mycobacterium tuberculosis*, fungal, spirochetes, malignant, sarcoid
CSF			
WBC	>1000 polymorphonuclear	<1000 lymphocytic, initially polymorphonuclear	<200 lymphocytic
Protein	>100 mg/dL	Mildly elevated or normal	High
Glucose	<50% of serum glucose	Normal	Low

3. Bacterial Meningitis

Bacterial meningitis presents acutely with fever >38.5°C, headaches, neck stiffness and mental status changes, followed by confusion, delirium and seizures, and can progress to coma. Photophobia, nausea and vomiting are common in the initial stage. Cranial nerve abnormalities may be observed. Increased intracranial pressure can cause a sixth nerve palsy. The classical triad of fever, neck stiffness and mental status changes is only present in approximately 45% of community-acquired meningitis (van de Beek, de Gans et al, 2004). Bacterial meningitis can be fulminant and if untreated may quickly result in coma and death due to septic shock or increased intracranial pressure. In neonates and in the elderly, symptoms may develop much more insidiously. Listlessness, irritability, refusal to feed, tachypnea and high-pitched crying can be the sole manifestations of bacterial meningitis in the neonate. Delirium and confusion may be the initial presentation of bacterial meningitis in the elderly.

If bacterial meningitis is suspected it is important to initiate antibiotic treatment immediately. Diagnostic evaluation of a patient with suspected meningitis should include immediate blood cultures and lumbar puncture. If the patient is immunocompromised or has a history of CNS disease, if there are new onset seizures, papilledema, abnormal level of consciousness or a focal neurological deficit, a CT scan should be performed before the lumbar puncture. However, obtaining a CT scan should not delay treatment with antibiotics (Tunkel, 2004). The CT scan will exclude other intracranial pathologies such as intracranial hemorrhage, subarachnoid hemorrhage or mass lesion. CSF analysis usually shows an elevated opening pressure (>200mm H_2O; normal: 100-200mm H_2O); an elevated white blood cell count >1000 cells/mm^3 (normal <7-10 cells/mm^3); elevated protein >100mg/dL (normal <45 mg/dL); and low glucose <50% of serum glucose. Early in the course, the white blood count may be lower. Polymorphonuclear cells are predominant. Gram stain is positive in 90% of pneumococcal, 86 % of *H influenza*, 75% of neisseria, 50% of Gram-negative and 25% of listeria menginitis. Sensitivity of a Gram stain is high (>97%) (Tunkel, 2004). CSF cultures could yield the final diagnosis.

Infections with *Neisseria meningitis* (meningococcus) and subsequent meningococcemia present with rash, which later evolves into typical petechial and purpuric lesions predominantly located at the extremities. If acute bacterial meningitis is preceded by sinusitis, mastoiditis, otitis media or pneumonia, *Streptococcus pneumoniae* (pneumococcus) is frequently the pathogen due to hematogenous or direct spread into the subarachnoid space. A foreign body, previous head trauma, or an immunocompromised state suggests certain underlying organisms (Table 3).

Age usually determines the causative organism of meningitis (Table 3). Direct open head trauma, previous neurosurgical procedure or a CSF leak with

Table 3

Most Common Organisms Responsible for Bacterial Meningitis in Various Populations

Population	Organisms
Newborn	Group B strep, *E coli, Listeria*
Children and Young Adults	*Streptococcus pneumonia, Neisseria meningitis, Haemophilus influenzae* (less common after vaccination program has been instituted)
Elderly (>50 years old)	*Streptococcus pneumonia, Listeria monocytogenes, Haemophilus influenzae*
Trauma, Iatrogenic (shunts, neurosurgical procedures)	*Staphylococcus aureus,* Gram-negative bacilli
Immunocompromised	*Listeria monocytogenes,* Gram-negative bacilli, *Streptococcus pneumoniae, Haemophilus influenzae*

rhinorrhea predisposes to certain organisms (Table 3). The presence of a ventricular shunt suggests infection with Gram-negative *bacilli*.

The spread of pathogens to the subarachnoid space can be direct invasion (trauma, sinusitis or mastoiditis). Colonization of the nasopharynx with meningococcus or pneumococcus leads to invasion of the nasal epithelial cells and subsequent spread to the blood stream. Hematogenous spread with breakdown of the blood-brain barrier results in CNS invasion. Exudation into the subarachnoid space, which is the result of inflammation of the pia, contributes to increased intracranial pressure.

If bacterial meningitis is suspected it is important to initiate antibiotic treatment immediately. Diagnostic evaluation of a patient with suspected meningitis should include a CT scan of the head and a lumbar puncture. The CT scan will exclude other intracranial pathologies such as intracranial hemorrhage, subarachnoid hemorrhage or mass lesion. CSF analysis usually shows an elevated opening pressure (>200mm H_2O); an elevated white blood cell count >1000 cells/mm^3 (normal <45 mg/dL); and low glucose less than 50% of serum glucose. Early in the course, the white blood count may be lower. Polymorphonuclear cells are predominant. Gram stain is positive in 60%-80% of cases; CSF cultures are positive in approximately 75%. Sterilization of the CSF occurs as early as one hour after initiation of antibiotic treatment in meningococcal meningitis and after four hours in pneumococcal disease. Therefore, the initiation of antibiotic therapy before a diagnostic LP is controversial, but the lumbar puncture should not delay treatment significantly (Kanegaye, Soliemanzadeh et al, 2001). Lactate and C-reactive protein in CSF may help to differentiate bacterial from viral meningitis (Tunkel, 2004). The Limulus assay, which detects endotoxin, identifies Gram-negative bacilli. Those tests are useful, but not generally recommended (Tunkel, 2004).

Antibiotic therapy in bacterial meningitis aims for effective blood-brain barrier penetration and should be directed towards the age of the patient and the probable pathogen. Antibiotic therapy should always be adjusted when the organism is identified and sensitivities confirmed. In the neonate, ampicillin and gentamycin are employed as initial therapy. In children and adults, ceftriaxone or cefotaxime are first-line therapy. Vancomycin should be added if penicillin resistant pneumococcus is suspected. In the elderly, ampicillin should be added to cover *Listeria*. In patients with head trauma, shunts or previous neurosurgical procedures, vancomycin plus ceftazidine are recommended to cover *Staphylococcus aureus* and Gram-negative *bacilli*. In the immunocompromised population, ampicillin and ceftazidine are recommended.

There is controversy whether steroids should be administered in the setting of acute bacterial meningitis (Tunkel, 2004). A recent study indicated that steroids decrease mortality and unfavorable outcomes in bacterial meningitis (de Gans and van de Beek, 2002). Dexamethasone is recommended in addition to antibiotics, especially in pneumococcal meningitis (de Gans and van de Beek, 2002).

In case of increased intracerebral pressure, head elevation (>30%), hyperventilation and mannitol should be started.

Mortality rate ranges between 17%-37%, with the elderly being at higher risk. Mortality rates are higher with streptococcal than meningococcal infections (van de Beek, de Gans, et al, 2004). Risk factors for an unfavorable outcome are advanced age, presence of otitis or sinusitis, absence of rash and initial coma (van de Beek, de Gans et al, 2004).

Pneumococcus, meningococcus and *Haemophilus influenzae* are transmitted by droplets; the prophylaxis of close contacts is always important. *S pneumoniae* does not require prophylaxis, but in cases of meningitis with *N meningitidis* and *H influenzae*, prophylaxis with rifampicin for two days is indicated to eliminate nasal carriage.

4. Viral CNS Infections

Viral (Aseptic) Meningitis

Viral meningitis presents less acutely and fulminantly than bacterial meningitis. Headache, malaise, low-grade fever and meningismus are common. Changes in mental status are unusual. Photophobia is often present. Many viruses are responsible for viral meningitis and it is usually not possible to identify the organism which led to the term "aseptic" meningitis. Echovirus, influenza and cocksackie are often common pathogens (Table 4).

CSF analysis shows a mildly elevated WBC >100 <1000 cells/mm^3, mildly elevated protein <100 mg/dL, and normal glucose. Viral meningitis is predominantly a lymphocytic response, but early in the course polymorphonuclear cells are present.

Treatment is symptomatic, with bed rest and anti-inflammatory agents. Prognosis is usually good, with complete resolution of symptoms.

Recurrent aseptic meningitis is referred to as Mollaret's meningitis, and common pathogens are HSV2, HIV and EBV (Tyler, 2004). Immunoglobulins and anti-inflammatory agents, such as ibuprofen, also cause recurrent aseptic meningitis.

Viral Encephalitis

Viral encephalitis presents similar to bacterial meningitis. High fever, headache, meningismus and photophobia are common. As there is direct invasion of the brain with the virulent agent and focal neurological, signs may occur early. Aphasia occurs especially in infection with herpes simplex type I. HSV I has a predilection for the temporal lobe (Figure 1). Seizures, confusion, changes in mental status, hemiparesis and coma occur.

Multiple organisms are responsible for viral encephalitis and are dependent on host and mode of transmission (Table 4). The most commonly occurring encephalitis is herpes simplex type I. Axoplasmatic transport of HSV from the trigeminal ganglia is responsible for CNS invasion (Tyler, 2004). Latent HSV in the trigeminal sensory ganglia is detectable in all seropositive persons. The close proximity of temporal lobes and trigeminal ganglion could explain the predilection for the temporal lobes. Another route of invasion into the central nervous system is via the olfactory pathways. Invasion of the temporal lobes with herpes simplex leads to hemorrhagic changes. HSV encephalitis can be due to primary infection or reactivation of HSV. Thirty percent of HSV I infections are primary infections.

Diagnosis is based on clinical presentation, CSF analysis, neuroimaging and EEG (Steiner, Budka et al, 2005). CSF analysis reveals a lymphocytic pleocytosis with <100 WBC, mildly elevated protein and normal glucose. Opening pressure is normal (100-200 mm H_2O) or elevated. The red blood cell count in CSF can be mildly elevated due to hemorrhagic changes. MRI reveals typical high signal intensities in the mesial temporal lobes on T2-weighted, FLAIR and diffusion-weighted imaging (Figure 1). EEG can be helpful with the presence of periodic lateralizing epileptiform discharges (PLEDS) in 80% of cases (Figure 2). PLEDS are not specific for herpes encephalitis and serial EEGs may be required. In the past brain biopsy was the gold standard for diagnosis, but it is now reserved for very rare cases. CSF herpes PCR can rapidly confirm the diagnosis and has a sensitivity of 96% and a specificity of 99% (Steiner, Budka, et al, 2005). Viral cultures are often unrevealing.

Bacterial meningitis and subarachnoid hemorrhage are the major differential diagnoses but CSF examination should easily distinguish between those diseases.

Treatment should be initiated as soon as possible with Acyclovir IV. The use of acyclovir has dramatically reduced the mortality of herpes encephalitis. Nonetheless, the mortality still remains 6%-11% (Tyler, 2004). Thirty-eight percent to 56% of patients recover without neurological impairment. Outcome is dependent on the delay between initial symptoms and initiation of treatment. Untreated mortality is over 70% (Tyler, 2004). HSV type 2 usually presents as a viral meningitis and has a good prognosis.

For encephalitis caused by other pathogens, refer to Table 4.

Table 4

Viral CNS Infections and Their Treatment

Infection/Vector	Clinical Manifestations (Neurologic)	Diagnosis	Associated Features	Treatment	Prognosis
Herpes simplex Type 1					
Respiratory and salivary secretions, reactivation	Encephalitis	CSF: herpes PCR, MRI: hyperintense signal temporal lobes, EEG: PLEDS		Acyclovir IV 14-21 days	30%-50% neurologic deficit 6%-10 % mortality
Herpes simplex Type 2					
Salivary secretions, reactivation	Meningitis	CSF: HSV2-PCR	Previous herpes genitalis	Acyclovir po x 10d or Famiciclovir po x 10d or Valacyclovir po x 10d	Recurrent
Varizella zoster					
Airborne, herpes zoster: Reactivation of dormant virus in dorsal ganglia	Herpes zoster (shingles), Encephalomyelitis after acute infection or may follow zoster eruption	CSF: VZV-PCR Culture of vesicles	Vesicular eruption in dermatomal distribution	Encephalitis: Acyclovir IVx 14-21 days Herpes zoster: Acyclovir po x 10 d or Famiciclovir po x 10d or Valacyclovir po x 10d	Good Postherpetic neuralgia after herpes zoster
CMV					
Secretions	Encephalitis or polyradiculitis in immunocompromised	Mononucleosis on peripheral smear CSF: CMV-PCR Serum IGM	Retinitis	Ganciclovir x 14-21d or Foscarnet x 14-21d	Variable
EBV					
Secretions	Encephalitis (<1% of mononucleosis)	Mononucleosis CSF: EBV-PCR Serum IGM	Lymphadenopathy, splenomegaly	Acyclovir IV x 14-21 days or symptomatic	Good

(continued)

Table 4

Viral CNS Infections and Their Treatment *(continued)*

Infection/Vector	Clinical Manifestations (Neurologic)	Diagnosis	Associated Features	Treatment	Prognosis
Human Herpes Virus 6 (HHV6)					
	Aseptic meningitis, encephalitis	CSF: HHV6-PCR	Diffuse maculopapular rash following four days of high fever (Exanthema subitum), febrile seizures in children	Symptomatic	Good
Mumps					
Airborne	Encephalitis	CSF: Viral culture	Orchitis, mastitis, parotidis, myocarditis	Symptomatic	Good
Measles					
Airborne	Postmeasles encephalomyelitis (2 weeks after rash), SSPE (subacute sclerosing panencephalitis) 2- 12 years after infection	SSPE: MRI: hyperintense lesions EEG: periodic pattern	Maculopapular rash beginning at face and extending downward	Ribavirin x 7days SSPE: interferon alpha	SSPE: fatal but rare due to vaccination program
Arbovirus *St. Louis encephalitis, Eastern equine encephalitis, Western equine encephalitis, California (La Crosse), Colorado tick fever*					
Mosquitos, ticks	Encephalitis	Viral culture or serologic	Conjunctivitis and urinary symptoms with St. Louis encephalitis, maculopapular rash with Colorado tick fever	Symptomatic	Mortality rate: St. Louis encephalitis: 2%-20% Eastern equine encephalitis: 50%-70% Western equine encephalitis: 3%-5% California (La Crosse): <1% Colorado tick fever: <1%

(continued)

Table 4

Viral CNS Infections and Their Treatment *(continued)*

Infection/Vector	Clinical Manifestations (Neurologic)	Diagnosis	Associated Features	Treatment	Prognosis
West Nile Virus					
Mosquitos	Encephalitis, myelitis	CSF: IGM, PCR		Symptomatic	Usually good, more severe in elderly population
Lymphocytic choriomenigititis virus (LCMV)					
Rodents	Aseptic meningitis or mild encephalitis	IGM in serum and CSF	Lymphadenopathy	Symptomatic	Good
Nonpolio enterovirus (Coxsackie, Echovirus)					
Enteral	Meningitis in hypogammaglobinemic patients and newborns	CSF: Enterovirus PCR	Macules/papules on palms, soles (hand-foot-mouth disease)	Pleconaril x 7d	Good
Poliomyelitis					
Enteral	Encephalomyeliltis	Eradicated from Western hemisphere	Anterior horn cell disease with flaccid paralysis		Postpolio syndrome possible
Rabies					
Saliva of infected animal	Encephalitis	Brain biopsy or autopsy		Postexposure vaccine and immunoglobuline	Fatal once disease is manifest

Herpes Zoster (Shingles)

Herpes zoster manifests with radicular pain and vesicular eruption in a dermatomal distribution. The vesicles are filled with a clear fluid and resemble the rash in acute varicella infection. The rash is pruritic and painful. Zoster oticus involves the facial nerve and has typical eruptions in the auditory canal and an associated Bell's palsy. Ophthalmic zoster involves the first branch of the trigeminal nerve. The vesicular rash is noted over the forehead and may involve the cornea, which affects visual acuity and can lead to permanent visual loss if not treated appropriately.

Shingles represent a reactivation of *Varicella zoster* virus that lays dormant in the dorsal root ganglion or trigeminal ganglion. Often it occurs in the immunocompromised or elderly population. It develops 8-10 times as frequently after 60 years of age than before (Gilden, Kleinschmidt-DeMasters, et al, 2000). Due to the introduction of the varicella vaccine and incomplete immunity, shingles are now also more commonly occurring in children and young adults.

Figure 1

Hyperintense mesial temporal lobe due to herpes encephalitis

FLAIR-MRI sequence

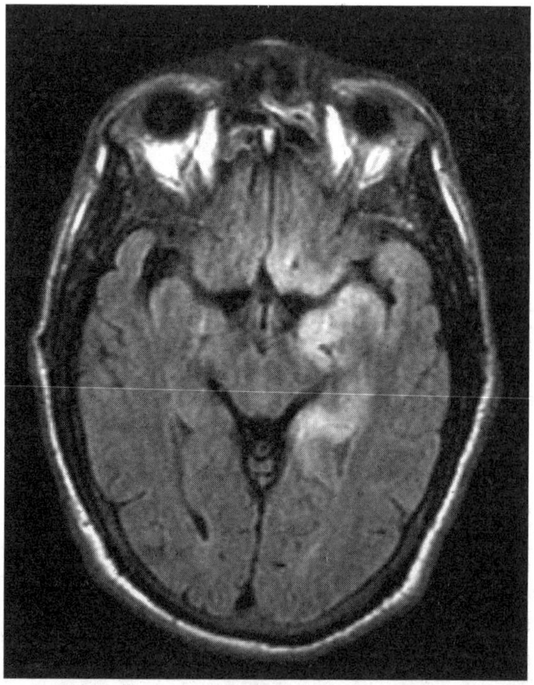

Treatment should be initiated as soon as possible. Acyclovir, famciclovir and valacyclovir are equally effective (Table 4). Prednisone is believed to reduce the incidence of postherpetic neuralgia (Wood, Johnson, et al, 1994). Postherpetic neuralgia is an acute pain syndrome which follows the vesicular eruption and follows the same dermatomal distribution. Treatment can be difficult. Gabapentin, amitriptyline, pregabalin, carbamazepine and opiates are commonly used (Gilden, Kleinschmidt-DeMasters, et al, 2000).

Varicella zoster is also responsible for myelitis and encephalitis in the immunosuppressed (Gilden, Kleinschmidt-DeMasters, et al, 2000) (Table 4).

West Nile Virus

West Nile virus infection has become more endemic in the US since the initial outbreak in New York in 1999. In 80% of infected persons the infection is latent. Of the 20% with symptoms, 50% develop a maculo-papular rash. Neuroinvasive disease consists of encephalitis as well as bilateral flaccid paralysis due to anterior horn cell invasion similar to poliomyelitis (Davis, 2006). Diagnosis is established by determining IGM-antibodies in CSF. Treatment is symptomatic.

5. Fungal and Parasitic Infections

Fungal infections frequently occur in the immunocompromised population and are only rarely seen in the immunocompetent. *Cryptococcal meningitis* is the most frequent fungal meningitis, especially in the HIV positive population. CNS infections with *Aspergillus* and *Candida* neoformans are less frequent. *Histoplasma capsulatum* and *Coccidioides immitis* can also invade the CNS (Gottfredsson and Perfect, 2000).

Patients present with insidious symptoms: headache, low-grade intermittent fevers, and mental status changes. The mental status changes can mimic dementia, but are usually more subacute in onset. Symptoms may wax and wane. Mild hydrocephalus develops as a consequence of disturbed CSF absorption. Fungi, especially *Aspergillus*, can present as an abscess with symptoms related to mass effect (Table 5).

Fungi invade the CNS either by inhalation of the agent or can be transmitted iatrogenically (eg, *Candida albicans* infection via implantation of ventriculo-peroneal shunts). In rare cases, sinus disease leads to invasion of the CNS with *Aspergillus*. Fungal infections occur if there is lack of an efficient cell-meditated response by CD4+ cells, cytotoxic lymphocytes and natural killer cells, as is typical in the AIDS population and other immunosuppressed patients.

Diagnosis is established by CSF examination and neuroimaging used to ascertain if an abscess is present. CSF shows lymphocytic pleocytosis, elevated protein and low glucose (Table 2). Eosinophilia is common. Fungal cultures can identify the organism, but are frequently negative. Ancillary tests in the CSF-like cryptococcal antigen (CrAg), and India ink stain for cryptococcus are very helpful for diagnosis.

Figure 2

Periodic lateralizing epileptiform discharges over the right hemisphere in herpes encephalitis

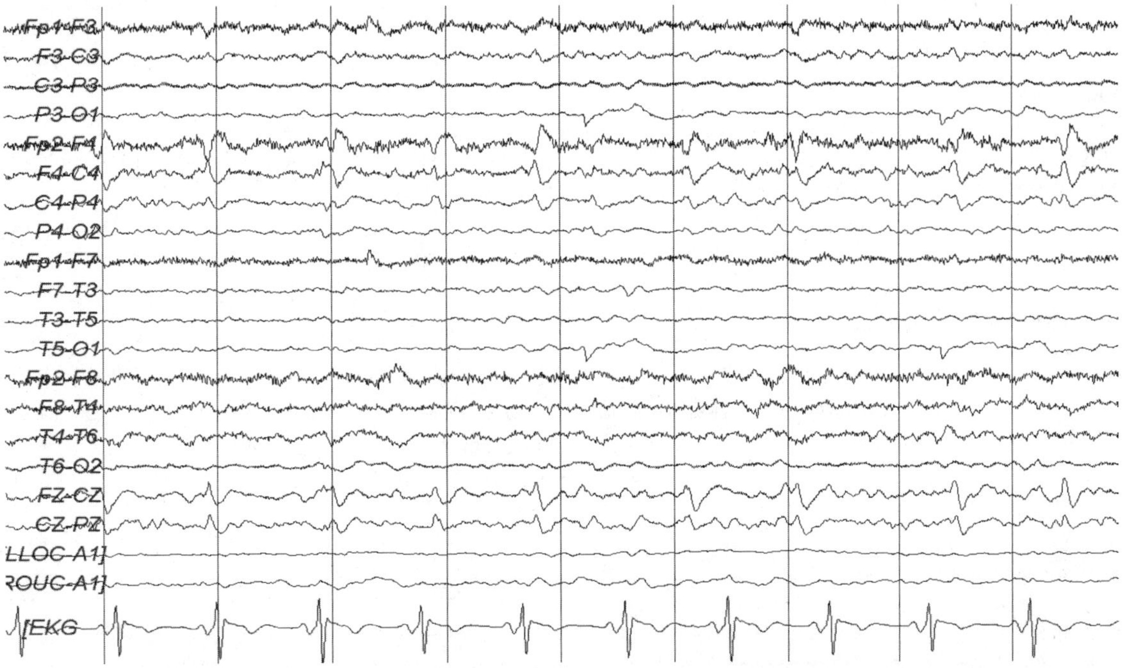

Neuroimaging can identify brain abscesses as ring-enhancing lesions. Blood cultures are helpful if there is disseminated disease, but are usually negative in *Aspergillus* infections.

Treatment is usually with amphotericin B alone or in combination with other antifungals (Table 5). Amphotericin B adversely affects kidney function, and BUN and creatinine should be monitored closely. Dosing should be adjusted with decreased kidney function. Treatment is often for the patients' lifetime, especially in the immunosuppressed. As fungal infection usually occurs in the immunocompromised, prognosis is often dependent on the underlying disease.

Table 5

Fungal Infections

Main Presentation	Associated Symptoms	Diagnosis	Treatment
Cryptococcus neoformans			
Subacute meningitis	Pulmonary disease cyptococcal skin lesions	CSF: Cryptococcal antigen India ink stain	Amphotericin B plus flucytosin for two weeks; then fluconazole high dose for 10 weeks; then fluconazole low dose for 1 year or for life
Aspergillus fumigatus			
Brain abscess Vascular thrombosis with stroke	Necrotizing bronchopneumonia	CSF: culture	Amphotericin B followed by Itraconazole 400-800 mg/d for life
Candida albicans			
Menigoencephalitis, microabscesses	Frequently in newborns and after VP shunt implantation	CSF: large volume required for positive culture Blood cultures	Amphotericin B plus flucytosin for 6 weeks
Histoplasma capsulatum			
Meningitis	Pulmonary involvement Erythematous skin eruption	CSF: culture positive in 10%-30% Histoplasma polysaccheride antigen	Amphotericin B followed by Itraconazole 400 mg/d for 6 months or life
Coccidioides immitis			
Meningitis Endemic in Southwest of United States	Lytic bone lesions Pulmonary and skin involvement	CSF: Cultures neg, Complement fixation antibodies	Amphotericin B followed by fluconazol for life

Cysticercosis

Cysticercosis is one of the most common fungal infections in the United States due to the migration of immigrants from endemic areas, especially Latin America.

Cysticercosis is the invasion of tissue by the larval stage of the pork tapeworm. Eggs of tapeworm are ingested by contaminated food or water. The eggs hatch to larvae that invade various tissues like the brain, muscles, liver and eyes. Cysticerci are oval cysts with an invaginated scolex, usually about 1 cm in size, but can be larger if located in the subarachnoid space or ventricles. The cysts undergo transformation from an active inflammatory stage to an inactive calcified stage (Figure 3).

Symptoms usually occur in the active inflammatory stage. Seizures are the most common presentation, but hemiparesis, hydrocephalus and mass effect occur due to compression by cysticerci. Cysticerci in the muscle present with painful hypertrophy and proximal weakness. Subcutaneous nodules indicate skin invasion.

Diagnosis is based on the history of possible exposure and neuroimaging. MRI or CT show cystic, enhancing lesions and parenchymal brain calcification (Figure 3). CSF studies for detection of cysticercal antibodies (ELISA or enzyme-linked immuno-electrotransfer blot) are helpful. The presence of cysticerci in muscle or skin is diagnostic and histological examination may reveal the diagnosis. Ophthalmological evaluation may reveal retinal, vitreous or conjunctival cysts.

Inactive disease does not require antiparasitic treatment but antiepileptic medications may be required to control seizures. Hydrocephalus should be treated with shunting. Patients with active disease are treated with praziquantel or albendazole. However, treatment may trigger an inflammatory response that can be more detrimental than the presence of relatively inactive cysts.

6. Mycobacterial and Spirochetal Infections

Tuberculous Meningitis

Tuberculous meningitis presents as subacute lymphocytic meningitis with headaches, low-grade fevers and mental status changes. General malaise and systemic symptoms such as night sweats and weight loss can be present. Obstructive hydrocephalus can develop as well as isolated cranial nerve palsies. Ischemic infarcts occur in 30% of cases. Since symptoms are variable, the time to diagnosis can be significant. Tuberculous meningitis may also present as a subacute dementia.

Mycobacterium tuberculosis usually invades the CNS per reactivation of a previous pulmonary infection in the setting of immunosuppression. With the HIV epidemic, tuberculous meningitis has significantly increased in incidence. It often manifests as basilar meningitis, but mass lesions in the form of tuberculous granuloma are also possible. Differential diagnosis includes other types of chronic meningitis such as fungal or syphilitic infections.

Figure 3

Calcification in the right frontal lobe due to cysticercosis on CT imaging

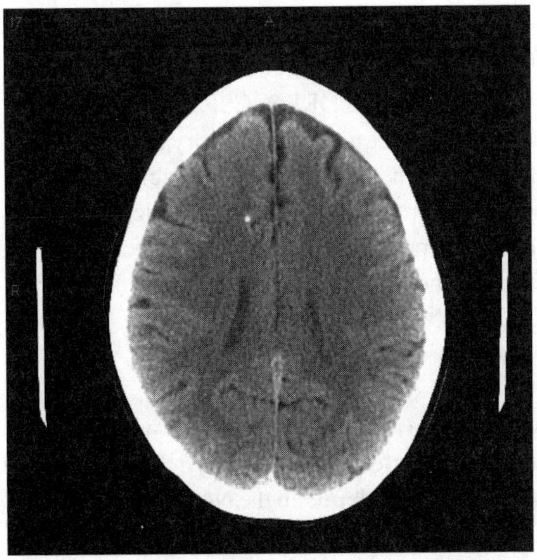

CSF analysis shows lymphocytic pleocytosis with an exceedingly high protein and low glucose. Eosinophilia may be present. PDD is negative in 25% due to the lack of a sufficient immune response to *Mycobacterium*. Acid-fast bacilli stain or culture can establish the diagnosis; however, it is time consuming and has significant delay. DNA amplification (PCR) has sensitivity between 33%-90% and specificity between 88%-100%, but allows rapid diagnosis.

Rifampicin, isoniazid, pyrazinamide and ethambutol for 6-12 months are recommended. Additional steroids improve mortality but not functional outcome. Prognosis is dependent on the initiation of treatment relative to disease progression as well as on the etiology of immunosuppression.

Neurosyphilis

Syphylitic infections caused by *Treponema pallidum* are increasing in incidence in the immunosuppressed population, especially HIV-positive individuals. Invasion of the CNS can occur early as asymptomatic meningitis. Symptomatic meningitis, cranial neuritis, ocular disease or cerebrovascular involvement are also manifestations of early neurosyphilis. Tertiary syphilis or late neurosyphilis manifests as tabes dorsalis or general paresis. General paresis is a progressive dementia with psychosis. Tabes dorsalis is a spinal cord disorder with sensory ataxia due to posterior column degeneration.

CSF shows lymphocytic pleocytosis with elevated protein. RPR and VDRL in CSF can indicate neurosyphilis but require confirmatory testing with FTA-ABS. A negative FTA-ABS excludes neurosyphilis. Treatment consists of penicillin G IV for 14 days. Repeat CSF examination is recommended after treatment.

Lyme Disease

Lyme disease is caused by infection with *Borrelia burgdorferi*. Infection occurs via tick bites. *Borrelia burgdorferi* is endemic in the Northeast United States.

Erythema migrans (round target lesion at the site of infection) is the initial presentation of *Borrelia* infection. Erythema migrans subsides and arthralgias may be the secondary stage of Lyme disease. If CNS invasion occurs—a polyradiculitis with dermatomal paralysis—sensory changes and pain is common (Bannwarth syndrome). Bilateral Bell's palsy, especially in children, is frequent (Gerber, Shapiro et al, 1996). Encephalitis is rare.

In Lyme disease, the CSF shows lymphocytic pleocytosis with protein elevation but normal glucose. Antibody testing in serum may suggest the diagnosis, but specificity is low. A positive Lyme IGG titer requires additional testing with Western blot to confirm the diagnosis. There is leukocytosis in the CSF with neuroborreliosis. Treatment of Lyme disease with nervous system involvement consists of ceftriaxone for two weeks. Penicillin, cefotaxime and oral doxycyclin have also shown to be effective. There is no evidence that prolonged treatment is beneficial. The prognosis is usually favorable.

7. Brain Abscess and Empyema

Brain Abscess

Brain abscesses present as mass lesions. Abscesses can be bacterial, fungal or parasitic. In bacterial brain abscesses, aerobe and anaerobe organisms are usually present. Direct hematogenous spread to the CNS from dental abscesses or endocarditis leads to initial cerebritis with subsequent encapsulation and eventual rupture of the abscess. Abscesses are also the result of direct invasion of the CNS via head trauma or neurosurgical procedures.

Abscesses present with focal neurological deficits such as hemiparesis, language difficulties or visual field impairment. Headache is common, but fever may be absent. Increased intracranial pressure can lead to herniation syndromes. Seizures can be the sole manifestation of brain abscess. The MRI reveals single or multiple ring-enhancing lesions. The differential diagnosis includes tumors and metastasis. The CSF is usually not diagnostic and may be completely normal including cultures.

The diagnosis is made by aspiration or biopsy and aerobe and anaerobe cultures. Surgical treatment of abscesses is indicated if there is impending herniation. Otherwise, depending on size or location, antibiotic treatment after biopsy for diagnosis is the recommended treatment. Initial antibiotic includes ceftriaxone and metronidazole. Antibiotics should be adjusted to antibiotic sensitivities. The mortality is 5%, but a significant number of patients, 20%-60%, are left with a subsequent neurological deficit (Davis, 2002).

Subdural Empyema

Invasion of the subdural space with aerobe and anaerobe bacteria leads to subdural empyema. Multiple organisms like *Streptococcus milleri*, *staphylococcus aureus*, *bacteroides* and enteric bacteria are present. Sinusitis, otitis or mastoiditis are the usual initial entry of infection with subsequent osteomyelitis. Subdural empyema also occurs in the setting of significant head trauma or neurosurgical intervention.

Symptoms are fulminant, with headaches, altered consciousness, hemiparesis and other focal neurological abnormalities due to mass effect. Fever is common.

The MRI or CT readily establishes the diagnosis. The LP is contraindicated due to increased intracranial pressure. Treatment is surgical to relieve intracranial pressure with the addition of antibiotic therapy (nafcillin, ceftriaxone and metronidazole).

Spinal Epidural Abscess

Hematogenous spread of bacteria, commonly *Staphylococcus aureus*, can lead to spinal epidural abscess with subsequent spinal cord compression. Endocarditis or dental abscesses are frequently the primary infections. Iatrogenic abscesses due to spinal anesthesia, surgical intervention or lumbar puncture are other etiologies. Therapy of rheumatoid arthritis with steroids or immunosuppressants are other predisposing factors. Patients present with cervical, thoracic or lumbar pain and fever, as well as with symptoms of spinal cord compression. There is typical percussion pain in the region of the spinal abscess. The thoracic region is most commonly affected. If there is spinal cord compression, surgical intervention is indicated but carries a poor prognosis. Medical treatment with antibiotic may be attempted if there are no neurological deficits.

8. HIV and AIDS

HIV is a neurotropic virus and has multiple peripheral and central nervous system manifestations. Opportunistic CNS infections are frequent in patients with HIV infection. Highly active antiviral therapy (HAART) reduces viral load and death rates from AIDS, but has significant neurological side effects.

Depending on the stage of the disease, different neurological manifestations are typical (Table 6). With seroconversion, mild aseptic meningitis or demyelinating polyneuropathy may occur. In the mid-stage of the disease (CD4+ count between 200-500), asymptomatic CSF abnormalities with lymphocytic pleocytosis and elevated protein are present. If the CD4+ cell count falls below 100, and with increasing viral load, certain opportunistic infections are common in HIV patients as T-cell function decreases. Typical opportunistic infections of the central nervous system include toxoplasmosis, progressive multifocal leukencephalopathy (PML), tuberculous and syphilitic meningitis, herpes virus and CMV infections (Table 6). CMV polyradiculitis is a common opportunistic peripheral nervous system infection. Direct invasion of the central nervous system with HIV can result in HIV dementia complex and vacuolar myelopathy.

Toxoplasmosis

Toxoplasma gondii is a parasite that is acquired by ingestion of undercooked meat or from cat feces. In the immunocompetent individual, infection is mild and toxoplasma survives but lays dormant in tissue macrophages. Ten to 40% of the population of the United States is infected with toxoplasma. Due to breakdown of T-cell immunity in HIV infection, the parasite is reactivated and can invade the CNS.

Cerebral toxoplasmosis presents with focal neurological deficits: hemiparesis, aphasia, dysarthria or other neurological deficits depending on the location of toxoplasma cysts in the brain. Headache, encephalopathy and seizures are common.

The MRI reveals multiple ring-enhancing lesions (Figure 4). CSF is generally not helpful but may show mild pleocytosis and mild protein elevation. As there is a high incidence of latent toxoplasma infection in the general population, toxoplasma IGG antibodies are helpful only if the patient is known to be previously negative. IGM-antibodies suggest a recent infection.

In the HIV population, the most common differential diagnosis is primary CNS lymphoma (PCNSL). PCNSL is radiologically and clinically indistinguishable from toxoplasmosis. PCNSL is due to reactivation of Epstein-Barr virus (EBV). EBV-PCR in the CSF corroborates the diagnosis but is not specific. Thallium-201 SPECT may support the diagnosis but usually brain biopsy is required for final diagnosis (Anonymous, 1998). The prognosis is dismal and palliative radiation therapy is the only established treatment.

As brain biopsy carries a significant risk in a HIV patient, a ring-enhancing lesion should be treated with antiparasitic treatment with pyrimethamine and sulfadiazine for two weeks. Folic acid should be added to prevent megaloblastic anemia. In case of sulfa intolerance, clindamycin is alternatively prescribed. If the patient responds to therapy with decreasing lesion load and significant clinical improvement, this confirms the diagnosis of toxoplasmosis. If there is no improvement, biopsy is recommended. Only if there is a negative toxoplasma titer and a single mass lesion is immediate brain biopsy indicated.

If the diagnosis of toxoplasmosis is established, lifelong suppressive therapy with pyrimethamine and sulfadiazine is mandatory. Primary prophylaxis in the HIV population is recommended if the CD4+ count falls below 100.

Progressive Multifocal Leukencephalopathy (PML)

PML is another late neurological opportunistic infection in AIDS, but also occurs in other types of immunosuppression. PML has been recently associated with the use of natalizumab in patients with multiple sclerosis and leads to restricted use of the natalizumab (Kappos, 2007). JC virus, a polyoma virus, is the responsible infectious agent. Asymptomatic JC virus infection is highly prevalent in the immunocompetent population. With impaired T-cell immunity, the virus is reactivated. CD4+ counts are usually less than 100 in patients with AIDS.

JC virus causes demyelination of the white matter, with predilection for the parieto-occipital regions. MRI shows demyelination with cortical sparing (Fig. 4). The onset is insidious with impairment of speech, sensory symptoms, cognitive impairment, ataxia and visual impairment. Cortical blindness is common.

AIDS Dementia Complex and Minor Cognitive Motor Dysfunction

As HIV is a neurotropic virus, invasion of the CNS is responsible for cognitive impairment at the later stages of AIDS. Pathology shows vacuolar changes, with white matter pallor and multinucleated cells. CD4+ count is low.

Table 6

Neurologic Manifestations of HIV Infection Dependent on Disease Stage

Stage/CD4 count	Peripheral Nervous System	Central Nervous System	Muscles
Early HIV CD 4>500	PNS seroconversion syndromes: Acute or chronic demyelinating polyradiculoneuropathy Ataxic neuropathy Bell's palsy	CNS seroconversion syndromes: Aseptic HIV meningitis or meningoencephalitis	Acute rhabdomyolysis with seroconversion myopathy
Midstage HIV CD4 between 200-500	Mononeuritis multiplex	Asymptomatic meningitis	Inflammatory myopathy
Advanced HIV CD4 <100	HIV related: Distal sensory polyneuropathy Opportunistic: CMV polyradiculomyelitis Tuberculous polyradiculitis Syphylitic polyradiculitis Herpes zoster	HIV related: Vacuolar myelopathy AIDS dementia complex Opportunistic: Toxoplasmosis Cryptococcal meningitis Tuberculous meningitis Syphylitic meningitis PML CMV encephalitis HHV6 infection Neoplastic: Primary CNS lymphoma	Inflammatory myopathy
HAART related	Distal sensory polyneuropathy		Mitochondrial myopathy with ragged red fibers

CD4 = CD4 cell count; PML = progressive multifocal leukencephalopathy; CMV = cytomegalovirus; HHV6 = human herpesvirus-Type 6; HAART = highly active antiretroviral therapy

Patients present with attention and concentration difficulties, which progresses to impairment in other cognitive domains or psychosis. Motor impairment usually follows the cognitive impairment and consists of ataxia and incoordination.

Neuropsychological testing quantifies cognitive impairment. CT and MRI shows diffuse atrophy. CSF analysis reveals mild pleocytosis and mildly elevated protein. Quantitative viral load in CSF can assist in the diagnosis.

The only therapy is highly active antiretoviral treatments (HAART). If the immune status or CD4+ counts improve, cognitive impairment may improve.

Vacuolar Myelopathy

Vacuolar myelopathy is caused by the direct effect of HIV virus on the spinal cord. It is pathologically equivalent to AIDS dementia complex. Vacuolar changes in the myelin with relative preservation of the axons are present. It is a late complication of HIV infection.

Figure 4

Multiple ring-enhancing lesions due to cerebral toxoplasmosis

Gadolinium enhanced T1-weighted MRI

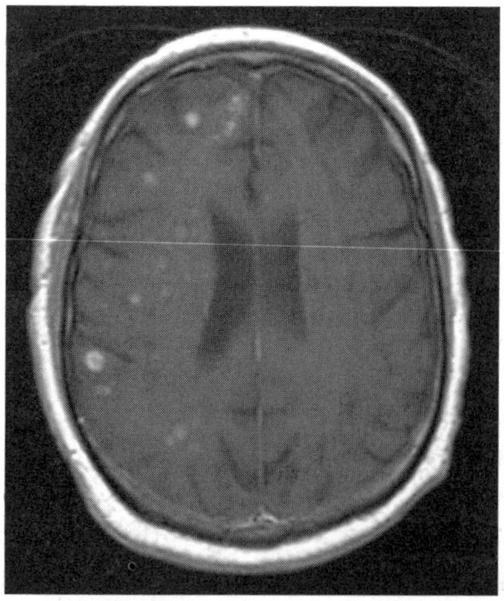

Over several months spasticity, paraparesis, impaired proprioception and impaired sphincter function evolve. The upper extremities are usually spared and there is no definite sensory level. In severe cases, MRI reveals major cord atrophy. Improvement is possible following HAART therapy.

Neurological Complications of HIV Treatment

Highly active antiretroviral therapy (HAART) has significantly improved prognosis of HIV. However, neurological side effects occur with treatment.

Nucleoside analogues like didanosine, stavudine and zalcitabine are associated with a painful toxic neuropathy with distal sensory loss and loss of reflexes. Nucleoside neuropathy can be distinguished from HIV-associated distal sensory neuropathy by the relatively subacute onset after initiation of treatment with nucleosides. Treatment consists of lowering the dose or using alternative retroviral therapy.

Zidovidudine can be responsible for a proximal myopathy by impairing mitochondrial function. Muscle biopsy shows ragged red fibers as typically seen in mitochondrial disorders. CK elevations can be variable. The condition may be difficult to distinguish from HIV-associated inflammatory myopathy.

Figure 5

Right frontal hyperintensities and hyperintensities in the cerebellar peduncles in a patient with PML

MRI-FLAIR images

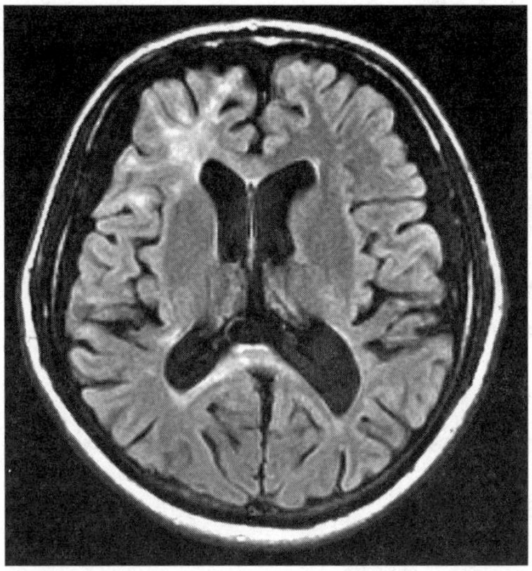

A.

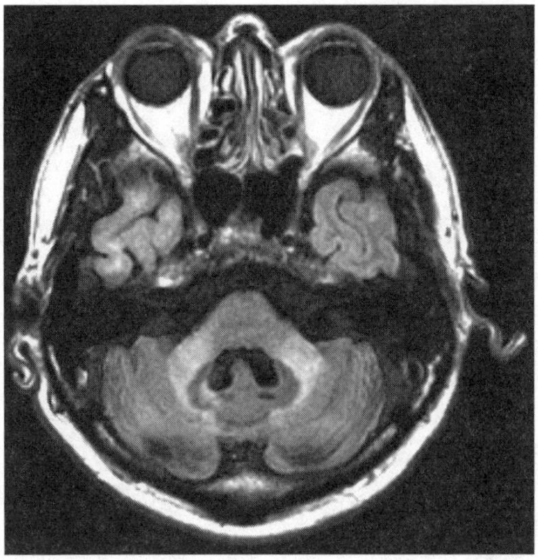

B.

9. Prion Diseases

Prion diseases are transmissible spongiform encephalopathies and present as neurodegenerative disorders. They include Creutzfeldt-Jakob disease (CJD), Gerstmann-Sträussler-Schenker syndrome, fatal insomnia and Kuru (Table 7). Those diseases are unique and can be sporadic, familiar or acquired (Table 7).

Prions are abnormal isoforms of the prion protein (PrP), which is a normal constituent of the neuronal cell membrane. PrP is encoded by the gene PRNP on the short arm of chromosome 20. Another related gene (doppel) may interact with PrP and may also be involved in the disease process.

Sporadic Creutzfeldt-Jakob disease usually affects older adults. Cognitive symptoms develop first, followed by ataxia and myoclonus. Startle myoclonus (stimulus-induced, eg, response to hand clapping) is especially typical. The Heidenhain variant begins with cortical blindness (Figure 6). Cognitive impairment progresses to severe dementia over months, and can be misinterpreted as rapidly progressive Alzheimer disease. Extrapyramidal symptoms, with rigidity, tremor and bradykinesia develop later in the disease. Eventually the patient becomes an akinetic mute. The time course is usually rapid, with time from onset to death usually within 4-6 months.

The MRI shows diffuse atrophy. Approximately 10% have hyperintensities in the basal ganglia on T2 weighted MRI imaging. Abnormalities on diffusion weighted MRI imaging are present in 92% of patients (Figure 6) . Diffusion weighted imaging abnormalities are present in the basal ganglia and/or the cerebral cortex. CSF is essentially normal, but 14,3,3 protein may support diagnosis, although it is not specific. Viral encephalitis and stroke also lead to 14,3,3 elevation. However, in rapidly progressive dementia without pleocytosis, the sensitivity is 96% and specificity is 99% for 14,3,3 protein (Table 8). The EEG has been used to establish diagnosis. Periodic bilateral 0.5-2 Hz discharges are the characteristic pattern, concomitant with the disappearance of organized background rhythms. However, only 50% of patients have these typical findings on their first EEG. In the new variant Creutzfeldt-Jakob disease, the EEG is less periodic.

The new variant Creutzfeldt-Jakob disease is thought to be related to bovine spongiform encephalopathy (BSE). If familiar CJD is suspected, direct sequencing of the PRNP gene can be diagnostic. The "definite" diagnosis can only be made by biopsy (Table 8), but neurosurgeons are hesitant to perform a biopsy due to the risk of contamination. Prions are not eliminated by sterilization.

Pathology shows spongiform abnormalities with vacuolation of the gray matter and neuronal loss. An inflammatory response is usually lacking. There is no effective treatment.

Table 7

Sporadic, Familiar and Transmissible Prion Diseases

	Infection	Clinical Manifestation	Other Features
Sporadic Creutzfeldt-Jacob disease	Polymorphism of PRNP gene codon 129 may raise susceptibility	Rapidly progressive dementia, ataxia, myoclonus	
Familiar Creutzfeldt-Jacob disease	Autosomal dominant mutation of PRNP gene on chromosome 20		
Iatrogenic Creutzfeldt-Jacob disease	Growth hormone, dura, neurosurgically, corneal transplant		
New variant Creutzfeldt-Jacob disease	Consumption of infected beef	Cerebellar signs, prominent behavioral and personality changes	Younger onset; EEG does NOT show typical periodic complexes; mainly in Britain
Gerstmann-Sträussler-Schenker syndrome	Autosomal dominant mutation of codon 102 of the PrP gene	Cerebellar signs more common than dementia	Death in 5-11 years; mean age 48
Familiar or sporadic fatal insomnia	Mutation of codon 178	Insomnia, autonomic dysfunction, minimal dementia	Selective atrophy of ventral and mediodorsal thalamic nuclei, death in 7-15 years
Kuru	Cannibalism	Cerebellar signs	Only in New Guinea

Figure 6

Diffusion weighted MRI imaging in a patient with the Heidenhain variant of Creutzfeldt-Jakob disease

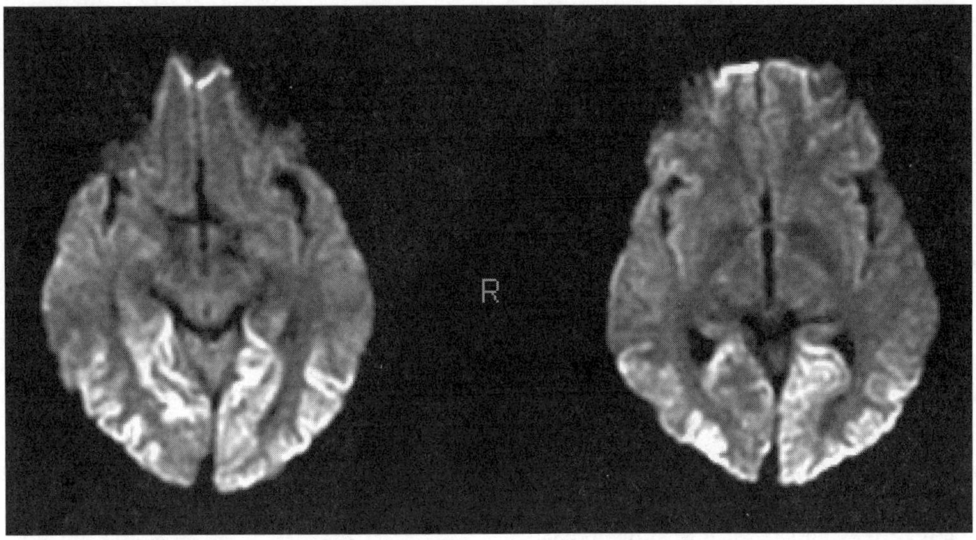

Table 8

WHO Criteria for Possible, Probable and Definite Creutzfeldt-Jakob Disease

Possible CJD	**Probable CJD**	**Definite CJD**
Progressive dementia	Progressive dementia	Diagnosed by standard neuropathologic techniques
And	*And*	*And/or*
At least two of the following four clinical features:	At least two of the following four clinical features:	Immucytochemically
Myoclonus	Myoclonus	*And/or*
Visual or cerebellar disturbance	Visual or cerebellar disturbance	Western blot confirmed protease-resistant PrP
Pyramidal/extrapyramidal signs	Pyramidal/extrapyramidal signs	*And/or*
Akinetic mutism	Akinetic mutism	Presence of scrapie-associated fibrils
And	*And*	
No EEG available or atypical	Periodic discharges on EGG	
Duration <2 years	*And/or*	
	A positive 14,3,3 CSF assay and a clinical duration to death <2 years.	
	Routine investigation should not suggest alternative diagnosis	

www.who.int/emc

10. References

1. Evaluation and management of intracranial mass lesions in AIDS. Report of the Quality Standards Subcommittee of the American Academy of Neurology. *Neurology*. 1998;50(1):21-6.

   (Guidelines for the management of ring enhancing lesions in AIDS.)

2. Davis L, ed. *Infectious Disease*. Philadelphia, Pa: Lippincott Williams and Wilkins; 2002.

   (Overview of the most important infectious diseases in neurology.)

3. Davis LE, DeBiasi R., Goade DE, Haaland KY, Harrington JA, Harnar JB, Pergam SA, King MK, DeMasters BK, Tyler KL (2006). West Nile virus neuroinvasive disease. *Ann Neurol*. 2006; 60(3): 286-300.

   (Review of West Nile Virus infection and neurologic disease.)

4. de Gans J, van de Beek D. Dexamethasone in adults with bacterial meningitis. *N Engl J Med*. 2002;347(20):1549-56.

   (Key study that proved the usefulness of steroids in bacterial meningitis.)

5. Gerber MA, Shapiro ED, et al. Lyme disease in children in southeastern Connecticut. Pediatric Lyme Disease Study Group. *N Engl J Med*. 1996;335(17):1270-4.

   (Describes the clinical manifestations of Lyme disease in children.)

6. Gilden DH, Kleinschmidt-DeMasters BK, et al. Neurologic complications of the reactivation of varicella-zoster virus. *N Engl J Med*. 2000;342(9): 635-45.

   (Describes the neurological complications of herpes zoster.)

7. Golden MR, Marra CM, et al. Update on syphilis: resurgence of an old problem. *JAMA*. 2003;290(11):1510-4.

   (Informs about the clinical manifestations of syphilis in the HIV population.)

8. Gottfredsson M, Perfect JR. Fungal meningitis. *Semin Neurol*. 2000;20(3):307-22.

   (This is a comprehensive review of fungal meningitis.)

9. Halperin JJ, Shapiro ED, Logigian E, Belman AL, Dotevall L, Wormser GP, Krupp L, Gronseth G Bever CT, Jr. (2007). Practice parameter: treatment of nervous system Lyme disease (an evidence-based review): report of the Quality Standards Subcommittee of the American Academy of Neurology. *Neurology*. 2007; 69(1): 91-102.

10. Johnson RT, Gibbs, Jr CJ. Creutzfeldt-Jakob disease and related transmissible spongiform encephalopathies. *N Engl J Med*.1998; 339(27):1994-2004.

    (Review of Creutzfeldt-Jakob and related diseases.)

11. Kanegaye JT, Soliemanzadeh P, et al. Lumbar puncture in pediatric bacterial meningitis: defining the time interval for recovery of cerebrospinal fluid pathogens after parenteral antibiotic pretreatment. *Pediatrics*. 2001;108(5):1169-74.

    (The authors examine the timing of the lumbar puncture in relation to sterilization of the CSF by antibiotic therapy.)

12. Kappos L, Bates D, Hartung HP, Havrdova E, Miller D, Polman CH, Ravnborg M, Hauser SL, Rudick RA, Weiner HL, O'Connor PW, King J, Radue EW, Yousry T, Major EO, Clifford DB 2007. Natalizumab treatment for multiple sclerosis: recommendations for patient selection and monitoring. *Lancet Neurol*. 2007; 6(5): 431-41.

13. Shiga Y, Miyazawa K, et al. Diffusion weighted MRI abnormalities as an early diagnostic marker for Creutzfeldt-Jakob disease. *Neurology*. 2004;63(3):443-449.

(The study explains why DWI is a good imaging study for Creutzfeldt-Jakob disease.)

14. Steiner I, Budka H, et al. Viral encephalitis: a review of diagnostic methods and guidelines for management. *Eur J Neurol*. 2005;12(5): 331-43.

(Review of viral encephalitis.)

15. Thwaites G, Chau TT, et al. Tuberculous meningitis. *J Neurol Neurosurg Psychiatry*. 2000;68(3): 289-99.

(This a comprehensive review of tuberculous meningitis.)

16. Tunkel AR, Hartman BJ, Kaplan SL, Kaufman BA, Roos KL, Scheld WM, Whitley RJ. Practice guidelines for the management of bacterial meningitis. *Clin Infect Dis*. 2004; 39(9): 1267-84.

17. Tyler KL. Herpes simplex virus infections of the central nervous system: encephalitis and meningitis, including Mollaret's. *Herpes*. 2004 ;11 Suppl 2: 57A-64A. Review of herpes simplex infections.

18. van de Beek D, de Gans J, et al. Clinical features and prognostic factors in adults with bacterial meningitis. *N Engl J Med*. 2004;351(18):1849-59.

(Defines prognostic factors in bacterial meningitis.)

19. Wood MJ, Johnson RW, et al. A randomized trial of acyclovir for 7 days or 21 days with and without prednisolone for treatment of acute herpes zoster. *N Engl J Med*. 1994;330(13): 896-900.

(Review of treatment of herpes zoster.)

20. Zunt JR. Central nervous system infection during immunosuppression. *Neurol Clin*. 2002;20(1):1-22.

(Review of CNS infections in HIV and immunosuppression.)

1. A 42-year-old patient with HIV on HAART presents with headaches and a focal motor seizure. MRI reveals multiple ring enhancing lesions.

A. An immediate brain biopsy should be performed

B. The patient's CD4+ count is likely to be above 200

C. Treatment with pyrimethamine and sulfadiazine should be initiated

D. Prognosis is dismal

E. CSF analysis is likely to reveal parasites

The differential diagnosis includes toxoplasmosis versus primary CNS lymphoma (PCNSL). Both usually occur with CD4+ counts < 100. Toxoplasmosis has a fairly good diagnosis if treated, while PCNSL does not. Empirical treatment is recommended; if the lesions improve, the diagnosis of toxoplasmosis is confirmed. If there is no response to treatment, a brain biopsy should be entertained. Parasites are usually not seen in the CSF, as lesions represent encapsulated abscesses.

2. AIDS dementia complex:

A. Is typically associated with ataxia

B. Is a direct effect of HIV invasion into the CNS

C. Causes vacuolar changes and neuronal loss

D. Is treated with HAART

E. All of the above

AIDS dementia complex is a direct effect of the HIV virus on the brain that results in vacuolar changes and neuronal loss. No other treatment is available besides treatment of the HIV infection itself. Ataxia is commonly associated with the disease.

3. Creutzfeldt-Jakob disease is:

A. A slow virus disease

B. Transmissible by neurosurgical procedures

C. Characterized by startle myoclonus and ataxia

D. B. and C.

E. A., B. and C.

Creutzfeldt-Jakob is a prion disease that is transmissible by cannibalism and direct contact with brain tissue, as in neurosurgical procedures. The pathogen is not destroyed by sterilization.

4. 14,3,3 protein is:

A. Only elevated in prion diseases

B. Moderately specific for prion disease in the setting of progressive dementia

C. Not helpful in familiar Creutzfeldt-Jakob disease

D. Measured in serum

E. All of the above

14,3,3 protein can be useful in the diagnosis of Creutzfeldt-Jakob disease in the appropriate clinical setting; however, is not entirely specific. 14,3,3 protein should be determined in CSF.

5. A 58-year-old patient presents with fever, meningismus, decreased consciousness and seizures. CT head is normal. CSF shows 58 WBC, 12 RBC, protein 87 and normal glucose.

The patient most likely suffers from:

A. Bacterial meningitis

B. Viral encephalitis

C. Subarchnoid hemorrhage

D. Aseptic meningitis

E. Tuberculous meningitis

The fever, seizures, meningismus and level of consciousness would suggest a meningoencephalitis. CSF examination reveals a viral picture with moderately elevated WBC, minimally elevated protein, and normal glucose. The most likely pathogen would be HSV 1 consistent with typical herpes encephalitis.

6. The most common organisms causing bacterial meningitis in the elderly are:

A. *Listeria monocytogenes*, *Staphylococcus aureus* and *Streptococcus pneumoniae*

B. Group B strep, *E coli* and *Listeria monocytogenes*

C. *Listeria monocytogens*, *Haemophilus influenzae* and *Streptococcus pneumoniae*

D. *Staphylococcus aureus*, *Streptococcus epidermidis* and Gram-negative *bacilli*

E. *Bacteroides* species, *Neisseria meninigitis* and *Streptococcus pneumoniae*

Listeria, *H influenzae* and pneumococcal infections are the most common in the elderly. *Staphylococcus aureus* and Gram-negative *bacilli* are common after neurosurgical procedures and head trauma. Group B *Streptococcus*, *E coli* and *Listeria* are typical for newborn bacterial meningitis.

7. Antibiotic treatment in an adult immunocompetent patient >50 years of age with bacterial meningitis of a not yet known organism should include:

A. Ceftriaxone, as it has good blood-brain barrier penetration

B. Dexamethason to decrease inflammation

C. Vancomycin to cover penicillin-resistant strains of *Streptococcus pneumoniae*

D. Ampicillin to cover *Listeria* monocytogenes

E. All of the above

Rational treatment of bacterial meningitis in the older population should include a third generation cephalosporin to cover pneumococcus, vancomycin to cover resistant strains, and ampicillin to cover Listeria. The addition of steroids is thought to be beneficial to reduce brain swelling and inflammation.

8. Low CSF glucose is typical for:

A. Bacterial meningitis

B. Viral meningitis

C. Tuberculous meningitis

D. A. and C.

E. A., B. and C.

Low CSF glucose is typical for bacterial, tuberculous, malignant and fungal meningitis, but is not typical for viral meningitis (Table 2).

9. An 8-year-old boy presents with sudden onset of bilateral Bell's palsy. The most likely diagnosis is:

A. Lyme disease

B. Moebius syndrome

C. Brain stem glioma

D. Arbovirus infection

E. West Nile virus infection

Moebius syndrome is an inborn bilateral or unilateral facial nerve palsy often due to calcified infarction of the tegmentum *in utero*. A brain stem glioma presents with more gradual symptoms. West Nile virus infection consists of encephalitis or bilateral flaccid lower extremity paresis due to myelitis. Arbovirus infections cause encephalitis. Lyme disease frequently affects the facial nerves or is the cause a polyradiculitis if there is nervous system involvement.

10. Cryptococcal meningitis:

A. Is common in the HIV-positive population

B. Is always fatal

C. Can only be diagnosed by fungal CSF cultures

D. Is treated with nystatin

E. Is associated with congestive heart failure due to antibiotic treatment

Cryptococcal meningitis is the most common fungal CNS infection in HIV-infected patients. It responds to treatment with amphotericin and is diagnosed in the CSF by determining the cryptococcal antigen titers. India Ink stain has also been used for diagnosis in the past.

11. A 45-year-old man with a history of lupus with antiphospholipid antibody syndrome and long-term treatment with prednisone presents to the emergency room for the second time with relentless headaches. The patient also reports chills but has no fever on admission. His wife obtained a temperature at home which was 103°. He lost 20 lbs. over 2 months. His neurological exam and CT scan showed minimally enlarged ventricles. How should the emergency room physician proceed?

A. Discharge him home with ibuprofen for his headaches

B. Obtain an MRI and MRA to rule out sinus venous thrombosis

C. Perform an LP and obtain blood cultures

D. Call neurosurgery to implant at VP shunt for the increased ventricular size

E. Admit, place a PPD and await results; in addition, obtain a chest X-ray to rule out malignancy

In an immunosuppressed patient, chronic meninigitis, like fungal or tuberculous meningitis, should always be suspected if the patient presents with severe headache, malaise, weight loss, and intermittent fevers. An LP should be performed to rule out a chronic infection. Mild hydrocephalus can be seen on the CT scan with fungal or tuberculous meningitis due to protein precipitation at the basal cisterns, and shunting will not be helpful without treatment of the underlying etiology. Sinus venous thrombosis should be in the differential diagnosis, especially as the etiology can be infectious in the immunosuppressed population, and the above patient also has a coagulopathy. However, the evaluation sinus venous thrombosis for this should be pursued after meningitis has been ruled out.

12. The above patient's CSF findings showed a white blood cell count of 204, a red blood count of glucose of 17mg/dL, and protein of 169 mg/dL; CRAG was positive.

A. The patient should be treated with antituberculostatic therapy until cultures return.

B. The patient has cryptococcal meningitis and should be started on amphotericin B and fluconazole.

C. The patient has Lyme disease and should receive oral doxycycline.

E. The patient has syphilitic meningitis and should be started on penicillin IV.

The CSF findings are consistent with a fungal meningitis and antifungal treatment with amphotericin B and fluconazaole should be initiated. The CSF white blood count is not sufficiently high enough to suggest bacterial meningitis. The CSF findings could be consistent with tuberculosis, but the positive CRAG (cryptococcal antigen) confirms the diagnosis of a cryptococcal infection.

13. How should the patient be treated further?

A. Amphotericin B should be continued for three months IV.

B. Amphotericin B and fluconazole should be continued for two weeks, then only fluconazole should be continued.

C. Kidney function should be monitored closely.

D. A and C

E. B and C

Amphotericin B is only indicated for two weeks as the initial treatment period for cryptococcal meningitis, then fluconazole alone should be continued for up to one year. Amphotericin is highly nephrotoxic.

14. A 67-year-old man is found unresponsive in his bathroom and brought to the emergency room. In the preceding two weeks he had severe headaches and was treated by his primary care physician with ciprofloxacin for presumed sinusitis. His temperature is 38.5° Celsius and he has meningismus. There are no focal signs on cranial nerve exam, he seems confused, does not follow any commands, moves all four limbs spontaneously, and has normal O_2 saturations. A head CT was normal. How should proceed?

A. Perform lumbar puncture and await results

B Start antibiotic treatment and then perform LP

C. Draw blood cultures, start antibiotics and steroids and then perform LP

D. Perform MRI

E. Draw blood cultures, start antibiotics. As the patient definitely has bacterial meningitis no lumbar puncture is necessary.

When bacterial meningitis is suspected, antibiotic treatment should be initiated as soon as possible and even before a lumbar puncture is performed. Blood cultures can aid identification of the pathogen. Steroids are now recommended in bacterial meningitis.

15. Lumbar puncture shows Gram stain was negative and CSF culture was negative; blood cultures showed Gram-positive cocci.

A. The patient does not have bacterial meningitis as the Gram stain was negative

B. The patient is likely to have herpes encephalitis; acyclovir started, and herpes PCR should be ordered

C. The patient has most likely has pneumococcal meningitis; vancomycin, third generation cephalosporin and steroids should be continued until sensitivities of blood cultures are back

D. The patient does not have bacterial meningitis, as CSF cultures are negative

E. It is unlikely that the preceding sinusitis was the nidus for bacterial invasion to the meninges

The Gram stain has a sensitivity of 25%-90%, depending on the organism. Bacterial cultures have a higher sensitivity than the Gram stain, but do not have a 100% sensitivity. The patient's history and CSF suggests bacterial meningitis and the blood cultures demonstrate the bacteremia has spread to the central nervous system. The most likely pathogen is *Streptococcus pneumoniae* (Gram-positive). The sinusitis was most likely responsible for direct hematogenous spread of the pathogens.

16. The next day the patient worsens, becomes comatose and requires intubation. This could be caused by:

A. Postinfectious vascultitis

B. Ventricultis and subsequent hydrocephalus

C. Pathogen resistant to antibiotics

D. Aspiration pneumonia

E. All of the above

Postinfectious vasculitis, ventriculitis, and hydrocephalus are all complications of bacterial meningitis. Aspiration pneumonia and resistance to antibiotics could account for clinical deterioration. In the case described, the deterioration was due to ventriculitis and subsequent hydrocephalus. Shunting was required.

17. A 65-year-old previously healthy man is brought to the neurologist due to rapid memory changes over the last three months. His family has noted intermittent twitching, especially to loud noises. The patient also has difficulties with expressive language and mild ataxia. No fevers or headaches were noted. The patient was a photographer at the pathology department of a medial school. How would you proceed?

A. The patient suffers from Alzheimer dementia; he should be placed on donezepil and nursing home care should be discussed with the family

B. A metabolic panel including TSH and B12 should be ordered. Imaging and lumbar puncture should be considered to search for etiologies

C. The patient definitely has typical Creutzfeldt-Jakob disease; this should be discussed with the family and end-of-life care considered

D. Non-convulsive status epilepticus is not in the differential diagnosis

E. The patient likely suffers from fungal meningitis due to the confusion

The history is suggestive of Creutzfeldt-Jakob disease due to the rapid deterioration, the startle myoclonus and the professional history. However, other etiologies of rapid dementia should be explored. This includes metabolic abnormalities, ischemic events and non-convulsive status epilepticus. Chronic meningitis like fungal meningitis is in the differential diagnosis in a person with rapidly progressive dementia, but certainly not the most likely diagnosis in a non-immunosuppressed person.

18. An MRI is performed on the patient above that shows hyperintensities in the basal ganglia on diffusion weighted imaging. An EEG shows periodic discharges. A routine metabolic panel including B_{12} and TSH is normal.

A. The patient has probable Creutzfeldt-Jakob disease as per WHO criteria

B. A brain biopsy should be performed

C. The patient has Gerstmann-Sträussler-Schenker syndrome

D. The patient has bovine spongiform encephalopathy associated with mad cow disease

E. The patient had an ischemic stroke

The patient meets WHO criteria for CJD with progressive dementia, myoclonus and periodic discharges on EEG. Determination of 14,3,3 protein in CSF could be helpful. A brain biopsy should be deferred as this carries a great risk of infection and the operative equipment has to be quarantined and discarded if diagnosis is confirmed. Bovine spongiform encephalopathy is assumed to be related to the new variant of CJD with more prominent ataxia and was mainly observed in Britain. Hyperintensities in the basal ganglia on diffusion weighted imaging are a prominent imaging feature of CJD.

19. A 54-year-old woman with diabetes mellitus is diagnosed with *staph aureus* endocarditis. She also complains of back pain that is improved with opoids. She is started on antibiotics. Ten days later her back pain gets worse and she notes right leg weakness and increasing constipation. An MRI of the spine is performed as shown below.

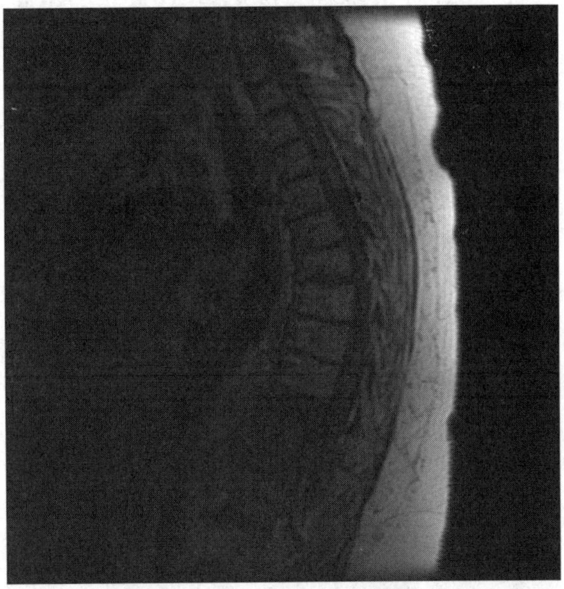

A. The patient's antibiotics should be changed

B. The patient has a herniated disk and should be continued on pain treatment and physical therapy

C. The patient should be referred for surgery

D. The most likely organism for this infection is *Streptococcus pneumoniae*

E. The leg weakness is most likely due to an embolic stroke from the infectious endocarditis.

The MRI shows an epidural abscess at the lower thoracic levels. As the patient has a clear neurological deficit and compression of the spinal, the patient should undergo surgery for evacuation of the abscess. The leg weakness is explained by the spinal cord compression. It is likely that the same organism (*Staphylococcus aureus*) that caused the endocarditis will also be found in the abscess. Antibiotics should only be changed after additional cultures are obtained from the abscess and the organism is clearly not sensitive to the current regimen.

20. A 60-year-old female with history of stage II breast cancer had been unwell for the previous 5-7 days. She has had progressive neurological symptoms during this time period. The symptoms have included a bi-temporal headache which she described as 10/10 in intensity. She has noted left-sided weakness both in her arm and leg, a left-sided facial droop and slurred speech. Her gait has become unsteady. The patient previously had undergone chemotherapy and radiation therapy. An MRI was performed as shown below.

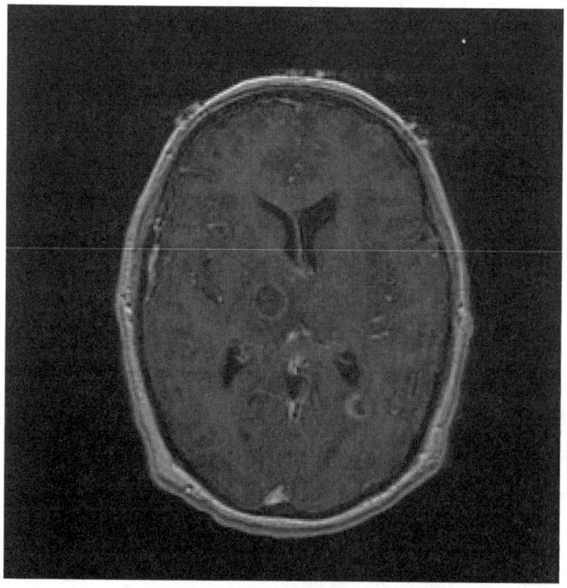

A. The differential diagnosis includes brain metastasis and infectious brain abscess. A brain biopsy with culture should be performed to establish a diagnosis.

B. The patient has progressive multifocal leukencephalopathy due to the immunosuppression, and prognosis is dismal

C. The patient is likely to have a glioblastoma multiforme as this has a predilection for the basal ganglia

D. As toxoplasmosis is common in patients in breast cancer; a treatment trial should be undertaken to assess whether lesions diminish in size

E. The patient should be immediately referred for brain radiation

The patient should be referred for biopsy to assess whether those lesions represent abscesses or metastases. A biopsy in this patient shown above showed *Streptococcus milleri*, and the patient improved with antibiotic treatment. Progressive multifocal leukencephalopathy is characterized by more diffuse white matter lesions, and glioblastoma multiform has a predilection for the cerebral hemispheres and the corpus callosum.

Answers

1. C.

2. E.

3. D.

4. B.

5. B.

6. C.

7. E.

8. D.

9. A.

10. A.

11. C.

12. B.

13. E.

14. C.

15. C.

16. E.

17. B.

18. A.

19. C.

20. A.

Chapter 10: Neurometabolic Diseases

James J. Filiano, MD

Contents

1. Introduction

Goals

This chapter is designed to be a basic introduction to neurometabolic diseases that present in the neonate. By neurometabolic disease, we mean inheritable inborn errors of metabolism, genetic disorders of developmental neural topography, and degenerative disorders of neural function. It is not intended for experts in genetics and metabolism, but those in training who seek to specialize in such disorders later may find it to be a useful introduction. It hopes to assist those who provide care for pediatric or adult patients who are suspected of having neurometabolic disease: to help the clinicians recognize signs and symptoms that signify neurometabolic disease; to teach how and when to initiate a neurometabolic diagnostic sequence; and to help neurologists and pediatricians interface with geneticists and metabolists. This chapter will not discuss the neuroanatomy and physiology of clinical findings of neurometabolic disease in detail. Nor will it discuss endocrine or renal disorders that affect electrolyte or glucose metabolism, nor myopathies. Because it is not meant for metabolists, pathways and concepts are presented in a simplified manner for deliberate educational purposes. As a conse- ience of that intent, this chapter does not discuss icate details of biochemical pathophysiology, ic diagnosis, and metabolic management, nor ınalyze each individual disorder of organic ino acids, the urea cycle, or peroxisomal ondrial diseases. Each such topic apter of its own for detailed discussion managers of those diseases. ions of treatments are described in nner in other texts. Instead, this us on the approach to diagnosis learning this skill.

rganize this chapter. Tra- the diseases based on d in urine or blood (eg, ect); or based on mitochondrial, pparatus dis- neuraxis is or leukodys- se are rea- on your st, neurologist, metabolic geneticist or general pediatrician). Each has its merit and each has its flaw. The primary flaw is that neurometabolic diseases usually have multisystem effects, and evolve over time to affect different parts of the neuraxis. For example, organic acidopathies can cause dementia, lactic acidosis, leukodystrophy and epilepsy at different times in the same patient. No one-dimensional organization plan is adequate.

This chapter incorporates elements of all those organization approaches, in an overlapping, multidimensional way. It starts by choosing the basic food groups to extract two parts from the universe of neurometabolic disease: diseases of small molecules (intermediary metabolism) vs. diseases of large molecules (eg, storage diseases). This keeps the reader's focus simultaneously on the etiology of characteristic symptoms, and also on a framework for management in the simplest and most familiar chemical framework we know – food. Next, this chapter incorporates other traditional categories of disease, because they have the merit of being recognizable and part of the standard literature. It will be noted that, of necessity, some disorders will be listed in more than one category. For example, elevated abnormal organic acids (including lactic acid) can be derived from either diseases of fatty acid oxidation, protein metabolism or mitochondrial dysfunction, because the pathways of intermediary metabolism are interwoven so intricately.

For efficiency, this chapter is constructed of many expanded lists and Tables. This is done so that each paragraph does not become an unreadable collection of biochemical and clinicopathological data. Instead, the paragraphs are designed to impart concepts, and the Tables to impart correlative facts in an efficient way. Read the paragraphs, but save the tables for rapid reference, or for comparing and contrasting diseases. Table 1 is the organization plan that will be used in this chapter, which will be subdivided according to the same subgroups of this list.

General Aspects of the Diagnostic Process

Why pursue a neurometabolic diagnosis? These are important diseases because they usually are severely debilitating. Often they can be treated effectively if diagnosed early. Diagnosis can be dif-

Table 1

Categories of Neurometabolic Disease

SMALL MOLECULE DISEASES
Inborn errors of small molecules

Diseases of sugar metabolism (non-storage)
- Diseases of simple sugar dysmetabolism
- Diseases of mitochondrial oxidative phosphorylation and lactic acidoses

Diseases of proteins (+ heme / porphyrin)
- Organic acid disorders
- Amino acid disorders
- Urea cycle diseases
- Diseases of glutathione metabolism
- The porphyrias

Diseases of fat metabolism
- Diseases of fatty acid oxidation (abnormal organic acids)
- Diseases of cholesterol metabolism

Diseases of purine and pyrimidine metabolism

Nutritional deficiencies

Toxins

LARGE MOLECULE DISEASES

Non-lysosomal disorders of large molecules
- Peroxisomal diseases
- Disorders of glycoprotein synthesis

Lysosomal and storage disorders
- Lipidoses
- Glycogen storage diseases

OTHER NEUROGENETIC DISORDERS
- Chromosomal disorders
- Subtelomeric disorders
- Nucleotide repeat disorders
- Other genetic mutations and deletions
- Heritable disorders of unknown cause

LEUKODYSTROPHIES

CAUSES OF NEURODEGENERATION

HEREDITARY ATAXIAS

ficult to make quickly, because presenting symptoms are protean, not specific, and may not be obvious until permanent damage has occurred. Diagnostic tests for neurometabolic diseases usually are sent away to specialty laboratories, so that results will not return promptly. These factors are why newborn screening is so important for this category of disease. However, many of these diseases have not yet been added to state newborn screens. Clinicians sometimes dismiss this category of diseases as being too rare to warrant committing aspects of these diseases to memory. However, although each individual disease is rare, this collective class of diseases is not rare among the causes of neurological impairment in pediatrics. The rarity of these diseases is vexing, because it makes diagnosis, triage, and cost containment during diagnosis quite difficult. Therefore, it may benefit our patients for all of us to become familiar with the modes of presentation of each subcategory of rare neurometabolic diseases, and to initiate the diagnostic and therapeutic sequence when one of these disorders is considered.

When should one pursue diagnosis of a possible neurometabolic disease? Neurometabolic disease can cause many symptoms. As a result, neurometabolic disease, as an etiological class, can be on the differential diagnosis for every undiagnosed disease. Usually, it should be at the bottom of the differential diagnosis list, because each neurometabolic disorder is rare. Neurometabolic etiology should be pursued with vigor when the patient's illness is associated with any of the following unexplained clues:

1.) Common etiologies excluded;

2.) Family history of similar symptoms, or of metabolic disease;

3.) Growth failure, especially with recurrent vomiting;

4.) Developmental delay;

5.) Intractable, severe symptoms;

6.) Recurrent, unexplained neurological events;

7.) Progressively degenerating course;

8.) Recurrent apparent severe infectious, without infectious agent identified;

9.) Movement disorder;

10.) Myoclonus;

11.) "Cerebral palsy" without prenatal or perinatal difficulties;

12.) A feature in the patient's history or physical examination that is pathognomonic for a particular disease.

The first of these characteristics is intrinsic to the diagnostic technique of "exclusion." This remains the first task of diagnosis, because each characteristic 2-11 in the above list can be caused by more common etiologies, such as trauma, infection, autoimmune disease or malignancy. Because the more common disorders are more probable (by definition), it is efficient, and therefore may be prudent, to pursue the common disorders first, and exclude them if they are not present. Occasionally, there are physical examination findings that point very strongly to a specific diagnosis, such as coarsening of facial features in lysosomal storage diseases, alopecia with trichorhexis nodosa in argininosuccinic aciduria, or external ophthalmoplegia in mitochondrial disease. Sometimes, there will be a particular diad, triad, or tetrad of findings that will establish a diagnosis, such as: cataplexy + loss of upgaze in Neimann-Pick disease type C; intractable epilepsy + alopecia + severe diaper dermatitis in biotinidase deficiency; or trismus + strabismus + retrocolis in neonatal Gaucher disease. These clustered findings add so much to improve the efficiency of our diagnostic pursuit, that more will be said of these later.

Usually, and unfortunately, our diagnostic efforts are not aided by fortuitous pathognomonic findings. Instead, a diagnosis is made by judicious and cross-correlated laboratory investigations, sometimes over a protracted time course. This reality does not please the patient or family, our colleagues who await our input, nor the third party payers and hospital business managers. The best we can do is to be attuned to clues of history and exam, mindful of cost, but aware that the cost of hospitalization or missing a treatable or familial disease in terms of human suffering, medical charges, and other fees is usually greater than the expense of a well-paced laboratory investigation. It may be most prudent to exclude treatable disorders first, while pursuing, simultaneously, some of the more common untreatable disorders that fit the patient's symptoms. Patients may benefit from us explaining to them how long it may be to make a full diagnosis, as they need courage to continue the diagnostic process. This is especially true of the emotional circumstance of when a baby is born with unexpected neurological symptoms.

The idea to pursue neurometabolic disease may come readily if there is an older sibling or other family member with neurological disease. However, if there is no such family history, then it is useful to keep in mind that neurometabolic disease may present masquerading as an acute or recurrent infection, or with unexplained low Apgar scores. If an infectious agent is not identified, the symptoms may be attributed to "a viral syndrome." That presumptive diagnosis usually is correct, because viral infections are common, after all. If, however, the clinical course of a "viral syndrome" or other infectious syndrome, such as pneumonia, is unusually severe or prolonged in the patient or her siblings, then it may be prudent to consider a neurometabolic explanation. For example, parents may say "One of her brothers gets the same viral illnesses as the other children, but the illnesses affect him much worse, last much longer, and he vomits and just won't eat." Similarly, parents may report that, "One of her brothers had somewhat low Apgar scores that were not explained, and he was very slow to feed for days after birth." Astute clinicians may take such comments about prolonged infections or unexplained low Apgar scores as clues to consider that the patient may have a disorder of fatty acid, organic acid, amino acid, or urea cycle metabolism. Such disorders are treatable, but, if not identified and treated early, they will cause developmental delay, future cognitive and motor impairment, and may cause a fatal Reye-like illness. Unfortunately, if is very difficult for even gifted clinicians to recall and apply the utility of these subtle clues, because so very many patients have viral illnesses and mildly low Apgar scores; "common things are common," as the adage says with truth.

Those two scenarios above highlight an important general feature of inborn errors of metabolism: the symptoms and laboratory abnormalities may worsen dramatically when the patient is stressed by any combination of birth, fasting, protein load, infection, surgery or exercise, and sometimes menstrual periods. The common features of these stressors are that they all cause catabolism, or drive a combination of impaired metabolic, mitochondrial, endocrine, and/or inflammatory pathways. This phenomenon can assist our efforts to make a diagnosis by using these circumstances as "stress testing" that occurs either naturally (as in the case of infection), or under our control (as when we perform newborn metabolic screening after feeding). Sometimes the patient may indeed have an infection at the time of neurometabolic presentation, but that infection may be the trigger for catabolism that makes an underlying metabolic disease manifest for the first time. In this situation, a usually mild infectious agent may cause a neurometabolic patient to have a severe illness, whereas the same infectious agent might manifest as an otherwise mild infection in a normal host. Alternately, the patient may have a mild but persistent acidosis substantially after the acute infection is treated and the patient's hemodynamic state has normalized.

Here is a diagnostic sequence that is convenient for a medical care provider who is pursuing a neurometabolic diagnosis. It employs a "biochemical modification" of the principles used in diagnosing other classes of neurological disorders. Although it is listed in sequence, logistics usually requires a sequential overlap of our thinking and testing. It asks the following questions:

1.) Where is the predominant lesion?

   a. Central vs. peripheral nervous system or both?

   b. White matter vs. gray matter or both?

   c. Brain vs. spinal cord or both?

   d. Disorder of small molecules vs. large molecules?

   e. In which food group is the involved pathway?

2.) What pathognomonic clues are found in history or physical exam?

3.) Do the symptoms fit a common, non-metabolic etiology?

4.) Screen for an abnormal metabolite in a tissue or body fluid (chemical or genetic test; magnetic resonance imaging or spectroscopy; microscopy – light or electron).

5.) Confirm the diagnosis by testing for a defect in a specific enzyme or gene (leukocytes; fibroblasts; chorionic villi; amniotic fluid).

6.) Restart the sequence if no diagnosis is found, mindful of circumstances that cause false positive and false negative results.

Classification based on symptoms and physical signs is one way to classify neurometabolic diseases. It is a time-tested aid to diagnosis, which used to be called pathognomy. It helps us assess probabilities as to the location of the lesion in the neuraxis, and this can help us focus our laboratory investigations. Many diseases can produce the same symptoms and signs, however, and there is much overlap among disease categories, so this method of classification can have low diagnostic specificity. Individual neurometabolic diseases can be multisystem, or affect many cell types in the neuraxis. This limits the value of diagnosis based on neuraxial location. Therefore, classification based on symptoms has only modest and partial utility. That utility is valid, nonetheless, because some of the clues add efficiency to our investigations.

Using the diagnostic approach of pathognomy and relative probabilities, the following are simple points to start the neurometabolic sequence:

1.) Metabolic acidosis may imply the patient has a small molecule disease;

2.) Hypoglycemia without ketones may imply the patient has a disorder of fatty acid oxidation;

3.) Organomegaly with coarse features may imply the patient has a storage disease;

4.) Organomegaly without coarse features can be caused by storage and non-storage disease;

5.) Severe spasticity, ataxia, and, later, peripheral neuropathy may imply the patient has a white matter disease, rather than a gray matter disease;

6.) Seizures may imply the patient has a gray matter disease rather than a white matter disease.

These rules of thumb are only starting probabilities. They can be misleading, so caution should be exercised. For example, small molecule diseases can cause hepatomegaly, and large molecule diseases can cause acidosis. Similarly, white matter diseases can present with seizures, and some neurometabolic diseases can affect combinations of white and gray matter, or cause both central and peripheral neuraxial disease.

Our two pathognomy Tables (2, 3) relate signs to specific diseases. Much of the Tables is not directly relevant to neonatal diagnosis. However, it might be a helpful background for the clinician who may use the information in questioning parents about family history, or in providing prognostic information after a neurometabolic diagnosis is made.

Table 2

Pathognomy: Using Signs and Symptoms to Facilitate Diagnosis

Growth failure:	Too non-specific to be a strong clue, but points toward an underlying systemic defect.
Dysmorphic features:	Chromosomal and subtelomeric disorders; peroxisomal disorders; 7-dehydrocholesterol reductase deficiency.
Coarsened features:	Lysosomal storage diseases (eg, mucopolysaccharidoses and oligosaccharidoses); coarsening results from "organomegaly" of the ground substance of cartilage and bone.
Cataracts:	Galactosemia; Marinesco-Sjögren syndrome (sometimes in mitochondrial neurodegeneration with ataxia and retinitis pigmentosa {NARP}); storage diseases; lipidoses with retinitis pigmentosa (Appendix Table 3).
Keyser-Fleischer rings:	Wilson disease.
Retinitis pigmentosa:	Mitochondrial disease, ceroid lipofuscinosis, lipidoses, metachromatic leukodystrophy; others (Appendix Table 4).
Optic pallor:	Mitochondrial or peroxisomal disease; lipidoses; others.
Cherry red macula:	Lipidoses.
Hepatomegaly:	Organic acidopathies and urea cycle defects; fatty acid oxidation disorders with or without cardiomyopathy; mitochondrial disorders with or without cardiomyopathy; peroxisomal disorders; storage diseases (lysosomal and non-lysosomal). (The association of coarse features and organomegaly raises the probability that the patient has a storage disease. Hepatomegaly with acidosis may imply a disorder of small molecules; hepatomegaly with profound hypoglycemia may imply glycogen storage disease.)
Skin lesions:	Eczema and/or alopecia in biotinidase deficiency. Angiokeratoma in several lipidoses (eg, Fabry disease, Appendix Table 2). Lipid deposits in Farber disease and cerebrotendinous xanthomatosis. Café au lait in neurofibromatosis and congenital disorders of glycoprotein synthesis. Ash leaf spots and chagrin patch in tuberous sclerosis. Jaundice in hepatopathy. Icthyosis in ceroid lipofuscinosis. Hyperpigmentation in adrenoleukodystrophy and some urea cycle defects; contractures, trismus, retrocolis found in spasticity, Gaucher disease, and mucopolysaccharidoses; lipodystrophy, wide spaced nipples, severe hypotonia and/or seizures and/or coagulopathy in congenital disorders of glycoprotein synthesis (Golgi apparatus disorders).
Alopecia:	With eczema in biotinidase deficiency; with trichorhexis nodosa in argininosuccinate lyase deficiency; with acrodermatitis enteropathica in zinc deficiency; with severe seizures and developmental stagnation, and pili torti in Menke disease; Thallium exposure; porphyria.

continued

Table 2 (continued)

Pathognomy: Using Signs and Symptoms to Facilitate Diagnosis

Dark hair with blond roots:	With painful myopathy and pail nail beds in selenium deficiency.
Hypospadius:	With 2-3 syndactyly in 7-dehydrocholesterol reductase deficiency; chromosomal and subtelomeric abnormalities; endocrine defects.
Unusual odor:	Small molecule diseases; see separate list.
Renal acidosis:	Mitochondrial diseases and organic acidopathies; Lowe syndrome.
Self-injurious behavior:	Lesch-Nyhan hyperuricemia; Smith-Magenis syndrome.
Dementia:	With psychosis may imply leukodystrophy; with seizures may imply gray matter disease; with chorea may imply mitochondrial disease or Huntington chorea; with spasticity and/or blindness, may imply storage diseases or leukodystrophy, or ceroid lipofuscinosis.
Epilepsy:	Gray matter disease: all small molecule diseases (including mitochondrial and peroxisomal diseases); ceroid lipofuscinosis; storage diseases; Glut-1 transporter and folate transporter defects; Rett syndrome; ARX and neuroligand gene defects; chromosomal and subtelomeric diseases; repetitive nucleotide expansion gene defects in myoclonic epilepsies.
Retinal blindness:	Gray matter diseases more than leukodystrophies; mitochondrial and peroxisomal diseases; ceroid lipofuscinosis; lipidoses; oligosaccharidoses.
Loss of upgaze:	With cataplexy + hepatomegaly +/- seizures in Neimann-Pick disease type C; with deafness and choreoathetosis in kernicteris.
Lateral gaze paresis:	With hepatomegaly in Gaucher disease type III; without hepatomegaly in mitochondrial defects.
Movement disorders:	Basal ganglion and cerebellar disorders: all small molecule diseases, especially mitochondrial diseases, cerebral folate deficiency and disorders of neurotransmitters and neopterin defects, kernicteris, neurodegeneration with brain iron deposition, repetitive nucleotide expansion gene defects.
Central ataxia:	Small molecule diseases, especially mitochondrial diseases; leukodystrophies; storage diseases; repetitive nucleotide expansion gene defects.
Spasticity:	Leukodystrophies more often than gray matter diseases; peroxisomal diseases; arginase deficiency; spinocerebellar degeneration gene defects.
Neuropathy:	Peroxisomal disease more often than mitochondrial disease; selenium toxicity; late metachromatic leukodystrophy and late Krabbe disease; inherited neuropathies from nucleotide repeat gene defects.
Myopathy/cardiomyopathy:	Disorders of fatty acid oxidation; mitochondrial oxidation/phosphorylation defects; taurine deficiency.

Table 3

Clues to the Cause of Coma from the Physical Exam

SITE	FINDING	DISEASE
HEAD	Contusion	Trauma, Coagulopathy
	Vasodilation	Sagittal sinus thrombosis
NECK	Rigid	Meningitis, Encephalitis, Subarachnoid hemorrhage, Neck or throat inflammation, Pneumonia
	Enlarged thyroid	Myxedema, Thyrotoxicosis
EYES	Chemosis	Cavernous sinus thrombosis
	Periorbital ecchymosis	Blow-out orbital fracture, Periorbital and cavernous sinus parameningeal infection
	Subhyaloid blood	Subarachnoid hemorrhage
	Vasospasm	Hypertensive encephalopathy
	Retinal hemorrhages	Shaken-baby syndrome
EARS	Hemorrhage	Basilar skull fracture
	Otitis media	Brain abscess, lateral sinnus thrombosis
NOSE	SCF rhinorrhea	Basilar skull fracture
MOUTH	Scarred tongue	Seizure disorder
	Pigmentation	Addison disease
	Lead lines	Lead intoxication
ODORS	Acetone	Diabetes mellitus
	Alcohol	Ingestion
	Almond	Cyanide poisoning
	Cabbage	Methioninemia, Tyrosinemia
	Feculent	Hepatic encephalopathy (fetor hepaticus)
	Fishy	Trimethylaminuria
	Fruity	Diabetic ketoacidosis
	Garlic	Selenium/paraldehyde/arsenic toxicity; also part of fetor hepaticus
	Hops	Oasthouse disease (methionine malabsorption)
	Maple syrup	Maple Syrup Urine Disease (branched chain ketoaciduria)
	Mouse urine	Phenylketonuria
	Musty	Glycine
	Sweaty feet	Glutaric Acuria (II) Isovalericacidemia
	Swimming pool	Hawkinsism (tyrosylauria, 5-oxoprolinuria hydroxycyclohexylacetic acid)

continued

Table 3 (continued)

Clues to the Cause of Coma from the Physical Exam

SITE	FINDING	DISEASE
ODORS	Tomcat urine	Methylcrotonyl acidemia or multiple carboxylase deficiency
	Uremia	Renal failure
HEART	Murmur	Endocarditis, Cerebral embolism/abscess
LUNG	Rales	Heart failure, Pneumonia, Respiratory distress syndrome
ABDOMEN	Hepatomegaly	Leukemia; Hepatic failure, Storage disease; Heart failure
	Vomiting	Organic acidemia, Galactosemia Hyperglycinemia, Beta-keto-thiolase deficiencies
LIMBS	Fracture	Trauma, Fat embolism
	Ecchymosis	Trauma, Coagulopathy
SKIN	Ash leaf spots	Neurophakomatoses (eg, TS) with seizures
	Butterfly rash	Lupus, Tuberous sclerosis (TS)
	Café au lait	Neurofibromatosis with seizures
	Cyanosis	Hypoxia, Congenital heart disease with Cerebral embolism/abscess
	Desquamation	Vitamin A toxicity, Scarlatina Toxic shock syndrome
	Dry	Dehydration, Myxedema, Adrenal insufficiency
	Erythema	Carbon monoxide, Atopine/mercury toxicity
	Periungual fibromoa	Tuberous sclerosis with seizures
	Petechiae/ Purpura	Sepsis, Endocarditis, Trauma Hemolytic Uremic Syndrome, Henoch-Schoenlein Purpura, Thrombocytopenia
	Hyperpigmentation	Addison disease
	Splinter hemorrhages	Endocarditis, Hypoparathyroidism
	Uremic frost	Uremia
	Wet	Syncope
	Needle tracks	Addiction, Chronic disease, Abuse/neglect Risk for HIV

Modified from Lockman LA, 1982.

2. Small Molecule Diseases

The disorders of small molecules are so named because the diseases are characterized by the accumulation of a small toxic molecule, or the deficiency of a small molecule whose presence is vital for health and whose absence causes disease. These disorders are important because, of all the neurometabolic diseases, they are most likely to be rapidly fatal. They are also most likely to be treated successfully by dietary management. In the neonatal period their clinical presentations may include low Apgar scores, marked hypotonia, vomiting and/or poor suck, neonatal seizures or epilepsy, coma or neonatal Reye-like syndrome (rarely recurrent), and unexplained jaundice. The patients may be born with intrauterine growth retardation, but this is not common because the infant's metabolism may be protected somewhat *in utero*. Later, they are likely to suffer growth failure, often with feeding difficulties or vomiting. Whether or not the infant escaped the prior symptoms, eventually patients with small molecule disease are likely to suffer any combination of developmental delay, mental retardation, movement disorder, or intermittent ataxia added to their prior symptoms. Those are the general clinical characteristics of small molecule diseases, but individual disorders may have unique clinical features; for example, non-ketotic hyperglycinemia often presents itself as refractory hiccups.

It is convenient to subclassify the small molecule disorders according to the relevant food group that is most likely to be the origin of the abnormal metabolites. Classifying the small molecule diseases by dysfunctional food group is convenient because it reminds us of the metabolites for which we must screen, and whose nutrient intake we must manage (either by regulating diet or intravenous intake):

1.) Sugars and energy metabolism:
   a. Galactosemia (and galactosurias)
   b. Fructosemia (and fructosuria, and pentosuria)
   c. Glut-1 cerebral transporter defect
   d. Cerebral creatine metabolism defects
   e. Mitochondrial disorders of the electron transport chain

2.) Proteins, (+ heme and porphyrin) metabolism:
   a. Amino acid and organic acid disorders
   b. Urea cycle defects (amino acid disorders causing hyperammonemia)
   c. Disorders of glutathione metabolism
   d. The porphyrias

3.) Fat metabolism:
   a. Disorders of fatty acid oxidation, with abnormal organic acids
   b. Disorders of cholesterol metabolism

4.) Disorders of purine, pyrimidine and uric acid metabolism

5.) Nutrient defects:
   a. Vitamin deficiencies
   b. Cerebral folate deficiency
   c. Metal metabolism defects (especially copper and selenium)
   d. Deficiencies of other micronutrients

6.) Toxins (including excess of vitamins or other micronutrients)

A cardinal feature of disorders of small molecules is that an enzyme in a pathway of intermediary metabolism is defective, either by genotype, or nutritional/vitamin deficiency, or toxic insult. This takes the general form of A → B →//→ C; where each letter represents a metabolite; each arrow represents an enzymatic reaction; and →//→ represents the dysfunctional enzymatic step. This produces two immediate outcomes: 1.) metabolite B (and perhaps its precursor) accumulates, and 2.) there is a deficiency of metabolite C, which cannot be synthesized because of the dysfunctional enzymatic step. The accumulated metabolite B may be toxic, or its precursor or one of its breakdown products may be toxic; that may cause symptoms. The body will be deficient in metabolite C and its breakdown products, and too may cause symptoms. The general approach to diagnosis of diseases of small molecules is to find the increased concentration of a diagnostic unmetabolized biochemical marker (metabolite B), and to confirm the diagnosis by proving the presence of a deficient enzyme or defective gene. The general approach to treatment is to minimize the dietary supply of substances B (and/or A), supplement the deficient substance C, and/or provide high doses of a vitamin that catalyzes the step from B to C.

The newborn care provider is usually not responsible for treating these diseases chronically, and usually not alone. Chronic management is usually left to geneticists and metabolists, unless the patient is far from such resources. However, a neonatal or neurological specialist may be one of the first to see the patient in consultation from a primary care provider. It may be useful for clinicians to consider the diagnostic possibility of disorders of small molecules in order to recommend proper screening laboratory studies. These studies are best obtained simultaneously with a work-up for infection, inflammation, toxin, trauma, hemorrhage, endocrine and other diseases. In addition, it may be prudent for the clinician to recommend the rudiments of emergency stabilization for these disorders (see below). To aid in the rapid diagnosis, it is useful to keep in mind the laboratory hallmarks of disorders of small molecules: acidosis and/or hypoglycemia, and/or hyperammonemia, at times of metabolic stress (Appendix Figures 2, 3, 4). Further clarification of a specific disorder requires a more detailed evaluation. The first queries and tests include the following:

1.) Review of systems:

   a. Any feeding intolerances (protein load intolerance in organic acidemias and urea cycle defects; fruit juices in fructosemia)?

   b. Seizures or tremor in the morning (fasting hypoglycemia)?

   c. Ravenous eater of sweets (disorder of fatty acid oxidation)?

   d. Slow developmental progress, or loss of milestones?

2.) Are there prior similar episodes, symptoms or lab abnormalities?

3.) Is family or ethnic history consistent with neurometabolic disease?

4.) Does the patient show any unique or salient physical findings?

5.) Test urinalysis for ketones, sugars, pH;

6.) Rapid glucose test;

7.) Blood electrolytes (hyponatremia and acidosis often occur in small molecule diseases);

8.) Blood ammonia (obtain from free-flowing blood, not a tourniqueted vessel);

9.) Liver enzymes, bilirubin;

10.) Blood L-lactate (on ice);

11.) Uric acid;

12.) Complete blood count (anemia and thrombocytopenia may be present);

13.) Urine organic acid screen;

14.) Urine amino acid screen;

15.) Urine acylglycines;

16.) Blood acylcarnitine profile;

17.) Blood filter paper newborn screen (especially the newer "expanded" screens);

18.) Specific vitamin levels, if indicated.

19.) Chromosomes and subtelomeric studies, especially if patient is dysmorphic, or if sex chromosome polyploidy is suspected;

20.) Heavy metal studies in blood or urine, if indicated: (eg, selenium if there are blond hair roots in otherwise dark hair, plus painful myopathy; thallium if alopecia is present; lead if anemia with basophilic stippling or lead lines on plain roentgenograms);

21.) Plain roentgenograms when appropriate, eg:

a. Patellar calcification in neonatal peroxisomal disease;

b. Dysostosis multiplex (beaked vertebrae, distal extremities) in storage disease;

c. Adrenal calcification in Wolman disease;

22.) Lumbar puncture for cerebrospinal fluid (CSF) specimens:

a Cells, protein, glucose, VDRL;

b. L-lactate (may be abnormal in mitochondrial disease even if blood lactate is normal);

c. Amino acids (may be abnormal even if blood and urine amino acids are normal);

d. Neurotransmitter metabolites and neopterin profile if spasticity, tremor or dystonia;

e. 3-methyltetrahydrofolate if seizures and motor signs are not explained by prior studies;

23.) Cerebral imaging;

24.) Electrophysiology (encephalogram or nerve/muscle studies) if indicated;

25.) Urine orotic acid should be added to tests of amino and organic acids if there is hyperammonemia. This test clarifies the specific subtype of urea cycle defect.

26.) Blood pyruvate can be added if blood L-lactate is elevated. If pyruvate is elevated, it implies the disorder is in the early phases of the electron transport chain, and less likely the result of sepsis or dehydration.

Each urine test requires approximately 10 ml of urine, each in its own separate frozen aliquot. These have greatest sensitivity when obtained promptly at the time of the patient's symptoms, prior to rehydration or prolonged treatment with dextrose. The results may be normal in a patient with an "intermittent" form of a disease, if the laboratory studies are obtained when the patient is no longer symptomatic. Therefore, if clinical suspicion is high that the patient has a disorder of small molecules, and tests done when the patient is not acutely ill return normal, the tests may yet be diagnostic if obtained at the next sign of illness. Thus, it may be prudent to obtain the urine at the time of acute illness, to freeze it, store it, and send it for analysis later if other studies do not reveal a non-metabolic diagnosis or if the patient has a marked acidosis. If, however, a diagnosis of a non-metabolic diagnosis is made, then the frozen specimen can be thrown away. Usually, urine "screening" amino acids and organic acids are sufficient to make a presumptive diagnosis, although quantitative versions are superior. The quantitative form of the tests, and blood quantitative amino acids, are most indicated for following the course of dietary management, or for clarifying a presumptive diagnosis.

Elevated blood lactate is a hallmark of disorders of the mitochondrial electron transport chain (oxidative/phosphorylation diseases; Ox/Phos diseases), although elevated lactate may not be observed in every patient with Ox/Phos disease. Lactate accumulates because of inability of dysfunctional mitochondria to metabolize pyruvate generated from the breakdown of sugars (glycolysis). However, in addition to the electron transport chain, many other biochemical reactions take place, at least in part, in mitochondria. As a result, disorders of small molecules may make mitochondrial function inefficient, which thereby increases blood lactate or ammonia as an epiphenomenon, even if the defective enzyme is not strictly part of the electron transport chain or urea cycle. Therefore, elevated blood lactate can be found in many diseases of small molecules (Appendix Table 3). It is very helpful, therefore, to obtain simultaneous correlated laboratory studies at the time of the acute illness in order to clarify the diagnosis; if possible, it is best not to rely on a single test, such as L-lactate. This is depicted by Figure 1 of a simplified view of the expansive role of mitochondria in intermediary metabolism:

The pivotal role of mitochondria is due to a great extent to the importance of energy metabolism for living things. (That is only part of the function of each mitochondrion, as will be discussed later.)

Figure 1

Simplified view of the expansive role of mitochondria in intermediary metabolism

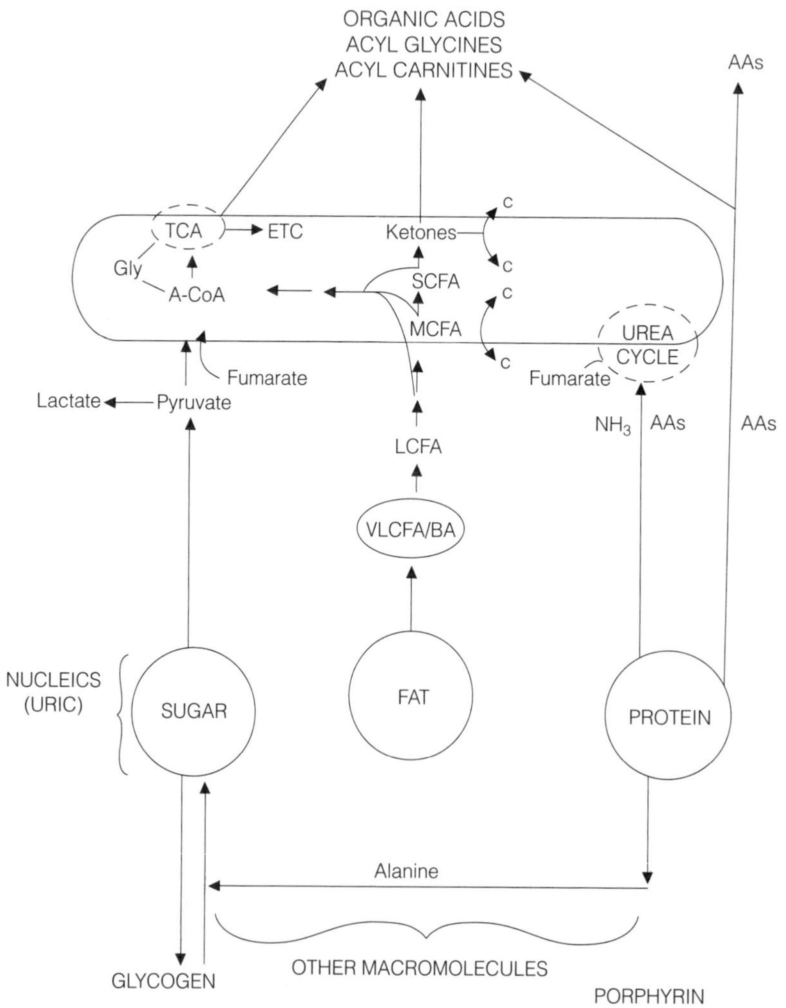

AAs = amino acids; A-CoA = acetyl CoEnzyme A; BA = bile acids; c = carnitine; ETC = electron transport chain; Gly = glycine; LCFA = long chain fatty acids; MCFA = medium chain fatty acids; NH3 = ammonia; Nucleics = nucleic acids; SCFA = short chain fatty acids; TCA = tricarboxylic acid cycle; VLCFA = very long chain fatty acids.

When mitochondrial energetics and the urea cycle fail, many pathways and many tissues are disrupted. One symptomatic outcome is the combination of hepatic and cerebral failure in the presence of lactic acidemia +/- hyperammonemia. In the neonate, this syndrome has been called several terms, including overwhelming neonatal metabolic coma. In older children, it sometimes takes the form of what has been called the Reye-like syndrome.

The Reye syndrome and the Reye-like syndrome may not be unique independent diseases. Rather, the Reye syndrome has been shown, in some cases, to be a presentation of several treatable neurometabolic disorders of small molecules. This was first recognized several decades ago when patients who had classic Reye syndrome were shown to have urea cycle defects during a catabolic decompensation. This hepato-cerebral dysfunction syndrome has been reported in the setting of a number of other small molecule diseases, most of which involve impairment of mitochondrial function. It is noteworthy that salicylic acid (aspirin), use of which was associated with Reye's epidemiological analysis of the syndrome, can uncouple oxidative phosphorylation. To accommodate this new information, some metabolists prefer the term "Reye-like syndrome" to encompass both classic Reye syndrome and those associated with a diagnosable metabolic disease. Symptoms can present late in the course of a viral syndrome, and may be made more likely to occur by the use of salicylate. Symptoms start with irritability, followed by stupor and then coma; hyperammonemia and fatty liver usually are present; death or severe disability from cerebral edema and herniation can occur. Known or suspected causes of the Reye-like syndrome, and those that "mimic" it, are listed as follows.

Causes of the Reye-like Syndrome

Urea Cycle Defects

Ornithine transcarbamylase deficiency (X-linked: males > females)

Argininosuccinic acid synthase deficiency (homozygote and heterozygote)

Acetyl glutamate synthetase deficiency

Citrullinemia

Triple H-syndrome (hyperornithinemia-hyperammonemia-homocitrullinuria)

Lysinuric protein intolerance

Organic Acidemias

3-methylcrotonyl CoA carboxylase

Glutaric aciduria type I (glutaryl CoA dehydrogenase deficiency)

Methylmalonic aciduria

Propionic aciduria

Isovaleric acidemia

Biotinidase deficiency

Disorders of Fatty Acid Oxidation and Ketogenesis

Medium chain acyl CoA dehydrogenase deficiency (MCAD)

Long chain acyl CoA dehydrogenase deficiency (LCAD)

Long chain hydroxy-acyl CoA dehydrogenase deficiency (LCHAD)

Short chain acyl CoA dehydrogenase deficiency (SCAD) (not confirmed definitively)

Multiple acyl CoA dehydrogenase deficiency

3-hydroxy-3-methylglutaryl CoA lyase (HMG CoA lyase) deficiency

Carnitine Metabolism Defects

Carnitine palmitoyl transferase I (CPT I) deficiency

CPT II deficiency

CPT translocase deficiency

3-ketoacyl CoA thiolase deficiency (not a definitively confirmed cause)

Mitochondrial electron transport chain defects and pyruvate carboxylase deficiency

Wilson disease

Carbohydrate metabolism disorders

Fructosemia

Fructose diphosphatase deficiency

Glycogen storage disorders

Alpha-1-antitrypsin deficiency

Neonatal jaundice can be associated with neurological disorders. Other than the important issue of applying the guidelines for phototherapy to prevent kernicteris, it is also valuable to pursue underlying causes of neonatal jaundice, including neurometabolic causes. Consider the following causes of neonatal jaundice:

1.) Hemolysis;

2.) Neonatal hemochromatosis;

3.) Alpha-1 antitrypsin deficiency;

4.) Crigler-Najjar syndrome;

5.) Wilson disease;

6.) Galactosemia;

7.) Fructosemia (rare, because neonates are usually not exposed to fructose);

8.) Tyrosinemia;

9.) Organic acidemias (eg, propionic acidemia);

10.) Urea cycle defects.

Treatment of Small Molecule Diseases

Early diagnosis, especially through newborn screening, is a mainstay of effective management. A complete exposition of treatments for all these disorders is beyond the scope of this chapter. However, the general approach listed below, with a few examples, may be instructive. The general plan of treatment for disorders of small molecules is as follows:

1.) Avoid catabolism if possible (eg, fasting, infections, surgery without dextrose);

2.) Avoid introducing the unmetabolized nutrient (metabolite B in the paradigm, above; for example, avoid excessive protein intake in urea cycle defects);

3.) Supply the vitamin/co-factor for the deficient enzyme;

4.) Supply the missing metabolite to bypass the metabolic block (metabolite C, eg, arginine in some of the urea cycle defects);

5.) Remove toxic metabolites (eg, chelation in Wilson disease; careful use of intestinal cathartics in organic acidemias and urea cycle defects in order to minimize production of unmetabolized toxins, such as propionic acid, from gut bacteria);

6.) Avoid toxic drugs if possible (eg, barbiturates in porphyria);

7.) Provide general medical and neurological therapies (eg, cardiorespiratory support, anticonvulsants, mannitol in Reye-like syndrome);

8.) Genetic counseling and family planning;

9.) Psychosocial interventions;

10.) Enzyme replacement (if available; eg, some storage diseases);

11.) Bone marrow transplant (if effective);

12.) Gene replacement (experimental);

13.) Phototherapy or dialysis when indicated;

14.) Referral to additional consultants, including nutrition, when feasible.

Effective therapy is available for many organic and amino acidopathies, urea cycle defects, and galactosemia. In some cases, treatment with a specific vitamin alone may be effective. For example, some cases of biotinidase deficiency and multiple carboxylase deficiency can be treated effectively with biotin supplementation alone. There are also rare forms of thiamine dependent branched chain ketoaciduria (Maple Syrup Urine Disease) that respond to thiamine alone. Usually, treatment for small molecule diseases is more involved than the fortuitous circumstance of a vitamin responsive disease.

An instructive example of therapy that involves all three aspects of small molecule enzyme dysfunction is found with disorders of the pyruvate dehydrogenase complex. Pyruvate dehydrogenase is a key enzyme in the utilization of pyruvate for energy metabolism at the beginning of the electron transport chain. Pyruvate dehydrogenase complex utilizes thiamine and lipoic acid in its processes. Pyruvate dehydrogenase function can be impaired by one of three mechanisms: 1.) mutations in genes involved in synthesis or assembly of its protein subunits; 2.) thiamine deficiency; or 3.) accumulation of a toxin, such as acetaldehyde, which is a breakdown product of ethanol and is toxic to the pyruvate dehydrogenase complex. Recall that small molecule diseases take the general form as follows: A → B →//→ C; where each letter represents a metabolite; each arrow represents an enzymatic reaction; and →//→ represents the dysfunctional enzymatic step. The general approach to treatment of small molecule diseases is to minimize the dietary supply of substances B (and/or A), supplement the deficient substance C, and/or provide high doses of a vitamin that catalyzes the step from B to C. In the case where the defective enzyme is pyruvate dehydrogenase (whether from gene mutation, cofactor deficiency, or toxin), symptoms may be improved by four steps: 1.) minimize excessive sugar intake (the source of pyruvate); 2.) provide thiamine and lipoic acid supplementation; 3.) avoid alcohol or other drugs that are toxic to pyruvate dehydrogenase; and 4.) use the ketogenic diet to provide energy substrate that bypasses dependence on pyruvate to drive the electron transport chain.

Patients with urea cycle defects develop hyperammonemia and symptoms after a high protein load, because it is the urea cycle that facilitates the excretion of nitrogen during protein metabolism. Treating urea cycle defects may require limiting protein intake to just the patient's basal needs; no greater, but also not less, because insufficient protein will cause the body to catabolize muscle in order to salvage essential amino acids. This essential amino acid recycling during "negative nitrogen balance" liberates other amino acids. When these amino acids are metabolized, they release nitrogen that forms ammonia, which cannot be removed efficiently in a patient with a urea cycle defect. Clinicians can also replace insufficient arginine or citrulline to restore the ability of the urea cycle to remove ammonia in some urea cycle defects. In addition, phenylbutyrate or phenylacetate may be given; these combine with excessive toxic metabolites to form harmless byproducts that are excreted in the urine. In the event that a patient with a urea cycle defect develops a Reye-like syndrome, vigorous urgent therapy is indicated, which may include management of increased intracranial pressure, cardiorespiratory stabilization, and sometimes dialysis.

Obviously, it is most productive to tailor treatment, when possible, to the needs of the individual patient and the managing institution. For example, newborns need not be counseled to avoid alcohol. Use of dialysis may be replaced with exchange transfusion, if that is what is best for a particular infant. Often, breast-feeding may be done by strict measurement of pumped breast milk, so that protein intake can be regulated. Nutrition consultation and genetic consultation is indicated.

Disorders of Sugar Metabolism (not storage)
The common pathogenic mechanism in these disorders is disruption of enzymes involved in the metabolism and utilization of a simple sugar, pyruvate, or the energy currencies of NADH/NADPH, ATP, or phosphocreatine. A diagnostic algorithm for disorders that cause hypoglycemia, and disorders that produce excessive urinary simple sugars reducing substances are listed in Appendix Figure 1 and Table 1. These disorders are summarized in the Table 4, which lists each disease name, its clinical and laboratory hallmark features, enzyme defect, gene defect, general prognosis and basic treatment.

Additional entities deserve mention. Galactosuria can occur from impaired galactokinase or epimerase enzymes. Galactosuria is detected by the same newborn screening techniques as galactosemia; patients may be assymptomatic, or develop cataracts or pseudotumor cerebri. Fructosuria (also called essential fructosuria) is a benign disorder characterized by excessive fructose in urine after ingesting foods high in fructose or sucrose. The fructose may be detected by test of urine-reducing substances. It is caused by deficiency of liver fructokinase and does not produce the clinical symptoms of fructosemia. Pentosuria is a benign disorder characterized by excretion of urinary L-xylulose, common in the Jewish population. Remember that testing urine with the glucose oxidase method (used for diabetes mellitus) will not detect galactose, fructose or other reducing substances.

The Glut-1 transporter defect causes a low concentration of glucose in the CSF, which results in intractable epilepsy and mental retardation, among other symptoms. Phenobarbital sometimes worsens the seizures. Noting that the CSF glucose is <1/3 the serum level makes the diagnosis. The ketogenic diet may be its best current remedy, perhaps by forcing cerebral metabolism to shift away from glucose as the preferred energy source.

Mitochondrial Diseases

This rich collection of disorders can be subdivided into several groups. Mitochondrial disease is commonly associated with disorders of pyruvate metabolism and the electron transport chain, so they are included in this section on disorders of sugar metabolism because pyruvate is the end product of sugar metabolism, and the beginning of the electron transport chain. However, the mitochondrion is involved in more functions than just the vital function of energy metabolism. It has been stated that oxidative phosphorylation may involve less than 10% of the role of the mitochondrion. Other aspects of its role in energy metabolism involve pyruvate metabolism and fatty acid beta-oxidation fats, such that there is valid reason to include mitochondrial disease among diseases of fat metabolism. Its other roles in intermediary metabolism include free radical detoxification, the citric acid cycle, the carnitine shuttle, the urea cycle, sterol and sex hormone synthesis, pyrimidine synthesis (dihydroorotate dehydrogenase involved in orotic aciduria), heme synthesis (via delta-amino levulinic acid synthetase), and even neurotransmitter metabolism. However, in the last two decades there has been a blossoming of molecular genetic diagnostic techniques. These have been used to identify electron transport chain disorders encoded in the maternally inherited mitochondrial genome. This has been a "celebrity marriage" of clinical and basic science that, in clinical literature, has overshadowed the importance of other roles of the mitochondrion. The other pathways are usually discussed amongst other classes of diseases, such as urea cycle defects and organic acidopathies. For the sake of completeness and order, they are listed separately. They are usually characterized by various degrees of acidosis (lactate and/or pyruvic and other organic or dicarboxylic acids), developmental delays, seizures, motor dysfunction, and dysfunction of other organ systems, especially liver, kidney and blood cells. Virtually all can present with some symptoms and signs in the neonatal period, although the full manifestation of certain syndromes depends on maturity, and some patients do not present until adulthood. Below is a fairly comprehensive summary, subdivided into related functional groups. The entities are listed first, then discussed:

The following acidemias (Tables 5b, c) have the common hallmark of excessive excretion of glutaric acid and its structural relatives, and dicarboxylic acids. Glutaric aciduria II can be considered a disorder of metabolism of fatty acids more than a disorder of protein metabolism. The challenge for the

Table 4

Small Molecule Disorders of Sugar Metabolism

Disease Name	Galactosemia	Fructosemia (Hereditary Fructose Intolerance)	Glut-1 Transporter Defect	Cerebral Creatine Defects	Mitochondrial Disorders of Electron Transport
Enzyme Defect	Galactose-1-phosphate uridyl transferase; several variants.	Hepatic fructose -1-phosphate aldolase.	Cerebral glut-1 transporter	Guanidine-Acetate-Methyl-transferase	See separate section
Clinical Features	Congenital hepatomegaly, jaundice, vomiting, neonatal sepsis, failure to thrive, microcephaly or infantile pseudotumor cerebri, hypoglycemia, acidosis, thrombocytopenia, urinary reducing substances, renal Fanconi syndrome, seizures; later cataracts, mental retardation, speech dyspraxia, hypergonadotropic hypogonadism.	Symptoms after ingestion of fructose or sucrose: hypoglycemia, tremor, disorientation, vomiting, +/- convulsions and coma. Chronic growth failure, vomiting, jaundice, hepatomegaly, proteinuria, aminoaciduria. Severe in infants; mild later because patients develop aversion to sweets.	Intractable epilepsy, mental retardation, other neurological signs. Seizures may be worsened by phenobarbital therapy.	Neonates +/- hypotonia and seizures; developmental delay; later extrapyramidal movement disorder.	See separate section
Hallmark Lab Findings	Urine reducing substances (galactosuria) and galactitol; blood galactose.	Fructosuria; +/- fructosemia, hypoglycemia, amino aciduria, hypophosphatemia, hypokalemia, hyperuricemia.	Low CSF Glucose (<40mg/dL).	Very low creatinine: serum, CSF urine, and brain MR spectroscopy. Urine guanidinoacetate.	See separate section
Genetics	9p13, recessive.	Autosomal recessive and autosomal dominant forms.	Autosomal recessive	Autosomal recessive	See separate section
Treatment	Galactose free diet + ophthalmologic, endocrine and educational assistance.	Avoidance of foods with fructose and sucrose; IV glucose during crisis.	Ketogenic diet	Creatine monohydrate.	See separate section
Prognosis	Normal, with diet and support.	Normal if sucrose and fructose are withheld; fatal if continued.	Good if treated early, otherwise mental impairment.	Amelioration on treatment.	See separate section

clinician is to be aware of the difference between the benign and the fatal forms of these diseases.

Subcategories of Mitochondrial Diseases

Electron transport chain defects of oxidative phosphorylation:
Many mitochondrial genome mutations and deletions (see syndromes in list below)

Nuclear gene mutations
X-linked gene mutations

Mitochondrial depletion syndromes and miscellaneous mitochondrial defects:
Alpers hepatocerebral degeneration (see gene defects below)

Mitochondrial DNA depletion syndromes caused by deficiencies of thymidine kinase, DNA polym gamma A1 or deoxyguanosine kinase.

Menke kinky hair disease (ATPase 7a, Xq12 mutation → copper deficiency → Cytochrome C dysfunction)

Enzyme defects in fatty acid oxidation:
CoA deficiency

Carnitine palmitoyl transferase I

Carnitine palmitoyl transferase II

Carnitine uptake defect

Carnitine depletion

(from exogenous or endogenous toxins; eg, valproate toxicity, organic acidopathy, or starvation)

Electron transfer flavoprotein (Complex II)

Very long chain acyl or hydroxy acyl CoA dehydrogenase

Long chain 3-OH-acyl CoA dehydrogenase

Medium chain acyl CoA dehydrogenase

Short chain acyl CoA dehydrogenase

3-OH-acyl CoA dehydrogenase

Enoyl-CoA hydratase

3-keto thiolase deficiency

Enzyme defects in pyruvate metabolism:
Monocarboxylase translocase

Pyruvate carboxylase complex

Pyruvate dehydrogenase complex

Phosphoenolpyruvate carboxykinase

Disorders of carnitine metabolism

Enzyme defects in the citric acid cycle:
Fumarase

Alpha-ketoglutarate dehydrogenase

Disorders of fatty acid oxidation often present as follows:
Short chain acyl CoA dehydrogenase deficiency as cyclic vomiting;

3-ketothiolase as cyclic vomiting and migraine;

Medium chain acyl CoA dehydrogenase as:

seizures with fasting (morning) hypoketotic hypoglycemia;

apparent life-threatening events;

sudden infant death.

Long chain disorders of fatty oxidation present as acute fatty liver with or without rhabdomyolysis. Most can present with intermittent lethargy, coma, cardiomyopathy, the Reye-like syndrome, and retinopathy.

Disorders of carnitine metabolism can present as cramps, rhabdomyolysis, acute fatty liver, myopathy, the Reye-like syndrome, and developmental delay.

Disorders of the oxidative phosphorylation (Ox/Phos) electron transport chain are caused by a defective enzyme complex, or deficient cofactor of electron transport, or mitochondrial depletion. Simplistically, electrons derived from pyruvate (from sugar) enter the chain preferentially through complex I; electrons from lipids enter preferentially via complex II. Thiamine and lipoic acid are cofactors for pyruvate dehydrogenase/complex I. Riboflavin is a cofactor involved in complex II. The hallmark of these disorders is high body fluid lactate or a lactate:pyruvate ratio >20. The simplified electron transport pathway is summarized below:

Pyruvate dehydrogenase / Complex I → CoQ ← Complex II

↓

Complex III → Cytochrome C

↓

Complex IV/V

Some Syndromes of Oxidative Phosphorylation Dysfunction

Alper disease
Hepatocerebral degeneration, often caused by mitochondrial depletion associated with defects of DNA polymerase gamma A1 (POLG1), deoxyguanosine kinase, or thymidine phosphorylase.

Ataxia
POLG1 and PEO1 twinkle C100RF2 nuclear mutations, and many mitochondrial deletions.

Barth
X-linked cardiomyopathy and leucopoenia.

Cardiomyopathy
Hypertrophic, dilated, histiocytoid, or fibroelastosis; mitochondrial mutations, thymidine kinase nuclear mutations causing mitochondrial depletion, and other nuclear gene mutations.

Childhood diabetes +/- deafness

CPEO
(Chronic Progressive External Ophthalmoplegia): POLG1 and PEO1 twinkle C100RF2 nuclear mutations, and mitochondrial deletions.

Cytochrome oxidase deficiencies

SCO1 nuclear gene; hepatopathy, encephalopathy

SCO2 nuclear gene; cardiomyopathy, encephalopathy

COX10 nuclear gene; proximal renal tubulopathy, encephalopathy, leukodystrophy

COX15 nuclear gene; Leigh syndrome; fatal neonatal cardiomyopathy

Deafness +/- aminoglycoside ototoxicity

DIDMOAD
Diabetes insipidus, D mellitus, optic atrophy, deafness = Wolfram syndrome; 3 gene defects.

Dystonia +/- LHON (Leber Hereditary Optic Neuropathy)

Hackett-Tarlow
Juvenile mitochondrial myopathy.

HAM
Hearing loss, ataxia, myoclonus.

HEADD
Hypotonia, epilepsy, autism, with developmental delay.

Kearns-Sayre
Chronic progressive external ophthalmoplegia (CPEO); several nuclear and mitochondrial mutations.

Leigh

Subacute necrotizing encephalomyelopathy; SURF1 nuclear gene and mitochondrial genome mutations.

LHON
(Leber Hereditary Optic Neuropathy)

Luft
Hypermetabolic uncoupling of oxidative phosphorylation.

MELAS
Myopathy, encephalopathy, lactic acidosis, stroke-like episodes.

Menke
ATPase 7a, Xq12 mutation → copper deficiency → Cytochrome C dysfunction.

MERRF
Myoclonus, epilepsy, with ragged red fibers.

MNGIE
Myopathy, neuropathy, gastrointestinal disorder, encephalopathy; nuclear DNA; ECGF1 gene thymidine phosphorylase deficiency; high blood thymidine and deoxyuridine.

Myopathy
Mitochondrial mutations and nuclear gene thymidine kinase mutation causing mitochondrial depletion.

NARP
Neurodegeneration, ataxia, retinitis pigmentosa.

Optic Atrophy
Nuclear gene OPA1; dynamin related GTPase defect; autosomal dominant.

Parkinsonism
Leigh mutations; also DNA polymerase gamma A1 (POLG1).

Pearson
Bone marrow depression, pancreatic dysfunction.

Sensory neuropathy
POLG1 and PEO1, twinkle C100RF2 nuclear mutations and mitochondrial deletions.

Sideroblastemia
X-linked sideroblastic anemia; ABCB7 nuclear gene mitochondrial iron transporter defect; also mitochondrial genome mutations.

Additional nuclear gene mutations causing ox/phos function:
Complex I nuclear genes: NDUFS1; NDUFV1; NDUFS4; NDUFS7; NDUFS8

Complex II nuclear genes: SDHA (flavoprotein subunit A)

SDHB (Iron sulfur protein)

SDHC (Integral membrane Protein C)

SDHD (Integral membrane protein D)

Complex III: BCS1L gene

In general, disorders of mitochondria, whether of electron transport chain or not, usually are multisystem disorders with slow, intermittently accelerated degeneration. Some can be so very slow as to be virtually static. They are often worsened during times of metabolic stress, such as during febrile illnesses. Mitochondrial diseases can be considered as rare causes for a variety of common symptoms. In the newborn, mitochondrial ox/phos diseases mimic hypoxic/ischemic encephalomalacia, or presents with any combination of the following symptoms: intrauterine growth retardation, hypotonia, seizures, apnea, cardiomyopathy, difficulties feeding and swallowing, lactic acidosis, sideroblastic anemia, or hepatopathy. A list of the most frequent presenting symptoms in older children and adults include the following:

Systemic Signs of Mitochondrial Disease

- Cardiomyopathy +/- cardiac pre-excitation and other dysrhythmias
- Esophageal dysmotility
- Intestinal dysmotility
- Fanconi nephropathy

- Acute fatty liver
- Reye-like syndrome
- Pancreatitis
- Hypoparathyroidism
- Childhood diabetes
- Multiple autoimmune endocrinopathies
- Blood dyscrasias, pancytopenia

Neurological Signs of Mitochondrial Disease

- Microcephaly
- Apnea
- Developmental delay
- Complicated migraine
- Retinitis pigmentosa
- Hearing loss
- Stroke-like episodes
- Parkinsonian symptoms
- Ataxia
- Chorea
- Epilepsy
- Myoclonic epilepsy
- Dorsal column dysfunction (in Leigh syndrome)
- Spinocerebellar degeneration
- Neuropathy / Leukodystrophy
- Myopathy
- Hypotonia
- Hepato-cerebral complications

Other Characteristics of Mitochondrial Ox/Phos Disease

- Necrosis in any tissue from acute or subacute energy deficiency;
- Acidotic disruption of intermediary metabolism (lactic, uric, organic, amino, ammonia);
- Catabolic or cytokine stress triggers symptoms (eg, infection, birth);
- Vulnerability to drug toxicity (chloramphenicol, valproate, adriamycin, aminoglycoside).

Mitochondrial diseases can be inherited by any inheritance pattern, not just maternally inherited mitochondrial genome inheritance. Mitochondrial genome maternal inheritance accounts for only 5% of mitochondrial disease presenting in pediatrics. However, 30% of adults that present with mitochondrial Ox/Phos disease are derived by maternal inheritance. Nuclear genome autosomal recessive inheritance is the most common form of inheritance of Ox/Phos disease, including causes of decreased mitochondrial number (from impaired mitochondrial replication). Autosomal dominant inheritance is less common, but has been found in some forms of progressive external ophthalmoplegia associated with nuclear gene deletions. X-linked dominant disease is found in Barth syndrome. Disordered intergenomic communication has been observed in cases of defects in nuclear DNA control of mitochondrial DNA repair.

Mitochondrial genome inheritance refers to diseases caused by deletions or mutations of the circular genome found in mitochondria, rather than Mendelian inheritance of nuclear chromosomes. Usually, there are approximately six different mitochondrial genomes in the oocyte, and each type is found in several copies. When the sperm unites with the egg, the mitochondria in the sperm's tail fall away, or are destroyed by the oocyte; usually, only the egg's mitochondria survive. (In some animals, and in rare situations in humans, it has been shown that some sperm mitochondria may enter the fertilized egg.)

As the fertilized egg replicates, multiple copies of each mitochondrial genome "segregate" randomly into different offspring cells. This process is called "replicative segregation." The mutant load necessary to produce symptoms is thought to be that at least 75% of the mitochondria in a cell must be defective for the cell to be defective. This means that any offspring cell in which at least 75% of its mitochondrial genome is defective will be a dysfunctional cell, and thus will convey symptoms in the person. For example, if most of the defective mitochondria is segregated into muscle, the patient will have a myopathy. Replicative segregation causes some cells to accumulate mutant mitochondrial genome, and others to have limited mutant copies; this is called heteroplasmy. This heteroplasmy accounts for variable presentation of diseases, such that one mitochondrial mutation or deletion can cause myopathy in one person, and encephalomyopathy with neurodegeneration in another person, sometimes even within the same family. For example, a mutation at site 3243 can cause the Kearns-Sayre symptom in one person, NARP in another, and MELAS in a third. Conversely, the Leigh syndrome can be caused by defects of complex I, cytochrome oxidase, mutations at 3243, or large-scale mutations. The determining feature is not which mutation causes the cellular dysfunction, but rather, which cell has inherited dysfunctional oxidative phosphorylation enzymes.

Another cause of variability lies in age dependent tissue energy requirements. For example, the basal ganglia are at risk for acute or subacute necrosis in childhood, but only for slow deterioration in adulthood. An additional cause of vulnerability is that some patients incur external stressors, whereas other children are fortunate to avoid them. For example, a patient who is treated with aminoglycocides for an infection may suffer profound hearing loss even at levels not usually considered toxic, whereas his sibling, with the same mitochondrial genome but who is not exposed to aminoglycocides, may not lose hearing. (See paragraph on Triple Risk Model of disease in this chapter.)

To confirm a diagnosis of most mitochondrial diseases, other than Ox/Phos diseases, eg, a disorder of fatty acid oxidation, the clinician need only demonstrate an enzyme dysfunction or a gene defect that matches the clinical syndrome of the patient. Confirming the diagnosis of a mitochondrial oxidative phosphorylation disease is made more difficult, however, by heteroplasmy. That is because heteroplasmy creates a situation whereby a disease may not be present even if a mitochondrial mutation is present; disease is only present if there is sufficient mutation load (>75% of the cells involved). Therefore, for oxidative phosphorylation diseases, the gold standard for definitive diagnosis is high. It requires clinicians to prove the presence of enzyme defect (usually in muscle) plus an appropriate gene defect, or enzyme defect plus definitive histological findings in muscle or other tissues, or appropriate gene defect plus definitive histological findings.

Because of this high standard for diagnosis, to enter into the "diagnostic sequence" (see above), one must first screen for more common disease. After that, one may initiate a diagnostic work-up for mitochondrial disease if the patient has any one of the following criteria:

- A characteristic mitochondrial disease syndrome;
- Maternal lineage disease (only found in some disorders of oxidative phosphorylation);
- Lactate elevation (+/- pyruvate) in blood, urine, or CSF;
- The combination of multisystem disease (three or more organs), common diseases excluded, and recurrent paroxysmal or progressive disease.

Tests for non-Ox/Phos mitochondrial disorders can be included when testing for other disorders of small molecules. If these are normal, one can pursue Ox/Phos diseases more invasively. Prior to obtaining a muscle biopsy, the following studies are helpful to indicate that a mitochondrial Ox/Phos disease may be present:

- Blood mitochondrial mutations and deletions (abnormal in <35% of confirmed cases of Ox/Phos diseases)

- CSF L-lactate and alanine elevation (from CSF amino acids);

- MRI to look for lesions of Leigh syndrome or MELAS syndrome;

- Magnetic resonance spectroscopy looking for a lactate peak and inversion at affected area;

- Urine organic acids and amino acids, urine orotic acid, and blood ammonia when ill;

- Urine methylglutaconic acid elevation;

- Skin biopsy (electron transport chain and other enzymes);

- ECG (pre-excitation; conduction block);

- Fanconi nephropathy;

- Liver biopsy if symptoms are appropriate;

Muscle biopsy, even if CPK and EMG are normal (microscopy, genome & enzyme analysis; fresh specimens are much more reliable than flash frozen).

It may be helpful to consult ophthalmology, genetics, cardiology, clinical pharmacology, nutrition, and/or rehabilitation services. Swallowing studies may be helpful.

There are a number of fallacious clinical pearls regarding mitochondrial diseases, and these must be addressed directly:

1.) Not all Ox/Phos disorders cause elevated blood lactate; some patients will have elevated CSF lactate with a normal blood lactate.

2.) As stated above, not all Ox/Phos disorders follow maternal inheritance; rather, of 100 proteins involved in oxidative phosphorylation, only 13 proteins, 22tRNA, and 2riboRNA are derived from the mitochondrial (non-nuclear) genome.

3.) Not all disorders fit a characteristic syndrome.

4.) Not all mitochondrial Ox/Phos myopathies manifest initially with histologic abnormalities such as ragged red fibers. These ragged red fibers are very rare in children under 4 years old, even those with pronounced multisystem dysfunction.

5.) Not all mitochondrial disorders require muscle biopsy; only the Ox/Phos disorders that present without the triad of characteristic syndrome, abnormal blood mitochondrial mutations and maternal lineage disease may require it.

6.) Collectively, Ox/Phos and non-Ox/Phos mitochondrial diseases are not rare, although each is rare, individually.

7.) Not all mitochondrial disorders cause noticeably progressive degeneration.

8.) The mitochondrial genome defect does not necessarily predict the syndrome, and the syndrome does not predict the genome defect.

Treatment for mitochondrial disease follows the same pattern as that for all diseases of small molecules (see above); viz., to replace the defective metabolite, avoid the precursors of the toxic metabolites, provide vitamins that improve the function of the dysfunctional enzyme, and provide symptom relief for affected organs. For disorders of fatty acid oxidation, the treatment is to arrange the dietary intake of selected fats that bypass the oxidation block. For example, in disorders of long chain oxidation (long chain acyl CoA dehydrogenase deficiency), treatment requires supplying medium chain fats, and avoiding long chain fats. Nocturnal cornstarch has been recommended to treat disorders of fatty acid oxidation to ameliorate early morning hypoglycemia. Ox/Phos disorders are difficult to treat. Treatment has emphasized use of vitamins to facility electron transport. Thiamine, riboflavin and lipoic acid are employed in cases of defects of electron transport complexes I and II and pyruvate dehydrogenase deficiency. The ketogenic diet has been recommended to treat pyruvate dehydrogenase deficiency. Co-enzyme Q (ubiquinone) and carnitine have been recommended for the treatment of all

Ox/Phos disorders. Dichloroacetate has been recommended for severe lactic acidosis. Idebenone and vitamin K have been recommended. Vitamins C and E have also been recommended, on general grounds of free radical scavengers, but current data showing that high doses of vitamin E is associated with increased cardiac risk must be factored in. There are some data to indicate that arginine supplementation may help prevent infarctions in MELAS. There are scant data to confirm that any of these treatments are effective in most patients with Ox/Phos disease, although there have been small studies of patients who have appeared to have dramatic improvement. There is theoretic reason to think that, in cases of mitochondrial disease associated with elevated methylglutaconic acid, supplementation with pantothenic acid (vitamin B_5) might reduce the level of methylglutaconic acid; this may have no impact on symptoms, however.

There are a few drugs that can exacerbate symptoms in mitochondrial diseases, and may be best avoided, when possible. These include aminoglycosides, valproate, chloramphenicol, doxorubicin, phenobarbital, salicylate, azothiaprine, ifosfamide, simvastatin, and pravastatin.

Diseases of Protein Metabolism

These can be subdivided into organic acidopathies, urea cycle defects, aminoacidopathies, and disorders of glutathione metabolism. The porphyrias are added to this category for mnemonic value; they are derived from the breakdown of proteins that contain the heme/porphyrin moiety. This is a convenient separation, but somewhat artificial, because there is much overlap, and some disorders present with both abnormal amino acids and abnormal organic acids. The glutathione disorders can be considered forms of aminoacidopathies. In disorders of protein metabolism, some metabolic steps occur in the mitochondria and some in the cytosol. These diseases share the common but variable feature of protein intolerance: symptoms and laboratory abnormalities worsen with protein load. Treatment of many usually involves feeding with formulas restricted in specific amino acids for each specific disease. Breast-feeding usually is stopped or modified. These diseases also share a tendency to cause various degrees of neonatal or infant growth failure, feeding intolerance and emesis, hepatopathy, anion gap metabolic acidosis, hypoglycemia, hyperammonemia, hyponatremia, moderate elevation of lactate, and propensity to develop the Reye-like syndrome and myelinolysis during infectious or catabolic stress, and hypotonia followed by movement disorder and/or seizures, and later mental impairment. Many have acute severe neonatal, infantile, and childhood forms, as well as intermediate or intermittent forms, depending on the specific gene mutation or the degree of residual enzyme function. Comparative Table 4 is a list of features for each disorder that are particularly prominent or distinctive. General principles of treatment are discussed in the section titled Treatment of Small Molecule Diseases. Cerebral intracranial pressure monitoring, mannitol therapy, cardiorespiratory stabilization and other treatments may be helpful in the Reye-like syndrome. In contrast to the other disorders of protein metabolism, the porphyrias often are not affected by protein load, generally do not require amino acid restriction formulas, and may not cause the Reye-like syndrome.

Disorders of Protein Metabolism that Cause Abnormal Urine Organic Acids (Table 5a)

This first group of acidemias is characterized by a tendency to present as a potentially fatal Reye-like crisis in infancy, and are characterized by elevated excretion of organic and amino acids specific for each disease. Some are treated very effectively with vitamin therapy alone, if diagnosed early. The neurologist may see the child for seizures, hypotonia, movement disorder, developmental delay, or coma.

Methylmalonic acidemia is the salient metabolic disturbance of a collection of defects of vitamin B_{12} (cobalamin) metabolism. Vitamin B_{12} undergoes modifications to function as a cofactor for methylation, in conjunction with folate. Some are designated by their complementation group title, termed cobalamin defect A – G (Cbl A, Cbl B, etc.). These include deficiencies of several enzymes and proteins: methylmalonyl CoA mutase (mutation 0, mutation -); adenosyltransferase (Cbl A); homocystinuria with methylmalonic acidemia (Cbl C, D); transcobalamin II; lysosomal B12 transporter (Cbl F); methionine synthetase (Cbl G); intrinsic factor (pernicious anemia); infantile B12 deficiency (from breast feeding vegan mother = "vegan child").

Depending on the variation, treatment may require cyano-, hydroxy-, or methylcobalamin, usually by frequent intramuscular injection, obtained via a compounding pharmacy. Patients may have delayed language development and have no convulsions and normal daytime EEG, but had non-convulsive, slow spike wave status epilepticus during sleep; their language may improve abruptly when treated with anticonvulsants.

The "ketones" found by urine indicator strips are usually ketoacids. This can serve as an early sign of organic acidopathy, and can be used to prompt the clinician to send urine organic and amino acids, and to start presumptive therapy.

The acidemias in Tables 5b, c have the common hallmark of excessive excretion of glutaric acid and its structural relatives, and dicarboxylic acids. Glutaric aciduria II can be considered a disorder of metabolism of fatty acids more than a disorder of protein metabolism. The challenge for the clinician is to be aware of the difference between the benign and the fatal forms of these diseases.

It is also possible to classify 3-hydroxy-3-methylglutaryl CoA lyase (HMG CoA lyase) deficiency among the autosomal recessive methylglutaconic acidurias (Table 6), because 3-methylglutaconic acid is elevated in the urine, and there is an associated hypoketotic hypoglycemia. It is also a disorder of fatty acid oxidation, because it is the last step in the formation of acetoacetate, which produces 3-hydroxybutyrate, and also causes increased urine glutaric acid. Infants present with hypoketotic hypoglycemia and hepatomegaly with elevated liver enzymes and ammonia; and metabolic acidosis and aciduria with the following acids: 3-OH-3-methylglutaric, 3-methylglutaric, glutaric, 3-OH-isovaleric, adipic and 3-methylglutaconic. Urine acetoacetate and 3-hydroxybutyrate are low. There may be considerable cerebral atrophy and hypomyelination or dysmyelination on MRI. Fatal Reye-like syndrome can occur. Treatment is supportive, and intensive care with sodium benzoate or phenylacetate, arginine, glucose, and respiratory care are indicated for the Reye-like syndrome. Avoid fasting, and consider frequent or continuous gastric carbohydrate infusions or cornstarch at night. Protein (leucine) and fat restriction, and carnitine supplementation are helpful.

Urea Cycle Defects and Hyperammonemias (Table 7)

They are characterized by their tendency to cause hyperammonemia, excessive excretion of urea cycle intermediates, and respiratory alkalosis.[5] However, many diseases cause hyperammonemia even if the defective enzyme is not in the urea cycle, eg, organic acidemias caused by dysfunctional enzymes within mitochondria, such as pyruvate carboxylase. Occasionally, disorders that cause excessive excretion of urea cycle intermediates may not cause hyperammonemia, such as hyperornithinemia with gyrate atrophy. In both situations, these disorders are listed in different sections of this chapter (Tables 8a, b, c).

Table 5a

Small Molecule Disorders of Protein Metabolism that Cause Abnormal Urine Organic Acids

Disease	**Propionic Acidemia (PPA)**	**Methyl Malonic Acidemia (MMA)**	**MMA and Homocystinuria (Cbl C,D)**	**Multiple Carboxylase Deficiency (2 types)**	**3-Methyl-Crotonyl-Glycinuria**	**Isovaleric Acidemia**
Enzyme Defect	Propionyl CoA carboxylase	Methylmalonyl CoA mutase 8 variations.	Methylmalonyl CoA mutase & methionine synthase.	Holocarboxylase synthase -> propionyl CoA carboxylase, 3-methyl-crotonyl-CoA & pyruvate carboxylase. Or biotinidase deficiency.	3-methyl-crotonyl CoA carboxylase	Isovaleryl CoA dehydrogenase
Clinical Features	Recurrent ketosis, acidosis, dehydration, Reye, osteoporosis, rash.	Recurrent hypotonia ketoacidosis, dehydration, Reye, hepatomegaly, monilia, growth failure. Later: osteoporosis, chorea, seizures, ataxia, tremor, mental impairment.	Recurrent hypotonia ketoacidosis, dehydration, Reye, hepatomegaly, monilia, growth failure. Later: osteoporosis, mental impairment, chorea, seizures, ataxia, tremor.	Infantile red scaly rash, alopecia, cyclic vomiting, coma, Reye. Same as PPA, MMA, Cbl disorders. Stupor, hypotonia, hydrocephalus, ataxia. Deafness, blindness, seizures in biotinidase defect.	Late infant Reye-like episodes, coma, growth failure, seizures, delays.	Neonatal Reye, Sweaty feet locker room smell. Cerebral hemorrhages. Vomiting mimics pyloric stenosis or bowel obstruction. Intermittent pancreatitis, fatty liver. Delays, microcephaly ataxia, tremor, seizures.

Table 5a *(continued)*

Small Molecule Disorders of Protein Metabolism that Cause Abnormal Urine Organic Acids

Disease	Propionic Acidemia (PPA)	Methylmalonic Acidemia (MMA)	MMA and Homocystinuria (Cbl C,D)	Multiple Carboxylase Deficiency (2 types)	3-Methyl-crotonyl-glycinuria	Isovaleric Acidemia
Hallmark Lab Findings	High propionic, glycine, methyl-citrate, tiglylglycine, neutropenia, thrombocytopenia, hyponatremia, ammonia. "Ketones" in urine. Spongiform brain.	High glycine, MMA, neutropenia, thrombocytopenia, megaloblastic anemia, hypersegmented polys +/- ammonia, homocystine, cystathionine. "Ketones" in urine. Spongiform brain.	High glycine, MMA in C&D neutropenia thrombocytopenia, megaloblastic anemia, hypersegmented polys, "ketones" in urine +/- ammonia, homocystine, cystathionine. MRI T2 lesion in basal ganglion.	Lactate, methylcitrate, 3-methyl-crotonylglycine, 3-OH-isovaleric, ammonia; urine "ketones." Abnormal EEG. Spongiform brain.	Ketoacidosis hypoglycemia, ammonia, hepatopathy, 3-methyl-crotonyl-glycinuria, 3-OH-isovalerate, low free carnitine.	Ketoacidosis hypoglycemia, ammonia, hepatopathy, leukopenia, thrombocytopenia, urine: isovalerylglycine, 3-OH-isovalerate, low free carnitine. Abnormal EEG. Spongiform brain.
Genetics	Autosomal recessive	Chromosome 6 recessive	Autosomal recessive	Autosomal recessive	Autosomal recessive	Autosomal recessive
Treatment	Restrict methionine, threonine, valine, isoleucine. Add carnitine, metronidazole. Reye management. Biotin for rash. Growth hormone.	B_{12}, +/- restrict isoleucine, threonine, methionine, valine. Add alanine, carnitine, metronidazole, growth hormone. Reye therapy when needed.	Hydroxy-B_{12} or methyl B_{12}. Rare restrict isoleucine, threonine, methionine, valine. Add alanine? Carnitine,? growth hormone. Reye therapy when needed.	Dramatic response to biotin. Prenatal biotin is helpful. Late biotin will not reverse loss of cranial nerve function.	Reduce intake of protein and leucine. Add carnitine. Reye therapy.	Reye therapy. Restrict dietary leucine. Add glycine + carnitine.
Prognosis	Neonatal fatality if not treated promptly. Older age presentations better prognosis.	Good if treated early (newborn screen).	Unsatisfactory compared to other cobalamin defects.	Good if treated early. Delays, dilated ventricles, deafness, blindness may stay.	Can be normal.	50% die in acute neonatal event. Normal if treated early.

Table 5b

Disorders of Protein Metabolism that Cause Abnormal Urine Organic Acids

Disease	Glutaric Aciduria I	Glutaric Aciduria II	D-2-hydroxy-Glutaric Aciduria	L-2-hydroxy-Glutaric Aciduria	Ethylmalonic Aciduria
Enzyme Defect	Glutaryl CoA de-hydrogenase	Electron transfer flavoprotein or its multiple acyl CoA dehydrogenase	D-2-hydroxy-glutaric acid dehydrogenase	Unknown	Cytochrome oxidase
Clinical Features	Megalencephaly, acute infant or childhood encephalitic-like crisis ≥ dystonia, degenerative spasticity ataxia, dyskinesia, seizures, profuse sweating. Cyclic vomiting.	Fatal neonatal acidosis, sweaty odor, dysmorphic. Later onset vomiting hypoglycemia, lipid storage, myopathy.	Macrocephaly, hypotonia, vomiting, seizures, delays, coarse features, later dystonia.	Moderate delays, hypotonia, ataxia, tremor, seizures, neonatal apnea. Mild spasticity.	Slow neuro-degeneration, petechiae, acrocyanosis, hypotonia with hyper-reflexia, epicanthal folds, torturous retinal vessels. May die in childhood, pulmonary and cerebral edema.
Hallmark Lab Findings	MRI: wide operculum, caudate/putamen signal. Urine glutaric acid. Mild acidosis. Spongy white matter. Mild fatty liver.	Lactate, glutaric, ethylmalonic, adipic, butyric, methylbutyric, isobutyric, isova-leric. Hypoketotic hypoglycemia, ammonia, urea cycle intermedi-ates in urine. Polycystic kidneys. Low carnitine.	D-2-hydroxy-glutaric and oxoglutaric acids. Cerebral atrophy.	L-2-hydroxy-glutaric acid. Cerebellar atro-phy. White matter and caudate hypoplasia.	Ethylmalonic, lactic pyruvic acids; episodic acidosis, T2 basal ganglion lesions.
Genetics	Autosomal recessive. Amish, Swedish, Ojibway, etc.	Autosomal recessive	Autosomal recessive	Autosomal recessive	Autosomal recessive; ETHE1 gene.
Treatment	Restrict tryptophan & lysine. Add riboflavin, carnitine, Baclofen; IV saline and dextrose for cyclic vomiting.	Dextrose fluids, comfort care in fatal neonatal form. Restrict protein and fat. Add riboflavin, carnitine, glycine.	Unknown	Unknown. Lab must distinguish D from L isomers for diagnosis.	Not known
Prognosis	Normal if early treatment.	Fatal in neonates. Impaired older.	Poor development	Moderately impaired	Usually fatal

Table 5c

Disorders of Protein Metabolism that Cause Abnormal Urine Organic Acids

Disease	3-Hydroxy-Isobutyric Aciduria	4 - Hydroxy-Butyric Aciduria	2-Methyl-3-Hydroxy-Isobutyric Aciduria	Malonic Aciduria	2-Oxo-Adipic Aciduria
Enzyme Defect	Defective oxidation of valine and B-alanine.	Succinic semialdehyde dehydrogenase	3-Oxo-thiolase = mitochondrial acetoacetyl CoA thiolase.	Not known in cases of normal malonyl CoA decarboxylase	2-oxoadipic acid dehydrogenase
Clinical Features	Recurrent ketoacidosis, cyclic vomiting, Russell-Silver growth failure, clinodactyly, hypospadius.	Mental impairment, hyperkinetic, intermittent lethargy, autism, hypotonia, motor delay, ataxia, hyporeflexia, seizures.	Recurrent severe ketosis, cyclic vomiting.	Global delay, growth failure, moniliasis, seizures, spasticity, severe dystonia, myoclonic seizures	Varies from normal to growth impairment, infantile global delay, hypotonia, edema, seizures, ventricular dilation, ataxia, ichthyosis.
Hallmark Lab Findings	3-hydroxy-isobutyric, 2-ethyl-3-hydroxy-propionic, lactic acids, hypoglycemia. Severe have dysmorphic brains.	Urine 4-hydroxy-butyric acid, cerebral atrophy.	2-methyl-3-hydroxy-isobutyric aciduria, hyperglycemia. Glycine may be high. T2 signal in basal ganglia.	Malonic acid, Methyl-malonic, 3-hydroxy-3-methylglutaric, dicar-boxylic, lactic acids, ammonia, +/- hypo-glycemia. Progressive atrophy of cortex, white matter, and basal ganglia.	Aminoadipic acids; 2-oxoadipic acid
Genetics	?X-linked	Autosomal recessive.	11q22 recessive.	Autosomal recessive or X-linked?	Autosomal recessive.
Treatment	Restrict valine. Add carnitine, growth hormone.	Benzodiazepine, Vigabatrine have been used.	Restrict isoleucine. Carnitine. IV resuscitation of emesis episodes.	Unclear. Support during episodes of ketoacidosis. Clon-azepam, carnitine.	Not known. Q? lysine restriction. Acute acidosis management.
Prognosis	Good on treatment.	Mild to moderately impaired.	Good if treated.	Poor.	Varies.

Table 6

Methylglutaconic Acidurias

Disease	Type I	Type II (Barth Syndrome)	Type III (Costeff Syndrome)	Type IV
Enzyme Defect	3-methylglutaconyl CoA hydratase	Deficient mitochondrial membrane protine tafazzin;impairs phospholipid metabolism	Indirect marker of mitochondrial dysfunction; mitochondrial membrain protein defect that impairs ATD Synthase.	Unclassified mitochondrial dysfunction.
Clinical Features	Speech delay; global neuro dysfunction or no symptoms	Cardiomyopathy, neutropenia and recurrent infections, growth failure, lipid myopathy.	Neurodegeneration; +/- optic atrophy, extrapyramidal sings, spasticity, mitochondrial cytopathy.	Dysmorphic features; cerebral dysfunction.
Hallmark Lab Findings	Fasting hypoglycemia, acidosis: 3-methylglutaconic, 3-methylglutaric, 3-hydroxyisovaleric acids in urine.	3-methylglutaconic, 3-methylglutaric aciduria, neutropenia, low carnitine, hypertrophic ventricular fibroelastosis.	+/- acidosis, +/- hypoglycemia, +/- sideroblastic anemia, (Pearson aplastic anemia), markers of disorders of oxidative phosphorylation.	Elevated urine methylgutaconic acid.
Genetics	Autosomal recessive	X-linked: Xq28: TAZ1/G4.5 gene	Autosomal recessive, and mitochondrial deletions.	Unclear
Treatment	? restrict leucine. ? pantothenic acid (vitamin B5)	Restrict protein. Add carnitine and cholesterol. Heart transplant, ? treat with pantothenic acid (vit B5).	Mitochondrial therapies. Vitamin B5 (?)	Mitochondrial therapies. ? treat with pantothenic acid (vit B5)
Prognosis	Mild impairment	Can be fatal	Variable	Variable.

Table 7

Urea Cycle Defects and Hyperammonenemia

Disease	Orotic Aciduria & Hyperammonemia	Ornithinemia	Citrullinemia and Orotic Aciduria	Arginino-succinic Aciduria	Argininemia	"HHH" Syndrome	Lysinuric Protein Intolerance
Enzyme Defect	Ornithine Transcarbamylase	Carbamyl phosphate synthetase	Arginino-succinate synthetase	(Arginino-succinase lyase).	Arginase	Ornithine transport into mitochondria	Transport of cationic amino acids
Clinical Features	Male infantile or childhood Reye-like hyperammonemic crisis, coma, seizures, stroke-like episodes; affected females.	Neonatal hyperammonemic crisis.	Neonatal seizures, hyperammonemia with or w/o Reye-like crisis; cyclic vomiting, recurrent emesis, headache, tremor, ataxia, seizures, all intermittently. Short hair.	Same as arginino-succinate synthetase deficiency, but more hepatomegaly, trichorrhexis nodosa.	Spastic quadriplegia. Opisthotonos, microcephaly, seizures.	Intermittent emesis or Reye	Growth failure, intermittent emesis, headache, diarrhea or Reye. Pulmonary fibrosis,nephritis, fractures, pancreatitis, liponecrosis, terminal liver failure.
Hallmark Lab Findings	Elevated glutamine, alanine, orotic acid, ornithine; low cit-rulline in fluids. Res-piratory alkalosis.	High ornithine. Low citrulline, orotic acid, arginine and low BUN. Respiratory alkalosis.	High citrulline, high orotic acid, low arginino-succinate.	High arginino-succinate, glutamine, ala-nine, moderate citrulline.	High arginine, cystine, lysine, ornithine, orotic and arginic acid.	Hyperornithine, ammonia, homocitrulline.	Low lysine and others in blood; high urine lysine, ornithine, arginine. Anemia, leukopenia.
Genetics	X-linked; also affected females.	Autosomal recessive.	Autosomal recessive.	Autosomal recessive.	Autosomal recessive.	Autosomal recessive.	Autosomal recessive.
Treatment	Protein restriction, benzoate, pheny-lacetate or phenyl-butyrate, arginine, citrulline, pyridox-ine, folate, IV dex-trose; mannitol +/- dialysis may be nec-essary. Keep glu-tamine normal.	Same as OTC, plus N-carbamyl-glutamate.	Same as OTC. Once stable, some may be managed with just argi-nine supplementation. Others need protein restriction.	Same as arginino-succinate synthetase deficiency.	Low arginine diet. Add lysine, ornithine, benzoate.	Restrict protein, add lysine, add ornithine.	Restrict protein. As for OTC, plus lysine, ornithine, arginine, citrulline, prednisolone for lungs.
Prognosis	Treatable, but potentially lethal acutely.	Treatable, but potentially lethal acutely.	Treatable, but potentially lethal acutely. 75% 10-year survival. Moderate mental impairment.	Same as arginino-succinate synthetase deficiency.	Good amelioration.	Good amelioration.	Guarded.

Table 8a

Disorders of Protein Metabolism that Cause Abnormal Urine Amino Acids (Deficient Tyrosine, Excess Phenylalanine and Homocystine)

Disease	Phenylketonuria	Hyperphenylalaninemia	Homocystinuria Type 1	Homocystinuria Type 2
Enzyme Defect	Phenylalanine hydroxylase and secondary: tyrosinase	GTP cyclohydrolase, or pyruvoyltetrahydro-bioperin or other defects of tetra-hydrobiopterin metabolism.	Cystathionine synthase	N(5,10)-Methylene-tetrahydrofolate reductase
Clinical Features	Blond hair, blue eyes, pale skin, eczema, infant vomiting, mousy odor, short, mental impairment, hyperactivity, seizures, spasticity, tremor, athetosis.	Microcephaly, hypotonia, growth impairment, mild vomiting, mental impairment, parkinsonian rigidity, dystonia, drooling, seizures.	Ectopia lentis, cataracts, glaucoma, detached retinae, vascular occlusions, malar flush, osteoporosis and bony dysplasia, aortic dilation, strokes, behavioral disturbances.	Vascular occlusions, strokes, variable mental delay and psychosis, infantile spasms. Strokes may occur if additional risk factors.
Hallmark Lab Findings	Phenylalanine high. Tyrosine low.	Phenylalanine. Tyrosine low. Prolactin high.	Homocystine, methionine both high.	Homocystine high. Methionine low or normal.
Genetics	12q recessive	Autosomal recessive.	Autosomal recessive.	Autosomal recessive.
Treatment	Restrict phenylalanine lifelong. Add carnitine. Treat pregnant patients to protect fetus.	Tetrahydrobiopterin, folinic acid.	Pyridoxine, folate, betaine.	Folate or folinic acid. with B_{12} to avoid spinal toxicity. Betaine and pyridoxine may help, but pyridoxine alone has caused deterioration.
Prognosis	Normal during treatment.	Good if treated.	Fair.	Variable.

Phenylalanine inhibits tyrosinase, causing the pale skin and hair in phenylalaninemias by interfering with melanin production. Genetic deficiency of tyrosinase itself, caused by several gene defects, causes albinism, translucent iris, retinal pallor, nystagmus, photophobia, and dysplastic optic chiasm. Tyrosinemias also benefit from reduction in dietary phenylalanine.

Diseases of Glutathione Metabolism

These are a subset of aminoacidopathies, because in these disorders there is an accumulation of individual amino acids, but they are listed here separately for educational convenience. They are thought to follow autosomal recessive inheritance. They usually do not express their full features in the neonatal

Table 8b

Disorders of Protein Metabolism that Cause Abnormal Urine Amino Acids

Disease	Tyrosinemia Type I (Oculocutaneous; Richner-Hanhart syndrome)	Tyrosinemia Type II (Hepatorenal)
Enzyme Defect	Tyrosine aminotransferase of cytosol, normal mitochondrial	Fumarylacetoacetate hydrolase
Clinical Features	Painful keratitis with inflammation, lacrimation, photophobia, painful keratosis of hands and feet. Usually very mild mental impairment, but can be severe, with hyperactivity, self injury, seizures.	Liver failure, cirrhosis, hepatocellular carcinoma, rickets, cabbage odor, Reye-like crisis rare, painful peripheral neuropathy. Uncommon: myopathy, cardiomyopathy, behavioral disorder, self-injury, seizures.
Hallmark Lab Findings	Tyrosine high, its crystals cause the keratoses.	High tyrosine and alpha fetoprotein. Succinylacetone is diagnostic. Fanconi nephropathy (aminoaciduria, phosphaturia, glycosuria).
Genetics	16q22 recessive	15q23 recessive; French-Canadians, etc.
Treatment	Restrict tyrosine and phenylalanine, add etretinate.	Restrict tyrosine and phenylalanine. Use of NTBC reverses liver failure, and may prevent need for liver transplant.
Prognosis	Excellent on treatment.	Excellent on NTBC treatment.

period. ***Pyroglutamic aciduria (5-oxoprolinuria)*** is caused by glutathione synthetase deficiency. It is associated with mental impairment, spasticity, ataxia, dysarthria, and intermittent acidosis and hemolytic anemia associated with febrile illnesses, and possibly with diaphragmatic hernia. When this enzyme defect is limited to red cells, there is intermittent hemolytic anemia and splenomegaly, but no 5-oxoprolinuria or neurological signs. ***Gamma-glutamylcysteine synthetase deficiency*** is associated with myopathy, peripheral neuropathy, spinocerebellar degeneration, intermittent hemolytic anemia and generalized aminoaciduria, and one patient had acute psychosis. 5-Oxoprolinase deficiency appears to be restricted to intestine and kidney, causing enterocolitis and urolithiasis. Glutathione peroxidase deficiency is associated with drug induced hemolysis and platelet dysfunction. This is a selenium dependent enzyme, and selenium deficiency impairs this enzyme and causes cardiomyopathy, painful skeletal myopathy and blond roots of dark hair, among other symptoms. ***Glutathione disulfide reductase deficiency causes hemolysis.***

The porphyrias (Table 9) are a collection of disorders characterized by abnormal heme metabolism, and excretion of porphyrins, which sometimes cause dark urine. They can be divided into hepatic

Table 8c

Disorders of Protein Metabolism that Cause Abnormal Urine Amino Acids

Disease	Maple Syrup Urine Disease (Branched-chain oxoaciduria)	Nonketotic Hyperglycinemia	Ornithinemia with Gyrate Atrophy
Enzyme Defect	Branched-chain ketoacids dehydrogenase 4 protein complex: E1 α, E1 β, E2, thiamine/ E3	Glycine cleavage 4 enzyme complex	Ornithine-5-aminotransferase
Clinical Features	Neonatal coma, hypotonia that leads to opisthotonus, seizures, delays, recurrent ataxia. Intermediate and intermittent forms also. Maple syrup odor of fluids and earwax if protein intake.	Severe neonatal coma, seizures, myoclonus, hiccups; hypotonia leads to spasticity, develop mental stagnation. Rare mild & slow degenerative forms.	Gyrate atrophy of choroid and retina, mental impairment, renal impairment.
Hallmark Lab Findings	Branched-chain amino and oxo acids. Acidosis is not common. Brain edema, myelinolysis.	High CSF/plasma glycine ratio (>.06, normal=.02), EEG burst-suppression, spongiform white > gray matter.	Ornithinemia but **normal** ammonia.
Genetics	E1α 19q13; E1β 6p21; E2 1p31; E3 7q31; all recessive.	Autosomal recessive	Autosomal recessive
Treatment	Restrict leucine, isoleucine, valine. Add thiamine. Dialysis, exchange transfusion. IV dextrose and nonbranched-chain amino acids to overcome catabolism.	Benzoate, dextromethorphan, pyridoxine, anticonvulsants.	Restrict protein. Add lysine.
Prognosis	Excellent if treated early.	Often fatal to neonate.	Variable

Table 9

The Porphyrias

Disease	Acute Intermittent (hepatic)	Coproporphyria (hepatic)	Variegate (hepatic)	Amino-Levulinic Aciduria (hepatic)	Cutanea Tarda (hepatic)	Congenital (Gunther) (erythropoietic)	Proto-Porphyria (erythropoietic)
Enzyme Defect	Porpho-bilinogen deaminase	Coproporphyrinogen oxidase	Protoporphyrinogen oxidase	Amino-levulinic dehydrase	Uroporphyrinogen decarboxylase	Uro-porphyrinogen III cosynthase (isomerase)	Heme synthase (ferrochelatase)
Neuro-logical Signs	3+	2+	2+	1-2+	0	0	0
Abdominal Signs	3+	3+	3+	2-3+	0	0-1	2+
Rash (light & trauma)	0	1+	2+	0	2+ childhood	3+ disfiguring	2+
Hemolytic Anemia	0-1	0-1	0-1	0-1	0-1	Infant, dark urine, 3+ hemolysis, splenomegaly, erythrodontia	Childhood, dark urine, 2+ hemolysis, splenomegaly, erythrodontia
Other	Teen, adult. Dark urine, back and chest pain. Acute psychosis.	Any age dark urine, back and chest pain.	Dark urine, back and chest pain.		Alopecia or hirsutism, hyper- or hypo-pigmentation, mild elevated transaminases	Alopecia or hirsutism. Later disfigured face and fingers.	Gallstones

(continued)

Table 9 *(continued)*

The Porphyrias

Disease	**Acute Intermittent (hepatic)**	**Coproporphyria (hepatic)**	**Variegate (hepatic)**	**Amino-Levulinic Aciduria (hepatic)**	**Cutanea Tarda (hepatic)**	**Congenital (Gunther) (erythropoietic)**	**Proto-Porphyria (erythropoietic)**
Hallmark Lab Findings	Hyponatremia, urine aminolevulinic acid, porphobilinogen + enzyme	Urine and stool coproporphyrin	Plasma porphyrin fluorescence	Urine Amino-levulinic acid + enzyme	Urine Uroporphyrin III + enzyme	Uroporphyrin & coproporphyrin in urine, blood, feces + enzyme.	Proto-porhyrin in blood and feces + enzyme
Genetics	11q23 dominant (Swedish)	3q12 Autosomal dominant	Autosomal dominant (South African)	Autosomal recessive	Autosomal dominant & sporadic	Autosomal recessive	18q dominant
Treatment	Avoid barbiturates, estrogens, etc. Add hematin, ?histrelin, ?hemin, ?zinc mesoporphyrin, other study drugs. Bromide for seizures. Saline + dextrose.	Avoid sun, barbiturates, estrogens, etc. Add ?histrelin, hemin, zinc mesoporphyrin. Bromide for seizures. Saline + dextrose.	Avoid sun, fasting, alcohol, drugs. Add ?histrelin, hemin, zinc mesoporphyrin. Bromide for seizures. Saline + dextrose.	Avoid sun, fasting, alcohol, drugs. Add hemin, zinc meso-porphyrin bromide for seizures. Saline + dextrose.	Avoid sun, alco-hol, chlorinated hydrocarbons, iron, estrogens. Add hemin, zinc meso-porphyrin, saline + dextrose.	Transfusion, splenectomy, hematin. Saline + dextrose. Avoid sun.	Avoid sun. Add Beta carotene, cholestyramine, ? L- cysteine, Saline + dextrose.

Table 10

Disorders of Cholesterol Metabolism

Disease	**Familial Hypercholesterolemia**	**Type I Hyperlipoproteinemia**	**Cerebrotendinous Xanthomatosis**	**Mevalonic Aciduria**	**Smith-Lemli-Opitz**	**A/hypobeta-lipoproteinemia**
Enzyme Defect	At least 4 defects in LDL receptor synthesis and processing.	Lipoprotein lipase or Apolipoprotein C-II	Mitochondrial C27 Steroid 26-hydroxylase	Mevalonic acid kinase	7-dehydro-cholesterol reductase	Post-translational modification of apo-B-100; several defects.
Clinical Features	Xanthomas, arcus senilis, multiorgan vascular disease. Homozygotes have xanthomas as children.	Infantile episodic abdominal pain, pancreatitis, eruptive xanthomas, hepatosplenomegaly, lipemia retinalis, scrotal swelling, some have anemia, leukopenia, or thrombocytopenia. Apolipoprotein C-II deficient patients present late adolescence, with abdominal pain or pancreatitis; sometimes with lupus, lymphoma or histiocytosis, but none with xanthomas or hepatomegaly.	Childhood cognitive delays, sometimes mental deterioration; adolescent white matter degeneration and xanthomas of cholestanol in tendons, lungs and brain, causing tendon pain, ataxia and spasticity, with gray and white matter degeneration of brain, and spinal cord.	Growth failure and malabsorption, recurrent fever, hepatosplenomegaly, lymphadenopathy arthralgia, rash, psychomotor retardation, cataracts, ataxia.	Microcephaly, dysmorphic face, small jaw, cleft palate, 2,3-syndactyly, hypospadius or ambiguous genitalia, Hirschprung's obstipation, pyloric stenosis, hypotonia, mental retardation, behavioral disorder; seizures are not common.	Childhood chronic diarrhea, vomiting, growth failure, oxalate stones, cardiomyopathy and myopathy, pigmentary retinopathy and visual impairment, nystagmus without cataracts, ataxia, head tremor, movement disorder, sensory neuropathy and dorsal column demyelination and hypotonia with Babinski sign.
Hallmark Lab Findings	High LDL cholesterol	Creamy fasting plasma from high triglycerides and chylomicrons.	High blood cholest*anol*, low cholesterol.	Urine mevalonic acid; elevated plasma IgD, anemia, elevated CPK during febrile crises, low plasma ubiquinone.	High blood 7-dehydro-cholesterol, low cholesterol	Acanthocytes, low vitamins A, E, and K (not D), low Prothrombin, low ApoB and LDL cholesterol.

(continued)

Table 10 *(continued)*

Disorders of Cholesterol Metabolism

Disease	**Familial Hypercholesterolemia**	**Type I Hyperlipoproteinemia**	**Cerebrotendinous Xanthomatosis**	**Mevalonic Aciduria**	**Smith-Lemli-Opitz**	**A/hypobeta-lipoproteinemia**
Genetics	Chromosome 19 dominant. Most common single-gene disease in humans.	Autosomal recessive	Autosomal recessive CYP27A1 gene	Autosomal recessive	Autosomal recessive	Autosomal recessive
Treatment	Liver transplant for homozygotes. Binding resins, and HMG -CoA reductase inhibitors, nicotinic acid and low-fat diet in heterozygotes.	Dietary restriction of fats; vigilance for pancreatitis	Oral chenodeoxycholic acid; surgical removal of xanthomas in tendons; cataract removal; others.	None known. Corticosteroids ameliorate febrile crises. HMG-CoA reductase inhibitors trigger rhabdomyolysis. Vitamins A, D, E, K ?	High doses of cholesterol, often via egg yolks; symptom management.	Vitamins A ,E, K, restrict long and medium chain triglycerides.
Prognosis	Poor for homozygotes	Amelioration	Amelioration	Poor	Guarded	Amelioration

Table 11

Disorders of Purine Metabolism

Disease	Lesch-Nyhan	Lesch-Nyhan Variants	Phosphoribosylpyrophosphate Synthetase Excess	Adenylosuccinate Lyase Deficiency	Adenine Phosphoribosyl Transferase Deficiency	Severe Combined Immune Deficiency
Enzyme Defect	Hypoxanthine-guanine phosphoribosyl transferase (HPRT)	Variants of HPRT deficiency	Phosphoribosylpyrophosphate synthetase excess.	Adenylosuccinate lyase	Adenine phosphoribosyl transferase.	Adenosine deaminase
Clinical Features	Motor delay, spasticity, dystonia, chorea, athetosis, mental impairment, severe self-injury, tophi, gouty arthritis, urate and xanthine nephropathy.	a) Renal stones alone, or b) Lesch-Nyhan without self-injury, or c) mild spasticity + mental retardation.	Hyperuricemia, uricosuria, hematuria, crystalluria and stone nephropathy, gouty arthritis, sensorineural deafness, variable mental impairment (rare absent lachrymal ducts, small teeth, hypospadius).	Developmental delay, autistic behavior, seizures.	Renal calculi and crystalluria, hematuria +/- nephropathy in children, rarely brown spots on cloth diapers; normal neurodevelopment.	Severe combined immune deficiency, diarrhea, pneumonia, moniliasis, skeletal defects.
Hallmark Lab Findings	Hyperuricemia, uricosuria, and calculi 3 mg uric acid/mg creatinine.	Serum uric acid >5mg/dL	Elevated uric acid and oxypurines in urine and blood.	Adenylosuccinate & succinylamino-imidazole carboxamide riboside in urine and CSF, **uric acid normal.**	Crystalluria, 2,8-dihydroxyadenine in urine, **uric acid normal.**	Enzyme or gene, deficient immune markers, **uric acid normal.**
Genetics	Xq26 recessive	Xq26 recessive	X-linked, with some lyonization symptoms in females	22q, recessive, some heterozygote effect.	16q24 subtelomere, Japanese, recessive.	ADA gene, autosomal recessive.

(continued)

Table 11 *(continued)*

Disorders of Purine Metabolism

Disease	**Lesch-Nyhan**	**Lesch-Nyhan Variants**	**Phosphoribosylpyrophosphate Synthetase Excess**	**Adenylosuccinate Lyase Deficiency**	**Adenine Phosphoribosyl Transferase Deficiency**	**Severe Combined Immune Deficiency**
Treatment	Allopurinol, 5-OH-tryptophan, carbidopa, dental extraction, lithotripsy, stone removal, hydration, ? deep brain stimulation	Allopurinol, lithotripsy, stone removal, hydration.	Allopurinol, hearing aids.	Anticonvulsants and behavior therapies.	Low purine diet, allopurinol, hydration, lithotripsy.	Enzyme replacement, bone marrow transplantation; gene replacement.
Prognosis	Some amelioration with treatment.	Amelioration with treatment, good to excellent.	Amelioration good.	Prolonged stable impairment.	Varies from asymptomatic to renal failure.	

and erythropoietic subclasses. All symptoms are acute and intermittent or subacute. Neurological signs include psychiatric changes from abnormal tryptophan metabolism and increased serotonin, Kluver-Bucy behavior, seizures, proximal or distal weakness and diaphragmatic weakness that can be mistaken for Güillain-Barré syndrome, sensory neuropathies, and seizures. Abdominal symptoms include pain, nausea, vomiting, diarrhea, and constipation. The intensity of abdominal symptoms can prompt surgical exploration. Some porphyrias produce photosensitive rash. Other less prominent symptoms include back or chest pain, hypertension and tachycardia. Most patients will have no symptoms unless triggered by menses, light exposure, or medications, including by anticonvulsants, sedatives, antidepressants and antibiotics that clinicians may prescribe for the presenting symptoms before the diagnosis of porphyria is made. Bromides are safe for treating seizures in this disorder. Given that several porphyrias are inherited with autosomal dominance, these are not very rare disorders; it may be prudent to test extended family members. Secondary porphyria occurs as an unexplained laboratory finding. Porphyria cutanea tarda may be the only disorder that presents in infancy, and can do so as a light-sensitive rash.

Small Molecule Diseases of Fat Metabolism

It is convenient to separate this category into disorders of fatty acid beta-oxidation and disorders of cholesterol metabolism. Disorders of fatty acid beta-oxidation can also be placed in the category of organic acidemias, because poorly metabolized fats produce unusual organic acids (eg, adipic acid, sebacic acid, suberic acid, octenedioic acid, etc.). Some of these fatty acids may be toxic. The patient may also have a deficiency of appropriate fatty acids downstream from the enzyme defect, and also may have energy depletion, because as much as 60% of our energy needs may be fulfilled by fat in ordinary circumstances. The body compensates for lack of fat by increasing utilization of sugars, but at times of fasting or energy need, the patient may develop nonketotic hypoglycemia. Disorders of fatty acid oxidation are, strictly speaking, "mitochondrial diseases" because of the role that mitochondria have in fatty acid beta-oxidation, even though fatty acid oxidation is not a direct part of the electron transport chain. Disorders of fatty acid beta-oxidation are discussed in more depth in the section on mitochondrial diseases.

Disorders of cholesterol metabolism cause either excess or deficiency of cholesterol and its precursors or metabolites. They cause neurological symptoms by any combination of disrupting neuronal cell membranes, disrupting fetal cerebral development and myelin formation, or causing atheromata with subsequent ischemic complications. Excess cholesterol is present in familial hypercholesterolemia, and Type I hyperlipoproteinemia. Types II-V hyperlipoproteinemia tend to present after childhood. Deficient cholesterol is found in mevalonic aciduria, Smith-Lemli-Opitz syndrome, abetalipoproteinemia, and cerebrotendinous xanthomatosis. Of the disorders in the table, only mevalonic aciduria and Smith-Lemli-Opitz syndrome present in newborns.

There are other, rarer, disorders of cholesterol metabolism that are not listed in Table 10, which are useful to mention for completeness: ***Hypobetalipoproteinemia and chylomicron retention disease*** are variants of abetalipoproteinemia and are caused by defects of posttranslational modification of Apo B. ***Tangier disease*** is a disorder with very low HDL, apo A-I and apo A-II in plasma, and is distinguished by tangerine colored, lipid-filled histiocytes in many tissues, especially in rectal mucosa and tonsils (use the mnemonic "tangerine tonsils of Tangier disease"). These findings, with hepatomegaly, can be present in the newborn. Its cause is not known. Autosomal recessive familial lecithin:cholesterol acyl transferase (LCAT) deficiency causes high unesterified cholesterol in the plasma, and very low levels of esterified cholesterol. Foam cells may be noted in bone marrow, as in Niemann-Pick C disease, but there is no organomegaly as is found in Niemann-Pick. A variant of LCAT deficiency causes only corneal opacity, and is called "fish eye disease." Cholesterol is stored within cells in other diseases, such as in ***cholesterol ester storage*** disease and ***Wolman disease***, but these are listed and discussed later in this chapter under the topic of large molecule lipid storage diseases.

Disorders of Purine and Pyrimidine Metabolism (Table 11)

These are important causes of developmental delay and spasticity. Some disorders of purine metabolism, especially adenosine deaminase deficiency, may have no neurological symptoms. Each disorder disrupts purine metabolism, but only some cause various degrees of hyperuricemia. Some variants of Lesch-Nyhan disease produce only mild elevation of uric acid in infancy, in a range that may be considered normal by adult standards (5mg/dl), and therefore can be misdiagnosed. For the sake of thorough comparison and contrast, some disorders are tabulated below. The most important for the neonatal care provider to recall are Lesch-Nyhan disease and adenosine deaminase deficiency. Lesch-Nyhan sometimes can present in the neonate as hypotonia and tiny stones that can be identified in a cloth diaper (rarely reported with modern diapers). Untreated, its outcome is severe spasticity, mental retardation, and severe self-injurious behavior. Adenosine deaminase deficiency causes severe combined immune deficiency, which can present as late neonatal infections, rash, and/or growth failure. Dihydropyrimidine dehydrogenase deficiency causes urinary excretion of uracil, thymine, 5-hydroxymethyluracil, and is associated with microcephaly, hypotonia, seizures, delayed myelination and mental retardation. Replacement of underproduced beta alanine has been proposed as a therapy; results are uncertain.

Nutrient Defects

Deficiencies or excesses of vitamins and trace minerals and micronutrients, or specific amino acids, are listed here for convenience (two of which can be considered amino acid disorders):

- AVED (Ataxia from vitamin E deficiency)
- Zinc deficiency (associated with dermatitis enteropathica; alopecia, moniliasis)
- Copper deficiency and X-linked Menke kinky hair disease (Xq12)
- Copper removal deficiency (Wilson hepatolenticular degeneration)
- Taurine deficiency (myopathy)
- Selenium deficiency (painful myopathy, cardiomyopathy, blond hair roots)
- Selenium toxicity (neuropathy)
- Carnitine deficiency (myopathy, hepatopathy)
- Hartnup disease (tryptophan transport and renal reabsorption defect; ataxia)
- Cerebral folate deficiency (movement disorder, seizures, neurological delay)
- Neurodegeneration with brain iron deposition (formerly Hallervorden-Spatz)
- Pyridoxine (vitamin B_6) deficiency, responsiveness, or dependency (ALDH7A1) gene on chromosome 5q; may cause pipecolic acidemia and α-amino-adipic semialdehyduria.

Cerebral folate deficiency can cause any combination of movement disorder, seizures, developmental delay or regression, anxiety, and sometimes basal ganglion calcifications. This disease is caused by one of three mechanisms: 1.) a deficiency of folate intake; 2.) defective cerebral folate receptor/transporter system; 3.) or antibodies to the cerebral folate receptor/transporter system. If the blood folate level is normal, the transporter defect is diagnosed by finding a deficiency of cerebrospinal fluid (CSF) 3-methyltetrahydrofolate. It is treated very effectively with folinic acid, which does not require a transporter to enter the CSF. This treatment can cause worsening of seizures, paradoxically, if given to a person who does not have cerebral folate deficiency, or if not accompanied by simultaneous vitamin B_{12} therapy.

Neurodegeneration with brain iron deposition is an autosomal recessive disorder characterized by childhood onset degenerative movement disorder, ataxia, seizures, spasticity, and dementia. It worsens inexorably to death. The MRI reveals a T2 signal of iron deposition in the pallidi that resembles "tiger's eyes." Bone marrow histiocytes and peripheral lymphocytes contain granular and multilaminated bodies similar to those in ceroid lipofuscinosis. Iron accumulates in basal ganglion and other neurons as well as in fibroblasts, and a cerebral neuroaxonal dystrophy is present. The PANK2 gene for pantothenate kinase, needed in the utilization of pantothenic acid (vitamin B_5), has been shown to contain a mutation in one kindred with this disease. It is thought that deficiency of pantothenate kinase may cause an accumulation of cysteine metabolites that will chelate iron in the affected cells, which causes toxicity. This is not likely to present in the neonate. Japanese authors have described a syndrome with many of the clinical features of neurodegeneration with brain iron deposition, but which manifests deficiency of N-acetylgalactosaminidase; this disorder has been called Hallervordern-Spatz type II. Its relationship to utilization of pantothenic acid has not been clarified.

Toxins

Toxins cause their symptoms by blocking the function of an enzyme, receptor or structural protein. When they impair the function of an enzyme of intermediary metabolism, they mimic metabolic disease or nutritional/vitamin deficiencies. An example is found in the way that acetaldehyde (a metabolite of ethanol) impairs pyruvate dehydrogenase, which is part of a thiamine dependent enzyme complex. In neonates, toxins will usually come via the mother's circulation, and include drugs of abuse, and rarely lead or methyl mercury. Neonatal symptoms are not specific, and usually include hypotonia or hypertonia, and seizures during drug withdrawal. Iatrogenic toxicity is another source of toxins. This class of disease is addressed in other chapters.

Diseases Causing Hypoglycemia

It is convenient, educationally, to take this moment to summarize small molecule diseases and anticipate our discussion of large molecule storage diseases by listing the differential diagnosis where both classes of diseases can present with a common symptom, namely hypoglycemia. Many diseases of small molecules cause hypoglycemia, as the body stores of glycogen or lipids are depleted during a fast. Glycogen storage disease is a class of storage disease that presents with hypoglycemia commonly. Causes of hypoglycemia are listed below, and many present during the neonatal period.

Hypoglycemic Disorders of Infants and Children

ENDOCRINE:

- *Hyperinsulinism*
  - *Transient Neonatal:*
    - Infant of diabetic mother
    - Erythroblastosis fetalis
    - Beckwith-Wiedemann syndrome
  - *Persistent:*
    - Islet cell dysplasia
    - Focal/diffuse adenomatosis
    - Nessidioblastosis / Insulinoma
  - *Drug-induced:*
    - Insulin
    - Oral hypoglycemic agents
  - *Other endocrine disorders:*
    - Growth hormone deficiency**
    - ACTH or cortisol deficiency**
    - Glucagon deficiency*
    - Somatostatin deficiency
    - Thyroid hormone deficiency

INSUFFICIENT SUBSTRATE:

- Post-operative hypoglycemia
- Ketotic hypoglycemia**
- Underlying liver disease
- Sepsis
- Hepatitis
- Starvation and small-for-gestational-age infants
- Cyanotic congenital heart disease

INBORN ERRORS OF METABOLISM:

- *Carbohydrate:*
  - Glycogen storage and synthesis diseases
  - Galactosemia
  - Fructosemia

Amino acidurias (eg, Tyrosinemia)

Organic acidurias

- Mitochondrial disorders
- Disorders of fatty acid oxidation and ketogenesis
- Carnitine metabolism disorders

Other causes of Reye-like syndrome (eg, urea cycle disorders)

TOXINS:

Alcohol
Salicylates
Oral hypoglycemic agents

*Hypoketotic syndromes: suppressed or defective ketogenesis

**Hyperketotic syndromes: excess ketogenesis or impaired ketolysis

3. Large Molecule Diseases

The hallmark of large molecule disease is the storage of large molecules in tissues or body fluids. They tend to produce dementia, epilepsy, movement disorders, gradual blindness, and spasticity, in the case of leukodystrophies. What constitutes "large molecules" is somewhat arbitrary, but in general, the dysfunctional molecules have a structural, membrane, receptor, or other function in cells, but are not usually involved directly in intermediary energy metabolism and removal of acid or nitrogen. Because the disorders produce their symptoms in tandem with gradual accumulation of stored material, there are only a few of these disorders that present in the neonatal period.

Subclassification of Large Molecule Diseases

Clues derived from phenotype have been incorporated in the Table of physical findings in the introduction of this chapter. Biochemically, once again, we can start from the perspective of "the food groups" to prompt our memory as to which tests to obtain. If a patient manifests no strong clues of a storage disease on history or physical exam, it may be economical to reserve testing for these disorders until after more common disorders and the small molecule diseases have been excluded. Currently, emergency newborn diagnosis is very helpful for some glycogen storage diseases, especially neonatal acid maltase disease (Pompe disease), for which there is now enzyme replacement therapy, and which can be fatal in the newborn period. Nevertheless, early diagnosis is helpful to the patient and family, and it is helpful to start enzyme replacement whenever possible. Below is an organization scheme of large molecule diseases, listed for educational purposes:

1.) Diseases characterized by storage of sugars, glycoproteins or glycolipids:

a. Glycogen storage diseases

b. Mucopolysaccharidoses

c. N-acetyl galactosaminidase deficiency (Schindler)
(discussed under lipidoses)

Table 12

Glycogen Storage Diseases

Disease Type	Enzyme Defect	Tissue Affected	Chromosome	Distinctive Feature
0	UDPG-Glycogen transferase	Liver, Muscle	17q23	No hepatomegaly. Fasting ketotic hypoglycemia; low lactate, low alanine. After a meal there is hyper glycemia and high alamine and low ketones; underdiag-nosed
Ia vonGierke	Glucose-6-phosphatase	Liver, kidney		
Ib	Glucose-6-Phosphate Transport Protein (translocase)	Liver, Neutrophils (later gut, kidney)		Uric acid high. Gout. Anemia. Short stature. Prolonged bleeding time. Hyperlipidemia, xanthomas. Lactic acidemia.
Ia sp	Stabilizing (regulatory) Protein	Liver		Neutropenia, anemia. Uric acid high. Gout. Inflammatory bowel disease.
Ic	Microsomal Phosphate Transporter	Liver		Short stature. Hyperlipidemia. Lactic acidemia.
Id	Microsomal Glucose Transporter	Liver		
II Pompe	a-1,4-glucosidase (acid maltase)	Generalized, Cardiac	17	Short PR interval, cardiomegaly. Fatal neonatal heart failure, Macroglossia, Severe hypotonia. Milder adult form with respiratory muscle failure.
III Cori Forbes	Amylo-1,6-glucosidase (debrancher)	Liver, Muscle (+/- red & white cell)	1	
IV Andersen	Amylo-(1,4-6)-transglucosidase (brancher)	Liver +/- (muscle, red & white cell)	3	Amylopectinosis
V McArdle	Muscle phosphorylase (Myophosphorylase)	Muscle	10; 11 14	Cramps, easy fatigue high CPK; myoglobinuria; liver rarely enlarged because mostly muscle disease.
VI Hers	Liver phosphorylase	Liver +/- (white cell)	10; 11 14	
VII	Muscle phosphofructokinase	Muscle, red cells	1; 10; 21	Hemolytic anemia
VIII/IX Tarui	Phosphohexosisomerase (inhibitor) Phosphoglycerate kinase Phosphorylase b kinase	Liver (+/- white cell)	X; 16q12; 7p12	The kinase form is X-linked
X	Phosphoglycerate kinase Phosphorylase kinase	Muscle	16q12; 7p12	
XI	Lactate dehydrogenase Phosphoglucomaltase	Liver, muscle	11; 12	Rhabdomyolysis
XII	Cyclic kinase; AMP-dependent	Liver		

d. Oligosaccharidoses (discussed under lipidoses)

e. Congenital Disorders of Glycoprotein synthesis (Golgi apparatus disorders)

2.) Diseases characterized by accumulation of cholesterol and complex lipids:

a. Intracellular cholesteroloses

b. Peroxisomal disorders of long chain fatty acid metabolism

c. Sphingolipidoses

d. Mucolipidoses

e. Glycoproteinoses (oligosaccharidoses)

f. Neuronal ceroid lipofuscinoses

3.) Miscellaneous storage diseases:

a. Glutamyl ribose-5-phosphate storage disease (ADP-ribosyl protein lyase deficiency)

b. N-acetylaspartate excess (aspartoacylase deficiency = Canavan disease)

c. Alexander disease

Diseases Characterized by Storage of Sugars, Glycoproteins or Glycolipids

Glycogen storage diseases (Table 12) are a collection of disorders characterized by abnormal synthesis or degradation of glycogen, resulting in lysosomal and/or cytoplasmic storage of unmetabolized glycogen in most forms of these diseases. Most are myopathic, hepatopathic, or both, but blood, kidney, and brain can be affected. Cerebral glycogenosis may be a form of myophosphorylase deficiency. Fasting ketotic hypoglycemia is common to many of the glycogen storage diseases; this may cause seizures prevented by feeding at bedtime of uncooked cornstarch at 2 grams/kg. Myopathic forms often cause muscle cramps and may cause rhabdomyolysis. When liver is involved, hepatomegaly can be massive. Diagnosis usually requires enzyme analysis from blood, muscle, or liver. Enzyme replacement is available for Pompe disease (Type II, neonatal acid maltase disease). All are autosomal recessive, except one form of phosphoglycerate kinase deficiency and two forms of phosphorylase b kinase, which are X-linked, whereas two other forms of phosphorylase b kinase are autosomal recessive. This depends on which subunit of the enzyme is affected. ***Aldolase deficiency*** is a newly described disorder of developmental delay, myopathy, rhabdomyolysis, hemolysis during febrile illness, and no glycogen found in muscle. Another syndrome has been described – mental retardation, cardiomyopathy, and autophagic vacuolar myopathy – but the enzyme defect is still under investigation. ***Lafora polyglucosan body disease*** occurs in adolescents and adults; it causes dementia, myoclonus and epilepsy; muscle biopsy reveals non-lysosomal, round, PAS-positive inclusions in the perikarya of liver, muscle, skin, and neurons. When glycogen storage diseases present in neonates, they do so usually as hypoglycemia, with or without seizures, sometimes with hypotonia, cardiomyopathy, and variable hepatomegaly. Pompe disease manifests a characteristic short PR interval, low voltage on electrocardiogram, and neonatal heart failure. Some classify Fanconi-Bickel disease as glycogen storage disease type XI. Its defect is a glucose transporter (GLUT2). It is characterized by renal Fanconi syndrome that causes rickets, small stature, malabsorption, hepatomegaly, nephromegaly, aminoaciduria, phosphaturia, glycosuria, fasting hypoglycemia, but with paradoxical glucose and galactose intolerance; it is treated by frequent feedings and at bedtime with uncooked cornstarch at 2 grams/kg.

Mucopolysaccharidoses

These are characterized by dysmorphic features, visceromegaly, bony dysostosis, which often leads to short stature, sometimes primary cerebral dysfunction and sometimes compressive neuropathies and myelopathies, depending on the specific disorder. All store mucopolysaccharides (glycosaminoglycans), and most excrete these in the urine. They follow an autosomal recessive inheritance, gener-

Table 13

Mucopolysaccharidoses (MPS)

Disease	**MPS I (Hurler) (Scheie milder)**	**MPS II (Hunter)**	**MPS III (Sanfilippo A-D)**	**MPS IV (Morquio)**	**MPS V (formerly Scheie)**	**MPS VI (Maroteaux-Lamy)**	**MPS VII (Sly)**
Enzyme Defect	Iduronidase	Iduronate sulfatase	Heparan N-sulfatase	Galactose 6-sulfatase	Obsolete	Aryl sulfatase B	β-glucuronidase
Clinical Features	Corneal clouding. Coarsening. Skeletal dysostosis. Visceromegaly. Heart disease. Delay and dementia. Seizures.	Cornea normal. Coarsening. Skeletal dysostosis. Joint restriction. Visceromegaly. Short stature. Delay and dementia. Seizures late.	Cornea normal. No coarsening. Mild visceromegaly. Delays and hyperactive.	Corneal clouding slight. Coarsening mild. Skeletal dysostosis is distinctive. Odontoid hypoplasia. Short stature. Viceromegaly. Normal mentation. Compression neuropathies and myelopathy.	Obsolete	Corneal clouding slight. Coarsening mild. Skeletal dysostosis is distinctive. Short stature. Visceromegaly. Normal mentation. Compression neuropathies & myelopathy.	Corneal clouding slight. Skeletal dysostosis is distinctive. Short stature. Visceromegaly. Wide range of mental function.
Hallmark Lab Findings	Dermatan sulfate, Heparin sulfate	Dermatan sulfate, Heparin sulfate	Heparin sulfate	Keratan sulfate, Chondroitin 6-sulfate	Obsolete	Dermatan sulfate	Dermatan sulfate, Heparan sulfate, Chondroitin 4-sulfate
Genetics	Autosomal recessive	X-linked recessive	Autosomal recessive	Autosomal recessive	Obsolete	Autosomal recessive	Autosomal recessive
Treatment	Enzyme replacement	Enzyme replacement	Supportive	Supportive	Obsolete	Supportive	Supportive

ally. Some of the lipidoses also have chemical and clinical characteristics of the mucopolysaccharidoses (eg, multiple sulfatase deficiency and Sandhoff disease); they are discussed in the section on lipidoses. Presentation in the newborn is rare, but may be recognized by hoarse cry, persistent stridor, short size, and rarely hypotonia, cataracts or odontoid hypoplasia; usually coarse features are not present yet. Other features are listed in Table 13.

Oligosaccharidoses are discussed under lipidoses.

N-acetyl galactosaminidase deficiency (Schindler disease) is discussed under lipidoses.

Glutamyl ribose-5-phosphate lysosomal storage disease is caused by ADP-ribosyl protein lyase deficiency, and is X-linked. The product is not excreted and diagnosis is made only by noting storage in renal or brain tissue. This disease causes infant onset dementia, progressive neuronal loss, and renal failure. Neonates may have hypotonia and renal impairment.

Congenital disorders of glycoprotein synthesis (CDGS) (Golgi apparatus disorders) were first called carbohydrate deficient glycoprotein syndromes. The new name preserves the initials of the original title, but expresses the pathophysiology better. These disorders are characterized by defective glycosylation of proteins in the Golgi apparatus. This is, in a way, the reverse of the oligosaccharidoses. The proteins are normal, but they are insufficiently glycosylated, so that their function, transport, and survival are impaired. The most common screening test is to identify hypoglycosylated transferrin isoforms (carbohydrate deficient transferrin) in plasma. Phosphomannomutase deficiency was the first form identified, and Dol-P-mannosidase deficiency was reported more recently. All tissues and organs can be affected. Common symptoms include microcephaly, seizures, apnea, hypotonia from combined neuropathy and myopathy, cerebellar hypoplasia and olivary gliosis in some forms, growth failure, diarrhea, mild hepatic and renal dysfunction, and mild coagulopathy from factor XI dysfunction. Fatal neonatal cases with apnea and infantile spasms have been noted. The diseases are autosomal recessive, and no treatment is successful, although addition of mannose to patients with phosphomannomutase deficiency may diminish diarrhea and aid growth.

Miscellaneous Storage Diseases

Canavan disease (N-acetylaspartate (NAA) excess from aspartoacylase deficiency) is characterized by megalencephaly, hypotonia, swallowing difficulties, optic atrophy, seizures and developmental delay that cause fatal neurodegeneration. Head MRI and CT scans reveal strikingly watery myelin. Pathology reveals spongy degenerative leukodystrophy. Head MR spectroscopy and urine demonstrate increased NAA. The disorder is autosomal recessive, with a moderate predominance in the Jewish population, and occurs in congenital, infantile, and juvenile ataxia forms. The gene defect is mapped to chromosome 17p. Gene therapy in this disease is being investigated currently.

Alexander disease is an autosomal recessive leukodystrophy characterized by megalencephaly and Rosenthal fiber hypertrophied astrocytes adherent to blood vessels in the white matter. This disease can present in the newborn or early infantile period. It causes megalencephaly, growth failure from feeding incapacity, spasticity, dementia and fatal neurodegeneration. In older presentations, it can resemble multiple sclerosis with megalencephaly. The most common forms are infantile, but juvenile and adult onset can occur. There is no treatment.

Diseases Characterized by Storage of Fats

Peroxisomal Diseases

A class of disorders characterized by dysfunction of the peroxisome. They bridge the categories of small molecule diseases and large molecule diseases. They cause fluid accumulation of unmetabolized long chain fatty acids in the plasma, but these are not "stored" in fixed intracellular collections, as occurs in other of large molecule diseases. The known roles of the peroxisome include: generation of hydrogen peroxide for biochemical reactions; synthesis of plasmalogens (eg, phosphatidylethanolamine); beta-oxidation of very long chain and long chain fatty acids; oxidation of phytanic acid and pipecolic acid; some steps of bile acid formation; and some steps of dicarboxylic acid metabolism. Defects of the peroxisome will lead to disruption of one or more of these steps. Therefore, the clinician's most efficient diagnostic screening test for peroxisomal disease is to measure the excessive relative accumulation of very long and long chain fatty acids in the blood. After that has been established, the metabolist can confirm a specific subtype of peroxisomal disease through analysis of enzymes in skin fibroblasts, or through gene tests. Inheritance is usually autosomal recessive, with the notable exception of X-linked adrenoleukodystrophy.

Peroxisomal diseases tend to present with signs of central +/- peripheral myelin dysfunction (leukodystrophy with or without demyelinating polyneuropathy), sometimes with liver or other organ dysfunction. In cases of newborn and infantile presentations, skeletal or other organ dysplasia is common. The most severe forms are neonatal. These newborn diseases include Zellweger cerebrohepatorenal syndrome and neonatal adrenoleukodystrophy, which are multisystem malformation syndromes of cortical dysplasia and hypomyelination, sometimes with renal microcysts and hepatic dysplasia (Zellweger), and chondrodysplasia with neonatal peripatellar calcifications (neonatal adrenoleukodystrophy). In these two diseases, optic pallor is often present, and seizures can be severe and intractable. Refsum disease is primarily a peripheral neuropathy presenting in early adulthood, characterized by accumulation of phytanic acid. Neonatal Refsum disease is severe, and does not have the same metabolic defect or treatment as the adult form, but does presently similarly with polyneuropathy and elevated phytanic acid.

Treatment is symptomatic, coupled with genetic counseling. A therapeutic diet contains the lipids glyceryl trioleate and glyceryl trierucate (variants of "Lorenzo's oil"). This diet bypasses the defective pathways and has been shown to delay demyelination in asymptomatic patients with X-linked adrenoleukodystrophy genotype. Adrenal hormone replacement is indicated if adrenal dysfunction is present. In Zellweger disease or neonatal adrenoleukodystrophy, supplementation with cholic and deoxycholic and docosahexanoic acids may be helpful. Supplementation with vitamin K is indicated if there is severe liver dysfunction. A diet low in phytanic acid, sometimes augmented with plasmapheresis, treats Refsum disease. It is noteworthy that some peroxisomal disorders are accompanied by secondary pyruvate dehydrogenase dysfunction. Bone marrow transplantation is being studied in X-linked adrenoleukodystrophy.

Some Inherited Disorders of the Peroxisome

Disorders of peroxisomal assembly (neonatal presentations):

- Zellweger cerebrohepatorenal syndrome
- Neonatal adrenoleukodystrophy
- Infantile Refsum disease
- Hyperpipecolic acidemia
- Rhizomelic chondrodysplasia punctata

Single peroxisomal enzyme deficiency:

- X-linked adrenoleukodystrophy / adrenomyeloneuropathy
- Acyl-CoA oxidase deficiency
- Bifunctional enzyme deficiency
- Peroxisomal thiolase deficiency
- Dihydroxyacetone phosphate deficiency
- Alkyl dihydroxyacetone phosphate deficiency
- Glutaric aciduria type III
- Refsum disease
- Hyperoxaluria type I
- Acatalasemia

Intracellular Cholesteroloses

For educational convenience, some diseases of cholesterol metabolism can be grouped among small molecule diseases, and some can be grouped

Table 14

Intracellular Cholesteroloses and Niemann-Pick

Disease Name	**Wolman Disease**	**Cholesterol Ester Storage**	**Niemann-Pick C**	**Niemann-Pick A**	**Niemann-Pick B**
Enzyme Defect	Lysosomal lipase	Lysosomal lipase	Lysosomal cholesterol esterification	Lysosomal sphingo-myelinase	Lysosomal sphingo-myelinase
Clinical Features	Vomiting, diarrhea, growth failure, hepatosplenomegaly, developmental delay.	Milder than Wolman	Infant hepatospleno-megaly, dementia, upgaze paraly-sis, cataplexy, narcolepsy, rare seizures, dystonia, ataxia.	Infant Liver > spleno-megaly, hydrops fetalis, growth failure, cherry red/black macula with halo, xan-thomas, neurodegener-ation.	Infant to adult. Same as type A, but milder.
Hallmark Lab Findings	Adrenal calcifications, foamy lymphocytes & marrow histiocytes; stored cholesterol esters. Blood cholesterol and triglycerides may be normal.	Same as Wolman, but no adrenal calcifications.	Foamy histio-cytes. Stored cholesterol. Poor fibroblast lysosomal cholesterol esterification, filipin stain +.	Foamy histiocytes. Stored choles-terol and sphingo-myelin all cells + pla-centa. High transaminases, microcytic anemia, pancytopenia, pulmonary disease.	Like Type A. Lung > liver > brain dis-ease, but "Lewis variant" has sea blue histio-cytes in spleen > liver.
Genetics	Chromosome 10 recessive	Chromosome 10 recessive	18q11 recessive	11p15 recessive Ashkenazi	11p15 recessive Ashkenazi
Treatment	None; ? liver & marrow transplant	None; ? HMG- CoA reductase inhibitors; liver and marrow transplant	Research studies. Anti-convulsants, protriptyline and clomipramine for cataplexy. Anticholiner-gics for dystonia.	None	None
Prognosis	Poor	Poor	Poor	Guarded	Good

Table 15

Sphingolipidoses

	Enzyme Defect	Accumulated Substances	Viscero-megaly	Cherry Red Macula	Special Feature	Enzyme Replacement
Niemann-Pick A, B	Sphingomyelinase	Sphingomyelin and cholesterol	3+	Red/black with halo	Organomegaly, Lung disease	0
Niemann-Pick C	Cholesterol esterification	Cholesterol	1-2+	0	Upgaze paresis Cataplexy Dystonia	0
Gaucher	β-Glucosidase (Glucocerebrocidase)	Glycosylceramide (Glucocerebroside)	1-3+ Spleen infarcts Pathologica l fractures	0	Trismus + strabismus + retrocollis in Type 2. Loss of voluntary lateral gaze in type 3.	+
Fabry	α Galactosidase A	Ceramide trihexoside	0	0	Lancinating pain Angiokeratoma, Renal failure, strokes	+
Farber Lipogranulomatosis	Ceramidase	Ceramide	+/-	+/-	Hoarse voice Lipid nodules	0
Gm1 Gangliosidosis	β Galactosidase	Gm1 ganglioside Galactosyl oligosaccharides Keratan sulfate	+/-	+	Dysostosis Organomegaly Morquio-like syndrome	0
Gm2 Gangliosidosis Tay-Sachs	Hexosaminidase α	Gm2 ganglioside	0	+	Startle. Blindness.	0

(continued)

Table 15 *(continued)*

Sphingolipidoses

	Enzyme Defect	Accumulated Substances	Viscero-megaly	Cherry Red Macula	Special Feature	Enzyme Replacement
Gm2 Gangliosidosis Sandhoff	Hexos-aminidase A and B/β	Gm2 ganglioside Oligosaccharides Glycosaminoglycans	+/-	+	Blindness, Startle	0
Gm2 Activator Deficiency	Gm2 activator	Gm2 ganglioside	0	+	Equal to Tay-Sachs	0
Schindler	α Galactosidase B N-acetyl galactose-aminidase	N-acetyl -galactosaminyl oligosaccharides & glycopeptides	0	0	Neuroaxonal dystrophy	0
Metachromatic Leukodystrophy (MLD)	Arylsulfatase A; sulfatide activator (saposin B)	Galactosylsulfatide Lactosylsulfatide	0	+/-	Leukodystrophy, Neuropathy	0
Krabbe Globoid Leukodystrophy	Galactosidase (Galactocylceramide β galactosidase)	Galactosylceramide	0	0	Leukodystrophy, very irritable infants, high CSF protein	0
Multiple Sulfatase Deficiency	Arylsulfatase A,B,C; other sulfatases	Galactosylsulfatide Lactosylsulfatide Oligosaccharides Mucopolysaccharides	3+	+	Like MLD + dysmorphic, osteodystrophy with spinal cord compression	0

Table 16

Mucolipidoses

	Enzyme Defect	Accumulated Substances Excreted in Urine
Mucolipidosis I (Sialidosis)	α- Neuraminidase	Sialylyoligosaccharides Sialylglycopeptides
Mucolipidosis II (I-cell disease)	UDP-N-acetylglucosamine: lysosomal enzyme, N-acetylglucosamine-1 phosphotransferase	Sialylyoligosaccharides Glycoproteins Glycolipids
Mucolipidosis III (Pseudo-Hurler polydystrophy)	Same phosphotransferase as Mucolipidosis I	Sialylyoligosaccharides Glycoproteins Glycolipids
Mucolipidosis IV (Sialolipidosis)	Gangliosialidase	Gangliosides Phospholipids Mucopolysaccharides

with the large molecule diseases, based on clinical presentation. Cholesterol metabolites may collect outside cells in familial hypercholesterolemias, mevalonic aciduria and cerebrotendinous xanthomatosis; those are listed in the small molecule disorders because the abnormal location of the lipid is predominantly extracellular. In contrast, diseases of intracellular storage of cholesterol metabolites (which this chapter calls intracellular cholesteroloses) are listed here, under large molecule diseases. This is done because the lipid is stored as large inclusions within cells and the defective enzymes are lysosomal; even though the stored metabolite is a small molecule, the clinical features are so similar to lipidoses that they must be evaluated, considered, and excluded together. The intracellular cholesteroloses include Niemann-Pick C, cholesterol ester storage disease, and its severe variant, Wolman disease. The intracellular cholesteroloses tend to cause dysfunction of gray matter, producing dementia, seizures and movement disorders, and also cause organomegaly. Niemann-Pick A and B are listed here for educational purposes, because their presentation is very similar to Niemann-Pick C, but sphingomyelin, rather than cholesterol, is the primary stored material in types A and B. Niemann-Pick D is no longer considered a separate entity, but is Type C in a French Acadian population. Table 14 compares these disorders, and highlights a few unique features. Presentation in the newborn period is extremely rare.

Sphingolipidoses (Table 15) and glycolipidoses are defects of lysosomal metabolism of sphingolipids that cause an intralysosomal > intracytoplasmic accumulation of complex sphingolipids, "glycolipids" and glycopeptides. (Glycolipid is a term that can be used to designate composites of oligosaccharides and lipid derivatives. Glycopeptide is a term that can be used to designate composites of oligosaccharides and peptide derivatives.) If the accumulation is in oligodendrocytes, or Schwann cell, the predominant features are those of a leukodystrophy (demyelinating dementia, spasticity, ataxia, and later

Table 17

Oligosaccharidoses (Glycoproteinoses)

	Enzyme Defect	Accumulated Substances Excreted in Urine
α-Mannosidosis	α-Mannosidase	α-Mannosyl-oligosaccharides
β-Mannosidosis	β-Mannosidase	β-Mannosyl-oligosaccharides
Fucosidosis	Fucosidase	Fucosyl-oligosaccharides Fucosyl-glycosphingolipids
Aspartylglucosaminuria	Aspartylglucosaminidase	Aspartylglucosamine
Galactosialidosis	Protective protein for α-Neuraminidase and β-Galactosidase	Sialyloligosaccharides Galactosyloligosaccharides
Sialic acid storage disease	Sialic acid transport	Free sialic acid

Table 18

Neuronal Ceroid Lipofuscinoses

	Enzyme Defect	Inclusions
Infantile (Haltia-Santavuori)	Palmitoyl-protein thioesterase	Granular osmiophilic deposits
Late Infantile (Jansky-Bielschowsky)	Tripeptidyl peptidase I	Curvilinear bodies; Subunit C of mitochondrial ATP synthase
Juvenile (Spielmeyer-Vogt-Batten)	438 amino acid membrane protein	Curvilinear and laminated (fingerprint) bodies; Subunit C of mitochondrial ATP synthase
Adult (Kufs)	?	Mixed osmiophilic and laminar inclusions

demyelinating neuropathy). If the accumulation is in gray matter neurons or astrocytes, the predominant features are those of a poliodystrophy (dementia, seizures, retinal dysfunction, movement disorder, axonal neuropathy). The substance accumulated in the cells may be different from that which is excreted in urine. Cell death is usually slow, caused by the accumulation itself, or by toxic or deficiency effects of metabolites in the affected pathways of normal sphingomyelin formation. Presentations occur as infantile, late childhood, and adult forms. They generally follow autosomal recessive inheritance, except for Fabry disease, which is X-linked.

Table 19

Diagnostic Algorithm for Infantile Storage Diseases and Leukodystrophies

I) Dysmorphic +/- mild organomegaly, +/- neurological symptoms

- Mucopolysaccharidoses (Urine berry spot positive):
  - Mental retardation:
    - Hurler
    - Hunter
    - Hunter-Scheie
    - Sanfilippo
    - β Glucuronidase deficiency
    - Mucosulfatidosis
    - Multiple sulfatase deficiency
  - No mental retardation:
    - Scheie
    - Morquio
    - Maroteaux-Lamy
- Oligosaccharidoses (Urine berry spot negative):
  - Urine sialic acid increased:
    - Mucolipidosis I
    - Mucolipidosis II
    - Mucolipidosis III
  - Urine sialic acid not present:
    - Fucosidosis
    - Mannosidosis
    - Aspartylglucosaminuria
    - Mucolipidosis IV
  - Peroxisomal diseases
  - Chromosomal diseases

II) Visceromegaly without dysmorphic features

- Disordered sugar metabolism:
  - Galactosemia
  - Fructosemia
  - Glycogen storage diseases
  - Childhood mucopolysaccharidoses
- Disordered metabolism without acidosis:
  - Wolman
  - Cholesterol ester storage disease
  - Niemann-Pick A-C
  - Farber disease
  - Tangier disease
  - Sandhoff (some)
  - Childhood mucolipidoses
  - Urea cycle defects
- Disordered metabolism with acidosis:
  - Sometimes in organic and amino acidurias
  - Mevalonic aciduria
  - Sometimes in disorders of fatty acid oxidation
  - Metabolic diseases with heart failure

III) Neurologic diseases without dysmorphic features or visceromegaly

- Predominantly gray matter disease:
  - Tay-Sachs
  - Sandhoff
  - Gm1 gangliosidosis
  - Alexander disease
  - Neuroaxonal dystrophy
  - Neuronal ceroid lipofuscinosis
  - Many mitochondrial diseases
  - Some organic and amino acidopathies
  - Urea cycle defects
- Predominantly white matter disease:
  - Canavan spongy degeneration
  - Adrenoleukodystrophy
  - Krabbe globoid-cell leukodystrophy
  - Metachromatic leukodystrophy
  - Pelizaeus-Merzbacher proteolipid protein mutation diseases

Modified from Lyon, Adams and Kolodny.

Treatment is usually supportive, and all are fatal, except for Gaucher and Fabry disease, which are responsive to enzyme replacement. All Niemann-Pick disorders have features similar to Gaucher disease, except the liver is usually more involved than the spleen in Niemann-Pick, whereas the spleen is usually larger than the liver in Gaucher disease. Niemann-Pick and Gaucher diseases produce histologically similar vacuoles and sea blue foamy histiocytes as a histological hallmark, but the accumulated stained lipid substance is different in each disease. There are three forms of Gaucher: Type 1 presents in childhood or teen years, sometimes progressing to parkinsonian rigidity in early middle age; Type 2 is a fatal neonatal and infantile form presenting with the tetrad of trismus, strabismus, and retrocolis along with hepatosplenomegaly; Type 3 causes massive splenomegaly with loss of voluntary lateral gaze. In the case of oligosaccharidoses and mucopolysaccharidoses, abnormal oligosaccharides and glycosaminoglycans (mucopolysaccharides) can be detected in urine; enzyme testing confirms a diagnosis. Sandhoff disease and multiple sulfatase deficiency combine features of oligosaccharidosis, mucopolysaccharidosis, and sphingolipidosis. The lipidoses that are most likely to present in the newborn period are Gaucher disease type 2, Krabbe globoid cell leukodystrophy, Tay-Sachs Gm2 gangliosidosis, Gm1 gangliosidosis, and multiple sulfatase deficiency. Krabbe disease presents as a very hypertonic infant who has a high CSF protein and is very irritable; the old mnemonic is "Krabbe kids are crabby."

Mucolipidoses (Table 16)

These are characterized by lysosomal storage and urinary excretion of mucolipid sialyloligosaccharides, sialylglycopeptides, glycolipids, and sometimes mucopolysaccharides. Clinical features include variable coarsening of features, visceromegaly, cloudy cornea, neural degeneration, and retinal degeneration. Diagnosis is made by combining clinical features, urinary screening, and enzyme assay in fibroblasts or leukocytes. All are autosomal recessive, all can present in the newborn, and the only current treatments are symptomatic management and genetic counseling.

Oligosaccharidoses (Glycoproteinoses) (Table 17)

Diseases caused by inability to disassemble glycoproteins. For educational simplicity, this can be considered the reverse of congenital disorders of glycoprotein synthesis, although the impaired degradation does not occur in the Golgi apparatus. They are also called oligosaccharidoses, because they are characterized often by lysosomal storage of products bound to oligosaccharides. Their symptoms include varying degrees of dysmorphic features, visceromegaly, dementia, seizures, global neurodegeneration with seizures, myoclonus, movement disorder, ataxia, progressive cerebral atrophy that can be severe, and storage in skin, endothelia, and all affected organs. All are autosomal recessive, all can present in the newborn, all are very rare, and the only proven treatments are symptomatic management and genetic counseling.

Neuronal Ceroid Lipofuscinoses (Table 18)

They cause dementia, intractable epilepsy, movement disorder and retinal blindness, global neurodegeneration and death. EEGs often show a photoconvulsive response, and the electroretinogram is nearly always abnormal. Their pathological hallmark is accumulation of complex osmiophilic inclusions, which, by light microscopy, were originally called lipofuscin. Patients can sometimes suffer icthyosis, especially in the adult form. These are not, strictly speaking, lysosomal storage diseases. They were considered lipidoses in the past, because of the accumulation of membranous structures that contain sphingolipids. Usually there is only slight organomegaly or coarse features, or none at all. They occur in four age presentations. There is no reliable diagnostic urinary product; the obsolete assay for urinary dolichols is not sufficiently predictive. The infantile form can present in the newborn as hypotonia, seizures, and little visual interest.

4. Other Neurogenetic Disorders

The following disease categories were listed in the introduction of this chapter, and are summarized as follows for completeness. Most are, strictly speaking, not metabolic disorders, but they are genetic, and must be included in the differential diagnosis of neurometabolic diseases in the newborn. Many will present well beyond the newborn period, and are listed for educational purposes.

- Chromosomal disorders
- Subtelomeric disorders
- Nucleotide repeat disorders
- Other genetic mutations and deletions
- Heritable disorders of unknown cause

Disorders of Small Mutations and Deletions

These are point mutations, expansion multinucleotide repeats, deletions, and rearrangements that usually affect only one gene product. These gene products are not usually part of energy/acid intermediary metabolism or detoxification, which distinguishes them from mutations that cause the disorders of small molecules. Clearly, however, there can be overlap in all classification of diseases. Usually, there is no circulating or excreted metabolite to serve as a hallmark of the disease, and usually no dietary therapy. Potentially, this class of disease may be as vast as the genome itself. Its ranks are expanding rapidly, and the next decades are likely to enlarge this category, such that it will need to be subdivided in future diagnostic algorithms. Because of this rapid and continuous accumulation of data, this chapter could become a fossil rapidly. Therefore, it seems prudent to refer the reader to the excellent Internet-based resources that provide continuously updated data on genes, enzymes, and presentations of neurogenetic diseases: *Genetests.com;* and *Online Manual of Inherited Disorders in Man (OMIM)*. The United States National Library of Medicine and the National Institute of Health run these web sites.

For the purpose of this chapter, it will suffice to list the most common such disorders. There are diagnostic gene probes available for all of these disorders. After the list, selected abnormalities are summarized. Fluorescence *in situ* Hybridization (FISH) probes are available for diagnosis of these disorders.

Dysmorphic Syndromes

- Prader-Willi syndrome (Chromosome 15)
- Angelmann syndrome (Chromosome 15)
- Miller-Dieker Lissencephaly
- Williams syndrome
- Smith Magenis syndrome
- Cri-duc-chat Microdeletion syndrome
- Wolf-Hirschhorn Microdeletion syndrome
- Chromosome 22 DiGeorge/Velocardiofacial syndrome
- Microdeletion Syndromes (eg, 4p- syndrome)

Epilepsies

- Rett syndrome (MECP2 gene)
- Rett-like syndrome (STK9 gene)
- Inherited Epilepsies (eg, Chromosome 6 mutations; Progressive myoclonic epilepsy)

(See Appendix Table 5)

Pelizeaeus-Merzbacher syndrome (proteolipid protein gene)

Movement Disorders (discussed elsewhere in this text)

- Huntington Disease
- Neuroacanthocytosis
- Dentato-Rubro-Pallido-Luysian Atrophy
- Torsion Dystonia
- Dopa Responsive Dystonias (see Small Molecule Diseases)

Inherited Spinocerebellar Atrophies

Inherited Polyneuropathies and Axonopathies

- SMN genes
- SMA gene

Inherited Myopathies and Muscular Dystrophies (discussed elsewhere in this text)

Neurocutaneous Disorders

- Neurofibromatosis
- Tuberous Sclerosis
- Xeroderma Pigmentosum
- Osler-Weber-Rendu
- Von Hippel-Lindau
- Incontinentia Pigmenti
- Giant Melanotic Nevus syndrome
- Hypomelanosis of Ito
- Ataxia-Telangiectasia (ATM gene)
- Chediak-Higashi syndrome
- Griscelli syndrome (melanophilin gene)

Prader-Willi syndrome is a multisystem, mental retardation syndrome caused by a contiguous gene deletion on paternal chromosome 15q11-q13. Characteristic features include hypotonia as a neonate, sometimes with hypoglycemia caused by feeding difficulties, and respiratory difficulties caused by poor airway protection. There may be a modest increase probability for seizure. The children reach milestones slowly, and by prepuberty have small genitalia, obesity and hyperphagia, behavioral difficulties and cognitive impairment; severity is variable. Patients may benefit from carnitine therapy in the neonate.

Angelmann syndrome is a multisystem, mental retardation syndrome caused by a contiguous gene deletion on maternal chromosome 15q. Characteristic features include hypotonia as a neonate, infantile onset epilepsy with characteristic parasagittal spikes, hyperactivity, anxiety, cognitive impairment, ataxia, and discontinuous jerky voluntary movements that prompted the old mnemonic of "happy puppet syndrome." Some patients with the STK9 mutation mimic the characteristics of Angelmann syndrome.

Williams syndrome: Patients present as neonates and infants with small size, failure to thrive, gastroesophageal reflux, hoarse voice, supravalvar aortic stenosis, truncal hypotonia and extremity hypertonia, and hypercalcemia. By school age, additional symptoms become prominent: short stature; dental abnormalities; hernias; hyperextensible joints; urinary frequency and enuresis; an "elfin face"; mild cognitive impairment that tests worse than a "cocktail party personality" conveys; hypersensitivity to sound; anxiety when walking on unstable or elevated surfaces; and strabismus. Some may have Chiari I malformation. Williams syndrome is caused by a submicroscopic deletion of one chromosome 7q11.23, disrupting the elastin and lim kinase 1 genes.

Miller-Dieker Lissencephaly: Symptoms include high wrinkled forehead, carp-shaped flat lip, small jaw, prominent occiput, clouded cornea, seizures, developmental stagnation, and lissencephaly noted on magnetic resonance imaging of the brain. The defect is a small autosomal recessive mutation at chromosome 17p13.3. Additional small mutations for other lissencephalic states have been identified.

Smith-Magenis syndrome: Infants have growth delay, flat face, wide nose, short wide digits, hoarse voice, and hearing loss. Later they present with mental retardation, hyperactivity, self-mutilating behavior as severe as patients with Lesch-Nyhan hyperuricemia, severe pica and placing objects in body orifices, high pain tolerance with absent reflexes and signs of neuropathy, and uncommonly, congenital heart defects. It is caused by a small deletion at chromosome 17p11.2.

Cri-duc-chat Microdeletion syndrome: The patients present as newborns with low birth weight, poor growth, a cry that sounds like a weak cat during the first weeks of life. Newborn exam reveals microcephaly, round face with hypertelorism, epicanthal folds, low and malformed ears, small chin, prominent nose and facial asymmetry, and strabismus. Less common features are bifid uvula, cleft lip or palate, structural abnormalities of abdominal viscera, or structural abnormalities of feet and digits. Ultimately, patients are cognitively impaired. It is caused by a small deletion at 5p; karyotype or FISH testing can confirm the diagnosis.

Wolf-Hirschhorn syndrome: Patients present with full or partial collection of low birth weight, microcephaly with a high forehead, wide nasal bridge, broad or beaked nose, epicanthal folds, hypertelorism, cardiac and renal defects, hypospadias, cryptorchidism, and urethrovaginal fistula, developmental delay, hypotonia, seizures and infantile spasms. It is caused by a deletion at 4p16.

Chromosome 22 DiGeorge/Velocardiofacial syndromes: Presentation is variable and can be subtle, and from neonatal to early adolescence. Diagnosis is suggested when two or more of the following symptoms and signs are noted: submucosal cleft, nasal speech, conotruncal congenital heart disease, narrow eyes, small abnormal ears, bulbous nose, micrognathia, long digits, feeding difficulties, developmental delay, mood disorder or schizophrenia, hypotonia, renal abnormalities, hypocalcemia with or without seizures, and T-cell dysfunction. This is the most common microdeletion syndrome (1/2000 – 1/4000 births), and is caused by a small deletion of chromosome 22q11.2 identified by fluorescence *in situ* hybridization (FISH).

Microdeletion syndromes: (eg, 4p- syndrome) may be caused by chromosomal microdeletions that are large enough to be seen by light microscopy, but most require FISH to identify. Many symptoms can be caused by these microdeletions, depending on the gene product coded for at the site of the genomic defect. Some laboratories screen for many defects simultaneously by using gene microarray technology.

Rett syndrome: By its classical definition, patients present with late toddler decline of language and hand function, autistic symptoms, and progressive cognitive decline; seizures can vary from absent to intractable. This was once thought to occur only in females, and the mutation in the male was thought to be fatal. Two genome defects have been identified recently at the MECP2 gene and the STK9 gene. With these discoveries has come the finding that some patients can present as severe as neonatal seizures or infantile spasms, or less severe, as a mimic of Angelmann syndrome. The MECP2 gene is a regulator that suppresses glutamate receptor expression. In the Rett mutation, glutamate receptor function persists excessively, leading to deterioration of function from toxic neural excitation.

Autistic Spectrum Disorder mutations: These are a collection of mutations, some of which are associated with X-linked mental retardation and autistic features. The value of identifying these genes in a given patient is that it can lead to genetic counseling and family planning, may identify patients for therapeutic trials, and can provide parents with an explanation for their child's symptoms to keep them from wasting time, money and unrequited hope in numerous dubious therapies. These genes include the neuroligand genes involved in neuronal and synaptic development and X-linked mental retardation genes. STK9 and ARX mutations have been associated with infantile spasms. ARX mutations have been associated with infantile spasms, Proud syndrome, and Partington syndrome, and X-linked lissencephaly with abnormal genitalia. PQBP1 mutations have been associated with the Renpenning, Sutherland-Haan, and Hamel cerebropalatocardiac syndromes. See Appendix Table 6 for a list of recently identified genes associated with autism and mental retardation.

Inherited Epilepsies: These are discussed in detail elsewhere. It suffices to state here that numerous genes have been identified and associated with epileptic syndromes (eg, Chromosome 6 mutations; Progressive myoclonic epilepsy). Some present in newborns, especially benign familial neonatal epilepsy. See Appendix Table 5 for a list of additional genes associated with severe or intractable epilepsy.

Pelizaeus-Merzbacher syndrome: This syndrome was originally described as global cerebral (and sometimes peripheral) hypomyelination. It occurs in 3 forms: autosomal recessive acute infantile (neonatal); X-linked infantile (Xq21.3-q22); and autosomal dominant adult onset. Symptoms include developmental delay or stagnation, hypotonia followed by spasticity and contractures, nystagmus, tremor, dysmetria, ataxia and seizures. After a mutation was found in the proteolipid protein (PLP) gene, patients are identified who present with acquired spastic paraparesis and spastic quadriplegia and occasional seizures who also have PLP mutations. Experimental therapy is available.

Inherited Ataxias: Very few of the following present in infants, except the Marinesco-Sjögren syndrome.

Spinocerebellar Atrophies Types 1-17, SETX and POLG1 gene mutations: These patients have variable presentations of ataxia, nystagmus or ophthalmoparesis, dysarthria, pyramidal and extrapyramidal signs. Some are caused by an autosomal dominant CAG nucleotide repeats in chromosome 6, 11, 12, 14, 16; additional forms have been found and await confirmation. Cognitive impairment, rare seizures, and peripheral neuropathy are found in a few patients.

Central Diabetes Insipidus followed by Progressive Spastic Cerebral Ataxia: The ataxia is of later onset than most spinocerebellar atrophies. Some patients have evidence of histiocytosis, which may be localized to the central nervous system only. Many have calcified cerebellar dentate nuclei.

Friedreich Ataxia: Patients usually present with intermittent clumsiness and loss of reflexes, followed by more prominent ataxia, then dysarthria, then tremor, scoliosis and finally fatal restrictive lung disease and cardiomyopathy. That classic sequence is not always observed. It is caused by an autosomal recessive mutation in the Frataxin gene, whose gene product is linked to mitochondrial function.

Spinocerebellar degeneration with retinal degeneration is caused by an autosomal dominant mutation in chromosome 3.

Dentatorubropallidoluysian Atrophy causes ataxia, choreoathetosis, dystonia, myoclonus, epilepsy and dementia. It is caused by autosomal dominant CAG repeat mutation in chromosome 12.

Machado-Joseph disease is characterized by ataxia with ophthalmoparesis and dysfunction of upper and lower motor neurons. It is caused by autosomal dominant CAG repeats in chromosome 14, most frequently in people of Portuguese ancestry.

Episodic Ataxia type 1 causes brief and non-progressive episodes of ataxia triggered by startle or exercise, accompanied by facial and hand myokymia. It is caused by autosomal dominant mutation to KCNA1 potassium channel coded on chromosome 12. It can be treated by phenytoin.

Episodic Ataxia type 2 causes ataxia and downbeat nystagmus that lasts for days. These events are triggered by stress and fatigue and eventually cause progressive cerebellar atrophy. It is caused by an autosomal dominant mutation in chromosome 19p and is treated by acetazolamide.

Marinesco-Sjögren syndrome has been found in some cases to be a presentation of mitochondrial ATP synthase deficiency from the NARP mutations. There may be other causes.

Inherited Polyneuropathies and Axonopathies: These can present from late neonatal period to adulthood.

- Spinal Muscular Atrophy genes (SMA genes)
- Inherited Motor and Sensory Neuropathy genes (HMSN genes, HMSN I-III)
- Inherited Motor and Sensory Neuropathy With Optic Atrophy (HMSN IV)

Disorders of Chromosomal and Subtelomeric Damage

This category is comprised of disorders that are caused by chromosomal duplications, large deletions, or rearrangements that sometimes may be identified by the standard Giemsa stain for karyotyping with light microscopy. It is a large category, but relatively fixed in size, as all the newest research is focused at the level of the single gene. We refer the reader to the classic reference originally written by Smith, cataloging all these disorders (see References). The clinical hallmarks of these diseases are dysmorphic features and multiple malformations noted in the newborn. In many cases, the disorders are caused by dysfunction of several genes that have been disrupted by the chromosomal defect, ie, they are often multigene defects. If a chromosomal disorder is identified, it is appropriate to enlist the services of geneticists for their expertise in prognosis, management and counseling of these disorders. Furthermore, if a patient has three minor malformations (eg, syndactyly + epicanthal folds + low set ears) the chance that the patient has an occult visceral malformation is approximately 60 percent. Therefore, when a chromosomal disorder is identified, imaging of brain, thorax and abdomen may be appropriate. Aneuploidy and polyploidy of the sex chromosomes, however, may have only subtle physical abnormalities, identifiable after puberty; their presenting symptoms may be only attention deficit and learning disabilities. It is common to defer or forget to check chromosomes when only such minimal signs are present.

A few of the prototypes of these diseases are listed below, along with a few important diagnostic or management issues:

- Down syndrome (Trisomy 21)
- Other chromosomal aneuploidies, polyploidies (eg, trisomy 13), deletions, translocations
- Fragile X syndrome
- Ring Chromosomes (eg, ring 20 syndrome)
- Russell-Silver syndrome (uniparental disomy)
- Turner syndrome
- Klinefelter syndrome
- 47, XYY syndrome
- 47, XXX syndrome

Down syndrome (Trisomy 21): This is one of the first, and one of the most common causes of mental retardation. Many years of study have produced a great body of knowledge about management of the patients' multisystem difficulties (see the two References by Cooley). One word of caution: the facial features of a neonate with trisomy 21 mosaicism can be subtle; one may consider testing for it in any infant with hypotonia.

Other chromosomal aneuploidies, polyploidies (eg, trisomy 13), deletions and translocations: Many of these diseases are catastrophic and can lead to neonatal death. Their hallmarks are dysmorphic features and multiorgan dysfunction, often with seizures and arthrogryposis. Pursuit of chromosome analysis in blood, cultured skin, or cells in saliva can be obtained post-mortem, if necessary. It is often difficult to keep in mind that parents who have balanced translocations can be normal, but may have a history of multiple miscarriages prior to bearing affected offspring.

Ring Chromosomes (eg, ring 20 syndrome): This disorder presents as developmental delay with epilepsy. Overnight or prolonged EEG may reveal extended periods of generalized non-convulsive spike-wave stupor that can be intractable. The diagnosis can be missed in standard chromosome analysis, but testing for ring 20 only, in 200 cells (leukocytes or fibroblasts), has excellent sensitivity. Its neonatal presentation is variable.

Turner syndrome: This presents with short stature, gonadal dysgenesis and lack of secondary sexual characteristics, sometimes with associated findings of congenital heart disease, renal abnormalities, hypothyroidism, and recurrent ear infections, but mental function is normal after thyroid replacement. It is associated with 7 different abnormalities of the X chromosome, identified by karyotype testing. It is usually not symptomatic in the newborn, except for mild non-specific hypotonia.

Klinefelter syndrome (47, XXY; 48, XXXY; 49, XXXXY): This common syndrome (1/600 males) causes tall stature, testicular dysgenesis, gynecomastia and language-based learning disabilities. It is associated with increased risk for breast cancer and extragonadal germ cell tumors. The prepubertal patient, prior to diagnosis, may present for evaluation of learning difficulties; so testing chromosomes may be useful if the above somatotype is present. It is usually not recognized in the newborn.

47, XYY syndrome: A male with this syndrome comes to the attention of the clinician, usually before diagnosis, because of attention deficit and sometimes slight cognitive impairment compared to his siblings. They are not at increased risk for violent behavior, as was once thought. They may be tall, but their physical phenotype is otherwise normal, and they have no particular symptoms as newborns.

47, XXX syndrome: These girls have a normal physical phenotype, but may have tall stature and learning difficulties.

Fragile X syndrome: This is the most common cause of mental retardation, so it can be considered in every case of developmental delay, male or female. It occurs in 1 in 1250 boys and 1 in 2500 females. Newborns may have mild hypotonia that is usually not investigated. They present again as prepubertal developmental delay (especially language delay) and autistic features, with attention deficit and hyperactivity, enuresis, and sometimes hypotonia and hyperextensible joints. Cerebral imaging may reveal cerebellar hypoplasia. Postpubertal enlargement of testes, a long face with a large jaw, and obsessive-compulsive behavior may be noted. It is caused by a CGG trinucleotide repeat at the "fragile X mental retardation 1 gene" located at Xq27. Diagnosis is now made by DNA-based testing because the older chromosomal method to find a "fragile site" produces too many false negative results.

Russell-Silver syndrome: These children have global somatic growth restriction, and frontal bossing, but otherwise often have a normal phenotype. They come to the attention of neurologists because of the frontal bossing. Uniparental disomy can be demonstrated in a minority of patients.

Heritable syndromes of unknown cause: This is a shrinking class, because the human genome project and related endeavors have led to the discovery of so many pathological gene mutations. In the following list, the inborn nature of some of the entities has not been established. One could presume that some form of any "idiopathic" disorder has a potential to belong to this category:

- Idiopathic Epilepsies
- Idiopathic Movement Disorders
- Idiopathic Cerebellar Degenerations
- Fazio-Londe syndrome
- Sudanophilic Leukodystrophy
- Some forms of Amyotropic Lateral Sclerosis

5. Leukodystrophies

Leukodystrophies are disorders characterized by disruption of myelin formation or by destruction of normal myelin. This class of disease can be subdivided into three groups: dysmyelination, myelinolysis and demyelination. Dysmyelination signifies inherited disorders of myelin chemistry, causing biochemical instability in myelin or defective myelin formation. Myelinolysis signifies disorders where there is normal myelin genotype chemistry, but assembly and water content is disrupted by toxic or metabolic factors that cause formation of vacuoles in myelin sheathes, producing a "spongy myelinopathy." Demyelination signifies disorders where the original myelin was normal, but was damaged by inflammatory processes, whether from infectious, immune or other etiologies. It is clear from this organization that leukodystrophies can be caused by disorders originating from the full panoply of etiologies (eg, small molecule or large molecule diseases). In some cases, such as in adrenoleukodystrophy or after trauma, as leukodystrophy progresses, demyelination may be added to dysmyelination or myelinolysis.

Dysmyelination

- Metachromatic Leukodystrophy (Aryl sulfatase A deficiency) and SAP-1 deficiency
- Congenital disorder of carbohydrate synthesis (previously called carbohydrate deficient glycoprotein syndrome)
- Krabbe Globoid Cell Leukodystrophy (galactosylceramide beta galactocidase deficiency)
- Peroxisomal Disorders (eg, adrenoleukodystrophy and others)
- Sudanophilic Leukodystrophy
- Pelizaeus-Merzbacher Disease (proteolipid protein deficiency)
- Alexander Disease
- Canavan Disease, perhaps
- Salla Disease (sialic acid storage disease)
- Sjogren-Larsson syndrome
- Aicardi-Gutieres pleocytosis syndrome
- Niemann-Pick Disease (Type A & B = sphyngomyelinase deficiency)
- GM2 Gangliosidosis
- Cockayne syndrome (periventricular clacification)

Type 1 = Classic type

Type 2 = Prenatal onset

- Cholesterol Metabolism Disorders

Cerebrotendinous xanthomatosis

Niemann-Pick disease Type C

Cholesterol Ester Storage Disease

Smith-Lemli-Opitz Syndrome (Cholesterol synthesis defect)

- Lipodystrophy
- Atypical Leprechaunism
- Dandy-Walker syndrome
- Myelinopathia centralis diffusa
- Childhood Onset Ataxia with Cerebral Hypomyelination (CACH) (previously called hypomyelination with atrophy in basal ganglia and cerebellum (H-ABC) and "vanishing white matter disease")

Myelinolysis

- Hexachlorophene toxicity
- Cuprizon toxicity
- B_{12} deficiency
- Amino acidopathies

Serine deficiency in CSF

Homocystinuria: methylenetetrahydrofolate reductase deficiency

Folate defects

Methioninemia

- Organic acidopathies

Methylmalonic aciduria

Maple syrup urine disease

L-2-hydroxyglutaric aciduria

Glutaric aciduria (II) (multiple acyl CoA dehydrogenase deficiency)

Ethylmalonic aciduria

4-hydroxybutyric aciduria

Carnitine deficiency

Riboflavin deficiency

- Urea Cycle defects (especially ornithine transcarbamylase deficiency)
- Lowe syndrome
- Reye syndrome
- Glycogen Storage Disease (cerebral glycogenosis)
- Central pontine myelinolysis
- Marchiafava-Bignami disease
  Spongy degeneration of infancy and childhood
- Canavan-Van Bogaert Bertrand disease (aspartoacylase deficiency)
- Coeliac disease
  Type II carbonic anhydrase deficiency (often with occipital calcification)
- Intrathecal Methotrexate toxicity
- Oculodentodigital dysplasia syndrome
- Hepatic encephalopathy
  18q- syndrome (never achieves true myelination)
- Acute calcific myelinolysis of Boltshauser
- Periventricular Leukomalacia
- Binswanger disease
- Hypoxic encephalopathy
- Diffuse axonal injury from trauma
- Congenital disorder of glycoprotein synthesis
- Smith-Lemli-Opitz syndrome (7-dehydrocholesterol reductase)
- Lipodystrophy
- Atypical leprechaunism
- Dandy-Walker syndrome
- Mitochondrial disorders (sometimes with periventricular calcification)
- Pyruvate dehydrogenase deficiency
- Leigh syndrome
- MELAS
- Cytochrome C oxidase deficiency
- Complex I deficiency
- Mitochondrial ATP Synthase deficiency
- Pyruvate Carboxylase deficiency
- Kearns-Sayre syndrome
- MNGIE

• MERRF (tRNA substitution)

• LHON

• Lactic acidoses

• Glutaric Aciduria

Demyelination

• Multiple sclerosis

• HIV encephalopathy

• Acute disseminated encephalomyelitis

• Progressive multifocal leukoencephalopathy

• Post-infectious (multifocal) leukoencephalopathy

(Periventricular leukomalacia)

(Binswanger disease)

(Hypoxic encephalopathy)

(Diffuse axonal injury from trauma)

(Idiopathic polyneuritis ((Landry-Güillain-Barré)) rarely is associated with focal CNS demyelination)

6. Causes of Neurodegeneration

Neurodegeneration is defined as the loss of milestones. The most common presentations of neurodegenerative disorders include:

• Severe developmental delay (motor or cognitive or loss of vision)

• Developmental stagnation

• Intractable or myoclonic seizures

• Ataxia or movement disorder

• Bizarre behavior

The causes are vast, although most are rare. The "universe" of neurodegenerative disorders can be divided into four categories: extraneural causes; simultaneous extraneural and neural causes; primary neural, but not destructive causes; and primary neural destructive causes.

Extraneural Causes (progressive neurological dysfunction caused by etiologies that first damage tissue outside the nervous system, which result in secondary neurological dysfunction or damage)

• Thyroid dysfunction (hypo- and hyperthyroidism)

• Adrenal insufficiency

• Coeliac disease

• Hepatic encephalopathies (Crigler-Najjar syndrome, organic and aminoacidopathies)

• Renal encephalopathies

• Porphyria

• Malnutrition and vitamin deficiencies

• Hypo-and pseudohypoparathyroidism and Fahr disease

• Galactosemia and fructosemia

• Sulfite oxidase deficiency

Simultaneous Extraneural and Neural Causes (damage simultaneously to neural and non-neural tissues)

- Vasculitides and connective tissue diseases
- Wilson disease
- Menke disease
- Syphilis
- Lyme disease
- Cerebral brucellosis
- Chronic cerebral parasites
- Chronic infections associated with immunodeficiency, and cerebral HIV infection
- Post-infectious encephalitides with demyelination
- Sydenham chorea and pediatric autoimmune neuropsychiatric disorders associated with *streptococcus* infections (PANDAS)
- Subacute Sclerosing Panencephalitis
- Neoplastic metastases
- Paraneoplastic syndromes (eg, neuroblastoma opsoclonus myoclonus syndrome)
- Toxins (heavy metals, chronic drugs of abuse, methylphenyltetrahydropyridine (MPTP))
- Chronic head trauma and chronic subdural hematomas
- Repeated child abuse
- Chronic inflammatory myopathy and demyelinating neuropathy
- Late onset radiation neurodegeneration
- Sarcoid
- Urea cycle defects
- Progressive vascular malformations and moyamoya disease
- Carbonic anhydrase I deficiency
- Purine nucleoside phosphorylase deficiency
- Cerebrotendinous xanthomatosis
- Abetalipoproteinemia
- Osteopetrosis

Primary Neural, Non-destructive Causes

- Intractable epilepsy
- Psychoses
- Behavioral disorders
- Severe depression

Primary Neural Destructive Causes (direct damage to any component of the nervous system directly)

- Lysosomal storage diseases
- Disorders of mitochondrial oxidative phosphorylation

Mitochondrial Encephalomyopathy with Lactic Acidosis and Stroke-like Episodes (MELAS)

Myoclonic Epilepsy with Ragged Red Fibers (MERRF)

Leigh Subacute Necrotizing Encephalomyelopathy

Barth syndrome

Progressive External Ophthalmoplegia and Kearns-Sayre Syndrome

Neurodegeneration Ataxia with Retinitis Pigmentosa (NARP)

Leber Hereditary Optic Neuropathy

Various mitochondrial encephalopathies, neuropathies, myopathies and multisystem disorders

Myopathies and encephalopathies of mitochondrial fatty acid oxidation with or without rhabdomyolysis

- Disorders of peroxisomal function

  Neonatal Adrenoleukodystrophy

  X-linked Adrenoleukodystrophy

  Adrenomyeloneuropathy

  Leber Hereditary Amaurosis

  Refsum Disease

  Neonatal Refsum Disease

  Zellweger Cerebrohepatorenal Syndrome

  Other Peroxisomal Disease Variants

- Disorders of organic and amino acids
- Disorders of the golgi apparatus (congenital disorders of glycoprotein synthesis)
- Disorders of purine and pyrimidine metabolism (eg, Lesch—Nyhan hyperuricemia)
- Leukodystrophies
- Disorders of expansion genes, neural survival genes, etc.

  Friedreich ataxia

  Dentatorubropallidoluysian atrophy

  Familial ataxias

  Spinocerebellar ataxias

  Familial and chronic demyelinating neuropathies (Charcot-Marie-Tooth, Dejerine-Sotas, etc.)

- Familial Dystonias
- Juvenile Parkinsonism
- Juvenile Huntington disease (often presents as parkinsonism before chorea)
- Lafora polyglucosan body disease (myopathy and myoclonus)
- Familial Spastic Paraplegia
- Muscular dystrophies, spinomuscular atrophies, and neuropathies (including Fazio-Londe disease)
- Neuroaxonal Dystrophies
- Schindler disease

Neurodegeneration with brain iron deposition (NBID; formerly Hallervorden-Spatz)

- Seitelberger syndrome
- Ataxia telangiectasia
- Ceroid Lipofuscinosis

  Infantile form (Haltia-Santavuori)

  Late Infantile form (Jansky-Bielschowsky)

  Juvenile form (Spielmeyer-Sjogren)

  Young adult form (Kufs)

- Disorders of Neurotransmitter Metabolism

  Dopa responsive dystonia

  GTP cyclohydrolase deficiency

  Tyrosine hydroxylase deficiency

  Disorders of Pterin metabolism

- Untreated hydrocephalus

- Cerebral and spinal malignancies
- Canavan disease
- Alexander disease
- Neurophakomatoses (eg, neurofibromatosis, tuberous sclerosis)
- Ectodermal dysplasia (eg, trichothiodystrophy)
- Primary Lateral Sclerosis
- Alper Spongioform Hepatoencephalopathy
- Neuroacanthocytosis
- Neurodegenerative disorders with progressive sensorineural hearing loss

7. Hereditary Ataxias

The hereditary ataxias are a list of disorders with the common salient symptom of ataxia. They are derived from many causes, thus each disorder is extracted from one of the etiological categories described above. They are arranged under their symptoms here, because that is another convenient way to remember them. It is also important to remember that ataxia itself can be caused by any combination of cerebellar disease, vestibular disease, upper motor neuron disease, lower motor neuron disease, or sensory neuropathy.

Metabolic Ataxias

Progressive Unremitting Ataxia

- Mitochondrial encephalomyopathies (including the Marinesco-Sjögren syndrome, which may be an early name for mitochondrial neurodegeneration with ataxia and retinitis pigmentosa)
- Refsum peroxisomal disease
- Abetalipoproteinemia
- Neuroacanthocytosis
- Cerebrotendinous xanthomatosis
- Hexosaminidase deficiency
- Leukodystrophies

Intermittent Ataxia

- Pyruvate dehydrogenase deficiency
- Hartnup disease
- Intermittent branched-chain ketoaciduria (maple syrup urine)
- Urea cycle defects

Chromosomal DNA Repair Failure

- Ataxia telangiectasia
- Xeroderma pigmentosa
- Cockayne syndrome

Table 20

Neurological Disorders Presenting as Psychiatric Symptoms

Disorders of small molecules and micronutrients

1. Hypocalcemic disorders
2. Wilson disease
3. Non-Wilsonian disorders of copper metabolism with dementia
4. Neurodegeneration with brain iron deposition (formerly called Hallervorden-Spatz)
5. Leigh disease
6. Tyrosinemia (with ALAuria)
7. Porphyria (with or without polyneuropathy)
8. B_{12} deficiency (with elevated methyl malonate and homocystine)
9. Niacin deficiency (dementia, diarrhea, dermatitis (pellagra))
10. Toxins (heavy metals; drugs of abuse; meds; plants)

Disorders of large molecules

1. Andrade polyneuropathy
2. Lafora-body myoclonic epilepsy
3. Neuronal ceroid-lipofuscinosis
4. Gaucher
5. Niemann-Pick disease
6. Mucopolylsaccharidoses
7. Schilder disease with or without adrenal atrophy
8. Refsum disease
9. Adrenoleukodystrophy
10. Nonspecific sudanophilic leukodystrophy
11. Metachromatic leukodystrophy
12. Globoid cell leukodystrophy (Krabbe disease)
13. Mucolipidosis type I (sialidosis type I)
14. Adult Gm2 Gangliosidosis

Other

1. Huntington chorea
2. Nonconvulsive status epilepticus and PLEDS (periodic lateralized epileptiform distarges)
3. Confusional migraine
4. Coeliac
5. Lupus cerebritis
6. Thyroid dysfunction (hypo- or hyper)

Infections

1. HIV encephalopathy
2. SSPE
3. Early pneumococcal sepsis/ meningitis
4. Shigella encephalopathy
5. EBV encephalopathy
6. Cat scratch encephalopathy
7. Tertiary syphilis

Chromosomal DNA Defects and Trinucleotide Repeats

- **Childhood onset:**

  Spinocerebellar ataxias

  Friedreich ataxia

  Ramsay Hunt syndrome

X-linked recessive and mitochondrial spinocerebellar ataxia

- **Adult onset:**

  Machado-Joseph disease

  Olivopontocerebellar atrophy

  Idiopathic cerebellar atrophy

8. Neurometabolic Causes of Neuropsychiatric Syndromes

When neurometabolic diseases present as psychiatric syndromes, they do so as attention deficit (with or without hyperactivity); atypical depression or abulia; irrational behavior; oppositional defiant disorder; or atypical psychosis, acute, intermittent or chronic. Clues to an underlying neurometabolic cause are the presence of an abnormal neurological sign, such as chorea or Babinski sign, or the coexistence of epilepsy. A list of neurological disorders that present with psychiatric symptoms is in Table 20.

9. Conclusions, Misconceptions and Hazardous Pearls

Over the years, "clinical pearls" were taught to help simplify diagnosis of neurometabolic disease. These did increase the efficiency of finding some of these rare diseases. The last two decades' progress of biochemical neurogenetics has shown some of these pearls to be unreliable, or potentially misleading. Some of the pearls can lead a clinician to exclude diseases prematurely. The following are a discussion of some of these hazards of differential diagnosis.

It was once taught that malformations imply large chromosomal defects, by virtue of the thought that the large portion of DNA disrupted by the large chromosomal defect affects many enzymes and structural proteins. It is true that large chromosomal defects often cause congenital malformations. However, it is also true that small molecule diseases can cause dysmorphic features. This is the concept known as metabolic dysplasia: whereby the presence in the fetus of a toxic metabolite, or the absence of a useful metabolite, can cause abnormality of organogenesis. Three examples are instructive, each of which has been presented above. The first example is that pyruvate dehydrogenase deficiency can cause the same facial features as fetal alcohol syndrome. This is probably because the primary toxic agent in fetal alcohol syndrome is acetaldehyde, which is toxic to the pyruvate dehydrogenase. Another example is that of Smith-Lemli-Opitz syndrome, which is a multisystem dysplastic syndrome manifested by characteristic facial features, hypotonia, hypospadias, 2-3 syndactyly, mental impairment, and a panoply of neurological symptoms. It is caused by a deficiency of 7-dehydrocholesterol reductase. This causes an excess of 7-dehydrocholesterol and a deficiency of cholesterol, which disrupts organogenesis and neural and myelin formation. Symptoms are improved by treatment with large doses of cholesterol. The third example is that of Zellweger cerebrohepatorenal syndrome. It is caused by defective peroxisomal function, and is described above. The lesson of all of these examples is that when one is called to diagnose the cause of a malformation syndrome, it may be prudent to check chromosomes and subtelomeric studies, but other disorders cannot yet be excluded by presumption. It is useful to look, also, for the hallmarks of small and large molecule diseases, such as metabolic acidosis, or organomegaly, and screen for these disorders. In short, ***malformations can be caused by small molecule diseases, large molecule diseases, or chromosomal defects.***

It has crept into the thoughts of clinicians that a protein load is the only way to find metabolic disease, and, by extension, that a newborn who has not yet fed will not display the neurological effects of an organic acidemia or aminoacidemia. As a result, it is generally advised to obtain a newborn screen (blood spot) test for metabolic disease after the child has been fed. This may be prudent, because diseases such as phenylketonuria and branched chain amino acidopathy (maple syrup urine disease) exhibit increased urinary excretion of their unmetabolized intermediates after the patient is given a protein load from milk. In contrast, however, for some diseases a fasting state can be the best stressor to make some diseases manifest, such as is found with the hypoketotic hypoglycemia of fatty acid beta-oxidation disorders. The lesson is that it may be necessary to obtain urine amino acids and organic acids during both the fasting and the protein loaded state if the diagnosis of a suspected metabolic disorder remains elusive. In short, ***some organic and amino acidopathies can be diagnosed on newborn screen during the fasting state.***

It was once taught to pediatricians that it was not necessary to test for neurometabolic disease unless the patient had loss of milestones. The truth is that neurodegenerative disease is often neurometabolic, but neurometabolic disease is not always degenerative. Often, the patient fails to develop well, and may have no loss of milestones ever, or perhaps only after a febrile illness or the onset of seizures many years later; an affected patient may thereafter stay at a diminished, but steady state. This is exemplified by glutaric aciduria type I, which is caused by glutaryl CoA dehydrogenase deficiency. These children may be born macrocephalic, but are otherwise normal. At some time, usually during a viral syndrome, they develop an acute encephalitic-like crisis. This crisis is characterized by acute necrosis of the caudate and putamen, sometimes also with frontotemporal atrophy, and they are left with severe dystonia, choreoathetosis, dyskinesia, seizures and spasticity. If, however, a person with glutaryl CoA dehydrogenase deficiency is treated with the proper diet and passes through the age of seven years without this encephalitic-like crisis, the child will have no deterioration and will be functionally normal. Similar phenomena are found in other diseases. The lesson is that if one waits to test for neurometabolic disease on only patients with neurodegeneration, it is possible that some patients will develop severe disease, and neurometabolic diseases will be missed. Instead, refer to the indications to test for neurometabolic disease, in addition to neurodegeneration, listed at the beginning of this chapter. In short, ***neurometabolic diseases do not always present as neurodegeneration.***

It is commonly taught to medical students that it is best to follow the principle of parsimony: look for a single cause of disease that accounts for all symptoms. In the case of neurometabolic disease, there is usually a nexus of causality that involves a "Triple Risk Model" of disease. In this model, three factors are required to bring on illness: 1.) A host factor (in this case, a genetic disorder of metabolism); 2.) A developmental proclivity (such as the pre-7 year old risk period for glutaric aciduria type I; and 3.) A trigger, such as a viral syndrome, birth, trauma, dehydration, or even menses, that causes a shift toward catabolism or dependence on the dysfunctional metabolic pathway that, in turn, leads to a deterioration of neural function. That deterioration can be sudden, as in the case of the Reye-like syndrome, or the encephalitic-like syndrome, or intermittent ataxia. Alternately, that deterioration can be slow or subacute, and lead to gradual neurodegeneration, or intermittent minor declines. With this triple-risk model in mind, the lesson is that if a patient has a severe form of a common viral illness, it may be prudent when possible to perform a few screening tests for metabolic disease, such as testing for unexplained or persistent acidosis. There is a corollary to this. Each individual neurometabolic disease can present with a variety of severities in different patients, depending on the severity of the underlying gene defect, social or other circumstances during the particular critical biochemical developmental period of presentation, or the severity of the trigger (viral or otherwise). Therefore, a laboratory or clinical test for a neurometabolic disease may be normal when the patient is not acutely ill, or when the child is young, as in the case of late childhood or adult onset disorders. The triple risk model of disease does not dispel the principle of parsimony, as the patient's neurometabolic disease still remains the fundamental cause of symptoms. However, the triple risk model modifies the principle of parsimony, and puts it into the broader context of developmental physiology, common exogenous triggers, and biopsychosocial complexities. Some will be uncomfortable with this idea of modifying the principle of parsimony, which has also been called "Occam's razor" or the "KISS" principle ("keep it simple, stupid"). However, Occam himself described the principle as follows: "Entities should not be multiplied more than necessary." There are many situations, however, where the simplest solution is not accurate and not sufficient, and it is necessary to modify the simple solution. (As if to symbolize that modification of his principle is often necessary, even the name "Occam" has been spelled in several official varieties, including "Occum," and "Ockham.") In short, ***the principle of parsimony can lead to missing the diagnosis of neurometabolic disease, if it is not coupled with an awareness of the triple-risk model of disease.***

The final note concerns the problem of missing one of these diagnoses. Each disease is rare. Most are complex. Most of them present non-specifically, or mimic more common diseases. They may be missed because they first become manifest during a simultaneous febrile illness or other stress, which obscures the coexistent neurometabolic disease. At the time that many of the readers of this chapter were in training, some of these diseases were not yet discovered, or their diagnosis was not provable without autopsy, or the disorders were not taught in our training institutions or textbooks. Progress has moved so rapidly in genomics and biochemistry that some of what is written in this chapter may be outdated by the time it is published. The reader will never encounter most of these diseases, or will be asked to assist with management only once or twice in a career. The barriers to sharing management over great distances are daunting, and we cannot expect that all such patients can be sent away to large academic centers for care. Moreover, we all feel loyalty to the people of our geographical region, and feel a strong obligation to provide as much service as we can to our fellow community members. Before a diagnosis is made, the patient's care is impeded severely without the guidance derived from a confirmed diagnosis. It is always very disturbing that it can take months before a diagnosis is known. This delay can occur even if the clinicians have a high suspicion that some neurometabolic disease is present, and even with expert and ardent diagnostic effort. All this occurs under constant urgent pressure to provide simultaneous care for the sick patient as well as all other patients under our care. Patients may benefit from us explaining to them how long it may be to make a full diagnosis; they need courage to continue the diagnostic process. Rarely is there a situation where the title of "patient" is more appropriate, because rarely does a patient and family require more patience than in the evaluation of a potential neurometabolic disease. Their strain against the disease is magnified by uncertainty. The effort is enough to make clinician, patient and family lament. With such burdens, it is unreasonable to expect that we would never miss one of these diagnoses, or miss an aspect of management. It is more unfortunate for our communities if anxiety over the risks associated with diagnosing and managing these diseases were to block us from engaging as active participants. Instead, it can be a goal of a compassionate, concerned, and competent clinical environment to keep these diagnoses in the differential diagnosis, to utilize newborn screens whenever they are available, to encourage the expansion of reliable newborn screening, and to share the load of diagnosis and management with colleagues. Despite our efforts, perfection is not possible. It is this chapter's intent, however, to assist you as you provide children and their families with your scientific acts of caring.

Appendix of Tables and Figures

Appendix Figure 1

Hypoglycemia

Diagnostic Algorithm

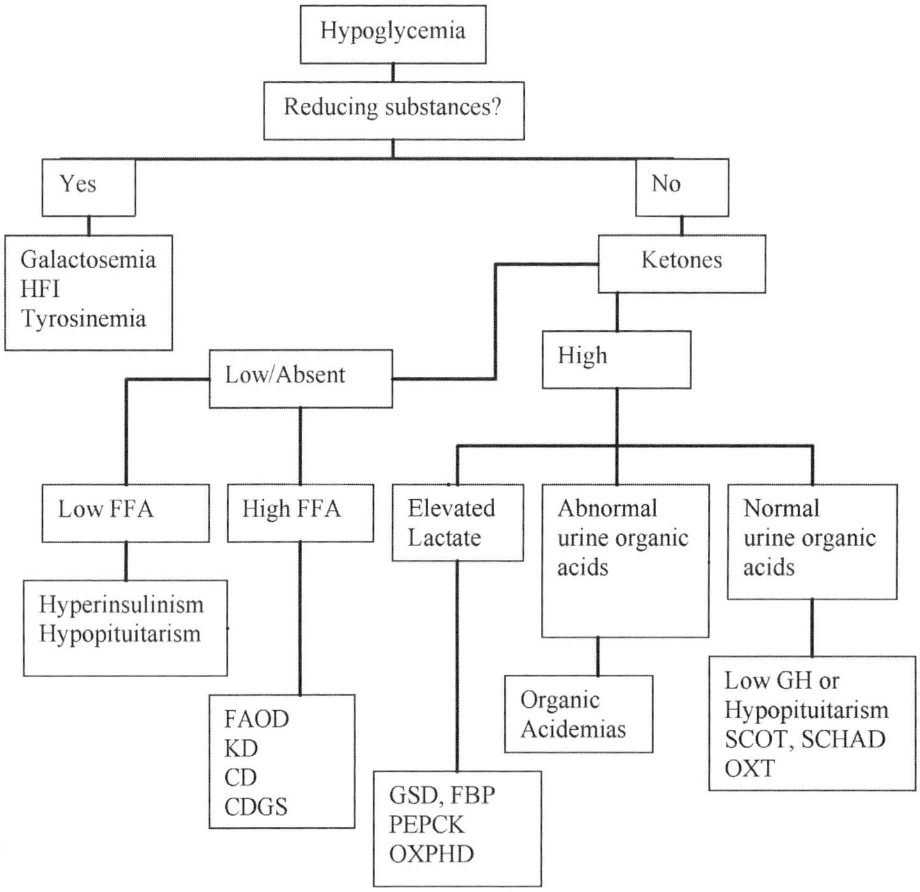

CD, carnitine shuttle disorders; CDG, Congenital disorders of glycoprotein synthesis; FAOD, fatty acid oxidation disorder; FBP, fructose 1,6 bisphosphatase deficiency; FFA, free fatty acids; GH, growth hormone; GSD, glycogen storage disease (especially types 0, 1 and 3); HFI, hereditary fructose intolerance; HMG, both 3-hydroxy 3-methylglutaryl CoA lyase and synthase deficiency; KD, ketogenesis disorders (eg, HMG CoA lyase deficiency); OXPHD, mitochondrial oxidation phosphorylation disorders including pyruvate carboxylase deficiency; OXT, 3 oxothiolase (acetoacetyl CoA lyase) deficiency; PEPCK, phosphoenolpyruvate carboxykinase deficiency; SCHAD, short chain 3-hydroxyacyl CoA dehydrogenase deficiency; SCOT, succinyl CoA:3 oxoacid CoA transferase deficiency. Test blood glucose, uric acid, ammonia, lactate, ketones, free fatty acids and insulin; test urine ketones, reducing substances, amino acids, organic acids.

Appendix Table 1

Causes of Urine Reducing Substances

Compound	Disorders or Source
Glucose	Diabetes mellitus Renal Franconi Syndrome
Galactose	Galactosemia Severe Liver Disease
Fructose	Hereditary Fructose intolerance Essential Fructosuria
Xylose	Pentosuria
4-Hydroxyphenylpyruvic acid	Tyrosinemia
Homogentisic acid	Alkaptonuria
Oxalic Acid	Hyperoxaluria
Uric Acid	Hyperuricosuria
Ascorbic acid	Exogenous administration
Salicylates	Exogenous administration

Appendix Figure 2

Metabolic acidosis

Diagnostic Algorithm

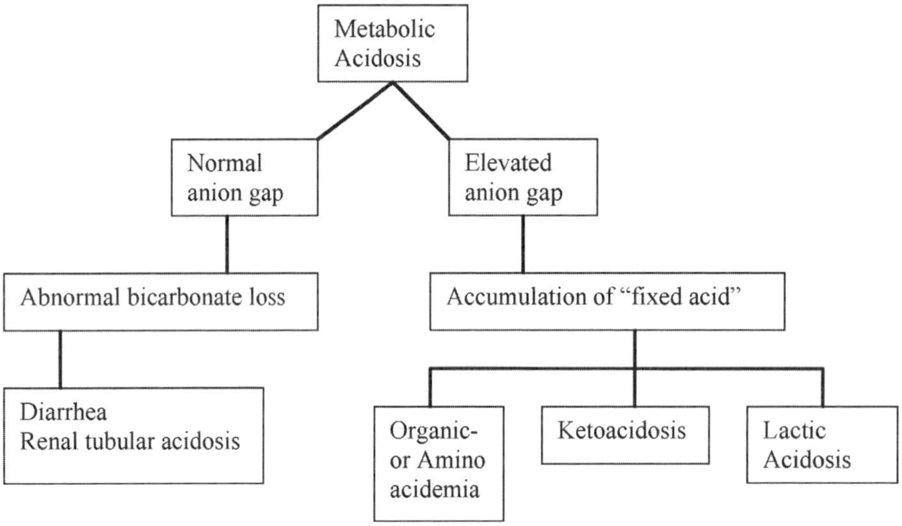

Appendix Figure 3

Lactic acidosis

Diagnostic Algorithm

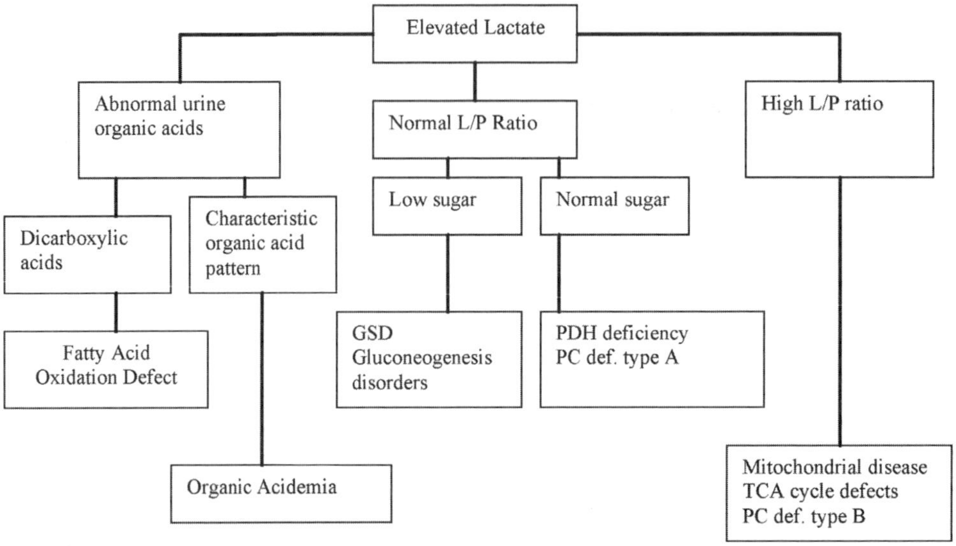

GSD, glycogen storage disease; L/P ratio, lactate/pyruvate ratio; PC def., pyruvate carboxylase deficiency; PDH, pyruvate dehydrogenase; TCA, tricarboxylic acid cycle.

Appendix Figure 4

Hyperammonemia

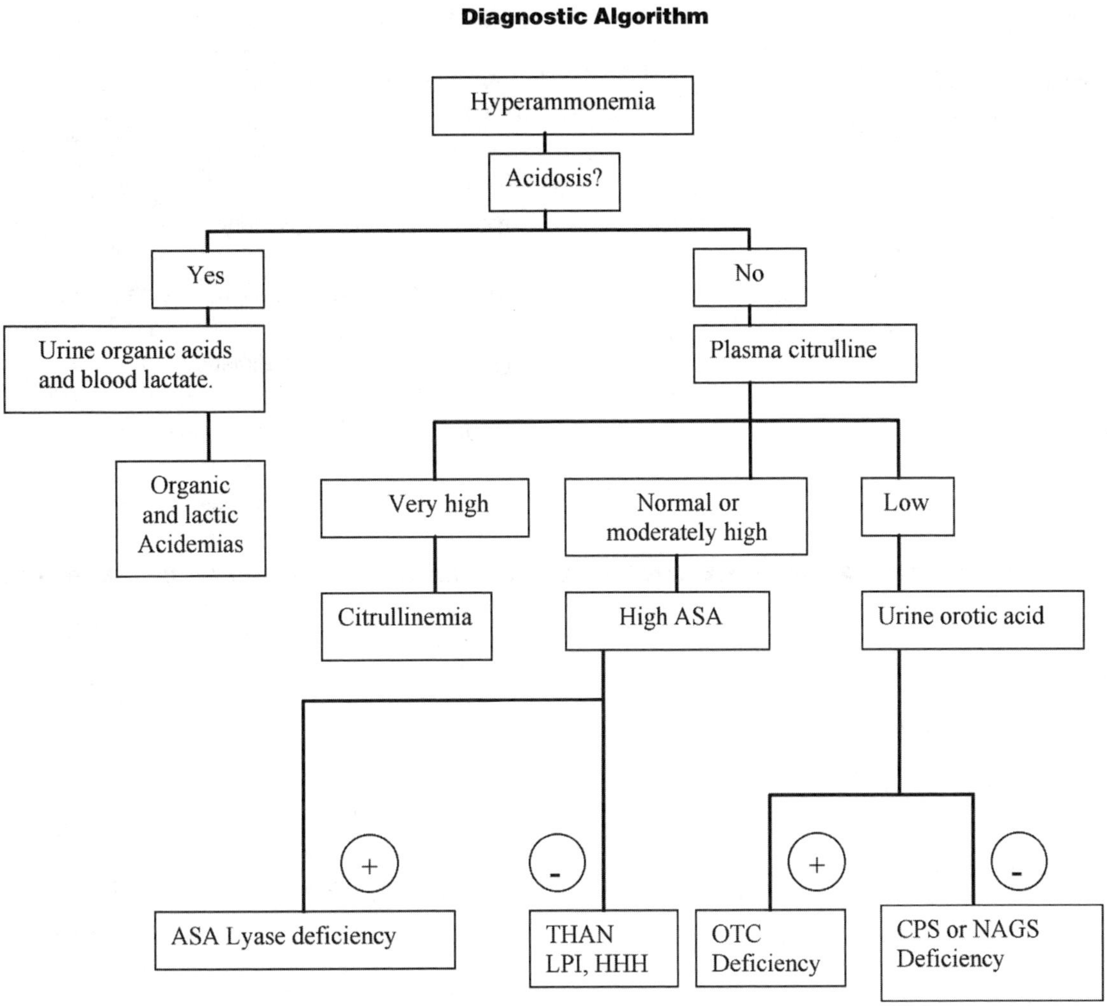

ASA, argininosuccinic acid; CPS, carbamyl phosphate synthase; HHH, hyperammonemia hyperornithinemia homocitrullinuria; LPI, lysinuric protein intolerance; NAGS, N-acetylglutamate synthase; OTC, ornithine transcarbamylase; THAN, transient hyperammonemia of the newborn. Test plasma and urine amino acids to find level of citrulline and low proline (fasting hyperammonemia), and high lysine in LPI and ASA; urine organic acids; blood lactate; urine orotic acid.

Appendix Table 2

Causes of Angioketatoma Corporis Diffusum

Fabry disease	(alpha-galactosidase A deficiency)
GM1 gangliosidosis	(acid beta-galactosidase deficiency)
Beta-Mannosidosis	(beta-mannosidase deficiency)
Galactosialidosis	(protective protein deficiency)
Sialidosis	(alpha-L-N-acetyl-neuraminidase deficiency)
Fucosidosis	(alpha-L-fucosidase deficiency)
Schindler disease	(N-acetylgalactosaminidase deficiency)
Hallervordern-Spatz disease type II	(Japanese N-acetylgalactosaminidase deficiency)

Appendix Table 3

Neurometabolic Causes of Cataracts

- Abetalipoproteinemia
- Alpha-mannosidosis
- Alport syndrome
- Cerebrotendinous xanthomatosis
- Cockayne syndrome
- Diabetes mellitus
- Galactosmia
- G6PD deficiency
- Hypoglycemia of various causes
- Hypoparathyroidism and Pseudohypoparathyroidism
- Lactose intolerance
- Lowe syndrome (X-linked)
- Lysinuric protein intolerance
- Menke disease
- Metachromatic leukodystrophy
- Mevalonic aciduria
- Mitochondrial Ox/Phos disorders
- Myotonic dystrophy (Steinert type)
- Neutral lipid storage disorders
- Nonketotic hyperglycinemia
- Ornithine aminotransferase deficiency
- Peroxisomal diseases
- Sialidosis
- Sjögren-Larsson fatty alcohol oxidoreductase deficiency
- Sorbitoldehydrogenase deficiency (isolated cataracts)
- Vitamin D deficiency
- Vitamin E deficiency
- Wilson disease
- Other neurogenetic syndromes

Appendix Table 4

Neurometabolic Causes of Retinitis Pigmentosa

- Abetalipoproteinemia
- Alsthom syndrome
- Ceroid lipofuscinoses
- Cobalamin metabolism defects
- Cockayne syndrome
- Congenital disorders of glycoprotein synthesis
- 3-hydroxy-acyl CoA dehydrogenase deficiency
- Joubert syndrome
- Laurence-Moon and Bardet-Biedl syndromes
- Mitochondrial Ox/Phos disorders
- Neurodegeneration with brain iron deposition
- Peroxisomal diseases
- Senior-Loken syndrome
- Sjögren-Larsson fatty alcohol oxidoreductase deficiency
- Usher syndrome type II
- Vitamin E deficiency (malabsorption)
- Other neurogenetic syndromes

Appendix Table 5

Additional Genes Associated with Severe or Intractable Epilepsy

SCN1A and SCN1B: "Generalized epilepsy with febrile seizures plus" (GEFS+). These genes code for voltage gated sodium channel subunits; they also involve gamma 2 subunits of the $GABA_A$ receptors.

KCNQ2 and KCNQ3: Benign familial neonatal convulsions (BFNC). These genes code for voltage gated K+ channels.

CHRNA4, CHRNB: Autosomal Dominant Familial Nocturnal Frontal Lobe Epilepsy (ADNFLE). These genes code for parts of the neuronal acetylcholine receptor.

Appendix Table 6

Genes Associated with Autism and Mental Retardation

- NLGN3; chromosome Xq28.3; neural synapse formation.
- NLGN4X; chromosome Xq28.33; neural synapse formation.
- ARX; chromosome Xp22.13; homeobox gene.
- X-linked mental retardation genes: PQBP1, JARID1C, TM4SF2, FACL4, DIG3, FTSJ1, ZNF41, and STK9.
- UBE3A gene; chromosome 15Q11-Q13; Angelman syndrome encodes ubiquitin protein ligase.
- ATP10C; chromosome 15q11.2-q12; phospholipid transporter for central nervous system developmental signaling.
- NF1; chromosome 17q11.2; RAS protein regulation.
- Chromosome 2q31-33; gene not specified; partially tested at 2q31.1; DLX1 and DLX2 gene of split hand/foot malformation 5; and also the HOXD gene cluster for synpolydactyly and syndactyly.
- SLC25A12 gene; chromosome 2q24; mitochondrial aspartate and glutamate carrier protein.
- Chromosome 2q31-33; gene not specified.
- Chromosome 3q25-27; gene not specified.
- Chromosome 6q14; gene not specified.
- C4B; chromosome 6p21; complement component.
- GLO1; chromosome 6p21; zinc metalloenzyme oxoaldehyde scavenger.
- GRIK2; chromosome 6p21; glutamate receptor 6 involved in neural development.
- HOXA1; chromosome 7p15-p14.2; homeobox gene for hindbrain development.
- RELN; chromosome 7q22.1; signaling protein for neural migration.
- WNT2; chromosome 7q31; signaling protein in embryonic patterning, cell proliferation and cell determination.
- FOXP2; chromosome 7q31; transcription factor in embryogenesis and neural function.
- UBE2H; chromosome 7q32; ubiquitin-dependent proteolysis enzyme.
- EN2; chromosome 7q36.2; homeobox gene in midbrain and cerebellum development.
- PTEN; chromosome 10q23.31; tumor suppressor.
- HRAS; chromosome 11p15.5; oncogene GTPase in cell division, differentiation and apoptosis.
- AVPR1A; chromosome 12q14-q15; arginine vasopressin receptor involved in social behavior.
- Chromosome 13q21; gene not specified.
- Chromosome 16p13; gene not specified.
- GABRB3, GABRA5, GABRG3; chromosome 15q11.2-q12; GABA receptor subunits.
- SLC6A4; chromosome 17q11.1-q12; serotonin transporter.
- HOXB1; chromosome 17q21-q22; homeobox gene for hindbrain development.
- Chromosome 17q31; gene not specified.
- APOE2; chromosome 19q13.2; lipoprotein receptor for neuronal migration and lipid transport.
- Chromosome 19q13.2; gene not specified.

10. References

Birnbaum DC, Shields D, et al. Idiopathic Central Diabetes Insipidus Followed by Progressive Spastic Cerebral Ataxia. *Arch Neurol*. 1989;46:1001-1003.

(This reference is a first clinical description of its topic.)

Cooley, WC. *Down Syndrome*. Elsevier, Philadelphia. 2005:1060-1064.

(This is a superb comprehensive summary of complications and management of this most common of chromosomal defects.)

Enns GM, Steiner RD. Diagnosis and Treatment of Children with Suspected Metabolic Disease in: *Pediatrics*. Osborn LM, et al, eds. Elsevier, Philadelphia. 2005:1866-1875.

(This summary explores the chemistry and laboratory confirmation of suspected diagnoses of diseases of small molecules, and is the source of several of the Appendix Tables.)

Filiano JJ, Kinney HC. A Perspective on Neuropathologic Findings in Victims of the Sudden Infant Death Syndrome: The Triple Risk Model. *Biol Neonate*. 1994;65:194-197.

(This reference elaborates on the concept of the triple risk model of disease, which is useful to modify a diagnostic process based on the principle of parsimony.)

Filiano JJ. Neurometabolic Disease in: Coffey J, Jenkyn L., eds. *Neurology Board Review Guide*. Greenwich, Clinical Communications; 1995.

(This is the original source of the study questions that accompany this chapter.)

Filiano JJ, Goldenthal MJ, Rhodes CH, Marin-Garcia J. Mitochondrial dysfunction in patients with hypotonia, epilepsy, autism, and developmental delay: HEADD syndrome. *J Child Neurol*. 2001;17(6):435-9.

(This reviews a syndrome associated with disorders of the mitochondrial electron transport chain, and helps clarify at what threshold to test for mitochondrial disease in a patient with autistic symptoms, so that patients do not undergo a fruitless search for the cause of autism in every affected child.)

Filiano J, Olson A. Neurodegenerative Diseases in: *Pediatrics*. Osborn LM, et al, eds. Elsevier, Philadelphia. 2005.

(This reference details the differential diagnosis of undiagnosed neurodegenerative disease in pediatric patients.)

Jess G. Thoene, Nancy P. Coker. *Physicians' Guide to Rare Diseases*, 2nd ed. Dowden Publishing, New Jersey; 1995.

(This is a classic, comprehensive reference that summarizes the presentation, diagnosis, prognosis, and treatment of many rare metabolic diseases and syndromes, and includes addresses of investigators and family support groups for each disease.)

Kim S, Westphal V, Srikrishna G, Mehta DP, Peterson S, Filiano J, Karnes PS, Patterson MC, Freeze HH. Dolichol phosphate mannose synthase (DPM1) mutations define congenital disorder of glycosylation Ie (CDG-Ie). *J Clin Invest*. 2000;105(2):131-2.

(This reference reviews the concept of congenital disorders of glycosylation in the context of describing the first elucidation of a new form of this class of disorders.)

Kuban KK, Filiano JJ. Neonatal Seizures in: *Manual of Neonatal Care*, 3rd ed. Cloherty JP, Stark AR, eds. Little Brown, Boston. 3rd ed. 1991:367-381.

(This reference is a summary of causes of neonatal seizures, with a discussion of metabolic causes. It clarifies the limits of attributing hypoxia-ischemia as the cause of "cerebral palsy," and discusses the data to support the use of the term of "neonatal encephalopathy.")

Leslie ND. Principles of Metabolism in: *Pediatrics*. Osborn LM, et al, eds. Elsevier, Philadelphia. 2005, 110-121.

(This is a relatively sophisticated summary of principles of metabolic disease written for pediatricians, from the perspective of a metabolic specialist.)

Lockman LA. Coma in: *The Practice of Pediatric Neurology*. Swaiman K., ed. CV Mosby, St. Louis; 1982:150.

(This is the source of the summary of physical findings as clues to the cause of coma.)

Lyon L, Adams RD, Kolodny EH. *Neurology of Hereditary Metabolic Diseases of Children*, 2nd ed. McGraw-Hill, New York, 1996.

(This is a classic reference on neurometabolic disease, with an emphasis on neurological presentation of lysosomal storage diseases and childhood dementia.)

Nyhan WL, Ozand PT. *Atlas of Metabolic Diseases*. Chapman & Hall Medical, London, 1998.

(This is a recent summary of clinical and biochemical aspects of metabolic disease written by people who have devoted their very productive professional lives to this topic. It is an excellent reference to read once a diagnosis is made, or when a neurologist is encountering a patient whose neurometabolic disease has been established.)

Steinlein OK, et al. Genes and mutations in idiopathic epilepsy. *Am J Med Gen*. 2001;106:139-145.

Rosenberg RN, Prusiner SB, DiMauro S, Barchi RL. *The Molecular and Genetic Basis of Neurological Disease*, 2nd ed. Butterworth-Heinemann, Boston, 1997.

(This is an authoritative reference that explores many neurometabolic diseases in depth.)

Jones KL. *Smith's Recognizable Patterns of Human Malformation,* 5th ed. Saunders, Philadelphia, 1997.

(This is the classic compendium of malformation syndromes and chromosomal disorders. It contains excellent photographs, and accessible summaries of the presentations and clinical course of these syndromes.)

Victor M, Ropper AH. *Principles of Neurology*, 7th ed. McGraw-Hill, New York, 2001; pp.983-1049;1106-1174.

(This is a superb textbook of neurology. It contains concise tables and descriptions of some pediatric neurometabolic disorders.)

Wilson G, Cooley WC. *Preventive Management of Children with Congenital Anomalies and Syndromes*. Cambridge University Press, Cambridge, 2000.

(This is an excellent text on the chronic management of patients with congenital anomalies, malformation syndromes, and neurometabolic disease. It covers the life history of many diseases. It is a valuable guide for long-term management for any neurologist who follows such patients.)

Genetests.com.

(This web-based reference is funded by the United States National Institutes of Health. It provides frequently updated information on the genetic diagnostic tests used to diagnose many neurometabolic diseases. It includes phone numbers and contact information, prices, specimen types, and web links.)

Pubmed.gov/OMIM.

(This is the web site of the United States National Library of Medicine's "Online Mendelian Inheritance in Man," accessed through the *Pubmed.gov* web site. It is an annotated literature search site specific for neurometabolic and genetic diseases. It provides up-to-date summaries and references, with an emphasis on molecular genetic aspects of these diseases.)

11. Questions

True or False

1. An infant is born with a low Apgar score (depressed respiration, heart rate, level of consciousness and responsiveness, and poor motor performance). This occurred after a prolonged labor, and the infant had a persistently slow heart rate during labor. Subsequently, the infant developed seizures. Septic work-up was begun; serologic studies were sent for intrauterine infection; maternal screening for drugs of abuse was unrevealing; cerebral imaging studies showed a small amount of subarachnoid blood; blood calcium, electrolytes, magnesium, glucose, phosphorus and thyroid studies were normal, except for the evidence of mild acidosis. This is an adequate and cost-effective work-up in the acute setting. True or false?

2. Regarding the above patient, you recommend testing for inborn errors of metabolism, and are told by the pediatrician that metabolic diseases will not cause intrauterine cerebral damage or seizures on the first day of life because the mother's metabolism will purge the abnormal metabolites. You are told that inborn errors of metabolism will present only after the infant has been fed a meal containing protein. The pediatrician elects to send a blood spot newborn screen that tests only for galactosemia, maple syrup urine disease, phenylketonuria, hypothyroidism, and toxoplasmosis after day three of life. This is an adequate and cost effective plan. True or false?

3. Consider again the patient from Question 1, except that you were not consulted at the time of birth. Instead, he was treated with anticonvulsants. He is then brought to you as an eight-year-old boy who has mild "cerebral palsy" with hyper-reflexia, stable seizures and educational difficulties, and now has a worsening ataxic gait. He has neither dysmorphic features nor organomegaly, but his head circumference is 7%, whereas his BMI is 15%. Head MRI scan reveals normal myelination and minimal or equivocal atrophy. CSF evaluation, infectious work-up and standard chemistries are negative. The etiology of his neurological dysfunction should be attributed to the evolution of cerebral palsy from hypoxic-ischemic encephalopathy during a difficult birth that caused his low Apgar scores. True or false?

4. A patient cannot have a mitochondrial disease if he or she does not have lactic acidosis. True or false?

5. Most organic acidopathies and amino acidopathies are very difficult to treat. True or false?

6. Most storage diseases have infantile, juvenile, and adolescent forms. The adolescent form may begin with very subtle symptoms which progress very slowly over many years into adulthood. True or False?

Match a Finding With a Disease

Answers can be used once, more than once, or not at all.

A. Disorders of mitochondrial pyruvate metabolism

B. Disorders of peroxisomal metabolism

C. Organic acidopathy

D. Amino acidopathy

E. Sphingolipidoses

F. Mucopolysaccharidosis

G. Gaucher disease type III

H. Neimann-Pick disease type C

7. Loss of voluntary upgaze, narcolepsy

8. Wolfe-Parkinson-White syndrome, cardiac conduction defect, pigmentary retinopathy or optic atrophy

9. Cerebral cortical gray matter migration defects, seizures, large anterior fontanel, multisystem dysfunction

10. Cherry red maculae, startle myoclonus, cognitive impairment

11. Dysostosis multiplex with varying degrees of cerebral dysfunction

12. Generalized amino aciduria and phosphaturia

13. Seizures stop after therapy with biotin

14. Mild acidosis, mild cerebral hypomyelination, mild hyperammonemia, mental retardation

15. Foamy histiocytes, hepatosplenomegaly, lateral gaze paresis

Match a Finding With a Disease

Answers can be used once, more than once, or not at all.

A. Medium and long chain acyl CoA dehydrogenase deficiency

B. Disorders of peroxisomal metabolism

C. Glycogen storage disease

D. Urea cycle defect

16. Nonketotic hypoglycemia, sudden death

17. Reye syndrome, abnormal amino acids in the urine

18. Abnormal signal in cerebral white matter in MRI

19. Hepatomegaly, ketotic hypoglycemia

Match Physical Exam or History With a Lab Test

Answers can be used once, more than once, or not at all.

A. Elevated urine oligosaccharides

B. Dysostosis multiplex on plain x-ray

C. Delayed nerve conduction, mitochondrial DNA mutation

D. Photoconvulsive response on EEG

E. Angiokeratoma

F. Storage granules in white cells on electron microscopy of the buffy coat

20. Liver disease, intestinal pseudo-obstruction, esophageal dysmotility

21. Cherry red maculae

22. Visual impairment, myoclonus, developmental delay

23. Flexion at the elbows, failure to grow

24. Family history of kidney failure, early stroke, lancinating pains in extremities

25. Hepatomegaly

Answers

1. False

Sigmund Freud coined the term "cerebral palsy" to describe childhood weakness caused by a cerebral lesion. He hypothesized its primary cause was perinatal hypoxia, because neonatal resuscitation methods were primitive. He did not, however, limit the cause of neonatal cerebral injury to hypoxia. Despite rapid bag/mask ventilation and quick return to spontaneous respiration and normal heart rate and blood pressure, infants were found with cerebral injury. This was attributed to hypoxic-ischemic injury caused by prepartum vascular compromise. Despite improved methods of detecting fetal distress and resuscitating mothers and newborns, and rapid delivery, unexplained "cerebral palsy" persists. In fact, only approximately 15% of patients with cerebral palsy can be explained by definite, documented hypoxic and/or ischemic circumstances. Progress in the fields of genetics, metabolism and magnetic resonance imaging indicate that nearly 25% of what was once thought to be hypoxic-ischemic injury is found to be caused by genetic, neurometabolic, infectious or malformative factors. This, of course, leaves 60% of cerebral palsy still not explained. It is only custom, and our presumption of probability, that leads us to attribute cases of "cerebral palsy" to birth asphyxia or perinatal hypoxic ischemic encephalopathy.

With regard to the child in this question, a small amount of subarachnoid bleeding occurs in many births, and should not be considered the cause of seizures until other causes have been excluded, including metabolic diseases.

The answer is false because the work-up was neither adequate, nor "cost effective," although it was "charge reductive." The urine can be tested for ketones; if present, that may indicate the presence of the ketoacids produced by an organic acidemia. Testing of blood spot tandem mass spectrometry as well as urine for organic acids and amino acids, and blood testing of lactate and ammonia are indicated to test for treatable inborn errors of metabolism that can cause neonatal seizures. Although testing for these diseases increases charges, the lifetime cost to the patient, family, and health care system of missing a treatable disease is one million dollars, in 1998 dollars. Other metabolic disorders, most of which are untreatable currently, can be considered and tested later.

2. False

The idea that metabolic disease only presents after feeding, and no damage occurs *in utero*, is an old belief. It applies to galactosemia, maple syrup urine disease, phenylketonuria, and sometimes in urea cycle defects, but some organic acidopathies can present even before the first ingestion of milk.

Therefore, this old concept is not correct enough to be trusted to exclude diagnosis of metabolic disease. For example, congenital peroxisomal disease, such as Zellweger cerebrohepatorenal syndrome or neonatal adrenoleukodystrophy, nearly always presents with cerebral dysplasia and dysmorphic features, and early onset seizures. This is the prototype of the concept of metabolic dysplasia. This concept states that a fetal neurometabolic disease can produce a teratogenic metabolite; or alternatively, the absence of a necessary metabolite has teratogenic effects that generate dysmorphic features and lifelong neurological disability. The same occurs in some mitochondrial diseases, such as pyruvate dehydrogenase complex deficiency. Patients with glutaric aciduria type I are born with marked underdevelopment of the operculum.

3. False

Attributing cerebral palsy to hypoxia-ischemia can be made as a diagnosis of exclusion after thorough evaluation that includes testing for inborn errors of metabolism. There are a number of ways in which the newborn metabolic screen may be falsely negative. First, not all states employ the expanded newborn screen that tests for more than just galactosemia, hypothyroidism, phenylketonuria or branched-chain ketoaciduria (maple syrup urine disease). Secondly, some disorders can remain stable, but worsen later and intermittently, during times when the patient is in a catabolic state, usually from infection. The classic examples include the intermittent and intermediate forms of branched-chain ketoaciduria.

The primary lesson is that the Apgar score indicates that a neonate is "in trouble" and requires resuscitative errors. It does not specify the cause of that "trouble" and a low APGAR score is not tantamount to a diagnosis of neonatal hypoxic ischemic encephalopathy. When evaluating such infants at birth or later, such as in a "cerebral palsy clinic," it is prudent for a neurologist to resist the tendency to attribute all "cerebral palsy" to hypoxic-ischemic injury, unless there is definitive proof of ischemia or hypoxia, such as occurs in severe placental abruption. To emphasize this point, and encourage equipoise in the pursuit of neonatal diagnosis of seizures and cerebral dysfunction, Kuban and Leviton advise using the term neonatal encephalopathy instead of hypoxic ischemic encephalopathy.

4. False

Lactic acidosis develops only if there is extensive mitochondrial myopathy or mitochondrial hepatic disease. There may be no lactic acidosis if the disease is restricted to the brain, as in Leber hereditary optic neuropathy or in a syndrome of intestinal pseudo-obstruction and peripheral neuropathy without myopathy.

5. False

Just the opposite is true. Although the symptoms are severe and often irreversible in untreated cases, dietary management can be successful in eradicating nearly all symptoms in some cases diagnosed early. This dietary management can include restriction of protein and certain amino acids, or supplementation with specific vitamins, eg, biotin in multiple carboxylase deficiency.

6. True

The prototype for this is late onset GM2 gangliosidosis, which can present as mental deterioration and be diagnosed and treated as mild schizophrenia. Later, signs of upper motor neuron or basal ganglion disease develop, which can be construed as extrapyramidal symptoms from antipsychotic medications.

7. H.

8. A.

9. B.
Particularly neonatal Zellweger cerebrohepatorenal syndrome. Congenital peroxisomal disorders are not exclusively leukodystrophies, but are metabolic dysplasias with gray and white matter disease and multisystem manifestations.

10. E.

11. F.

12. A.
These features are often referred to as the renal Fanconi syndrome.

13. C.
The specific organic acidemia caused by biotinidase deficiency or multiple carboxylase deficiency.

14. A., C. or **D.**
This is a trick question meant to show that in early or even later stages, it may be difficult to separate those three categories of disease. This necessitates testing amino acids, organic acids, and lactate simultaneously.

15. G.
The foamy histiocytes are often called Gaucher cells but can also be found in Neimann-Pick disease, as can hepatosplenomegaly. What distinguishes Gaucher from Neimann-Pick disease here is that presentation with strabismus is common in Gaucher and rare in Neimann-Pick disease.

16. A.
Nonketotic hypoglycemia in a young child or infant is the hallmark of disorders of beta-oxidation of lipids: the patient consumes glycogen; attempts to mobilize fats for energy production, but ketones cannot be generated because the complete oxidation of the fats cannot be accomplished.

17. D.
This is a trick question. Both A. and D. have been associated with Reye syndrome. However, the presence of citrulline and ornithine in the urine, determined by amino acid analysis in some laboratories, implies a urea cycle defect.

18. B > D > A > C.
This is a trick question. B is the best-fit answer, because progressive, severe white matter damage is a classic finding in peroxisomal disorders, such as adrenoleukodystrophy. It must be remembered, however, that all metabolic diseases can affect myelin formation to varying degrees.

19. C.
The presence of ketosis distinguishes glycogen storage disease from forms of fatty acid oxidation disorders that have hepatomegaly but nonketotic hypoglycemia.

20. C.

21. A.

22. D.
This finding is usually present early in ceroid lipofuscinosis.

23. A., B.
These are common characteristics of mucopolysaccharidoses, caused by dysostosis. Dysostosis multiplex can be found, in varying degrees, in many forms of lipidoses and oligosaccharidoses.

24. E.
Along with this history, angiokeratoma are a hallmark of Fabry disease. The lancinating pains in the limbs may be caused by lipid infiltration in the endothelium of the vaso nervorum of peripheral nerves. Angiokeratoma can be found in other lipidoses and oligosaccharidoses, but without family history of kidney failure, early stroke, and lancinating pains.

25. F.
Sometimes light microscopy also can reveal vacuoles in buffy coat white cells or bone marrow in storage diseases and ceroid lipofuscinosis.

Chapter 11: Cerebrovascular Disease

Timothy G. Lukovits, MD

Contents

1. Introduction

The field of cerebrovascular disease has evolved into a separate specialty within adult neurology. It covers an extremely diverse number of diseases, each with a unique pathophysiology, epidemiology, management, and prognosis. There have been many advances in neuroimaging, endovascular therapy, secondary prevention, and rehabilitation, making this a very interdisciplinary and exciting field. This review only superficially touches on many important aspects of cerebrovascular disease and emphasizes more practical clinical areas.

2. Basic Anatomy of the Cerebral and Spinal Cord Circulation

A basic understanding of the vascular supply of the brain and spinal cord is needed to properly identify the site of arterial occlusion based on the lesion location, understand the consequences of arterial occlusion and properly interpret imaging studies. Figures 1-3 show the arteries on the base of the brain, the vascular territories of the hemispheres, and the vascular supply of the spinal cord, respectively.

Figure 1

Arteries at the base of the brain

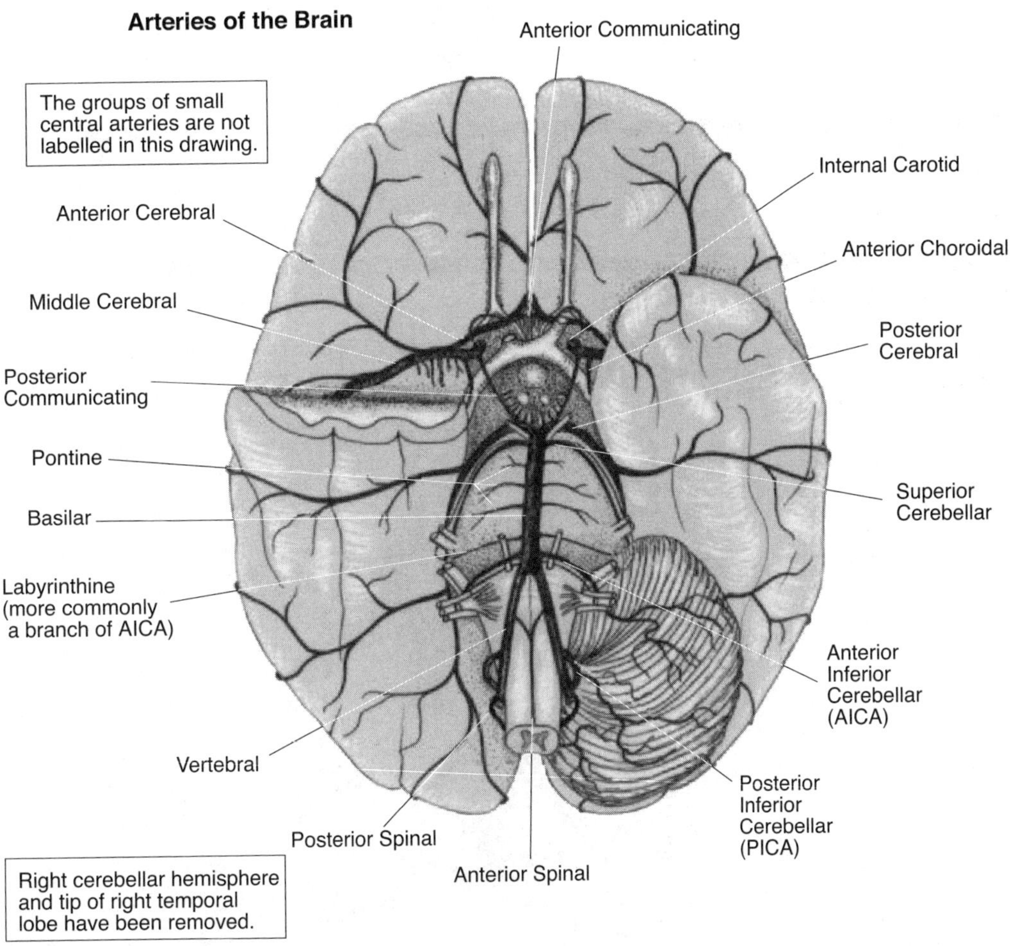

http://instruct.uwo.ca/anatomy/530/350notes.htm

Figure 2

Vascular territories of the cerebral hemispheres

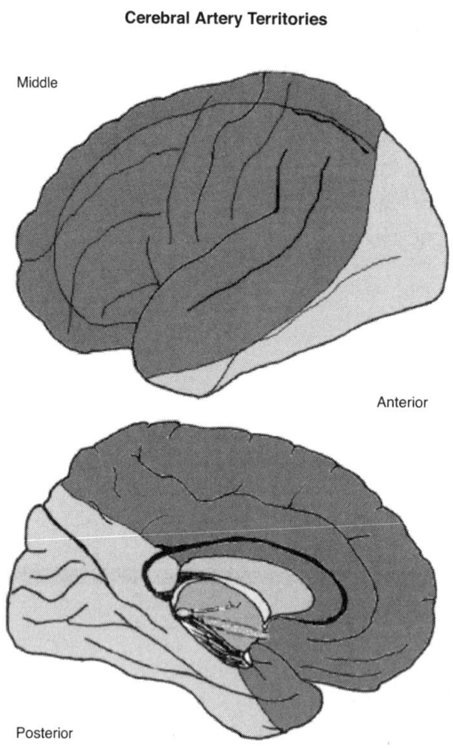

http://instruct.uwo.ca/anatomy/530/350notes.htm

Figure 3

Vascular supply of the spinal cord

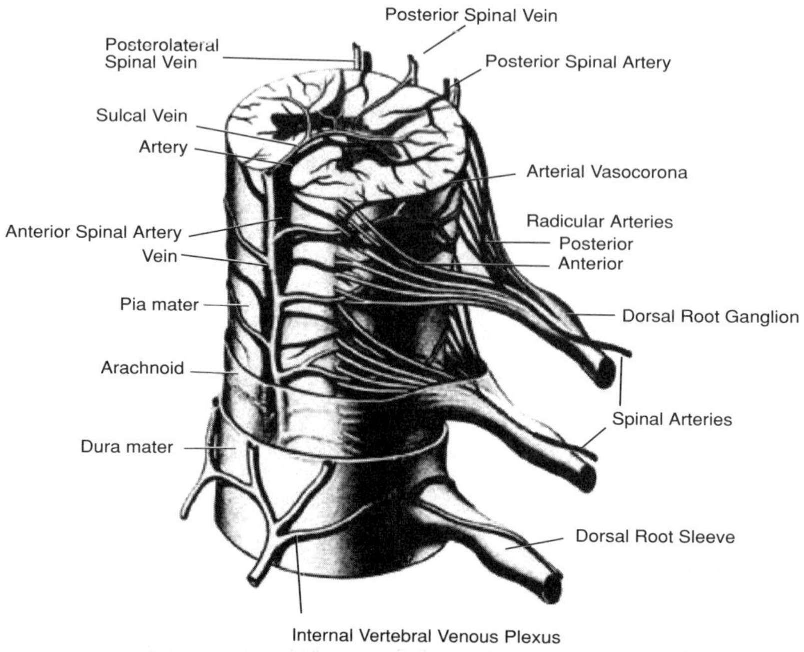

http://www.anatomy.dal.ca/Human_Neuroanatomy/Labs/Lab1.html

3. The Pathophysiology of Cerebral Infarction

The key pathophysiologic aspects of cerebral infarction include excitotoxicity, inflammation, edema, and apoptosis.

Excitotoxicity

Hypoxia and hypoglycemia cause the release of glutamate from presynaptic nerve terminals and astrocytes, which leads to the overstimulation of NMDA and glutamate receptors, sodium influx and excessive release of intracellular calcium stores. Calcium activates catabolic enzymes that lead to the breakdown of cell membranes, proteins and DNA, and eventually, neuronal necrosis.

Inflammation

Tissue damage induces the expression of transcription factors in glial and endothelial cells and increased production of cytokines, chemokines, and adhesion molecules, leading to the migration of polymorphonuclear cells and lymphocytes. This causes microvascular obstruction and neurotoxicity related to the release of reactive oxygen species and nitric oxide.

Edema

Both cytotoxic and vasogenic edema occur following brain infarction and can worsen ischemia by raising intracranial pressure. Glutamate-mediated influx of sodium and lactic acidosis have been implicated in the development of cellular edema. Damage to the microvascular endothelium and disruption of the blood-brain barrier leads to vasogenic edema.

Apoptosis

Excitotoxicity and excessive oxygen free radicals leads to mitochondrial damage and the induction of cytochrome c. This leads to the activation of caspases and the induction of gene-programmed cell death in neurons. Similar processes seem to result in endothelial cell apoptosis.

4. Stroke Mechanisms

Identifying the specific cause of stroke is a critical step that is required before one can determine the prognosis and the most appropriate acute management and secondary prevention strategy. For example, two patients may present with the identical neurologic deficit, but in one case the stroke is caused by paradoxical embolism through a patent foramen ovale (PFO), and in the other, by carotid stenosis. The risk of recurrence, the proper management of acute blood pressure elevations, and appropriate long-term interventions obviously differ greatly in these two situations.

The causes of stroke are extremely varied and complex and so are usually categorized broadly according to the site of vessel occlusion, the source of embolism, or the systemic process leading to arterial occlusion (eg, carotid artery disease or cardioembolism). These categories are then subdivided into more specific pathophysiologic mechanisms or diseases (eg, arterial dissection related to fibromuscular dysplasia). However, there are some important limitations to this traditional method of classification. The first is that signs, symptoms and CT scan results obtained on admission frequently do not identify the cause of stroke and more comprehensive testing is needed. Failure to recognize this limitation can lead to premature exclusion of many potential mechanisms of stroke. Furthermore, multiple pathophysiologic factors may simultaneous contribute to stroke in a given patient. For example, a patient with a hematologic disorder leading to hypercoagulability (eg, anticardiolipin antibodies) may develop a DVT after falling out of a tree and then experience paradoxical embolism through a PFO. In this case, hematologic, traumatic, and congenital cardiac etiologies are all present. However, a shotgun approach to diagnosis often identifies many irrelevant laboratory abnormalities and leads to confusion.

Large Artery Disease

Large artery disease atherosclerosis is a common cause of stroke and can involve the extracranial or intracranial circulation. The most common sites are the carotid bifurcation, proximal vertebral arteries, carotid siphon, middle cerebral artery trunk, distal vertebral arteries, and the midbasilar artery. Nonatherosclerotic causes of large artery disease are also common and include a variety of diseases such as arterial dissection, fibromuscular dysplasia, radiation arteriopathy, vasospasm, and inflammatory conditions including the vasculitides. Large artery diseases cause infarction through distal atherothromboembolism, occlusion of the ostia of perforating vessels, hypoperfusion, or a combination of these mechanisms.

Cerebral Small Artery Disease

Intracranial small artery disease is usually due to lipohyalinosis, which consists of atherosclerosis of the penetrating arteries 100-500 microns in size and arteriolosclerosis of the smaller arteries. This most commonly leads to small, deep infarctions in the basal ganglia, hemispheric white matter, pontine base, and lateral thalamus.

Cerebral Venous Thrombosis

A basic awareness of cerebral venous thrombosis (CVT) is important since it has a varied and nonspecific presentation and is potentially treatable. The most common sites of thrombosis are the superior sagittal and transverse sinuses. Symptoms are caused by venous hypertension with subsequent cerebral edema and hemorrhagic infarction, intracranial hypertension, and seizures. Causes are as varied as the clinical presentation and include hypercoagulable states, severe dehydration, and intracranial infection (mastoiditis). Specific systemic conditions associated with CVT include pregnancy and the postpartum period, inflammatory bowel disease, nephrotic syndrome, Behçet's disease, and hematologic conditions (see below).

Hematologic Disorders Associated with Ischemic Stroke

Sickle cell disease is an important cause of pediatric stroke that leads to intracranial large artery stenoses, most commonly at the carotid siphon and the proximal anterior and middle cerebral arteries. In adults with sickle cell disease, intracranial hemorrhage is more common than infarction. Stroke has also been reported with polycythemia vera, essential thrombocythemia, leukemia, numerous solid organ malignancies, disseminated intravascular coagulation, nephrotic syndrome, antiphospholipid antibodies, and the postpartum state. Inherited and acquired deficiencies of coagulation inhibitors (protein C and S), and activated protein C resistance, usually from the Factor V Leiden mutation, have been associated with venous thrombosis and only weakly with arterial thrombosis.

Antiphospholipid antibody syndrome is associated with both arterial and venous thrombosis, and one of the most common manifestations is stroke. Anticardiolipin (ACL) antibodies and the lupus anticoagulant are the most studied. Beta-2 glycoprotein-1 are gaining increased recognition and elevated antibody titers are thought to be more specific than ACL titers. This is a cofactor required for antiphospholipid antibodies to bind to phospholipids and this normally inhibits the prothrombinase activity of platelets and the intrinsic pathway. Antiphospholipid antibodies are thought to cause stroke by several mechanisms including valvular lesions (nonbacterial vegetations and myxomatous changes), an intracranial endotheliopathy, and hypercoagulability. The specific mechanisms leading to hypercoagulability are unclear but binding to activated platelets and effects on protein C and S have been documented.

Cardiac and Aortic Sources of Embolism

The most common cardiac causes of stroke include left atrial appendage, left ventricular, and prosthetic valvular thromboembolism. Other causes include atrial myxomas, calcific valvular embolism, bacterial and nonbacterial endocarditis, and embolism associated with patent foramen ovale and atrial septal aneurysms. Aortic atheroembolism, a previously unrecognized but important cause of stroke, is likely responsible for many of the strokes that occur during coronary artery bypass grafting and coronary and cerebral angiography. Plaque thickness greater than 4 mm or complex atheroma has been consistently associated with an increased risk of stroke.

Spinal Cord Stroke

Although all rare, the varied causes of spinal cord stroke are important to recognize. Aortic atherosclerosis, thoraco-abdominal aortic aneurysm surgery, global hypoperfusion from cardiac arrest, decompression sickness, fibrocartilaginous embolism, and vertebral artery dissection are recognized causes of infarction. Spinal aneurysms and spinal cavernous malformations are potential causes of spinal subarachnoid and intermedullary hemorrhage.

Intracranial Hemorrhage

Intracranial (intracerebral) hemorrhage can be caused by a variety of diseases and exposures. The most common causes are small artery disease from hypertension, trauma, anticoagulation, thrombolysis, thrombocytopenia, amyloid angiopathy, arteriovenous malformations, hemorrhagic metastasis, and cocaine. Presumably lipohyalinosis and vessel rupture underlies most hypertensive hemorrhages. Venous infarction commonly is associated with parenchymal hemorrhage. Cavernous malformations, mycotic aneurysms, vasculitis, eclampsia, hypertensive encephalopathy, disseminated intravascular coagulation and hyperperfusion syndrome are less common causes. In addition to the direct mass effect of the hematoma, secondary damage from delayed edema and toxicity from hemoglobin degradation products are also believed to contribute to brain injury.

Subarachnoid hemorrhage (SAH) is primarily caused by saccular aneurysm rupture, trauma and extension of intraparenchymal hemorrhage. SAH causes sudden elevations in intracranial pressure, hydrocephalus, parenchymal hemorrhage, and delayed cerebral infarction secondary to cerebral vasospasm.

5. Common Clinical Stroke Syndromes

Recognizing common stroke syndromes is often helpful in determining prognosis, the most likely etiology and the most appropriate diagnostic testing strategy. For example, a Wallenberg syndrome in a young person is usually due to a vertebral artery dissection and an infarction in the postero-lateral medulla and is associated with a good prognosis unless a large cerebellar infarction is present. Below (Table 1) are some of the more important syndromes.

Table 1

Summary of Important Changes in Nomenclature of Lower Extremity Veins

Syndrome	Usual Site(s)
Classic lacunar syndromes	
Pure motor hemiplegia	Internal capsule, pons, corona radiata
Ataxic hemiparesis	Internal capsule, pons, corona radiata
Dysarthria-clumsy hand syndrome	Internal capsule, pons, corona radiata
Pure sensory stroke	Postero-lateral thalamus
Brainstem syndromes	
Wallenberg (ataxia, vertigo, ptosis, crossed loss of pain and temperature)	Postero-lateral medulla
Foville (conjugate gaze paresis, ipsilateral facial weakness, contralateral weakness)	Pontine tegmentum and base
Millard-Gubler (ipsilateral facial palsy and contralateral weakness)	Pontine tegmentum and base
"Locked-in" syndrome	Pontine base, bilateral
Weber (3rd nerve and contralateral weakness)	Midbrain base
Benedict (3rd nerve palsy and contra ataxia)	Midbrain tegmentum
Parinaud (decreased upward gaze, ptosis, fixed pupils)	Midbrain tectum
Hemispheric syndromes	
Alexia without agraphia	Dominant occipital lobe and splenium of corpus collosum
"Top of the basilar" syndrome	Midbrain, thalami, temporo-occipital
Anton syndrome	Bilateral occipital lobes
Spinal cord syndromes	
Anterior spinal artery syndrome (paraparesis, sensory level sparing, posterior column function, incontinence)	Anterior spinal cord

6. Evaluation and Management of Stroke and TIA Patients

The evaluation and treatment of the patient experiencing an acute stroke or transient ischemic attack (TIA) is a complex and rigorous process. This process requires coordinated and collaborative, multidisciplinary management that optimally begins with proper triage, characterization of the pathophysiology and etiology of symptoms, and concludes with the initiation of rehabilitation and secondary prevention (Adams, 2003; Albers, 1999).

It is recommended that all patients with the diagnosis of ischemic stroke be admitted under the inpatient designation to a dedicated stroke unit. Randomized controlled trials have demonstrated that stroke units reduce mortality, dependency and institutionalization and improve quality of life when compared to general medical wards (Indredavik, 1998). Essential features of stroke units are nurses who are trained to closely monitor a patient's neurologic status, psychiatrists, rehabilitation therapists, and physicians trained to diagnose and treat cerebrovascular disease.

Inpatient Treatment Goals

1. To determine the etiology of stroke or TIA, treat the acute consequences of stroke, and to initiate an appropriate treatment plan aimed at preventing recurrent stroke.

2. To determine the patient's clinical deficit and care needs and to establish a plan for rehabilitation.

3. To prevent and/or treat the subacute complications of stroke including deep venous thrombosis, aspiration, and urinary tract infection.

4. To educate the patient and caregivers.

General Measures

Rapid evaluation and treatment of those eligible for thrombolysis is encouraged. There is general agreement to institute airway support and ventilatory assistance for patients with a depressed level of consciousness, oxygen supplementation to correct hypoxemia, assessment and treatment of hypoglycemia, hyperglycemia and fever, as these measures may reduce the degree and volume of infarction.

Blood Pressure Management

Arterial hypertension is common in the setting of acute stroke and there is no evidence that the use of agents to artificially lower or raise blood pressure improves outcome. Many authors have expressed concerns about the use of antihypertensive agents, which may deleteriously affect the ischemic penumbra or cause recurrent ischemia in patients with large artery stenoses.

There is general consensus that blood pressure treatment should be considered when the systolic blood pressure remains consistently above 220 mm Hg, the diastolic blood pressure remains consistently above 120 mm Hg, and the mean arterial pressure (MAP) remains above 130 mm Hg, or in the setting of emergencies such as myocardial infarction or aortic dissection. In situations where blood pressure needs to be reduced it should be done gradually in 10%-20% decrements in the MAP while observing the patient for clinical deterioration. Recommended agents include intravenous labetolol, nicardipine, hydralazine, and enalaprilat with the appropriate level of physiological monitoring if used. Persistent arterial hypotension can be managed with volume replacement with normal saline, correction of arrhythmias, and vasopressor agents including dopamine (Adams, 2003).

Anticoagulation

There is a growing consensus against the *routine* use of anticoagulants in the management of acute ischemic stroke. Unfractionated and low molecular weight heparins in lower doses are effective agents for the prophylaxis and treatment of DVT following stroke. Nonpharmacologic treatments for preventing DVT including early mobilization, anti-embolic stockings, and intermittent compression boots should also be considered (Coull, 2002).

In recent large randomized trials evaluating unfractionated heparin (International Stroke Trial), low-molecular weight heparins (FISS, FISS bis, Heparin in Acute Embolic Stroke Trial, and TAIST) and a heparinoid (Trial of ORG 10172 in Acute Stroke Treatment), these agents were not helpful in patients with acute ischemic stroke (Bath, 2000). Subgroup analysis of the TOAST study showed a benefit at 3 months among patients with large artery atherosclerotic stroke and severe stenosis or occlusion of the internal carotid artery after treatment with a heparinoid.

At this time, anticoagulation in specific stroke subtypes has received inadequate attention. Experts suggest that anticoagulation should be considered ONLY for patients who have an unstable course consisting of recent recurrent episodes of brain ischemia and in patients believed to be at high risk of recurrent embolism or thrombus extension. These patients include those with a high-risk cardiac source of embolism (ie, atrial fibrillation, recent anterior wall myocardial infarction, dilated cardiomyopathy, or valvular heart disease), noninfectious cerebral vein thrombosis, or severe stenosis or recent occlusion of a large extracranial or intracranial artery (Albers, 2004).

Recently, the results of the WASID (Warfarin-Aspirin Symptomatic Intracranial Disease) trial were published and found that long-term anticoagulation was no better and somewhat riskier than aspirin alone for patients with angiographically-defined intracranial disease. However, approximately 40% of the subjects were enrolled after having only a TIA, after a mean of greater than 14 days; only half were taking any antithrombotic medication at the time of the initial event; and less than 40% had stenoses >70%.

The RAPID (Rapid Anticoagulation Prevents Ischemic Damage) trial is testing acute anticoagulation with unfractionated IV heparin versus aspirin in patients with nonlacunar stroke. ESPRIT (European/Australian Stroke Prevention in Reversible Ischemia Trial) is comparing oral anticoagulation with an INR of 2-3 with aspirin in the secondary prevention of noncardioembolic stroke.

A modified protocol for intravenous unfractionated heparin is often used for stroke patients. This modified protocol is also weight-based and allows one to avoid the use of a heparin bolus. This strategy may reduce the risk of hemorrhagic complications. Low molecular weight heparins including enoxaparin have not been shown to be superior to unfractionated heparin in the prevention of early stroke recurrence or progression, but potential advantages include the ease of administration and the avoidance of administering boluses, and may allow certain patients to be discharged to home as they start Coumadin®. Low molecular weight heparins have been accepted as first-line therapy for patients with unstable angina/non-ST-elevation myocardial infarction, and have several pharmacological advantages over unfractionated heparin. Unfractionated heparin is preferred over low-molecular weight heparins in the setting of renal failure and if surgery or invasive procedures are expected in the near future.

Anticoagulants are contraindicated for 24 hours after intravenous t-PA is used. Anticoagulants are also contraindicated for large cerebral infarcts, small or medium-sized infarcts with significant hemorrhagic transformation (with the exception of venous thrombosis), uncontrolled severe hypertension, bacterial endocarditis, and sepsis.

Antiplatelet Agents

Aspirin started within 48 hours of cerebral infarction modestly lowers the risk of death and recurrent stroke at 6 months. On the basis of the International Stroke Trial and the Chinese Acute Stroke Trial, aspirin can prevent an estimated 9 fewer deaths or nonfatal stroke per 1000 patients treated. Based on these studies, aspirin 160-325 mg/day is recommended on admission for patients able to take aspirin (Coull, 2002).

Dipyridamole with aspirin (available as Aggrenox®) and clopidogrel (Plavix®) have been shown to be effective in the secondary prevention of stroke, but their role in acute ischemic stroke is undefined. Clopridogrel is the drug of choice in patients who are unable to take aspirin. Glycoprotein IIb/IIIa agents have not been studied sufficiently after acute ischemic stroke and are not recommended. Antiplatelet agents are contraindicated for 24 hours after t-PA is used.

Seizures

The reported frequency of seizures following acute ischemic stroke has most consistently been estimated to be from 5% to 10%, and occur less often than following acute hemorrhagic stroke. Most often, seizures complicating brain infarction occur after the acute period. Most are partial and the incidence of status epilepticus is very rare. Recurrent seizures are observed in only a minority of patients who experience a first seizure. Phenytoin, fosphenytoin, gabapentin, leviteracetam, and carbamazepine are appropriate anticonvulsants for patients with post-stroke seizures. There is no data to support the prophylactic use of anticonvulsants following ischemic stroke.

Elevated Intracranial Pressure

Clinical deterioration as a result of focal "compartmentalized" or generalized elevated intracranial pressure occurs in 10%-20% of patients, usually as a complication of large hemispheric infarction associated with extensive cerebral edema. Large cerebellar infarctions can also lead to hydrocephalus and increased intracranial pressure. Edema usually peaks at 3-5 days following the initial stroke (Adams, 2003).

Conservative measures include elevating the head, avoiding neck rotation and compression of jugular vein flow, avoiding hypo-osmolar intravenous fluids, and treating conditions such as hypoxia and hyperthermia that may increase intracranial pressure. Hypotension can further decrease cerebral perfusion and can be treated with intravenous fluids and, if associated with clinical deterioration, pressors such as phenylephrine (2-10 micrograms/kg/min) or dopamine (2-20 micrograms/kg/min). Therapies that can be used to reduce intracranial pressure in patients whose condition is deteriorating include osmotherapy (eg, mannitol, glycerol, and hypertonic saline), hyperventilation and ventriculostomy. Mannitol 20% is most commonly used and is given as 0.25-0.50 grams/kg over 20 minutes and is often given with furosemide 10 mg intravenous push to encourage diuresis and avoid volume overload. Doses are repeated up to every 6 hours based on the response, but serum osmolality should remain less than 310 mOsm/L. Craniotomy with partial temporal lobectomy and hemicraniectomy are sometimes considered in massive hemispheric infarction with deterioration, and hemicraniectomy is currently under investigation. Corticosteroids have been shown to be ineffective (Adams, 2003).

Surgical decompression and evacuation can be effective in the management of large cerebellar infarctions that compress the brain stem if extensive brainstem infarction has not already occurred.

Dysphagia

It has been estimated that up to 45% of all strokes are complicated by dysphagia.

More than half of patients with dysphagia improve by the end of the first week. Improvement, however, may still not mean that they are able to eat a non-modified diet, or consume enough to maintain their caloric needs.

Feeding should be done cautiously and under the direction of a Speech Language Pathologist if any of the following are present: lethargy; dysarthria; gurgling vocal quality; hypophonia; aphasia; severe neglect; obvious weakness of face, tongue or palate; confusion; significant apraxia; difficulty handling secretions; or drooling.

For patients for whom the decision has been made to provide supplemental enteral nutrition, initial feeding is usually through a soft, small bore nasogastric feeding tube until the degree of, and or, resolution of dysphagia is determined. Because initial recovery from dysphagia may occur spontaneously, decision making regarding percutaneous gastrostomy (PEG) placement is generally best delayed for 2-4 weeks except in special patient populations. These include those with brainstem infarction or large hemispheric infarction and severe bulbar dysfunction with little clinical improvement.

Serial evaluations by a speech and language pathologist and, as recommended by speech pathology, a modified barium swallow examination, are helpful when making clinical decisions related to nonoral or modified oral means of nutrition. Decisions regarding the management of dysphagia will be based on the clinical presentation of the patient, the length or time the dysphagia is expected to persist, and the caloric intake required.

Initial Diagnostic Evaluation

In addition to a thorough neurological examination, the initial evaluation of the patient with an acute stroke should include a comprehensive history and physical examination. Special attention should be paid to identifying any prior history of brain ischemia and physical evidence of cardiac murmurs, rhythm disturbances and carotid bruits (Adams, 2003).

Initial imaging should be carried out by non-contrast head CT to determine whether the stroke is ischemic or hemorrhagic, since this carries immediate implications for further treatment.

Initial laboratory testing should include an ECG, chest x-ray, complete blood count including platelets, PT, PTT, serum electrolytes, glucose, BUN, and creatinine. For patients with known or suspected diabetes, a glycosylated hemoglobin (HbA1C) is recommended. A fasting lipid panel should be ordered on admission if a recent one is not available.

Extracranial Doppler ultrasonography should be considered in all cases to screen for internal carotid and proximal vertebral artery disease. Transcranial Doppler ultrasonography can be used to evaluate patients for intracranial stenosis and abnormal blood flow patterns related to extracranial disease.

MRI and MRA of the brain are recommended when causes of symptoms other than stroke are being considered or when the cause of stroke is not evident after the above tests are obtained. MRI may provide useful information on possible mechanism of stroke and prognosis. MRA of the cervical arteries can be useful when ultrasonographic evaluation is limited, not available, or needs corroboration, or if disease of the extracranial vertebral or common carotid arteries is suspected. Despite the resolution of symptoms, TIA patients often have abnormalities on MRI (DWI) sequences. These changes can be useful in confirming the vascular nature of the symptoms and providing useful clues that can help establish the potential pathogenic mechanism.

The use of hyperacute multi-modal MRI with diffusion-weighted imaging (DWI), perfusion-weighted imaging, and gradient-recalled echo (GRE) or susceptibility-weighted MRI sequences is currently under investigation and, at this time, is not recommended for most patients. These techniques may allow one to distinguish tissue with potentially reversible ischemia from tissue with irreversible infarction while having adequate sensitivity for detecting hemorrhage. Axial T1-weighted images with fat suppression of the neck and brain can detect changes of arterial dissection.

CT angiography can provide information on the intracranial and extracranial vasculature and should be considered when MRI is contraindicated, technically limited, or not tolerable. CT angiography of the intracranial vasculature can be obtained on admission, when decisions regarding intravenous and intra-arterial thromobolysis and anticoagulation need to be made rapidly.

Echocardiography should be ordered on admission if a cardiac or aortic source is strongly suspected, and in other cases, after the above investigations fail to identify the probable cause of stroke and a cardiac or aortic source is suspected. For patients with recent anterior wall myocardial infarction or a known cardiomyopathy, transthoracic echocardiography (TTE) is the appropriate initial study to order. Transesophageal echocardiography (TEE) is indicated when TTE results are technically inadequate.

TEE is often performed *before* TTE in patients less than 50 years of age, and when sources of embolism usually not adequately detected by TTE are strongly suspected. These sources include: left atrial enlargement and thrombus, atrial septal aneurysms, patent foramen ovale, aortic arch atherosclerosis, and valvular vegetations from endocarditis. For stroke patients with brain embolism attributed to atrial fibrillation, echocardiography is not always required unless the results would assist decision making about anticoagulation or cardioversion. Telemetry or 24-hour Holter monitoring should be considered if the history or cardiac examination suggests increased risk of arrhythmia or cardiac ischemia.

When routine testing or clinical factors fail to establish a likely etiology of stroke or TIA, additional laboratory tests (eg, thrombosis screen, urine drug screen, RPR), and occasionally, conventional angiography, and cerebrospinal fluid analysis, may be helpful in select cases. Thrombosis screen testing, including antiphospholipid antibodies, should be tailored to the presumed etiology. For venous thrombosis (eg, cerebral vein thrombosis, patent foramen ovale), testing for Factor V Leiden mutation, prothrombin gene mutation, protein C and S, anti-thrombin III and Factor 8 levels should be considered. However, these have questionable relevance for arterial thrombosis in adults (Bushnell, 2001).

Preventive Measures

Early Mobilization and Return to Self Care

Early mobilization should be encouraged as soon as possible after admission, if medically and neurologically feasible, as this can prevent the complications discussed below. Patients should also be encouraged to resume self-care activities including eating, toileting, dressing, and grooming, and participate in mental and social activities as soon as possible after admission, as this enhances recovery and the patient's sense of control and well-being (Adams, 2003).

Stroke patients are at high risk of developing deep vein thrombosis (DVT) and nonambulatory patients should receive an effective regimen for DVT prevention. Acceptable measures include intermittent pneumatic compression sleeves, low-dose unfractionated heparin (5,000 units subcutaneously twice a day), and low-molecular weight heparins.

Urinary tract infection is a common complication of stroke and often relates to the use of indwelling urinary catheters. The use of catheters should be avoided if possible. For patients unable to void independently, intermittent catheterization is an alternative to indwelling catheterization that is associated with a lower risk of infection.

Daily bowel programs should be started from admission to allow appropriate regulation of bowels. Bowel movements slow as a result of immobility, illness, and change in routine. Maintaining rectal vault evacuation daily will assist in avoiding obstipation which can delay recovery. Symptoms of obstipation include anorexia, fatigue, and nausea, progressing to abdominal pain and vomiting.

Assessment of Stroke Severity

A number of valid instruments have been developed to assess stroke severity and predict prognosis. These scales can also be used to measure the impact of medical interventions on stroke outcomes.

In a recent analysis by the TOAST investigators, the baseline NIHSS score strongly predicted outcome, with one additional point on the NIHSS decreasing the likelihood of an excellent outcome at 3 months by 17% (Adams, 1999). At 3 months, excellent outcomes were noted in 46% of patients with scores of 7 to 10 and in 23% with scores of 11 to 15 (Table 2). A score of greater than or equal to 16 predicts a high probability of death or severe disability, whereas a score of 6 or less predicts a good recovery. In another recent series, the initial NIHSS score predicted hospital disposition. A score of <5 was associated with discharge home, 6-13 with rehabilitation, and >13 with long-term nursing facility. An admission score of >7 has been associated with a higher risk of deterioration.

Table 2

NIHSS Outcomes at Three Months

	Good or Excellent	Excellent
0-3	95%	80%
4-6	87%	64%
7-10	78%	45%
11-15	56%	23%
16-22	41%	18%
23+	19%	5%

Discharge Timing and Planning and the Risk of Early Deterioration

Stroke severity, risk of deterioration, and the degree of long-term disability can be estimated within the first 48 hours after stroke onset. However, stroke is a very complex disease with an extremely variable presentation and course, so early deterioration, recurrent stroke, and life-threatening complications can occur unpredictably. We therefore generally recommend close observation and neurological monitoring in an inpatient setting for a minimum of 3 days for patients with a significant functional deficit.

Neurological deterioration, either focal or global, has been reported to occur in 20%-40% of patients within the first week of ischemic stroke and can occur despite initial improvement. Of 92 patients presenting with a severe motor deficit, 24% had worsening of motor function during the first 5 days after stroke onset, and interestingly, these worsening patients tended to have small "lacunar" infarctions. Predictors of deterioration include large hemispheric or cerebellar infarctions, severe large artery occlusive disease, pure motor stroke from lacunar infarction, chronic hypertension and diabetes. The admission NIHSS score has been shown to predict early deterioration. In one study, 66% of patients with a score >7 worsened within 48 hours versus 15% of those with score greater than or equal to 7.

Deterioration can be due to recurrent infarction or enlargement of infarction, hemorrhagic transformation, delayed cerebral edema, brainstem compression, hydrocephalus, seizures, medical complications (eg, infection, myocardial infarction, pulmonary embolism, hyperglycemia, hypoglycemia, hyponatremia, withdrawal states) and medications (eg, benzodiazepines, opioids, and neuroleptics).

This deterioration may be amenable to specific therapies if initiated early. Blood pressure elevation and hydration and urgent revascularization may improve cerebral perfusion; osmotherapy, hyperventilation and sedation can decrease intracranial pressure; more aggressive antithrombotic agents may lessen the chance of thrombus propagation and recurrent embolism; ventriculostomy relieves hydrocephalus; and surgical resection is indicated for large cerebellar infarction with brainstem compression. Recent studies suggest there is a benefit from hemicraniectomy that can be lifesaving in select cases (Vahedi, 2007). Also, treatment of fever and hyperglycemia may lessen ischemic damage and improve outcome.

The risk of early stroke following a TIA may be higher than previously estimated. In one study from California emergency departments, approximately 10% of TIA patients suffered a stroke within 90 days and half of those occurred in the first 48 hours after TIA (Johnston, 2000). A recent review of patients presenting with TIA in Oxford found that certain clinical characteristics increased the risk of stroke in the next 90 days and were used to create the "ABCD" score (age > 60 years, blood pressure elevation on presentation, clinical features of speech disturbance and weakness, duration of symptoms > 10 minutes, and diabetes mellitus (Johnston, 2007).

Discharge should be considered when the patient is judged to be clinically stable after a reasonable period of close observation has passed. A minimum hospitalization of 3 days is recommended for most patients with ischemic stroke and a longer period should be considered for patients at higher risk for deterioration and those with an unstable course or complications. In some cases, discharge needs to be delayed until diagnostic studies are completed so that high-risk sources of stroke recurrence can be identified or excluded and the most appropriate therapy can be initiated (eg, angiography to assess for severe stenosis of the internal carotid, basilar or middle cerebral artery). Discharge should not occur until functional status has been assessed, a stroke prevention and rehabilitation plan has been established and the patient and the family have been educated.

Prevention of Recurrent Stroke

Initiation of measures to prevent recurrent stroke, with the exception of aggressive lowering of blood pressure in the acute phase, are encouraged during the hospitalization following ischemic stroke or TIA (Albers, 1999). The timing of anticoagulation for prevention of stroke from atrial fibrillation and endarterectomy for symptomatic carotid artery disease is controversial and is based on many factors, including the size of infarction, neurologic status, medical comorbidities, and the estimated risk of recurrent stroke.

Risk Factor Management

Hypertension should be treated to maintain systolic blood pressure below 140 mm Hg and diastolic blood pressure below 90 mm Hg. For persons with diabetes, blood pressure levels <130/85 mm Hg are recommended. The most recent guideline from The Seventh Report of the Joint National Committee on Prevention, Detection, Evaluation, and Treatment of High Blood Pressure (JNC-7) recommends that individuals with a systolic BP of 120 to 139 mm Hg or a diastolic BP of 80 to 89 mm Hg should be considered as prehypertensive and require health-promoting lifestyle modifications to prevent CVD, including dietary changes and regular physical exercise (Chobanian, 2003). JNC-7 also recommends the use of thiazide-type diuretics and ACE-I to treat hypertension following stroke. Adjustment of these blood pressure goals may be necessary in some patient subgroups (eg, those with severe carotid stenosis and possible hemodynamic impairment).

Cigarette smoking should be discontinued. Counseling, nicotine replacement therapies, bupropion, and formal smoking cessation programs should be made available.

Excessive use of alcohol should be eliminated. Formal alcohol cessation programs are recommended. Mild-to-moderate use of alcohol (1 to 2 drinks per day) has been associated with a reduction in stroke rates.

Treatment of hyperlipidemia is recommended. The AHA dietary guidelines for those with elevated LDL or pre-existing cardiovascular disease (formerly known as the Step II diet) are recommended. These consist of <30% of calories derived from fat, <7% from saturated fat, and <200 mg/d cholesterol consumed is recommended, along with maintenance of ideal body weight and engagement in regular physical activity. If lipid levels remain elevated (LDL >130 mg/dL), use of a lipid-lowering agent, preferably a statin, is recommended. The goal of therapy should be an LDL level <100 mg/dL. Recent studies have found that these medications reduce the risk of stroke in patients with systemic vascular disease, diabetes, or hypertension (absolute risk reduction 1.4%), and the risk of major vascular events but not stroke alone in patients with cerebrovascular disease with low LDL levels.

Additional dietary changes, including increased intake of fruits,vegetables and fish, should be encouraged as they have been associated with improvement in vascular disease risk factors and a decreased risk of stroke.

Fasting blood glucose levels <126 mg/dL are recommended. Diet and oral hypoglycemics or insulin should be prescribed as needed to control diabetes.

Physical activity (at least 30 minutes per day, most days of the week) is recommended.

Analysis of data from the Stroke Prevention by Aggressive Reduction in Cholesterol Levels trial (SPARCL) shows that patients with a history of stroke or TIA who had a recurrent ischemic stroke during the study had a less severe recurrent stroke if they were receiving treatment with atorvastatin.

Antiplatelet Therapy

In general, aspirin at a dosage range of 50 to 325 mg/d is recommended as initial therapy for patients who are not allergic or intolerant to aspirin. Clopidogrel and the combination of aspirin and extended-release dipyridamole are acceptable options for initial therapy following a stroke or TIA, although their cost-effectiveness has been questioned.

Although the combination of aspirin and clopidogrel has become popular, there is little evidence supporting its routine use for stroke prevention. The MATCH (Management of ATherothrombosis with Clopidogrel in High-risk patients) trial recently showed that adding aspirin to clopidogrel in patients at high risk of vascular events was not beneficial. Potential limitations of this study included the large percentage of patients with small vessel disease, and the delay between the qualifying event and enrollment. These factors may have diluted any beneficial effect present. The CHARISMA (Clopidogrel for

High Atherothrombotic Risk and Ischemic Stabilization, Management and Avoidance) trial is currently comparing clopidogrel and aspirin versus aspirin alone in the primary and secondary prevention. The PRoFESS (the Prevention Regimen for Effectively avoiding Second Strokes) trial is comparing clopidogrel and Aggrenox® (extended release dipyridamole with aspirin).

Anticoagulation

Anticoagulation with warfarin remains a powerful and underused means of preventing stroke in patients with atrial fibrillation. Clinical factors that increase the risk of stroke from atrial fibrillation include age >75 years or a history of congestive heart failure, hypertension, diabetes mellitus, or prior stroke or TIA (Albers, 2004). It was thought that ximelagatran, a direct thrombin inhibitor, might replace warfarin but it was recently turned down by the FDA following the release of the SPORTIF trials in atrial fibrillation. Left atrial appendage occluder devices are now under investigation.

Several ongoing trials will address the role of anticoagulation in specific situations, including aortic arch atherosclerosis (Aortic Arch Related Cerebral Hazard trial), PFO (CLOSURE-I and RESPECT), and ischemic cardiomyopathy (Warfarin-Aspirin Reduced Cardiac Ejection Fraction study).

Carotid Endarterectomy

The two large clinical trials of carotid endarterectomy, the NASCET (North American Symptomatic Carotid Endarterectomy Trial) and the European Carotid Surgery Trial (ECST) have shown that surgery is very effective in preventing stroke in selected patients with symptomatic carotid stenosis >50% (Rothwell, 2003). The benefit is greatest for those with hemispheric events (versus retinal), stroke (versus TIA), men (versus women), older age, short delay between event and surgery, irregular or ulcerated plaques (Barnett, 2002). Degree of stenosis was also directly correlated with benefit, up to the point of "near occlusion," and then little or no benefit was seen. The ACAS (Asymptomatic Carotid Atherosclerosis Study) and the ACST (Asymptomatic Carotid Surgery Trial) found a small reduction in stroke with surgery in asymptomatic patients.

Carotid Stenting and Angioplasty

Despite the success of carotid endarterectomy, there is a great deal of interest in the endovascular treatment of carotid artery disease. Patients that may be appropriately treated with endovascular therapy rather than endarterectomy include those with surgically inaccessible bifurcations, restenosis following endarterectomy, radiation-induced atherosclerosis, and severe stenosis due to arterial dissection and fibromuscular dysplasia.

SAPPHIRE (Stenting and Angioplasty with Protection in Patients at High Risk for Endarterctomy) found that carotid stenting was superior to endarterectomy for symptomatic patients judged to be at high-risk for surgery based on anatomic or clinical factors. This trial was unique in that it was the first trial to use both a stent designed for the carotid artery and an embolism protection device. Much of the benefit was related to a reduction in perioperative non-ST segment myocardial infarction. Some limitations of this trial include the lack of a medical arm, a majority of asymptomatic patients, and a significant number of patients with recurrent stensosis following carotid endarterectomy. Based on this trial, in March of 2005 the Centers for Medicare and Medicaid Services expanded coverage of carotid stenting for some high-risk patients.

CREST (Carotid Revascularization Endarterectomy versus Stent Trial) is now enrolling subjects who are judged to be of average risk for surgery, and uses a different stent system and embolism protection device. Results from the lead-in phase included an unexpected high rate of complications for those over 80 years, and these patients are now excluded.

Closure of Patent Foramen Ovale

The role of surgical and transcatheter closure of patent foramen ovale is unclear and is currently under investigation in clinical trials (CLOSURE-I and RESPECT).

7. Thrombolysis for Acute Ischemic Stroke

Intravenous t-PA for Ischemic Stroke

In 1996, the Food and Drug Administration (FDA) approved the use of t-PA for acute ischemic stroke after the report of a randomized, two-part trial sponsored by the National Institute of Neurological Disorders and Stroke (NINDS). The committees of the American Heart Association (AHA) and the American Academy of Neurology (AAN) then published guidelines endorsing the use of t-PA for acute ischemic stroke under strict inclusion and exclusion criteria (Adams, 2003; Albers, 2004). The NINDS trial results were recently reanalyzed by an independent panel because of persistent questions about the trial's design. This panel reaffirmed the benefit of t-PA despite these questions.

Coordination of the acute stroke response team is critical to success. Each team member is responsible for a designated component of care. The Emergency Medical System (EMS) and Emergency Department Staff will identify potential candidates and begin the determination process. Neurologists, and other members of an Acute Stroke Response Team, need to respond immediately to consult on a potential candidate (Alberts, 2000).

Minimum Inclusion Criteria for IV t-PA

- Age ≥18 years.
- Clinical diagnosis of acute ischemic stroke causing a measurable neurological deficit.
- Time of symptom onset well established to be less than 180 minutes before infusion would begin. Patients thus awakening with stroke are generally ineligible.
- Potential benefits and risks discussed with patient, family, and/or legal guardian before treatment begun.

Exclusion Criteria

- Only minor or rapidly improving stroke symptoms. Examples of such exclusions are: ataxia alone; sensory loss alone; dysarthria alone; minimal weakness.
- Evidence of intracranial or subarachnoid hemorrhage on pretreatment Computerized Axial Tomography (CT).
- Clinical presentation suggestive of subarachnoid hemorrhage, even with normal CT.
- Awakening with stroke and ≥3 hours has passed since patient last seen at baseline.
- Active internal bleeding.
- History of intracranial hemorrhage.
- Known bleeding diathesis, including but not limited to:
- Platelet count <100,000/mm^3.
- Patient has received unfractionated heparin and has an elevated aPTT (greater than upper limit of normal for laboratory).
- Patient has received low molecular weight heparin in past 24 hours.
- Current use of oral anticoagulants (eg, warfarin sodium) or recent use with an elevated INR >1.7.

In patients without recent use of oral anticoagulants or heparin, treatment with t-PA can be initiated prior to the availability of coagulation results but should be discontinued if either the INR is greater than 1.7 or the aPTT is elevated.

- Current pregnancy.
- Within 3 months of any intracranial surgery, serious head trauma, or previous stroke.
- Major surgery or truncal trauma within the preceding 14 days.
- History of gastrointestinal or urinary tract hemorrhage within 21 days.
- Recent arterial puncture at a noncompressible site.
- Recent lumbar puncture.

- On repeated measurements, systolic blood pressure >185 mm Hg or diastolic blood pressure >110 mm Hg at the time treatment is to begin and patient requires aggressive treatment to reduce blood pressure to within these limits.

- Abnormal blood glucose (<50 or >400 mg/dL).

- Postmyocardial infarction pericarditis.

- Seizure near the time of onset of stroke symptoms.

- History of severe dementia or severe pre-existing neurologic impairment.

Note: Current or recent use of aspirin, ticlopidine, or clopidogrel is not a contraindication.

Warnings/Relative Contraindications

- Age ≥85 years

- Severe neurologic deficit (eg, National Institutes of Health Stroke Scale Score >20).

- Baseline CT scan evidence of extensive ischemic changes. This includes early evidence of sulcal effacement, herniation, mass effect, or edema.

- Recent myocardial infarction (given risk of post-myocardial infarction pericarditis and LV thromboembolism), recent dysfunctional uterine bleeding, or active menstruation.

Intra-arterial and Mechanically-assisted Thrombolysis for Ischemic Stroke

Direct thrombolysis with catheter-based approaches has several theoretical advantages over intravenous t-PA. Since the arterial occlusion and pattern of collateral flow can be visualized, the need and adequacy of treatment can be immediately determined. More rapid and effective lysis with a lower dose of thrombolytic may be achieved with these direct methods. Although the PROACT-II (Prolyse in Acute Cerebral Thromboembolism-II) trial showed that intra-arterial lysis with pro-urokinase was effective, it was not approved by the FDA (Albers, 2004). Combined intravenous and intra-arterial treatment is gaining favor since treatment can begin sooner at less specialized hospitals and then patients can be transferred to more specialized centers for "rescue" intra-arterial treatments. Other mechanical methods to enhance lysis including balloon angioplasty, snares, intravascular ultrasound catheters and transcranial ultrasound are being studied. The MERCI trial using the corkscrew-like retriever device that extracts thrombi was recently completed and led to the approval of this device, but its role is still to be determined.

Treatment of Primary Intracerebral Hemorrhage

Trials attempting to demonstrate a role for urgent surgical evacuation of parenchymal hemorrhage have failed. However, surgical evacuation is usually considered for cerebellar hematomas larger than 3 cm in diameter given the high risk of brainstem compression and deterioration, and for younger patients with nondominant hemispheric hemorrhages with neurologic deterioration. External ventricular drainage is commonly performed for hydocephalus from ventricular compression or associated intraventricular hemorrhage (Broderick, 1999). Preliminary trials have shown that recombinant factor VIIa may prevent hematoma expansion; however, a recently-completed phase 3 trial showed no benefit in outcome (Mayer, 2007).

Treatment of Subarachnoid Hemorrhage

Early clipping or coiling of ruptured aneurysms and treatment of hydrocephalus with ventriculostomy can be life-saving. Preventing and managing the complications of SAH are also critical, including vasospasm, pneumonia, deep venous thrombosis, hyponatremia, and seizures. The ISAT (International Subarachnoid Aneurysm Trial) compared endovascular coiling and surgical clipping of ruptured aneurysms and found a 7% absolute reduction in the risk of disability in the coiling group. However, the study has been criticized because the population was skewed towards lower grade hemorrhages from smaller aneurysms mostly in the anterior circulation, and so the results may not be generalizable. Also, the surgical group did poorer than expected and the long-term durability of coiling was not assessed (Johnston, 2002).

8. Rehabilitation of Stroke Patients

Organized inpatient stroke units have been shown to reduce disability following stroke and much of the benefit of this organization is attributed to early rehabilitation (Indredavik, 1998). In order to be eligible for inpatient rehabilitation, patients typically need to be disabled in 2 or more areas of daily activities and cognitively and physically be able to participate in at least 3 hours of rehabilitation each day. The early phase of rehabilitation focuses on functional assessment, compensatory strategies, and the use of task-related movements. Depression, pain and cardiopulmonary disease are common in this population and may limit rehabilitation efforts (AHCPR, 1995; Dobkin, 2005).

Constraint-induced therapy is a newer technique that attempts to overcome the learned non-use of a weak hand by constraining the unaffected limb, but this is only beneficial for patients able to extend the wrist and fingers greater than 10 degrees. Treatment of spasticity with medications or botulinum toxin injections does not usually improve function but can relieve spasms and passive range of motion if combined with physical therapy. Treadmill training with partial body-weight support, peripheral and transcortical electrical stimulation are under investigation (Dobkin, 2005).

9. References

1. Adams HP Jr, Adams RJ, Brott T, et al. Guidelines for the early management of patients with ischemic stroke: a scientific statement from the Stroke Council of the American Stroke Association. *Stroke*. 2003;24:1056-1083.

2. Adams HP, Jr., Davis PH, Leira EC, et al. Baseline NIH Stroke Scale score strongly predicts outcome after stroke: A Report of the Trial of Org 10172 in Acute Stroke Treatment (TOAST). *Neurology*. 1999;53(1):126-31.

3. Albers GW, Hart RG, Lutsep HL, et al. Supplement to the Guidelines for the management of transient ischemic attacks. *Stroke*. 1999;30:2502-2511.

4. Albers GW, Amarenco P, Easton JD, et al. Antithrombotic and thrombolytic therapy for ischemic stroke. *Chest*. 2004;126:483S-512S.

5. Alberts MJ, Hademenos G, Latchaw RE, et al. Recommendations for the establishment of primary stroke centers. *JAMA*. 2000;283:3102-3109.

6. Barnett HJM, Meldrum HE, Eliasziw M. The appropriate use of carotid endarterectomy. *Canadian Medical Association Journal*. 2002;166(9):1169-1179.

7. Bath PMW, Iddenden R, Bath FJ. Low molecular-weight heparins and heparinoids in acute ischemic stroke: a meta analysis of randomized controlled trials. *Stroke*. 2000;31:1770-1778.

8. Broderick JP, Adams HP, Barsan W, et al. Guidelines for the management of spontaneous intracerebral hemorrhage. *Stroke*. 1999;30:905-915.

9. Bushnell CD, Siddiqi Z, Goldstein LB. Improving patient selection for coagulopathy testing in the setting of acute ischemic stroke. *Neurology*. 2001;57(7):1333-1335.

10. Chobanian AV, Bakris GL, Black HR, et al. The Seventh Report of the Joint National Committee on Prevention, Detection, Evaluation, and Treatment of High Blood Pressure: The JNC-7 Report. *JAMA*. 2003;289:2560-2572.

11. Coull BM, Williams LS, Goldstein LB, et al. Anticoagulant and antiplatelet agents in acute ischemic stroke. *Stroke*. 2002;33:1934-1942.

12. Dobkin B. Rehabilitation after stroke. *N Engl J Med*. 2005;352:1677-84.

13. Indredavik B, Bakke F, Slordahl SA, Rokseth R, Haheim LL. Stroke unit treatment improves long-term quality of life: a randomized controlled trial. *Stroke*. 1998;29(5):895-9.

14. Johnston SC, Gress DR, Browner WS. Short-term prognosis after emergency department diagnosis of TIA. *JAMA*. 2000;284(22):2901-2906.

15. Johnston SC, Higashida RT, Barrow DL, et al. Recommendations for the endovascular treatment of intracranial aneurysms. *Stroke*. 2002; 33:2536-2544.

16. Johnston SC, Rothwell PM, Nguyen-Huynh MN et al. Validation and refinement of scores to predict very early stroke risk after transient ischaemic attack. *Lancet*. 2007;369(9558):283-92.

17. Mayer SA, and the FAST Steering Committee. Complications in patients with intracerebral hemorrhage treated with recombinant factor VIIa. *Neurology*. 2007;69(3): 319-320.

18. Rothwell PM, Eliasziw M, Gutnikov SA, et al. Analysis of pooled data from the randomized controlled trials of endarterectomy for symptomatic carotid stenosis. *Lancet*. 2003;361:107-116.

19. Smith WS. Safety of mechanical thrombectomy and intravenous tissue plasminogen activator in acute ischemic stroke. Results of the multi Mechanical Embolus Removal in Cerebral Ischemia (MERCI) trial, part I. *AJNR*. 2006;27(6):1177-82.

20. U.S. Department of Health and Human Services Agency for Health Care Policy and Research. *Post-stroke Rehabilitation*. AHCPR Publication No. 95-0662. May 1995.

21. Vahedi K, Hofmeijer J, Juettle E, et al. Early decompressive surgery in malignant infarction of the middle cerebral artery: a pooled analysis of three randomised controlled trials. *Lancet Neurology*. 2007;6(3):215-222.

10. Questions

1. In which circumstance is intravenous tissue plasminogen activator (t-PA) definitely contraindicated?

A. CT scan shows possible subtle hypodensity in the white matter of the left hemisphere

B. Time from symptom onset 120 minutes

C. Age 80 years

D. Platelet count of 90,000

E. Isolated incomplete aphasia

2. In a 50-year-old man, which of the following conditions would you NOT consider a risk factor for ischemic stroke?

A. Patent foramen ovale

B. Antiphospholipid antibodies

C. Atrial fibrillation

D. Elevated protein C levels

E. Nephrotic syndrome

3. An 80-year-old woman presents with transient loss of vision in the right eye associated with a 70% internal carotid artery stenosis. All of the following clinical factors have been associated with more benefit from carotid endarterectomy except:

A. Female gender

B. Severity of stenosis

C. Ulcerated or irregular plaque

D. Hemispheric event rather than retinal

4. A 70-year-old woman with diabetes presents to the emergency department after transient slurred speech and hand weakness. Which of the following is a factor that increases the estimated risk of subsequent stroke following TIA according to the ABCD score?

A. Diplopia

B. Diabetes

C. Babinksi sign

D. Aortic stenosis

5. The family of a patient who had a severe ischemic stroke 2 months ago asks whether constraint-induced therapy would be helpful. What seems to be required for patients to benefit from this therapy?

A. Independent mobility

B. At least mild cognitive impairment

C. Spasticity

D. Voluntary extension of the wrist and fingers greater than 10 degrees

6. Following a large hemispheric infarction, one would expect neurologic deterioration from delayed cerebral edema to peak at approximately what time point?

A. 3-12 hours

B. 10 days

C. When diffusion perfusion mismatch is maximum

D. 3-5 days

E. Soon after recanalization occurs

7. Following an ischemic stroke resulting in hemiplegia, effective ways to prevent deep venous thrombosis include all of the following except:

A. Low-molecular weight heparins

B. Bedrest

C. Compression stockings

D. Intermittent pneumatic compression sleeves

E. Unfractionated subcutaneous heparin

8. A 30-year-old with a history of oral ulcers and kidney disease presents with headache and a hemorrhagic infarction in the left temporal lobe. Which of the following HAS NOT been associated with cerebral vein thrombosis?

A. Pregnancy and the postpartum period

B. Inflammatory bowel disease

C. Nephrotic syndrome

D. Behçet's disease

E. Insulin resistance

9. An 80-year-old presents with a large right thalamic hemispheric hemorrhage. Which of the following is clearly indicated for this patient?

A. Factor VIIa

B. FFP if the INR is elevated

C. Platelet transfusion if count is <100,000

D. Immediate evacuation

10. Approximately 24 hours after a patient is admitted with an ischemic stroke, the blood pressure is elevated. Recommended agents to lower severe elevations in blood pressure for such a patient include all of the following except:

A. Intravenous labetalol

B. Sublingal nifedipine

C. Nicardipine

D. Hydralizine

Answers

1. D.
Thrombocytopenia with a platelet count below 100,000 predisposes to bleeding and is an absolute contraindication to administering intravenous tissue plasminogen activator. Time of onset > 180 minutes, not 120 minutes, is an absolute contraindication. In the NINDS trial, advanced age interacted with severity of deficit in predicting outcome, but is not considered an absolute contraindication. A limited but disabling deficit such as an isolated aphasia is not considered an absolute contraindication.

2. D.
Protein C has anticoagulant properties so deficiency rather than an elevation is a risk factor for venous thrombosis.

3. A.
Large randomized trials of carotid endarterectomy (NASCET and ECST) have shown that women typically benefit less from surgery than men because of a lower risk of ipsilateral stroke with medical treatment and a higher risk of perioperative complications. The other factors have all been shown to increase the benefit from surgery.

4. B.
Recent studies from Oxford and California have quantified the early risk of stroke following TIA. A risk stratification system, called the ABCD, has shown that clinical factors including diabetes increase this risk.

5. D.

Constraint-induced therapy aims to overcome "learned non-use" of a weak limb by constraining the use of the normal limb, usually with a mitt, combined with very intense, short-term, therapist-supervised rehabilitation.

6. D.

Deterioration following large hemispheric infarction can be related to extension of the infarction, recurrent infarction in other regions, seizures, concomitant infection and metabolic derangements, and delayed cerebral edema. This edema typically peaks at 3-5 days after onset.

7. B.

Bedrest promotes the formation of lower extremity deep venous thrombosis (DVT). All of the other agents are reasonable options for preventing DVT following ischemic stroke.

8. E.

Insulin resistance is considered a possible risk factor for atherosclerosis and ischemic stroke but not stroke related to venous thrombosis.

9. B.

Factor VIIa did not improve outcome after intracerebral hemorrhage (ICH) in the recently completed FAST trial. Platelet tranfusions are not usually given for ICH unless the count is in the severely low range (ie, < 30,000). Surgical evacuation has not been shown to improve outcome in deep hemispheric hemorrhage.

10. B.

Agents that precipitously and unpredictably lower blood pressure, such as sublingual nifedipine, are not recommended after ischemic stroke. The other agents listed can be given intravenously in low doses or as steady infusions and offer more predictable blood pressure control.

Chapter 12: Movement Disorders

Stephen L. Lee, MD, PhD
David J. Coffey, MD

Contents

1. General Principles

The control and refinement of movement relies on two systems, the cerebellum and the basal ganglia, which act in concert to provide feedback to the motor cortex via the thalamus. Disruption of these feedback pathways results in movement disorders. This chapter focuses primarily on disorders of the basal ganglia, but in broader terms it deals with disorders of cerebellar pathways.

Anatomical Organization

The basal ganglia nuclei are anatomically organized into four major nuclei—the substantia nigra, striatum, globus pallidus, and subthalamic nucleus (Figure 1). The substantia nigra contains two physiologically and anatomically distinct parts, the pars compacta (SNc) and pars reticulata (SNr). The striatum is divided anatomically into the caudate nucleus and the putamen. The globus pallidus consists of two important subnuclei, the globus pallidus extern (GPe) and globus pallidus internus (GPi) nucle.. The basal ganglia nuclei send and receive important connections between the cerebral cortex, thalamus, cerebellar and brainstem nuclei.

The connectivity of the basal ganglia can be considered both integrative as well as segregated and parallel. In addition to motor information, cognitive and emotional information passes through distinct territories in the striatum. Somatotopically organized motor information from the premotor and postcentral somatosensory cortex projects to motor areas in the basal ganglia and projects back to the primary motor, SMA, and premotor cortex. Cognitive function is subserved by the associative territory, located in the dorsal caudate nucleus and projecting to the prefrontal cortex. Emotional or motivational information is subserved by the limbic territory, located in the ventral striatum and projecting to the anterior cingulate cortex, and medial orbitofrontal cortical output projects back to the frontal cortex and supplementary motor area, whereas nigral output projects to the dorsolateral prefrontal cortex.

In motor function, cortical projections to the striatum synapse on dense dendritic spines of medium spiny neurons, which make up greater than 90% of the neurons in the striatum (Figure 2a). The output from these medium spiny neurons segregates into two pathways, termed "direct" and "indirect", which carry information from the striatum to the globus pallidus internus and substantia nigra pars reticulata. Dopaminergic projections from the substantia nigra pars compacta contact the dendritic shafts of these neurons, where they modulate output depending on the dopamine receptor expressed. In the indirect pathway, dopaminergic input is inhibitory by way of D2-dopamine receptors. These neurons express GABA and enkephalin, and project to the GPi and SNr indirectly first by means of GPe and STN projections. In the direct pathway, GABAergic neurons containing D1-dopamine receptors are stimulated by dopaminergic modulation and project directly to the GPi and SNr. Inhibitory projections from the GPi and SNr project to the subthalamic nucleus, which is then output to the V_A/V_L nuclei of the thalamus.

Figure 1

Basal ganglia nuclei

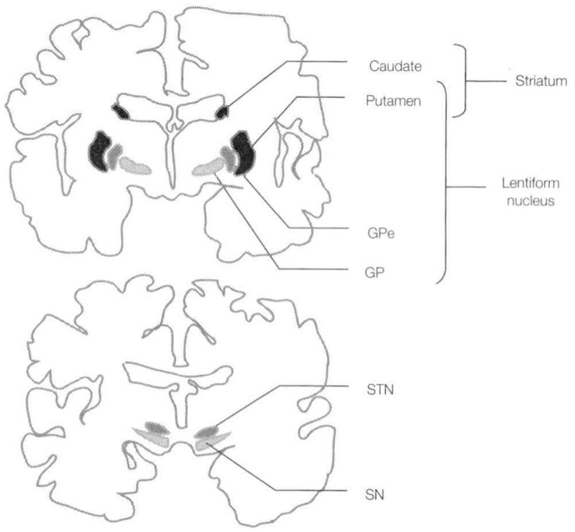

The anterior limb of the internal capsule divides the striatum into two anatomically distinct but functionally similar caudate and striatum. The lentiform nucleus is an anatomical group of three functionally distinct nuclei, the striatum (putamen), globus pallidus externus (GPe), and the globus pallidus internus (GPi). The substantia nigra (SN) and the subthalamic nucleus (STN) are depicted in a separate coronal section.

Figure 2a

Basal ganglia connectivity diagram (normal)

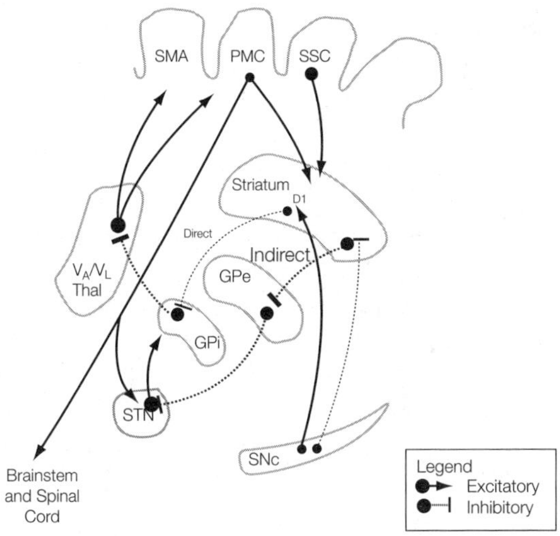

A simplified view of basal ganglia connectivity. Excitatory projections from the primary motor cortex (PMC) and the Somatosensory cortex (SSC) synapse at the striatum. Dopaminergic terminals from the substantia nigra (SN) exert excitatory influence via D1 receptors on striatal neurons in the direct pathway, whereas effects via D2 receptors are achieved through inhibiting the indirect pathway. The direct pathway synapses directly with the main output of the basal ganglia, the inhibitory projections from the globus pallidus internus (GPi). The indirect pathway synapses first in the globus pallidus externus (GPe), which in turn sends inhibitory projections to the subthalamic nucleus (STN), which sends excitatory projections to the GPi. The net result is an alteration of inhibitory output from the globus pallidus internus nucleus (GPi) to the ventral anterior and ventrolateral nucleus of the thalamus (V_A/V_L.Thal).

The balance between the direct and indirect pathway is mediated by dopaminergic input from the substantia nigra pars compacta to the striatum and, to a lesser degree, the globus pallidus and STN. Important feedback on striatal activity is mediated by projections from the GPi to the centromedian nucleus, to the sensorimotor putamen; whereas the SNr projects its medial part of the parafascicular nucleus, then back to the caudate. Other circuits to the basal ganglia include connections from the GPi to the pedunculopontine nucleus, which projects back to the SNc and the STN.

Synaptic Organization

The synaptic organization and neurochemical phenotype of neurons and supporting cells of the basal ganglia provide clues to their function. Over 90% of the neurons in the striatum are medium spiny neurons, which are densely covered by dendritic spines. Glutamatergic efferents from the cortex synapse at these dendritic spines. Dopaminergic input from the substantia nigra pars compacta occur at the dendritic shafts, suggesting a modulatory role. The medium spiny neurons send out local inhibitory collaterals to other medium spiny neurons, in addition to sending an inhibitory efferent axon to tonically active GABAergic neurons in the globus pallidus and substantia nigra pars reticulata. Medium spiny neurons are GABAergic, but also contain neuropeptides substance P, dynorphin, whereas others contain enkephalin. The other striatal neurons are small GABAergic and large cholinergic interneurons. The small GABAergic neurons, together with the local collateral arborization, provides the structural basis for a local surround inhibition.

Inhibitory striatal output converges on pallidal and nigral neurons, which are about 100 times less numerous than striatal neurons, are also GABAergic, and unlike the striatum are tonically active.

Dopaminergic projections from the substantia nigra (pars compacta) impinge on the caudate and putamen by direct and indirect pathways. The direct pathway results in inhibition of the internal segment of the globus pallidus with projection in turn to the thalamus. The indirect pathway is via the external segment of the globus pallidus to the subthalamic nucleus (itself strongly influenced by cortical input), then back to the internal segment of globus pallidus. In this way the indirect pathway exerts a modulatory effect upon the direct pathway. There are also, of course, abundant connections between the basal ganglia and cortex – association cortex directly influences the putamen and caudate; while output from globus pallidus through thalamus project to premotor cortex.

Prior to molecular cloning technology, two subtypes of dopamine receptors were recognized pharmacologically and functionally by their ability to stimulate (D1 type) or inhibit (D2 type) cyclic AMP production. Subsequently, molecular cloning techniques identified five unique dopamine receptor genes, D1 (D1a), D2, D3, D4 and D5, that have either D1 type (D1 and D5) or D2-type (D2, D3, and D4) activity. D1 type receptors are concentrated in the striatal cells, whereas D2 type receptors are in matrix. D1 type receptors predominate in the direct output pathway, while D2 type predominate in the indirect pathway. In Parkinson disease, striatal dopamine is diminished and both pathways are affected. The direct pathway is underactive and the indirect pathway is overactive (Figure 2b).

Figure 2b

Basal ganglia connectivity diagram (Parkinson disease)

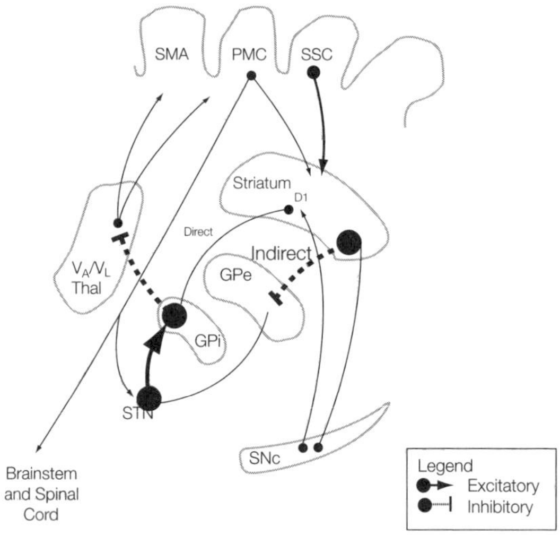

A simplified view of changes in basal ganglia activity due to Parkinson disease. Loss of dopaminergic input to the striatum results in changes in both direct and indirect pathways, with the net result being increased inhibitory output from the globus pallidus internus (GPi). This in turn reduces excitatory projections to the cortex resulting in overall hypokinesia.

2. Approach to the Patient with Movement Disorders

History Taking

It is helpful to recall the basic approach to history taking by allowing the patient to describe the symptoms in their own words. However, additional questions may be necessary to obtain the clinical history that may not be volunteered by the patient. What part of the body is affected? Are there other parts of the body involved? Is one side affected more than the other? Are the movements stereotypical or are they random and different? Are there associated sensory symptoms? Can the movements be suppressed? Do certain postures or tasks or actions elicit, aggravate, suppress or improve the severity of the movements? What is the effect of alcohol, caffeine, sleep, rest, fatigue, stress, or anxiety on the movements? Do they occur during sleep? Do they tend to occur during a particular time of day? Are there associated symptoms affecting mood or behavior? Is speech, swallowing or other neurological function affected, such as vision and balance? Is handwriting affected?

Physical Exam

A thorough physical examination is conducted with additional attention to causes of movement disorders. For example, the eye exam should include an evaluation for the presence of a Kayser-Fleischer ring. This can be seen by the unaided eye as a brownish pigment at the limbus of the cornea, but often requires a slit-lamp examination by an ophthalmologist. The presence of this ring is almost always associated with neurological manifestations of Wilson disease. An exam for movement disorders should consist of a thorough vascular exam, evaluation of autonomic function, and dermatologic signs of autoimmune disease. Indirect observation is as important as the directed examination. Observe as the patient enters and leaves the clinic, stands up and navigates through a crowded waiting area, or during the interview as the patient speaks casually. In the directed examination, spontaneous movement or lack of it at rest is evaluated. Conditions that are reported to elicit the movement disorder such as writing, or holding a glass to drink, are reproduced. At the end of the examination, classification based on description is attempted (Table 1).

Diagnostic Studies

Imaging by computed tomography (CT) or magnetic resonance imaging (MRI) can help narrow the differential diagnosis but it is seldom diagnostic in movement disorders. In the majority of cases, these studies are helpful in excluding structural lesions. Evaluation of ventricular size to rule out normal pressure hydrocephalus may be helpful.

Functional neuroimaging studies such as positron emission tomography (PET), and single photon emission computed tomography (SPECT), permit the evaluation of metabolic demands, relative cerebral blood oxygen content, and neurochemical changes that occur as a consequence of changes in basal ganglia function. These imaging methods provide more specific functional information with respect to metabolic or molecular markers relevant to the neuronal pathway in question. Measures of neuronal activity as it is correlated with cerebral blood flow may provide support for overall cerebral function, as in the case for frontotemporal dementia with parkinsonism. In Parkinson disease, the extent of loss of dopaminergic nerve terminal function is measured by uptake of radioactively tagged ligands (18F Dopa for PET and ^{123}I tropanes for SPECT). Use of these modalities for differentiating between different forms of parkinsonism suffers from insufficient specificity and sensitivity, although in specific cases, they can be helpful in confirmation. For example, PET and SPECT are useful for the differentiation of dopa-responsive dystonia from PD. Ultrasonography is another imaging method that despite its limitations of penetration through the skull has been successfully applied to image the substantia nigra pars compacta in Parkinson disease. The quality of the ultrasound images are highly operator dependent but may offer substantial noninvasive and relatively inexpensive information in the future.

Electroencephalography is a necessary adjunctive study to evaluate seizures in the setting of myoclonic movement disorders. Simple motor status epilepticus (epilepsia partialis continua) may appear as tremor-like movements. Electromyography (EMG) can document rhythmic muscular contractions at 11-18 Hz in orthostatic tremor, as well as detect timing and sequence of agonist/antagonistic muscle groups. Accelerometry has been reported to be helpful in distinguishing between psychogenic tremor from essential tremor or the tremor of Parkinson disease.

Laboratory studies are sought to identify potentially treatable causes of secondary movement disorders, such as the tremor associated with hyperthyroidism, a low serum ceruloplasmin and elevated urinary copper excretion in Wilson disease, autoantibodies in Lupus, and paraneoplastic antibodies anti-

Table 1

Descriptive Terminology

Terms used to describe abnormal movement

Bradykinesia

Decreased ability to initiate movement, resulting in slowing of motor activity. Its extreme form, akinesia, results in no movement.

Tremor

Rhythmical movements of limbs, head, voice, or tongue that may be distinguished into groups based on rate, regularity, distribution and effect of posture/action.

Chorea

Quick ("dance-like") movements that are rapid, jerky and irregular, usually affecting muscles of the face, orobuccal cavity, and limbs.

Rigidity

Increase in resting muscle tone. In parkinsonism, it is consistent throughout the range of motion, unlike the "clasp-knife" effect of spasticity. When rigidity and tremor are both present "cogwheeling" results.

Athetosis

Involuntary slow writhing ("worm-like") movements flowing from one to the next, sometimes associated with chorea, hence "choreoathetosis".

Dystonia

Abnormal sustained, repetitive muscle contractions resulting in twisting motions or unusual postures, often painful. Dystonia can be focal, segmental or generalized.

Myoclonus

An involuntary, sudden, and brief muscle jerk.

Ballismus

Flinging, large amplitude movements often involving leg and arm, most often on one side only, hence "hemiballismus".

Tics

Muscle movements or vocalizations that are compulsive and largely involuntary, but may be voluntarily suppressed for short periods – they can be very disruptive of normal activity and are purposeless.

CRMP-5, and anti-GAD65. Anti-streptolysin-O titers can support a diagnosis of Sydenham chorea. Acanthocytes on peripheral blood smear are required for a diagnosis of neuroacanthocytosis.

The number of molecular genetic studies for movement disorders continues to expand rapidly. With the appropriate family history and age at onset, there is a moderate chance for a diagnostic yield for detecting gene mutations for parkin and other genetic forms of Parkinson disease. Generalized dystonia is often the result of mutations in the DYT1 gene. Neurodegeneration with brain iron accumulation I (NBIA-I), formerly known as Hallervorden-Spatz syndrome, is caused by homozygous mutations in the pantothenate kinase 2 gene (PANK2). The majority of familial dominant choreas is due to CAG trinucleotide repeat expansion of the IT15 gene in Huntington disease.

Neuropsychiatric testing serves to evaluate the psychiatric aspect of movement disorders where a single office visit evaluation is insufficient. This is especially important in surgical procedures where changes can occur afterward. Neuropsychiatric testing is also useful to assess cognitive impairment and depression, or to support the possible role of psychogenic movement disorders.

3. Diseases Presenting with Movement Disorders

Movement disorders were classified historically as pyramidal or extrapyramidal. They can be further subdivided into hyperkinetic or hypokinetic movement disorders.

Hypokinetic Movement Disorders

Parkinson Disease

By far the most studied of the movement disorders, the pathophysiology of idiopathic Parkinson disease centers on the loss of greater than 70%-80% of dopaminergic input to the corpus striatum. Most of the pharmacologic therapies for parkinsonism rely on promoting dopamine, either by replacing its precursor levodopa, directly agonizing the dopamine receptors, by inhibiting breakdown of dopamine, or by opposing dopamine's antagonist, acetylcholine.

Surgical treatment for parkinsonism has entailed pallidotomy (fixed lesion in globus pallidus), thalamotomy (fixed lesion in thalamus), or direct stimulation of thalamus (for tremor), or subthalamic nuclei (for bradykinesia/rigidity) using indwelling deep-brain stimulator electrodes.

James Parkinson is credited with the first description in the medical literature of the disease. His essay, "On the Shaking Palsy", published in 1817, denoted the basic clinical triad of bradykinesia/akinesia, rigidity and tremor. Associated features may also include postural instability, shuffling gait, reduced eye-blink rate, paucity of facial expression, flexion posture, drooling, hypophonia and micrographia (Table 2).

The etiology of Parkinson disease is still not clear. Most cases are still considered sporadic (cohort studies of identical twins show incomplete concordance) but there may be genetic predisposition that can be triggered by some environmental influence. The NINDS is sponsoring a large DNA registry to explore candidate genes. Rarely, Parkinson disease can be a truly inherited disease. More than ten genetic loci (Park 1 through Park 13) have been identified in isolated families worldwide (Table 3).

The environmental trigger in most cases is unknown. Growing up in a rural area may predispose to Parkinson disease, raising questions about agricultural chemicals/pesticides. When a group of young people became severely parkinsonian after injecting themselves with a contaminant of illicit meperidine production (MPTP-N-methyl-4-phenyl1,2,3,6-tetrahydropyridine) it became clear that specific toxins could produce all manifestations of the condition. By the same logic, the disease might be prevented (or its natural history modified) by agents that could prevent such toxicity. A large series of multi-center NINDS-sponsored clinical trials (NETPD Neuroprotection Exploratory Trials in Parkinson disease) is underway to find such agents.

For now, treatment of Parkinson disease remains symptomatic. In general, current medications all have the property of promoting dopamine in some way. The mainstay treatment is dopamine replacement, as the combination carbidopa-levodopa (CD/LD). This combination is available in varying strengths, as is a long-acting preparation. Levodopa enters the bloodstream via an amino acid transporter and therefore must compete with dietary amino acids for transport. This forms the basis for diet manipulation for patients on CD/LD. Carbidopa prevents amino acid decarboxylase from converting levodopa to dopamine until after it enters the brain. Enzyme inhibition is part of the function of several medications (Table 4).

Table 2

Parkinson Disease: Clinical Features

Primary Characteristics (usually unilateral, or at least asymmetric)

Bradykinesia (akinesia)
Rigidity
Tremor
(Gait disorder)

Secondary Characteristics

Gait disorder (*"marche a petit pas"*)
Reduced arm swing postural instability, freezing spells, start hesitation
Flexion posture
Seborrhea
Masked facies ("reptilian stare")
Reduced eye-blink rate
Excessive saliva production (drooling, especially at night)
Difficulty with fine motor tasks (utensils, buttons, toothbrush)
Micrographia (handwriting, spiral drawing)
Difficulty arising from chair, rolling over in bed
Speech difficulty (hypophonia, aprosody, tachyphemia)

Table 3

Genetic Parkinsonism

Name	Locus	Gene
Park 1	4q 21.3	α-synuclein
Park 2	6q 25.2-q 27	Parkin
Park 3	2p 13	Unknown
Park 4	4q	Multiple copies of synuclein
Park 5	4p14	Ubiquitin C-terminal hydrolase l1
Park 6	1p 35-p 36	Pink-1
Park 7	1p 36	DJ-1
Park 8	12p 11.2-q 13.1	LRRK2
Park 9	1p 36	(Not confirmed as Parkinson disease)
Park 10	1p 32	Unknown
Park 11	2q 36-q 37	Unknown

Controversy remains about whether the oxidative byproducts of dopamine (endogenous or exogenous) may be injurious to the striatum, thereby worsening the disease or contributing to the motor fluctuations seen in many patients as years go by. Often, patients enjoy a honeymoon period of symptom relief with CD/LD, only to later develop less predictable effects. "Wearing off" of each dose can occur late in the course and can be addressed by using long-acting CD/LD, or by varying dose and/or interval of short-acting CD/LD. "On/off" phenomenon is more problematic since it is not predictable. As time goes by, dyskinesias (initially indicative of too high a dose) may occur even at doses only minimally effective. In other words, the therapeutic window narrows with time and can become a moving target.

Figure 3

Metabolic pathway for levodopa

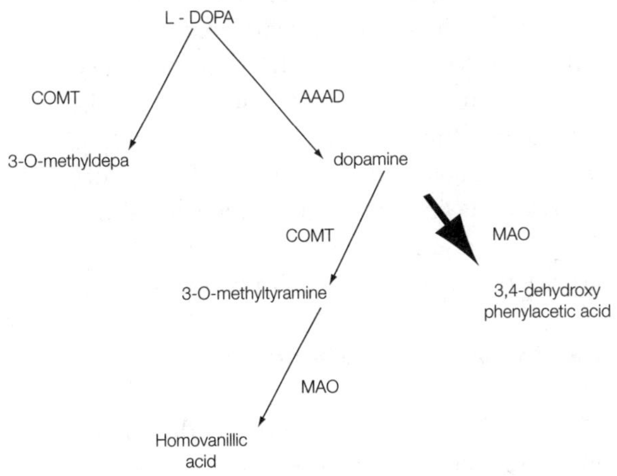

Possibly, complications like these can be delayed or avoided by adopting a levodopa sparing strategy. Delaying levodopa treatment and keeping dosage low can be accomplished by expectant management (frequent visits to monitor clinical condition) and by use of other agents—however, it is less effective than dopamine in general.

Synthetic direct-acting dopamine agonists have been designed to initiate the action of dopamine at its receptors and may have other pharmacologic properties as well (Table 4). Ropinirole and pramipexole are more specific than bromocriptine mesylate and pergolyde mesylate for the D2 and D3 receptors and are nonergoline in derivation, thus avoiding ergotamine side effects.

Nondopaminergic agents may also be useful for symptoms of parkinsonism. Amantadine is an antiviral agent that has an uncertain mechanism,

Table 4

Drugs Whose Mechanism of Action Includes Specific Enzyme Inhibition

Drug	Enzyme Inhibited	Effect of Inhibition
Carbidopa (CD)	Amino acid decarboxylase	Prevents peripheral conversion of levodopa to dopamine
Selegeline	Monoamine oxidase, type B (MAO-B)	Prevents breakdown of monamines incuding dopamine (?reduces harmful oxidation products)
Tolcapone, entacapone	Catechol-O-methyltransferase	Prevents degradation of catecholamines including dopamine, thereby increasing area under time-concentration curve

with some dopaminergic, anticholinergic and antiglutaminergic properties. It can sometimes be useful as initial treatment in mild Parkinson disease, or to diminish dyskinesias. Limiting side effects can include ankle edema and livedo reticularis. Anticholinergic agents such as benztropine, trihexyphenidyl or biperiden HCl were the first synthetically produced drugs to treat Parkinson disease. They are useful in early disease (especially tremor-predominant patients) but are less effective for bradykinesia / rigidity than dopaminergic drugs. They can cause dry mouth, constipation, dizziness, urinary retention, or even delirium/hallucinations.

Parkinson-Plus Syndromes

There are a number of other primary disorders that may resemble or share some clinical characteristics with Parkinson disease but are otherwise distinct entities (Table 5). At the time of presentation, they may be extremely difficult to distinguish from Parkinson disease. Later on, it may become clear that additional symptoms develop that are not parkinsonian, hence the term "parkinson-plus". Also, the rate of decline tends to be worse than in idiopathic Parkinson disease, and anti-parkinson medications may be ineffective. Like Parkinson disease, the diagnosis is made clinically, as there is no definitive radiologic or laboratory testing (Table 6).

Table 5

Parkinson-Plus Syndromes

Progressive supranuclear palsy (PSP)
Corticobasal ganglionic degeneration (CDBG)
Multiple system atrophy (MSA)
Striatonigral degeneration (SND)
Olivopontocerevellar atrophy (OPCA)
Shy-Drager syndrome (SDS)
Parkinsonism-dementia-ALS complex of Guam (PDACG) (also called Lytigo-Bodig)

Table 6

Clinical Clues that Suggest Parkinson-Plus Syndromes vs. Parkinson Disease

Lack of tremor
Poor response to dopaminergic treatment
Symmetry or persistent asymmetry of signs; Asymmetry early is usual in Parkinson disease
Prominent autonomic dysfunction (eg, orthostatic hypotension, incontinence)
Early hallucinations / dementia
Frequent falls at time of diagnosis
Myoclonus
Nuchal dystonia, torticollis
Alien limb phenomenon
Cerebellar signs with bulbar dysfunction
Upper / lower motor neuron signs
Impaired extraocular movement (especially vertical gaze)

Table 7

Radiologic Findings Sometimes Seen in Parkinson-Plus Conditions

Condition	Finding
Dementia with Lewy bodies	Relative sparing of hippocampi compared with Alzheimer disease
Multiple system atrophy-SND type	Putamenal rim hyperintensity in T2-weighted MRI images
Multiple system atrophy-OPCA type	Infratentorial atrophy
Progressive supranuclear palsy	Reduced midbrain diameter

However, some radiologic findings can be suggestive of certain diagnoses (Table 7). Also, CT or MRI can reveal some causes of secondary parkinsonism, such as tremor, stroke, manganese and carbon monoxide poisoning (lesions in globus pallidus and/or white matter), or communicating hydrocephalus, erroneously called "normal pressure" hydrocephalus.

Secondary parkinsonism can uncommonly be caused by toxins/medications (Table 8). Of these, neuroleptic-induced parkinsonism is the most common and ought to be obvious in the clinical setting by simple review of the patient's medications. Other toxic exposures may be occult or remote in time from presentation of symptoms, so are often difficult to prove. Infections of the central nervous system can sometimes produce parkinsonism as part of a larger clinical picture (Table 9).

Pathologically, the Parkinson-plus syndromes are different from Parkinson disease. Tau protein is hyperphosphorylated in progressive supranuclear palsy (PSP), corticobasal ganglionic degeneration (CBGD), and frontotemporal dementia with parkinsonism linked to chromosome 17 (FTDP-17), leading to deposition of neurofibrillary tangles. In multiple system atrophy, there are glial cytoplasmic inclusions composed of insoluble aggregates of α-synuclein.

Clinically, while up to one-fourth of all parkinsonism cases referred to movement disorders centers may actually be parkinsonism-plus in type, distinguishing these remains difficult. As mentioned earlier, emergence of atypical symptoms and signs may provide clues, as does diminished or absent response to dopamine replacement (Table 6).

Dementia with Lewy Bodies (DLB)

Parkinsonism with dementia and dementia with Lewy bodies may be part of the same spectrum of illness as idiopathic Parkinson disease, but some experts define them differently. By current consensus, three cardinal characteristics of DLB are: 1) fluctuations in cognitive performance; 2) visual hallucinations; and 3) parkinsonism. Presence of only one or two of these make the diagnosis possible or probable, respectively. The parkinsonism of DLB is less likely than Parkinson disease to be asymmetric at onset and less likely to include typical resting tremor. DLB patients are prone to falling even early in the course of illness, and may have syncope, delusions, and hypersensitivity to antipsychotics.

Table 8

Toxic-Metabolic Causes of Parkinsonism

Neuroleptics (including anti-emetics)
Heavy metal intoxication (manganese, lithium, mercury)
Carbon disulfide
Cyanide
Carbon monoxide
Methanol
Hypothyroidism
Parathyroid abnormalities

Table 9

Infections That Can Manifest Parkinsonism

AIDS
Postencephalitic (mainly of historical interest, related to von Economo encephalitis, 1916-1927)
Subacute sclerosing panencephalitis
Creutzfeldt-Jakob
Other prion diseases

Multiple System Atrophy

Historically, terms such as striatonigral degeneration, olivopontocerebellar atrophy (up to six subtypes), and Shy-Drager were all applied to different patients with this category of illness. These older designations are now considered variants of multiple systems atrophy (MSA) because of the shared pathologic abnormality of α -synuclein glial cytoplasmic inclusions (also sometimes in neurons). Neuronal cell loss and gliosis may be found in many structures from spinal cord (Onuf's nucleus, corticospinal tracts, anterior horns, intermediolateral cell columns) to vestibular structures, vagal nuclei, cerebellar Purkinje cells, olivary nuclei, locus ceruleus, thalamus, substantia nigra, caudate and putamen. Hence, different patients may show to variable degrees symptoms of akinetic rigidity, autonomic insufficiency (eg, orthostatic hypotension, impotence, urinary incontinence), cerebellar ataxia, and pyramidal tract signs. Dystonia, tremor, dysarthria and vocal stridor can sometimes be seen.

Progressive Supranuclear Palsy (PSP)

The hallmark feature of PSP is loss of vertical gaze (downgaze abnormality usually is the first to appear), followed eventually by difficulty with eye movements in all directions. Eye movement problems may only appear after several years, however, so these patients may initially be given a diagnosis of Parkinson disease based upon their rigidity and bradykinesia. These parkinson-like features are: poorly responsive to treatment, and patients are more prone to falling and early postural instability than patients with Parkinson disease. Rigidity is more symmetric and axial than in Parkinson disease, while tremor is often absent or kinetic rather than static. Neck hyperextension, dystonia and blepharospasm/blepharotonus may occur. Unlike the flexed posture of Parkinson disease patients, modified hyperextension may be seen when standing. Dysarthria and dysphagia are often present, but autonomic abnormality is uncommon. The prognosis and course are worse than Parkinson disease, with earlier impairment and death within a decade or so. When present, cognitive dysfunction appears late in the course.

Frontotemporal Dementia with Parkinsonism Linked to Chromosome 17 (FTDP-17)

Another of the tauopathies, this condition leads to atrophy of frontal and temporal lobes and associated impairment of judgment and behavior. Disinhibited, apathetic and inappropriate behaviors can be quite severe even when memory, attention and visuospatial functions are still preserved. Psychotic symptoms can include paranoia, fixed delusions and threatening auditory hallucinations. Only later do the parkinsonian symptoms occur, with bradykinesia and rigidity more often than tremor. Because this condition is caused by any of a number of mutations of a tau gene on 17q21, patients often have multiple affected relatives in an autosomal dominant pattern. As with other Parkinson-plus conditions, prognosis is worse than Parkinson disease and no treatment offers lasting benefit.

Corticobasal Ganglionic Degeneration (CGBD)

This tau-related disease may have distinctive cortical characteristics, most notably limb apraxia/dystonia, that can progress to the "alien limb" phenomenon. In some instances an affected upper extremity can seem to function entirely on its own, even exhibiting groping or manipulation approach behaviors. CBGD appcars spontaneously with no known genetic or environmental cause. It may initially be misdiagnosed as Parkinson disease until the limb apraxia, dystonias and cortical sensory changes (sometimes with cortical myoclonus) distinguish themselves. Progression from unilateral to bilateral disease occurs rapidly and treatment is generally ineffective, though botulinum toxin injections can partially relieve dystonia. Pathology in CBGD is loss of cells and enlargement of neuronal ("ballooned") cells in frontal and parietal cortex

Table 10

Tremor Types by Frequency and Etiology

Type	Frequency	Etiology
Kinetic (action)	1-5 hz	Cerebellar degeneration
Static (resting)	3-10 hz	Parkinsonism
Task specific	3-10 hz	?Dystonia
Essential	4-8 hz	Unknown
Orthostatic	16-25 hz	Unknown / neuropathic

with degeneration of corpus striatum and depigmentation/cell loss in substantia nigra. Lewy bodies are not seen.

Lytigo-Bodig/Parkinsonism-dementia Amyotrophic Lateral Sclerosis Complex of Guam (PDALS)

Essentially restricted in time and geography to post-World War II Guam, this condition has been fascinating to researchers because it might teach us about genetic and environmental causes of similar conditions. Unfortunately, early theories about possible causative agents (including locally made flour from the seeds of Cycas circinalis) have not held up. The coincidence of Parkinson disease dementia and ALS does suggest some overlap in etiology, however yet unexplained.

Though uncommon tremors of various frequencies have been associated with specific structures and conditions (Table 10), the most common clinical distinction that neurologists are asked to make is between essential tremor and parkinsonism. A number of factors can aid in that differential diagnosis (Table 11).

Essential Tremor (ET)

By far the most common tremor is essential tremor, ten to twenty times more common than Parkinson disease. Other terms used to describe this condition include "benign" and "familial", but many authors point out that neither is fully accurate. Sporadic cases can occur and some individuals can have significant impairment. Typically, however, essential tremor is mild, only worsening slowly over decades. When this tremor is first recognized in elder years it is called "senile" tremor. Essential tremor is symmetric, fine and irregular in frequency. It is not present at rest but comes out with posture (hands held out in front) and with action (finger-to-nose testing).

Table 11

Distinguishing Features of Parkinson vs. Essential Tremor

Parkinson Tremor	vs.	Essential Tremor
Static ("resting")		Postural / action
Usually sporadic		Often familial
Typically unilateral at onset		Bilateral, symmetric
May progress rapidly		Slowly progressive
Hand / leg		Hands / head / voice

Many patients who seek medical attention for tremor are satisfied only to learn that they don't have Parkinson disease. If their ET is neither embarrassing to them nor disabling, they may choose to have return visits annually or semiannually for reassessment rather than taking medical or surgical treatment. Roughly three-quarters of ET patients find that their tremor is measurably suppressed by small amounts of alcohol. This observation can occasionally prove useful, but of course there are potential hazards to alcohol use.

Though ET is widely recognized and studied, remarkably little is known about the underlying mechanism/substrate. There are relatively few established effective medical treatments. Beta-blockers and primidone are the two primary medications with adequate evidence for efficacy from clinical trials. Some patients are refractory to benefit from any medication and may require surgical treatment in the form of continuous high-frequency electrical stimulation of the ventral intermediate (VIM) nucleus of the thalamus via deep brain stimulating electrodes.

While the upper extremities are the most often affected areas, essential tremor can also affect (sometimes later in the course) head, voice or lower extremities. The pattern of inheritance is likely autosomal dominant but may show incomplete penetrance or variability in expression, given the wide range of reported incidence within families, from 17%-100%.

Other less common causes of tremor may mimic essential tremor, including drug effects, anxiety, psychogenic tremor, primary orthostatic tremor, or hyperthyroidism.

Myoclonus

Myoclonus is an involuntary, sudden, and brief muscle jerk. It can be the only symptom or part of a larger syndrome. The many causes and associated conditions of myoclonus can be organized categorically (Table 10). Caviness and colleagues conducted the only study thus far in a defined population (Olmsted County, Minnesota), and estimated the annual incidence of pathological and persistent myoclonus for 1976 to 1990 was 1.3 cases per 100,000 person years. The lifetime prevalence was 8.6 cases per 100,000. A useful approach to the patient with myoclonus is to determine whether the context is physiological, epileptic, symptomatic, or essential. Although myoclonus can result from lesions anywhere along the neuraxis, knowledge of its probable location can help narrow the differential and treatment options.

Physiologic myoclonus describes the normal phenomenon that almost everyone experiences. Sleep related myoclonus (hypnic jerks) occurs during transition between wakefulness and sleep. Another situation where myoclonus may occur normally is hiccoughs. Physiologic myoclonus can increase in the setting of exercise or anxiety.

In epileptic myoclonus, or myoclonic epilepsy, both myoclonus and seizures are the main neurological presentations. The clinical presentation is usually in childhood. Either seizures or myoclonus can be the initial presenting symptom but eventually epilepsy is the dominating presentation. Juvenile myoclonic epilepsy is the prototypic myoclonic epilepsy, in which myoclonus occurs in the setting of generalized tonic-clonic or absence seizures, without other neurological disability. Myoclonus often precedes the onset of seizures. Electroencephalography will often reveal generalized ictal epileptiform discharges associated with the myoclonus.

Symptomatic myoclonus, secondary to a known condition, is by far the most common and is often accompanied by additional neurologic or medical findings. The myoclonus may be only a minor feature in the overall clinical presentation. Attention is paid to screening for causes that can be easily treated or corrected. The motor cortex is the area most commonly involved in symptomatic myoclonus, but subcortical, brainstem, spinal and peripheral nervous system lesions can also occur. Drug-induced myoclonus is increasingly recognized. Lithium, quinolone antibiotics, and paradoxically, gabapentin and pregabalin, have been reported to cause myoclonus.

Essential myoclonus is a diagnosis of exclusion. When myoclonus is the only presenting complaint, the examination is normal, and the other causes of myoclonus have been eliminated, the most likely diagnostic consideration is essential myoclonus. Psychogenic myoclonus is a consideration when other possibilities have been eliminated. Distinguishing between these usually becomes evident after careful observation.

Treatment principles can be guided by etiologic and anatomic classification. In symptomatic myoclonus, the inciting cause should be pursued if possible. When the underlying etiology cannot be addressed, symptomatic therapy is guided by the anatomical source for the myoclonus. In cortical myoclonus, the main pathophysiology is a relative gamma-aminobutyric acid (GABA) deficiency. Medications aimed at correcting this are often effective. Valproate has the property of increasing GABA concentration in the cortex as well as potentiating GABA-postsynaptic inhibition. Effective doses range from 1200-2000 mg per day. Well known adverse effects of this medication may be limiting, including weight gain, tremor, hepatotoxicity, and drowsiness. Alternatively, benzodiazepines and barbiturates may be useful. Clonazepam is the most effective of this class of medications, but as high as 15 mg per day may be required for therapeutic effect, which can seldom be achieved without the cost of side effects such as drowsiness and imbalance. As with most medications, but especially with benzodiazepines, caution against abrupt cessation of the medication is required. Piracetam, a derivative of GABA, and the structurally similar levetiracetam, are well tolerated and effective for myoclonus. Doses for piracetam range from 2.4-21.6 g per day, and for levetiracetam 1000-3000 mg per day. Frequently, combination therapy is required to achieve adequate control of myoclonus. Given their minimal side effect profile, these medications are useful as adjunctive medications. For cortical-subcortical myoclonus, typified by juvenile myoclonic epilepsy and other myoclonic epilepsies, treatment is often successful with valproic acid or lamotrigine monotherapy.

Effective therapy is lacking in subcortical/supraspinal myoclonus, of which myoclonus dystonia, reticular reflex myoclonus, and opsoclonus-myoclonus are thought to be examples. Anticonvulsants are not effective and response to clonazepam is often only partial. Palatal myoclonus, a controversial term in itself because it has been debated whether this movement disorder represents tremor or myoclonus, localizes to the subcortical-brain stem area involving connections between the dentate nucleus, red nucleus, and inferior olivary nuclei (the Güillain-Molleret triangle). Effective treatment is lacking. Limited anecdotal reports suggest clonazepam, carbamazepine, baclofen (lioresal), anticholinergics, tetrabenazine, valproic acid, phenytoin, lamotrigine, sumatriptan, and piracetam as possible therapy. Botulinum toxin injection to the tensor veli palatini muscle may provide symptomatic relief in some cases. Effective treatment is also lacking for spinal myoclonus. Clonazepam, at doses as high as 6 mg per day, offers partial symptomatic relief and is the drug of first choice in propriospinal and spinal segmental myoclonus.

For peripheral myoclonus, of which hemifacial spasm is prototypical, the etiology is often secondary to direct or indirect compression or distortion of the root exit zone of the seventh cranial nerve. This is most commonly compressed by an arterial loop, but also may be compressed by any mass including tumor, cyst or aneurysm. Therefore, all patients must undergo MRI and vascular imaging either by MRA, CTA, or conventional angiography. Oral medications, typically anticonvulsants such as carbamazepine, may be useful. Local injection of botulinum toxin is also very successful and has the lowest rate of complications. When medication and botulinum toxin injections are inadequate, microvascular decompression should be considered as it offers definitive treatment.

Dystonia

Dystonia is used to describe contortions and bizarre postures caused by involuntary muscle contractions. The clinical presentation is highly variable and may mimic other movement disorders. For example, when dystonia is brief, it may resemble myoclonus but with more prolonged bursts of muscle activity. When dystonia is irregular, it can resemble chorea, but usually has more of a directional component in contrast to chorea, which is more random. When associated with voluntary or involuntary resistance, dystonia can resemble essential tremor, but usually is more irregular in frequency and amplitude and is less oscillatory.

An important clinical feature unique to dystonia is the phenomenon of gestes antagonistes or sensory trick, in which the dystonia can be suppressed by touching an affected or adjacent body part. Patients may describe these tricks without their awareness. It is also important to characterize the dystonia in relation to normal voluntary movement. For example, rest dystonia occurs without associated movement; task-specific dystonia occurs in association with specific movement, such as writing or a well-learned movement; and overflow dystonia overlies normal movement.

Dystonia can be classified on the basis of etiology (primary vs. secondary), anatomical distribution, and age at onset. Some causes of dystonia are readily treatable with specific therapy, and evaluation should be directed toward identifying these. Dopa-responsive dystonia (Segawa disease), for example, should be considered in the appropriate age group by a brief trial of low-dose levodopa (up to 300 mg levodopa per day). Wilson disease frequently presents as dystonia or tremor. Autoimmune, vascular and other conditions that can damage the basal ganglia can present with dystonia and are detectable by brain imaging. Clues to suggest a secondary dystonia include hemidystonia or rest dystonia at symptom onset. Clues to suggest a dystonia of psychogenic origin include an abrupt onset of symptoms, and extreme variability of symptoms. However, these conditions may be indistinguishable from primary dystonia and therefore must be carefully screened.

Generalized dystonia tends to present in childhood up to the third decade with rare exceptions. A three-nucleotide deletion in the DYT1 gene on chromosome 9q34 accounts for approximately three-fourths of typical early-onset generalized dystonia. The inheritance pattern is autosomal dominant with variable penetrance in which approximately two-thirds with the mutation are unaffected. A typical presentation begins with dystonia in the lower extremity and progresses to generalized dystonia. The differential diagnosis includes dopa-responsive dystonia and parkin gene mutation carrier status.

Focal dystonias encompass several distinct dystonic syndromes, including blepharospasm, oromandibular dystonia, cervical dystonia (spasmodic torticollis), laryngeal dystonia (spasmodic dysphonia), and limb dystonia. Common features shared by these syndromes include age at onset, usually becoming apparent in the fourth or fifth decade, and affecting women more frequently than men. The onset of symptoms is usually insidious, first appearing only with stress.

Cervical dystonia is the most common form of focal dystonia. The age at onset is typically younger than other focal dystonias, but can appear at any age between 20 and 60 years. The dystonia often begins intermittently and when accompanied by an opposing reaction results in a head tremor that may resemble essential tremor. Progression leads to more sustained muscle contractions, resulting in several characteristic patterns of cervical musculature involvement and abnormal postures, including rotation of the head (torticollis), tilt of the head to a side (laterocollis), front (anterocollis), or back (retrocollis). Shoulder elevation is often seen in combination with torticollis and retro or anterocollis. Segmental involvement of the upper extremity is sometimes seen. Clinical features of cervical dystonia, as in other dystonias, include exacerbation with stress or other activity, improvement with sleep, and very often with a sensory trick, by touching the side of the face opposite to the direction of the head turning. About two-thirds of patients have associated neck pain, and one-third have a tremor. About one-fifth of patients have involvement of adjacent body parts.

Blepharospasm is the involuntary closure of the muscles of the eye. The onset is typically insidious and attributed initially to dry eyes or an irritation. For this reason an ophthalmologist is usually seen first. Onset is usually bilateral. Sensory trick phenomenon can often be elicited by the touch to an adjacent part of the face. The pattern is usually focal, but can involve other facial musculature, resulting in squinting and nose wrinkling. Oromandibular dystonia affects the jaw, mouth, and lower face, causing symptoms of jaw closure, jaw opening, teeth clenching, or teeth grinding. Meige syndrome refers to segmental dystonia involving oromandibular dystonia and blepharospasm.

Treatment for dystonia follows three broad categories: pharmacologic therapy, chemodenervation, and surgery. In childhood or early onset dystonia, dopa-responsive dystonia results in dramatic improvement after low-dose levodopa (at least 300 mg levodopa per day). A trial of an anticholinergic medication, typically trihexyphenidyl (Artane®) can be helpful. The side effects can be avoided by starting at a low dose (half of a 2 mg tablet taken two to three times daily), and titrated very slowly to a goal of 15-20 milligrams per day, or the onset of significant side effects, whichever comes first. Unfortunately, the side effects of dry mouth, constipation, and cognitive impairment are significant and limit its usefulness, especially in the older patient population. Medications affecting other neurotransmitter classes include benzodiazepines, dopamine depleters (tetrabenazine), and GABAergics, and atypical neuroleptics.

In focal or segmental dystonia, local injections of botulinum toxin are effective in selective weakening of the over-active muscles. For generalized dystonia, pallidotomy and deep brain stimulation to the globus pallidus internus are considerations. However, selective lesioning of the GPi in pallidotomy or DBS is not explained well by current models. Nevertheless, the role of surgery will likely continue to expand, and increasing numbers of case reports describe successful application in cervical dystonia and other focal dystonias. Adjunctive therapy such as physical therapy and supportive therapy are important components for a comprehensive treatment program.

Chorea

Chorea was first named in the 16th century by Paracelsus to describe uncoordinated dance-like movements. Chorea can be caused by genetic and nongenetic causes. The most common genetic cause of chorea is Huntington disease, named after George Huntington, who characterized the clinical manifestations and noted its familial nature in 1872. The gene for HD was discovered in 1993. The disease results from abnormally long CAG trinucleotide repeats in the IT15 gene, and is the prototypical nucleotide repeat disease, which includes bulbospinal muscular atrophy, dentatorubropallidoluysian atrophy (DRPLA), and the spinocerebellar ataxias (SCAs), among others.

Prevalence estimates of HD vary considerably because of founder effects and difficulty with ascertainment, but may be as high as 10 per 100,000, and those at 50% or 25% risk are thought to be 5 and 11 times that number. The mean age at symptom onset typically ranges from 35-42 years, and mean age at death is 50-56. When onset is in the juvenile age, an akinetic-rigid syndrome called the Westphal variant predominates. This variant is characterized by parkinsonism, dystonia, more severe cognitive decline, seizures and myoclonus. Late-onset cases, seen in one-third of cases, begin after age 50. There is no upper age limit to the diagnosis of HD. As a result, a negative family history in the parents does not exclude the possibility of HD.

The molecular pathogenesis of HD is not fully understood. It is a true dominant mutation in which having two abnormal copies does not differ from having one abnormal copy. The CAG repeats encode glutamine, which forms a polyglutamine tract in the Huntingtin protein. A CAG repeat length less than 32 is considered normal, while 32-39 is indeterminate, and greater than 39 is definitely abnormal. Repeat length correlates with disease severity, but there is considerable variability, which implicates other environmental or genetic influences.

Treatment for Huntington disease remains symptomatic. Chorea can be treated with neuroleptic medications or the dopamine depleter tetrabenzine. However, there is a risk for depression and tardive dyskinesia with these agents. Hallucinations and behavioral disorders may be controlled with neuroleptic medications. Behavioral disorders may also respond to neuroleptic medications, as well as carbamazepine. Depression is common and treatable with antidepressants. In the early and middle stages, suicide is high risk. Obsessive compulsive symptoms may respond to clomipramine or an SSRI. The akinetic rigid symptoms are not responsive to levodopa or dopamine agonists, but may respond to amantadine or anticholinergic medication.

Huntington disease is a prototypical genetic disease that has helped establish concepts in genetic counseling and testing. An important distinction to be made early is whether testing is performed for presymptomatic vs. symptomatic reasons. While symptomatic diagnostic testing can be performed on individuals at any age with appropriate consent, presymptomatic testing can still only be offered to adults. One potential area of difficulty in genetic testing is the testing of presymptomatic offspring of an at-risk parent who does not want to know their genetic status. Predictive testing should take the interest of the at-risk offspring over the wish of the at-risk parent not to know. Fortunately, these issues can be effectively addressed with genetic counseling.

Other hereditary choreas include dentatorubral-pallidoluysian atrophy (DRPLA), neuroacanthocytosis, and benign hereditary chorea. The clinical presentation of DRPLA is similar to HD and is caused by a CAG trinucleotide repeat expansion in the ATN1 gene. Neuroacanthocytosis can be caused by mutations in the chorea-acanthocytosis (CHAC) gene, or by the absence of the Kell-binding erythrocyte membrane protein Kx, referred to as McLeod syndrome. Onset is usually in the fifth decade. Lip biting and facial tics are characteristic of choreoacanthocytosis, whereas facial grimacing and involuntary vocalization may occur in McLeod syndrome. Dysphagia is uncommon in McLeod syndrome, but psychiatric signs and symptoms may be present. Benign hereditary chorea has been associated with mutations in the TITF-1 gene, a transcription factor essential for the organogenesis of the lung, thyroid, and basal ganglia.

Of the nongenetic causes of chorea, Sydenham chorea is the most common cause of childhood onset. Molecular mimicry is thought to result from the postinfectious condition associated with betahemolytic streptococcal infection. The age at onset is 8-9 years on average with a range between age 5 up to the third decade. The typical presentation is the onset of chorea preceded 4-8 weeks by a history of pharyngitis. Subsequent antibody titers to antistreptolysin-O confirm infection with group A betahemolytic streptococcus. Interestingly, streptococcal infection of the skin does not produce this syndrome. The typical course is a focal onset with rapid generalization, although hemichorea can occur in a fifth of cases. Examination shows motor impersistence upon testing of prolonged tongue protrusion or ocular fixation. The spectrum of disorders in Sydenham chorea also extends to Gilles de la Tourettes, including tics, obsessive compulsive, as well as attention deficit hyperactivity disorders. Case studies estimate that as much as one-quarter to one-third of cases can manifest with tics, OCD, or ADHD symptoms. No controlled studies are available to guide symptomatic treatment. The conventional approach uses anticonvulsants valproic acid or carbamazepine as first-line agents. Dopamine blocking agents, usually pimozide, are used in refractory cases. The association with specific antibodies form the rationale for immunosuppressive therapy, although its use is not well established. Cardoso reported that methylprednisilone, at 25 mg/kg per day in children and 1 g/kg in adults, for 5 days followed by 1 mg/kg per day of prednisone was effective and well tolerated in patients refractory to conventional treatment. Rarely is the cost and risk of plasma exchange or IVIG justified, but it has been used in the most severe cases.

Chorea gravidarum (CG) is another nongenetic chorea that is seen in relatively small but significant cases of pregnancy. A prior history of chorea in childhood was observed in more than half of cases. Like Sydenham chorea, CG is much less common today, suggesting a link between the two.

Other autoimmune conditions such as lupus and primary anti-phospholipid antibody syndrome are well recognized to cause movement disorders, including chorea. A small percentage of SLE can present with chorea. Other autoimmune paraneoplastic antibodies have been associated with chorea, including anti-Hu and anti-CRMP5 associated with small lung cancer.

In adults, the most common cause of nongenetic chorea is stroke. It is a rare manifestation of stroke, accounting for less than 1% of acute stroke presentations. The vascular territories that usually result in chorea are the basal ganglia and surrounding white matter in the middle or posterior cerebral artery territory.

Medications are well known to cause chorea, the most common being dopaminergic therapy for Parkinson disease. Lithium, lamotrigine, and methadone can also cause chorea. Estrogens, which in experimental animals can upregulate dopamine receptors, may account for the association seen between oral contraceptive-induced chorea and chorea gravidarum.

In contrast to the postinfectious effect of betahemolytic streptococcus, other infections cause chorea via direct changes to the basal ganglia. These include HIV and tuberculosis.

Tics and Stereotypies

Tics are stereotypic, brief, repetitive, purposeless, nonrhythmic, involuntary movements or sounds. Tics tend to involve facial, pharyngeal, and shoulder musculature, manifesting as both motor stereotypies and vocalizations. Other characteristics of tics include a tendency to occur in bursts or clusters. They can be suppressed temporarily—to accommodate a social situation, for example—but involuntarily resume with increased intensity and severity. The stereotypies can be simple, involving only a single muscle group, such as the orbicularis oculi (blinking), shoulder musculature (head jerking, or shrugging), or orbicularis oris (grimacing). They can also be complex, involving more than one muscle group, such as touching objects or people, jumping, spinning, or more complex motor sequences such as imitating other's actions (echopraxia), or manifesting inappropriate behavior (copropraxia) or vocalizations (coprolalia); or repeating a phrase that was last heard over and over (echolalia), or that was last spoken (palilalia). Other stereotypies can occur under both normal and abnormal circumstances. Repetitive head banging, thumb sucking and other behaviors are seen in normal children. However, many stereotypies often indicate a brain disorder, including static encephalopathy due to any central nervous system injury, as well as diseases across the autism spectrum, including Rett syndrome, Angelman and Prader-Willi syndrome.

The prototypical tic disorder is the syndrome of Gilles de la Tourette, named after the neurologist who first provided the most comprehensive description. It is defined as the childhood onset of multifocal, motor and vocal tics of more than one year duration, occurring in a waxing and waning course. Tics are only a part of a broader spectrum of clinical manifestations that includes obsessive compulsive disorder (OCD), attention deficit hyperactivity (ADHD), impulsive and self-destructive behaviors, and sleep abnormalities. Estimates of prevalence are difficult, and were initially low but now are considered to be relatively high, with many children undiagnosed because of mild symptoms. One review of epidemiological prevalence data in children estimated a range from 0.5 to 50 per 10,000 population.

The etiology of tics is unknown. Genetic factors are likely to play a role, because a family history can be found in more than 60% of cases of GTS. The mode of inheritance is complex and in some cases appears autosomal dominant, whereas in other GTS families a bilineal (from maternal and paternal lines) pattern is present. No specific genetic marker has been identified. Dopamine has been implicated in pathophysiology because dopamine-depleting drugs and neuroleptic DA receptor antagonists are effective in treating tics. Serotoninergic pathways may also play a role because serotonin reuptake inhibitors are effective in treating the obsessive-compulsive symptoms often associated with GTS. Other neurotransmitter systems (opiate) have also been proposed.

GTS is diagnosed by history and verified by neurological observation. Video is helpful to document observations when they are sufficiently rare to make office observations difficult. Past history, birth and developmental history may suggest a history of neonatal or perinatal injury. At least a three-generation family history with careful screening for tics, unusual habits, rituals, and obsessive-compulsive symptoms should be screened. Unless associated neurologic findings suggest a secondary tic disorder, neuroimaging and other studies are seldom required. Other laboratory testing should be directed toward screening secondary tic disorders.

Nonpharmacological therapy is the rule for most cases of tic disorders. Education and recognition of waxing and waning symptoms help with adjustment, coping and understanding. Supportive counseling may help with coping strategies. Neuropsychological testing may help thoroughly assess an individual profile. The local and national Tourette Syndrome Association can serve as an important resource for educational material and as a patient advocate in the school and work environment.

Assessment of the particular aspect of GTS is important to direct appropriate treatment when necessary. GTS may at times require temporary treatment because of the highly fluctuating nature. Tics are responsive to DA antagonists such as pimozide, fluphanzine, haloperidol, and risperidol. Clinicians often favor pimozide and fluphenazine, which are less sedating. All carry a risk for tardive dyskinesia, and discussion with the family is necessary. Dopamine depletion by tetrabenazine (not available in the United States) is also effective without the long-term risks of dyskinesia carried by the other treatments. Obsessive compulsive symptoms requiring treatment respond to tricyclics such as clomipramine, and SSRIs such as sertraline, fluoxetine, and paroxetine. ADHD symptoms respond to clonidine, guanfacine, and methylphenidate. Severe mood changes and problems with impulse control respond to lithium carbonate and carbamazepine.

The majority of patients with GTS will improve after adolescence and few will have clinically significant tics as adults. However, approximately one-third continue to be symptomatic throughout early adulthood.

4. References

1. Goetz C. *Textbook of Clinical Neurology*. 2nd ed. Oxford: Elsevier; 2003.

   (A definitive text with excellent emphasis on movement disorders.)

2. Watts RL, Koller WC, eds. *Movement Disorders: Neurologic Principles and Practice*. 2nd ed. New York, NY: McGraw-Hill; 2004.

   (Very thorough and current, incorporating extensive research evidence.)

3. Royden Jones H Jr. *Netter's Neurology*. Oxford: Elsevier; 2005.

   (Wonderful text, appropriately enhanced by Dr. Frank Netter's classic illustrations.)

4. LP Rowland, ed. *Merritt's Neurology*. 11th ed. Philadelphia, Pa: Lippincott, Williams and Wilkins; 2005.

   (A classic textbook for reference and board review.)

5. Coffey DJ. Neurological therapeutics: Parkinsonism. In: Melmon & Morelli's *Clinical Pharmacology: The Principles and Practical Application of Therapeutics*. 4th ed. New York, NY: McGraw-Hill; 2001.

   (Short review chapter about medications used to treat Parkinson disease.)

6. Hauser RA, Pahwah R. Current treatment challenges and emerging therapies in Parkinson disease. *Neurol Clin*. 2004;22(3s).

   (This supplement deals with a number of current concepts, including possible disease-modifying strategies such as neuroprotection.)

7. Mark MH. Lumping and splitting the Parkinson plus syndromes: dementia with Lewy bodies, multiple system atrophy, progressive supranuclear palsy, and cortical-basal ganglionic degeneration. *Neurol Clin*. 2001 Aug vi;19(3):607-27.

(A thoughtful explanation concerning the differential diagnosis of these parkinsonian syndromes.)

8. Louis ED. Essential tremor. *Lancet Neurology*. 2005 Feb;4(2):100-10.

(Emphasizes the current approaches to better understanding of this disorder.)

9. Pahwa R, Lyons KE. Essential tremor: differential diagnosis and current therapy. *Am J Med*. 2003 Aug 1;115(2):134-42.

(Brief, clear summary of important aspects of essential tremor and differential diagnosis.)

10. Caviness J, Brown P. Myoclonus: current conceptsand recent advances. *Lancet Neurology*. 2004;3:598-607.

(Provides an organized, rational approach toward diagnosis and treatment of myoclonus.)

11. Brewer GJ. Neurologically presenting Wilson disease: epidemiology, pathophysiology and treatment. *CNS Drugs*. 2005;3:185-92.

(A concise review on the neurological manifestations of Wilson disease, with a practical discussion on current treatment.)

12. Tepper JM, Abercrombie ED, Bolam JP. Basal ganglia macrocircuits. [Review] [19 refs] *Progress in Brain Research*. 2007; 160: 3-7.

(An introductory chapter to a volume dedicated to the basal ganglia, reviewing the basal ganglia nuclei, cellular structure, connections and function.)

13. Vitek JL. Pathophysiology of dystonia: a neuronal model. *Mov Disord*. 2002;17 Suppl 3:S49-62.

(Controversies and deficiencies of the current model in accounting for dystonia.)

14. Bradley WG, Daroff RB, Fenichel G, Jankovic J, eds. *Neurology in Clinical Practice*. 4th ed. London: Butterworth-Heinemann; 2004.

(Clinically oriented; detailed and thorough discussion.)

5. Questions

1. Which of the following exhibit characteristics of D1-type dopamine receptors?

   A. D1, D2 and D3

   B. D1 (D1a) and D5

   C. D4 and D5

   D. D1 only

2. When striatal dopamine is diminished in Parkinson disease:

   A. The direct pathway is overactive

   B. The indirect pathway is underactive

   C. The direct and indirect pathways are over-active

   D. The direct pathway is underactive and the indirect pathway is overactive

3. You are seeing a 50-year-old accountant with a 3-month history of progressive right hand tremor of insidious onset, which has been a source of concern during staff meetings. Examination reveals resting tremor of the right hand, isolated right wrist rigidity, and diminished amplitude and frequency of repetitive movements. Reflexes and coordination are normal. Gait and turn are normal with the exception of a decreased arm swing and enhanced tremor of the right hand. Which of the following is (are) true of this patient?

   A. This patient has three cardinal features of Parkinson disease: resting tremor, rigidity and bradykinesia

   B. As much as 70%-80% of striatal dopamine is already lost in this patient

   C. Genetic and environmental factors may contribute to the cause of this patient's symptoms

   D. All of the above

4. The patient informs you that tremor is the most concerning symptom. Which of the following medications might be considered first?

   A. Levodopa/carbidopa

   B. Amantadine

   C. Trihexyphenidyl

   D. All of the above

5. The patient asks you for therapy that has proven to slow the progression of Parkinson disease. What can you tell him?

   A. Several agents have been proven to slow progression of Parkinson disease

   B. Only amantadine can slow progression in Parkinson disease

   C. At present only symptomatic treatment is available for Parkinson disease

   D. In general Parkinson-plus conditions progress more slowly than idiopathic Parkinson disease

6. You are seeing a 79-year-old retired school teacher with a six-month history of gradual decline in function, now with difficulty with independent living. The following clinical characteristics are supportive of a diagnosis of dementia with Lewy bodies EXCEPT:

A. Parkinsonism

B. Fluctuations in cognitive performance

C. Auditory hallucinations

D. Visual hallucinations

7. The patient declined rapidly over the next four years despite best therapeutic efforts. Early discussion with the patient and family about postmortem diagnosis has subsequently led to the family's request for pathological analysis. Specialized studies were sent and came back positive for hyperphosphorylation of tau protein. The LEAST likely diagnosis is:

A. Multiple system atrophy

B. Frontotemporal dementia linked to chromosome 17

C. Progressive supranuclear palsy

D. Corticobasal ganglionic degeneration

8. You are asked to consult on a 75-year-old man with 3-year history of progressive left-sided stiffness and decreased arm swing that was diagnosed as Parkinson disease but has not been responsive to escalating doses of carbidopa/levodopa. Examination revealed that in addition to rigidity and bradykinesia, the patient seemed to exhibit grasping actions of the left hand unbeknownst to him. What is this phenomenon and what condition is this associated with classically?

A. This is the "geste antagoniste" phenomenon seen in focal limb dystonia of rapid onset dystonia-parkinsonism

B. This is the "alien limb" phenomenon seen in corticobasal ganglionic degeneration

C. This is the "echopraxia" phenomenon seen in tic disorders

D. This is "motor impersistence" phenomenon seen in the Westphal variant of Huntington disease

9. C.H. is a 35-year-old woman with a lifelong history of tremor. What features in the history would support a diagnosis of essential tremor?

A. Usually begins unilaterally

B. Typically improves with age

C. May be suppressed after alcohol ingestion

D. Is primarily a static tremor

10. Trials of propranolol and primidone have failed to provide adequate control of the tremor. She inquires about surgical options. What would you suggest?

A. Deep brain stimulation of the thalamus

B. Deep brain stimulation of the globus pallidus

C. Deep brain stimulation of the subthalamic nuclei

D. There is no evidence for efficacious surgery for tremor

11. A 20-year-old college student presents with involuntary movements. She provides examples where she suddenly claps her hands together for no apparent reason. Other times she accidently sends her pen off the notebook flying across the room in class. Lesions in which of the following structures can cause this?

A. Motor cortex

B. Spinal cord

C. Peripheral nerve

D. All of the above

12. Most neurons in the following nuclei are considered GABAergic EXCEPT:

A. Striatum

B. Subthalamic nucleus

C. Globus pallidus externus

D. Globus pallidus internus

13. The following statements about dystonia are true EXCEPT:

A. Childhood generalized dystonia typically begins in the upper extremity

B. A trial of levodopa should be tried in childhood onset dystonia

C. Early onset Parkinson disease can present as distal dystonia

D. Dystonia can be classified by age at onset and anatomical involvement

14. Dystonia is unique from other movement disorders in that:

A. Botulinum toxin therapy can provide symptomatic benefit

B. There are both childhood and adult onset forms

C. Sensory stimulation can modulate its severity

D. It can be responsive to levodopa

15. The first anatomical site involved in Huntington disease is located in the:

A. Striatum

B. Subthalamic nucleus

C. Globus pallidus externus

D. Globus pallidus internus

16. You are asked to evaluate an 8-year-old boy who presents with involuntary movements preceded by a recent upper respiratory tract infection. The following statements concerning his condition are true EXCEPT:

A. It is associated with post-streptococcal infection.

B. Genetic testing will reveal a trinucleotide repeat expansion of the IT15 gene.

C. The prognosis is good and symptoms are expected to resolve in their own in time

D. Treatment is not necessary unless the movements are excessively intrusive

17. The movements are interfering with the boy's ability to attend class. First line therapy to consider include the following:

A. Carbamazepine

B. Valproic acid

C. Both A and B

D. None of the above

18. During a follow-up appointment, the child's parents note frequent sniffing, and repetitive eye blinking. The most likely explanation is that:

A. This child also has a diagnosis of Gilles de la Tourette syndrome.

B. The Post-streptococcal antibody syndrome can mainifest in a spectrum including vocal and motor tics.

C. This patient is experiencing medication-related side effects

D. The patient has a lingering nasal and conjuctival infection and should be referred to a specialist in infectious disease.

19. A 19-year-old female presents with bilateral random involuntary finger movements. The remainder of the exam is normal. Possible explanations for this condition include the following EXCEPT:

A. Lithium, lamotrigine, or methadone therapy may cause this

B. The patient takes oral contraceptives

C. HIV infection may manifest as this condition

D. Post-infectious manifestation of streptococcal infection may cause this

E. All are correct

20. You are asked to see a 12-year-old child with a 2-year history of repetitive vocalizations and involuntary facial movements. Past history is significant for attention deficit and a tendency for impulsive behavior. Which of the following statements about this child are most likely true?

A. The impulsive behavior and OCD are likely coincidental and not part of the clinical syndrome

B. Diagnosis is verified by serologic testing for anti-streptolysin-O antibodies

C. Nonpharmacological therapy such as education and supportive counseling may help as first-line therapy.

D. Selective serotonin reuptake inhibitors are useful for treating the vocalizations and involuntary movements.

E. Prognosis is poor with the majority (two-thirds) continuing to be symptomatic into adulthood.

Answers

1. B.

Five unique dopamine receptors have been cloned in the study of dopamine pharmacology, D1 through D5. All five can be categorized as either D1 type or D2 type, depending on the population of striatal cells they affect and whether they increase or decrease cyclic AMP production. D1 (also called D1a) receptors and D5 are of the D1 type, while D2, D3 and D4 receptors are of the D2 type. D1 type receptors are concentrated in the striatal cells, whereas D2 type receptors are in matrix. D1 type receptors predominate in the direct output pathway, while D2 type predominate in the indirect pathway.

2. D.

If striatal dopamine is diminished as in Parkinson disease, both pathways are affected. The loss of dopamine stimulation of D1 type receptors in the direct pathway results in decreased cyclic AMP production and is underactive. The loss of dopamine stimulation of D2 type receptors in the indirect pathway results in increased cyclic AMP production and is therefore overactive.

3. D.

James Parkinson 1817 essay, "On the Shaking Palsy", denoted the basic clinical triad of bradykinesia/akinesia, rigidity and tremor. The pathophysiology of idiopathic Parkinson disease centers on the loss of greater than 70%-80% of dopaminergic input to the corpus striatum. The etiology of Parkinson disease is still not clear. Most cases are still considered sporadic (cohort studies of identical twins show incomplete concordance), but there may be genetic predisposition that can be triggered by some environmental influence.

4. C.

Anticholinergic agents such as benztropine, trihexyphenidyl or biperiden HCl were the first synthetically produced drugs to treat Parkinson disease. They are useful in early disease (especially tremor-predominant patients) but are less effective for bradykinesia / rigidity than dopaminergic drugs. They can cause dry mouth, constipation, dizziness, urinary retention or even delirium/hallucinations.

5. C.

For now, treatment of Parkinson disease remains symptomatic. In general, current medications all have the property of promoting dopamine in some way. Parkinson-plus conditions usually progress more rapidly.

6. C.

Dementia with Lewy bodies is characterized by: (1) fluctuations in cognitive performance, (2) visual hallucinations, and (3) parkinsonism. Auditory hallucinations are not likely.

7. A.

A. Multiple system atrophy, which includes striatonigral degeneration, olivopontocerebellar atrophy (up to six subtypes), and Shy-Drager, is characterized pathologically by project to the subthalamic nucleus, which is then output to the VA/VL nuclei of the thalamus.

8. B.

The geste antagoniste or sensory trick phenomenon seen in dystonia is characterized as the ability to diminish the dystonia simply by touching near or adjacent to the affected body part. The "alien limb" phenomenon is seen in corticobasal ganglionic degeneration and is characterized by the inability to recognize one's own limb. The "echopraxia" in tic disorders characterizes the tendency to imitate observed motor actions. "Motor impersistence" or the inability to maintain a fixed position for a period of time can be seen in Huntington disease.

9. C.

Essential tremor usually begins bilaterally, and typically worsens with age. It may be suppressed after alcohol intake and can serve as a diagnostic clue. It is primarily a slowly progressive tremor.

10. A.

Deep brain stimulation of the ventral intermediate nucleus of the thalamus has been shown in clinical trials to be efficacious in the treatment of essential tremor. The globus pallidus (internus) and subthalamic nucleus are sites favored in Parkinson disease deep brain stimulation therapy.

11. D.

She most likely is describing myoclonus, which can result from lesions anywhere along the neuraxis from the motor cortex to the brain stem, spinal cord and peripheral nerve.

12. B.

The subthalamic nucleus is unique in that its output neurons are glutamatergic rather than GABAergic.

13. A.

Childhood onset dystonia can begin anywhere in upper or lower extremity or in the neck or trunk. However, generalization usually occurs when dystonia initially affects the lower extremity. Dopa-responsive dystonia cannot be missed and therefore a trial of levodopa should be tried in childhood onset dystonia. Early onset Parkinson disease can present as distal dystonia. Dystonia can be classified by age at onset and anatomical involvement.

14. C.

A generally well-recognized feature of dystonia is the ability to modulate the severity with sensory stimulation. Botulinum toxin can be used in many movement disorders. Dystonia is not unique in its onset in both childhood and adulthood, nor is it unique in its responsiveness to levodopa.

15. A.

The first anatomical site of involvement in Huntington disease is the striatum, in particular the caudate. However, neuronal loss is not restricted to these areas, but all areas of the brain are broadly affected.

16. B.

This child most likely has a post-streptococcal choreoathetosis. Trinucucleotide repeat expansion identifies Huntington disease patients, not post-streptococcal choreoathetosis. The condition usually resolves on its own, and treatment is not usually indicated unless it is severe.

17. C.

Limited clinical evidence suggests that carbamaepine and valproic acid, traditional first line agents for Sydenham chorea, are equally efficacious.

18. B.

While motor and vocal tics are necessary for the diagnosis of Gilles de la Tourette syndrome, post-streptococcal infections may lead to a wide spectrum of disorders termed pediatric autoimmune neuropsychiatric disorders associated with streptococcal infection (PANDAS), that includes vocal and motor tics as well as OCD type behavior.

19. E.

Medications are well known to cause chorea, the most common being dopaminergic therapy for Parkinson disease. Lithium, lamotrigine, and methadone can also cause chorea. Estrogens, which in experimental animals can upregulate dopamine receptors, may account for the association seen between oral contraceptive-induced chorea and chorea gravidarum. In contrast to the postinfectious effect of betahemolytic streptococcus, other infections cause chorea via direct changes to the basal ganglia. These include HIV and tuberculosis.

20. C.

The impulsive behavior and OCD are likely part of the Gilles de la Tourette syndrome. Serologic testing is important to support a post-infectious streptococccal autoimmune disorder but not for establishing a diagnosis of Gilles de la Tourette syndrome. Nonpharmacological therapy such as education and supportive counseling is first line therapy. Selective serotonin reuptake inhibitors are useful for treating the obsessive-compulsive symptoms. The prognosis is good in the majority of cases with the majority (two-thirds) subsiding as they enter adulthood.

Chapter 13: Cerebellar Disease and Ataxia

Stephen Alan Berman, MD, PhD

Contents

1. Introduction

Ataxia refers to incoordination, unsteadiness, or instability of movement, which cannot be explained by simple loss of strength. The word "ataxia" itself derives from a combination of Greek roots. The "a" means "not" or "lack of." "Tax" comes from "taxis" or "tassein," meaning "order," and "ia" is a suffix used to represent a condition. So via the Greek derivation it is a "condition characterized by a lack of order," eg, disordered or unorderly movements.

Cerebellar lesions and cerebellar disease are prominent causes of ataxia. But lesions in other parts of the brain or brainstem or in the spinal cord can cause ataxia by disrupting the flow of information into or out of the cerebellum. Lesions in the peripheral nerves, especially those which carry sensory proprioceptive (position sense) data as well as vestibular lesions, can cause ataxia.

2. Anatomical Basis of Cerebellar Syndromes

Located in the posterior fossa, the cerebellum integrates sensory input from the periphery to help regulate voluntary movements. It modulates, coordinates, and regulates the rate, direction, timing and other related aspects of movement, as well as the muscle tone. Numerous animal studies and human anatomical, pathophysiological and clinical correlations have helped define specific areas in the cerebellum that regulate certain aspects of movement. There is, however, no exact correspondence between the animal data and human cerebellum disorders. Even the best attempts to apply clinical correlative knowledge of cerebellar localization may fail to agree with results of MRI scans. Nonetheless, the study of cerebellar disease and ataxia frequently gives the clinician the ability to make sophisticated diagnoses from a good history and physical exam.

Cerebellar Input (Afferent) Tracks

Most sensory information enters the cerebellum through the juxtarestiform body in the inferior cerebellar peduncle. Some enters through the superior cerebellar peduncle. Proprioceptive (position sense) data informs the central nervous system of the position of joints and muscle activity.

Vestibular information (from middle ear sensory receptors) also enters through the juxtarestiform body. Inputs from the cerebral cortex synapse in the pons prior to relaying via the middle cerebellar peduncle to reach the cerebellum.

Output (Efferent) Tracks

Information leaves the cerebellum largely through the superior cerebellar peduncle (brachium conjunctivum). The output arises from deep cerebellar nuclei and mostly terminates in the contralateral ventral lateral thalamic nucleus. Some fibers terminate in the red nucleus, which then sends projections to the thalamus via the rubospinal tract and also to the brain stem and the spinal cord.

Microscopic Anatomy and Neurotransmitters

On the microscopic level, there are five major types of neurons in the cerebellum: Purkinje, granule, stellate, basket and Golgi cells. Cerebellar granule cells use the excitatory neurotransmitter glutamate. The others use the inhibitory neurotransmitter gamma amino butyric acid (GABA).

Neuroanatomical Correlations

There are numerous systems for cerebellar anatomy nomenclature and cerebellar neuroanatomical correlations. The neuroanatomical system I find the most clinically useful is based on the two simple types of neuroanatomical categories illustrated in Figure 1. The Longitudinal Divisions consist of a central vermis and two cerebellar hemispheres on each side. The Transverse Divisions consist of an Anterior Lobe, a Posterior Lobe, and a Floculonodular Lobe. As noted on the Figure, vermal lesions affect postural stability. The rostral vermis, which is affected early by alcohol and related nutational problems, has a particularly strong influence on gait. Alcoholic vermal damage causes gait ataxia acutely and long-term chronic damage causes the typical "wide-based cerebellar gait" seen in alcoholics. Among the cerebellar cell types mentioned above, the Purkinje cells are exquisitely sensitive to alcohol toxicity, which causes dysfunction acutely and neuronal cell death chronically. The fact that individuals often can somewhat increase the amount they drink without staggering is not due to cerebellar adaptation but to increased alcohol metabolism by the liver. The caudal vermis controls truncal stability and is most commonly affected by tumors, paraneoplastic syndromes, or as part of a more generalized pancerebellar degeneration.

The floculonodular lobe has a major involvement with vestibular sensations. In fact, the floculonodular lobe is sometimes called the vestibulocerebellum. Thus, floculonodular lesions can cause nystagmus, eye deviations, and other eye movement abnormalities. The most common causes are either direct tumor invasion, paraneoplastic involvement, or as part of a larger pancerebellar syndrome.

Damage to a cerebellar hemisphere causes ataxia in the ipsilateral extremities. The ataxia can take the form of dysnergia (poor synchronization of movement, decomposition of movement); dysmetria (difficulty reaching to and stopped at a specific point); dysdiadochokinesia (difficulty with rapidly alternating

Figure 1

Anatomical divisions of the cerebellum

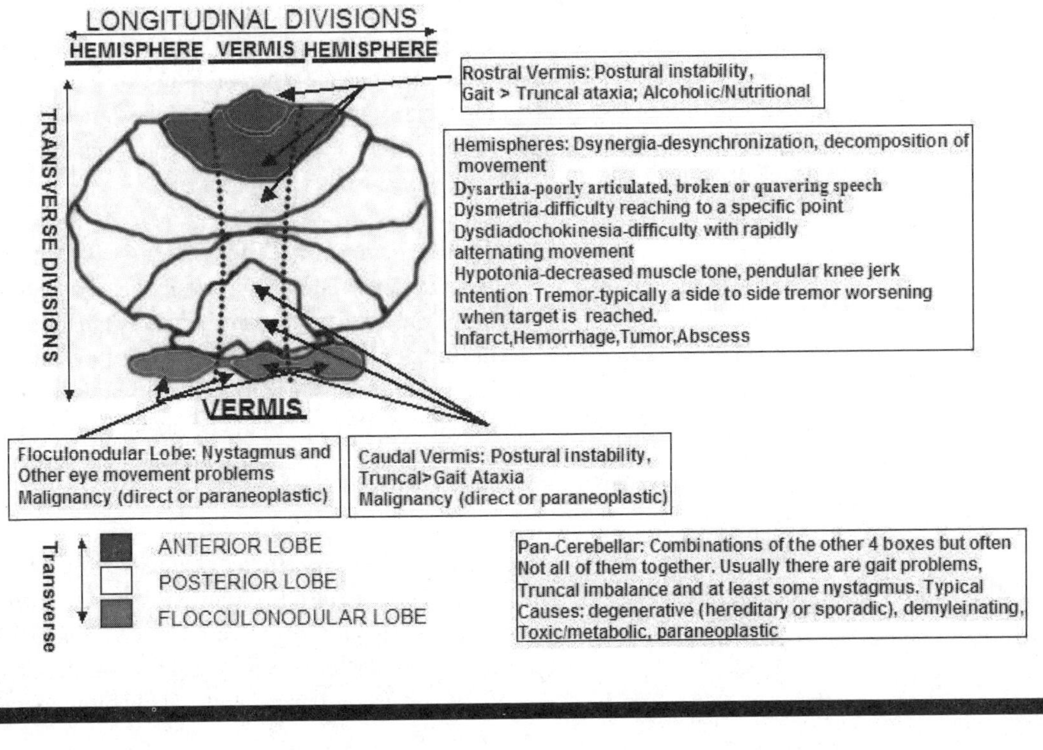

movements); or tremor (typically a side-to-side tremor worsening when the target is reached.) Hypotonia is sometimes seen, especially with acute lesions. In addition, dysarthria (poorly articulated, broken or quavering speech) and difficulties swallowing (due to problems coordinating the swallowing process) may be seen. Typical causes are infarct, hemorrhage, tumor, and abscess.

Finally, there is the pancerebellar syndrome, which implies dysfunction of all (or a reasonably large subset) of the above mentioned components. Most commonly, this is caused by a neurodegenerative disease, such as a spinocerebellar degeneration, or an autoimmune (eg, paraneoplastic) attack on the cerebellum. Demyelination (eg, multiple sclerosis) and toxic/metabolic problems may also cause a pancerebellar syndrome. Generally, a familial pancerebellar syndrome would come on gradually, whereas autoimmune or demyelinating (in the sense of multiple sclerosis, which is actually also thought to be autoimmune), or toxic/metabolic cases would present more rapidly. As one might expect, one sees a combination of the cerebellar problems mentioned above, typically including gait ataxia, truncal instability, and nystagmus. In the discussion below, I will explain the terminology of cerebellar deficits in further detail.

3. Terminology of Cerebellar Deficits and Ataxia

Neurologists use numerous clinical terms to describe cerebellar dysfunction. The phenomena they describe overlap somewhat and are not always well defined. Ataxia is perhaps the most frequently used term to described cerebellar dysfunction. It is also a more general term and includes many of the others. Dysmetria is the inability to correctly gauge the velocity or amplitude of a movement. Thus, the patient tends to miss the target. Dysnergy or asynergy implies a loss of coordination with the muscles not working together harmoniously. Intention tremor is best seen in cerebellar disease when an individual attempts to hit a target. As the individual comes closer and closer to the target, the tremor shows an increasing side-to-side movement perpendicular to the line of motion. However, the actual character of the tremor as seen in cerebellar disease can be quite variable in clinical practice. Cerebellar dysfunction also produces various eye movement abnormalities, such as nystagmus, described below.

Coordination

Coordination, as described by Gordon Holmes (one of the founders of modern neurology), involves the rate, range and force of movement. Common tests to assess coordination include the well-known finger-to-nose and heel-to-shin test. In these tests, problems with coordination become evident, particularly toward the end of the movement with a side-to-side motion. Other tests of coordination include rapidly inverting one hand upon the other, or taking the index finger and repeatedly tapping the crease of the thumb. Damage to the cerebellar hemispheres typical impair coordination of the ipsilater extremities.

Dysdiadochokinesia. This is a long word for impairment of rapid alternating movements. For example, the normal individual can alternately tap his palm and the back of the same hand against his thigh or on the back of the opposite hand. The individual with cerebellar disease (particularly hemispheric cerebellar disease) performs such alternating movements clumsily, if at all.

Abnormal Rebound or Loss of Checking Ability. If a normal individual pulls against resistance and the resistance is suddenly released, he can "check" or stop his output of strength quickly. The arm snaps back only a bit and he can generally avoid hitting himself.

In cerebellar disease, this checking ability is lost or reduced. Thus, the patient may hit himself because he will not be able to stop or check his output of power quickly enough. This phenomenon is often called "rebound." Similarly, if a patient stretches his arms out horizontally and the examiner pushes down, the arms usually rebound upwards only slightly when the examiner lets go. In cerebellar disease, this rebound is accentuated.

Arm Drift (Difficulty Sustaining the Arms in a Level Outstretched Position). The normal person can close his eyes, stretch both arms forward in front of him parallel to the floor, and keep them relatively level with little movement for at least a minute. In cerebellar disease, one arm or the other, generally the one on the side of the cerebellar problem, drifts either upward or downward. An upward drift with a slight turning out of the palm is a reasonably strong indicator of cerebellar dysfunction on the same side. A downward drift could also indicate cerebellar disease but the more likely cause would be weakness. This is a rather indefinite sign and this phenomenon can be seen in cases of proprioceptive loss as well as psychogenic problems. But the experienced examiner can often diagnose cerebellar dysfunction from this sign.

Dysynergia and asynergia. Another aspect of incoordination is a breakdown in the normally smooth motion produced by reaching for an item. Many jerky movements replace one continuous movement.

Past Pointing or Hypermetria. To detect past pointing, the subject is shown an object and instructed to point at it. Then he is asked to point at it again with his eyes closed. Frequently the individual with cerebellar disease will miss the object, with the arm often pointing somewhat to one side of it or sometimes a little down or up. Similar to the test of maintaining arm position, this can be hard to interpret. Typically, the deviation is toward the side of the cerebellar lesion, assuming the lesion is unilateral. We also see this in vestibular disease.

Incoordination of Speech (Dysarthria). Incoordination of speech is also characteristic of cerebellar disease. This can consist of slurring of words together or variability in the force or intonation of speech (scanning speech or scanning dysarthria).

Balance, Equilibrium, and Truncal Stability

Romberg test. The Romberg test is mainly a test for sensory or proprioceptive ataxia, but it reveals some clues about cerebellar disease. The examiner asks the patient to stand with his feet together and stretch out his arms in front of him. Assuming the patient can perform this at all, the examiner notes how steady the patient is and to the extent to which he sways or loses his balance. Then the examiner asks the patient to close his eyes and reassesses the stability of the stance. The patient with cerebellar disease often shows difficulty performing the test with the eyes open and sways when attempting to stand with his feet together. With the eyes closed, the swaying may increase somewhat. If the instability is such that the patient falls or would fall if the examiner does not catch him, this is usually considered to be an indication of severe loss of position sense or proprioceptive ability, ie, this is a sensory ataxia, not cerebellar ataxia. Vestibular lesions can also cause similar problems, but usually the accentuation of swaying with the eyes closed indicates a proprioceptive ataxia. Thus, the neurological lesion usual revealed by an abnormal Romberg test is an abnormality of the peripheral nerves, the dorsal root ganglia, and/or the dorsal columns of the spinal cord leading to a deficit in proprioceptive ability.

Truncal Ataxia. With the patient sitting, the examiner may observe instability of the trunk. This suggests a midline lesion in the caudal part of the vermis. Patients with cerebellar disease often have head or truncal titubation, a tremor of the head or trunk.

Heel-Shin Test. This is generally performed with the patient sitting. One asks the patient to place one heel on the knee of the opposite leg and slide it smoothly down. One looks in particular for exaggerated side-to-side movement as the heel slides down the shin. Some examiners ask the patient to slide the shin back up and sometimes request that the patient slide it up and down several times. The patient is asked to do the same with the opposite heel and shin. This actually combines some of the truncal control with the extremity control and is therefore not as specific for a given part of the cerebellum as some of the other tests. Also, patients commonly have musculoskeletal problems (eg, arthritis, pain knees) that diminish their ability to perform this test.

Gait Abnormalities

The person with cerebellar problems, particularly a lesion in the rostral vermis, will manifest a broad-based and unstable gait. He may also complain of instability or dizziness but generally not of spinning or true vertigo. Alcoholic cerebellar degeneration is a prototype for this problem. In chronic alcoholics, there is often a wide-based gait with difficulty even standing still with the feet together. Interestingly, the gait of the chronic alcoholic is similar to that of a person acutely intoxicated with alcohol, because the acute and chronic effects of alcohol involve much the same regions.

A standard technique to detect cerebellar dysfunction is to have the patient walk on a straight line heel-to-toe. This is often called the test of ability to perform a "tandem walk." The patient with cerebellar disorder, particularly a mid-line (especially rostral vermal) cerebellar disorder, has great difficulty with this task or, perhaps, cannot perform it at all. Such a patient has a "cerebellar gait," a wide-base gait because he cannot walk well unless his feet are separated from each other further than normal. Even with the wide base, the individual often is unsteady on his feet and sways from side-to-side. He may make irregular and uncertain steps. Sometimes police use this as the "drunk test."

Tremor and Other Abnormal Movements

Several types of tremors are seen in cerebellar disease. In the finger-to-nose maneuver, as previously mentioned, side-to-side movement is seen when the patients comes close to the target. This is often called intention tremor. A postural tremor occurs with attempts to maintain a specific posture. This is also common in cerebellar disease. Sometimes a more coarse or gross irregular tremor is seen with movement, a "wing-beating" tremor. Disruption of outflow through the superior cellebellar peduncle produces a coarse resting tremor (which worsens with posture maintenance and movement) in the ipsilateral upper limb. Gordon Holmes called this a rubral tremor because of his belief that it involved the red nucleus. It is now believed to involve nearby structures but not the red nucleus itself. It is also now called Holmes tremor in his honor.

Another type of sudden jerky movement can be seen in cerebellar disease: myoclonic movements or myoclonic jerks. Sometimes these movements break up otherwise normal movements, giving the impression of a tremor.

Eye Movement Abnormalities

Cerebellar dysfunction can cause a breakdown of the normal gaze mechanisms. The saccades can deteriorate and become shorter. One can also see overshoot of the target with corrections needed afterwards.

Nystagmus. The most commonly recognized eye movement disorder is nystagmus. Nystagmus is a drift of the eyes in one direction with a rapid attempted correction in the other direction. Usually the rapid phase is the most noticeable part, and the direction of the rapid phase usually defines the direction of the nystagmus. Typically, cerebellar nystagmus is coarse, and the fast phase is toward the side of the lesion. If the patient is asked to look laterally toward the side of the lesion, the amplitude increases.

Macro-Square-Wave jerks. These are sudden jerks away from and then back to the fixation point, and sometimes occur in ataxia. One may also see ocular flutter and opsiclonus. Ocular flutter consists of rapid horizontal conjugate saccades, which lack a specific fixation point. Opsiclonus is similar, but it is multidirectional rather than exclusively horizontal. Both may be seen in cerebellar disease caused either by a paraneoplastic reaction to cancer (such as in neuroblastoma), or in viral or autoimmune encephalitis. They can also been seen in drug intoxications.

Ocular Myoclonus. Ocular myoclonus consists of pendulum-like back and forth eye movements, often accompanied by myoclonus of nearby muscles such as the palate or other muscles in the facial region. This is thought to result from abnormalities in neuronal circuits involving the dentate nucleus of cerebellum and/or nearby structures, such as the red nucleus or inferior olive.

Disorders of Tone. Patients with cerebellar disease often show hypotonia. This tends to be most marked with acute cerebellar lesions such as infarcts or hemorrhages. The hypotonia in such cases is ipsilateral to the lesion.

4. Non-Cerebellar Causes of Ataxia

Peripheral Nerve Disease

Peripheral nerve disease may affect the large proprioceptive fibers, part of which ultimately feed into the spinal cerebellar system. We can see ataxia in severe diabetic peripheral neuropathy, including a condition called diabetic pseudotabes, in which there is heavy involvement of the dorsal root ganglion. We can also see ataxia in the variant of Güillain-Barré syndrome called Miller Fisher syndrome. This is presumably due to the severe involvement of nerves carrying spinal cerebellar input in the cranial distribution.

The gait in sensory ataxia differs from the cerebellar variety in that it is not so wide-based. There is a strong tendency for sensory gait instability to worsen in the dark or when the eyes are closed. This is the basis for the Romberg test, which is most sensitive to proprioceptive or sensory ataxia. This condition was most commonly associated with neurosyphilis (tabes dorsalis). Now it is most commonly associated with diabetic peripheral neuropathy.

Vestibular Disease

Vestibular problems can cause ataxia because of vertigo. Ataxia due to vertigo can usually be distinguished from ataxia due to cerebellar disease. The simplest way to distinguish it is if there is the subjective complaint of vertigo, either a spinning sensation or a rocking sensation on the part of the patient. Frequently the patient will list to one side and will display prominent past pointing. Nystagmus, which can sometimes be seen in cerebellar disease, is more severe in vertigo. Often there is a rotatory component to the nystagmus.

Thalamic or Parietal Damage

Thalamic or parietal injury, either via infarction, hemorrhage, trauma, or tumor can sometimes cause a contralateral unilateral ataxia. Presumably, the damage impairs processing of sensory information. Frequently, the effects of infarct, hemorrhage or trauma are transient.

5. Diseases or Conditions that Can Cause Cerebellar Ataxia

Infectious Causes of Cerebellar Dysfunction

Viral and Mycoplasmal Infections

Viral illnesses, such as chickenpox, can cause cerebellar ataxia, especially in children. The onset is gradual with a progressively worsening gait and frequently nystagmus. Other eye movement disturbances, tremor and truncal titubation appear as well. Usually such cases resolve spontaneously but sometimes leave residual cerebellar deficits. Presumably, the cause is either an encephalitis or an immunological reaction to the viral infection. Similar problems may occur in adulthood, but they are much more rare.

A transient cerebellar dysfunction can be seen in infectious mononucleosis and Mycoplasma pneumonia infection, probably as an immune reaction. Viral and mycoplasmal ataxias usually resolve or at least ameliorate with time. Brain abscesses from bacterial infections can also affect the cerebellum. Abscesses are more likely to leave permanent sequelae than viral or mycoplasmal infections.

Prion Diseases (Kuru, Creutzfeldt-Jacob, Bovine Spiniform Encephalopathy)

Kuru originally appeared in New Guinea, predominantly among young women who ate brains of infected patients during tribal rituals. Unsteady gait, tremor and other cerebellar signs, along with a severe dementia, develop rapidly and death occurs in three to six months. Though this prion disease is rare, more common forms such as Creutzfeldt-Jakob disease and bovine spongiform encephalopathy (BSE or Mad Cow Disease) have similar manifestations.

Post-Infectious Problems

The generally transient ataxia previously mentioned as part of the Miller Fisher syndrome, which is a specific type of Güillain-Barré (acute inflammatory demyelinationg polyneuropathy or AIDP), in which patients have areflexia, ataxia and abnormalities of oculomotor function, exemplifies post-infectious ataxia. As in the more usual Güillian-Barré syndrome, the spinal fluid usually shows a high protein but a normal cell count. Interestingly, patients with Miller Fisher syndrome almost always harbor antibodies to GQ1b (or sometimes GT1b) gangliosides (which are part of the myelin of peripheral nerves).

Patients with Miller Fisher syndrome may also have facial sensory loss and facial weakness and sometimes weakness in other parts of their bodies, including the respiratory muscles. But these other areas of weakness are typically milder than in other types of Güillain-Barré. Other forms of Güillain-Barré and other post-infectious conditions also may cause ataxia, possibly even by a direct effect upon the cerebellum in addition to the peripheral nerves. Post-infectious ataxia usually resolves with time.

Toxic and Metabolic Causes of Cerebellar Disease

Alcohol intoxication is probably the most common cause of acute ataxia. The ataxia generally lasts for the period of the alcohol intoxication, but chronic alcoholism can permanently damage the cerebellum. Other intoxicants that affect the cerebellum include anticonvulsants (such as dilantin, carbamazepine and barbiturates), lithium, haldol and sometimes other sedating or tranquilizing drugs. Lithium, in particular, can cause ataxia at therapeutic levels. Usually these problems are reversible if the dose of the offending medication is lowered. However, prolonged intoxication can lead to permanent cerebellar damage. A number of cytotoxic or cytostatic medications used in the treatment of cancer or as immunosuppressive agents can cause cerebellar ataxia. Among these are vincristine, cytosinearabinoside, 5-fluorouicil, procarbazine and cyclosporine. The carbonic anhydrase inhibitor, Diamox® or acetazolamide, is capable of causing ataxia in some patients. Heavy metals such as mercury, various organic solvents and chemicals such as DDT and acrylamide and ciguatera fish poisoning can cause ataxia. Children with conditions that raise the ammonia level frequently exhibit ataxia. Hypothyroidism, including myxedema, may cause cerebellar signs and symptoms.

Prolonged alcohol abuse may lead to chronic cerebellar atrophy. This affects mainly the midline regions, especially the vermis (and the rostral vermis more than the caudal vermis). There is mainly an ataxia of gait affecting the legs. Truncal ataxia can be seen in more advanced stages of the disease (as the caudal vermis becomes more affected). Another type of alcohol-induced ataxia is seen in Wernicke's encephalopathy. This condition is due to a thiamine deficiency. There is an acute or subacute onset of eye movement disturbances, ataxia, short-term memory problems, and an acute delirium. The memory problems, which often become chronic, are separately called Korsakoff syndrome. High doses of thiamine are useful in treatment. If the patient receives thiamine promptly and afterwards refrains from alcohol, the condition can be reversible.

Hereditary Causes of Cerebellar Disease

There are numerous hereditary causes of cerebellar dysfunction. These include:

Friedreich's ataxia, various cerebellar cortical ataxias including what is often called the pure cerebellar cortical ataxia of Holmes, olivopontocerebellar atrophy, Machado-Joseph-Azorean disease, dentatorubropallidoluysian atrophy, dentatorubral degeneration, and a number of other genetic cerebellar degenerations. Recently, genetic scientists have discovered many specific genes in which mutations can cause specific cerebellar syndromes.

For example, Friedreich's ataxia (FA), is one of the classic hereditary spinocerebellar syndromes. An autosomal recessive degeneration of the spinal cord, peripheral (mainly sensory) nerves, and cerebellum, FA progresses gradually but relentlessly to render most patients unable to walk by mid-to-late adult life. We now know that FA is caused by a GAA expanded repeat on chromosome 9q. This is located in the gene coding for a protein, now called frataxin.

Many of the genetic forms of cerebellar disease are denoted with the term SCA (spinocerebellar ataxias). Most of these are autosomal dominant. The list of specific genes is ever growing. There are 27 known and accepted specifically numbered SCAs: SCA1 through SCA28, with SCA9 omitted and unassigned. There are also some additional autosomal dominant ataxias without SCA numbers.

For example, SCA1 is due to a mutation on chromosome 6p. SCA2 is caused by a defect on chromosome 12q, and is distinguished by eye movements with slow saccades. The locus for dentatoruborubropallidoluysian atrophy is chromosome 12p. SCA3 (the Machado-Joseph syndrome) has a locus on 14q. SCA4 is located on chromosome 16q. Patients have upper motor neuron signs as well as a sensory neuropathy. SCA5 is caused by a defect in the centromeric portion of chromosome 11. SCA7 is caused by a mutation at 3p. Retinal degeneration is among the prominent findings. SCA 6 involves the mutation at 19p, which involves the voltage gaited calcium channel. There is also a separate mutation of the voltage gated calcium channel, which causes an episodic ataxia (EA2), which is improved frequently by acetazolamide (Diamox, the same medication which causes ataxia in some people–see above). Another episodic ataxia (EA1) involves a potassium channel encoded on chromosome 12p. Also, there is a form of hereditary ataxia and myoclonus often called the Ramsay-Hunt syndrome, or dyssynergia cerebellaris myoclonica. The Rett syndrome produces progressive ataxia, autism and dementia. It affects only females. Recently the gene for the Rett syndrome has been identified. Multisystem atrophies, which are sometimes dominant, sometimes sporadic and very rarely recessive, typically present with combinations of cerebellar involvement including olivopontocerebellar atrophy, autonomic dysfunction, and signs and symptoms similar to those found in Parkinson disease.

Table I lists many of the autosomal dominant spinocerebellar ataxias (SCAs plus several other that are not technically considered to be SCAs but which are very similar).

To make the categorization of the ataxias a bit more complicated, there are at least two other numbered classification systems for predominantly dominant ataxias. One of these is the OPCA classification system. This system derives from pathological observations that frequently the pons and the inferior and/or superior olives are involved in cerebellar ataxias. The most commonly recognized OPCA numbers are OPCA I (or OPCA1), OPCAII, OPCA2 (note that OPCA2 is different than OPCAII, even though for the other numbers the Roman numeral designation is equivalent to the English number designation), OPCA III (or OPCA3), OPCA IV (or OPCA4), OPCA V (or OPCA5), and OPCA X (and this is not also called OPCA10 because the X means x-lined, not the number 10). There are many problems with this system. The actual clinico-pathological correlation with regions in the pons and olives is not precise and many other structures are involved. Many old cases from the literature have been classified inconsistently. It is probably fair to say that all cases which can be reasonably well-classified using the OPCA system can be better classified using the SCA system. So, in my opinion, and in the opinion of almost all geneticists, neurogeneticists, and neurologists who frequently see such cases, there is no reason to continue using these designations.

The third numbered classification system is the ADCA system. ADCA stands for "autosomal dominant cerebellar atrophy." One virtue of this system is its simplicity. There are three main types: ADCA I (ataxia plus involvement of other parts of the nervous system, including sometimes peripheral); ADCA II (like ADCA I plus retinal degeneration); and ADCA III (pure cerebellar ataxia—no involvement of other systems). Sometimes a fourth ADCA is defined and that is when seizures are combined with cerebellar ataxia. The ADCA system lumps the larger number of genetically defined syndromes into larger groups. It can be considered a phenotypic classification. Some geneticists recommend discontinuing this system as well, because the phenotypic classifications are not perfect. They argue that it is best simply to try to learn what each separate disease entails, phenotypically and genetically. Others feel that the ADCA system is still useful.

Table II gives the correspondences between the ADCA classification system and that of the SCAs. Enzyme deficiencies and other hereditary diseases can cause pathology in the cerebellum. These are frequently autosomal recessive.

Bassen-Kornzweig disease, or abetalipoproteinemia, is an abnormality of lipid transport due to a problem with synthesis of apolipoprotein B. The patient has extremely low cholesterol and triglyceride concentrations, and there is a deficiency of vitamin E and other vitamins that depend upon lipids for synthesis. The vitamin E deficiency causes damage to the nervous system including the cerebellum. Hexosaminidase deficiency, or GM2 gangliosidosis, causes cerebellar damage. Pyruvate dehydrogenase deficiency, glutamate dehydrogenase deficiency, and glutaric acid decarboxylase dysfunction also cause cerebellar damage or dysfunction. Intermittent ataxias are seen with Hartnup disease, an autosomal recessive condition in which there is a defect in the transport of several amino acids, tryptophan, alanine, and histidine in the renal tubules and in the intestines. In addition to

Table 1

Dominant Ataxias

Disease Names	Locus	OMIM #[1]	Gene Product (OMIM #)	Clinical Signs and Symptoms	Genetic Lab Test
SCA1 *ADCA1*	ATXN1, 6p23	#164400	Ataxin-1 (*601556)	• Onset 30s • Ataxia, spasticity, dysarthria, ophthalmoplegia, slow saccades, nystagmus, optic atrophy, pyramidal tract signs, rare extrapyramidal signs. Some have dementia. Neuropathy occurs late.	Genetic Test available
SCA2 *ADCA1*	ATXN2, 12q24	#183090	Ataxin-2 (601517)	• Onset 30s • Ataxia, dysarthria, muscle cramps Slow saccades/ophthalmoplegia Peripheral neuropathy, hyporeflexia, dementia in some, no pyramidal or extrapyramidal features.	Genetic Test available
SCA3/ Machado Joseph Disease (MJD) ADCA1	ATXN3, 14q24.3-q31	#109150	Machado-Joseph disease protein 1(ATXN3). (607047)	• All have ataxia, dysarthria, ophthalmoplegia • Type I onset in mid-20s • Facial-lingual myokymia, pyramidal+ extrapyramidal features; • Type II onset 40s • Type III onset mid-40s • Peripheral neuropathy (weakness and atrophy).	Genetic Test available
SCA4 *ADCA I*	Gene Unknown, 16q22.1 (same region as #117210 below)	%600223		• Onset average about 40 (19-72) • Pure ataxia in some, deafness in some, most have sensory axonal neuropathy.	

Table 1 (Continued)

Dominant Ataxias

Disease Names	Locus	OMIM #[1]	Gene Product (OMIM #)	Clinical Signs and Symptoms	Genetic Lab Test
Spinocerebellar Ataxia, 16q22-linked ADCA III	PLEKHG4, 16q22.1	#117210	Puratrophin-1 (609526)	• Cerebellar ataxia with gait ataxia, cerebellar dysarthria, limb ataxia, decreased muscle tone, and horizontal gaze nystagmus. • Similar to SCA4, but lacks deafness and neuropathy (but may actually be SCA4).	
SCA5 ADCA III	SPTBN2, 11p13	#600224	Spectrin beta chain, brain 2 (604985)	• Onset mid-30s • Downbeat nystagmus, ataxia, dysarthria, impaired smooth pursuit, and gaze-evoked nystagmus. Slow progression; both vermal and hemispheric cerebellar atrophy, normal life expectancy.	
SCA6 ADCA1 ADCA III	CACNA1A, 19p13	#183086	Voltage-dependent P/Q-type Ca^{+2} channel α-1A subunit (601011)	• Onset 20–40 • Ataxia, dysarthria, nystagmus, distal sensory loss, normal life expectancy.	Genetic Test available
SCA7 ADCAII	ATXN7, 3p21.1-p12	#164500	Ataxin-7 (607640)	• Onset mid-20s • Pigmentary retinal degeneration, ataxia, dysarthria, ophthalmoplegia, slow saccades, pyramidal tract signs.	Genetic Test available
SCA8 ADCAII	KLHL1AS, 13q21	#608768		• Onset 20s to 70s • Ataxia, dysarthria, nystagmus, impaired smooth pursuit.	Genetic Test available
SCA9	unassigned category			• unassigned category.	

Table 1 (Continued)

Dominant Ataxias

Disease Names	Locus	OMIM #[1]	Gene Product (OMIM #)	Clinical Signs and Symptoms	Genetic Lab Test
SCA10 ADCA III	ATXN10, 22q13	+603516	Ataxin-10	• Onset 20s • Ataxia, dysarthria, nystagmus, epileptic seizures, so far only found in Mexican families.	Genetic Test available
SCA11	SCA11, 15q14-q21.3	%604432		• Onset in patients aged 20–40 years • Ataxia, dysarthria, nystagmus.	
SCA12	PPP2R2B, 5q31-q33	#604326	Serine/threonine protein phosphatase 2A, 55-kd regulatory subunit B, beta isoform	• Onset 8–55 years, commonly 30s • Upper extremity and head tremor, gait ataxia, ophthalmoplegia, hyperreflexia, bradykinesia, dementia.	Genetic Test available
SCA13 (sometime considered ADCA I or III)	KCNC3, 19q13.3-q13.4	#605259	Voltage-gated K^+ channel, subfamily C member 3	• Onset in childhood • Ataxia, dysarthria, mental retardation. Slow progression.	Genetic Test available
SCA14	PRKCG, 19q13.4	#605361	Kinase C, gamma type	• Onset in most > 39 • Ataxia, dysarthria, nystagmus • Earlier patients < 27 years old, also had intermittent axial myoclonus prior to the ataxia.	Genetic Test available
SCA15	Gene Unknown, 3p26.1-p25.3	%606658	Unknown	• Similar to SCA6 and SCA8. MRI-cerebellar atrophy. • Onset 10 to 50 years. • Slowly progressive pure cerebellar ataxia, ataxic dysarthria. tremor, May have head titibation, nystagmus, occulo-vestibular reflex abnormalities, mild hyperreflexia (no spasticity or Babinski signs).	

Table 1 (Continued)

Dominant Ataxias

Disease Names	Locus	OMIM #[1]	Gene Product (OMIM #)	Clinical Signs and Symptoms	Genetic Lab Test
SCA16	SCA16, 8q22.1-q24.1	%606364		• MRI–cerebellar atrophy without brainstem involvement • Onset 20-66 • Pure cerebellar ataxia, some with head tremor, slow progression.	
SCA17	TBP, 6q27	#607136	TATA-box binding protein	• Onset 3-55 • Ataxia and involvement of the pyramidal, extrapyramidal, and possibly autonomic system and intellectual impairment dementia, psychosis, chorea, looks like Huntington disease. Degeneration of caudate, putamen, thalamus, frontal cortex, temporal cortex, and cerebellum.	Genetic Test available
SCA18	SCA18 7q22-q32	%607458		• Onset teens, 20s and 30s • Sensorimotor neuropathy with ataxia (SMNA), gait abnormality, dysmetria, hyporeflexia, muscle weakness and atrophy, axonal neuropathy, decreased vibratory and proprioceptive sense.	
SCA19	1p21-q21	%607346		• Onset 12-40 • Gait and limb ataxia, hyporeflexia, dysphagia, dysarthria, and gaze-evoked horizontal nystagmus. cerebellar atrophy by MRI.	

Table 1 (Continued)

Dominant Ataxias

Disease Names	Locus	OMIM #[1]	Gene Product (OMIM #)	Clinical Signs and Symptoms	Genetic Lab Test
SCA20	SCA20, 11cen	%608687		• Onset 19-64 • Dysarthria, gait ataxia, upper limb, slow progression; more variable features: mild pyramidal signs, hypermetric saccades, nystagmus, palatal tremor, slow cognitive decline, CT scan: dentate calcification.	
SCA21	SCA21, 7p21-15	%607454		• Onset 6-30 • Cerebellar ataxia, limb ataxia and akinesia, dysarthria, dysgraphia, hyporeflexia, postural tremor, resting tremor, rigidity, cognitive impairment, cerebellar atrophy.	
SCA22	1p21-q21	%607346		• Now believed to be identical to SCA19 (Schelhaas et al. (2004) though Chung & Soong 2004 have disputed this.	
SCA23	20p13-12.3	%610245		• Onset 40s, 50s • Slow progression, gait and limb ataxia, dysarthria (varies), slow saccades and ocular dysmetria, and decreased vibratory sense, severe cerebellar atrophy.	

Table 1 (Continued)

Dominant Ataxias

Disease Names	Locus	OMIM #[1]	Gene Product (OMIM #)	Clinical Signs and Symptoms	Genetic Lab Test
SCA25	SCA25, 2p21-p13	%608703		• Onset childhood • Invariable feature: cerebellar ataxia • Variably present: lower limb areflexia, peripheral sensory neuropathy, nystagmus, decreased visual acuity, facial tics, extensor plantar responses, urinary urgency, and gastrointestinal symptoms.	
SCA26	19p13.3	%609306		• Onset 25-60 • Pure cerebellar signs, including ataxia of the trunk and limbs, dysarthria, and irregular visual pursuit movements. Intelligence normal. MRI showed atrophy of the cerebellum sparing the pons and medulla.	
SCA27	FGF14, 13q34	#609307	Fibroblast growth factor 14 (601515)	• Onset childhood • Cerebellar ataxia, tremor, low IQ, aggressive behavior, eye movement abnormalities incl. nystagmus, cerebellar dysarthria, head tremor, orofacial dyskinesias, cerebellar atrophy, pes cavus, axonal sensory neuropathy, neuronal loss in cerebral cortex, amygdala, and basal ganglia.	

Table 1 (Continued)

Dominant Ataxias

Disease Names	Locus	OMIM #[1]	Gene Product (OMIM #)	Clinical Signs and Symptoms	Genetic Lab Test
SCA28	18p11.22-q11.2	%610246		• 19.5 years (range 12 to 36) • Imbalance and mild gait incoordination. Gaze-evoked nystagmus, slow saccades, ophthalmoparesis, and often ptosis. Frequently lower limb hyporeflexia.	
DRPLA	DRPLA, 12p13.31	#125370	Atrophin-1 related protein (607462)	• 20s to 30s • Myoclonic epilepsy, dementia, ataxia, and choreoathetosis, degeneration of the dentatorubral and pallidoluysian systems.	Genetic Test available
Episodic ataxia, type 1 EA1	KCNA1, 12p13	#160120	K^{+1} voltage-gated channel (A1) (600111)	• Usually starts in childhood • Continuous muscle movement (myokymia) and periodic ataxia.	Genetic Test available on research basis
Episodic ataxia, type 2 EA2	CACNA1A, 19p13	#108500	Voltage-dependent P/Q-type Ca^{+2} channel alpha-1A subunit (601011)	• Onset childhood • Ataxia, downbeating nystagmus, dizziness, helped by acetazolamide, no progression after childhood, cerebellar atrophy.	Genetic Test available on research basis
Episodic ataxia, type 3 EA3	1q42	%606554	(unknown)	• 1 to 42 years • Vestibular ataxia, vertigo, tinnitus, and interictal myokymia.	

Table 1 (Continued)

Dominant Ataxias

Disease Names	Locus	OMIM #[1]	Gene Product (OMIM #)	Clinical Signs and Symptoms	Genetic Lab Test
Episodic ataxia, type 4 EA4	(unknown)	%606552	(unknown)	• Onset 3rd to 6th decade • Recurrent attacks of vertigo, diplopia, and ataxia, slowly progressive cerebellar ataxia in some; periodic vestibulocerebellar ataxia in an autosomal dominant pedigree pattern, defective smooth pursuit, gaze-evoked nystagmus, ataxia, and vertigo.	
Episodic ataxia, type 5 EA5	CACNB4, 2q22-q23	+601949	Voltage-dependent L-type calcium beta-4 subunit (+601949)	• 3rd or 4th decade • Mutation: C104F • French-Canadian family • Ataxia similar to EA2 • Episodic severe ataxia–hours to weeks • Treatment: Acetazolamide • Interictal ataxia: gait and truncal, mild dysarthria, • Nystagmus (downbeat, spontaneous, gaze evoked); plus seizures.	

Table 1 (Continued)

Dominant Ataxias

Disease Names	Locus	OMIM #[1]	Gene Product (OMIM #)	Clinical Signs and Symptoms	Genetic Lab Test
Choreoathetosis Spasticity, episodic (CSE)	12p13 (near potassium channel gene KCNA1)	%601042	(unknown)	• Onset 2-15 • Paroxysmal choreoathetosis with episodic ataxia and spasticity.	
Hereditary (autosomal dominant) Spastic ataxia	SAX1, 12p13	%108600	(unknown)	• Onset 10-20 years • Lower-limb spasticity, generalized ataxia with dysarthria, dysphagia, impaired ocular movements, gait abnormalities; brain and cord MRIs have been normal; neuropath has shown midbrain neuronal loss.	

Footnotes:

[1] *OMIM# is from Online Mendelian Inheritance in Man, http://www.ncbi.nlm.nih.gov/sites/entrez?db=OMIM.*

Table 2

ADCA Phenotypic Classification

ADCAs	**ADCA I**	**ADCA II**	**ADCA III**	**ADCA IV**
ADCA Phenotypic Description	Ataxia plus involvement of other parts of the nervous system, including sometimes peripheral	Ataxia plus pigmentary retinal degeneration, as well as sometimes macular degeneration	Pure cerebellar ataxia–no involvement of other systems	Cerebellar ataxia plus seizures and or myoclonus. Sometimes deafness is also included.
SCAs	SCA1,2,3 8, 12, 17, 25, 27, 28, (13)1	SCA7, (2)[2]	SCA 4, 5, 6, 10, 11, 14,15, 22 , 26, (13)[1]	SCA 10, 17 Also DRPLA[4]

Footnotes:

[1] SCA 13 is frequently said not to fit any of the ADCA phenotypes but sometimes can be put into I or III.

[2] Uncommonly SCA 2 manifests retinal degeneration

[3] ADCA IV is not universally accepted as a category

[4] Dentatorubral-Pallidoluysian atrophy, see Table I

ataxia, there is nystagmus, a gait defect, dementia, and spasticity.

There are several diseases of DNA synthesis that cause cerebellar symptoms: xeroderma pigmentosum, Cockayne syndrome, and ataxia telangiectasia or Louis-Bar syndrome. Recently the gene for ataxia telangiectasia has been identified.

Table 3 lists a number of recessive ataxias.

The reader should be aware that Tables listing genetic disorders become outdated quickly. It is good to be aware of online sources that are updated regularly. Here are some good sources:

1. The Washington University web page on neuromuscular disease in the section on ataxia: *http://www.neuro.wustl.edu/neuromuscular/ataxia/aindex.html*

2. A web page by Dr. Thomas Bird from the University of Washington in Seattle: *http://www.geneclinics.org/profiles/ataxias/details.html*

3. Online Mendelian Inheritance in Man (OMIM), developed, authored, and edited by Dr. Victor A. McKusick and his colleagues at Johns Hopkins, gives a broad coverage of genetic disease, including most neurogenetic diseases: *http://www.ncbi.nlm.nih.gov/sites/entrez?db=OMIM.*

4. Gene Cards, from the Weismann Institute: *http://www.genecards.org/*

Table 3

Some Recessive Ataxias

Disease Names	Gene and Locus	Disease OMIM #	Clinical Signs and Symptoms (in addition to the ataxia)	Genetic Lab Test or other tests
Friedreich's ataxia	X25/FRDA (9q13)	229300	Adolescent onset; despite absent lower limb reflexes (axonal neuropathy) plantars are extensor, other systems involved, eg, cardiomyopathy, impaired glucose tolerance, skeletal abnormalities such as pes cavus.	Gene test available
Ataxia telangiectasia	ATM (11q22.3)	208900	Early onset (1–6); immune deficiency (recurrent infection, malignancies) malignancy, oculomotor apraxia, telangiectasias of skin and conjunctiva, chorea, dystonia, hypogonadism, memory loss, neuropathy (absent lower limb reflexes), flexor plantars.	Raised serum α-fetoprotein Low IgA and IgG Gene test available
Ataxia with oculomotor apraxia type 1	Aprataxin, APTX (9p13.3)	208920	Early onset (1–6); oculomotor apraxia, chorea, cognitive impairment and mental retardation, sensorimotor axonal neuropathy (areflexia), flexor plantars.	Hypoalbuminaemia Hypercholesterolaemia Elevated LDL Low HDL Gene test available
Ataxia with oculomotor apraxia type 2	Linkage only (9q34); gene Not available	606002	Adolescent to young adult onset (10-early 20s) oculomotor apraxia, choreoathetosis, dystonia, absent lower limb reflexes, sensory neuropathy, extensor plantars.	Gene test not available
Abetalipo-proteinaemia	Microsomal triglyceride transfer protein, MTP (4q22-q24)	200100	Childhood to adolescent or young adult onset (2-20), similar to Friedreich's neurologically; distal amyotrophy, plus steatorrhoea, retinitis pigmentosa.	Acanthocytes (spiky red cells), low serum cholesterol, VLDL/LDL are absent, low Vitamin A, E, K; no commercial gene test yet

Table 3 (Continued)

Some Recessive Ataxias

Disease Names	Gene and Locus	Disease OMIM #	Clinical Signs and Symptoms (in addition to the ataxia)	Genetic Lab Test or other tests
Ataxia with vitamin E deficiency	a-tocopherol transfer protein, a-TTP (8q13.1-q13.3)	277460	Onset childhood to adolescent or young adult (2–20) similar to Friedreich's but no cardiomyopathy or impaired glucose tolerance; about one-quarter have head titubation.	Low vitamin E levels in serum; no commercial gene test yet
Autosomal recessive spastic ataxia of Charlevoix-Saguenay	SACS (13q12)	270550	Onset childhood to adolescent or young adult (1–20); similar to Friedreich's, extensor plantars, and brisk reflexes generally except for areflexia at ankles (axonal neuropathy).	Gene test available
Cerebrotendinous xanthomatosis	sterol 27-hydroxylase (CYP27) 2q33-qter	213700	Onset generally post-puberty. Frequently involves a sensory ataxia due to peripheral neuropathy and a cerebellar ataxia. Also can include upper motor neuron signs, brainstem dysfunction, mental retardation, and myoclonus.	Can test for increased cholestanol in serum & tissues and bile alcohol in urine: Increased
Early onset cerebellar ataxia with retained tendon reflexes (EOCARR)	13q11-12	212895	Onset first or second decade, somewhat similar to Friedreich's ataxia but with preserved deep tendon reflexes.	Gene test not available
Infantile onset spinocerebellar ataxia (IOSCA)	10q22.3-q24.1	271245	Onset in infancy. Ataxia, athetosis, hypotonia and decreased or absent deep tendon reflexes. Ophthalmoplegia, hearing loss, and seizures can occur.	Gene test not available
Marinesco-Sjögren syndrome (MSS)	SIL1 (also called BAP) 5q31	248800	Noticeable beginning in childhood. Ataxia, cognitive deficiency, hypotonia, cataract, short stature.	Commercial gene test not yet available

Table 3 (Continued)

Some Recessive Ataxias

Disease Names	Gene and Locus	Disease OMIM #	Clinical Signs and Symptoms (in addition to the ataxia)	Genetic Lab Test or other tests
Spinocerebellar ataxia with axonal neuropathy	Tyrosyl-DNA phosphodiesterase 1 (TDP1) 14q31	607250	Ataxia is secondary due to neuropathy. Both motor and sensory neuropathy with distal muscule atrophy and sensory loss, pes cavus and steppage gait.	Commercial gene test not yet available
Coenzyme Q10 deficiency with cerebellar ataxia		607426	Generally it starts in childhood but this may vary. In addition to ataxia there is usually epilepsy and often upper motor neuron signs, mental retardation, myopathy, delayed motor development.	Gene test not available
Posterior column ataxia and retinitis pigmentosa (PCARP)	1q31	176250	Sensory ataxia and loss of proprioception (posterior column involvement), visual impairment (retinitis pigmentosa), diminished or absent deep tendon reflexes.	No genetic test yet available
Joubert syndrome	9q34	213300	Congenital cerebellar agenesis. Ataxia, nystagmus and other eye movement abnormalilties, ptosis, retinopathy, breathing problems and abnormalities of other organs including skin, and heart. Mental retardation.	No genetic test yet available
Cockayne syndrome type I	CKN1 Chromosome 5	216400	Evident by year 1. Mental retardation. Premature aging, growth failure, spasticity, contractures, retinal degeneration, cataracts.	Genetic test potentially available, mainly still on research basis

Paraneoplastic Syndromes

Individuals with cancer, particularly breast cancer, ovarian cancer, small-cell lung cancers, and Hodgkins and non-Hodgkins lymphomas may exhibit a subacute paraneoplastic cerebellar degeneration. Typically, the cerebellar cortex is involved in a symmetrical fashion, causing mild-to-moderate ataxia involving the limbs and ultimately the trunk. There can also be associated brain stem involvement causing dysphagia and dysarthria. Sometimes vertigo and other eye movement disorders such as nystagmus, ocular flutter, and opsoclonus can be seen. In addition, there can be even more widespread nervous system problems including upper motor neuron signs, loss of proprioception, generalized peripheral neuropathy, dementia and diplopia. Typically, MRI and CT scans show cerebellar atrophy. Inflammatory cells can be seen in the cerebral spinal fluid, especially early in the syndrome. But they do not necessarily have to be found. Sometimes specific anti-neuronal antibodies can be demonstrated in such conditions. Anti-Yo antibodies in association with this condition are highly suggestive of a cancer, especially ovarian (or possibly breast) cancer. If these antibodies are found in cases of subacute cerebellar degeneration, a thorough malignancy workup is indicated because one may find the cancer in an early curable stage. Sometimes multiple attempts, including exotic high tech tests such as PET scans, or somewhat invasive methods such as laporoscopy, are employed in order to find a tumor which will be present in about 2/3 of such cases. In small cell carcinoma of the lung, the antibody type is more commonly anti-hu. With this type of antibody, the syndrome is often more broad, involving dementia (due to limbic system involvement), eye movement problems, myoclonus (often the opsoclonus-myoclonus syndrome), sensory neuropathy, and a general encephalomyelitis, as well as ataxia. Treatment of the cancer, though important, may not cure the paraneoplastic condition. In fact, the cerebellar syndrome seen with anti-Yo antibodies usually improves only slightly when a tumor is found and treated. This is true even with complete eradication of the tumor. In the case of anti-hu antibodies, if the oncologists manage to cure the lung cancer, then major improvement in the neurological syndrome is more common than in the case of the anti-Yo syndromes. Intravenous immunoglobulins or plasmaphoresis can promote improvement in some cases. Infantile myoclonic encephalopathy can also be seen as a paraneoplastic condition in children with neuroblastoma. Some cases, however, are idiopathic. Affected children show cerebellar dysfunction and myoclonus, as well as irregular eye movements including opsoclonus.

Tumors Affecting the Cerebellum

Meduloblastoma, astrocytoma, and hemangioblastoma are not uncommonly seen in the cerebellum, and these can cause cerebellar ataxia.

Cerebellar astrocytomas commonly arise in childhood. They are less malignant than astrocytomas in other parts of the brain and often are quite well circumscribed. They cause gradually worsening cerebellar problems including incoordination, nystagmus, and dysfunction in other parts of the brain by virtue of their pressure. Surgical cures are possible.

Ependymomas may affect the cerebellum, particularly in children. They obstruct cerebral spinal fluid flow causing hydrocephalus. In addition to cerebellar signs the patient frequently complains of headache. Histologically, the ependymomas are usually rather benign or of low-grade malignancy. However, they are frequently positioned in such a way that it is quite difficult to remove them surgically. Radiation therapy is frequently necessary. The completeness of removal generally governs the long-term outlook.

Medulloblastomas are also seen in childhood. These are often found in the region of the vermis; however, they may arise in the cerebellar hemispheres or the nearby pons. These tumors are generally very malignant and even after what seems to be complete surgical resection and radiation therapy they tend to recur. Chemotherapy may also be used in an attempt to increase the rate of survival.

Meningiomas, which are usually histologically benign, may also affect the cerebellum. They mainly exert their effects due to pressure. If they can be completely removed, it is rare for them to recur.

Schwannomas of the eighth cranial nerve produce pressure in the region of the cerebellopontine angle. This can cause deafness, tinnitus and cerebellar dysfunction. It may also cause loss of function in the fifth and seventh cranial nerves and sometimes upper motor neuron signs, and signs of intercranial hypertension. Other tumors including metastatic tumors may also affect the cerebellar pontine angle. Indeed, brain metastasis from primary tumors in other parts of the body may also affect the cerebellum.

Cerebellar Strokes

Strokes, both infarcts and hemorrhages, may affect any part of the cerebellum. Virtually any cerebellar sign or symptoms may occur in such cases including ataxia, tremor, dysequilibrium or eye movement abnormalities. In cases of cerebellar infarction, typically the brainstem may be affected as well and thus the patient may display motor and sensory loss of both the face and the body. Cerebellar hemorrhages may be confined to the cerebellum, or they may involve the ventricular system, therefore causing other problems including coma and death. For both cerebellar infarcts and hemorrhages, swelling and the ensuing brainstem compression and herniation is a potentially life-threatening problem.

Other Causes of Cerebellar Degenerative Diseases

In congenital cerebellar ataxia, gait disorder and impaired coordination may be seen. This is often combined with other congenital syndromes including problems in motor development, dysarthria and sometimes other neurological problems. Agenesis of the cerebellum may sometimes occur. Heat stroke can cause cerebellar damage. A combination of cerebellar dysfunction and polyneuropathy may be caused by sprue as well as by macroglobulinemia. In the Marie-Foie-Alajouanin syndrome, the midline region of the cerebellum, principally the vermis, gradually degenerates with a loss of both Purkinje and granule cells. This is usually evident by the fifth decade.

There are also many other gradually progressive cerebellar atrophies, which occur at various ages in adult life that yet are not clearly delineated.

6. Treatment for Cerebellar Dysfunction and Other Forms of Ataxia

Specific medical treatments for cerebellar dysfunction and ataxias are quite limited and supportive, and compensatory care such as can be obtained through physical and occupational therapies are the mainstays. In small numbers of cases, neostigmine, ondansetron, and amantadine have been reported to ameliorate some of the symptoms of ataxia. Vestibular ataxia may be helped by meclizine, various vestibular exercises, and a type of head rotation called the Epley maneuver, which can remove the debris that accumulates in the vestibular system. Ibedone, an antioxidant, may somewhat slow the progression of Friedriech's ataxia. In at least two of the genetically determined, autosomal dominant episodic ataxias, EA-1 and E1-2, the medication acetazolomide is very helpful. Intravenous immunoglobulin may help speed recovery in the Miller Fisher syndrome, other post infectious immune mediated ataxias, and paraneoplastic ataxias. Of course, for the paraneoplastic ataxias, finding and removing accessible tumors is very important, but tumor removal does not guarantee cure of the ataxia.

7. References

1. Aggerbeck LP, Mc Mahon JP, Scanu AM. Hypobetalipoproteinemia: clinical and biochemical description of a new kindred with Friedreich's ataxia. *Neurology*. 1974; 24:1051-1063.

2. Amarenco P. The spectrum of cerebellar infarctions. *Neurology*. 1991; 41:973-979.

3. Baloh RW, Yue Q, Furman JM, Nelson SF. Familial episodic Ataxia: clinical heterogeneity in four families linked to chromosome 19p. *Ann Neurol*. 1997; 41:8-11.

4. Beirne P, Taylor P, Chodhury RP, Somerville J. Cerebellar syndrome complicating mycoplasma pneumoniae pneumonia. *JR Soc Med*. 2000; 93:28-29.

5. Bidichandani SI, Ashizawa T, Patel PI. The GAA triplet-repeat expansion in Friedreich ataxia interferes with transcription and may be associated with an unusual DNA structure. *Am J Hum Genet*. 1998; 62(1):111-121.

6. Bird TD, Tapscott SJ. Clinical neurogenetics. In: *Neurology in Clinical Practice*. Edited by Bradley WG, Daroff RB, Fenichel GM, Jankovic J. 4th Ed. Butterworth, 2004.

   (Good chapter for genetic ataxias. But also see Bird's web page: *http://www.geneclinics.org/profiles/ataxias/details.html*)

7. Botez MI, Botez-Marquard Th, Elie R, et al. Amantadine hydrochloride treatment in heredodegenerative ataxias: a double blind study. *J Neurol Neurosurg Psychiatry*. 1996; 61:259-264.

8. Bouchard JP, Richter A, Mathieu J, Brunet D, Hudson TJ, Morgan K, Melancon SB. Autosomal recessive spastic ataxia of Charlevoix-Saguenay. *Neuromuscul Disord*. 1998; 8:474-9.

9. Brazis P W, Masdeu J C, Biller J. *Localization in Clinical Neurology*. 3rd ed. Boston: Little Brown; 1996.

10. Brusco A, Gellera C, Cagnoli C, Saluto A, Castucci A, Michielotto C, Fetoni V, Mariotti C, Migone N, Di Donato S, Taroni F. Molecular genetics of hereditary spinocerebellar ataxia: mutation analysis of spinocerebellar ataxia genes and CAG/CTG repeat expansion detection in 225 Italian families. *Arch Neurol*. 2004; 61:727-33.

11. Burk, K, Bosch, S, Muller, CA, et al. Sporadic cerebellar ataxia associated with gluten sensitivity. *Brain*. 2001; 124(5):1013-1019.

12. Campuzano, Montermini L, Molto MD, Pianese L, Cossee M, Cavalcanti F, Monros E, Rodius F, Duclos F, Monticelli A, et al. Friedreich's Ataxia: Autosomal recessive disease caused by an intronic GAA triplet expansion. *Science*. 1996; 271:1423-1427.

13. Cavalier L, Ouahchi K, Kayden HJ, Di Donato S, Reutenauer L, Mandel JL, Koenig M. Ataxia with isolated vitamin E deficiency: heterogeneity of mutations and phenotypic variability in a large number of families. *Am J Hum Genet*. 1998; 62:301-310.

14. Chung MY, Lu YC, Cheng NC, Soong BW. A novel autosomal dominant spinocerebellar ataxia (SCA22) linked to chromosome 1p21-q23. *Brain*. 2003; 126:1293-1299.

15. Combaross O, Infante J, Lopez-Hoyos M, et al. Celiac disease and idiopathic cerebellar ataxia. *Neurology*. 2000; 54(12):2346.

16. Conolly AM, Dodson WE, Prensky AL, Rust RS. Course and outcome of acute cerebellar ataxia. *Ann Neurol*. 1994; 35:673-679.

17. Counsell CE, McLeod M, Grant R. Reversal of subacute paraneoplastic cerebellar syndrome with intravenous immunoglobulin. *Neurology*. 1994; 44:1184-1185.

18. Dalakas MC. Chronic idiopathic ataxic neuropathy. *Ann Neurol*. 1986; 19:545-554.

19. DeMyer, WE. *Technique of the Neurological Examination*. 5th ed. New York: McGraw Hill; 2003.

(Interesting programmed learning textbook.)

20. Dixon-Salazar T, Silhavy JL, Marsh SE, et al. Mutations in the AHI1 gene, encoding jouberin, cause Joubert syndrome with cortical polymicrogyria. *Am J Hum Genet*. 2004; 75:979-87

21. Durr A, Cossee M, Agid Y, Campuzano V, Mignard C, Penet C, Mandel JL, Brice A, Koenig M. Clinical and genetic abnormalities in patients with Friedreich's ataxia. *New England Journal of Medicine*. 1996; 335:1169-1175.

22. Fine EJ, Ionita CC, Lohr L. The history of the development of the cerebellar examination. *Semin Neurol*. 2002; 22:375-384.

23. Gilman S, Quinn NP. The relationship of multiple system atrophy to sporadic olivopontocerebellar atrophy and other forms of idiopathic late-onset cerebellar atrophy. *Neurology*. 1996; 46:1197-1199.

24. Gotoda T, Arita M, Arai H, Inoue K, Yokota T, Fukuo Y, Yazaki Y, Yamada N. Adult-onset spinocerebellar dysfunction caused by a mutation in the gene for the alpha-tocopherol-transfer protein. *New England Journal of Medicine*. 1995; 333: 1313-1318.

25. Hadjivassilious M, Grünewald RA, Chattopadhyay AK, Davies-Jones GA, Gibson A, Jarratt JA, Kandler RH, Lobo A, Powell T, Smith CM. Clinical, radiological, neurophysiological, and neuropathological characteristics of gluten ataxia. *Lancet*. 1998; 352:1582-1585.

26. Hausse AO, Aggoun Y, Bonnet D, et al. Idebenone and reduced cardiac hypertrophy in Friedreich's ataxia. *Heart*. 2002; 87(4):346-349.

27. Higgins JJ, Morton DH, Loveless JM. Posterior column ataxia with retinitis pigmentosa (AXPC1) maps to chromosome 1q31-q32. *Neurology*. 1999 Jan 1; 52(1):146-50

28. Holmes, G. Clinical symptoms of cerebellar disease and their interpretation. The Croonian lecture III. *Lancet*. 1922; 2: 59-65.

(This is one of the really classical articles on the cerebellum. It is amazing and humbling how much Holmes knew in the 1920's.)

29. Holmes, G. The cerebellum of man. *Brain*. 1939; 62:1-30.

(A more complete article than the earlier *Lancet* piece on the cerebellum by one of the masters of early 20th Century neurology.)

30. Harding AE. Classification of the hereditary ataxias and paraplegias. *Lancet*. 1983; I:1151-1155.

31. Hurko O. Recent advances in heritable ataxias. *Ann Neurol*. 1997; 41:4-6.

32. Jellinger K, Heiss W D, Deisenhammer E. The ataxic (cerebellar) form of Creutzfeldt-Jakob disease. *J Neuro*. 1974; 207:289-305.

33. Klockgether T, ed. *Handbook of Ataxia Disorders*. New York: Marcel Dekker; 1999.

34. Klockgether T, Döller G, Wüllner U , Petersen D, Dichgans J. Cerebellar encephalitis in adults. *J Neurol*. 1993; 240:17-20.

35. Leggo J, Dalton A, Morrison PJ, Dodge A, Connarty M, Kotze MJ, Rubinsztein DC. Analysis of spinocerebellar ataxia types 1, 2, 3, and 6, dentatorubral- pallidoluysian atrophy, and Friedreich's ataxia genes in spinocerebellar ataxia patients in the UK. *J Med Genet*. 1997; 34:982-985.

36. Lubbers WJ, Brunt ER, Scheffer H, Litt M, Stulp R, Browne DL, van Weerden TW. Hereditary myokymia and paroxysmal ataxia linked zu chromosome 12 is responsive to acetazolamide. *J Neurol Neurosurg Psychiatry*. 1995; 59:400-405.

37. Marsden CD, Harding AE, Obesoet JA, Lu CS. Progressive myoclonic ataxia (The Ramsay Hunt Syndrome). *Arch Neurol*.1990; 47:1121-1125.

38. Nagafuchi S, Yanagisawa H, Sato K, et al. Dentatorubral and pallidoluysian atrophy expansion of an unstable GAG trinucleotide of chromosome 12p. *Nat Genet*. 1995; 6:14.

39. Nechiporuk A, Lopes-Cendes I, Nechiporuk T, Starkman S, Andermann E, Rouleau GA, Weissenbach JS, Kort E, Pulst SM. Genetic mapping of the spinocerebellar ataxia type 2 gene on human chromosome 12. *Neurology*. 1996; 46:1731-1735.

40. Pandolfo M: Molecular pathogenesis of Friedreich Ataxia. *Arch Neurol*. 1999; 56:1201-1208.

(This is a good, clear explanation of the underlying molecular genetics of one of the classical ataxic disease.)

41. Penney JB Jr. Multiple system atrophy and nonfamilial olivopontocerebellar atrophy are the same disease. Editorial. *Ann Neurol*. 1995; 37: 553-554.

(John Penney was a great late 20th Century neurologist who made many contributions to movement disorders and ataxia. His idea that nonfamilial olivopontocerebellar atrophies of somewhat different types will ultimately converge to multiple system atrophy is quite helpful in understanding this group of diseases.)

42. Pierrot-Deseilligny C, Gray F, Brunet P. Infarcts of both inferior parietal lobules with impairment of visually guided eye movements, peripheral visual attention and optic ataxia. *Brain*. 1986; 109:81-97.

43. Posner JB, Dalmau JO: Paraneoplastic syndromes of the nervous system. *Clin Chem Lab Med*. 2000; 38(2):117-222.

(Jerome Posner and his colleagues probably did more than everyone else put together to define the paraneoplastic syndromes of the nervous system. This article is well worth reading.)

44. Pulst SM. Inherited ataxias. In: Pulst SM, ed. *Genetics of Movement Disorders*. Amsterdam: Academic Press; 2002: 19-34.

(Pulst's book can be considered the Bible on the topic of genetics of movement disorders.)

45. Ouahchi K, Arita M, Kayden H, et al. Ataxia with isolated Vitamin E deficiency is caused by mutations in the alpha-tocopherol transfer protein. *Nat Genet*. 1995; 9:141-145.

46. Rice GPA, Lesaux J, Vandervoort P, Macewan L, Ebers GC. Ondansetron, a 5-HT3 antagonist, improves cerebellar tremor. *J Neurol Neurosurg Psychiatry*. 1997; 62:282-284.

47. Rolak LA, ed. *Neurology Secrets*. 4th ed. Philadelphia: Mosby; 2004.

48. Rosenberg RN. Spinocerebellar ataxias and ataxins. *New England Journal of Medicine*. 1995; 333:1351-1353.

49. Rosenberg RN, Paulson HL. The inherited ataxias. In: *The Molecular and Genetic Basis of Neurologic and Psychiatric Disease*. 3rd ed. RN Rosenberg, et al, eds. Philadelphia: Elsevier Science, and Boston: Butterworth-Heinemann; 2003.

50. Saiz A, Arpa J, Sagasta A, Casamitjana R, Zarranz JJ, Tolosa E, Graus F. Autoantibodies to glutamic acid decarboxylase in three patients with cerebellar ataxia, late-onset insulin-dependent diabetes mellitus, and polyendocrine autoimmunity. *Neurology*. 1997; 49(4):1026-1030.

51. Santillan A, Bristow RE. Paraneoplastic cerebellar degeneration in a woman with ovarian cancer. *Nature Clinical Practice Oncology*. 2006; 3:108-112.

52. Savitsky K, Bar-Shira A, Gilad S, Rotman G, Ziv Y, Vanagaite L, Tagle DA, Smith S, Uziel T, Sfez S, et al. A single ataxia telangiectasia gene with a product similar to PI-3 kinase. *Science*. 1995; 268:1749-1753.

53. Savoiardo M, Bracchi M, Passerini A, Visciani A. The vascular territories in the cerebellum and brainstem: CT and MR study. *Am J Neuroradiol*. 1987; 8:199-209.

54. Selhorst JB, Kaufman B, Horwitz SJ. Diphenylhydantoin-induced cerebellar degeneration. *Arch Neurol*. 1972; 27:453-456.

55. Senderek J, Krieger M, Stendel C, et al. I. Mutations in SIL1 cause Marinesco-Sjögren syndrome, a cerebellar ataxia with cataract and myopathy. *Nat Genet*. 2005 Dec; 37(12):1302-3.

56. Sobue G, Yasuda T, Kachi T, Sakakibara T, Mitsuma T. Chronic progressive sensory ataxic neuropathy: clinicopathological features of idiopathic and Sjögren's syndrome-associated cases. *J Neurol*. 1993; 240:1-7.

57. Subramony SH, Filla A. Autosomal dominant spinocerebellar ataxias ad infinitum? *Neurology*. 2001; 56:287-289.

58. Tagliatti M, Simpson D, Morgello S, et al. Cerebellar degeneration associated with human immuno-deficiency virus infection. *Neurology*. 1998; 50:244-25.

59. Tan EK, Ashizawa T. Genetic testing in spinocerebellar ataxias: defining a clinical role. *Arch Neurol*. 2001; 58:191-5.

(Ashizawa and his colleagues are outstanding neurologists and neurogeneticists. This article is well worth reading.)

60. Tsukamoto T, Mochizuki R, Mochizuki H, Noguchi M, Kayama H, Hiwatashi M, Yamamoto T. Paraneoplastic cerebellar degeneration and limbic encephalitis in a patient with adenocarcinoma of the colon. *J Neurol Neurosurg Psychiat*. 1993; 56:713-716.

61. Vahedi K, Joutel A, van Bogaert P, Ducros A, Maciazeck J, Bach JF, Bousser MG, Tournier-Lasserve E. A gene for hereditary paroxysmal cerebellar ataxia maps to chromosome 19p. *Ann Neurol*. 1995; 37:289-293.

62. Zoghbi HY, Orr HT. Glutamine repeats and neurodegeneration. 2000; 23:217-247.

(Huda Zoghbi continually breaks new ground in neurogenetics. Though this article is now a little old, it is still worth reading for its insights.)

8. Questions

1. Willlie Fall is a 21-year-old college student. He left a fraternity party at 2 am and attempted to drive home. A policeman noticed his car weaving noticeably on the highway and pulled him over. The officer asked Willie to walk heel to toe on a straight line but he was unable to perform this simple task. Dysfunction in what structure is mainly responsible for Willie's inability to "walk the straight and narrow."

A. Caudal vermis of the cerebellum

B. Rostral vermis of the cerebellum

C. Left and right cerebellar hemispheres, sparing the vermis

D. Left cerebellar hemisphere

E. Right cerebellar hemisphere

2. Which of the major cell types in Willie's cerebellum was probably the most affected by the alcohol due to its exquisite sensitivity to alcohol toxicity?

A. Basket cells

B. Granule cells

C. Purkinje cells

D. Smirnoff cells

E. Golgi cells

3. In counseling Willie about his drinking, his primary care physician might honestly inform him that:

A. Sooner or later, his cerebellum will become "immune" to the toxic affects of alcohol. Thus, if he gradually increases his ethanol consumption he will avoid such problems in later life.

B. The Purkinje cells in his cerebellum are very sensitive to alcohol toxicity acutely. Though continued drinking may induce liver enzymes that metabolize alcohol a bit faster, thus lowering acute levels for a given amount of consumption, the cerebellar cells will remain sensitive to alcohol throughout life and with repeated exposure they may degenerate, leaving him with a chronic, irreversible wide-based gait and ataxia.

C. His staggering gait had little to do with the alcohol and may have been the result of food poisoning.

D. As long as he does not fall over, he doesn't have a problem.

4. In the transverse organization of the cerebellum there are three lobes:

A. Anterior, posterior, and vermal

B. Anterior, middle, and posterior

C. Anterior, posterior and flocculonodular

D. Anterior, middle, and rubral

E. Exterior, interior, and middle

5. In the longitudinal organization of the cerebellum, there are three parts:

A. Left hemisphere, right hemisphere, and vermis

B. Anterior, hemispheric, and flocculonodular

C. Posterior, left hemisphere, and anterior

D. Upper, middle, and lower

E. Inner, outer, and vermal

6. Which of the following is NOT a common feature of cerebellar dysfunction?

A. Postural tremor

B. Resting tremor

C. Intention tremor

D. Hypotonia

E. Titubation

F. Nystagmus

7. A long word for incoordination of rapid alternating movements is:

A. Antidisestablishmentarianism

B. Dysdiadochokinesia

C. Olivopontocerebellarism

D. Dysynergia cerebellaris myoclonica

E. Dolichocephaly

8. You are examining Mr. Jones, a 52-year-old man with a complaint of problems walking. His gait is not particularly wide-based, and he can do a creditable job of performing the tandem walk and the heel-shin maneuver. You then perform the following test: you ask him to stand up straight with his feet together and his arms outstretched. When he does so he sways slightly. Then you ask him to close his eyes. His swaying increases markedly and as he starts to fall over, you catch him and tell him to open his eyes again, but he would have fallen had you not caught him.

What is the name of the last test you have performed?

A. Steinberg test.

B. Pittsburgh test.

C. Romberg test.

D. Holmes test.

E. Guttenberg test.

9. What would be the most likely source of Mr. Jones' problem walking?

A. Cerebellar dysfunction, mainly the temporal lobe of the cerebellum.

B. Cerebellar dysfunction, mainly posterior lobe.

C. Proprioceptive sensory loss, probably due to dorsal root ganglia and/or dorsal column involvement or severe peripheral neuropathy.

D. Cerebellar dysfunction involving the caudal vermis.

E. Disruption of the connections between the parietal lobe and the cerebellum.

10. Ms. Johnson is a 58-year-old woman previously in good health who has experienced a gradually worsening problem with coordination and gait for the last 6 months. She has been a lifetime teetotaler (ie, non-drinker). She has had, in particular, no complaints of gynecological problems or breast masses, and her Pap smear and breast exam, done slightly less than one year ago, were normal. Presently she can walk only with great difficulty using a walker and she experiences significant truncal titubation and limb ataxia. She is moderately dysarthric and dysphagic. Cranial nerve examination shows bilateral nystagmus in all directions of gaze. Speech is dysarthric and she has mild difficulty drinking a glass of water. Somatic strength and muscle bulk are normal. Cerebellar testing shows an impairment of the finger-nose-finger test, clumsiness in finger tapping, impaired heel shin exam, and a wide-based wobbly gait. Deep tendon reflexes are 1+ and symmetrical. Toes are down-going. On Romberg exam, she has difficulty standing on a narrow base but there is only mild worsening with the eyes closed. MRI scan of the brain is essentially normal (in particular, no signs of demyelination) but there is a suggestion of symmetrical cerebellar atrophy. Routine blood tests, including toxic/metabolic screen and CSF exam are normal. There is no family history of cerebellar problems.

Which of the following is the best next step?

A. Reassure the patient that no abnormalities were found, and her problems are probably a part of normal aging.

B. Accuse her of lying to you about her lack of drinking.

C. Without being accusatory, tell her rather firmly that such cerebellar dysfunction is almost always caused by alcoholism and that you suspect she is a closet alcoholic.

D. Order some additional tests, including those which detect antibodies suggestive of paraneoplastic syndromes.

E. Order a lie detector test to verify that she is indeed a non-drinker.

11. When Ms. Johnson's antibody testing comes back from the lab, there is a very strongly positive anti-Yo antibody level present. What is the next step in management of the patient?

A. Anti-Yo antibodies are highly suggestive of alcoholic cerebellar degeneration. You should now confront her with this information in the hopes that she will admit to her drinking problem.

B. Anti-Yo antibodies are highly suggestive of gynecological malignancy or breast cancer. But she had a normal Pap smear and breast exam less than a year ago, so this is not a possibility. Suggest to her that this may be a transient inflammation of the cerebellum and schedule her for follow up in 6 months to see if she gets better.

C. Anti-Yo antibodies are highly suggestive of lung cancer. Order a CT scan of the chest and send her to a pulmonary specialist for bronchoscopy.

D. Anti-Yo antibodies are highly suggestive of gynecological malignancy or breast cancer. Despite a reasonably recent normal Pap smear and breast exam, she could still have a malignancy in these areas. Do or have done a thorough gynecological and breast exam, including a mammogram if the other testing is negative.

E. Anti-Yo antibodies are highly non-specific and not one of the informative antibody results. Suggest to her that this may be a transient inflammation of the cerebellum and schedule her for follow-up in 6 months to see if she gets better.

12. Ms. Johnson's gynecological and breast exam are normal. But the neurological consultant now suggests a PET scan and/or possibly a laparoscopy in order to check even more thoroughly for malignancy. What is your response?

A. This has gone far enough. We are now getting into the area of throwing ridiculously expensive tests at obscure problems. Have her return in a few months for follow-up.

B. Given the high likelihood of a malignancy, further testing, especially a PET scan, is reasonable. You order the scan.

C. You still suspect alcoholism and you send the patient to Alcoholics Anonymous.

D. You consider that the patient may be malingering.

E. Given the high likelihood of malignancy, you recommend a hysterectomy with bilateral salpingo-oophorectomy

13. The PET scan was done on Ms. Johnson. It showed a small area of increased glucose uptake in the left adnexal region corresponding to the left ovary. A diagnostic laparoscopy with multiple biopsies revealed an ovarian carcinoma. After appropriate tumor staging, it was determined that a total hysterectomy with bilateral salpingo-oophorectomy followed by chemotherapy was appropriate, and these were done. The treating gynecologist stated that she had a reasonably high degree of optimism that long-term cure or control of the cancer may be achieved thanks in part to the fact that the diagnosis was reached earlier than it might have been by the standard preventive screening alone. What is the likelihood of cure or amelioration of the neurological syndrome?

A. Assuming that the tumor has been thoroughly removed or killed by the chemotherapy, there is a virtual certainty that the paraneoplastic syndrome will remit.

B. Once started, paraneoplastic syndromes never remit.

C. Usually, for gynecological malignancies causing anti-Yo neurological syndromes, the best one can hope for is mild-to-moderate improvement of the cerebellar syndrome, even if there is a total cure of the cancer. For cerebellar syndromes caused by lung cancer, complete remission of the cerebellar syndrome is fairly common if the cancer is cured completely.

D. It's a moot point because by the time a person has the cerebellar syndrome, the cancer is incurable anyway.

14. Friedreich's ataxia is:

A. An autosomal dominant cerebellar syndrome caused by a point mutation in the alpha tocopherol transfer protein (handles vitamin E).

B. An autosomal dominant cerebellar syndrome caused by a point mutation in the gene for frataxin.

C. A sporadic cerebellar syndrome which is sometimes associated with vitamin E deficiency and other times associated with autoantibodies to frataxin.

D. An autosomal recessive cerebellar syndrome cause by an expansion repeat mutation in the frataxin gene.

E. An X-linked cerebellar syndrome caused by an expansion repeat in the frataxin gene.

F. None of the above.

15. Which of the following are known molecular mechanisms for episodic ataxias? (pick 2)

A. Point mutation in a potassium channel gene.

B. Point mutation in a voltage-gated calcium channel gene.

C. Point mutation in the alpha tocopherol transfer protein (handles vitamin E).

D. Expansion repeat in ataxin-1.

E. Expansion repeat in ataxin-2.

16. Which of the following is NOT commonly thought to be in the differential diagnosis of cerebellar dysfunction?

A. Hypothyroidism

B. Gluten sensitive enteropathy or adult celiac-sprue

C. Vitamin E deficiency

D. Whipple disease

E. Muscular dystrophy

17. Most sensory information enters the cerebellum through:

A. The juxtarestiform body in the inferior cerebellar peduncle

B. The superior cerebellar peduncle (brachium conjunctivum)

C. The middle cerebellar peduncle

D. The spinothalamic tract

E. The corpus callosum

18. Most output leaves the cerebellum via:

A. The juxtarestiform body in the inferior cerebellar peduncle

B. The superior cerebellar peduncle (brachium conjunctivum)

C. The middle cerebellar peduncle

D. The spinothalamic tract

E. The corpus callosum

19. Assuming a unilateral cerebellar lesion:

A. Past pointing would be to the side of the lesion, but the fast phase of nystagmus would be to the opposite side.

B. Past pointing would be opposite to the side of the lesion, but the fast phase of nystagmus would be to the same side.

C. Both past pointing and the fast phase of nystagmus would be to the side of the lesion.

20. Ralph N. is a 34-year-old cab driver who noticed the progressive onset of a reeling, staggering gait over about a week. When seen in the emergency room he has ophthalmoplegia, ataxia, and areflexia. He also has mild facial weakness. Otherwise his neurological exam is normal. His lumbar puncture yields spinal fluid with no cells but with a high protein. His routine blood workup including toxin screen is normal. He has no history of heavy drinking and is otherwise in good health. Which of the following syndromes represent Ralph's most likely diagnosis?

A. Millard-Gubler syndrome

B. Miller Fisher syndrome

C. Carrie Fisher syndrome

D. Arthur Miller syndrome

E. Fisher-Katz syndrome

21. Which of the following tests can be used to confirm the above diagnosis?

A. Test for anti-GQ1b antibodies

B. Test for myelin basic protein

C. Test for anti-linoleum antibodies

D. Functional MRI scan

E. PET scan with gadolinium enhancement

22. Match the phenomena on the left with the cerebellar anatomy on the right:

1.) Truncal ataxia and truncal titubation. — a.) rostral vermis

2.) Wide-based stance and gait. Poorly coordinated walking. — b.) caudal vermis

3.) Poorly coordinated movements of (ipsilateral) extremities. — c.) cerebellar fine hemispheres

23. In the episodic ataxias EA-1 and EA-2, which of the following medications are effective in reducing or abolishing the attacks of ataxia?

A. Carbamazepine

B. Neurontin

C. Acetazolamide

D. Allopurinol

E. Hydrocholorothiazide

24. What is the most common known mutation in the group of spinocerebellar atrophies whose genetic causes have been elucidated?

A. Point mutation in the gene for neurofilament protein

B. Deletion mutation in the gene for tubulin

C. Expansion repeat of CAG in various genes

D. Expansion repeat of ATG in various genes

E. Mutant prion protein gene

25. True or False. Friedreich's ataxia is essentially a non-progressive or minimally progressive ataxia. The patients very rarely ever worsen to the point of needing a wheelchair.

26. The five major neuronal cell types of the cerebellum are:

A. Purkinje, granule, stellate, basket, and Golgi

B. Purkinje, granule, stellate, lunate, and basket

C. Purkinje, Golgi, Cajal, lunate, and basket

D. Purkinje, granule, pyramidal, basket, and Golgi

E. Purkinje, pyramidal, basket, oblate, and Golgi

27. Cerebellar granule cells use the neurotransmitter glutamate. The other cerebellar neuronal cell types use which neurotransmitter?

A. Serotonin

B. Epinephrine

C. Dopamine

D. Gama amino butyric acid (GABA)

E. Norepinephrine

28. True or False. Most types of cerebellar dysfunction are readily curable by a specific medical therapy.

29. Choose the two answers that are true:

A. Acetazolamide is a cure for Friedreich's ataxia.

B. Acetazolamide can cause ataxia in certain patients.

C. Acetazolamide toxicity causes the mutation found in Holmes ataxia.

D. Acetazolamide can treat some of the genetic episodic ataxias.

E. Acetazolamide has no effect on ataxias whatsoever.

30. Frataxin is:

A. A form of ataxia seen in college fraternity members when they are drunk (soroataxin is similar).

B. The gene involved with Frodo's ataxia.

C. The gene involved with Friedreich's ataxia.

D. The gene involved in French ataxia.

E. None of the above.

31. The ADCA classification system, in which cerebellar degenerations are organized in three or four groups (ADCA I, II, III, and sometimes IV), is now primarily looked upon as:

A. An obsolete system that should be abandoned

B. A system which completely defines the genetic characteristics of the ataxia.

C. A system which roughly describes the phenotype. More than one genotype can fit the phenotypic pattern.

D. A method for categorizing how much grant money is collected for research on the ataxias in each group.

E. None of the above.

Answers

1. B.
The rostral vermis is significantly involved in gait stability as noted in Figure 1. It is affected by alcohol, other toxins, and nutritional deficits.

2. C.
Purkinje cells, as noted in the text in the first paragraph under Neuroanatomical Correlations.

3. B.
As noted in the first test paragraph under Neuroanatomical Correlations.

4. C.
This is given in Figure 1 and in the discussion related to that Figure.

5. A.
This is given in Figure 1 and in the discussion related to that Figure. Actually, the figure does not specifically say right and left hemispheres. It shows two hemispheres and it should be obvious that one is on the right and the other is on the left.

6. B.
Only resting tremor is not a commonly seen feature of cerebellar disease. Resting tremor is commonly seen in Parkinson disease, however.

7. B.
Dysdiadochokinesia may be found by having the patient rapidly tap the front and then the back of his hand on the back of the other hand or on the thighs. Other rapid alternating movements may be tested.

8. C.
The Romberg test as stated in the text in section 3, Terminology of Cerbellar Deficits and Ataxia.

9. C.

It is a common misconception that the Romberg test is essentially a test of cerebellar function. Sometimes it is even taught that way in physical diagnosis courses, but the major pathology detected by this test is proprioceptive sensory dysfunction, usually due to a lesion in the peripheral sensory nerves, dorsal root ganglia and/or dorsal columns as stated in the text in section 3, Terminology of Cerbellar Deficits and Ataxia.

10. D.

Such a pervasive pancerebellar syndrome is not really typical of alcoholism. Possibly an "end-stage" advanced alcoholic might have many of these problems but it would take many years to gradually develop. This syndrome is much more suggestive of a parneoplastic cerebellar degeneration.

11. D.

About 2/3 of patients with positive anti-Yo and a cerebellar syndrome have an occult malignancy. This is surely high enough to push on and do more testing. A Pap smear and a normal breast exam certainly do not definitely rule out the possibility of malignancy and her's were done almost a year ago. Though a Pap smear was mentioned, this does not necessarily imply a thorough pelvic exam with palpation of ovaries. But even if this had been done, there are some tumors that can escape detection on physical exam.

12. B.

Though I generally discourage the "shotgun" use of expensive tests, this case is still at a stage where there is an extremely high chance of a serious yet possibly curable malignancy being present. Given that there are some non-invasive and/or less invasive means available, I do not think I would do the hysterectomy and salpingo-oophorectomy at this juncture. The PET scan, if available, is actually a reasonable test for malignancy at this point. Another approach might have been ultrasound and/or pelvic MRI scan. But one way or the other, some further non-invasive testing is necessary at this point. Also note that initially one might have expected some cells to be present in the CSF. It can be either way. Very early there are often cells present, which then go away. In her case, there were none at the time she was tapped, but serial spinal taps might have been a good idea.

13. C.

Unfortunately, the clinical response of the cerebellar syndrome is usually not very good. But frequently it does stop worsening and perhaps gets a little better over time. For some reason, cerebellar syndromes due to lung cancer seem to do a little better if the cancer can be cured. It is important to realize that picking up this constellation of signs and symptoms as early as possible can sometimes lead to a cure of the cancer. That part is definitely not hopeless, and the cerebellar syndrome can ameliorate somewhat.

14. D.

In Friedreich's ataxia there is an expansion repeat in what is now called the frataxin gene. Such expansion repeats are a recurring motif in neurogenetics.

15. A., B.

There is a mutation of the voltage-gated calcium channel encoded on chromosome 19p, which causes an episodic ataxia (EA2), which is frequently improved by acetazolamide. Another episodic ataxia (EA1) involves a potassium channel encoded on chromosome 12p.

16. E.

All of the others can cause cerebellar dysfunction and they were mentioned in the chapter. Muscular dystrophy has nothing to do with the cerebellum.

17. A.

This answer comes from the brief review of anatomy at the beginning of the chapter.

18. B.

This answer comes from the brief review of anatomy at the beginning of the chapter.

19. C.

As noted under the subheading Past Pointing or Hypermetria, past pointing due to cerebellar disease is generally toward the side of the cerebellar lesion. In the subsection Eye Movement Abnormalities, it was noted that the fast phase of nystagmus is generally toward the side of the cerebellar lesion.

20. B.
The Miller Fisher syndrome is a type of Güillain-Barré syndrome, ie, it is an acute demyelination inflammatory polyneuropathy. Unlike the typical Güillain-Barré Syndrome, which typically starts with lower extremity weakness, which then ascends, Miller Fisher Syndrome starts with opththalmoplegia and ataxia. Like the typical Güillain-Barré, there is also areflexia. This is discussed in the text under Post-Infectious Problems.

21. A.
Patients with the Miller Fisher syndrome generally have positive antibodies to the GQ1b (or less commonly the GT1b) ganglioside epitope.

22. 1.) B.
2.) A.
3.) C.
These facts were mentioned in various places in the chapter, including Figure 1 which gives the clino-anatomic correlations. The most basic categories should be simple to remember. The vermis is a midline structure, and vermal damage impairs the midline functions of truncal stability and gait. The hemispheres are anatomically more peripheral, so it seems logical that a right hemispheric lesion would impair right extremity (especially finger and hand coordination). How do you remember that the rostral vermis mainly involves gait stability and the caudal vermis mainly involves truncal stability? I guess you just have to memorize it.

23. C.
This was stated in the text. This must have something to do with the fact that EA-1 and EA-2 involve defects in a potassium channel and a calcium channel, respectively. Acetazolamide tends to influence the body's handling of potassium, so it tends to make sense that this might affect EA-1. The affect on EA-2 must be less direct.

24. C.
This was covered in the text. It is an interesting fact that many neurogenetic diseases involve expansion repeats of CAG. There are certain susceptible places in the chromosomes in which the CAG tracts can start to mutate and gradually get larger each generation. Eventually a critical point is reached and the abnormality causes clinical disease.

25. False.
Friedreich's ataxia is a very serious disease and causes significant impairment in mobility. It is hoped that gene therapy approaches may eventually produce some good treatments.

26. A.
This was mentioned in the text. I include it as a question because someone else may include it as a question on a test.

27. D.
This was mentioned in the brief review of microscopic anatomy and neurotransmitter. Actually, most of the circuits in the cerebellum are inhibitory to and rely on the inhibitory neurotransmitter GABA.

28. False.
Note how small the section on therapy is. Maybe this will inspire some of the readers of this chapter to do research on cerebellar diseases.

29. B.
As stated in the text, acetazolamide can cause ataxia in some individuals. Yet in individuals with EA-1 or EA-2 episodic ataxias it is generally quite helpful.

30. C.
This was mentioned in the discussion of Friedreich's ataxia. As of this writing, it is not clearly understood how the mutation in frataxin actually produces the disease.

31. C.
As mentioned in the text, the ADCA numbers divide the ataxias into broad groups of phenotypes. As can be seen in Table II, more than one genotype can show a given phenotype.

Chapter 14: Dementia

Christopher M. Filley, MD

Contents

1. Introduction

Background

The syndrome of dementia has recently emerged as a major medical challenge in society. In part, this development stems from the dramatic expansion of the human lifespan over the last century, rendering more people at risk for neurodegenerative diseases because of their increased longevity. It is well to remember, however, that dementia can occur in persons of any age who experience a decline of mental ability from a previously normal level. A persistent loss of intellectual capacity is a devastating condition that is being better appreciated as a manifestation of a great variety of neurologic, medical, and psychiatric etiologies, and a comprehensive approach to prevention, diagnosis, and management is increasingly important for physicians in a wide range of clinical settings.

Dementia has become the subject of vigorous study in both the clinical and basic neurosciences, and the understanding of its definition, classification, etiology, pathophysiology, diagnosis, treatment, and prognosis is rapidly evolving. While it is clear that dementia is neither synonymous with senility, an outdated and imprecise term, nor an inevitable accompaniment of aging,[1] much remains to be learned of this multifaceted syndrome. In this chapter, the emphasis will be on primary concepts that incorporate current thinking and help to organize the topic from a clinical perspective. Central to this approach will be the notion of how different disorders of the brain produce dementia by disrupting its normal function in recognizable ways, enhancing the clinician's appreciation of how each dementia syndrome, like each person in which dementia develops, is unique.

Definition

Dementia is an acquired and persistent syndrome of intellectual dysfunction characterized by impairment in three or more domains that include memory, language, visuospatial skills, executive function, and personality or emotional behavior, and that compromise ordinary social and occupational function.[1] This definition excludes patients with congenital mental retardation, who never attain normal mental function, and those with acute confusional state or delirium, who typically have a short-lived disorder with salient attentional impairment. In comparison to the definition of dementia given in the well-known *Diagnostic and Statistical Manual of Mental Disorders*, 4th edition (*DSM-IV*),[2] memory dysfunction is not required as a core deficit; the *DSM-IV* definition is thus less useful because it fails to capture those dementias that do not manifest with memory loss in the early phase of the disorder. In addition, it is important that the definition given above does not imply that dementia is either progressive or irreversible; in fact, dementias may be static, as in severe traumatic brain injury (TBI), or reversible, as in some cases of hypothyroidism. Dementia simply describes a clinical syndrome that has a range of presentations, etiologies, neuropathologies, treatments, and prognoses, and given this variability, the clinician's task is to make a secure diagnosis and proceed with the best available treatment as soon as feasible.

Epidemiology

Precise data on the incidence and prevalence of dementia are unavailable, in part due to uncertainties about diagnosis and classification. However, recent years have clearly witnessed a rising prevalence of dementia in industrialized countries that is largely related to the well-documented aging of the population. For example, Alzheimer disease (AD), typically cited as the most common dementia, afflicts some 4-5 million Americans and increases in prevalence with age so that about 30% of those over 85 are affected.[3] While these figures will grow higher because of increased longevity over the next several decades, it is important to remember that AD accounts for only 50%-70% of late-life dementias.[1] Another sobering statistic is that TBI, a disorder with peak incidence at age 15-24, and therefore an enormously high prevalence, produces yearly 70,000 to 90,000 new cases of severely injured persons who have long-term disability, including dementia,[4] and that are not ordinarily included in standard data collections of the dementias. Although AD alone is a serious threat to public health, the entire range of dementias—from all etiologies—merits vigorous medical, scientific, and societal attention.

2. Pathophysiology

The dementia syndrome encompasses a broad and diverse spectrum of neurologic, medical, and psychiatric entities, numbering several dozen at present and continually expanding. Faced with this formidable array of diagnostic possibilities, the clinician can usefully consider the dementias using a foundation of neuropathological changes that disrupt brain structure and function in a manner that predicts the clinical phenomenology of the illness. That is, every dementia has a distinct neuropathology that manifests as a recognizable clinical presentation. Although diagnosis is often complicated by more than one etiology of dementia, the schema presented herein serves to structure the conceptual approach to this area and simplify clinical reasoning. This approach involves a classification of dementias based on the sites of most prominent neuropathology: the cerebral cortex, the subcortical gray matter, the white matter, and combinations of all three. These categories are necessarily blurred to some extent because of unavoidable clinical and neuropathological overlap, but they do serve to organize the most important disorders that can produce the dementia syndrome. Tables 1, 2, 3, and 4 provide a listing of the clinical entities within each of these categories.

Alzheimer Disease

AD is the most common dementia of aging, and represents a major threat to older individuals and society because of the enormous emotional and financial losses associated with the progressive and thus far irreversible neurobehavioral decline experi-

Table 1

Cortical Dementias

Alzheimer disease Posterior cortical atrophy
Frontotemporal lobar degeneration Frontotemporal dementia Primary progressive aphasia Semantic dementia

Table 2

Frontal-Subcortical Dementias

Parkinson disease
Huntington disease
Progressive supranuclear palsy
Wilson disease
Depression
Manic-depressive illness
Schizophrenia

Table 3

White Matter Dementias

Category	Example
Genetic	Metachromic leukodystrophy
Demyelinative	Multiple sclerosis
Infectious	AIDS dementia complex
Inflammatory	Systemic lupus erythematosus
Toxic	Toluene leukoencephalopathy
Metabolic	Cobalamin deficiency
Vascular	Binswanger disease
Traumatic	Traumatic brain injury
Neoplastic	Gliomatosis cerebri
Hydrocephalic	Normal pressure hydrocephalus

Table 4

Mixed Dementias

Vascular dementia
Dementia with Lewy bodies
Corticobasal degeneration
Neurosyphilis and other conventional infections
Creutzfeldt-Jacob disease
Subdural hematoma
Toxic and metabolic disorders

enced by patients and witnessed by their families.[3] First described in a 51-year-old woman (Figure 1) and called "presenile dementia" by Alois Alzheimer in 1907, AD has since come to be recognized as affecting mostly older adults, although the disease has the same neuropathology regardless of age of onset. Diagnosis is based on consensus criteria that distinguish between "definite" AD, in which histologic confirmation of the neuropathology is available from biopsy or autopsy, and the more common "probable" AD, in which typical clinical features are present but histology is unavailable.[5] In the clinical setting, a diagnosis of probable AD is typically sufficient, and is likely to be about 90% accurate[1] if made using standard criteria.[2,5]

AD usually begins with the insidious loss of memory, and progressive amnesia is typically prominent throughout the disease course. At the earliest stage, this problem may be exceedingly subtle, and easily confused with normal aging or mild cognitive impairment (MCI; see below). As time passes, however, what was once mild forgetfulness advances to severe amnesia, and other cognitive deficits gradually develop. At the terminal stage of the disease, patients are severely demented, with global aphasia or mutism, rigidity, and incontinence, and nursing home placement becomes inevitable in most cases.

Figure 1

August D.

The original case of Alzheimer disease.

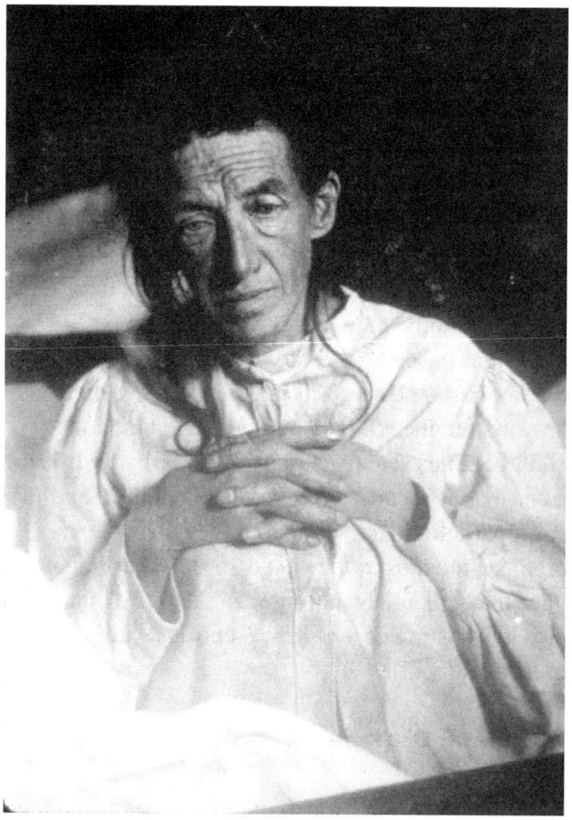

Table 5 provides a listing of characteristic clinical features of AD throughout its course, which is usefully divided into three stages.[1]

The neuropathology of AD is well known: grossly, the cerebral hemispheres show atrophy that reflects cortical neuronal loss (Figure 2), and microscopically, large numbers of characteristic neuritic (amyloid) plaques and neurofibrillary tangles appear, as described by Alzheimer a century ago (Figure 3). Neuronal loss is first apparent in the hippocampal regions of the medial temporal lobes and in the parietotemporal cortices, patterns that explain the early amnesia, and the language and visuospatial deficits that typify the clinical onset of AD (Figure 2). Synapse loss occurs , and neurons degenerate to worsen the cognitive decline. With time, additional neocortical areas become affected, especially the frontal lobes, and continued loss in cognitive ability occurs; notably, however, the primary motor, sensory, and visual cortices are spared until very late in the disease (Figure 2). The characteristic microscopic changes appear in parallel with the neuronal loss. Neuritic plaques are extracellular deposits of β-amyloid surrounded by degenerating dendrites and axons, and neurofibrillary tangles are intracellular deposits of abnormally phosphorylated tau protein that interfere with intraneuronal trafficking (Figure 3). In AD, both histologic features are found far in excess of the small numbers associated with normal aging. Although much attention has been devoted to both plaques and tangles in efforts to understand the pathogenesis of the disease,[3] a clear understanding of the pathogenic sequence involved in the complex cascade of events leading to synaptic and neuronal loss in AD is not yet available. Nevertheless, much effort is proceeding to exploit these neuropathological abnormalities in discovering new treatments.

With the exception of rare familial cases, the etiology of AD is not known. Most cases seen clinically are considered to have "sporadic" AD, as no clear family history is evident, but occasional patients present in whom a genetic origin can be invoked.[1] The first clue to a genetic cause was the observation that people with Down syndrome, a chromosomal disorder involving trisomy [21], typically develop the neuropathological changes of AD in midlife. As the 21st chromosome harbors a gene for amyloid precursor protein (APP), it was reasoned that expression of this gene in triplicate produces excessive amyloid deposition identical with that which occurs in sporadic AD. Other clues came later as it was recognized that three distinct gene mutations—presenilin-1 (PS1) on chromosome14, presenilin-2 (PS2)

Table 5

Clinical Stages of Alzheimer Disease

Stage 1 (1-3 Years)
Amnesia
Anomia
Indifference
Stage 2 (2-10 Years)
Severe amnesia
Fluent aphasia
Visuospatial deficits
Apraxia
Agnosia
Neuropsychiatric features
Stage 3 (8-12 years)
Severe dementia
Global aphasia or mutism
Rigidity
Incontinence

Figure 2

Medial aspect of the right hemisphere from a patient with Alzheimer disease

Showing marked cortical atrophy, particularly in temporal, parietal, and frontal regions subserving higher brain function.

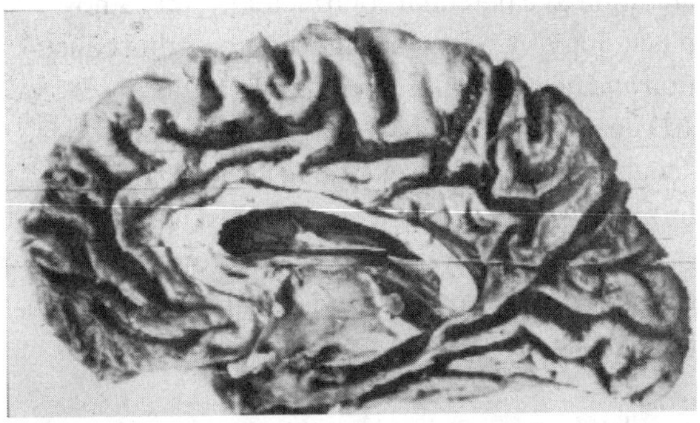

Figure 3

Neuritic plaques and neurofibrillary tangles from the cerebral cortex of a patient with Alzheimer disease (silver stain)

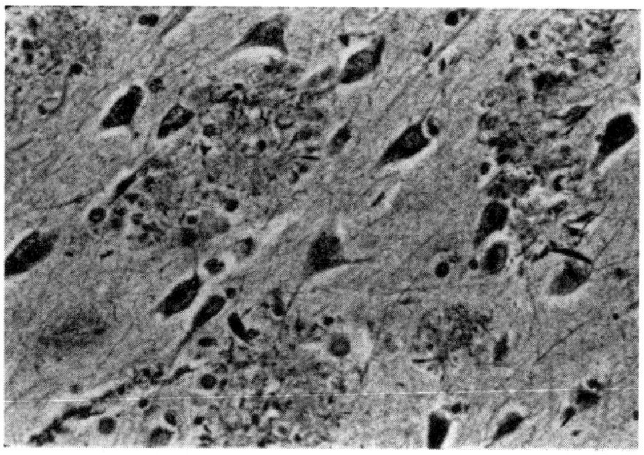

on chromosome 1, and APP on chromosome 21—are linked with autosomal dominant AD.[1] In addition, a gene called apolipoprotein E apo E)4 has been discovered to confer susceptibility to AD, especially if homozygous.[1] It is noteworthy that all of these conditions are characterized by the increased deposition of β-amyloid, leading many authorities to endorse the "amyloid hypothesis" of AD.[3]

However, genetics may not provide a complete explanation for the etiology of AD. Considerable evidence indicates that environmental variables may combine with genetic factors to influence the expression of the disease. TBI, for example, may be associated with an increased risk for later development of AD, and vascular disease is receiving more attention as a potential contributor to AD pathophysiology.[1] Conversely, higher premorbid education and occupational level may delay the onset of AD, leading to the theory that in some patients a "neuronal reserve" may exist in the brain that confers some degree of protection against neurodegeneration.[1] Much current opinion therefore favors a genetic etiology for AD that is modified by environmental factors.

Another important development in research on AD has been the observation that the cholinergic system originating in the basal forebrain is heavily damaged early in the disease.[1] Neurons producing acetylcholine project from the basal forebrain to widespread areas of the hippocampus and neocortex, and because acetylcholine has an important role in normal memory and cognitive function, loss of cholinergic cells contributes to the dementia of AD patients. The cholinergic hypothesis has been exploited to impel much drug development in AD, as it has been assumed that potentiating cholinergic function will improve cognition in a manner analogous to the improvement in motor function in patients with Parkinson disease (PD) that receive dopaminergic therapy. Unfortunately, cholinergic treatment of AD is not as effective as dopaminergic treatment of PD, at least in part because additional neurochemical deficits also contribute to dementia in AD and are not addressed by drugs designed to augment the cholinergic system.

Although the great majority of AD cases fit the above model, occasional cases of so-called posterior cortical atrophy (PCA) come to clinical attention. Also known as the visual variant of AD, PCA involves prominent occipitoparietal degeneration that results in higher visual impairments such as Balint syndrome (simultanagnosia, ocular apraxia, and optic ataxia), visuospatial dysfunction, environmental disorientation, visual agnosia, and alexia. Importantly, memory loss is not a typical initial feature of PCA, again pointing out the inadequacy of the *DSM-IV* definition of dementia.[2] Although when first described PCA was not well understood neuropathologically, it has come to be known as a variant of AD because more than half of cases prove to have the histologic changes of AD at autopsy.[1] The next most common cause of PCA is the Heidenhain variant of Creutzfeldt-Jakob disease (CJD1; see below).

Frontotemporal Lobar Degeneration (FTLD)

This disorder has a long and confusing history beginning with the entity Pick disease, which appeared in 20th-century textbooks as an unusual dementia involving lobar degeneration of the frontal and temporal lobes combined with histologic features of intracytoplasmic Pick bodies and ballooned neurons called Pick cells.[1] Pick disease has now been largely superceded in modern terminology by the concept of FTLD, a broad category including the entities frontotemporal dementia (FTD), primary progressive aphasia (PPA) or progressive nonfluent aphasia (PNFA), and semantic dementia (SD). The neuropathology of FTLD is evolving, and it is now thought that most of these patients demonstrate either: 1) tau-positive inclusions, including Pick bodies is some cases, 2) ubiquitin-positive inclusions (FTLD-U), or 3) dementia lacking distinctive histology.[6] The most common neuropathology is tauopathy, which links this form of FTLD with other tauopathies: tangle-predominant AD, progressive supranuclear palsy (PSP), dementia with Lewy bodies (DLB), corticobasal degeneration (CBD), and the very rare argyrophilic grain disease.[6] Some cases of FTLD-U also have motor neuron disease, and a disease protein called TDP-43 has been identified, different forms of which may influence clinical features. Mutations on chromosome 17—microtubule-associated protein tau (MAPT) and progranulin (PRGN)—are associated with tau-positive FTLD and FTLD-U, respectively.[6] The recognition of clinical overlap between FTLD-U and motor neuron disease is important clinically, as it is clear that motor features of amyotrophic lateral sclerosis (ALS) may occur in some people with FTD, and that, conversely, behavioral features of FTD may develop in some patients with ALS.[1]

The distinguishing neurobehavioral feature of all FTLD variants is that behavioral or language alteration is the first presentation, in contrast to the memory disorder that is typically the initial manifestation of AD.[6] In FTD, the most common of the FTLD diseases, behavioral abnormalities may be striking, and because of the prominent disturbances that may ensue, many such patients are first seen psychiatrically and receive diagnoses such as bipolar disorder and schizophrenia. Disturbances of social and personal conduct are common, and a central feature is disinhibition, which manifests as impulsive or inappropriate behavior, including loss of social tact, poor personal hygiene, hypersexuality, aggressiveness, a tendency to overeat, and impaired judgment. Although complaints of memory disturbance are frequent, amnesia is not encountered when formal testing is performed at the onset of disease, and a disorder of comportment is instead the salient

Figure 4

Drawing of the brain of a patient with frontotemporal dementia

Drawing shows marked atrophy of the frontal and temporal lobes.

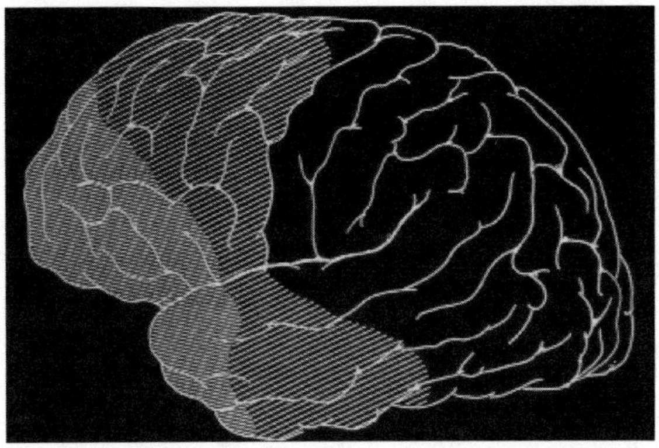

deficit. Grossly, the brain is atrophic in frontal and temporal regions (Figure 4), in keeping with the typical neurobehavioral presentation of the illness.

Language disorders constitute the other major manifestation of FTLD. The two FTLD types that present with language disturbance are PPA/PNFA7and SD.[8] PPA/PNFA is a syndrome of nonfluent aphasia that gradually evolves to dementia over several years. Affected individuals first develop subtle naming deficits, and then nonfluent aphasia, with sparing of other cognitive domains before generalized dementia appears. In contrast, SD involves fluent aphasia with a characteristic loss of knowledge of the meaning of words. Like PPA/PNFA, SD advances to dementia with time as other cognitive domains become affected. These diseases provide further illustration of the principle that the topography of cortical degeneration predicts the pattern of the clinical presentation and disease course.

Frontal-Subcortical Dementias

This group of diseases has been the subject of considerable debate since the 1970s, when the idea of subcortical dementia was championed as a category that could be differentiated from cortical dementia, mainly AD.[9] Subcortical dementia initially referred to a number of diseases that predominantly affect the subcortical gray matter structures of the basal ganglia, thalamus, and brainstem. The first entities listed in this category were PD, Huntington disease (HD), PSP, and Wilson disease (Table 3), and similar clinical profiles were noted in these diseases that contrasted with that of AD. In brief, the distinction between subcortical and cortical dementia is that the former is characterized by disturbances in the fundamental functions of arousal, attention, mood, and motivation, whereas the latter features deficits in the instrumental functions of memory, language, praxis, and perception. As time went on, the term "frontal-subcortical dementia" came to be preferred by many in light of a deeper understanding of neuroanatomy that established the existence of multiple cortical-subcortical circuits linking the subcortical regions to the frontal lobes.[9] Regardless of the terminology, clinical and research evidence suggests that the frontal-subcortical dementias may be more similar to each other than to AD.[9] At present, despite lingering uncertainty resulting from the both clinical and neuropathological overlap between cortical and frontal-subcortical diseases, the distinction between cortical and frontal-subcortical dementias continues to be useful for both clinical and research purposes.

Parkinson Disease

PD is well known to physicians as the most important movement disorder of late life and a major neurologic cause of disability. The characteristic neuropathology of PD involves depigmentation of the pars compacta of the midbrain substantia nigra, with neuronal loss and subsequent deficiency of dopamine in the striatum.[1] Lewy bodies, the pathognomonic histologic feature of PD, are also seen in the substantia nigra, and have recently been recognized to contain the abnormal protein α-synuclein. The classic features of bradykinesia, rigidity, and resting tremor are the clinical hallmarks of the disease, which typically begins asymmetrically and progresses slowly over many years. The dementia of PD is less well recognized, but occurs at some point in 40%-60% of patients, usually in the older age ranges.[1] Controversy has existed around the pathogenesis of dementia in PD, as it is unclear whether cognitive impairment can be ascribed to subcortical dopaminergic pathology, the presence of Lewy bodies elsewhere in the brain, or coexistent AD. Perhaps the most reasonable resolution of this debate at present is that each of these explanations pertains to certain patients, depending on their specific neuropathology. Thus dementia in PD appears to be heterogeneous, and some affected individuals do in fact have a true frontal-subcortical dementia related to substantia nigra Lewy bodies, whereas others have additional neuropathology that alters the clinical expression of the disease.[10] Detailed clinical-neuropathological studies will be required to further understand these various conditions.

Huntington Disease

This is an autosomal dominant disease in which dementia and chorea are the classic clinical features. HD is now known to result from an abnormally high number of trinucleotide repeats of cytosine, adenine, and guanine (CAG) on the short arm of chromosome 4.[1] Caudate atrophy is a consistent neuroimaging and neuropathological feature of the disease,[1] securely placing HD within the neuropathological spectrum of frontal-subcortical dementia. With onset in midlife, nearly 100% penetrance, and the absence of reversibility with current interventions, this disease presents a difficult challenge for asymptomatic persons who may carry the gene that is not yet expressed. Presymptomatic HD testing is now available and can help guide decisions about bearing children in such instances. The dementia of HD involves slowed cognition, attention and concentration deficits, impaired memory, executive dysfunction, and spared language, and a range of neuropsychiatric problems including depression, anxiety, disinhibition, and antisocial behavior.[1] In general, the cognitive problems of HD patients reflect core deficits in frontal-subcortical circuits.[11] The memory dysfunction of HD differs from that of AD in that deficits are present in memory retrieval, not encoding, and in procedural learning.[1] This profile has allowed the differentiation of HD dementia from both the cortical dementia of AD and the white matter dementias (see below).

Progressive Supranuclear Palsy

PSP has come to be a rather frequent diagnosis in both movement disorder and dementia clinics because it features a combination of motor and cognitive features. Often confused with PD because of the prominence of parkinsonism, PSP is a distinct disorder regarded by some as a "Parkinson plus" syndrome that includes a wide array of neurologic features. The principle components of PSP are supranuclear gaze palsy, especially of vertical gaze, axial rigidity, parkinsonism, pseudobulbar palsy, and dementia.[1] Neuropathologically, there is marked atrophy of the upper brainstem, and abundant tau deposition within neurofibrillary tangles in numerous brainstem and basal ganglia structures. Cortical tau deposition is present but is less abundant, qualifying PSP as a predominantly frontal-subcortical disorder.[1] The dementia has a characteristic frontal-subcortical quality, with cognitive slowing, inattention, and executive dysfunction.[1] One important clinical feature of PSP is that there is little or no response to standard PD drugs such as levodopa and the dopamine agonists. In this respect, PSP is similar to other "Parkinson plus" disorders such as dementia with Lewy bodies (DLB) and corticobasal degeneration (CBD; see below).

Wilson Disease

This is an autosomal recessive disease of copper metabolism in which dementia develops in association with a movement disorder in adolescence or young adulthood.[1] Copper is deposited in the basal ganglia, leading to the neurologic features of the disease, and also in the liver, where it can cause hepatic dysfunction, and the cornea, where slit lamp examination may disclose the pathognomonic Kayser-Fleischer ring. Serum ceruloplasmin and copper levels may be low, and urinary copper excretion is high. The dementia is often mild, and resembles the other fronto-subcortical dementias; neuropsychiatric problems may be prominent.[1] The clinical recognition of this rare disease is particularly important because chelation of copper may result in effective treatment.

Another group of diseases relevant to the concept of frontal-subcortical dementia is the major psychiatric disorders (Table 3). Initial formulations of the idea of subcortical dementia noted the frequency of personality and behavioral changes with these diseases, and disordered mood and motivation are more prominent in frontal-subcortical diseases.[1] Although depression, manic-depressive illness, and schizophrenia are not typically considered dementias, subgroups of patients within all three categories can develop dementia in the course of their disease, and available evidence suggests a frontal-subcortical origin for these disorders.[1,9] For the clinician, maximization of cognitive function by comprehensive treatment of these disorders and any associated problems is indicated, but there are some patients who nevertheless develop dementia as one aspect of their psychiatric problem.

White Matter Dementias

In recent years, it has been recognized that disorders of the brain white matter may alter cognition and behavior to the point where a diagnosis of dementia is justified.[12] To some extent, this notion is implicit in the dichotomy of cortical and frontal-subcortical dementia reviewed above, as cerebral white matter is clearly another subcortical region affected by many neuropathologies, but lists of frontal-subcortical dementias commonly exclude or minimize the white matter disorders. However, the importance of white matter in neurobehavioral function cannot be ignored; white matter constitutes about one-half the brain volume, contains about 135,000 km of myelinated axons, and is responsible for the vast connectivity of the brain (Figure 5). More than 100 diseases, injuries, and intoxications exert their neuropathological effect primarily or exclusively on the brain white matter, and all of these disorders are associated with some form of neurobehavioral impairment.[12] Many individuals with marked white matter involvement—regardless of the specific neuropathology—experience cognitive impairment that is sufficient to merit the definition of dementia by standard criteria.[1,2] This syndrome has been termed white matter dementia,[12] and its major etiologies are listed in Table 4. Although white matter dementia is closely related to frontal-subcortical dementia because these categories share prominent deficits in sustained attention and memory retrieval, preliminary evidence indicates that differences may exist. In contrast to the frontal-subcortical dementias, in which extrapyramidal disorders and procedural memory dysfunction occur, the white matter dementias manifest few movement disorders and no impairment of procedural memory.[12] Both of these profiles differ from that of cortical dementia, in which memory encoding is primarily affected,

Figure 5

Drawing of major white matter tracts in the human brain

CC = corpus callosum
UF = U fiber
SOFF = superior occipitofrontal fasciculus
IOFF = inferior occipitofrontal fasciculus
AF = arcuate fasciculus
C = cingulum
UnF = uncinate fasciculus

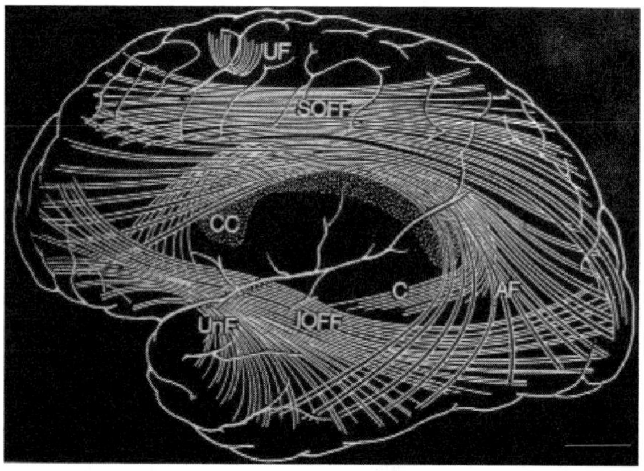

movement disorders are uncommon, and procedural memory is spared.[12] A comprehensive account of all white matter dementias is beyond our scope, but a brief survey of selected entities can highlight the clinical diversity of this group.

Multiple Sclerosis (MS)

Although not traditionally recognized as a dementing disease, MS has come to be known as causing cognitive impairment in more than half of affected patients, and up to 20% may develop dementia. MS and other demyelinative diseases involve the inflammatory destruction of myelin—and sometimes axonal degeneration in addition—that leads to neurobehavioral as well as neurologic disability.[12] Considerable research is establishing that the burden of white matter disease and cerebral atrophy shown by modern neuroimaging correlates with the degree of dementia, and that neurobehavioral syndromes constitute a major component of the disability experienced by MS patients.[12] Treatment with immunomodulatory agents and drugs for cognitive loss are showing promise in addressing this aspect of the disease.[12]

AIDS Dementia Complex (ADC)

A number of infectious diseases that produce cognitive decline may affect the white matter, including the acquired immune deficiency syndrome (AIDS) dementia complex.[12] Although the pathogenesis of ADC is not fully clarified, and subcortical gray matter regions are affected to some extent, neuropathological and neuroimaging studies of ADC clearly disclose early and prominent changes in the cerebral white matter,[1] and medical treatment of affected individuals may result in resolution of white matter changes in parallel with cognitive improvement.[12]

Toluene Leukoencephalopathy (TL)

The introduction of magnetic resonance imaging (MRI) in the 1980s led to a number of observations regarding the neurotoxic disorders. Among the large and growing number of white matter toxins recently identified,[12] the common industrial and household solvent toluene stands out. Toluene (methylbenzene) in spray paint may be inhaled as an abusable substance, and prolonged, intense exposure in this fashion has been associated with a prominent leukoencephalopathy that correlates with the severity of dementia produced.[12] Remarkably, toluene appears to exert its toxic effect exclusively on central myelin, sparing axons and cell bodies.[12] TL is an excellent example of a pure white matter disorder leading to a profound disorder of cognition.

Cobalamin Deficiency

One of the most commonly performed tests in the routine dementia work-up is the vitamin B_{12} (cobalamin) level. Although classically associated with pernicious anemia, cobalamin levels may be low in the presence of normal hematologic studies. Clinically significant cobalamin deficiency is rarely detected, but well documented cases demonstrate that metabolic demyelination in the cerebral white matter can produce dementia that can be reversible with vitamin B_{12} replacement.[12] MRI may also show impressive improvement in patients receiving such treatment.[12]

Figure 6

MRI scan of a patient with Binswanger disease

MRI demonstrates extensive periventricular ischemic white matter disease.

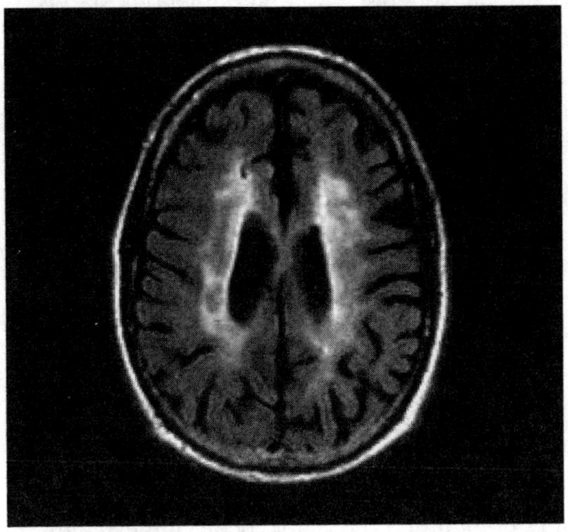

Binswanger Disease (BD)

First described in the 1890s, BD is a controversial vascular disorder that has been proposed to be one of the most common dementias of aging, or alternatively, a clinical entity of dubious legitimacy because of its vague nosological status. With the advent of MRI showing a high prevalence of white matter hyperintensities in old people that likely represent ischemia, interest in BD was rekindled, and the disease has gradually gained acceptance among many as one of the vascular dementias (see below). BD is a progressive dementing disease of older people that features widespread white matter ischemia that appears as T2 hyperintensity on MRI (Figure 6). More work will be necessary to clarify what is meant by the term BD, but there is little doubt that ischemic white matter disease, however classified, presents an important clinical problem with many neurobehavioral and therapeutic implications.[12]

Cerebral Autosomal Dominant Arteriopathy with Subcortical Infarcts and Leukoencephalopathy (CADASIL)

This is a genetic disease clinically similar to BD except that cerebrovascular risk factors are typically insignificant and the age of onset is generally younger. Patients with CADASIL have migraine, depression, stroke, and early-adult onset dementia, but the MRI findings of white matter disease may be indistinguishable from those of BD. Dementia is the major clinical problem, and diagnosis can be made by recognition of the clinical picture and genetic testing.[12]

Traumatic Brain Injury

In the classification system used in this chapter, TBI qualifies as a white matter disorder because of the common lesion in TBI patients known as diffuse axonal injury.[12] Cortical contusions and intracranial hemorrhages also occur in TBI and impact neurobehavioral outcome, but the most important neuropathological finding that produces long-term disability and dementia in TBI patients is the axonal shearing in the cerebral white matter that has permanent effects on attentional, executive, and memory systems.[12] TBI represents a major public health risk, as when all degrees of severity are considered—including the common concussion—the annual incidence of TBI exceeds that of AD, PD, and MS combined.[4]

Normal Pressure Hydrocephalus (NPH)

This poorly understood disorder has been recognized since the 1960s as a potentially reversible cause of dementia.[12] Presenting with the triad of dementia, urinary incontinence, and gait disorder, NPH can be further suspected by the finding of enlarged ventricles on computed tomography (CT) or MRI, and the observation of transient clinical improvement after removal of large volumes (30-50 cc) of cerebrospinal fluid (CSF) at lumbar puncture. NPH produces its major damage on the periventricular white matter, and reversibility likely relates to the normalization of ventricular volume affected by neurosurgical insertion of a shunt.[12]

Mixed Dementias

As with most classification systems in medicine, there are some entities that do not fit cleanly into any of the above categories. Many diseases do not show a predilection for one category of neuroanatomy, and rather involve a variety of sites.

Vascular Dementia (VaD)

The concept of VaD has a long and confusing history, but this group of diseases collectively represents the second most common dementia in the elderly, with up to 30% of patients falling into this category.[1,13,14] In the mid-20th century, vascular disease was assumed to account for most cases of dementia in old people, as implied by the designation "arteriosclerotic dementia" and the common but unscientific term "hardening of the arteries". As knowledge of the dementias evolved, a distinction between AD and VaD emerged, and for many years the major form of VaD was endorsed as the entity multi-infarct dementia (MID). However, with advances in modern neuroimaging, neuropathology, and genetics, the picture has become more complicated, and at present VaD is seen as a heterogeneous group of disorders that includes MID and several other entities.

MID has traditionally been used to describe patients who become gradually demented as a result of multiple recurrent strokes that erode cognitive function in a step-wise fashion.[1] These strokes are usually large vessel occlusions involving infarcts of the cortex and subcortical regions.[13] Uncertainties abound in this area, among them how many strokes are necessary for MID, what size they must be, and how much their location matters. Nevertheless, MID can be diagnosed in many patients, and stands as one variant of VaD.

Another important type of VaD is strategic infarct dementia, which implies that a single infarct may produce dementia by itself if localized in a brain region that is particularly eloquent for neurobehavioral function.[13] Such lesions include those in the left angular gyrus (producing fluent aphasia, apraxia, alexia, and Gerstmann syndrome), the distribution of the anterior cerebral arteries (causing various features of frontal lobe dysfunction), the right parietal lobe (leading to acute confusional state, psychosis, and inattention), and the basal forebrain (resulting in severe amnesia and behavioral disturbances).[13]

Perhaps most important in the development of recent thinking about VaD has been the concept of subcortical ischemic vascular dementia (SIVD),[14] often known as small vessel disease with dementia.[13] The widespread use of MRI disclosed that ischemic changes are very common in older people, being observed in about 70% of those 70 and older, and SIVD may therefore be the most common of the VaD subtypes. Currently, SIVD has come to include both the category of BD, considered above, in which white matter ischemic disease produces a progressive dementia, and the lacunar state, characterized by widespread subcortical lacunar infarcts in both the deep gray and white matter.[14] Both forms of SIVD produce a frontal-subcortical dementia, with BD proposed as having specific features of white matter dementia.[12] It has also been suggested that many more people are affected by a milder syndrome of vascular cognitive impairment,[14] analogous to MCI preceding AD.

The notion of SIVD has stimulated interest in the possibility that much of the dementia occurring in modern society may be preventable. If primary prevention of cerebrovascular disease by attention to factors such as hypertension, diabetes mellitus, cigarette smoking, obesity, and hypercholesterolemia can be achieved, the reduction in incidence of VaD, particularly SIVD, might be enormous.[14] Questions remain, however, about how successful such efforts may be; it is clear, for example, that many cases of VaD occur with coexistent neuropathological features of AD, and in addition, SIVD may be caused by the nonatherosclerotic disease cerebral amyloid angiopathy.[14]

Dementia With Lewy Bodies

This disease overlaps to a considerable extent with PD because both conditions are idiopathic degenerative diseases involving the accumulation of Lewy bodies containing α-synuclein. As opposed to PD, however, dementia with Lewy bodies (DLB) is primarily a dementing disease because of the diffuse distribution of Lewy bodies in a range of cortical and subcortical areas.[15] DLB is now thought to be the second most common neurodegenerative dementia in older people, accounting for 10%-15% of cases and ranking behind only AD.[15] The disease is characterized by recurrent confusional states in the setting of progressive cognitive decline, parkinsonism, and visual hallucinations.[15] Unlike PD, dementia occurs early, and an arbitrary rule of one year has been used to distinguish DLB; that is, dementia occurring within less than 12 months of the onset of parkinsonism argues for DLB and not PD with dementia.[15] However, clinical diagnostic criteria for DLB are not well standardized, and premortem diagnosis can be difficult, in part because of the frequent co-occurrence of AD changes in many patients.[15] A diagnostic clue is often evident from initial efforts at treatment, as patients with DLB typically have less response to levodopa and the dopamine agonists than those with PD.[15]Another important clinical feature of DLB is neuroleptic sensitivity, or the development of marked parkinsonism with the use of neuroleptic drugs for psychotic manifestations. This problem may be seen in as many as 50% of DLB patients,[15] but the use of atypical antipsychotic drugs in low dosage may be less likely to cause this complication.[15]

Corticobasal Degeneration

This disease is a degenerative disorder of the cerebral cortex and basal ganglia that produces core features of progressive asymmetric apraxia and rigidity.[16] A distinct feature of the disease is the asymmetry of clinical signs, which may involve either side and include a combination of cortical and extrapyramidal findings contralateral to the hemisphere primarily involved. Thus patients may have aphasia if there is right side apraxia and parkinsonism, or left hemineglect if these findings occur on the left side. Other features may include the alien hand sign, dystonia, myoclonus, and tremor. The dementia that occurs is often mild, and tends to involve frontal systems dysfunction in addition to the lateralized cognitive deficits predicted by the assymetry of motor signs. Similarities to both FTD and PSP have been noted, but it is uncertain whether these three disorders can be considered related.[16] The disease is typically unresponsive to levodopa therapy, and treatment is confined to symptomatic therapy as indicated.

Neurosyphilis and Other Conventional Infections

Infection of the brain with the spirochete *Treponema pallidum* still occurs, largely related to the AIDS epidemic, and most patients in the United States with neurosyphilis are infected with human immunodeficiency virus (HIV).[1] The two forms of neurosyphilis with the most potential to cause dementia are general paresis, in which involvement of the frontal and temporal lobes causes a variety of neuropsychiatric manifestations, and meningovascular syphilis, in which inflammatory arteritis affects the meninges, the cerebral cortex, and various subcortical structures to produce dementia.[1] Penicillin remains the mainstay of treatment and can be highly effective if used early. Another spirochete, *Borrelia burgdorferi*, produces Lyme disease, which occasionally involves the brain and can produce cognitive deficits or even dementia. Serologic tests for Lyme disease can be conducted on blood and cerebrospinal fluid, and treatment with ceftriaxone or penicillin is indicated. Other infections of the brain can produce dementia, but these diseases usually reveal themselves because of their unique clinical features: tuberculous meningitis, fungal infections including cryptococcal meningitis, parasitic disease such as neurosyticercosis, Whipple disease, and herpes simplex encephalitis and related viral infections.

Creutzfeldt-Jakob Disease

In some respects, this is the most feared of all the dementias because of its alarmingly fast course to death and its potential transmissibility. CJD is a rapidly progressive dementia that classically presents with myoclonus and periodic high amplitude sharp wave bursts on electroencephalography (EEG), and invariably results in death within a median duration of four months.[17] CJD is the best known of the human prion diseases, the others being variant CJD, Gerstmann-Straussler-Scheinker (GSS) disease, and fatal familial insomnia (FFI); all are caused by novel proteinaceous particles without nucleic acid called prions. Occurring at an annual incidence of about one per million, most CJD cases are sporadic, but a minority are caused by a mutation in the prion protein gene on chromosome[21], and a very small number have been iatrogenically caused by corneal transplantation, depth electrode insertion, pituitary gland grafts, dura mater grafts, and possibly the use of contaminated neurosurgical instruments.[17] The diagnosis can be established by brain biopsy, but this procedure is rarely undertaken because of neurosurgical risk and the absence of intervention to alter the clinical course. The characteristically rapid clinical course strongly suggests the diagnosis, and supportive features including myoclonus, a periodic EEG, MRI abnormalities in the putamen, caudate, or cerebral cortex, and the 14-3-3 protein in the CSF can be helpful.

Variant CJD is a less common type of CJD that appeared in England in the 1990s and was caused by the ingestion of beef containing the prion responsible for bovine spongiform encephalopathy ("mad cow disease").[17] These cases are usually younger than CJD patients (the mean age at death is 29 versus 66), experience more psychiatric impairment, and have a somewhat longer course of around 14 months until death.[17] GSS and FFI are rare autosomal dominant prion diseases producing prominent ataxia and sleep disturbance, respectively.[17]

Brain Tumors

Neoplasms of the brain are well-known causes of dementia, and may be primary or metastatic, benign or malignant. Following headache, neurobehavioral alterations are the most frequent presentations of brain tumors,[1] and the dementia produced may be subtle at first and variably progressive. These tumors typically exert pressure on or destroy the normal brain tissue, producing local effects at first and then diffuse damage that may proceed to herniation and death. Primary glial cell tumors originate in the white matter and spread along white matter tracts,[12] a feature that limits the prospect of effective treatment. Meningiomas, in contrast, are tumors lying outside the brain that can often be surgically extirpated with excellent results. Early identification of all tumors with neuroimaging is essential for diagnosis and prompt treatment.

Subdural Hematoma

This is an extra-axial mass lesion that exerts its effects by compression of one or both sides of the brain and may be associated with diffuse neuropathological and neurobehavioral sequelae.[1] Trauma is often found to be responsible, but in many older people this lesion may develop with only trivial head injury, or even spontaneously. When the blood clot is unilateral, lateralized cognitive deficits can be seen as highlights of the dementia, such that aphasia occurs with left and neglect with right hemisphere lesions. Removal of the hematoma by surgical drainage can lead to full recovery, and many patients can be treated conservatively with the same outcome.

Toxic and Metabolic Disorders

Most toxic and metabolic disorders affect the brain in a nonspecific fashion so that their neurobehavioral effects cannot be clearly categorized, although in some cases, such as TL and cobalamin deficiency, the white matter can be implicated (see above). For the most part, the toxic and metabolic disorders exert diffuse effects, and the clinical picture resembles a chronic confusional state from which recovery after treatment can be quite variable. Regardless of the uncertainty about pathogenesis and localization, chronic toxic and metabolic disorders are often readily treated by eliminating a culpable medication, for example, or by addressing a metabolic disturbance. Hypothyroidism is a common problem in many older patients, and others may merit evaluation for Hashimoto's encephalopathy, an autoimmune disorder characterized by the presence of antithyroglobulin and antithyroperoxidase antibodies and considered responsive to corticosteroid therapy.[1]

3. Differential Diagnosis

The diagnosis of dementia is a matter of grave concern for patients and their families, and much care need be taken to ensure this term is justified in any case where dementia is suspected. As the prognosis for most dementia syndromes remains poor, it is imperative for the clinician to be certain that dementia—and not some related condition—is present. This section will present a comprehensive approach to differential diagnosis of the syndrome so that nondementing conditions can be confidently excluded, and conversely, the dementia syndromes that merit clinical attention can be identified.

Dementia versus Normal Aging

One of the most common clinical questions in older people is whether cognitive symptoms represent the effects of normal aging or the first manifestations of dementia. Many older individuals experience changes in cognition that are recognized as normal, including mild slowing of information processing, decreased concentration ability, and occasional inability to recall names because of inefficient retrieval.[1] These changes are inconsequential if they involve no loss of functional ability, and reassurance can be most beneficial in allaying concerns that AD is imminent. Dementia from AD or any other cause is not an inevitable consequence of aging, and in fact normal older people can be encouraged that some aspects of cognition, such as verbal ("crystallized") intelligence, vocabulary, and accumulated knowledge ("wisdom") remain stable and may even improve with aging.[1] For those cases in which uncertainty persists, neuropsychological testing can be helpful in distinguishing dementia from normal aging.

Dementia versus Mild Cognitive Impairment

The transition to dementia has attracted much interest in recent years because of the possibility that detection of the earliest cognitive changes in AD may afford an opportunity for more effective intervention. In an effort to clarify this transition from normal aging and dementia, the category of mild cognitive impairment (MCI) has been invoked.[18] MCI is defined as the presence of memory complaints, memory impairment confirmed by objective testing, and the absence of other cognitive decline, problems with daily living activities, and dementia (Table 6).[18] Although the precise neuropathology of MCI is not well understood and may involve a variety of conditions, its importance lies in the observation that people over 65 with MCI develop dementia or AD at a rate of 10%-15% per year compared to 1%-2% for those without MCI.[18] Monitoring those with MCI for the transition to dementia, which often represents AD, is an important clinical objective, although no medical intervention to date has been shown to delay the transition to AD in those who are destined to acquire the disease.

Table 6

Mild Cognitive Impairment
Memory complaints, preferably corroborated by an informant
Objective evidence of memory impairment
Largely normal general cognitive function
Essentially intact activities of daily living
No dementia

Dementia versus Amnesia

This distinction is important because not all disorders of memory represent a dementing disease. Memory complaints are almost universal in clinics devoted to the assessment of cognitive function, but careful history and examination will disclose that some patients do not have dementia, but rather an isolated amnesia that reflects prior TBI, herpes simplex encephalitis, Korsakoff amnesia, or another source of damage to the medial temporal lobes. The key to this distinction lies in finding that all other realms of cognition and behavior are preserved. Recognition of amnesia is crucial because the treatment of the disorders causing this syndrome differs considerably from that of the dementias.

Dementia versus Acute Confusional State

Individuals in a wide range of medical practices are routinely seen with acute confusional state (ACS), a rapidly evolving disorder of attention that results in an inability to maintain a coherent line of thought.[1] The attentional disorder may produce hyperaroused states such as restlessness and agitation or, more commonly, hypoaroused states such as lethargy and somnolence, and fluctuations between these two extremes are frequent. These changes are not encountered in dementia, which is a chronic state of altered mentation in which attention is not primarily affected. Alternate terms for the ACS include delirium, which implies the hyperactive state of autonomic instability and visual hallucinations associated with delirium tremens; and toxic-metabolic encephalopathy, which points to the most typically identified causative factors in this syndrome—drugs (licit or otherwise) and metabolic derangements. Whatever the terminology, it is important to remember that ACS is often partially or completely reversible with prompt identification and treatment of the etiological factor(s) involved.

Dementia versus Aphasia

Although there is little difficulty in identifying patients with nonfluent aphasias such as Broca's or global aphasia, the distinction of dementia from fluent aphasia can be difficult. In fact, fluent aphasias such as transcortical sensory and Wernicke aphasia are routinely seen in the early and middle stages of AD.[1] In most cases, aphasia as an isolated syndrome can be distinguished from dementia by its onset, which is typically abrupt with the development of a stroke or other acute neurologic event, and associated with other neurologic symptoms and signs that identify the disorder as distinct from the dementias. Care should be taken, however, in the diagnosis of PPA/PNFA and SD, in both of which early aphasia is followed by dementia as progressive neurodegeneration occurs (see above).

Dementia versus Depression

A frequent request for consultation in the neurology clinic is the distinction of dementia from depression. Although in some patients this is a straightforward task, the approach taken in this chapter recognizes that in some cases no distinction between these two conditions is either possible or necessary; that is, depression may in fact cause dementia by the definition given herein.[1] In these cases, a multitude of cognitive deficits may produce a dementia syndrome, typically of a frontal-subcortical type, that may be fully reversible with appropriate treatment. Clues to the presence of depression include psychomotor slowing, tearfulness or other affective displays of sadness, frequent "I don't know" answers, and overall poor effort. In some cases, neuropsychological testing can be used to help clarify the diagnostic picture, and at times a trial of an antidepressant drug may be indicated while other possible causes of dementia are being investigated.

4. Diagnostic Testing

The diagnosis of dementia is founded on the history and physical examination. The history establishes the onset, tempo, course, and associated features of the illness, and the physical examination determines the impact of the disorder on bodily function. The sine qua non of this physical examination is the mental status examination (MSE), which requires special skill and often considerable patience and perseverance. In addition, accurate diagnosis typically requires the use of laboratory and neuroimaging tests that are chosen carefully and interpreted in light of the clinical picture. In this section, the diagnosis of dementia will be discussed with an overview of the history and physical examination, and then a consideration of the diagnostic tests most useful in this process.

History and Physical Examination

Central to any medical evaluation is a focused yet comprehensive history and physical examination. In the evaluation of dementia and the many syndromes for which it may be mistaken, the history is vital for establishing that dementia is in fact present, and there is no substitute for pursuing the distinction between dementia and related syndromes discussed above. Similarly, when dementia is detected, it is usually possible with detailed history-taking to acquire some idea of which dementia may be present. In many cases, the patient will be unable to disclose historical information with sufficient accuracy to allow an appropriate clinical evaluation, and informants such as a spouse, family member, companion, friend, or assistant may be required for additional data. For others, review of the previous medical records will prove most helpful. With experience exploiting these avenues of inquiry, the various dementias become more familiar, and a characteristic clinical profile often reveals itself to the physician without significant doubt.

The physical examination is important for identifying findings that suggest the specific cause of the dementia syndrome. General medical examination may detect signs of cardiac, pulmonary, hepatic, renal, or endocrinologic disease that may affect the brain, and evidence of trauma may be apparent. The neurologic examination plays a vital role in diagnosis, and despite the major advances made recently in neuroimaging, lesion localization remains a crucial process in identifying all types of neurologic disease. The elemental neurologic exam—that which is not concerned with higher function—can detect many signs of central nervous system dysfunction including head trauma, meningismus, cranial nerve signs, paresis, spasticity, rigidity, involuntary movements, ataxia, and gait disturbances that point toward specific neurologic disorders.

The MSE is the core procedure both for establishing that dementia is present and for distinguishing between the different disorders that may be responsible (Table 7). Following from the history after patient rapport is gained, the MSE should survey several domains of cognition and behavior, including attention, memory, language, visuospatial function, executive function, and emotion and personality.[1] Tests of praxis and perception can be useful in many cases, but care must be taken as these tests are not well standardized. The MSE is a time-consuming and detailed examination for which no brief substitute is completely satisfactory. Short screening

Table 7

Mental Status Examination

Domain	Tests
Attention	Digit span, serial sevens
Memory	Orientation, 3 word recall after five minutes, remote (semantic) memory
Language	Fluency, comprehension, repetition, naming, reading, writing
Visuospatial skills	Clock drawing, design copy
Executive function	Alternating programs, go - no go task, Luria 3-step manuever
Emotion and personality	Inquiries and observations of the patient, with informant assistance

Table 8

Routine Diagnostic Tests for Dementia

Metabolic survey
Complete blood count
Erythrocyte sedimentation rate
Thyroid function tests
Vitamin B_{12}
Syphilis serology
Brain CT scan or MRI

examinations such as the Mini-Mental State Examination (MMSE) are useful in many cases, but cannot be expected to capture the full range and depth of the neurobehavioral disorder.[1,12] Once the nature of the dementia is established, however, measures such as the MMSE can be usefully employed as markers of disease progression and response to treatment.

Laboratory Tests

For many years, a standard "dementia work-up" has been taught as an almost reflexive way to detect the reversible causes of dementia. Whereas such an approach carries the risk of not thinking in detail about the peculiar issues of an individual patient, the value of routinely checking for problems that can potentially be addressed by medical or surgical treatment must be acknowledged. This caveat is especially important in busy clinics where an efficient and timely group of tests can be obtained without delay to avoid overlooking a reversible disorder. Recent practice guidelines have clarified the tests that should be included.[19] A typical panel (Table 8) includes a survey of metabolic function (electrolytes, glucose, blood urea nitrogen, creatinine, calcium, liver function tests), hematologic status (complete blood count), erythrocyte sedimentation rate, thyroid function tests, vitamin B_{12} level, and syphilis serology (rapid protein reagin or Venereal Disease Research Laboratory test).

Neuroimaging

Another commonly employed component of the dementia work-up has been a scan of the brain (Table 8). CT and MRI have dramatically altered the evaluation of dementia because of their ability to detect structural lesions that might be amenable to medical or surgical treatment. CT is less expensive and preferred for detecting hemorrhagic disease, but reveals less neuroanatomic detail and entails some radiation exposure. MRI is more costly and cannot be used for those with cardiac pacemakers or intracorporeal metal, but demonstrates brain structures in excellent detail and involves no radiation risk. The major findings revealed by CT or MRI are brain tumors, subdural hematomas, hydrocephalus, and strokes, and the importance of detecting a reversible lesion when significant recovery is still possible cannot be denied.[19] Even for those patients who meet criteria for AD, in whom it is uncommon to detect a structural lesion, unexpected neuroimaging findings can often help guide management.[19] For these reasons, a CT scan or MRI is recommended at least once in every case of dementia.[19]

Clinical experience also teaches that interpretation of the scan from a neurologic perspective can be additionally helpful; the presence of bilateral frontal and temporal atrophy, for example, can help confirm a clinical diagnosis of FTD in a patient with profile of neurobehavioral deficits suggesting frontal and temporal lobe degeneration.

Additional Tests

Other tests may prove useful in selected cases of dementia (Table 9). The clinical picture dictates the need for these tests, although some restraint is in order because the yield of extensive evaluations is often low and the cost can be high. In the appropriate setting, the routine procedures of chest roentgenogram, electrocardiography, and urinalysis may be useful, and tests for HIV, ceruloplasmin, heavy metals, and porphyrin screening can occasionally assist in diagnosis. EEG may help in ruling in CJD if periodic complexes are observed. Lumbar puncture is now considered a low-yield test in dementia, and reserved for individuals with a clinical course suggesting infection with neurosyphilis, Lyme disease, tuberculosis, fungal infection, parasitic disease, Whipple disease, viral diseases, and prions.[19] Cerebral arteriography may be indicated for suspected vasculitis contributing to VaD. Functional neuroimaging with positron emission tomography (PET) and single photon emission computed tomography (SPECT) can be considered, but is not widely employed at present. These procedures can sometimes be used to define patterns of cortical hypometabolism that distinguish between AD and FTD. Brain biopsy is rarely performed, but can be justified if the diagnosis cannot be made by other means and there is a possibility of providing definitive treatment; central nervous system vasculitis and unusual brain neoplasms are examples of this principle.

Table 9

Additional Diagnostic Tests for Dementia

Chest roentgenogram
Electrocardiogram
Urinanalysis
Human immunodeficiency virus test
Ceruloplasmin
Heavy metal screen
Porphyrin screen
Electroencephalography
Lumbar puncture
Cerebral angiography
Positron emission tomography
Single photon emission computed tomography
Brain biopsy
Neuropsychological testing
Genetic testing for AD
Genetic testing for HD

Neuropsychological Evaluation

While not considered a required procedure, neuropsychological testing can be helpful in many ways during the process of making a diagnosis in people suspected of having dementia.[19] First, this kind of detailed testing may prove that dementia is not actually present, which can provide enormous relief for individuals who are concerned that normal memory and cognitive changes are the harbingers of AD. Similarly, neuropsychological testing can often discern whether a person's cognitive problem is related to depression or another emotional disorder which, if true, will significantly alter the treatment approach. Other cases can benefit from the delineation of specific features of the dementia, so that, for example, AD can be distinguished from FTD, PPA, SD, PD, HD, PSP, DLB, or CBD based on the specific profile of cognitive strengths and weaknesses. Finally, neuropsychological testing can be helpful in cases where there are important questions about a person's competency to make personal, medical, or financial decisions.

Genetic Testing

Although the possibility that clinical diagnosis may be enhanced by genetic testing remains intriguing, there are few dementing diseases in which genetic testing is regularly helpful. In AD, testing for PS1 mutations is commercially available, and testing for PS2 and APP mutations can be obtained in specialized centers for families seeking detailed information. The use of (apo) E4 testing is not recommended for patients or unaffected family members because of the presence of both falsely positive and falsely negative results.[1] Other tests of the blood and CSF for markers of AD have also not proven clinically useful.[1] In HD, testing for the CAG triplet repeat expansion can be valuable for families planning for childbearing. In all cases, genetic testing should be accompanied by appropriate counseling and psychological support.

The treatment of dementia has often been regarded with a certain nihilism, and assumptions may persist that the syndrome is invariably progressive and untreatable. One reason for adopting the definition of dementia in this chapter is that it bears no implications about either progressiveness or treatability. In this light, dementia can be seen as a syndrome of intellectual impairment with a variable course that may respond favorably to treatment, similar to other chronic disorders in medicine. Patients with dementia need proper management with the understanding that a cure is unlikely. Thus, whereas dementia may be irreversible, it is not untreatable.

Reversible Dementias

In the fortunate circumstance that a dementia is found to have a reversible cause, prompt attention to that etiology is warranted. The treatment of these diseases can be found in standard textbooks of neurology and medicine. In general, the earlier the etiologic problem is detected, the better the chance for full or good recovery. In many cases, particularly involving older individuals, decisions about the nature of treatment may need to include consideration of other medical problems such as coronary artery disease and diabetes mellitus, and extra caution is prudent to assure that medical or surgical treatment does not prove prohibitively hazardous.

Irreversible Dementias

In these cases, still far more numerous than the reversible dementias, the physician must rely upon the art of managing a disease that will persist for the foreseeable future and quite possibly prove to be the cause of the patient's demise. Although such a task may pose formidable obstacles, sympathetic, informed counseling and avoidance of medical problems that exacerbate symptoms of dementia can themselves be highly gratifying for the patient, their families, and the physician. The assistance of other professionals, including social workers, psychologists, nurses, and attorneys may prove invaluable in dealing with the many disruptions in life brought about by a dementing illness. Referral to an external agency such as the Alzheimer Association is another option that can offer much guidance and support.

The frequent behavioral problems that result from neuropsychiatric complications of dementia can be especially troubling, often more so than the memory or cognitive losses. Agitation, belligerence, delusions of infidelity or theft, wandering, and sleep disorders are some of the most disruptive behaviors that can be encountered. These problems can often be addressed by the judicious use of drugs such as the atypical antipsychotic agents (quetiapine, risperidone, or olanzapine), anticonvulsants (valproate or carbamazepine), sedatives (benzodiazepines), anxiolytics (buspirone), and sleep agents (trazodone or zolpidem).[1] "Starting low and going slowly" is an important principle for dosing, and the drug should be stopped when the target symptom or sign has subsided.

In terms of specific therapy for the irreversible dementias, the last 15 years have seen the emergence of several drugs for AD that have provided the first opportunity for pharmacologic treatment that can directly address symptoms of the neurodegenerative process (Table 10). These drugs may also find use in the treatment of other dementias, although less information about these disorders is available.

Alzheimer Disease

Based on the cholinergic hypothesis, a major effort in drug development was undertaken in the 1980s and 1990s that led to the introduction of a class of agents known as the cholinesterase inhibitors (CIs).[3] These drugs act to block the degradation of acetylcholine and therefore potentiate the activity of the cholinergic system that is so seriously damaged early in the disease. Four CIs are currently available: tacrine, donepezil, rivastigmine, and galantamine.[3] The efficacy of these drugs is roughly equivalent, and benefits in slowing cognitive decline as well as in ameliorating certain neuropsychiatric features may be seen.[3] The major distinction between these drugs lies in their toxicity and adminstration. Tacrine, for example, is rarely used because of hepatotoxicity and frequent gastrointestinal distress. The other drugs have no hepatotoxicity, but nausea, vomiting, and diarrhea may still occur. A transdermal form of rivastigmine has recently been released and may reduce gastrointestinal side effects for some patients. Enthusiasm for

Table 10

Drug Treatment of Alzheimer Disease

Medication	Dosage	Side Effects
Cholinesterase Inhibitors		
Tacrine	10 mg PO QID, advancing every four weeks to 20 mg QID, 30 mg QID, and 40 mg QID as tolerated	Nausea, vomiting, diarrhea, hepatotoxicity (liver function tests required every two weeks during titration and every three months thereafter), bradycardia
Donepezil	5 mg PO QD, advancing after four weeks to 10 mg QD as tolerated	Nausea, vomiting, diarrhea, bradycardia
Rivastigmine	1.5 mg PO BID, advancing every four weeks to 3.0 mg BID, 4.5 BID and 6.0 mg BID as tolerated	Nausea, vomiting, diarrhea bradycardia
Galantamine	4 mg PO BID, advancing every four weeks to 8 mg BID and 12 mg BID as tolerated	Nausea, vomiting, diarrhea bradycardia
NMDA-Receptor Antagonist		
Memantine	5 mg PO QAM for first week, 5 mg BID for second week, 5 mg QAM and 10 mg QPM for third week, then 10 mg BID	Confusion, constipation, headache, dizziness

these drugs should be tempered, however, by published data showing only modest effects over 6-12 months, and no possibility of reversibility.[1]

More recently, another agent was added to the armamentarium for treating AD: memantine, an N-methyl-d-aspartate receptor antagonist that may retard neuronal cell death related to glutamate excitotoxicity.[3] Approved for patients with moderate to severe AD, memantine can be used in conjunction with a CI and provide additional benefit. Although data on the use of memantine in mild AD are not yet available, the drug is likely to be at least as efficacious early in the disease as in its later stages.

Frontotemporal Lobar Dementia

In contrast to AD, current opinion holds that there is no role for the CIs in the treatment of FTLD.[3] Instead, the selective serotonin reuptake inhibitor (SSRI) class of antidepressants is recommended by most authorities on the basis of the relatively severe involvement of the serotonergic system and the relative sparing of cholinergic function in FTLD.[3] SSRI drugs may help with many aspects of frontal lobe disturbance including disinhibition and impaired executive function, but controlled trials are needed to establish the role of SSRI and other drugs with more certainty.

Vascular Dementia

The primary approach to VaD is preventive, as there is currently no means of restoring neurons destroyed by inadequate blood flow. This task falls largely to the primary care medical community, and control of hypertension and other common cerebrovascular risk factors is crucial. Secondary prevention of stroke is mainly the task of neurologists, and involves such interventions as antiplatelet drugs, anticoagulants, and referral for carotid artery or other surgical procedures. Emerging data are available, however, to support the use of CIs such as donepezil in treating the cognitive sequelae of stroke and VaD,[1] and these drugs may play a greater role in the years ahead.

Parkinson Disease and Dementia With Lewy Bodies

The treatment of diseases in the Lewy body spectrum has been evolving. PD is well known to respond to dopaminergic therapy for motor features, and the mild but measurable benefit of levodopa for certain cognitive features such as attention and executive function supports the notion that dopamine dysfunction alone can produce a cognitive disorder that may reach the level of frontal-subcortical dementia.[10] For both PD with dementia and DLB, however, it has recently been shown that cholinergic deficits exist, and that use of CIs may be helpful for cognitive and behavioral disturbances in some patients.[1] The treatment of DLB, however, is often challenging because of the limited efficacy of PD agents and the problem of neuroleptic sensitivity (see above).

Future Prospects

AD serves as paradigm for the neurodegenerative dementias, and most of the work on finding a cause, prevention, and cure for dementia focuses on this common disease. As discussed above, the cause of most dementias is poorly understood at best. This vexing reality explains why prevention of AD and similar diseases is not feasible, and why treatment is so limited. However, some progress has occurred, as reviewed above, and recent years have also witnessed the appearance of other potential treatments, including high-dose vitamin E, estrogen, prednisone, a variety of nonsteroidal anti-inflammatory drugs, statins, and nerve growth factor. Whereas these ideas are intriguing, none of these agents has gained widespread acceptance, and controlled studies often show no benefit at all.[1] Much effort is now focused on strategies for addressing the accumulation of example, Alzheimer disease (AD), typically cited as the most common dementia, afflicts some 4-5 million Americans and increases in prevalence with age so that about 30% of those over 85 are affected.[3] While these figures will grow higher because of increased longevity over the next several decades, it is important to remember that AD accounts for only 50%-70% of late-life dementias.[1]Another sobering statistic is that TBI, a disorder with peak incidence at age 15-24 and therefore an enormously high prevalence, produces yearly 70,000 to 90,000 new cases of severely injured persons who have long-term disability, including dementia,[4] and that are not ordinarily included in standard data collections of the dementias. Although AD alone is a serious threat to public health, the entire range of dementias—from all etiologies—merits vigorous medical, scientific, and societal attention.

6. Prognosis

The prognosis of dementia must realistically be seen as guarded in most cases. Medical science has only recently been accurately classifying the dementias, and this descriptive stage has not been readily followed by a thorough understanding of the etiology of disease that could lead to curative treatment. The few cases of reversible dementia seen in clinical practice are far outnumbered by those for whom the outlook is less hopeful.

Reversible Dementias

This category remains distressingly small in comparison to the irreversible dementias. Certainly there are dementias that reverse with medical or surgical treatment, but opinion has differed about how common these are, ranging from less than 1%-23% of all patients.[20] Much of the difficulty with this area rests on varying definitions of what dementia may be and what is meant by reversibility. A trend toward lower percentages in recent years is evident, in large measure due to the improved diagnosis of AD that increases the percentage of dementia patients in the irreversible category.[20] Nevertheless, if the most common causes of reversible dementia—depression and drug intoxication[20]—are included, it may be that partially or completely reversible dementia may occur in 10%-20% of patients in clinical practice. As many problems are found and corrected in primary care settings, neurologists and other specialists may have a biased impression that underestimates the number of reversible cases. In any event, the prompt and comprehensive evaluation of suspected dementia will optimize the likelihood that a reversible etiology will in fact be detected.

One of the areas in which a more optimistic prognosis can often be considered is the white matter dementias. As a general rule, disorders that do not involve lasting structural damage have a better prognosis than those in which neuronal loss occurs. Disorders of myelin display this principle particularly well; unless there is axonal loss, the possibility that myelin may be restored confers a better prognosis than in diseases such as AD or FTLD where gray matter disease results in neuronal dropout. The treatment of white matter disorders is of course quite diverse because of all the various neuropathological processes involved; treatment may involve interventions as varied as prescription of an immunomodulatory agent in MS, use of highly active antiretroviral therapy in ADC, removal of a toxic insult, treatment of primary risk factors in BD, and insertion of a lumboperitoneal shunt in NPH.[12] Intriguing options for the treatment of specific cognitive deficits in patients with these disorders are also appearing, such as CIs and stimulants for attentional and memory disturbances.

Irreversible Dementias

The prognosis for the irreversible dementias depends on the specific etiology. In few cases does the onset of dementia leave life expectancy unaltered. AD has a mean survival after symptom onset of about 10 years, but patients have been noted to live less than two or more than 20 years.[1] Conversely, the mean life expectancy after the onset of CJD is 4 months.[17] One of the many reasons for obtaining an accurate diagnosis is to be able to advise patients and their families about what might be expected in the future, as decisions about health care, financial settlements, and other personal matters are best made when a person's competency is relatively well preserved. Until treatments appear that significantly alter the disease course or render an irreversible disease reversible, an understanding of prognosis is one of the most helpful contributions the physician can make.

7. References

1. Mendez MF, Cummings JL. *Dementia: A Clinical Approach*. 3rd ed. Philadelphia, Pa: Butterworth-Heinemann; 2003.

   (A comprehensive, clinically-oriented textbook that has been an invaluable guide for physicians dealing with dementia for more than 20 years.)

2. American Psychiatric Association. *Diagnostic and Statistical Manual of Mental Disorders*. 4th ed. Washington, DC: American Psychiatric Association; 1994.

   (The major diagnostic manual for psychiatry, with important sections on neurobehavioral disorders including dementia.)

3. Cummings JL. Alzheimer disease. *N Engl J Med*. 2004;351:56-67.

   (An excellent current review of Alzheimer, with an emphasis on drug treatment.)

4. Kelly JP. Traumatic brain injury and concussion in sports. *JAMA*. 1999;282: 989-991.

   (A trenchant editorial about the "silent epidemic" of traumatic brain injury, in sports and elsewhere, which renders large numbers of young adults severely brain injured each year.)

5. McKhann G, Drachman D, Folstein M, Katzman R, Price D, Stadlan EM. Clinical diagnosis of Alzheimer disease: report of the NINCDS-ADRDA Work Group under the auspices of Department of Health and Human Services Task Force on Alzheimer Disease. *Neurology*. 1984;34:939-44.

   (The essential consensus statement that has served to standardize the diagnosis of Alzheimer disease.)

6. Bian H, Grossman M. Frontotemporal lobar degeneration: recent progress in antemortem diagnosis. *Acta Neuropathol*. 2007;114:23-29.

   (A recent summary of progress in the understanding of frontotemporal lobar degeneration.)

7. Mesulam M-M. Slowly progressive aphasia without generalized dementia. *Ann Neurol*. 1982;11:592-598.

   (The initial description of what has come to be known as primary progressive aphasia, or progressive nonfluent aphasia.)

8. Hodges JR, Patterson K, Oxbury S, Funnell E. Semantic dementia. Progressive fluent aphasia with temporal lobe atrophy. *Brain*. 1992;115:1783-806.

   (A seminal article describing clinical details of this variety of frontotemporal lobar degeneration, characterized by progressive fluent aphasia.)

9. Turner MA, Moran NF, Kopelman MD. Subcortical dementia. *Br J Psychiatry*. 2002;180:148-151.

   (The strengths and limitations of the concept of subcortical dementia, as described in a recent review.)

10. Levin BE, Tomer R, Ley GJ. Cognitive impairments in Parkinson Disease. *Neurol Clin*. 1992;10:471-485.

    (A thoughtful discussion of the diverse cognitive features of dementia in Parkinson disease, highlighting the concept that there may be subcortical and cortical subtypes of this syndrome.)

11. Zakzanis KK. The subcortical dementia of Huntington disease. *J Clin Exp Neuropsychol.* 1998;20:565-578.

(The prominence of fronto-subcortical dysfunction in producing the cognitive profile of HD patients, developed from a meta-analysis of neuropsychological studies.)

12. Filley CM. *The Behavioral Neurology of White Matter.* New York, NY: Oxford University Press; 2001.

(A description of cerebral white matter and its disorders from a neurobehavioral perspective, including the syndrome of white matter dementia.)

13. Román GC, Tatemichi TK, Erkinjuntti T, et al. Vascular dementia: Diagnostic criteria for research studies. Report of the NINDSAIREN International Workshop. *Neurology.* 1993:43:250-260.

(One of many consensus statements on vascular dementia, highlighting the complexities of this syndrome.)

14. O'Brien JT, Erkinjuntti T, Reisberg B, et al. Vascular cognitive impairment. *Lancet Neurology.* 2003;2:89-98.

(A recent commentary on vascular dementia, invoking the term vascular cognitive impairment.)

15. McKeith I, Mintzer J, Aarsland D, et al. Dementia with Lewy bodies. *Lancet Neurology.* 2004;3:19-28.

(The concept of dementia with Lewy bodies, and how it differs from Parkinson disease dementia.)

16. Boeve BF, Lang AE, Litvan I. Corticobasal degeneration and its relationship to progressive supranuclear palsy and frontotemporal dementia. *Ann Neurol.* 2003;54 (Suppl 5): S15-S19.

(A description of corticobasal degeneration highlighting the similarity of this disease to other neurodegenerative diseases.)

17. Knight RSG, Will RG. Prion diseases. *J Neurol Neurosurg Psychiatry.* 2004; 75(Suppl 1): i36-i42.

(The human prion diseases described, with an emphasis on Creutzfeldt-Jakob disease.)

18. Petersen RC, Doody R, Kurz A, et al. Current concepts in mild cognitive impairment. *Arch Neurol.* 2001;58:1985-1992.

(A consensus statement on the current status of mild cognitive impairment.)

19. Corey-Bloom J, Thal LJ, Galasko D, et al. Diagnosis and evaluation of dementia. *Neurology.* 1995;45:211-218.

(How a neurologist approaches the diagnosis and evaluation of patients with suspected dementia.)

20. Weytingh MD, Bossuyt PMM, van Crevel H. Reversible dementia: more that 10% or less than 1%? A quantitative review. *J Neurol.* 1995;242:466-471.

(A provocative study of the problem of ascertaining how many patients with dementia actually have a reversible disorder.)

8. Questions

1. Dementia is an increasingly important medical and social problem because:

   A. The population in industrialized countries is aging

   B. Traumatic brain injury is a "silent epidemic"

   C. The prevention of Alzheimer disease is not yet possible

   D. No cure is yet available for most dementias

   E. All of the above

2. A characteristic histopathologic feature of Alzheimer disease is:

   A. The Pick body

   B. The neuritic plaque

   C. The Lewy body

   D. Prion protein staining by immunocytochemistry

   E. Demyelination

3. A 62-year-old right-handed man has the insidious onset of word-finding difficulty over several months followed by dysarthria and labored, effortful speech. His elemental neurologic examination and comportment remain normal. What is the most probable cause of this clinical picture?

   A. The dementia syndrome of depression

   B. Alzheimer disease

   C. Primary progressive aphasia

   D. Neurosyphilis

   E. Stroke with Broca aphasia

4. In a 72-year-old woman with Alzheimer disease it is likely that:

   A. Liver function tests are abnormal

   B. Recent memory and language function are affected early

   C. A hemiparesis is present

   D. Seizures are frequent

   E. Autosomal dominant inheritance will be present

5. A 45-year-old man with Down syndrome has a decline in functional status and new incontinence. Histopathologic findings of which disease are likely developing?

   A. Alzheimer disease

   B. Pick disease

   C. Creutzfeldt-Jakob disease

   D. Wilson disease

   E. Progressive supranuclear palsy

6. Which of the following is not considered a frontal-subcortical dementia?

   A. Parkinson disease

   B. Progressive supranuclear palsy

   C. Wilson disease

D. Huntington disease

E. Semantic dementia

7. A previously healthy 62-year-old woman develops a progressive dementia syndrome over three months and then begins to have myoclonic jerks of all extremities. What is the most likely diagnosis ?

A. Alzheimer disease

B. Wilson disease

C. Creutzfeldt-Jakob disease

D. HIV infection

E. Hypothyroidism

8. A 55-year-old-woman is admitted to a psychiatric hospital after being noted to be progressively grandiose, hypersexual, and socially inappropriate for two years. She has no previous medical or psychiatric history. What is the most likely diagnosis?

A. Bipolar disorder

B. Alzheimer disease

C. Stroke with fluent aphasia

D. Frontotemporal dementia

E. Variant Creutzfeldt-Jakob disease

9. The most helpful CT finding in a case of suspected Huntington disease is:

A. Cortical atrophy

B. Ventricular enlargement

C. Cavum septum pellucidum

D. Caudate atrophy

E. Basal ganglia calcification

10. A college senior presents with new academic difficulties and episodic involuntary twisting of his arm. Which of the following are the most important to pursue first?

A. Family history, serum ceruloplasmin, brain MRI

B. Psychiatric consultation

C. EEG

D. Echocardiogram

E. Lumbar puncture

11. Progressive supranuclear palsy is characterized by:

A. Autosomal recessive inheritance with low penetrance

B. An asymmetric movement disorder

C. Normal cognition

D. Supranuclear gaze palsy, most marked for vertical movements

E. Seizures

12. Reversible causes of dementia include:

A. Neurosyphilis

B. Vitamin B_{12} deficiency

C. Hypothyroidism

D. Depression

E. All of the above

13. A 75-year-old man presents with fluctuating cognitive impairment, parkinsonism, and visual hallucinations for the past year. What is the most likely explanation for this presentation?

A. Multiple sclerosis

B. Dementia with Lewy bodies

C. Gerstmann-Straussler-Scheinker disease

D. Corticobasal degeneration

E. Frontotemporal dementia

14. Which of the following may produce white matter dementia?

A. Multiple sclerosis

B. Chronic, intense exposure to toluene

C. Binswanger disease

D. CADASIL

E. All of the above

15. A 78-year old woman has had the recent onset of gait disorder, dementia, and urinary incontinence. A large volume spinal tap results in more steady gait and mild improvement in cognitive function. What disease is suggested by this clinical picture?

A. The dementia syndrome of depression

B. Alzheimer disease

C. Normal pressure hydrocephalus

D. Neurosyphilis

E. Binswanger disease

16. An 82-year-old man is admitted to a medical ward with disorientation, restlessness, visual hallucinations, and seizures developing over the past five days. He has an extensive medical history including hypertension, diabetes mellitus, coronary artery disease, and alcoholism. What is the appropriate syndrome diagnosis?

A. Dementia

B. Aphasia

C. Acute confusional state

D. Depression

E. Mild cognitive impairment

17. A 74-year-old man is in excellent health and on no medications, but three weeks following a motor vehicle accident he is admitted for subacute confusion. Neurologic examination is normal except that he is disoriented and can only recall 1 of 3 words after 3 minutes. What is the most likely diagnosis?

A. Subdural hematoma

B. Alzheimer disease

C. Epidural hematoma

D. Alcohol intoxication

E. Normal pressure hydrocephalus

18. Which of the following tests is the least useful in the routine evaluation of dementia?

A. MRI scan

B. Thyroid stimulating hormone

C. Genetic testing for presenilin 1

D. Vitamin B_{12}

E. Rapid protein reagin

19. In a 68-year-old man with probable Alzheimer disease that began six years ago, what is the most efficacious treatment regimen for cognitive decline?

A. Reassurance and counseling

B. A cholinesterase inhibitor

C. An SSRI drug

D. A cholinesterase inhibitor and memantine

E. Memantine alone

20. Which disorder has the best prognosis for improvement in cognitive function with treatment?

A. Frontotemporal dementia

B. Huntington disease

C. Alzheimer disease

D. Vascular dementia

E. Depression

Answers

1. E.

Dementia represents a major challenge because is it increasingly common and mostly irreversible. Traumatic brain injury reminds us that dementia is not only a problem of older people.

2. B.

The neuritic plaque was first recognized by Alzheimer in 1907, and its amyloid core has captured most attention as a focus of research on finding the etiology of the disease.

3. C.

Primary progressive aphasia is one of the frontotemporal lobar degenerations and features progressive nonfluent aphasia (an alternate name) that leads in time to dementia.

4. B.

The early stage of Alzheimer disease is typically characterized by amnesia and often mild aphasia in the absence of systemic disease or elemental neurologic dysfunction.

5. A.

Individuals with Down syndrome regularly develop Alzheimer disease neuropathology when they reach midlife. Often this change can be detected by a decline in functional status.

6. E.

Semantic dementia is included under the rubric of frontotemporal lobar degeneration (FTLD), and thus qualifies as a cortical dementia. Whereas this classification is useful, it also true that subcortical pathology occurs to some extent in FTLD. The important point is that the major clinical manifestations of FTLD are thought to result from primary cortical degeneration.

7. C.

Creutzfeldt-Jakob disease is the classic rapidly progressive dementia, and myoclonus occurs in about 80% of patients at some point in the course.

8. D.

This case describes a two-year course of progressive frontal lobe disturbance. Given the relatively young age and absence of prior psychiatric history, a neurodegenerative disease is likely, and frontotemporal dementia best fits the clinical profile.

9. D.

Caudate atrophy is commonly seen on neuroimaging in patients with Huntington disease, reflecting prominent neuronal loss in these nuclei. Even before atrophy develops, caudate hypometabolism can be observed in HD patients using functional neuroimaging.

10. A.

At the young age of this patient, the onset of a neuropsychiatric syndrome and a movement disorder should always raise the possibility of Wilson disease.

11. D.

Progressive supranuclear palsy is an idiopathic degenerative dementia without focal motor signs or seizures. Supranuclear vertical gaze palsy is prominent, and downgaze is typically more affected.

12. E.

The routine dementia workup should include tests for neurosyphilis, vitamin B_{12} deficiency and hypothyroidism, and screening for depression may also disclose cases of reversible dementia that can be treated effectively.

13. B.

Dementia with Lewy bodies can be a difficult diagnosis to make because of clinical features suggesting acute confusional state, Parkinson disease, and psychiatric disorders. A helpful sign is neuroleptic sensitivity, whereby the use of neuroleptic agents for visual hallucinations results in marked worsening of parkinsonism.

14. E.

Whereas these disease entities (A-D) are indeed neuropathologically diverse, they can all produce a similar dementia syndrome, and the white matter damage in each can be easily seen with MRI.

15. C.

The "tap test" is used to assess whether removing a large volume of cerebrospinal fluid improves neurologic features of normal pressure hydrocephalus (NPH). The test is not always definitive, but if transient improvement does occur, and the clinical and neuroimaging findings are also typical of NPH, a shunt procedure can be considered. Typically, gait is more likely to be improved by the tap test than cognition.

16. C.

This man has acute confusional state, with the onset of encephalopathy over a period of days. A toxic-metabolic etiology will likely be found in view of his multiple medical problems.

17. A.

The history of this case is typical of subdural hematoma, and the recent motor vehicle accident is an important detail that argues against other etiologies. An epidural hematoma could be present, but typically this is a more fulminant form of intracranial hemorrhage.

18. C.

Testing for presenilin 1 (PS1) can be performed commercially, but is not relevant in the routine evaluation of dementia. PS1 mutations are very rare, and should only be considered in young-onset patients who have a strong family history of dementia. Even then, this testing must be understood as making no contribution to the treatment of the patient.

19. D.

The standard approach to pharmacologic treatment of cognitive dysfunction in Alzheimer disease is the use of a cholinesterase inhibitor and memantine. This regimen is usually well tolerated, and data exist supporting the combined use of these drugs.

20. E.

Depression clearly deserves a place among the reversible dementias. Whereas only a minority of depressed patients become cognitively impaired to the point where dementia can be diagnosed, the dementia syndrome of depression can be readily and effectively treated in most cases if recognized.

Chapter 15: Sleep Disorders

Glen Greenough, MD

Contents

1. Introduction

Sleep can be defined as a reversible behavioral state of unresponsiveness to the environment associated with perceptual disengagement. Sleep, however, is not a homogenous state. Sleep is divided into non-rapid eye movement (NREM) sleep and rapid eye movement (REM) sleep. NREM sleep is further separated into three stages. Stage one sleep is traditionally thought of as a transitional stage as one progresses from wake to sleep. Stage one sleep is characterized by theta frequencies in the electroencephalogram (EEG), a decrease in motor tone, and slow rolling eye movements. Stage two sleep has as its hallmarks sleep spindles (waxing and waning waves at 7-14 Hz that last 1-2 seconds and recur periodically) and K-complexes (large biphasic waves). Stage three or slow wave sleep (SWS) has as its defining feature high amplitude waves at a frequency of less than 2 Hz. REM sleep is characterized by theta rhythms in the EEG as well as rapid eye movements, as its name implies. Atonia of skeletal muscles is also a feature of this sleep stage, as well as autonomic instability manifesting as variability in tidal volume and heart rate.

Each night, sleep is entered through NREM. NREM and REM sleep cycle across the night at approximately 90-minute intervals. A reduced REM latency during nocturnal sleep would be a latency of less than 60 minutes and can be seen in some pathologic conditions. SWS predominates in the first third of the night and REM sleep predominates in the last third of the night. With so much happening physiologically during sleep it is no wonder that there are a number of pathologies associated with sleep.

Sleep disorders and their consequences are gaining greater recognition in all disciplines of medicine including neurology. Neurologists may be directly referred patients with sleep complaints. A good sleep-related history is essential for correct diagnosis. When taking a sleep history one must not only ask the patient about nocturnal symptoms but one should ask any other observers, such as the patient's bed partner. Assessment of the consequences of sleep problems either at night or the next day is also essential to making the correct diagnosis. Sleep disorders can generally be grouped into one of three categories, depending on the primary complaint: 1) excessive daytime sleepiness (EDS); 2) insomnia, and 3) parasomnias. EDS is suggested if the patient naps either voluntarily or involuntarily. Patients with this complaint are at risk for dozing off while driving or in other inappropriate situations. An insomnia complaint is one of difficulty initiating or maintaining sleep, or experiencing unrefreshing sleep with consequences the next day. Patients with a primary insomnia may not be able to nap even if they try, but often do complain of fatigue. Parasomnias are nocturnal behaviors or events such as sleepwalking. This division into three broad categories is useful but imperfect as there is often overlap.

Polysomnography (PSG) is the primary diagnostic tool for the diagnosis of many sleep disorders but is not required to make the diagnosis of all sleep disorders. Polysomnography consists of a multi-channel recording of multiple physiologic parameters and direct observations made by the recording technician (Table 1). Electro-oculograms (EOG), chin electromyograms (EMG), and EEG are primarily used to

Table 1

Polysomnography

EEG: electroencephalogram, typically C3 or C4 and O1 or O2
EOG: electro-oculogram which records near the left and right outer canthus
Chin EMG: electromyogram of submentalis in the chin
EKG: electrocardiogram, typically a modified lead II
Airflow: nasal and oral airflow are typically measured by temperature or pressure based nasal/oral sensors
Respiratory effort: typically measured from belt transduction over the chest and abdomen
Pulse oximetry: typically through a finger probe
Tibialis EMG: electromyogram of anterior tibialis bilaterally
Continuous video and audio monitoring by a trained technologist

determine sleep stage. Surface EMG of the tibialis anterior is used to record periodic limb movements (PLMs). Measure of respiratory flow and effort in conjunction with oximetry are used to measure respiratory events such as apneas or hypopneas. The polysomnographer will synthesize all of these recorded physiologic parameters with the patient's history and exam to make a correct diagnosis.

An objective assessment of EDS is usually necessary to diagnose disorders of primary hypersomnolence. The Multiple Sleep Latency Test (MSLT) provides a quantitive measure of a patient's drive to sleep. The MSLT is most accurate when performed the day after a PSG, since the PSG will provide a context for the interpretation of the MSLT. EEG, EOG, electrocardiogram and chin EMG recordings are made for the MSLT. Subjects are asked to lie in a bed in a dark room and to try to fall asleep on five occasions across the day at two-hour intervals. Their latencies to sleep are then calculated and which sleep stages are entered is also recorded. Mean latencies to sleep of less than eight minutes are generally considered indicative of excessive sleepiness. Latencies of 10 minutes or more are generally considered normal with latencies between eight and 10 minutes falling into a gray zone. A sleep onset REM period (SOREMP) is defined as the presence of REM sleep within 20 minutes of sleep onset. Context, however, is key in the interpretation of MSLT results. For example, a pathologic latency to sleep in a person who had 8 hours to sleep the night before might suggest a sleep disorder, but the same latency in a person who was awake all night would not necessarily be diagnostic of anything other than sleep deprivation. A medication history is important when interpreting MSLTs, as well in the usage or abrupt discontinuation of certain medications which may alter the test results. For example, the abrupt cessation of a REM-suppressing medication, such as an antidepressant, shortly before an MSLT could lead to the appearance of SOREMPs. The Maintenance of Wakefulness Test (MWT) is a variation on the MSLT, in which a subject is asked to maintain wakefulness sitting up in bed in dim light for 40 minutes on four occasions across the day at two-hour intervals. Normative values are yet to be clearly determined for this test. The average latency to sleep among normals is approximately 30 minutes. A patient probably has a normal level of alertness if able to stay awake for the entire 40-minute test all four times. The MWT can be helpful as a guide in assessing treatment outcome, particularly prior to returning to an activity requiring alertness, such as driving.

Table 2

Symptoms of Obstructive Sleep Apnea

Nocturnal Symptoms	**Daytime Symptoms**
Disruptive snoring	Sleepiness
Observed apneas	Fatigue
Waking short of breath	Depression
Restlessness	Irritability
Nocturia	Inattention
Gastric reflux	Impotence
Diaphoresis	

2. Sleep Disordered Breathing

Obstructive Sleep Apnea Syndrome

The obstructive sleep apnea syndrome (OSAS), as defined in the International Classification of Sleep Disorders (ICSD), is characterized by repetitive episodes of upper airway obstruction that occur during sleep, usually associated with a reduction in blood oxygen saturation. Characteristically, family or friends complain of loud, disruptive snoring, possibly punctuated by observed episodes where breathing stops (apneas). The patient may occasionally hear their own snoring but is often unaware of the severity or the pauses in breathing. EDS and dozing off inadvertently are typical presenting complaints. The patient, however, may be completely unaware of any symptoms, and only is evaluated because of concerned family members. Symptoms of sleep apnea can be divided into daytime and nocturnal symptoms (Table 2). Approximately 2% of women and 4% of men between the ages of 40 and 65 years may have OSAS. The prevalence may be even higher in high-risk groups such as patients with Down syndrome or stroke. Patient education, especially in regard to the health risks of obstructive sleep apnea, is important. Common risk factors for OSAS include obesity, age and male gender, but any factor that works to promote airway collapse can lead to OSAS.

A number of forces act upon the upper airway to promote collapse. The negative pressures generated in the pharynx during inspiration, along with extraluminal pressures, often from fat deposition, promote airway collapse. The reduction in genioglos-

Figure 1

A polysomnogram revealing an obstructive apnea

Note the absence of airflow but the persistence of respiratory effort. The apnea is terminated by an arousal and associated with a desaturation.

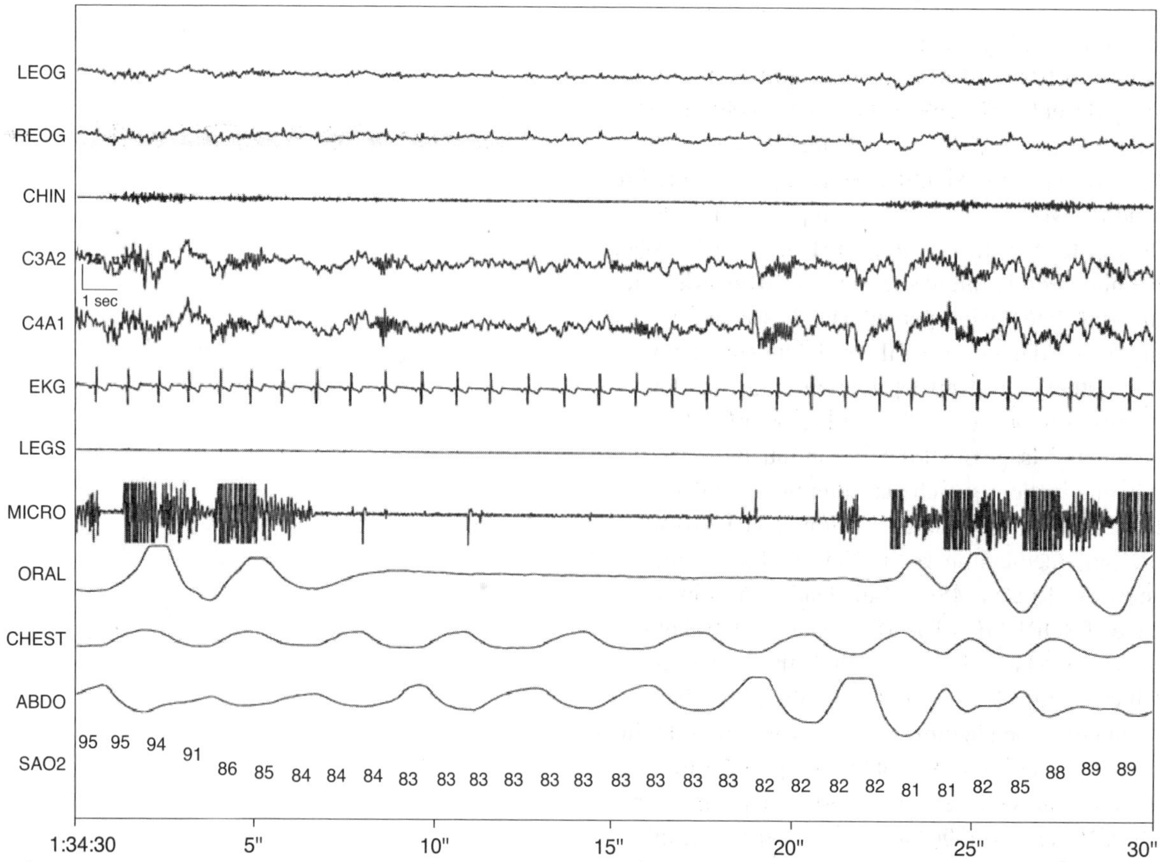

Courtesy of Dr Michael Sateia

Table 3

Differential Diagnosis of Excessive Daytime Sleepiness

Insufficient sleep	
	Insufficient sleep syndrome
	Inadequate sleep hygiene
	Long sleeper
Impaired sleep quality	
	Obstructive sleep apnea syndrome
	Upper airway resistance syndrome
	Central sleep apnea syndrome
	Restless legs syndrome-periodic limb movement disorder
	Parasomnias
Intrinsic sleepiness	
	Narcolepsy
	Idiopathic hypersomnia
	Other hypersomnia
Irregular timing of sleep-wake pattern	
	Circadian rhythm disorder
Other	
	Medications
	Medical conditions
	Psychiatric conditions – perception of EDS

sus (an airway dilator) activity that normally occurs with sleep onset makes the airway more collapsible during sleep. Patients with OSAS often have excessive genioglossus activity during wakefulness to maintain airway patency, but this compensatory increase in muscle tone is lost with the onset of sleep. In patients with OSAS, with the onset of sleep there is upper airway narrowing, often at multiple levels that leads to the reduction or absence of airflow. The effort to breathe against a critically narrowed or obstructed airway leads to arousal and sleep fragmentation accompanied by a sympathetic outflow. This sympathetic outflow leads to increases in heart rate and blood pressure at the termination of the respiratory event. The reduction in ventilation often leads to hypercapnia and hypoxemia.

Table 4

Differential Diagnosis of Chronic Insomnia

Psychiatric disorders	
Medications/substances	
Shift work	
Circadian rhythm disorder	
	DSPS – sleep onset insomnia
	ASPA – sleep maintainence insomnia
	Chronic illness/medical condition
Primary sleep disorder	
	RLS/PLMD
	Sleep disordered breathing
	Narcolepsy
	Psychophysiologic insomnia
	Idiopathic Insomnia
Poor sleep hygiene	

The consequences of sleep apnea are multiple. There are a number of neurobehavioral consequences. The excessive daytime sleepiness, which results from the sleep fragmentation, has been associated with an increase in the risk of motor vehicle and workplace accidents. Mood disturbance is common as well in patients with obstructive sleep apnea syndrome. OSAS has been associated with a number of cardiovascular consequences, including daytime hypertension. The intermittent hypertension associated with the termination of obstructive respiratory events evolves into sustained hypertension, presumably through chronically heightened sympathetic activity and arterial baroreceptor dysfunction. OSAS is now considered a potentially reversible cause of hypertension. Large population-based studies such as the Sleep Heart Health Study have linked OSAS with stroke, heart failure and myocardial infarction. Prospective data indicating treatment of obstructive sleep apnea leading to reduction in cardiovascular morbidity or mortality are sparse. There is some recent data suggesting that continuous positive airway pressure (CPAP) treatment of

OSAS leads to improved ejection fractions in patients with OSAS and to reduced ejection fraction.

Polysomnography is the gold standard for the diagnosis of OSAS. Overnight oximetry alone is inadequate as patients may not have significant desaturation but may have significant sleep fragmentation. OSAS can be graded as to its severity based on the apnea-hypopnea index (AHI). The AHI reflects the number of apneas and hypopneas per hour. Obstructive apneas represent the cessation of airflow for at least 10 seconds with continued respiratory effort (Figure 1). Hypopneas represent the attenuation of airflow for at least 10 seconds associated with a terminal arousal or desaturation. One grading criteria grades OSAS as mild if the AHI is 5-20, moderate if 20-40, and severe if greater than 40. The differential for OSAS is that of patients with excessive daytime sleepiness (Table 3).

Obstructive sleep apnea is a chronic disease that generally requires long-term treatment. Conservative measures such as weight loss, avoidance of alcohol or sedative medication before bed, smoking cessation, and position control (attempting to sleep with the head of the bed elevated or avoiding the supine position) may be helpful. Oral appliances, which advance the mandible or tongue, may lead to resolution of the OSAS in approximately 50% of cases. Surgical treatments for OSAS are available. The uvulopalatopharyngolplasty in which the uvula, part of the soft palate, and tonsils are removed leads to a cure less than 50% of the time, and relapse may be problematic. Other procedures are available but rarely performed. Tracheotomy is often effective but is now used rarely since the advent of continuous positive airway pressure (CPAP) devices. CPAP machines act to pneumatically splint open the upper airway. CPAP is very effective, and compliance as far as 5 years out is between 65%-90%.

A recently recognized variant of OSAS is the upper airway resistance syndrome (UARS). In this disorder the AHI is normal but episodes of airway narrowing lead to an increasing effort to breathe, which results in an arousal. The best way to document this disorder is with esophageal manometry during sleep to document the building effort to breathe prior to the arousals.

Central Sleep Apnea

Central sleep apnea syndrome (CSAS) is a heterogeneous group of disorders whose unifying characteristic is the episodic cessation of respiration as a result of the absence of output from the brain to breathe. Central apneas are defined as the absence of airflow for at least 10 seconds with an accompanying lack of respiratory effort. During sleep the wakefulness drive to breathe and behavioral control of breathing are lost. Breathing becomes dependent on metabolic control through pCO_2. Central apneas then result with the onset of sleep if the pCO_2 is below the apneic threshold. This is the physiology behind the normal phenomenon of sleep onset central apneas (central apneas that occur at sleep-wake transition) as well as the genesis of central apneas in a number of pathologic states. Like OSAS, CSAS is diagnosed using overnight polysomnography. The differential diagnosis of CSA is usually that of EDS. The prevalence of CSAS is difficult to tabulate as it represents a heterogeneous group of disorders and can occur in association with OSAS. Certainly, CSAS is much less common than OSAS. CSAS can be further classified as hypercapnic or nonhypercapnic CSAS.

Hypercapnic Central Sleep Apnea

In hypercapnic CSAS, there is a severe reduction of ventilatory motor output that leads to decreased alveolar ventilation and central apneas during sleep. This group of disorders have daytime steady-state hypercapnia that worsens with sleep onset. One subset of disorders that lead to hypercapnic CSAS are those whose common feature is the failure of automatic or metabolic control of breathing with the onset of sleep. This chronic alveolar hypoventilation occurs in the setting of normal pulmonary function. The problem can be genetic in origin as is the case in congenital central hypoventilation, or acquired as can be the case in a number of brainstem or spinal cord injuries. Therapies for this group of disorders often consists of ventilatory support or possibly diaphragmatic pacing. A second group of disorders associated with hypercapnic CSAS are neuromuscular disorders that affect respiratory muscles. These patients may also benefit from ventilatory support either in the form of assisted ventilation through a tracheostomy or bilevel ventilation. Opioids may also lead to hypercapnic CSAS.

Nonhypercapnic Central Sleep Apnea

Nonhypercapnic CSAS represents a diverse group of disorders. Cheyne-Stokes respiration (CSR) is the prototypical nonhypercapnic CSAS. CSR is characterized by regular cycles of crescendo-decrescendo tidal volume with a central apnea occurring at the nadir of ventilatory drive and arousal occurring at the zenith. Congestive heart failure (CHF) is the setting in which this disorder is most common. The etiology of CSR remains unclear but the resting pCO_2 in CHF patients is closer to the apneic threshold than in normals. If arterial pCO_2 is lowered below the apneic threshold, breathing ceases until pCO_2 rises. On this basis, even modest hyperventilation may lead to a central apnea. CSR has also been observed following stroke (discussed later) and in association with idiopathic pulmonary hypertension (not to be confused with OSAS which may cause secondary pulmonary hypertension). A pattern of breathing similar to CSR is also observed after ascent to high altitudes. Patients with nonhypercapnic CSAS may present with EDS or an insomnia complaint. Patients may report waking, gasping or choking. CSAS patients differ from OSAS patients in that snoring, if present, is mild and CSAS patients are less likely to be obese.

The best mode of therapy for nonhypercapnic CSR is not always clear and varies among the subtypes. Supplemental oxygen, positive pressure therapy, theophylline and acetazolamide may be useful in some situations. In the setting of CHF, improvement in control of the CHF is the best first step. The best form of positive pressure therapy remains controversial in that there is some data indicating increased early mortality in patients treated with CPAP for CSR in the setting of CHF. Newer bilevel positive pressure machines with servoventialiton technology may be helpful in this setting.

3. Primary Hypersomnolence

Narcolepsy

The cardinal and initial symptom of narcolepsy is typically EDS. Patients may report drowsiness or may doze off involuntarily. The overwhelming urge to sleep may occur suddenly, leading to what has been described as sleep attacks. Daytime sleep episodes usually last from minutes to hours and are transiently refreshing. Diagnosis of narcolepsy, however, cannot be made solely based on a patient's description of their EDS, as patients with other sleep disorders such as OSAS may have profound sleepiness as well. As with daytime sleepiness from other causes, narcolepsy patients may report difficulties with memory or concentration.

Ancillary symptoms in narcolepsy include cataplexy, sleep-related hallucinations and sleep paralysis. These ancillary symptoms, much like EDS, can be viewed as the inappropriate intrusion of REM sleep into wakefulness, as they share many features with normal REM sleep except for their timing during waking hours. Cataplexy is the transient reduction or loss of skeletal muscle tone often triggered by strong emotion. Other triggers might include stress, meals or fatigue, although not every episode has a clear trigger. Up to 70% of narcolepsy patients experience cataplexy. The cataplectic event itself can vary in form. The event may range from a brief sagging of the jaw to complete collapse to the floor. The weakness is typically bilateral. Occasionally, superimposed on the reduced muscle tone are bursts of phasic muscle activity. The weakness may be maximal at onset or evolve over seconds. The episodes can last from seconds to 30 minutes, but most last seconds to a few minutes. A key feature is that awareness and memory are retained during the episode, although dream-like images or hallucinations may accompany longer episodes.

Episodes of paralysis of voluntary muscles occurring upon awakening or at sleep onset represent sleep paralysis. Single or occasional episodes are common among the normal population with up to 50% of normal individuals reporting sleep paralysis at least once in their lives. Sleep paralysis occurs repetitively in up to 40% of patients with narcolepsy. The episodes last from one to several minutes and resolve either spontaneously or in response to external stimuli. Much like in REM sleep, muscles controlling respiration and eye movement, despite their voluntary nature, are spared. The episodes may be accompanied by hallucinations but consciousness is otherwise normal.

Hallucinations at sleep onset (hypnagogic) or upon awakening (hypnopompic) are reported in narcolepsy. The hallucinations are typically visual or auditory but tactile hallucinations also may occur. The hallucinations may be simple (ie, shapes) or complex (ie, figures, music).

Other features of narcolepsy include insomnia, with many narcoleptics reporting sleep maintenance, and less often sleep initiation difficulties. The total amount of sleep in a 24-hour period for narcoleptics is not increased but just inappropriately distributed with intrusion during the daytime and fragmentation of sleep at night. Narcolepsy patients may experience REM sleep behavior disorder (RBD) as well as PLMs.

The etiology of narcolepsy has remained elusive. There is a strong HLA association with narcolepsy. DQB1*0602 and DQA1*0102 appear to confer susceptibility to narcolepsy. However, genetic factors alone cannot explain the onset of this disorder, as indicated by the low concordance rate of narcolepsy (25%-30%) among identical twins. It has been postulated that there is some factor that triggers the onset of the disease in genetically susceptible individuals. Given this HLA association some have postulated an autoimmune trigger but one has yet to be identified. Recent studies have identified a neuropeptide thought to play an important role in narcolepsy. Hypocretin, also called orexin, is a neuropeptide found in the hypothalamus that comes in two forms. The cell bodies of hypocretin producing neurons are found in the dorso-lateral hypothalamus and have extensive projections, especially to the brainstem. It is believed that these neuropeptides play a role in multiple physiologic functions including food intake, endocrine function, thermoregulation, cardiovascular regulation, and the sleep-wake cycle. In narcolepsy, the connection between these hypocretin neurons and the locus ceruleus may be pivotal. The locus ceruleus is typically active during wakefulness but ceases firing prior to and during REM sleep. Hypocretin neurons appear to normally excite the locus ceruleus. If there were a functional defect in hypocretin transmission there would be less opposition to REM sleep, thereby possibly allowing the inappropriate intrusion of REM sleep.

Narcolepsy symptoms may begin at most any age but peak onset occurs in the second decade with a secondary peak in the fourth decade. EDS is usually the initial symptom. The ancillary symptoms (cataplexy, sleep paralysis, hypnogogic hallucinations) typically develop over the ensuing months to years.

A good clinical history is important in the diagnosis of narcolepsy. In particular, a history of clear-cut cataplexy in the setting of excessive daytime sleepiness is strongly suggestive of narcolepsy. PSG followed the next morning by an MSLT are important tests in the diagnosis of narcolepsy. The PSG is useful in excluding other causes of EDS and to establish adequate sleep was obtained before an MSLT. The PSG typically reveals fragmented sleep with multiple awakenings and possibly a shortened REM latency (the appearance of REM in less than 20 minutes after sleep onset). The MSLT typically reveals EDS with a sleep latency of less than 8 minutes, typically less than 5 minutes, and sleep onset REM periods on the naps. The ICSD suggests that at least two sleep onset REM periods are required to make the diagnosis of narcolepsy if cataplexy is absent.

The differential diagnosis for narcolepsy is that of excessive daytime sleepiness (Table 3). The differential diagnosis of cataplexy is narrower. Some degree of weakness associated with anger, stress, sexual activity or physical activity can be normal. Weakness triggered by laughter, especially of head and neck muscles, is more likely cataplexy. Atonic seizures and syncope can be confused with cataplexy but consciousness is retained in cataplexy unlike in the other two scenarios. The differential diagnosis of sleep paralysis includes atonic seizures, hypokalemic periodic paralysis, posterior circulation transient ischemic attack, and psychiatric disorders. The brevity of the paralysis, the absence of other features and the relation to sleep-wake transition can usually distinguish sleep paralysis from these disorders.

Narcolepsy is a chronic disorder. While the EDS may have a gradual onset, once established the symptoms are persistent. Patients can at least be reassured that narcolepsy is not progressive, but rarely do symptoms resolve. Narcolepsy is a relatively rare disorder with prevalence of 0.05% in the United States but of 0.18% in Japan. Genders are equally affected.

Treatment in narcolepsy focuses on symptom control. Stimulants or wakefulness promoting agents are prescribed to counter the EDS. The stimulants amphetamines, methylphenidate, pemoline, and now the alertness promoting agent modafinil, all may offer some benefit. Pemoline has been less widely used in recent years because of concerns about hepatic toxicity. While it is prudent to start at low doses and titrate upward, narcolepsy patients may require high doses of these medications. Up to 60 mg per day of methylphenidate or dextroamphetamine can be used in divided doses, or up to 400 mg of modafinil daily. Common side effects of these medications include nervousness, headache, tremor, palpitations and gastrointestinal symptoms, among others. Modafinil may be the best tolerated of this group of medications, although the traditional stimulants may have some modest benefit in treating cataplexy, which is not the case with modafinil. For years, the tricyclic antidepressants, typically imipramine, protriptyline and clomipramine, were the principal treatments for cataplexy. These medications presumably counter cataplexy by preventing uptake of norepinephrine. Side effects commonly associated with tricyclic antidepressants (dry mouth, weight gain, sexual dysfunction, etc.), limited the utility of these medications. Newer antidepressants such as fluoxetine and venlafaxine have been efficacious, with fewer side effects. Gammahydroxybutyrate has recently been demonstrated to help consolidate nocturnal sleep and improve cataplexy as well as EDS.

Idiopathic Hypersomnia

Idiopathic hypersomnia (IH) is a disorder presumably of central nervous system origin characterized by EDS in the absence of the ancillary symptoms of narcolepsy. IH may be the result of multiple etiologies, making diagnosis and treatment challenging. Patients may report long nonrestorative naps despite long nocturnal sleep times. Patients may also be hard to awaken. During long periods of drowsiness, automatic behavior may occur in which the patient continues to perform an activity in a semicontrolled way despite the intrusion of short periods of sleep (1-4 seconds) into wakefulness. During these episodes the patient may appear to behave inappropriately, such as wandering or putting dirty clothes in the dishwasher.

The pathophysiology of this disorder is unclear, as it seems to include a heterogeneous group of disorders. One small group of patients with this disorder have a family history of IH. Other clinical features of this subgroup include headaches, syncope, orthostatic hypotension and Raynaud's phenomena. Another group of patients with IH consist of patients who have a viral syndrome of some type prior to the onset of the EDS. The fatigue persists after the rest of the viral symptoms resolve. Mononucleosis, hepatitis, or atypical viral pneumonia are the most common preceding syndromes. A third subgroup represents subjects with IH but no family history and no antecedent viral illness.

Clinical history and PSG followed by MSLT are the standard diagnostic tools in this disorder. The PSG typically demonstrates long nocturnal sleep, with a possible increase in SWS percentage. The MSLT demonstrates brief latencies to sleep without sleep onset REM periods on the naps. The differential diagnosis is that of EDS. The age of onset is usually between 15-30 years. The EDS is thought to be lifelong once present. Treatment is similar to that of narcolepsy, with stimulants or modafinil as the principal treatments. Good sleep hygiene can also be helpful.

Post-Traumatic Hypersomnia

This is a poorly described condition of excessive sleepiness that occurs after trauma to the CNS either as a blow to the head or as the result of a neurosurgical procedure. It may occur directly after the inciting event and then resolve over weeks to months. It may be associated with postconcussive symptoms such as headache and memory dysfunction. This disorder should be distinguished from sleep-related breathing disorders in particular, as they may occur as the result of a whiplash injury.

4. Syndromes of Episodic Hypersomnolence

Kleine-Levin Syndrome

The Kleine-Levin syndrome typically presents in adolescence and consists of episodes of hypersomnia lasting from one day to several weeks (typically 4-7 days). Total daily sleep times can reach 20 hours. Hyperphagia, hypersexuality and behavioral or mood changes may also occur. Afflicted individuals return to normal between episodes. The constellation of symptoms suggest hypothalamic dysfunction but the etiology has yet to be determined. Diagnosis is typically made on clinical grounds. PSGs when performed have revealed high sleep efficiency but a reduced percentage of delta sleep. MSLT during an episode may reveal a shortened latency to sleep as well as sleep onset REM periods. The long-term course is unclear but the frequency of attacks may decline over time. Treatment has not been well established. Carbamazapine and lithium may help prevent attacks. Pemoline has been used to directly address the EDS. Menstrual related hypersomnia is characterized by EDS that has a temporal association to menses, and is thought by some to be a variation of the Kleine-Levin syndrome. Symptoms may improve with medication to suppress ovulation.

Idiopathic Recurrent Stupor

Idiopathic recurrent stupor, as its name suggests, is characterized by episodes of stupor that last from hours to days. It typically presents in middle age but a characteristic clinical course or pattern has yet to be established. EEG may reveal a diffuse 13-16 Hz rhythm without normal sleep stages. Some patients with this disorder have been found to have elevated blood and CSF levels of a naturally occurring endogenous benzodiazepine-like substance called endozepine-4. Interestingly, flumazenil, a benzodiazepine agonist, has been shown to be helpful, suggesting a role for the GABAergic system in this disorder.

Figure 2

A polysomnogram showing PLMs

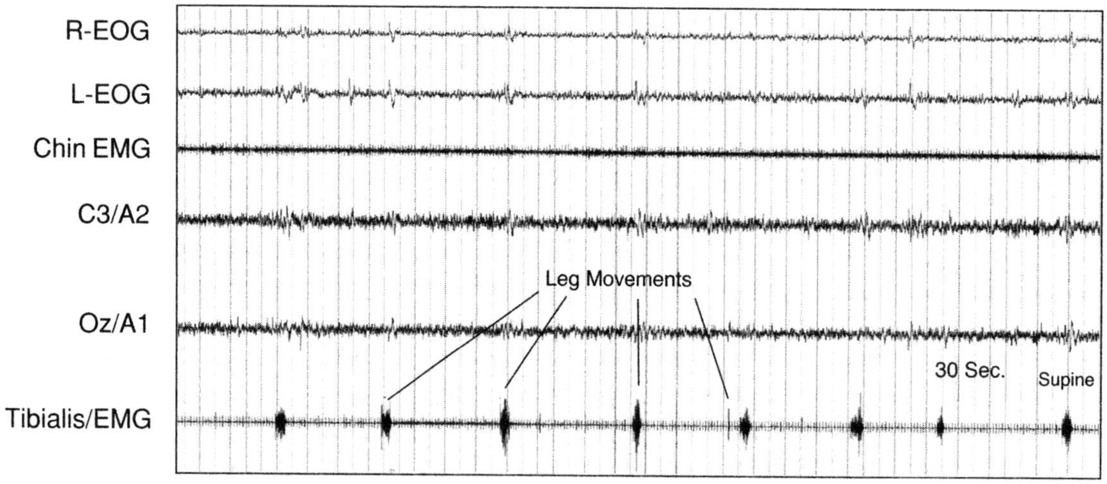

Courtesy of Dr Michael Sateia

5. Restless Legs Syndrome and Periodic Limb Movements

The restless legs syndrome (RLS) is a disorder characterized by an irresistible urge to move the legs, usually accompanied by an uncomfortable or unpleasant sensation in the legs. Arms can be affected in severe cases. The urge to move or uncomfortable sensation is brought on by or made worse by rest or inactivity, and typically worsens at night. Both the urge and sensation are partially or totally relieved by movement such as walking or stretching. Periodic limb movements (PLMs) are an associated but distinct phenomena from RLS. PLMs are triple flexion movements that occur while asleep or awake. They last 0.5-10 seconds and occur with a periodicity of 5-90 seconds (Figure 2). They tend to cluster in the first half of the night in NREM sleep. They may lead to sleep fragmentation and thereby to excessive daytime sleepiness. PLMs are present in 80%-90% of patients with RLS. It should be noted that the reverse is not always the case. Patients can have PLMs without RLS.

The RLS is a chronic disorder that may start in childhood and worsen over time. The prevalence increases with age. RLS is common in populations derived from Western Europe with a 5.8%-13% prevalence in these groups. RLS is less common in Asia with a 3% prevalence in Japan and a less than 1% prevalence in Singapore. Symptoms may wax and wane over time. Many but not all patients will have a family history of RLS. Familial RLS may have an autosomal dominant mode of inheritance with linkage to chromosome 12q, 14q and 9p. Renal failure, pregnancy, and iron deficiency are three conditions with the best-documented associations with RLS. Vitamin B_{12} deficiency, magnesium deficiency, Parkinson disease and neuropathy also may be associated with RLS. RLS and PLMs can be made worse by or be caused by a number of medications including lithium carbonate, tricyclic antidepressants and selective serotonin reuptake inhibitors. Withdrawal from benzodiazepines, barbiturates, and anticonvulsants may also worsen or induce RLS and PLMs. RLS secondary to medical or neurological conditions is clinically indistinguishable from the idiopathic and familial forms. There are a number of theories as to the pathophysiology of RLS and PLMs. There is some evidence for a defect in a dopaminergic system in the brain. The strongest evidence for this hypothesis is the strong positive response of this disorder to dopaminergic agents. A central nervous system iron deficiency also has some support, especially in light of the observed response to iron supplementation in subjects with RLS and low ferritin levels. Possibly linking the two hypotheses is the observation that iron is a cofactor in the production of dopamine.

RLS is diagnosed clinically as there is no objective test specific for RLS. Other information that might support the diagnosis is the presence of a family history of RLS, PLMs on polysomnography, the presence of a disorder known to be associated with RLS, or a positive response to dopaminergic agents. RLS must be distinguished from neuropathy. Unlike many neuropathy patients, patients with RLS have a normal physical exam, have a strong desire to move, and their symptoms improve with movement. The one caveat is that neuropathy and RLS can coexist, as neuropathy patients may have an increased risk for RLS. Patients with leg cramps may have a desire to move and have relief with movement but they may report contracture of a muscle. Leg cramps are also not predictably brought on by a sedentary posture. Claudication typically occurs in the legs like RLS but is brought on by walking and relieved by rest. Leg cramps, claudicatory pain and neuropathy pain generally would not respond to dopaminergic agents unlike the RLS. Given its relation to other medical disorders, when diagnosing RLS one should consider checking at a minimum long-term iron stores (ferritin).

There are multiple therapies available for RLS with PLMs. In general, good sleep hygiene, maintenance of a regular sleep schedule and avoiding medications or substances known to trigger RLS and PLMs is prudent. Exercise, massage and hot baths can be helpful. Iron replacement, in particular if the ferritin level is less than 45-50 ng/mL, may lead to improvement in symptoms. If a medication is required, as is usually the case in moderate to severe disease, dopaminergic agents are the gold standard of treatment. Carbidopalevodopa is effective but rebound (symptom recurrence when the medication wears off) and augmentation (the earlier appearance of symptoms in the day) are problematic. Rebound and augmentation may be less of an issue if one combines immediate and slow-release carbidopa-levodopa. The ergot-based dopamine agonist pergolide is effective but nausea may be problematic.

The rare but serious complication of pleuropulmonary fibrosis and cardiac valvulopathy also limits the utility of this medication. The dopamine agonists pramipexole and ropinrole are usually effective and well tolerated, making these medications the typical first line therapy. Other medications such as benzodiazepines, opioids, and anticonvulsants (specifically gabapentin) have utility in the treatment of this disorder.

6. Circadian Rhythms

Biologic rhythms are seen in the simplest to the most complex of organisms. The frequency of a biologic rhythm reflects the number of repetitions of the oscillation per unit of time. A circadian frequency, for example, represents one oscillation in 24 hours. Other features of rhythms include amplitude (maximal excursion from a reference point) and phase (temporal position of an oscillation in relation to an external cue such as the light-dark cycle). Physiologic, biochemical and anatomic variables *in vivo* are characterized by circadian fluctuations with a nadir and zenith in each 24-hour or circadian period. For example, body temperature reaches its peak during the active phase and its nadir during sleep. The timing of sleep-wake states as well as the quality of sleep are determined by not only an individual's circadian rhythm but also by an individual's homeostatic drive to sleep. The homeostatic drive reflects prior amounts of sleep and wakefulness. For example, sleep deprivation increases the homeostatic drive to sleep.

Circadian rhythms are endogenous in that they persist under a wide array of environmental conditions or situations. The suprachiasmatic nucleus (SCN) located in the anterior hypothalamus acts as the master generator of circadian rhythms in mammals. The SCN exerts influence over a wide variety of physiologic functions ranging from hormone levels to body temperature, to the sleep-wake cycle. Photic information is transmitted to the SCN via the retinohypothalmic tract from the retina. The SCN sends projections to the pineal gland to regulate the output of melatonin. Melatonin secretion is inhibited by exposure to light.

While a circadian rhythm is genetically preprogrammed, it can be modulated by external cues. In the absence of environmental cues a rhythm is said to be free-running. When environmental cues modulate the phase of an endogenous pacemaker, this is labeled entrainment. The primary environmental cue that works to entrain the circadian pacemaker is light. The intensity, duration and timing of the light exposure determines its effect on the circadian pacemaker. There are a variety of nonphotic stimuli (food, social cues, exercise, etc.), which may modulate the circadian rhythm, but their effects tend to be less than that of photic stimulation. A phase delay occurs when sufficient light is presented near the start of the subjective night (ie, bright light in the evening), and a phase advance occurs when sufficient light is presented near the end of the subjective night (ie, bright light in the morning).

There are four major disorders of the circadian sleep-wake cycle, as follows: delayed sleep phase syndrome (DSPS); advanced sleep phase syndrome (ASPS); irregular sleep-wake pattern; and non-24 hour sleep-wake pattern. We will focus on DSPS and ASPS.

7. Circadian Rhythm Disorders

Delayed Sleep Phase Syndrome

DSPS has as its hallmark the inability to get to sleep at conventional bedtimes and the inability to arise at conventional wake times. Typically, patients with this disorder describe an inability to get to sleep until the early morning hours (1-6 AM). If left to their own devices, they would sleep until the late morning or early afternoon. When forced to awaken at a conventional wake time, they describe significant sleepiness, especially in the morning hours. They function fine if allowed to sleep normal to extended amounts on this delayed schedule, but societal demands do not allow them to maintain such a schedule.

The precise prevalence of DSPS is unknown, but in sleep clinics it may represent up to 10% of chronic insomnia cases. The disorder is most common among adolescents and young adults, with no reported gender difference. There are reports of increased psychopathology among afflicted patients.

The diagnosis is typically an historical one. Sleep logs and actigraphy can be used to support the history. PSG is not required unless other disorders such as narcolepsy or OSAS are suspected as well. The results of PSG in the DSPS will vary depending upon the timing of the study. If studied under their habitual delayed schedule, sleep parameters are generally normal. The primary differential is that of a sleep onset insomnia (see Table 4 for insomnia differential). One of the major distinguishing features from other causes of sleep onset insomnia is that in DSPS the patient reports normal sleep and daytime functioning if allowed to sleep with a delayed pattern. Some individuals may choose a late bedtime, not because of their circadian rhythm, but because they elect to stay up late and then have a hard time arising. These patients really suffer from voluntary sleep restriction and not from a circadian rhythm disorder.

The essential abnormality in patients with DSPS is that of a phase delay of their circadian pacemaker. Why an individual might have this shift has yet to be fully elucidated. Treatment of DSPS consists of advancing the circadian rhythm through chronotherapy, phototherapy and pharmacotherapy.

Chronotherapy in this situation can be implemented in one of two ways. The wake time can gradually be advanced by 30 min. every week (get up 30 min. earlier each week) until a desired wake time is reached. Alternately, bedtime can be delayed by 3 hours per day (go to bed 3 hours later each day) until an appropriate schedule is achieved. Phototherapy with bright light upon awakening may have some utility but the timing, duration and intensity of light therapy have not been clearly established. From a pharmacotherapy standpoint, evening melatonin may have some utility but has not been well established. The utility of other pharmacological treatments such as hypnotics are even less well established in this syndrome.

Advanced Sleep Phase Syndrome

ASPS is a shift in the circadian rhythm in the opposite direction from that found in DSPS. Patients have trouble delaying bedtime to a socially acceptable time and awaken in the early hours. Bedtimes between 6-9 PM are typical with wake times between 1 and 3 AM. As in DSPS, the sleep itself is normal but it is the timing of the sleep that is abnormal. Patients may complain of evening sleepiness and/or sleep maintenance insomnia with early morning awakening.

ASPS is believed to affect 1% of middle-aged adults, with the prevalence increasing with age. Men and women are equally affected. The circadian pacemaker in patients with ASPS is by definition advanced but the reason for this remains unexplained. The diagnosis is an essentially historical one. Actigraphy and sleep logs can help reveal the sleep pattern, especially when the history is unclear. The differential is that of a sleep maintenance insomnia (Table 4). Psychiatric evaluation for depression leading to early morning awakenings can be helpful. Therapy may consist of bright light therapy in the evening (7-9 PM) to delay their circadian rhythm. Theoretically, morning administration of melatonin may be helpful but evidence is lacking and there is the added drawback of the potential direct sedating effect of the melatonin.

8. Parasomnias

Slow Wave Sleep Parasomnias

The SWS parasomnias, which consist of confusional arousals, sleep terrors and somnambulism, are best viewed as part of a continuum. All three primarily arise from SWS and all can be induced in predisposed individuals by a forced awakening during SWS. Therapies for these disorders then are often focused on allowing the patient to awaken more readily during the night or eliminating the triggering arousals. Based on the description of the event, it can usually be categorized into one of these three types of parasomnias. Some patients, however, describe events with overlapping features. SWS parasomnias may run in families but not all family members will have the same form. Because these events typically arise from SWS they most often occur in the first third of the night. The differential of SWS parasomnias is that of behavioral parasomnias (Table 5).

Table 5

Differential Diagnosis for Behavioral Parasomnias

Confusional arousals
Somnambulism
Sleep terrors
REM sleep behavior disorder
Nocturnal seizures
Partial arousal secondary to OSAS, PLMD, GERD or other fragmentary process
Malingering
Conversion hysteria/disassociative disorder
Nocturnal panic attacks
Post-traumatic stress disorder

Confusional Arousals

Confusional arousals consist of episodes of confusion during and after an arousal, typically from SWS. During an episode the subject is only partially awake, with slowed mentation and disorientation. An EEG during an episode reveals the incomplete awakening (theta or delta slowing may be noted, as well as sleep fragments intermingled with wakefulness or a poorly responsive alpha rhythm). The confusion usually lasts several to dozens of minutes. Most patients are amnestic to the episodes. Confusional arousals can occur in adults but are most common before the age of 5 and usually resolve over time. Any factor that deepens sleep or impairs the ability to arouse may lead to a confusional arousal. Recovery sleep after sleep deprivation or hypnotics are common culprits. Pathophysiologically, confusional arousals represent incomplete awakening from SWS leading to an intense period of sleep inertia before complete wakefulness is reached. In children, reassurance is the primary treatment. Avoidance of precipitating factors such as stress, hypnotics, or insufficient sleep leading to rebound is a helpful strategy.

Sleep Terrors

During a sleep terror the patient sits up from sleep and screams and appears to be terrified, with tachypnea, tarchycardia, dilated pupils and increased muscle tone. Attempts to console the subject are ineffective. The episodes last 30 seconds to 3 minutes and may be followed by some confusion. Subjects may have a vague recollection of the event. This disorder affects 3% of children and 1% of adults. In addition to the differential for behavioral parasomnias, night terrors must be distinguished from nightmares. Because nightmares are REM-related events, the time of night for nightmares is typically the last third of the night. Nightmares are also often not associated with the high degree of autonomic arousal and terror as seen with sleep terrors. Subjects who experience a nightmare often recall a storyline that became frightening, which differs from the vague recall of a patient with a sleep terror. Most children and parents should be reassured, as these episodes dissipate with age. Strategies to reduce stress or prevent arousals (hypnotics) can be helpful.

Somnambulism

Sleepwalkers arise from a deep sleep and without awakening display complex automatic behaviors including ambulation. The events usually last 1-5 minutes but can last up to one hour. Occasionally a sleep terror may evolve into a sleepwalking episode, further reinforcing that these disorders are part of a continuum. If awakened, the subject is confused. Most patients have little to no recall of the event. Somnambulism is most common in children around the age of 5 and usually resolves in adolescence although adult cases are not rare. Just as with the other SWS parasomnias, factors that deepen sleep or blunt arousal may predispose to these events. EEG during an event reveals lightening from SWS to stage one sleep or a slow alpha rhythm. Treatment, especially in childhood, consists mainly of reassurance and avoidance of precipitating factors. Benzodiazepines and tricyclics have been shown to have some efficacy in preventing attacks.

REM Sleep Parasomnias

REM Sleep Behavior Disorder

REM sleep behavior disorder (RBD) consists of recurrent dream enactment of typically violent dreams. This enactment may include such limited activities as verbalization or reaching, to as complex a behavior as jumping out of bed and running across the room. There is a strong male predominance. RBD has a prevalence rate of 0.5% in the general population.

Typical age of onset is in the 50s and 60s, although approximately 25% of affected individuals will have a prodrome for years of talking, hollering, limb twitching or jerking. Injury to the spouse or patient because of the violent nocturnal activities is typically what lead patients to seek out evaluation. Significant injuries including fractures may result because of this disorder. The parasomnias typically occur no earlier than 2 hours after sleep onset, which is not surprising since REM sleep occurs predominantly in the second half of the night. The frequency of events range from several episodes nightly to a few episodes per month. Despite this sleep disruption, EDS is not typically a complaint in this disorder. It has been postulated that the relative increase in SWS for age in RBD patients may compensate for the sleep disruption, thereby minimizing any EDS. Polysomnography may also reveal increased motor tone in REM sleep. This motor dysregulation may also spill over into NREM sleep in that both PLMs and nonperiodic limb movements are more common in NREM sleep in patients with RBD. The pathophysiology of RBD consists of the loss of REM atonia in conjunction with enhancement of phasic motor drive. Structural neuropathology is lacking, however, when one evaluates subjects with the idiopathic form of the disease.

RBD must be distinguished from other parasomnias and nocturnal seizures (Table 6). The PSG can be helpful given the EMG abnormalities often seen in RBD. Elevated submental EMG tone and/or excessive phasic submental or limb EMG twitching may be seen in RBD. In contrast to sleep terrors, there is generally an absence of autonomic hyperactivity (ie, tachycardia) in RBD. RBD events are often accompanied by violent or aggressive dreams, unlike nocturnal seizures or the SWS parasomnias.

RBD may occur as a secondary phenomenon or as an idiopathic disorder. The primary and secondary forms of RBD are clinically and polysomnographically indistinguishable. From a sleep disorders standpoint, RBD may occur in the setting of narcolepsy. RBD-like events can also occur in the setting of OSAS and resolve with treatment of the sleep disordered breathing. From a neurological standpoint, RBD appears to be associated with the synucleinopathies, which include Parkinson disease, multisystem atrophy and dementia with Lewy bodies. The RBD symptomatology may precede the development of the neurodegenerative disorder by

Table 6

Differentiating Nocturnal Frontal Lobe Epilepsy from SWS Parasomnias

	SWS Parasomnias	**NFLE**
Age of onset	Childhood	Adolescence (any possible)
Episodes per month	Up to a few	Often >10
Episodes per night	One	Often >1
Episode characteristics	Nonstereotypic	Stereotyped
Episode duration	Minutes	Seconds
Time of occurrence	First Third of Night	Random
Sleep stage of occurrence	SWS	Stage 2
Ictal EEG	Delta activity	Rare epileptic activity
Family history of SWS		
Parasomnias	80%	40%
Natural history	Remission	Persistence

Malow BA, Plazzi G. Nocturnal seizures. In: Chokroverty S, Hening WA, Walters AS, eds. Sleep and Movement Disorders. *1st ed. Woburn, Mass: Butterworth-Heinemann; 1999.*

many years. Acute RBD may develop in the context of alcohol or drug abuse and withdrawal, and also with the use of certain medications. Tricyclic antidepressants, selective serotonin reuptake inhibitors and venlafaxine all have been associated with RBD. RBD typically responds well to clonazepam. Clonazepam presumably works by suppressing phasic EMG activity during REM sleep but does not appear to restore the normal atonia. Other therapies that may be helpful include melatonin and dopaminergic agents.

9. Nocturnal Epilepsy

Most nocturnal seizures are easily recognized as such by a neurologist given the history and association with daytime events. The diagnostic difficulty often presents itself if the seizures are exclusively nocturnal. One form of nocturnal epilepsy is benign Rolandic epilepsy (benign childhood epilepsy with centrotemporal spikes) which is characterized by unilateral facial parasthesias with tonic or tonic-clonic movements of the facial musculature as well. Centrotemporal spikes may be noted in NREM sleep in the EEG. As the name implies, the course is typically benign with resolution of seizures in adulthood.

Nocturnal frontal lobe epilepsy (NFLE) is often challenging to diagnose because this disorder is characterized by bizarre behavioral manifestations that occur exclusively at night, for which the EEG, even ictally, is often normal. NFLE may be inherited in an autosomal dominant fashion. Men are more likely to be affected than women. Most attacks arise from NREM sleep. Imaging and neurological exam are usually normal. There is often a family history for epilepsy and parasomnias, further adding to the diagnostic difficulty.

NFLE has three primary subtypes: paroxysmal arousals (PAs), nocturnal paroxysmal dystonia (NPD), and episodic nocturnal wanderings (ENWs). PAs are a stereotyped sequence of movements lasting 2-20 seconds. Most commonly, the subject raises their head, sits up looking frightened, and screams. The upper limbs may be held in a dystonic posture. In NPD, there is a sudden arousal followed by a complex pattern of movements lasting 25-100 seconds. Patients may make cycling or kicking motions with their limbs. Rocking of the trunk may occur. Tonic asymmetric or dystonic posture of the limbs may also occur. ENWs last up to three minutes and consist of the patient jumping out of bed, moving around, talking unintelligibly or screaming, with a terrified expression. Dystonic posturing may occur.

Because of these unusual features, NFLE is often misdiagnosed as a nonepileptic seizure or as SWS parasomnias. NFLE can be distinguished, however, from SWS parasomnias by historical features (Table 6). One of the most important distinguishing characteristics of NFLE is the stereotypic nature of these behaviors, unlike most SWS parasomnias. An important distinction with nonepileptic seizures is that in NFLE and SWS parasomnias the episodes arise from sleep, whereas nonepileptic seizures may occur nocturnally but arise from a waking EEG. A good response to carbamazepine before bed, even at low doses, can be useful in distinguishing NFLE from alternative diagnoses; however, up to one-third of patients with NFLE may be resistant to antiepileptic drug treatment. It should be noted that occasionally patients with temporal lobe seizures might have exclusively or predominantly nocturnal seizures as well.

10. Insomnia

Insomnia is the subjective report by a patient of the inability to initiate sleep, maintain sleep, or of nonrestorative sleep with daytime consequences. Insomnia is best viewed as a symptom rather than a diagnosis. Rates of insomnia in general medical practice range from 10%-34%. Acute insomnia commonly occurs in the setting of stress or time zone change and can be managed with behavioral treatments and in certain instances with the judicious transient use of hypnotics. Chronic insomnia most commonly occurs in the setting of psychiatric disease, especially in the form of depression. Other common causes of insomnia include shift work, medical conditions that disrupt sleep (ie, chronic lung disease), pain that disrupts sleep, or medications that may disrupt sleep (ie, beta-blockers). Insomnia may be a symptom of a primary sleep disorder such as RLS, or less commonly OSAS. Poor sleep hygiene such as the consumption of evening caffeine or watching television in bed can also lead to insomnia.

Psychophysiologic insomnia is the principal form of primary insomnia encountered by sleep specialists. The essential feature of the disorder is conditioned arousal to efforts to sleep accompanied by negative expectations about sleep. When entering the bedroom, patients become increasingly anxious because of their concern or fear of their inability to sleep. Patients may report they sleep better in environments outside their own bedroom or may doze off involuntarily but be unable to sleep when they intend to fall asleep. Fatigue rather than excessive daytime sleepiness, however, is more likely to be the daytime complaint.

In the treatment of chronic insomnia it is important to address any underlying triggers or causes, such as pain or depression if present. Any underlying sleep disorders that might lead to insomnia should be treated as well, such as RLS. Good sleep hygiene is also important in that patients should reserve the bedroom for sleep and sex, avoid caffeine after noon, wind down in the evening, maintain a regular schedule, avoid napping, and avoid watching the clock. Behavioral treatments, beyond good sleep hygiene, can be helpful in the treatment of insomnia from a number of different causes and are particularly helpful in psychophysiologic insomnia. Stimulus control therapy consists of instructing the patient that, once in bed trying to sleep, to get up after 20 minutes if sleep is not achieved. They should do something that is relaxing in a different room, then return to bed when feeling sleepy. Sleep restriction therapy involves limiting time in bed so that once a subject gets to bed the sleep drive overwhelms the hyperarousal so that sleep is achieved. Other strategies such as progressive muscle relaxation may also be of some benefit. The role of medication in the treatment of chronic insomnia is unclear, but it may be a useful adjunct to behavioral therapies in certain patients.

11. Sleep in Specific Neurological Disorders

Stroke

There appears to be a bi-directional relationship between cerebrovascular accidents (CVA) and sleep-disordered breathing. Large population-based studies such as the Sleep Heart Health Study have linked OSAS with stroke, heart failure and myocardial infarction. The increased incidence of OSAS among TIA patients would suggest OSAS may be a risk factor for stroke. The means by which OSA may cause stroke or TIA is probably multifactorial. Many mechanisms have been proposed, such as elevated catecholamine levels leading to thrombosis, nocturnal desaturations directly leading to ischemia, or increased intracranial pressure after an apnea leading to decreased cerebral perfusion. The daytime hypertension that has been associated with OSAS may also mediate some of the increase in stroke risk among patients with OSAS.

Stroke, depending on location, may also lead to sleep-disordered breathing. As mentioned previously, there is an elevated incidence of OSAS in patients studied after stroke. Damage to the nucleus ambiguous or its outflow to the upper airway has been shown to cause OSAS. Bihemispheric strokes, as well as increased intracranial pressure, have been shown to cause CSR. In the waking state, CSR has been identified among patients with unilateral hemispheric or infratentorial strokes. Several unusual breathing patterns have been identified after brain stem stroke. Rare breathing disturbances, which can be seen after some types of brainstem strokes, include apneustic breathing (inspiratory breath holding), Biot's breathing (ataxic breathing) or Ondine's curse (failure of automatic breathing).

There is an interplay between circadian rhythms and stroke. Stroke, like myocardial infarction, occurs most frequently between the hours of 6 AM and noon. The reason for this variation is probably multifactorial. This relationship varies with the type of stroke as well. Ischemic stroke is more likely than intracerebral hemorrhage or subarachnoid hemorrhage to occur at night. Stroke may also alter circadian rhythms. Autonomic functions, which follow circadian patterns, can have their patterns disturbed by stroke, especially if the right hemisphere and insula are involved. Circadian related endocrine functions may also be disrupted by stroke. Cortisol-axis abnormalities have been identified acutely after stroke.

Hypersomnolence syndromes have been described after stroke in many different locations. Hypersomnia after stroke is most often seen as the result of bilateral or occasionally unilateral damage to the paramedian thalamus. The hypersomnia related to paramedian thalamic infarcts may be mild, especially in unilateral infarcts, or severe (ie, sleep behavior lasting over 20 hours per day). Some patients may recover within a few months and some may have persistent hypersomnia for over one year. Even if there is recovery from the hypersomnia there may be residual apathy, psychomotor slowing, attentional deficits and amnesia. L-dopa, methylphenidate, bromocriptine or mazindol may result in some improvement. Rather than true hypersomnia, a pseudohypersomnia consisting of compulsive pre-sleep behavior and increased behavioral sleep as opposed to true sleep has also been reported in bilateral paramedian thalamic infarcts as well.

Insomnia is a common complaint after a stroke. The etiology is often multifactorial. Stroke patients are usually in a different environment, less active, and may have difficulty emotionally adjusting to the stroke. Stroke patients may have pre-existing medical disorders, such as congestive heart failure, which could precipitate insomnia. Mood disorders or infections may also contribute to insomnia in the poststroke period. Medications given after a stroke may also play a role. Beta-antagonists and antidepressants are two classes of drugs commonly used after stroke that may cause insomnia. Insomnia directly related to damaged brain tissue is thought rare. Thalamic, thalamomesencephalic and large tegmento-basal pontine strokes have been reputed to cause depressive symptoms and insomnia via an inversion of the sleep-wake schedule. Good sleep hygiene, restoration of normal environmental cues, regularization of the sleep schedule, treating underlying mood disorders, and avoiding medications known to cause insomnia may all be helpful strategies.

Myotonic Dystrophy

Myotonic dystrophy is a disorder inherited in an autosomal dominant fashion, characterized by degeneration in multiple organ systems. Characteristic features include myotonia, progressive muscular weakness (particularly in the face, jaw and neck), gonadal atrophy, frontal balding, cataracts, and cardiac dysrhythmia. Patients with this disorder potentially have multiple sleep disorders. Alveolar hypoventilation, as well as central and obstructive apneas, have been described in these patients. Daytime sleepiness, however, may occur in the absence of sleep disordered breathing in these patients, suggestive of a primary disorder of hypersomnolence. The presence of SOREMPs in these patients supports this hypothesis. There appears to be a loss of serotinergic neurons in the dorsal raphe nucleus and superior central nucleus in myotonic dystrophy patients with hypersomnia, when compared to myotonic dystrophy patients without hypersomnia and controls. This hypersomnolence has been shown to respond to methylphenidate and modafinil.

12. References

1. *International Classification of Sleep Disorder: Diagnostic and Coding Manual*. 2nd ed.

2. Badr MS. Central sleep apnea syndrome. In: *Sleep Medicine*. 1st ed. Philadelphia, Pa: Hanley & Belfus; 2002:357-363.

3. Brooks SN, Mignont E. Narcolepsy and idiopathic hypersomnia. In: *Sleep Medicine*. 1st ed. Philadelphia, Pa: Hanley & Belfus; 2002:193-202.

4. Broughton RJ. Behavioral parasomnias. In: Chrokroverty S, ed. *Sleep Disorders Medicine*. 2nd ed. Woburn, Mass: Butterworth-Heinemann; 1999:635-660.

5. Burns RE, Sateia MJ, Lee-Chiong TL. Basic principles of chronobiology and disorders of circadian sleep-wake rhythm. In: *Sleep Medicine*. 1st ed. Philadelphia, Pa: Hanley & Belfus; 2002:245-254.

6. Carskadon MA, Dement WC. Normal human sleep: an overview. In: Kryger MH, ed. *Principles and Practice of Sleep Medicine*. 3rd ed. Philadelphia, Pa: WB Saunders; 2000:15-25.

7. D'Ambrosio CM. Miscellaneous syndromes causing excessive daytime sleepiness. In: *Sleep Medicine*. 1st ed. Philadelphia, Pa: Hanley & Belfus; 2002:193-202.

8. Fantini ML, Ferni-Strambi L, Montplaisir J. Idiopathic REM sleep behavior disorder: Toward a better nosologic definition. *Neurology*. 2005;64(5):780-786.

9. Greenough GP. Miscellaneous Neurological Disorders and Sleep. In: *Sleep Medicine*. 1st ed. Philadelphia, Pa: Hanley & Belfus; 2002:533-539.

10. Guilleminault C, Pelayo R. Idiopathic central nervous system hypersomnia. In: Kryger MH, ed. *Principles and Practice of Sleep Medicine*. 3rd ed. Philadelphia, Pa: WB Saunders; 2000:687-692.

11. Hening WA, et al. Motor functions and dysfunctions of sleep. In: Chrokroverty S, ed. *Sleep Disorders Medicine*. 2nd ed. Woburn.

12. Javaheri S. Central Sleep Apnea. In Lee-Chiong T, ed. *Sleep, A Comprehensive Handbook*. Hoboken, NJ. Wiley-Liss; 2006: 249-262.

13. Nieto JF, et al. Association of sleep-disordered breathing, sleep apnea, and hypertension in a large community-based study. *JAMA*. 2000;283(14):1829-1836.

14. Malow BA, Plazzi G. Nocturnal seizures. In: Chokroverty S, Hening WA, Walters AS, eds.

15. Olson EJ, et al. Obstructive sleep apnea hypopnea syndrome. *Mayo Clin Proc*. 2003;78:1545-1552.

16. Sateia MJ, Nowell PD. Insomnia. *Lancet*. 2004;364:1959-1973

17. Schenck CH. REM-sleep-associated parasomnias. In: *Sleep Medicine*. 1st ed. Philadelphia, Pa: Hanley & Belfus; 2002:215-224.

13. Questions

1. A 19-year-old female presents with a history of excessive daytime sleepiness. She reports the irresistible urge to take naps during the day. The naps, about 20 minutes in length, are somewhat restorative. Sleep time at night is adequate. She also reports frequent episodes of visual hallucinations sometimes accompanied by a feeling of being paralyzed upon awakening. Her physical exam is unremarkable. Body mass index is 22, blood pressure 110/70 and heart rate is 65 and regular. After history and physical exam the next diagnostic option(s) should be:

A. Polysomnography with MSLT if the polysomnogram is nondiagnostic

B. Polysomnography with MWT if the polysomnogram is nondiagnostic

C. MSLT only

D. MWT only

E. HLA typing

2. A diagnosis of narcolepsy is made in the patient in question one. Initial treatment for the excessive daytime sleepiness could include:

A. Modafinil, methylphenidate or dextroamphetamine

B. Modafinil, clomipramine or imipramine

C. Modafinil, fluoxetine or venlafaxine

D. Modafinil, pramipexole or ropinirole

E. Nasal CPAP

3. A 56-year-old male presents for evaluation of a daytime sleepiness complaint. He lives alone, so there is no bed partner. He allows regularly a seemingly adequate amount of sleep time. The most likely diagnosis in this setting is:

A. Narcolepsy

B. Idiopathic hypersomnia

C. Obstructive sleep apnea

D. Nocturnal epilepsy

4. A 52-year-old female presents complaining of difficulty getting to sleep. On questioning she reports an uncomfortable feeling in her calves in the evening when sedentary, associated with a strong desire to move her legs that prevents sleep onset. She is up pacing for two hours each night as that is the only thing that offers her some relief. The most likely diagnosis is:

A. Obstructive sleep apnea

B. Central sleep apnea

C. Psychophysiologic insomnia

D. Restless legs syndrome

E. Agitated depression

5. What further evaluative procedure or test would you offer to the woman in question four?

A. Ferritin level

B. Psychiatry consultation

C. Polysomnography

D. Polysomnography with MSLT

E. MWT

6. After completing your testing, what treatment would you offer to the woman in question four?

A. Nasal continuous positive airway pressure

B. Acetazolamide

C. Cognitive behavioral therapy

D. A dopamine agonist

E. An antidepressant

7. A 77-year-old male presents to the emergency department with a facial laceration after jumping out of bed and hitting his face on a lamp. On questioning, it is revealed that he dreamt he was fighting off alien invaders and awoke in the midst of the fight, finding himself at his bedside. Similar episodes occur once or twice a week. The most likely sleep disorder in this patient is the following:

A. REM sleep behavior disorder

B. Sleepwalking

C. Nocturnal seizures

D. Sleep terrors

E. Confusional arousals

8. You are concerned that the patient in question 7 might have another associated condition with his sleep disorder. Which of the following disorders is most closely associated with the most likely diagnosis in the patient in question seven?

A. Frontotemporal dementia

B. Progressive supranuclear palsy

C. Alzheimer disease

D. Dementia with Lewy body disease

9. After confirming your diagnosis by polysomnography in the patient in question 7, what treatment do you offer the patient?

A. Cognitive Behavioral Therapy

B. CPAP

C. Clonazepam

D. Carbamazapine

E. Reassurance

10. A four-year-old wakes from sleep one night screaming, with his heart racing, and tachypnea. He is inconsolable. The episode lasts a few minutes then he goes back to sleep. He has no memory of the event the next day. This happened once before two months ago in the setting of a few days with later than normal bedtime. The distraught parents bring him to your office for evaluation. Your therapeutic or diagnostic recommendation would be which of the following:

A. Avoidance of sleep deprivation and reassurance

B. Nightly benzodiazepines

C. Polysomnography

D. MSLT

E. A nightly tricyclic antidepressant

11. A 63-year-old female has been diagnosed with moderate obstructive sleep apnea. The most effective treatment would be:

A. Uvulopalatopharyngoplasty

B. Nasal continuous positive airway pressure

C. Oral appliance

D. Modafinil

12. A 17-year-old female presents with a two-year history of excessive daytime sleepiness, cataplexy, hypnogogic hallucinations and sleep paralysis. The symptom most specific for narcolepsy is:

A. Sleep paralysis

B. Excessive daytime sleepiness

C. Hypnogogic hallucinations

D. Cataplexy

13. Central apneas may develop in all of the following situations EXCEPT:

A. Upper airway collapse

B. Congestive heart failure

C. Multisystem atrophy

D. Neuromuscular disease

E. Idiopathic hypersomnia

14. The endogenous circadian pacemaker is the:

A. Dorsal raphe nucleus

B. Suprachiasmatic nucleus

C. Pineal gland

D. Medial thalamus

E. Locus ceruleus

15. Which of the following statements about seizures in the syndrome of nocturnal frontal lobe epilepsy (NFLE) is true?

A. Seizures in NFLE are stereotyped within an individual

B. Seizures in NFLE always have an abnormal surface EEG ictally

C. Seizures in NFLE usually resolve after adolescence

D. Seizures in NFLE characteristically last 5-10 minutes

E. Seizures in NFLE always respond to carbamazepine

16. Stroke of the bilateral paramedian thalamus has been associated with which of the following syndromes:

A. Obstructive sleep apnea syndrome

B. Central sleep apnea syndrome

C. Hypersomnolence syndrome

D. Restless legs syndrome

E. Delayed sleep phase syndrome

17. Bright light in the morning in an individual with a normal circadian rhythm would have what effect?

A. Phase delay

B. Phase advance

C. Development of a non-24-hour circadian rhythm

D. Pseudo-hypersomnolence

18. The hypothalamic neuropeptide thought to play an important role in narcolepsy is which of the following:

A. Hypocretin

B. Glutamate

C. GABA

D. Narcoleptin

E. Leptin

19. A 67-year-old male with a history of dilated cardiomyopathy (ejection fraction of 25%) presents to your office with complaints of daytime sleepiness and restless sleep. He and his wife (a keen observer) deny snoring but she reports pauses in his breathing at night. On exam his BMI is 24 and his lungs reveal bibasilar crackles. The best test or tests to make the diagnosis in this patient is/are:

A. MSLT

B. Actigraphy

C. Polysomnography

D. Overnight oximetry

20. The most likely diagnosis to be revealed by the testing on the patient in question 19 is:

A. Central Alveolar Hypoventilation

B. Cheyne-Stokes Respiration

C. Narcolepsy

D. Acromegaly

E. Opioid abuse

Answers

1. A.

Given the complaint of excessive daytime sleepiness despite adequate nocturnal sleep time, polysomnography is a prudent next evaluative step. The patient's age, and normal body mass index coupled with the complaints of excessive daytime sleepiness raise the question of a primary disorder of hypersomnolence. The sleep-related hallucinations, sleep paralysis and brief refreshing naps are suggestive but not diagnostic of narcolepsy. Given the likelihood of narcolepsy, MSLT the day after the polysomnogram would be useful. In the absence of cataplexy, sleep onset REM periods on the MSLT are needed to make the diagnosis of narcolepsy.

2. A.

Modafinil and the traditional stimulants (methylphenidate and dextroamphetamine) may help relieve the excessive daytime sleepiness associated with narcolepsy. Chlomipramine, imipramine, fluoxetine and venlafaxine through their noradrenergic action may be helpful for cataplexy. Pramipexole and ropinirole are dopamine agonists and have a role in the treatment of the restless legs syndrome but not narcolepsy. Nasal CPAP is useful for the treatment of obstructive sleep apnea.

3. C.

Excessive daytime sleepiness has many etiologies including sleep disorders. Of the sleep disorders listed in this question obstructive sleep apnea is the most common; hence, the most likely cause of this patient's sleepiness. Given the absence of a bed partner the physician is unlikely to be able to elicit many historical features suggestive of sleep apnea, such as snoring or observed apnea.

4. D.

Discomfort in the lower extremities, associated with a desire to move the legs and temporary relief with movement that occurs primarily in the evening or when sedentary, is highly suggestive of the restless legs syndrome. Sleep disordered breathing (central or obstructive sleep apnea) may be associated with an insomnia complaint but should not directly lead to leg discomfort. In psychophysiologic insomnia or depression, patients may describe difficulty "shutting their minds off," but not specifically leg discomfort limited to the evening.

5. A.

Ferritin levels less than 50 ng/mL have been associated with the restless legs syndrome. In patients with low or low normal ferritin levels iron replacement may help alleviate the symptoms. Polysomnography is not necessary for the evaluation of straightforward restless legs complaints.

6. D.

The most effective treatments for the restless legs syndrome are the dopamine agonists. Other treatment options might include opiates, benzodiazapenes, or some anticonvulsants.

7. A.

Nocturnal dream enactment, especially with violent content, is suggestive of REM sleep behavior disorder. Most patients with this disorder are older males. Slow wave sleep parasomnias (sleep walking, sleep terrors and confusional arousals) are more common in pediatric populations and are not typically associated with violent dream content. Nocturnal seizures are most likely to arise from NREM sleep, so associated dream content would not be characteristic.

8. D.

RBD appears to be associated with the synucleinopathies, which include Parkinson disease, multisystem atrophy and dementia with Lewy bodies. The RBD symptomatology may precede the development of the neurodegenerative disorder by many years.

9. C

The treatment shown to be most efficacious for RBD is clonazepam. Melatonin and dopaminergic agents may also be helpful.

10. A

The event described is most suggestive of a night terror given the age, autonomic arousal, and amnesia to the event. Sleep extension and reassurance are the first line of therapy. Medication is not usually necessary.

11. B

Nasal CPAP is the most effective therapy for obstructive sleep apnea. Oral appliance and uvulopalatopharyngoplasty are less likely to normalize the breathing at night. Modafinil can help address a consequence of sleep apnea (the sleepiness) but does not address the underlying airway obstruction or the other consequences of sleep apnea (hypertension, etc.).

12. D.

Sleep paralysis, sleep-related hallucinations and excessive daytime sleepiness are nonspecific symptoms and can be seen in a number of sleep disorders. Cataplexy, if present in the setting of excessive daytime sleepiness, is highly suggestive of narcolepsy.

13. E.

Central apneas may have many different causes. Congestive heart failure may lead to Cheyne-Stokes respirations. Upper airway obstruction may lead to central apneas. Neuromuscular disease may lead to hypercapnia and central apneas. Disorders characterized by autonomic dysfunction such as multisystem atrophy may lead to central apneas. Idiopathic hypersomnia is not associated with any respiratory abnormalities.

14. B.

Circadian rhythms are endogenous in that they persist under a wide array of environmental conditions or situations. The suprachiasmatic nucleus (SCN) located in the anterior hypothalamus acts as the master generator of circadian rhythms in mammals. The SCN exerts influence over a wide variety of physiologic functions ranging from hormone levels to body temperature to the sleep-wake cycle. Photic information is transmitted to the SCN via the retinohypothalmic tract from the retina. The SCN sends projections to the pineal gland to regulate the output of melatonin. Melatonin secretion is inhibited by exposure to light.

15. A.

NFLE typically starts in adolescence and persists. NFLE events occur multiple times per month and sometimes more than once per night. The episodes tend to be stereotyped but variable from individual to individual. The seizures in NFLE last seconds and typically arise from stage two sleep. Rarely does an ictal EEG capture an abnormality.

16. C.

Hypersomnia after stroke may be seen as the result of bilateral or occasionally unilateral damage to the paramedian thalamus. The hypersomnia related to paramedian thalamic infarcts might be mild, especially in unilateral infarcts, or severe. Some patients may recover within a few months and some may have persistent hypersomnia for over one year. Even if there is recovery from the hypersomnia there may be residual apathy, psychomotor slowing, attentional deficits and amnesia. Rather than true hypersomnia, a pseudohypersomnia consisting of compulsive pre-sleep behavior and increased behavioral sleep as opposed to true sleep has also been reported in bilateral paramedian thalamic infarcts as well.

17. B.

The primary environmental cue that works to entrain the circadian pacemaker is light. The intensity, duration and timing of the light exposure determines its effect on the circadian pacemaker. There are a variety of nonphotic stimuli (food, social cues, exercise, etc.), which may modulate the circadian rhythm, but their effects tend to be less than that of photic stimulation. A phase delay occurs when sufficient light is presented near the start of the subjective night (ie, bright light in the evening), and a phase advance occurs when sufficient light is presented near the end of the subjective night (ie, bright light in the morning).

18. A.

In narcolepsy, the connection between hypocretin-containing neurons and the locus ceruleus may be pivotal. The locus ceruleus is typically active during wakefulness but ceases firing prior to and during REM sleep. Hypocretin neurons appear to normally excite the locus ceruleus. If there were a functional defect in hypocretin transmission there would be less opposition to REM sleep, thereby possibly allowing the inappropriate intrusion of REM sleep.

19. C.

CSR is the most likely disorder in this case and is best demonstrated on polysomnography. MSLT and MWT are measures of daytime sleepiness. Overnight oximetry would not reliably detect a sleep-related breathing disorder and would not be able to differentiate between a central or obstructive sleep apnea syndrome.

20. B.

CSR is characterized by regular cycles of crescendo-decrescendo tidal volume with a central apnea occurring at the nadir of ventilatory drive and arousal occurring at the zenith. Congestive heart failure is the setting in which this disorder is most common. The etiology of CSR remains unclear but the resting pCO_2 in CHF patients is closer to the apneic threshold than in normals. If arterial pCO_2 is lowered below the apneic threshold, breathing ceases until pCO_2 rises. On this basis, even modest hyperventilation may lead to a central apnea.

Chapter 16: Neuro-oncology

Denise M. Damek, MD

Contents

1. Common Signs and Symptoms of Brain Tumors

The clinical presentation of brain tumors varies widely and depends upon the location of the tumor mass and its growth rate. Signs and symptoms may be nonlocalizing or focal. In some cases, brain tumors are discovered as an incidental finding.

Nonlocalizing signs and symptoms include: headache, nausea/vomiting, lethargy, confusion/disorientation, generalized seizures, and papilledema. These symptoms are most commonly seen in the setting of a rapidly growing, space-occupying lesion causing increased intracranial pressure or obstructive hydrocephalus. In most brain tumor patients, headaches are the result of increased intracranial pressure, and do not lateralize to the site of the tumor. These headaches increase in severity over days to weeks, are intermittent, more prominent in the early morning and with supine body positioning, and are aggravated by maneuvers that can increase intracranial pressure such as coughing, sneezing, or Valsalva maneuvers. They are frequently accompanied by other nonlocalizing signs and symptoms. In contrast, headaches that result from focal pressure on nerve endings in the dura and blood vessels may indicate tumor location. For example, tumors in the anterior and/or middle cranial fossa may produce frontal, in particular, supraorbital headaches, while those in the posterior fossa may present with suboccipital pain.

Nausea and vomiting are generally a manifestation of increased intracranial pressure; however, in rare instances they may represent tumor invasion of the area postrema or vagal nucleus in the posterior fossa. Rapid increases in intracranial pressure due to acute obstructive hydrocephalus can result in projectile vomiting. Nausea may also occur in conjunction with disequilibrium and vertigo due to increased pressure on medullary nuclei and the vestibular apparatus.

Seizures commonly herald the diagnosis of slow growing or low-grade superficially located tumors, such as oligodendrogliomas, brain metastases, and meningiomas. Moreover, approximately 30% of all brain tumor patients develop seizures at some point in time during their disease course, irrespective of tumor type. Focal seizures and complex partial seizures are most commonly reported, but primary and secondarily generalized seizures are also seen.

Roughly 10% of adults presenting with new onset seizures are found to harbor a tumor. In contrast, intracranial tumors are found in less than 1% of cases of new onset seizures in children. Neuroimaging should be pursued in all adults with new onset seizures, and in children with difficult to control partial seizures.

Brain tumors may cause any focal neurological deficit, depending upon their location. Symptom onset is generally subacute with progression over days to weeks. The symptoms result from the tumor location itself, local mass effect, or as a consequence of surrounding vasogenic edema.

Endocrine dysfunction is common in parasellar tumors, in particular those involving the pituitary gland and hypothalamus. Tumors that result in pituitary hormone hypersecretion produce symptoms such as gigantism, Cushing disease, galactorrhea, and precocious puberty. Alternatively, tumors that destroy normal gland tissue, thus reducing hormone production, lead to syndromes such as hypothyroidism, diabetes insipidus, syndrome of inappropriate antidiuretic hormone secretion, infertility, loss of libido, and amenorrhea.

2. Establishing the Diagnosis

The diagnostic suspicion of a brain tumor begins with the neurological history and physical examination. All patients with symptoms or signs of increased intracranial pressure or new focal neurological deficits should undergo a brain imaging study. Brain imaging will delineate the location and extent of the lesion, and will identify specific imaging characteristics such as the presence or absence of enhancement. This information, along with that provided during the history and physical examination, will help exclude other diagnostic possibilities and guide further evaluation.

The patient's age and lesion location can provide valuable diagnostic clues. Certain tumors demonstrate a predilection for a specific age group. For example, in adults, no tumors arise in the neurons themselves, and in children, meningiomas and metastatic tumors are distinctly uncommon. Seventy percent to 80% of childhood tumors arise infratentorially or within midline brain structures. However, in adults, tumors occur more frequently within the brain parenchyma or lateral brain structures.

A noncontrast head CT, which is often the screening examination of choice in the emergency room setting, is not sensitive enough to exclude a CNS lesion. However, with the addition of contrast-enhanced images, a head CT can detect most tumors >1 cm in diameter. There are inherent limitations to CT imaging, primarily beam hardening artifact caused by adjacent cranial bone. This manifests as obscurations across brain structures that are in close proximity to the skull, such as the cerebellum, brain stem, anterior temporal lobes and inferior frontal lobes. Brain magnetic resonance imaging (MRI) provides many advantages over head CT, and has become the standard imaging choice for evaluation and follow-up of brain tumors. With brain MRI, patients are not exposed to radiation or iodinated contrast agents, multiplanar images are available, skull-based and posterior fossa lesions are much better visualized, and the anatomical extent of the tumor and its related effects on surrounding brain are better delineated. However, not all patients can undergo brain MRI. Absolute contraindications to brain MRI include the presence of a cardiac pacemaker or other implanted electrical device, the presence of metal implants or fragments in soft tissue (ie, metal fragments in the eye, some aneurysm clips, etc.) and morbid obesity. Many heart valves, in particular those produced in the last decade, are MR compatible. MRI is not hazardous to patients with middle ear prosthesis per se; however, the device itself can be damaged. Pregnancy, in particular the first trimester, is a relative but not absolute contraindication to MRI. It should be emphasized that while brain MRI is very sensitive for the detection of CNS lesions, it lacks specificity. Tissue is always required to confirm the diagnosis.

The decision to biopsy or resect the tumor depends on many factors. If the suspected tumor is generally very sensitive to treatment, such as germ cell tumors or lymphomas, often a diagnostic biopsy is pursued. If the suspected tumor is potentially curable by surgery, a resection may be pursued. For other tumors, resection is often pursued if the majority of the tumor can be surgically removed with minimal risk of causing a new or worsened neurological deficit. Biopsies do not always provide a definitive diagnosis. The majority of primary brain tumors are microscopically heterogeneous. As a consequence, the biopsy sample, which generally is a tiny fraction of the entire lesion, may not be representative of the most aggressive component of the tumor. This is referred to as sampling error and is a potential pitfall of biopsy.

All pathologic specimens are subjected to routine histological assessment, immunocytochemical analysis, and more frequently, genetic analysis. Histological assessment evaluates the morphology of the lesion. Immunocytochemistry identifies specific proteins within tumor cells that can help differentiate tumors of similar morphology. For instance, the most helpful immunostain for confirming a diagnosis of meningioma is epithelial membrane antigen (EMA). Gliomas and schwannomas stain positively for S-100. Glial fibrillary acidic protein (GFAP) is useful to identify astrocytoma and ependymal tumors, and synaptophysin labels neurons within brain, spine, and retinal tissue. Genetic changes can identify distinct tumor subtypes within tumors of similar morphological appearance, and certain genetic characteristics may portend prognosis and response to therapy. For example, loss of heterozygosity (LOH) of the long arm of chromosome 19q is seen in 50%-80% of oligodendrogliomas. Furthermore, LOH of chromosome 1p in these tumors correlates with prognosis in patients with anaplastic oligodendrogliomas. Patients whose tumors have loss of heterozygosity (LOH) on 1p or combined LOH on 1p and 19q survive substantially longer (mean 10 years) than patients whose tumors lack these genetic changes (mean 2 years).

3. Staging

It is exceedingly rare for primary brain tumors to spread outside of the central nervous system, so staging evaluations of organs in the rest of the body (ie, CT scans of the chest/abdomen/pelvis, bone scans, etc.) are not routinely performed. Certain tumors, however, tend to spread within the central nervous system to the cerebrospinal fluid, leptomeninges, and spinal cord. These include lymphoma, medulloblastoma, pineoblastomas, germinomas, ependymomas, choroids plexus tumors, and rarely, malignant astrocytomas. In these cases, the entire neuroaxis (brain and spinal cord) is imaged and cerebrospinal fluid is obtained for cytologic examination. In addition, in patients with primary central nervous system lymphoma, an ophthalmologic slit lamp examination is pursued to exclude tumor spread to the vitreous.

4. Classification of Primary Brain Tumors

The World Health Organization (WHO) classification system, last updated in 2000, is the most commonly used classification system for primary brain tumors (Table 1). Brain tumors are generally, but not always, named according to the cell or tissue of origin. For example, gliomas are a group of primary brain tumors arising from the supporting tissue of the nervous system, or glial cells. These include astrocytes, oligodendrocytes, and ependymal cells. Uncontrolled growth of these cells gives rise respectively to astrocytomas, oligodendrogliomas, and ependymomas. Tumors containing a high proportion of more than one cell type are classified as mixed gliomas, and the name—for example, oligoastrocytoma—reflects each component.

In some instances, the cell of origin is not intuitive based on the name. An example is craniopharyngiomas, which are tumors that arise from small nests of cells located near the pituitary stalk. Furthermore, some tumors are classified based upon location. For instance, primitive neuroectodermal tumors (PNETs) located in the cerebellum are called medulloblastomas, while those occurring in the pineal region are called PNETs of the pineal gland or pineoblastomas, and those involving the cerebral hemispheres are called supratentorial PNETs. Likewise, when gliomas are located in areas that are not easily biopsied for a histopathological diagnosis, they are labeled by location rather than by specific glial cell type. Examples are optic tract glioma and brainstem glioma.

Table 1

World Health Organization Brain Tumor Grading System

WHO Grade	Aggressiveness/ Growth Rate	Microscopic Appearance	Examples	Typical Treatment
I	Least malignant Slow growing	Almost normal appearance	Pilocytic astrocytoma Craniopharyngioma Gangliocytoma Ganglioglioma Meningioma	Observation Surgery
II	Relatively slow growing Can invade adjacent normal tissue Can recur	Slightly abnormal appearance	Astrocytoma Oligodendroglioma	Surgery Radiation therapy
III	Malignant Intermediate growth rate Infiltrate adjacent normal brain tissue Tend to recur, often as a higher grade	Actively reproducing abnormal cells	Anaplastic astrocytoma Anaplastic oligodendroglioma Atypical meningioma	Surgery Radiation therapy Chemotherapy
IV	Highly malignant Infiltrate widely	Bizarre appearance Induce new blood vessel proliferation (endothelial proliferation) Often contain areas of necrosis	Glioblastoma multiforme Medulloblastoma Lymphoma	Surgery Radiation therapy Chemotherapy Experimental therapies

Primary central nervous system lymphomas are unique in that their cell of origin may not arise within the nervous system or adjacent tissues, yet they are still considered primary brain tumors. Because the central nervous system is devoid of lymphoid tissue, it has been postulated that these tumors likely arise within the lymphoid tissue of the body and migrate into the central nervous system. However, only 5%-10% of patients with CNS lymphoma will manifest systemic lymphoma during their lifetime or at autopsy.

5. Grading System for Primary Brain Tumors

Brain tumors are graded in order to facilitate communication between the patient and multiple physicians, in order to plan treatment, and to assess prognosis. The grade of the tumor reflects the degree to which its cells are different from normal cells, its tendency to spread, and its growth rate. Unlike the TNM (Tumor, Node, Metastasis) grading schema applied to most systemic cancers, brain tumor grading schema do not consider lymph node involvement or the presence of metastases, since these are exceedingly rare in primary brain tumors. The WHO 2000 classification system is the most commonly used grading system for primary brain tumors (Table 2). It provides an estimate of tumor malignancy using a scale of one to four. Other grading systems are also widely used for some tumor subtypes. For example, infiltrating astrocytomas are also commonly graded by the St. Anne/Mayo and the modified Ringertz systems. Not surprisingly, the natural history of many primary brain tumors is amenable to only a benign or malignant behavior designation, not a four-point scale. In these cases, the grading is generally based on the tumor subtype itself rather than a specific scale.

WHO grade I tumors are the least aggressive and slowest growing tumors. Microscopically they have an almost normal appearance and are usually associated with long-term survival. Observation only is warranted in many cases. In others, surgery alone can be effective treatment and might even be curative. Examples of grade I tumors are pilocytic astrocytomas, craniopharyngiomas, and meningiomas.

WHO grade II tumors are relatively slow growing and have a slightly abnormal microscopic appearance. They invade adjacent normal brain tissue and can recur or behave aggressively. Long-term survival is common. Treatment is maximally feasible surgical resection, possibly followed by radiation therapy. Examples include low grade gliomas.

WHO grade III tumors demonstrate an intermediate growth pattern and are considered malignant. Microscopically, these tumors are easily identified as abnormal and active tumor cell division is seen. These tumors are clinically aggressive, and tend to recur, often as a higher grade. Treatment is maximally feasible surgical resection, radiation therapy, and possibly chemotherapy. Examples include anaplastic astrocytoma and anaplastic oligodendrogliomas.

Table 2

World Health Organization Classification of CNS Tumors

Category	Approximate Percentage of Primary Brain Tumors	Major Subcategories
Neuroepithelial tumors	51%	Astrocytic tumors Oligodendroglial tumors Ependymal tumors Mixed gliomas Choroid plexus tumors Neuronal tumors Pineal tumors Embryonal tumors (includes primitive neuroectodermal tumors)
Tumors of cranial and spinal nerves	7%	Schwannoma Neurofibroma Malignant peripheral
Tumors of the meninges	25%	Meningioma Tumors of uncertain origin (includes hemangiopericytoma and capillary hemangioblastoma)
Hemopoietic tumors	4%	Lymphoma
Germ cell tumors	<1%	Includes germinoma, embryonal carcinoma, yolk sac tumor, coriocarcinoma, teratoma
Cysts and tumor-like lesions	<1%	Includes Rathke's cleft cyst, epidermoid cyst, dermoid cyst, colloid cyst, lipoma
Anterior pituitary tumors	9%	Pituitary adenoma Pituitary carcinoma
Local extensions of regional tumors	<1%	Craniopharyngioma Chordoma
Metastatic tumors	N/A	

WHO grade IV tumors are the most aggressive and fastest growing tumors. They have a bizarre appearance microscopically and widely infiltrate normal tissues. Because these rapidly growing tumors need more oxygen and food than the brain's existing blood vessels can supply, they secrete proteins that promote the growth of new blood vessels or angiogenesis. If angiogenesis cannot keep pace with tumor growth, focal areas of necrosis develop. Treatment is maximally feasible surgical resection, radiation therapy, chemotherapy, and possibly experimental protocols. While current treatments may prolong survival, they are generally ineffective at realizing long-term survival. For this reason, experimental treatments are often offered in hopes of improving the outcomes of standard therapy. Examples include glioblastoma multiforme tumors and medulloblastomas.

6. Treatment Overview

The symptomatic treatment of brain tumors includes treatment of increased intracranial pressure, pain, nausea/vomiting, and seizures. Corticosteroids are provided to control vasogenic edema prior to surgery, during radiation therapy, or at tumor recurrence. They are tapered as soon as possible to avoid side effects.

While the ultimate goal of surgery is the acquisition of diagnostic tissue, surgery is also frontline therapy for primary brain tumors. The goal of surgery is to establish the diagnosis and to remove the maximally feasible amount of tumor without causing a new neurological deficit. Potential benefits of tumor resection include possible cure, decreased intracranial pressure, improvement or resolution of neurological deficits caused by edema or tissue compression, improved seizure control, increased efficacy of additional therapies, and the provision of additional therapies such as the intraoperative placement of biodegradable wafers impregnated with chemotherapy.

Radiation therapy is provided for most brain tumors that are not cured by complete surgical resection. Radiation therapy damages DNA, which interferes with the tumor cell's ability to divide and ultimately survive. Some primary brain tumors, such as germinomas and lymphomas, are very sensitive to radiation therapy. In other tumors, such as grade IV astrocytomas (glioblastoma multiforme), radiation therapy increases survival but does not produce long term disease control or significant radiographic responses. Likewise, brain metastases from lymphomas, testicular cancers, and breast cancers have better response rates than the so-called "radio-resistant tumors" such as colon cancer, melanoma, and renal cell carcinoma. However, isolated clinical and radiographic responses in these tumors has led to the general practice of offering radiation therapy to all brain metastases patients irrespective of primary tumor type.

Chemotherapy is provided either before or after radiation in chemosensitive tumors such as oligodendrogliomas, germinomas, and lymphomas. For other primary brain tumors it is provided at initial diagnosis for tumors with a poor prognosis, or at disease recurrence or progression following surgery and radiation therapy. While surgery and radiation therapy are local treatment modalities, systemic chemotherapy is a more global therapy that has the potential to target microscopic tumor deposits distant from the primary lesion. Actively dividing cells, including most tumor cells and some normal cells, are the most vulnerable to chemotherapy. The main limitations of chemotherapy are its inability to adequately cross the blood-brain barrier, and systemic toxicity.

7. Selected Tumor Profiles

Tumors of Neuroepithelial Tissue

Diffuse Astrocytomas

Diffusely infiltrating astrocytomas account for more than 50% of all primary brain tumors, and are the most common primary brain tumor in both children and adults. These tumors may develop in essentially any region of the nervous system, reflecting the widespread distribution of their cell of origin, the astrocyte cell. Astrocytomas most commonly develop in the cerebral white matter in both children and adults. The brainstem is the second most commonly affected site. Localization in the cerebellum and spinal cord is uncommon. Mutations of the p53 gene on chromosome 17p occur in 40% of all astrocytic tumors, particularly in young adults. While astrocytomas are associated with some familial tumor syndromes (Table 3), familial clustering is rare and these tumors are not generally considered inheritable.

Diffuse astrocytomas have a wide range of histopathological features and biological behaviors, diffusely infiltrate brain structures, and have a tendency to progress to a more malignant phenotype (Table 4). Males are affected more than females. The age range at peak incidence increases with increasing tumor grade. Under the WHO 2000 criteria, diffuse astrocytomas that exhibit nuclear atypia and marked mitotic activity are classified as anaplastic astrocytomas (WHO grade III). If either vascular proliferation or necrosis is present, the neoplasm is upgraded to a glioblastoma multiforme tumor (WHO grade IV).

Oligodendrogliomas

Oligodendrogliomas arise from oligodendrocyte cells. These tumors are relatively uncommon, comprising only about 10% of all gliomas and less than 5% of all primary brain tumors. Mixed tumors, or oligoastrocytomas, are more common than pure oligodendroglial tumors. These tumors are typically located superficially within the cortex and white matter, and they often infiltrate overlying leptomeninges. Not surprisingly, they generally present with seizures, and up to 80% of patients with oligodendroglial tumors will have seizures at some point in their disease course. Oligodendrogliomas may be diagnosed at any age but occur most commonly in young and middle-aged adults, with a median age at diagnosis of 40-50 years. In children, only 6% of gliomas are diag-

Table 3

Familial Tumor Syndromes

Disease	Gene	Chromosome	Affected Protein/ Proposed Mechanism	Mode of Inheritance	Nervous System Manifestations	Skin Manifestations	Other Tissue Involvement
Neurofibromatosis Type I	NF1	17q11	Neurofibromin; inhibits the ras-oncogene pathway via activation of ras-GTPase	AD Variable penetrance Sporatic in 50%	Neurofibromas Plexiform neurofibromas MPNST Optic nerve gliomas Astrocytomas Hamartomas	Café-au-lait spots Axillary freckling Dermal neurofibromas	Iris hamartomas Osseous lesions Pheochromocytoma Leukemia Vascular dysplasias
Neurofibromatosis Type II	NF2	22q12	Merlin; a cytoskeletal protein of unknown oncogenic mechanism	AD Sporatic in 50%	Bilateral vestibular schwannomas Schwannomas and neurofibromas of cranial nerves/spinal roots Meningiomas Spinal ependymomas Astrocytomas Glial hamartias Cerebral calcifications Meningioangiomatosis	<6 café-au-lait spots	Posterior lens opacities Retinal hamartoma
Tuberous sclerosis	TSC1 TSC2	9q34 16p13	Hamartin, possible tumor suppressor function Tuberin; tumor suppressor function	AD Sporatic mutation in ~50%	Subependymal giant cell astrocytoma Cortical tubers	Cutaneous angiofibroma (adenoma sebaceum) Subungual and periunual fibromas Hypomelanotic macules Shagreen patch	Cardiac rhabdomyomas Hamartomas in multiple organs Renal adenomas and cysts

(continued)

Table 3 *(continued)*

Familial Tumor Syndromes

Disease	Gene	Chromosome	Affected Protein/ Proposed Mechanism	Mode of Inheritance	Nervous System Manifestations	Skin Manifestations	Other Tissue Involvement
von Hippel-Lindau	VHL	3p25	Unknown	AD	Hemangioblastomas		Rentinal hemangioblastomas Renal cell carcinoma Pheochromocytoma Visceral cysts Endolymphatic sac tumor
Bathing trunk epidermal nevus syndrome					Melanoma	Cutaneous melanoma	
Li-Fraumeni	TP53	17q13	Unknown; tumor suppressor function	AD	Astrocytomas PNET		Breast carcinoma Bone and soft tissue sarcomas Adrenocortical carcinoma leukemia
Cowden	PTEN (MMAC1)	10q23	Unknown; possible regulation of cell growth and differentiation	AD	Dysplastic gangliocytoma of the cerebellum (Lhermitte-Duclos) Megalencephaly	Multiple trichilemmomas Fibromas	Hamartomatous polyps of the colon Thyroid neoplasms Breast carcinoma
Turcot	APC hMLH1 hPSM2	5q21 3p21 7p22	Unknown	AD AR	Medulloblastoma Glioblastoma	 Café-au-lait spots	Colorectal polyps Colorectal polyps
Gorlin (Nevoid basal cell carcincoma syndrome)	PTCH	9q31	Unknown	AD	Medulloblastoma	Multiple basal cell carcinomas Palmar and plantar pits	Jaw cysts Ovarian fibromas Skeletal abnormalities

Table 4

Astrocytomas

Astrocytoma Type	**Pilocytic Astrocytoma**	**Low-Grade Astrocytoma**	**Anaplastic Astrocytoma**	**Glioblastoma Multiforme (GBM)**
WHO Grade	I	II	III	IV
Peak Incidence		30-40 years (mean age at biopsy 34 years)	30-40 years (mean age at biopsy 41 years)	45-70 years
Common Locations	Cerebellum Optic nerves Third ventricle Medial temporal lobe Brainstem	Cerebral hemispheres Brainstem Cerebellum Spinal cord	Cerebral hemispheres Brainstem Cerebellum Spinal cord	Frontotemporal region and parietal lobes predominate
MRI Characteristics	Well-circumscribed contrast-enhancing lesion, often cystic with a mural nodule	Hypointense on T1 Hyperintense on T2 Expansion of tissue No edema No enhancement	Hypointense on T1 Hyperintense on T2 Expansion of tissue/mass effect +/- edema +/- partial enhancement	Irregularly shaped lesions with heterogenous enhancement, often nodular peripheral rim enhancement with hypointense central necrosis and associated vasogenic edema
Histopathologic Features	Biphasic pattern of alternating micro-cysts and compact fiber-producing spindle cells Focal accumulation of Rosenthal fibers Nuclear atypia not associated with anaplasia	Increased number and size of normal-appearing astrocytes	Increased cellularity Nuclear atypia Mitotic activity	Bizarre-appearing astrocytes Mitotic activity Vascular proliferation Necrosis
Median Survival After Diagnosis		6-8 years	3-5 years	12 months

nosed as oligodendrogliomas. Radiographic features generally associated with more aggressive biological behavior such as necrosis, cyst formation, and hemorrhage may be present but are not associated with poor prognosis. Calcification is often present. Histopathologically, well-differentiated oligodendrogliomas have a characteristic fried egg or honeycomb appearance due to fixation artifact, and are associated with capillary sized blood vessels arranged in an acutely branching or chicken wire pattern. Overall, these tumors have a more favorable prognosis compared to astrocyte tumors. This is in part attributed to their indolent inherent biological behavior as well as an increased responsiveness to chemotherapy. Combined loss of heterozygosity for chromosomes 1p and 19q in anaplastic oligodendrogliomas is associated with a favorable response to chemotherapy.

Juvenile Pilocytic Astrocytoma

As the name suggests, juvenile pilocytic astrocytomas typically affect children and young adults. These tumors arise from astrocytes and may occur anywhere astrocytes are present. However, they have a predilection for cerebellum, brainstem, hypothalamic region, and optic pathways. In fact, they account for 80%-85% of cerebellar astrocytomas and 60% of optic nerve gliomas in children. The classic radiographic appearance of a cerebellar pilocytic astrocytoma is a well-circumscribed cystic lesion with a focal mural nodule. In other locations, lesions may appear more solid. Unlike diffuse astrocytomas, pilocytic astrocytomas are well demarcated and do not infiltrate surrounding brain tissue. In addition, they do not degenerate to a more malignant phenotype. When tumor location is amenable to surgery, complete surgical resection may be curative.

Dysembryonic Neuroepithelial Tumor

The dysembryonic neuroepithelial tumor (DNET) is composed of neurons and oligodendroglial-like cells clustered with intracortical nodules. They are indolent tumors and are frequently associated with cortical migration abnormalities. The majority arise within the temporal or frontal lobes and present with intractable partial epilepsy. Surgery is curative.

Pleomorphic Xanthoastrocytoma

Pleomorphic xanthoastrocytoma tumors are rare, usually benign tumors that affect children and young adults. Individuals typically present with intractable partial seizures or, less commonly, focal neurological deficits. Most lesions arise within the temporal or parietal lobes with a predilection for superficial cortex and leptomeningeal involvement.

Typical radiographic appearance is a large cyst with a superficially positioned mural nodule.

Ependymomas

Ependymomas arise from the ependymal cells that line the ventricles and the central canal of the spinal cord. They can present at any age, but are most common in childhood and adolescence. In children, ependymomas most commonly occur in children within the posterior fossa, in particular the fourth ventricular region. In fact, fourth ventricular region ependymomas represent 10% of all childhood brain tumors. In adults, these tumors are the most common primary neoplasm of the spinal cord, generally occurring in the fourth and fifth decades. Supratentorial ependymomas occur along the lateral ventricles or within the brain parenchyma adjacent to the ventricular surface. Spinal cord ependymomas occur anywhere along the length of the spinal cord and the filum terminale. Ependymomas may also extend along the leptomeninges or nerve roots, and may occur free-floating within the cerebrospinal fluid. Despite their tendency to disseminate, 85% of ependymomas are low-grade tumors. The neuroimaging characteristics of ependymomas are nonspecific, but some findings may suggest the diagnosis, such as calcification associated with a fourth ventricular mass. Ependymomas are potentially surgically curable; however, their location often precludes complete surgical resection.

Central Neurocytoma

Central neurocytoma is a mature neuronal intraventricular tumor, microscopically indistinguishable from oligodendroglioma. Its cell of origin is unknown. It typically occurs in a lateral ventricle near the foramen of Monroe, and occasionally extends into the third ventricle. Most tumors called intraventricular oligodendrogliomas in the past were probably central neurocytomas. Confirmation is provided by immunohistochemical demonstration of neuronal antigens or electron microscopic identification of neuronal features, such as cytoplasmic dense core granules.

Medulloblastoma

The medulloblastoma is a highly malignant embryonal tumor of predominantly neuronal differentiation. The exact cell of origin is unknown. Medulloblastomas are considered a subtype of primitive neuroectodermal tumor (PNET), and by definition are always located in the cerebellum. The vast majority of medulloblastomas are sporadic; however, several familial tumor syndromes have been linked to medulloblastomas, including p53 germ cell line mutations, Gorlin syndrome, and Turcot syndrome. Medulloblastomas are the most common malignant primary brain tumor in the pediatric population, but they can also occur in young to middle-aged adults. The majority of childhood medulloblastomas arise in the vermis of the cerebellum and often project into the fourth ventricle. Involvement of the cerebellar hemispheres is seen more frequently as the age of the patient increases. Medulloblastomas have an inherent tendency to metastasize via CSF pathways. Tumor cells may exist free floating in the cerebrospinal fluid, or may form nodular tumor deposits anywhere within the neuraxis. Disseminated disease is present in approximately one-third of patients at initial diagnosis. Rarely, disease may spread beyond the central nervous system to bone, lymph nodes, and/or soft tissue structures. Staging evaluations are routinely pursued. Medulloblastomas are fast-growing, aggressive tumors that require a multimodality treatment approach with surgery, radiation therapy, and chemotherapy.

Tumors of Cranial and Spinal Nerves

Schwannomas

Schwannomas are benign peripheral nerve sheath tumors that arise from Schwann cells. Schwannomas most commonly occur in peripheral nerves in the head and neck region and extensor aspects of the extremities, but they also can arise from spinal and cranial nerves. They account for roughly 8% of intracranial tumors and 29% of primary spinal tumors. Most schwannomas are solitary neoplasms that arise *de novo*. The exception is bilateral vestibular schwannomas, which are considered pathognomonic for neurofibromatosis type 2.

Grossly, schwannomas are discrete, well-encapsulated tumors that displace the nerve eccentrically. Histologically, schwannomas are composed of Antoni type A and type B regions. Type A tissue has elongated spindle cells arranged in irregular streams and is compact in nature. Type B tissue has a looser organization, often with cystic spaces intermixed within the tissue. Verocay bodies, characterized by palisades of nuclei separated by fibrillar anuclear zones, are typically seen in Antoni A areas of schwannomas. Immunohistochemically, schwannomas are invariably positive for the S-100 protein. These tumors are surgically curable if a complete tumor resection is feasible. Tumor location and extent of the lesion may preclude resection. Radiation may also play a role in treatment.

The most common intracranial schwannoma is the vestibular schwannoma or acoustic neuroma, followed in incidence by trigeminal and facial nerve schwannomas, and then glossopharyngeal, vagus, and spinal accessory nerve schwannomas. Schwannomas involving the oculomotor, trochlear, abducens, and hypoglossal nerves are rare.

Vestibular schwannomas, or acoustic neuromas, affect females more than males and typically occur in middle-aged adults. However, in patients with neurofibromatosis type II, vestibular schwannomas occur earlier , presenting in young adults or, less commonly, children. The most common presenting symptoms include progressive unilateral hearing loss, tinnitus, and gait imbalance. Vestibular schwannomas can compress vital structures such as cranial nerves, the brainstem, and the brain. A complete surgical resection is often possible.

Neurofibromas

Neurofibromas are benign, infiltrative peripheral nerve sheath tumors. Their cell of origin is unknown, but they are thought to possibly derive from Schwann cells, fibroblasts, and/or perineural cells. Neurofibromas are generally solitary, sporadically occurring tumors unrelated to any syndrome. However, multiple neurofibromas and plexiform neurofibromas are often associated with neurofibromatosis type I.

Unlike schwannomas, which tend to eccentrically displace the nerve, neurofibromas cause a fusiform enlargement of the nerve itself. Neurofibromas can occur in essentially any nerve with the exception of cranial nerves. However, they typically involve small nerves of the skin and present as a cutaneous nodule. Less commonly, they involve larger peripheral nerves or a nerve plexus. Malignant degeneration of a neurofibroma is rare. However, plexiform neurofibromas and neurofibromas of major nerves are antecedent to approximately two-thirds of all malignant peripheral nerve sheath tumors.

Because of the intimate involvement of neurofibromas with the nerve itself, these tumors cannot be dissected away from the nerve. Complete resection involves sacrificing the parent nerve. This is easily done if the neurofibroma is not involved with a major nerve. However, if a major nerve is involved, observation alone or subtotal resection may be considered.

Malignant Peripheral Nerve Sheath Tumors (MPNST)

Malignant peripheral nerve sheath tumors most commonly arise in a neurofibroma, often of the plexiform type. They may also arise *de novo* in any normal nerve. However, MPNSTs arising from cranial nerves or cranial nerve neuofibromas are exceedingly rare. Neurofibromas in neurofibromatosis type 1 may undergo malignant degeneration in 3%-10% of patients. Malignant transformation of a schwannoma is extremely rare; however, when it occurs, it is associated with neurofibromatosis type 1 in 75% of patients.

Tumors of the Meninges

Meningiomas are tumors that arise from arachnoidal cap cells associated with the arachnoid villi at the dural venous sinuses, cranial nerve foramina, cribriform plate, and the medial middle cranial fossa. Not surprisingly, frequent sites of tumor involvement include the parasagittal region, the convexity, the cerebellopontine angle, and the skull base. Intraventricular and spinal meningiomas are thought to arise respectively from meningothelial cells, which are present in the choroid plexus and arachnoid villa at the spinal nerve exit zones. Overall, meningiomas account for approximately 20%-25% of all primary brain tumors and an estimated 35% of all primary tumors of the spinal canal. Meningiomas are more common in women, with a 1.4-2.8:1 female-to-male ratio in intracranial meningiomas and a 10-20:1 female-to-male ratio in spinal meningiomas. The incidence of intracranial meningiomas increases with advancing age, with most occurring during the fourth through sixth decades of life. Meningiomas are rare in children. Approximately 90% of meningiomas are benign, solitary lesions. Multiple meningiomas are frequently, but not exclusively, seen in patients with neurofibromatosis type II.

Meningiomas are typically slow growing dural-based masses that cause symptoms due to compression of adjacent structures. Seizures, headache, and focal neurological symptoms are commonly reported. Many meningiomas are recognized as incidental findings on neuroimaging studies or at autopsy. Radiographically, on brain MRI, meningiomas appear as extra-axial broad-based dural lesions that are isointense to brain and show dense, uniform contrast enhancement. A "dural tail sign" is often seen on post-contrast imaging, reflecting the broad-based dural attachment. Often, focal expansion of the inner table of the skull overlying the mass can be seen. Histologically, nine subtypes of meningioma are recognized. The most helpful immunostain for confirming a diagnosis of meningioma is epithelial membrane antigen (EMA). Cytogenetically, meningiomas are associated with loss of chromosome 22, but this has little diagnostic utility. Standard therapies for benign meningiomas include observation for asymptomatic lesions and complete surgical resection, which can be curative. Recurrent meningiomas or higher-grade meningiomas are treated with surgical resection and radiation. The role of chemotherapy is unclear.

Under the WHO 2000 classification system, meningiomas are graded as WHO grade I meningioma, WHO grade II atypical meningioma, and WHO grade III anaplastic (malignant) meningioma. Seemingly contrary to its WHO grade I designation, invasion of mesenchymal tissues (dura, cranial bone, muscles, and scalp) is an intrinsic property of benign meningiomas and does not constitute criterion for upgrading to an atypical or anaplastic tumor. On the other hand, brain invasion in the absence of prior surgical procedures warrants upgrading to a diagnosis of atypical (WHO grade II) meningioma. Four of the nine recognized meningioma subtypes are automatically upgraded to WHO grade II tumors based on their potential for early recurrence and/or aggressive clinical behavior. These include the clear cell, chordoid, rhabdoid, and papillary histological subtypes.

Hemopoietic Neoplasms

Primary central nervous system lymphoma (PCNSL) is considered an extranodal malignant lymphoma that arises within the central nervous system in the absence of systemic disease. The exact tissue of origin of PCNSL is unknown. Presumably PCNSL arises within lymphoid tissue of the body and selectively migrates into the central nervous system, analogous to the MALT lymphomas of the gut—but this is only one of many theories and it remains unproven to date. Approximately 98% of PCNSL are diffuse large cell B-cell lymphomas. While PCNSL most commonly affects immunocompromised individuals, it is also seen in immunocompetent individuals. In patients with an intact immune system, the peak incidence of PCNSL is during the sixth and seventh decades. However, in individuals with an inherited immunodeficiency syndrome, the peak incidence is during childhood, while the peak incidence in transplant recipients and acquired immunodeficiency syndrome (AIDS) patients is during the fourth decade. For unclear reasons, the incidence of PCNSL is increasing in all patient populations; however, it remains a rare tumor. It is the most common central nervous system neoplasm in AIDS patients.

PCNSL usually occurs as single (25%-50%) or multiple masses within the cerebral hemisphere white matter, typically in proximity to the ventricular system. Multiple lesions are more common in immunocompromised patients. Secondary spread throughout the neuraxis is common, with involvement of cerebrospinal fluid or leptomeninges in 30%-40%, ocular disease in 20%, and other distant sites within the CNS in about 10%-20% of the cases. Disease outside of the nervous system is found in only 5%-10% of patients throughout the disease course, or at autopsy. All patients undergo a complete staging evaluation of the nervous system at diagnosis, but the extent of staging for systemic disease remains highly variable and physician dependent.

Germ Cell Tumors

Primary intracranial germ cell tumors are a rare group of diverse tumors that are homologous to germinal tumors arising in the gonads and in extragonadal sites such as the mediastinum. They account for less than 5% of childhood tumors and less than 1% of adult tumors. Approximately 90% of these tumors occur in individuals less than 20 years of age. Germ cell tumors may arise from developmental nests of primitive germ cells in midline structures. Not surprisingly, the majority of these tumors occur around the third ventricular region, in particular the pineal gland and suprasellar compartment. The spectrum of germ cell tumors in decreasing frequency includes germinoma, teratoma, embryonal carcinoma, endodermal sinus tumor, and choriocarcinoma. A considerable number of these tumors consist of mixed elements, and are designated mixed germ cell tumors. With the exception of benign teratoma, all germ cell tumors are malignant neoplasms, with the potential to disseminate throughout the neuraxis. Generally, germ cell tumors are grouped into germinoma and non-germinoma categories because germinomas are highly radiosensitive, while the remaining germ cell tumors are not.

Most non-germinomas are located in the pineal region, whereas germinomas generally occur within either the pineal or suprasellar region. Only 10% of germ cell tumors arise elsewhere in the brain. The majority of pineal region germ cell tumors affect males, while suprasellar germ cell tumors are seen predominately in females.

Germ cell tumors are the only primary brain tumor that might be diagnosed by the presence of oncoproteins, or tumor markers, in the cerebrospinal fluid and blood. The most useful markers are fetoprotein (AFP), placental alkaline phosphatase (PAP), and - human chorionic gonadotrophin (HCG). An elevated level of any of these tumor markers provides compelling evidence for a germ cell tumor diagnosis, and the pattern of marker elevation may implicate tumor histology (Table 5). Clinically, these markers are also used to monitor response to therapy and to detect tumor recurrence.

Cysts and Tumor-like Lesions

Epidermoid Cyst

Epidermoid cysts are thought to result from ectopic inclusion of epithelial cells during closure of the neural tube. They are benign, slow-growing tumors composed of an inner stratified epithelium and covered by an external capsule. Growth occurs through the accumulation of desquamated epithelial cells and their breakdown products, keratin and cholesterin. Unlike the dermoid variety, epidermoid cysts occur more frequently in the brain than the spine, with a predilection for the cerebellopontine angle, pituitary region, subarachnoid cisterns, and diploe of frontal and parietal bone. They have a bimodal peak incidence in the second and fifth decades, but are most common in middle-aged adults. Standard treatment is surgical removal. Despite their benign nature, the cysts tend to recur if not removed completely.

Dermoid Cyst

Dermoid cysts are benign lesions arising from ectoderm. They generally occur in the pediatric population. In children under ten, they tend to arise within the brain with a predilection for cerebellar vermis, fourth ventricle, and inferior frontal lobes. In the second decade, involvement of the cauda equine is more common. Midline cerebellar and cauda equine lesions may be associated with a dermal sinus, predisposing the affected individual to pyogenic meningitis. In addition, dermoid cysts may rupture, expelling lobules of fatty material, which can cause aseptic meningitis. Dermoid cysts are slow growing as a result of desquamation and secretion. They generally "flow" into any available space and can become quite extensive before becoming symptomatic.

Colloid Cyst of the Third Ventricle

Colloid cysts are benign, round circumscribed grape-like lesions typically attached to the roof of the third ventricle and the choroid plexus. Despite its benign growth pattern, ball-valve obstruction of the foramen of Monroe may produce position dependent CSF obstruction, leading to acute hydrocephalus and sudden death. This cyst almost always occurs in adults. Magnetic resonance imaging characteristics help differentiate colloid cysts from other third ventricular region lesions. Approximately 60% of colloid cysts are hyperintense on T1-weighted imaging and hypointense on T2-weighted images, which is attributable to their heavy protein or mucin content. Surgical resection without untoward residual deficits can be very difficult in this location. Often, cyst drainage or shunting is pursued.

Table 5

Tumor Markers in Germ Cell Tumors

Germ Cell Tumor	Alpha Fetoprotein	β-Human Chorionic Gonadotrophin	Placental Alkaline Phosphatase
Germinoma	-	-	+
Teratoma	+	-	-
Embryonal carcinoma	+	-	+/-
Endodermal sinus tumor (Yolk sac tumor)	-	-	+
Choriocarcinoma	-	+	+/-

Lipoma

Lipomas are rare, benign tumors composed of adipose tissue. They commonly occur near the midline, usually along the corpus callosum, third ventricle, or midbrain. They may also occur in other areas in the brain and within the spinal canal. Midline lipomas are thought to represent a form of dysraphism. The pathogenesis of a pericallosal lipoma is believed to result from abnormal resorption of the primitive meninx, which then differentiates into lipomatous tissue. Often lipomas are asymptomatic and only discovered as incidental findings in individuals undergoing neuroimaging for other medical reasons. On brain MRI, lipomas are hyperintense on both T1 and T2 weighted sequences, and do not enhance. When symptomatic, intracranial lipomas generally produce seizures, and intradural spinal lipomas most commonly present with spinal cord compression syndrome.

Table 6

Clinical Manifestations of Pituitary Adenomas

Hormone	Symptom
Prolactin	In males: impotence, loss of libido, obesity In females: amenorrhea, galactorrhea, infertility, obesity
Growth hormone	In children: gigantism In adults: acromegaly
ACTH	Cushing disease
Nonsecreting adenoma (most are thought to secret follicle stimulating hormone or lutenizing hormone)	Asymptomatic. Tumors become known due to symptomatic mass effect, incidental radiographic findings, or at autopsy.

Tumors of the Anterior Pituitary

Pituitary Adenoma

Pituitary adenomas are benign, slow-growing tumors of epithelial origin. They represent about 15% of all primary brain tumors. While they can occur at any age, they are rare before puberty. Most of these tumors grow in the anterior two-thirds of the pituitary, called the adenohypophysis. Tumors of the pituitary gland may produce hormonal disturbances or compress adjacent structures. The optic chiasm lies approximately 8-13mm above the pituitary gland and is particularly susceptible to tumor compression. Pituitary adenomas are classified as either secreting or nonsecreting. The majority of these tumors are secretory, and are further classified according to the specific hormone secreted (Table 6). Pituitary adenomas are also differentiated by size. Microadenomas are less than 1 cm in diameter and do not cause sellar enlargement. These tumors have no effect on vision and little effect on gland function. Macroadenomas are greater than 1 cm, are associated with generalized sellar enlargement, and commonly present with symptoms of mass effect. Standard therapy includes appropriate hormonal intervention and surgical resection.

Rarely, patients with pituitary adenomas experience a sudden onset of headache, visual loss, ophthalmoplegia, altered mental status, and hormonal dysfunction due to acute hemorrhage or infarction of the pituitary gland. This syndrome, called pituitary apoplexy, occurs in less than 1% of patients with pituitary adenomas. However, radiographic evidence of intratumoral hemorrhage or infarction in the absence of clinical symptoms occurs in up to one-fourth of patients. The pituitary gland's unusual vascular supply may predispose it to hemorrhage or infarct. The blood supply to the anterior pituitary gland is mainly from its portal venous system, which traverses down the pituitary stalk and is particularly vulnerable to compression or distortion.

Local Extension from Regional Tumors

Craniopharyngioma

Craniopharyngiomas are benign tumors thought to arise from embryonic remnants of Rathke pouch epithelium, which normally develops into the adenohypophysis as well as oral mucosa and tooth primordial. They most often occur near the pituitary stalk in the suprasellar region and frequently have an intrasellar component. Rarely, they occur at ectopic sites, including optic nerve, sphenoid bone, and cerebellopontine angle. They represent 2%-3% of all primary brain tumors and 5%-10% of childhood brain tumors.

There are two main types of craniopharyngiomas: adamantinomatous and papillary. Adamantinomatous craniopharyngiomas occur in children and tend to be fairly cystic and calcified. The cysts contain a cholesterol rich, machine oil-like fluid. Of interest, this fluid can cause aseptic meningitis in the event of cyst rupture. Papillary craniopharyngiomas occur in adults and tend to be more solid. Standard treatment is a complete surgical resection. Radiation may be recommended for incompletely resected tumors or recurrent tumors.

Chordoma

Chordomas arise from remnants of the embryonic notochord, which is a mesodermal derivative. They occur at the skull base, or at the end of the spine. While these tumors are benign, slow-growing, extradural tumors, they often behave aggressively, invading adjacent bone, growing into the sinuses, and compressing the brainstem. Chordomas occur at any age, but are most frequent in younger and middle-aged adults. Males are affected more than females. The most common presenting symptoms of clivus chordomas are double vision and headache. Radiographically, the normal, high-signal marrow cavity of the clivus is replaced by lower signal intensity tumor. Complete surgical resection might be possible for the spinal chordoma; however, the skull base location is very difficult to fully access surgically. Nonsurgical interventions are pursued for radiographically progressively lesions, but the results are often unsatisfactory.

Central Nervous System Metastases

Metastatic brain tumors outnumber primary brain tumors greater than ten to one. Brain metastases occur in approximately 25% of all cancer patients, and the incidence is expected to increase since cancer patients are often now living longer. Metastatic cancer to the nervous system most commonly presents as brain metastases, epidural spinal cord compression, or leptomeningeal carcinomatosis. Virtually any primary cancer can spread to the nervous system, although many have a predilection to involve a particular site (Table 7).

Brain Metastases

Brain metastases result from the hematogenous spread of tumor cells which lodge within blood vessels of the brain and subsequently extend into the brain parenchyma. Not surprisingly, brain metastases are multiple in approximately three-fourths of cases. The location of metastases within the brain is proportionate to the blood volume received by each area. Eighty percent are located in the cerebral hemispheres, 15% in the cerebellum, 3% in the basal ganglia, and 2% in the brainstem. In the cerebral hemispheres, brain metastases typically occur near the grey-white matter junction and at the arterial border zone regions. Similarly, cerebellar metastases generally occur at the arterial border zone between the superior and inferior cerebellar arteries. Metastases are the most common tumor of the posterior fossa in adults. Virtually any tumor can metastasize to the brain, but lung, breast, lymphoma, testicular, kidney, and melanoma are the most common. Brain metastases frequently herald the diagnosis of lung cancer. However, in other primary tumors, such as breast, brain metastases most often occur late in the disease course in the setting of widespread systemic disease. Solitary metastases are commonly seen with breast, colon, and renal carcinomas, while multiple metastases are associated with lung carcinoma and melanoma. Brain metastases from renal cell carcinoma and melanoma are often hemorrhagic; however, by virtue of sheer numbers, hemorrhagic brain metastases are more commonly seen in lung cancer.

In patients with established cancer, the diagnosis of brain metastases is generally based upon radiographic findings. Brain metastases are well demarcated, with significant surrounding edema. The enhancement pattern may vary from discrete uniform enhancement to rim enhancing. Some lesions may be obscured by hemorrhage. If a patient has a single brain lesion and a systemic cancer that usually does not metastasize to the brain, such as prostate, bladder, and ovarian carcinoma, a biopsy or surgical resection should be consid-

Table 7

Central Nervous System Metastatic Disease

Site	Pathologic Mechanism	Most Common Associated Primary Tumors
Brain	Hematogenous Direct extension from skin/bone/along cranial nerves	Lung (50%) Breast (15%-20%) Unknown (10%-15%) Melanoma (10%) Colon (5%) Renal cell carcinoma (5%)
Dura	Hematogenous	Breast Prostate Lymphoma
Epidural spinal canal	Bony spread (Hematologic malignancies can spread through vascular supply)	Solid tumors (50%-60%): Breast Lung Prostate Kidney Hematologic malignancies (10%-20%) Lymphoma Myeloma
Spinal cord	Hematogenous	Lung (49%) Breast (15%) Lymphoma (9%) Colorectal (7%) Renal cell carcinoma (6%) Head and neck (6%)
Leptomeningeal	Arterial Venous (through vertebral veins or Batson's plexus) Extension from bone Retrograde invasion along nerves Direct extension from parenchymal disease	Hematologic malignancies: Lymphoma Leukemia Solid tumors: Breast (12%-34%) Lung (9%-25%) Melanoma (17%-25%) Carcinomas of the GI tract (4%-14%) Primary brain tumors
Pituitary	Hematogenous	Breast

ered for diagnostic confirmation. Likewise, a tissue diagnosis should be pursued if imaging study characteristics are atypical for metastases.

The cause of death for nearly three-fourths of patients with brain metastases is uncontrolled systemic disease. In this setting, the median survival is around three months and standard therapy is palliative whole brain irradiation. Here the goal of therapy is to decrease or reverse neurological deficits due to the tumor(s) and surrounding edema. A more aggressive treatment approach may be pursued in patients with brain metastases and controlled systemic disease. Solitary and sometimes multiple lesions may be treated surgically or with focal irradiation (stereotactic radiosurgery). Whole brain irradiation is offered to patients with innumerous metastases, and those considered to be at high risk for developing progressive or recurrent brain metastases following focal brain irradiation.

Epidural Cord Compression

Epidural metastases typically result from the extension of a metastatic deposit in the vertebral bodies or paravertebral tissues into the epidural space. Tumors rarely metastasize directly into the epidural space. As such, epidural spinal cord compression is most commonly seen in cancers that metastasize to bone. These include breast, lung, prostate, and hematologic malignancies. Epidural metastases are the most common spinal tumors in the elderly. Patients often present with focal pain over the site of metastases and/or radicular pain. Neurological symptoms are initially due to the distortion of nerve fibers within the spinal cord; however, if treatment is delayed, spinal cord infarction and permanent disability may result. Standard therapy consists of steroids and emergent radiation therapy. Surgical resection is considered in those patients with well-controlled systemic disease, limited vertebral body metastases, and tumor histology generally refractory to radiation therapy. Surgical resection requires the placement of rods to stabilize the spine and is associated with a fairly lengthy rehabilitation period.

Leptomeningeal Carcinomatosis

Leptomeningeal carcinomatosis, or neoplastic meningitis, refers to the spread of tumor cells into the cerebrospinal fluid and/or tumor infiltration of the leptomeninges. It is most commonly seen in cancer patients with widespread systemic disease. Similar to brain metastases, most patients succumb to their systemic disease. Median survival is 6 weeks. Leptomeningeal tumor spread occurs through arterial, venous, or boney spread, or via direct extension from parenchymal brain lesions. The clinical presentation of leptomeningeal carcinomatosis is highly variable and may include symptoms suggestive of obstructive hydrocephalus or meningeal irritation, cranial nerve palsies, radicular or segmental pain, or lower motor spinal nerve dysfunction.

The gold standard of diagnosis is positive cerebrospinal fluid cytology. However, not all patients will have positive CSF cytology. The diagnostic yield from a single lumbar puncture is around 55%, increasing to 80% following a second procedure.

Typically there are other abnormalities in the CSF profile, including leukocytosis, an elevated CSF protein level, and occasionally a reduction in glucose. Contrast enhanced MRI often demonstrates linear or nodular enhancement of the leptomeninges. However, there is a high incidence of false negative studies and a normal MRI does not exclude the diagnosis. In the absence of positive cytology or leptomeningeal enhancement on contrast-enhanced MRI, a presumptive clinical diagnosis can be established in a known cancer patient with a clinical syndrome consistent with neoplastic meningitis.

The mainstay of therapy is the provision of chemotherapy into the spinal fluid either via lumbar puncture or an Ommaya reservoir. In patients with solid tumors, a radionucleotide cerebrospinal fluid flow study may be done to identify areas in the CSF compartment that intrathecal chemotherapy would not reach, otherwise known as CSF flow block. CSF flow block is most commonly seen at the base of the brain, the subarachnoid space of the lumbosacral spine, and over the cerebral convexities. These areas of abnormal CSF flow are additionally treated with focal irradiation, which restores normal CSF flow in approximately 50% of patients.

8. Familial Tumor Syndromes Involving the Nervous System

Approximately 5% of primary brain tumors are thought to be associated with hereditary factors. Patients with Li-Fraumeni syndrome, p53 deficits (usually associated with Li-Fraumeni syndrome), tuberous sclerosis, neurofibromatosis type I and II, von Hippel-Lindau disease, Turcot syndrome, and familial polyposis have a higher incidence of brain tumors than the general population (Table 3).

Neurofibromatosis

Neurofibromatosis denotes a group of autosomal dominantly inherited, multisystem neurocutaneous disorders that likely originate from neural crest and affect all three germinal layers. As such, it can involve any organ system. Two distinct types are recognized, neurofibromatosis type 1 (NF1), or von Recklinghausen disease, and neurofibromatosis type 2 (NF2). NF1 is most commonly seen, affecting 85% of patients, whereas NF2 is seen in approximately 10% of patients.

NF1 is one of the most common autosomal dominant genetic disorders, with an incidence of approximately 1 case per 3000 people. In familial cases, expressivity of the disorder is variable, but the penetrance is 100%. One half of cases are caused by new mutations. The responsible gene, the NF1 gene, has been localized to the long arm of chromosome 17. Only one NF1 gene needs to be deleted or mutated to produce the condition. NF1 is caused by decreased production of the protein neurofibromin, which plays a role in cellular development and function, and has a putative tumor suppressor function.

The clinical hallmark of NF1 is the presence of multiple café-au-lait spots and neurofibromas. However, diverse cutaneous, neurologic, skeletal, and neoplastic manifestations are typically present. Intracranial manifestations of NF1 may include optic gliomas, cerebral gliomas, schwannomas of the cranial nerves, vascular dysplasias, hamartomas, and craniofacial plexiform neurofibromas. NF1 can involve the spine, musculoskeletal system, and the gastrointestinal (GI) tract, and is associated with neural crest tumors.

The manifestations of NF1 generally occur at predictable time points in the affected individual's lifespan. Bone manifestations, such as cortical thinning, are congenital. Café-au-lait spots are generally present at birth and increase in number during subsequent years. Diffuse plexiform neurofibromas of the face and neck rarely appear after one year of age, and plexiform neurofibromas of other parts of the body rarely develop after adolescence. On the other hand, cutaneous and subcutaneous neurofibromas infrequently occur before puberty, but continue to develop throughout adulthood. Optic gliomas generally manifest in childhood. Other malignant tumors can develop at any point in life.

Neurofibromatosis type 2 (NF2) is an uncommon inherited autosomal dominant syndrome with an incidence of 1 case per 30,000-40,000 people. Similar to NF1, one half of cases are the result of *de novo* NF2 gene mutations. The manifestations of NF2 result from mutations of the NF2 gene located on the long arm of chromosome 22, leading to decreased function or production of the protein merlin. Merlin has a putative tumor suppressor function.

NF2 is characterized by neoplastic and dysplastic lesions of Schwann cells, meningeal cells, and glial cells. Despite its name, neurofibromas are rare in NF2. The cutaneous and spinal nerve lesions of NF2, which are often clinically and radiographically indistinguishable from neurofibromas, are actually schwannomas. This has led some to propose the term schwannomatosis or MISME syndrome, an acronym for multiple inherited schwannomas, meningiomas, and ependymomas. Despite the large number of tumor types found in NF2, malignant transformation is rare.

The diagnosis of NF2 is usually made as a result of symptoms associated with vestibulocochlear schwannomas (cranial nerve eight schwannomas or acoustic neuromas), which generally present in the second or third decade of life. Consequently, patients with NF2 are typically diagnosed later in life than those with NF1. NF2 may be diagnosed earlier in children with a family history of the disease, as a result of early screening, or in those who initially present with vision loss due to posterior subcapsular lens opacities or "juvenile cataracts." The cranial nerve schwannomas and meningiomas of NF2 are indistinguishable clinically and histopathologically from those occurring spontaneously in the absence of an inherited syndrome; however, they present at a much younger age than their *de novo* counterparts. NF2 should be considered in any patient with cranial nerve schwannoma or meningioma prior to age 30.

Lesions of the brain and spine eventually occur in almost all patients with NF2. Intracranial tumors seen in NF2 include cranial nerve schwannomas, multiple meningiomas, ependymomas, and, rarely, gliomas. Vestibulocochlear schwannomas are the hallmark of the disease, but schwannomas can be found involving any cranial nerve. Ependymomas are the most common intraparenchymal tumor in NF2. Spinal tumors seen in NF2 include meningiomas, ependymomas, and schwannomas. Schwannomas may present as intradural extramedullary masses or may involve the exiting nerve roots. Meningiomas present as intradural extramedullary masses and are typically located in the thoracic spine region. Most intramedullary spine tumors in NF2 are ependymomas, which generally arise in the upper cervical cord or the conus. Cutaneous manifestations are limited to cutaneous schwannomas that resemble skin tags, and rare café-au-lait spots.

von Hippel-Lindau Syndrome

von Hippel-Lindau syndrome (VHL) is an autosomal dominant inherited multisystem disorder characterized by abnormal growth of blood vessels producing angiomas or hemangioblastomas. These lesions may develop in the retina, certain areas of the brain, the spinal cord, the adrenal glands and other parts of the body. In the brain, hemangioblastomas most commonly involve the cerebellum. Individuals with VHL are also at a higher risk than normal for certain types of cancer, especially kidney cancer. The von Hippel-Lindau gene is a tumor suppressor gene found on chromosome 3. Individuals affected with a germline mutation in the von Hippel-Lindau gene can develop hemangioblastomas in childhood; however, the mean age at diagnosis is 29 years of age. Central nervous system symptoms vary widely and depend upon lesion location. The goal of therapy is to address symptomatic lesions prior to the development of permanent neurological deficits. Surgery is the treatment of choice, although radiation therapy may be provided to incompletely resected lesions.

Tuberous Sclerosis

Tuberous sclerosis complex (TSC) is an autosomal dominant genetic disorder affecting cellular differentiation and proliferation, which results in hamartia and hamartoma formation in the brain and on other vital organs such as the kidneys, heart, eyes, lungs, and skin. Hamartias and hamartomas both consist of circumscribed groups of cells that are misaligned or disrupted from their normal architecture. The underlying cell type may have dysplastic features but are otherwise appropriate for the tissue in which they are found. Hamartias lack growth potential and include lesions such as cortical tubers, retinal flat lesions, and renal cysts. Hamartomas, on the other hand, have the potential to grow. Hamartomatous lesions include facial angiofibromas, subependymal giant cell astrocytomas, and renal angiomyolipomas.

Three types of brain tumors are associated with TSC, including cortical tubers, subependymal nodules and subependymal giant cell astrocytomas. Subependymal giant cell astrocytomas arise in the vicinity of the foramen of Monro, and may produce CSF obstruction. They rarely undergo malingnant degeneration. The skin lesions of tuberous sclerosis include hypopigmented macules, facial angiofibromas, shagreen patch, and subungual and periungual fibromas. Common symptoms include seizures, mental retardation, and behavior problems. Mental retardation occurs as the result of poorly controlled seizures; intellect is generally normal in the absence of seizures. TSC results from mutations in one of two tumor suppressor genes, TSC1 or TSC2, encoding for hamartin and tuberin respectively.

9. Differential Diagnosis of Central Nervous System Tumors by Location

Supratentorial Tumor

- Glioma (approximately 50%)
  - Glioblastoma multiforme
  - Astrocytoma
  - Oligodendroglioma
  - Ependymoma
- Metastasis (20%-30%)
- Meningioma (16%)
- Pineal gland tumors
- Lymphoma

Multiple Lesions of the Cerebral Hemispheres

- Metastases
- Multifocal glioma
- Lymphoma
- Infection
- Demyelinating lesions
- Infarcts
- Inflammatory lesions

Posterior Fossa Tumors in Children

- Medulloblastoma
- Ependymoma
- Pilocytic astrocytoma
- Brainstem glioma

Posterior Fossa Mass in Adults

- Metastasis
- Hemangioblastoma
- Glioma
  - Ependymoma
  - Astrocytoma
- Medulloblastoma
- Lymphoma
- Infarct/hemorrhage
- Infection

Brainstem Lesion

- Brainstem glioma
- Infarction
- Hemorrhage
- Pontine myelinolysis
- Multiple sclerosis
- Metastasis
- Basilar artery aneurysm/dolichoectasia

Cerebellopontine Angle Region Tumors

- Schwannoma (7 out of 9)
- Meningioma (1 out of 9)
- Epidermoid cyst (1 out of 16)
- Metastasis

- Ependymoma
- Choroid plexus papilloma

Lateral Ventricle Masses (Above Foramen of Monroe)

- Central neurocytoma
- Subependymal giant cell astrocytoma
- Subependymoma
- Choroid plexus papilloma
- Meningioma
- Metastases to choroid plexus

Third Ventricular Region Masses

- Colloid cyst
- Craniopharyngioma
- Hypothalamic/thalamic glioma
- Choroid plexus papilloma
- Ependymoma
- Basilar tip aneurysm
- Neurocytoma

Suprasellar Masses

- Craniopharyngioma
- Aneurysm
- Meningioma
- Pituitary adenoma
- Dermoid cyst
- Chiasmal glioma
- Germinoma
- Ependymoma
- Sarcoid
- Histiocytosis X
- Local tumor spread (nasopharyngeal tumors, carcinoma of the sinuses, etc.)
- Sellar masses
- Pituitary adenoma
- Craniopharyngioma
- Meningioma
- Mestastasis
- Epidermoid
- Abscess
- Sarcoid
- Rathke cleft cyst
- Germinoma

Pineal Region Tumors

- Germ cell tumor
- Pineal cell tumors
- Gliomas
- Dermoid cyst

- Lipoma
- Arachnoid cyst
- Meningioma
- Vein of Galen malformations

Skull Base Tumors

- Chordomas
- Meningiomas
- Glomus jugulare
- Schwannomas
- Metastatic tumors

Intramedullary Spinal Cord Lesions

- Ependymoma
- Astrocytoma
- Medulloblastoma (CSF seeding)
- Lipoma
- Dermoid
- Epidermoid
- Hemangioblastoma
- Metastasis
- Syringomyelia/hydromyelia
- Myelitis
- AVM

Extramedullary/intradural Spinal Cord Lesions

- Meningioma
- Schwannoma
- Neurofibroma
- Drop metastases
- Dermoid
- Epidermoid
- Lipoma

Extradural Spinal Cord Lesions

- Herniated disk
- Osteophyte
- Metastasis
    - Breast carcinoma
    - Lung carcinoma
- Lymphoma
- Primary bone tumor
    - Chordoma
    - Osterosarcoma/blastoma
    - Myeloma
- Neurofibroma
- Dermoid/epidermoid

Lumbar Cistern Tumors

- Schwannoma

- Meningioma
- Myxopapillary ependymoma
- Paraganglioma of the filum terminale
- Solitary metastasis

10. Paraneoplastic Syndromes

Paraneoplastic syndromes are a group of symptom complexes that occur in cancer patients that cannot be explained by the tumor itself, metastases, or the hormones, which are normally secreted by the tissue from which the tumor arose. Paraneoplastic syndromes occur in approximately 10% of cancer patients and can affect any organ or tissue. In most cancer patients, they represent the effect of substances secreted by the tumor that mimic normal hormones or interfere with circulating proteins. Rarely, paraneoplastic syndromes are immune mediated. However, this is the case for the vast majority of neurological paraneoplastic syndromes. These syndromes are thought to result from the presence of onconeural antigens, or antigens common to both neoplastic and normal neural tissue (Table 8). As a result, autoantibodies attacking the tumor inadvertently recognize normal cells in the nervous system as foreign.

Neurologic paraneoplastic syndromes typically affect middle-aged to older individuals with lung, ovarian, hematologic, or breast cancer. Symptoms vary widely and generally develop subacutely over days to weeks. While symptom onset can occur during any point in the cancer course, neurological symptoms often precede tumor detection by months to years. Because the clinical features of neurologic paraneoplastic syndromes are often nonspecific and generally occur in patients without an established cancer diagnosis, the recognition and diagnosis of these disorders is difficult. However, many patients will develop specific serum or spinal fluid antibodies that can be instrumental in establishing the diagnosis. Early diagnosis can lead to tumor identification at a disease stage when the tumor may be curable. Moreover, treatment of the underlying cancer is considered the most effective therapeutic intervention for the neurologic paraneoplastic syndromes. Additional therapeutic approaches target the autoimmune response through steroids, high-dose intravenous immunoglobulin (IV IG), or plasmapheresis. If initiated early on in the disease process, symptom improvement or resolution can result. In addition, there are scattered reports of spontaneous symptom resolution. However, most patients have permanent neurological sequelae. In most cases, the overall prognosis is determined by the underlying cancer.

Table 8

Paraneoplastic Syndromes of the Nervous System

Autoantibody	Alternate Autoantibody Names	Most Common Clinical Presentation	Commonly Associated Cancer(s)
Anti-Hu	Type 1 antineuronal nuclear autoantibodies (ANNA-1)	Encephalomyelitis Sensory neuronopathy	Small cell lung cancer (90%) Neuroblastoma Breast Ovarian Lymphoma
Anti-Yo	Anti-Purkinje cell cytoplasmic autoantibodies	Cerebellar ataxia	Gynecologic Breast
Anti-Ri	Type 2 antineuronal nuclear autoantibodies (ANNA-2)	Cerebellar ataxia Opsoclonus Brainstem encephalitis	Gynecologic Breast Small cell lung cancer
Anti-Ma		Cerebellar dysfunction Brainstem dysfunction	Breast Lung Colon
Anti-Ta	Anti-Ma2 autoantibody	Limbic encephalitis Brainstem dysfunction	Testicular
Anti-CAR	Cancer associated retinopathy autoantibodies	Photoreceptor degeneration	Small cell lung cancer Gynecologic malignancies
Anti-MAR	Melanoma associated retinopathy autoantibodies	Photoreceptor degeneration	Melanoma
Anti-VGCC	P/Q-type voltage-gated calcium channel autoantibodies	Lambert-Eaton myasthenic syndrome	Small cell lung cancer
Anti-amphiphysin		Stiff-man syndrome Encephalomyelitis	Breast
Anti-K^+ channel		Limbic encephalitis	Lung

11. References

1. Bradley WG, Daroff RB, Fenichel GM, et al, eds. *Neurology in Clinical Practice*. 3rd ed. New York: Butterworth-Heinemann; 1999.
2. Kleihues P, Cavenee WK, eds. *Pathology and Genetics of Tumours of the Nervous System*. Lyon: International Agency for Research on Cancer; 2000.
3. Burger PC, Scheithauer BW, Viogel FS. *Surgical Pathology of the Nervous System and its Coverings*. 4th ed. New York: Churchill Livingston; 2002.
4. Hill JR, Kuriyama N, Kuriyama H, et al. Molecular genetics of brain tumors. *Arch Neurol*. 1999;56:439-441.
5. Czervionke LF, Daniels DL, Meyer GA, et al. Neuroepithelial cysts of the lateral ventricles: MR appearance. *AJNR*. 1987;8:609-613.
6. Greenberg JO. *Neuroimaging: A Companion to Adams and Victor's Principles of Neurology*. New York: McGraw-Hill; 1999.
7. Ellison D, Love S. *Neuropathology: A Reference Text of CNS Pathology*. Chicago: CV Mosby; 1998.
8. Fuller GN, Goodman JC. *Practical Review of Neuropathology*. Philadelphia, Pa: Lippincott, Williams & Wilkins; 2001.
9. Gomez MR, ed. *Tuberous Sclerosis Complex*. 3rd ed. New York: Oxford University Press; 1999.
10. Graham DI, Lantos PL. *Greenfield's Neuropathology*. 6th ed. London: Arnold; 1997.
11. Bakshi R, Lindsay BD, Kinkel PR. Brain magnetic resonance imaging in clinical neurology. In: Joynt RJ, Griggs RC, eds. *Clinical Neurology*. Philadelphia, Pa: Lippincott, Williams & Wilkins; 1998.

12. Questions

1. A 42-year-old female presents with a chief complaint of visual loss. Examination findings are limited to decreased visual acuity (20/50 in the right eye and 20/70 in the left eye), and a bitemporal hemianopia. A pituitary adenoma is suspected. Which additional endocrinologic symptom would the patient most likely have?

A. Amenorrhea

B. Galactorrhea

C. Change in ring and shoe size

D. Moon facies and weight gain

E. None

2. Calcification may be seen on neuroimaging in all of the following tumors except:

A. Oligodendroglioma

B. Craniopharyngioma

C. Ependymoma

D. Low grade astrocytoma

E. Pineoblastoma

3. Identifying placental alkaline phosphatase in the blood or CSF of a patient with a brain tumor suggests that the patient has a:

A. Germinoma

B. Pineoblastoma

C. Medulloblastoma

D. Choroid plexus papilloma

E. Pituitary adenoma

4. A 24-year-old male with neurofibromatosis type 2 presents to establish care after moving to your city. One might expect this patient to have all of the following except:

A. Plexiform neurofibromas

B. Schwannomas

C. Multiple meningiomas

D. Café-au-lait spots

E. Spinal cord ependymoma

5. A 45-year-old female presented to the emergency room with sudden onset incapacitating headache associated with nausea and vomiting. Head CT demonstrates a hemorrhagic lesion. The least likely diagnosis is:

A. Metastatic melanoma

B. Pituitary adenoma

C. Glioblastoma multiforme (grade IV astrocytoma)

D. WHO grade 2 astrocytoma

E. Hemangioblastoma

6. A series of patients with known systemic cancer and a solitary brain lesion are presented at a tumor board conference. A diagnosis of brain metastasis was established on the basis of radiographic findings in all but one patient. A diagnostic brain biopsy is recommended to this patient. Which one of the following primary tumors did this patient likely have?

A. Breast carcinoma

B. Prostate carcinoma

C. Lung cancer

D. Melanoma

E. Renal cell carcinoma

7. A 6-year-old child presents to the emergency room with headache and projectile nausea and vomiting. The most likely diagnosis is:

A. Meningioma

B. Medulloblastoma

C. Brain metastases

D. Large vestibular schwannoma

E. Lipoma

8. A 65-year-old male presents to the emergency room with a two-week history of progressive headache, and left hemiparesis. The most likely diagnosis is:

A. Medulloblastoma

B. Low grade astrocytoma

C. Glioblastoma multiforme

D. Colloid cyst

E. Pineoblastoma

9. A couple have a 6-year-old son with a diagnosis of neurofibromatosis type I. They are considering having a second child and present for preconception counseling. Both the husband and the wife were adopted and do not know their family history. They are both healthy 35-year-olds with no major medical illnesses and neither have cutaneous stigmata of neurofibromatosis type I. Which of the following statements is true?

A. Neurofibromatosis type I has an autosomal dominance inheritance pattern.

B. There is a 100% chance that a second child will have NF1.

C. Either the mother or father must have NF1 because every affected individual has an affected parent.

D. The mother must be an asymptomatic carrier for this X-linked trait.

E. The father must be an asymptomatic carrier for this X-linked trait.

10. A 24-year-old female presents with diplopia. Which one of the following tumors is the least likely?

A. Pituitary adenoma

B. Craniopharygioma

C. Lipoma

D. Hypothalamic histiocytosis X

E. Brainstem glioma

11. Which of the following statements concerning tumor location is correct?

A. Primary brain tumors in pediatric patients are generally infratentorial.

B. Primary brain tumors in pediatric patients generally arise from midline structures.

C. Primary CNS lymphoma commonly occurs in peri-ventricular white matter.

D. Primary brain tumors in adults never occur in the posterior fossa.

E. Brain metastases are the most common posterior fossa tumor in adults.

12. An 18-year-old female presents with intractable headache and vomiting precipitated by bending over and coughing, and made worse by lying down. Which of the following diagnoses is the least likely?

A. Colloid cyst

B. WHO grade 2 astrocytoma

C. Glioblastoma multiforme

D. Medulloblastoma

E. Subependymal giant cell astrocytoma

13. Which of the following tumors is the least likely to involve midline structures?

A. Primary CNS lymphoma

B. Glioblastoma multiforme

C. Raphke pouch cyst

D. Brain metastases

E. Mixed germ cell tumors

14. A staging evaluation to detect metastasis to the leptomeninges at the time of diagnosis is warranted for all tumor types except:

A. Lymphoma

B. Germ cell tumor

C. Medulloblastoma

D. Pineoblastoma

E. Oligodendroglioma

15. A 32-year-old male presents with new onset headaches. Neuroimaging reveals a left lateral ventricular mass. The least likely diagnosis is:

A. Neurocytoma

B. Meningioma

C. Subependymal giant cell astrocytoma

D. Colloid cyst

E. Brain metastases

16. Which of the following tumors would be unlikely to be located in the posterior fossa?

A. Pleomorphic xanthoastrocytoma

B. Hemangioblastoma

C. Medulloblastoma

D. Ependymoma

E. Central neurocytoma

17. Chemical meningitis is a possible complication of which of the following tumors?

A. Dermoid cyst

B. Craniopharyngioma

C. Epidermoid cyst

D. All of the above

E. None of the above

18. A 54-year-old female presents with a three month history of progressive neurological symptoms including vertigo, oscillopsia, dyarthria, appendicular ataxia, and unsteady gait. Serum and CSF contain high titer anti-Purkinje cell antibodies (anti-Yo antibodies). The most likely tumor diagnosis is:

A. Adenocarcinoma of the lung

B. Diffuse large cell B-cell lymphoma

C. Ovarian carcinoma

D. Melanoma

E. Neuroblastoma

19. Each of the following statements concerning gliomas is correct except:

A. Ependymomas are the most common primary neoplasm of the spinal cord.

B. Vascular proliferation is a histopathologic finding in WHO grade IV astrocytomas.

C. Loss of heterozygosity (LOH) of 1p19q is associated with favorable response to chemotherapy and favorable prognosis in oligodendrogliomas.

D. WHO grade II tumors classically show nuclear atypia and mitotic activity.

E. Optic nerve gliomas are frequently associated with neurofibromatosis type I.

20. A 66-year-old man with metastatic lung cancer develops a left peripheral facial palsy. Additional findings on examination are absent deep tendon reflexes in the lower extremities bilaterally and the right bicep tendon, and weakness in a right C6 nerve root distribution. Contrast enhanced MRI of the brain is normal. MRI of the cervical spine demonstrates contrast enhancement of several cervical nerve roots and linear enhancement along the cord surface. Examination of the CSF reveals 85 mg/dL protein, 66mg/dL glucose, and 30 white blood cells. The cytology is negative. The most likely diagnosis is:

A. Bell's palsy.

B. Paraneoplastic syndrome

C. Viral meningitis

D. Leptomeningeal carcinomatosis

E. Brain metastases

21. A 65-year-old male with prostate cancer has retro-auricular head pain and dysphagia. Neurological examination reveals asymmetric palate elevation. The most likely diagnosis is:

A. Metastasis to brain stem

B. Leptomeningeal carcinomatosis

C. Paraneoplastic syndrome

D. Metastasis to jugular foramen

E. Brainstem glioma

22. A 66-year-old female with a history of diabetes mellitus and hypertension presents with mid-thoracic back pain, lower extremity weakness, and urinary incontinence. MR imaging of the spine reveals an extradural mass at the T8 vertebral body level. The most likely diagnosis is:

A. Metastatic breast cancer

B. Ependymoma

C. Meningioma

D. Dermoid cyst

E. Lipoma

Answers

1. E.

Pituitary adenomas are typically benign, slow growing neoplasms arising from the anterior lobe of the pituitary gland. Symptoms result from hypo- or hypersecretion of pituitary hormones, or mechanical distortion of surrounding tissues. Symptoms from abnormal hormonal production frequently lead to medical evaluation and diagnosis prior to significant tumor growth. However, non-secretory pituitary tumors are typically diagnosed only after the tumor extends outside of the sella, producing symptoms of mass effect, such as headache and compression of the optic chiasm.

2. D.

Low grade astrocytomas are not associated with calcification. The remaining tumors listed are frequently associated with calcification on neuroimaging.

3. A.

Germ cell tumors are the only primary brain tumor that might be diagnosed by the presence of oncoproteins, or tumor markers, in serum and CSF. The most useful markers are alpha-fetoprotein, beta-HCG, and placental alkaline phosphatase. Elevation of levels of any of these markers strongly suggests that a CNS mass is a germ cell tumor. The pattern of marker elevation may predict tumor histology. Germ cell tumors include germinoma, teratoma, embryonal carcinoma, endodermal sinus tumor, and choriocarcinoma.

4. A.

Patients with neurofibromatosis type 2 may have <5 café-au-lait spots, schwannomas, multiple meningiomas, and spinal cord ependymomas. While the spinal cord tumors of NF1 and NF2 may appear similar radiographically, the pathology is neurofibroma in NF-1 and schwannoma in NF-2. Plexiform neurofibromas are only seen in NF-1.

5. D.

WHO grade 2 tumors are characterized histologically by increased cellularity and nuclear atypia. These slow growing tumors are not associated with vascular proliferation and do not have a propensity to bleed. Metastatic melanoma, glioblastoma multiforme tumors, and hemangioblastomas are vascular tumors with the potential for intra-tumoral hemorrhage. Hemorrhage or hemorrhagic infarction in a pituitary adenoma, or pituitary apoplexy, is a rare, but well recognized entity.

6. B.

In patients with established cancer, the diagnosis of brain metastases is generally based upon radiographic findings. However, if a patient has a solitary brain lesion and a systemic cancer that does not commonly metastasize to the brain, a biopsy or surgical resection should be considered for diagnostic confirmation. Lung, breast, testicular, and renal carcinomas, as well as lymphoma and melanoma commonly metastasize to brain. Prostate cancer most commonly spreads to dura or to the epidural space via local extension from boney mestastases, and rarely involves brain.

7. B.

Meningiomas, brain metastases, and vestibular schwannomas occur in older individuals. Lipomas are rarely symptomatic, but may cause seizures. Pilocytic astrocytomas have a predilection for midline structures and frequently present with obstructive hydrocephalus, in particular cerebellar pilocytic astrocytomas.

8. C.

Glioblastoma multiforme tumors, also known as grade 4 of 4 astrocytomas, are the most common primary brain tumor in adults. These rapidly growing tumors frequently present with symptoms of increased intracranial pressure. Medulloblastomas, low grade astrocytomas, colloid cysts, and pineoblastomas are generally pediatric primary brain tumors.

9. A.

Neurofibromatosis type I is a common autosomal dominant genetic disorder. In familial cases, penetrance is 100%, but expressivity of the disorder is variable. Children of an affected individual have a 50% chance of inheriting the disorder, but the extent of clinical disease manifestations may differ greatly from one generation to another. One half of the cases of NF1 are caused by new mutations. In this particular scenario it would be very unlikely that either parent is a genetic carrier in the absence of cutaneous stigmata or other disease manifestations at the age of 35 years. Their son's disease is likely the result of a new mutation and risk of a second afflicted child is no greater than that of the general population.

10. C.

Lipomas are rarely symptomatic and do not occur in proximity to optic nerve/tracts. All of the other tumors listed occur in the parasellar/skull base region and may compress the optic chiasm/optic nerves, causing visual symptoms.

11. D.

Primary brain tumors in adults most commonly occur in supratentorial locations. However, some primary brain tumors, such as medulloblastomas and brainstem gliomas, can occur in the posterior fossa in adults.

12. B.

Presenting symptoms suggest increased intracranial pressure. Colloid cysts and subependymal giant cell astrocytomas commonly obstruct ventricular outflow pathways leading to hydrocephalus. Glioblastoma multiforme and medulloblastoma tumors are rapidly growing tumors that cause increased intracranial pressure symptoms as a result of expanding mass lesions and/or ventricular obstruction. Grade 2 astrocytomas are slow growing tumors that typically present with seizures or focal neurological deficits.

13. D.

Brain metastases most commonly occur near the grey-white matter junction or at the arterial border zone regions. These sites are located peripherally, not centrally, within the brain.

14. E.

Widespread dissemination throughout the neuroaxis, including cerebrospinal fluid dissemination, is commonly found in patients with lymphomas, germ cell tumors, medulloblastomas, and pineoblastomas. Oligodendrogliomas may focally infiltrate the leptomeninges, but do not spread throughout the cerebrospinal fluid.

15. D.

Lateral ventricular masses (above the Foramen of Monroe) include central neurocytoma, subependymal giant cell astrocytoma, subependymoma, choroid plexus papilloma, meningioma and metastases to choroid plexus. Intraventricular meningiomas arise from meningothelial cells present in the choroid plexus. Colloid cysts typically occur with the third ventricular region.

16. E.

Central neurocytoma is a mature neuronal intraventricular tumor that most often arises in a lateral ventricle near the foramen of Monroe. The remaining tumors listed commonly occur in the posterior fossa.

17. D.

Cyst rupture or fluid leakage from dermoid cysts, epidermoid cysts, and craniopharyngiomas can all cause a chemical meningitis.

18. C.

Paraneoplastic cerebellar degeneration is associated with carcinomas of the breast, ovary, and female genital tract, as well as small cell lung cancer and Hodgkin's disease. However, anti-Purkinje cell antibodies (anti-Yo antibodies) are nearly entirely restricted to carcinomas of the breast, ovary, and female genital tract.

19. D.

WHO grade II tumors show increased cellularity and nuclear atypia, but generally not mitotic activity.

20. D.

The definitive diagnosis of leptomeningeal carcinomatosis requires identification of malignant cells in the CSF. However, the diagnostic yield from a single lumbar puncture is about 55%, increasing to 80% following a second procedure. Not all patients will have positive CSF cytology. A presumptive diagnosis can be established based on suggestive clinical picture in a patient with known systemic cancer, elevated CSF cell count and protein, and appropriate neuroimaging findings. The clinical hallmark of leptomeningeal carcinomatosis is multi-level disease. In this patient there is cranial nerve and spinal nerve root dysfunction.

21. D.

Prostate cancer most commonly metastases to bone and spreads to the dura or epidural space. It rarely metastases directly to the central nervous system and is not associated with neurological paraneoplastic syndromes. Metastatic disease to bone at the base of the skull commonly causes neurologically symptoms and signs due to compression of cranial nerves.

22. A.

Ependymoma, meningioma, dermoid cysts, and lipomas are all intradural, extramedullary tumors. Epidural metastases are the most common spinal tumors in the elderly. Breast, lung, prostate, and hematologic malignancies commonly metastasize to bone and can result in epidural tumor spread and spinal cord compression.

Chapter 17: Peripheral Neuropathy

Jeffrey A. Cohen, MD
John Taylor, DO

Contents

1. Peripheral Neuropathy

Peripheral neuropathy is a general term that encompasses all disorders of the peripheral nervous system. Peripheral neuropathy is subdivided into the various more specific disorders as discussed below. Terms applied to peripheral neuropathy can be general with no localizing context, or have more specific connotations such as mononeuropathy, mononeuropathy multiplex, radiculopathy or plexopathy.

Anatomical Considerations

The nervous system is made up of two main divisions: the central nervous system (CNS) consisting of the brain and spinal cord, and the peripheral nervous system (PNS) consisting of portions of neurons (axons) outside the CNS with cell bodies located in the CNS and neurons entirely within the PNS. PNS neurons are both sensory and autonomic.

It is important to remember the basic parts of the neuron in evaluating peripheral neuropathies. In the simplest terms, nerves have a cell body, processes (axons and dendrites), and myelin. Depending on the type of neuropathy and the pathophysiology, one or more of these components may be affected.

The cell body is the most common site of damage due to poisons, toxins, and metabolic disturbances. These interfere with intracellular processes that the neuron uses to maintain its integrity. Axons can be damaged by diseases that interfere with their blood supply or by direct immune mediated attack. Blood vessels are affected in diabetes, which is the most commonly encountered disease with small vessel arteriopathy. Other diseases which may affect the blood vessels and cause arteritis or inflammation of the arterioles include: systemic lupus erythematosis, polyarteritis nodosa, Sjögren syndrome, and Wegener arteritis.

Defective myelin can occur in inherited disorders, the most common being hereditary sensory motor neuropathy Type I (Charcot-Marie-Tooth disease (CMT)). In this condition there is a genetic abnormality causing a defect in myelin. This leads to demyelination, and as a result slowed nerve conduction velocities. Autoimmune disorders such as Güillain-Barré syndrome, chronic inflammatory demyelinating polyneuropathy (CIDP), multifocal motor neuropathy, and anti-MAG neuropathy may cause demyelination. In these disorders the immune system mounts an attack on myelin and/or axolemmal membrane. Targets for this attack include myelin-associated glycoprotein (MAG), GM1, GM2, and sulfatide.

Sensory neurons have cell bodies located in the dorsal root ganglion or cranial nerve ganglion (CNV), with one axonal process to the peripheral receptor and one that enters the CNS, synapsing on a second order neuron. The exceptions to this are the mesencepalic nucleus of the trigeminal nerve, which contains the only unipolar neurons within the CNS and specialized sensory neurons. Specialized receptor types carry nerve impulses for pain, touch, joint position, vibration and specialized senses. Sensory nerve fibers vary in both diameter and degree of myelination and can therefore be characterized electrophysiologically based on speed of conduction and amplitude of the action potential.

Lower motor neurons—alpha motor neurons—have their cell bodies located within the CNS, ventral horn of the spinal cord and cranial nerve motor nuclei. Their axons enter the PNS through spinal and cranial nerves, making the final common pathway to muscle fibers. At the level of the muscle cell there is a cholinergic synapse. The recruitment pattern of muscle fibers, the synapse of the terminal button on the muscle fiber, and loss of muscle innervation are important characteristics when evaluating diseases of muscle, diseases of the neuromuscular junction, and diseases of the motor neuron, respectively.

Autonomic neurons of the CNS are located in both specific cranial nerve nuclei and the lateral horns of the thoracolumbar region. Autonomic neurons of the PNS are located in the sympathetic chain ganglia and in parasympathetic ganglia associated with cranial nerves and splanchnic beds. The autonomic nervous system and its relationship to neuropathy may be overlooked. Autonomic nerves control involuntary functions such as breathing, regulation of blood pressure, sweating, digestion, bladder and bowel control, sexual function, pupillary changes, and cardiac rhythm. It is important to keep this in mind when evaluating peripheral neuropathy, since autonomic dysfunction may cause significant morbidity and mortality (Table 1).

Table 1

Neuropathies Commonly Associated with Autonomic Neuropathy

Diabetes mellitus
Amyloidosis (Familial and acquired)
Güillain-Barré syndrome
Vincristine-induced PN
Porphyria
HIV-related autonomic neuropathy
Idiopathic pandysautonomia

Epidemiology

The epidemiology of peripheral neuropathy is difficult to ascertain because the diseases involved are variable in severity, etiology, and pathology within a given population. In general, the overall prevalence is about 2400 (2.4%) per 100,000 United States population, but in people older than 55 years, the prevalence rises to about 8000 (8%) per 100,000. In contradistinction to the United States, leprosy is still highly prevalent in Southeast Asia, India, Africa, and Central and South America. In global terms, leprosy and HIV (though figures are unclear) are major causes of neuropathy. Other common acquired causes of peripheral neuropathy include metabolic disorders, infectious agents, vasculitis, toxins, and drugs. Autoimmune neuropathies and inherited polyneuropathies (PN) also constitute a substantial proportion of neuropathies, mostly chronic. Currently in the United States, the most commonly recognized cause of PN is diabetes mellitus Type II.

Diagnostic Considerations

As with all medical conditions, careful consideration of the history of the disease process is very important. Concomitant medical illnesses and past medical and family history can point to specific diagnostic considerations, such as painful small fiber neuropathies with diabetes mellitus, or past exposure to chemotherapeutic agents such as cisplatin (proprioceptive loss) or vincristine (sensorimotor neuropathy), or foot deformities within a family (CMT). The time course of illness and symmetry of symptoms is also very helpful. The acute symmetrical weakness of acute inflammatory demyelinating PN (AIDP) is diagnostic.

The history combined with neurological examination and electrophysiological studies will help define the type of neuropathy and its treatment.

2. Review of Electrodiagnostics: Nerve Conduction Studies (NCS) and Electromyography (EMG)

Sensory Nerve Conduction

As mentioned, the cell bodies of sensory neurons are located in the dorsal root and cranial nerve ganglia. The peripherally transduced sensory stimulus is transmitted along the axon toward the cell body and then through the dorsal root and into the spinal cord to synapse in the dorsal horn or medulla for spinal nerves and CNV nucleus for cranial nerves. The peripherally propagated impulse is called a sensory nerve action potential (SNAP). In performing a NCS, the nerve is electrically stimulated with electrodes along its course. This creates both orthodromic and antidromic conduction in the nerve, and either can be studied (Figure 1).

One must remember that mixed peripheral nerves consist of both myelinated and nonmyelinated sensory nerve axons as well as motor axons. Only the largest, fastest myelinated axons are recorded. For example, the small C-type, nonmyelinated axons cannot be measured by standard NCS. Two main assessments are made when testing the sensory component of the nerve. The number of axons is estimated by measuring the amplitude of the SNAP and the state of myelination of the axons is estimated by the conduction velocity. Therefore, in patients with primary axonal degeneration neuropathies, the primary feature of the NCS is reduced sensory action potential amplitudes, and in primary demyelinating neuropathies the primary feature is slowing of conduction velocity.

Figure 1

Typical set-up for median nerve motor conduction study

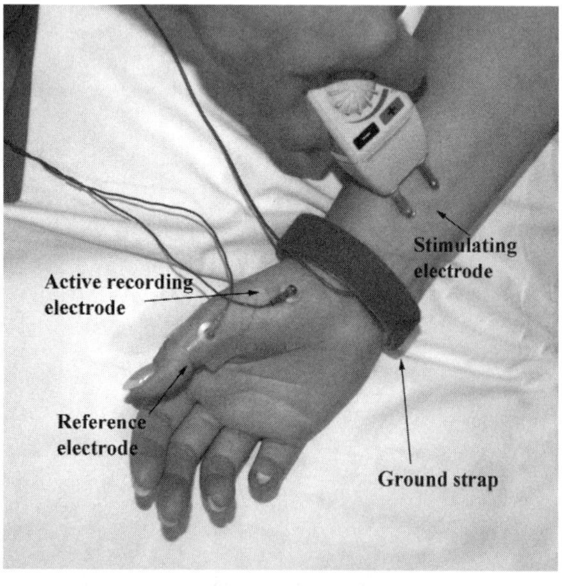

Motor Nerve Conduction

There are significant anatomical differences between sensory and motor nerves. The ability to study the motor component of mixed peripheral nerves in isolation of the sensory fibers is due to their innervation of muscles. One may stimulate the nerve and record from the muscle to determine the termination of the motor action potential, called the compound muscle action potential (CMAP). The time required to depolarize the neuromuscular junction and muscle must be kept in mind when interpreting the recording. Changes, secondary to diseases such as myasthenia gravis, (MG) may alter the study. This can be specifically studied when performing repetitive nerve stimulation in MG patients.

The amplitude of the CMAP is much larger than the SNAP, since each motor axon typically innervates a large number of muscle fibers, each contributing to the depolarization captured by the recording electrode. The amplitude of the muscle action potential is indicative of the number of activated muscle fibers.

The number of axons can be diminished and the CMAP can remain normal if the process of collateral reinnervation of muscle fibers by the remaining axons has been successful. Conversely, the number of axons can be normal and the action potential diminished if there is diminished synaptic transmission at the neuromuscular junction or if there is loss of muscle fibers. If a neuropathy progresses and collateral reinnervation fails to keep pace, the size of the CMAP declines.

Motor Neuron Conduction Velocity

Synaptic transmission between nerve and muscle is required to produce a CMAP. The delay associated with this process is referred to as the distal motor latency. This represents the time for the nerve action potential to travel down the axon, release acetylcholine from the nerve terminal and subsequently depolarize the muscle.

The actual motor nerve speed of conduction can then be measured by stimulating at two points along a given nerve and recording from a muscle innervated by that nerve. The distances from the point of stimulation to the recording electrode can then be subtracted for a distance divided by the time to give the conduction velocity of the motor nerve. Again, this is a measurement of the largest and most myelinated axons.

Certain disorders such as multifocal motor neuropathy (MMN) may show significant conduction block. Conduction block is defined as a 50% reduction in the CMAP at proximal as compared with distal sites of stimulation. Conduction block is usually present in acquired demyelinating neuropathies such as Güillain-Barré syndrome (GBS) or AIDP.

Late responses—H-reflex and the F-response—are useful to study the proximal segments of a nerve. Proximal segment diseases such as radiculopathies or AIDP are outside of the "view" of usual motor and sensory nerve conduction studies. These responses are recorded by applying an electrical stimulus to a peripheral nerve. These "late" responses appear after the orthodromic action potential travels to the muscle directly from the electrical stimulus.

The H-reflex is a monosynaptic reflex response that is the electrophysiologic equivalent of the tendon jerk. The electrical stimulus travels the same pathway from the Ia afferent to the alpha motor neuron and back to the muscle. An H-reflex depends upon the ability to stimulate the Ia afferents without stimulating the motor axons using a submaximal stimulus. In clinical practice, it is possible to use submaximal stimulation and produce an H-reflex by stimulating the posterior tibial division of the sciatic nerve and recording from the tibial nerve innervated gastrocnemius and soleus muscles.

The F-response, or F-wave, is a manifestation of recurrent firing of an anterior horn cell after it has been stimulated by an antidromic action potential. After a motor nerve is stimulated, an action potential runs antidromically as well as orthodromically, causing a small percentage of anterior horn cells to produce an orthodromic action potential recorded as the F-response. Thus, to produce an F-response, an action potential must travel twice through the ventral root of a spinal nerve. The F-wave is produced by a supramaximal stimulus (Table 2).

Electromyography

The physiology of electromyography (EMG) is based upon the function of the motor unit. A motor unit consists of all the muscle fibers innervated by a single alpha motor neuron. Characteristics of the firing of motor units such as amplitude, duration and configuration can be recorded with needle examination of muscle. Each motor unit action potential (MUAP) in a given muscle has a normal range of characteristics. The numbers of phases above and below the baseline are counted; more than four phases is polyphasic (Table 3).

After an EMG needle is inserted into a normal resting muscle there is no spontaneous electrical activity within the muscle. If there is spontaneous activity, its appearance may be either random or patterned. The "dive bombing" whine of activity with needle insertion into a myotonic dystrophy muscle is a patterned activity. The appearance of sharp waves and fibrillation potentials is characteristic of denervated muscle. In this condition the loss of innervation of muscle leads to membrane instability and dysregulation of acetycholine receptors. Insertion of the needle records this spontaneous activity. With increasing levels of contraction it is possible to see the individual MUAPs and evaluate their parameters and the recruitment of additional motor units. When maximal effort is reached, MUAPs cannot be discerned from the dense electrical pattern created. This interference pattern can be characterized by its density and peak-to-peak amplitude.

Table 2

NCS Characteristics of Axonal Degeneration Versus Segmental Demyelination of NCS and Late Responses

	Axonal Degeneration	Segmental Demyelination
CMAP amplitude	Decreased	Normal (except with CB)
Distal latency	Normal	Prolonged
Conduction velocity	Normal	Slow
Conduction block	Absent	Present
Temporal dispersion	Absent	Present
F wave	Normal	Prolonged or Absent
H reflex	Normal	Prolonged or Absent
SNAP amplitude	Decreased	Normal
Distal latency	Normal	Prolonged
Conduction velocity	Normal	Slow

Table 3

EMG Differences Between Axonal Degeneration and Segmental Demyelination

	Axonal Degeneration	Segmental Demyelination
Fibrillations	Present	Absent
Fasciculations	Present	Absent
Recruitment	Decreased	Decreased
Morphology	Long duration/ polyphasic	Normal

3. Mononeuropathies

A mononeuropathy is the term given to focal lesions of individual peripheral nerves. The commonest of these are the entrapment neuropathies. Individual entrapment neuropathies are discussed separately below. Mononeuropathies are asymmetric in presentation and must be distinguished from other disorders that present focally. These include plexopathies, mononeuritis multiplex (MM), and asymmetrically presenting hereditary neuropathies such as hereditary liability to pressure palsies. It is important to recognize that metabolic disorders or altered physiological states can predispose one to mononeuropathies. A common example is the association of carpal tunnel syndrome with diabetes, hypothyroidism, and pregnancy.

The phrase compressive mononeuropathy implies that the peripheral nerves are being impinged upon by adjacent anatomic structures. The injury may be related to decreased epineural blood flow decreasing axonal transport affecting the nerve's ability to conduct impulses or pressure on the nerve causing disruption of the myelin wrapping. Long-term changes may produce irreversible damage.

Electrophysiological studies are important in characterizing the site and extent of injury, as well as distinguishing a mononeuropathy from the other asymmetrically presenting neuropathies mentioned above. The examination should always include another extremity and in particular a lower extremity if a generalized PN is suspected.

4. Mononeuropathy (Mononeuritis) Multiplex

By definition, this describes a process involving multiple separate peripheral nerves either simultaneously or serially. The history is usually of a seemingly random and multifocal neuropathy that may have evolved into a symmetric or contiguous process that can resemble a PN. This is usually a late feature. Nerve involvement does not follow a pattern and may present distributed unilaterally or bilaterally, distally or proximally throughout the body.

Mononeuritis multiplex is usually secondary to systemic disorders such as diabetes, vasculitis or amyloidosis. Many rheumatological disorders may be associated with MM, such as polyarteritis nodosa, Wegener granulomatosis, Sjögren syndrome, rheumatoid arthritis, and systemic lupus erythematosus. MM can occur with both direct tumor invasion and paraneoplastic syndromes. Infectious diseases such as Lyme disease, leprosy, acute viral hepatitis, and acquired immunodeficiency syndrome also may cause a multifocal mononeuropathy. Up to a third of patients thought to have MM have electrodiagnostic studies consistent with a chronic inflammatory demyelinating polyneuropathy.

Workup in addition to EMG/NCS is directed at the potential etiologies suggested by history and examination. Imaging studies are usually not helpful. Routine laboratory studies looking for the more common causes should include an ESR, hepatitis panel, fasting blood sugar, Lyme titer, sural nerve biopsy, HIV test, serum protein electrophoresis, urine protein electrophresis, and rheumatological markers.

EMG and NCS characteristics may reveal either axonal disruption/degeneration or abnormal axonal conduction. Sensory nerve conduction studies show abnormalities of decreased amplitude in the presence of axonal disruption.

Results of needle electrode examination can vary, depending on the time course of the disorder. Findings are typically neuropathic and may include abnormal spontaneous membrane activity (positive sharp waves and fibrillation potentials) and increases in MUAP duration, amplitude, and polyphasia. Additionally, the loss of motor axons may generate a reduced number of MUAPs firing at high rates, manifest as reduced recruitment. Abnormal findings directly depend on the severity and aggressiveness of the underlying disease.

Nerve biopsy is used less in diagnosis of PN; although in mononeuropathy multiplex it may be useful in the evaluation of individual cases based on the suspected underlying disorder. It is particularly useful in the evaluation of vasculitis or amyloid disease (Figure 2), (Table 4).

Table 4

Causes of Mononeuropathy Multiplex

Vasculitis
Multifocal motor neuropathy
Multifocal acquired demyelinating sensory and motor neuropathy
Lyme disease
Sarcoid
Leprosy
HIV infection
Hereditary neuropathy with liability to pressure palsy

Figure 2

Sural nerve biopsy demonstrating vasculitis with fibrinoid necrosis

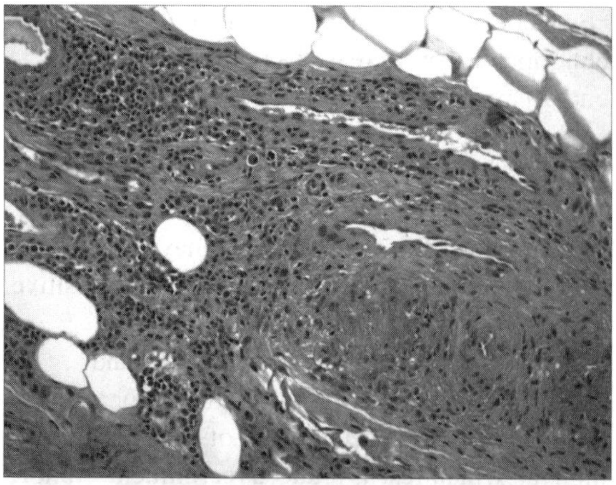

Courtesy of Dr. Brent Harris

5. Polyneuropathy

PN is usually characterized by symmetric distal sensory loss, burning, or weakness. It can, however, occur with only motor involvement, may be asymmetrical and involve any aspect of the peripheral nervous system, including the cranial nerves and autonomic nerves. The causes of polyneuropathies are protean.

Acute, subacute and chronic neuropathies indicate different pathophysiological processes and help tailor the work-up. The acute loss of motor function in GBS clearly requires a different level of urgency than a slowly progressive neuropathy associated with diabetes (usually most common). A history of other medical conditions, symptoms of systemic disease, infectious diseases, medications (including supplements and vitamins), and exposure to toxins are all important. A careful family history may indicate a heritable disorder and should never be discounted, even in the elderly. Electrodiagnostic studies in conjunction with the history and judicious use of laboratory testing will aid greatly in determining the etiology of the PN. NCS can determine whether the process is primarily axonal or demyelinating (Table 5).

Acute Peripheral Neuropathy

Acute Demyelinating PN

The most important PN to diagnose and treat urgently is the acute symmetrical PN, presenting as rapid progressive paralysis with areflexia. This clinical picture is usually one of the acute inflammatory demyelinating polyneuropathies (AIDP), of which GBS is the most common. The Miller Fisher variant (characterized by ophthalmoplegia, ataxia, and loss of tendon reflexes) is much less common. Familiarity with this illness is important since the disease can progress rapidly to respiratory insufficiency. Respiratory insufficiency requiring ventilatory support can occur in up to a third of patients. For this reason patients are hospitalized and respiratory function is monitored. The vital capacity, negative inspiratory and expiratory force, is monitored frequently to ensure proper timing of potential respiratory intervention. Early in the course of disease, symptoms such as paraesthesias, extremity weakness, and cranial nerve findings are often mild and overlooked. Most cases, as the name implies, are demyelinating. Electrophysiological studies show slowed MNCV and delayed SNAPs, conduction block, prolonged or absent F-waves and

Table 5

Specialized Tests for Peripheral Neuropathy

Sensory or Sensorimotor Neuropathies

1. Anti-MAG – PN with demyelination, IgM monoclonal proteins, if positive suggests immune mediated disease

2. Anti-Hu – Pure sensory syndrome, if positive suggests a paraneoplastic syndrome

3. Anti-Sulfatide – Unclear but may suggest distal, axonal, sensory-predominant peripheral neuropathy

Motor Neuropathies

1. Anti-GM1 – Multifocal motor neuropathy, IgM antibodies specific for motor neuropathies if present in Güillain-Barré syndrome suggests a more severe course

2. Anti-GQ1b – Associated with Miller Fisher variant of Güillain-Barré syndrome.

Genetic Testing

1. CMT testing – Highest yield with demyelinating forms, Important in special situations (child with PN, chemotherapy, other associated PN)

2. Hereditary sensitivity to pressure palsies, multiple mononeuropathies

Amyloidosis – Small Sensory Fiber Loss, Autonomic Neuropathy, Possibly CTS

1. Congo red positive deposits on nerve, muscle, fat pad, rectal, gingival, biopsy

H-reflex. There is a variant of AIDP with axonal damage and a poorer prognosis. EMG examination demonstrates active denervation. A lumbar puncture is usually required for proper diagnosis. The cerebrospinal fluid (CSF) demonstrates high protein and few cells. These findings may not be present in the acute stage, and may take many days to a week to develop. When white cells are present, this may suggest infection, such as HIV. There is an association of the Miller Fisher variant of AIDP with campylobacter infection and the presence of serum antibodies to GQ1b ganglioside. GBS is often associated with an upper respiratory prodrome and antibodies to the GM1 ganglioside. Autonomic neuropathy may be present: therefore, monitoring heart rate, blood pressure, bowel and bladder function is essential.

Treatment of AIDP is with either intravenous immunoglobulin or plasmapheresis. Treatment should begin as soon as the syndrome is recognized. Earlier treatment may lead to better outcome. Intravenous immunoglobulin is well tolerated and is as effective as plasmapheresis. Plasmapheresis can be associated with infection and clotting disorders, while intravenous immunoglobin (IVIG) is associated commonly with headaches, myalgias, and fatigue, as well as the potential problems of receiving blood products. It is important to carefully consider the side effects of plasma exchange if autonomic neuropathy is present.

Other less common causes of acute symmetrical or asymmetrical neuropathic weakness must be considered when considering a diagnosis of AIDP. These include toxins, viruses and CNS infection (Table 6).

Acute Axonal PN

The symptoms are similar to the chronic form of axonal neuropathy, but present with more fulminant symptoms. Pain is a predominant component, although it can be absent. These neuropathies are associated mostly with medication and toxins. Thallium, lead, organophosphates, and arsenic are the most commonly associated toxins, among many others. A variety of antineoplastics, antibiotics and cardiac medications may be the cause (Table 7). The PN tends to worsen over two to three weeks, plateau, and then recover over months, depending on the exposure duration and type.

Table 6

Causes of Acute Weakness

Category	Causes
Porphyria Toxins	Arsenic Thallium Organophosphates Lead Buckthorn
Marine Toxins	Ciguatoxin Tetrodotoxin Saxitoxin
Inflammatory Meningoradiculopathies	Lyme disease Human immunodeficiency virus Cytomegalovirus
Metabolic Disturbance	Hypophosphatemia Hypokalemia Hypermagnesemia
Disorders of Neuromuscular Junction	Botulism Myasthenia gravis
CNS Infection	Poliomyelitis West Nile virus poliomyelitis Rabies

Chronic Polyneuropathies

Chronic polyneuropathies are more common than the acute variety and have a different clinical picture. These polyneuropathies develop over months to years and are generally classified as being primarily axonal, demyelinating or mixed. The type of the polyneuropathy is determined with electrodiagnostic testing. The clinical course of progression, relative contribution of motor or sensory symptoms, and characterization of nerve fiber types as small or large fiber, can refine the differential diagnosis to two or three possible etiologies.

Chronic Demyelinating Polyneuropathies

Chronic demyelinating polyneuropathies represent one of the easier categories to define. They are generally either acquired or genetically linked. The hereditary motor sensory neuropathy (HMSN), also known as Charcot-Marie-Tooth disease, with subclasses and hereditary liability to pressure palsies, are the most common genetic neuropathies. HMSN represents an array of genotypic and phenotypic presentations, so genetic testing is indicated for a more refined diagnosis. The acquired chronic demyelinating polyneuropathies are chronic inflammatory demyelinating PN (CIDP), multifocal motor neuropathy (MMN), and those associated with paraproteins.

Electrodiagnostic and clinical features are helpful in making the distinction between genetic and acquired demyelinating chronic PN. The uniform symmetrical slowing of genetically determined neuropathy is distinct from the multifocal slowing and conduction block, indicating an acquired demyelinating neuropathy. Clinically CIDP is usually slowly progressive, although it can have a relapsing course. The neuropathy is usually primarily motor, affecting both proximal and distal muscles, but can have sensory symptoms as well. MMN is characterized by partial conduction block in motor axons, usually presents with weakness and atrophy of muscles in the forearms and hands, and can be mistaken for early motor neuron disease. Neuropathies associated with paraproteins have a pattern of slowing in distal nerve segments with prolongation of distal latencies. Clinically they present with slowly evolving distal symmetrical sensory abnormalities in the feet. The most common paraprotein is an IgM directed against myelin-associated glycoprotein (anti-MAG).

Treatment of these chronic demyelinating PN is supportive and directed at the underlying cause if amenable. In the case of CIDP high-dose corticosteroids (tapering dose), IVIG (400mg/kg/d over 5 days), and plasma exchange biweekly are the standard therapeutic options. Immunosuppressive agents may be used in selected cases. In the case of paraproteinemia and MMN, the treatment is similar to CIDP, though the evidence is more anecdotal. In all cases, physical therapy and use of assistive devices can aid in maintaining patient independence and mobility.

Figure 2

Distribution of sensory change in polyneuropathy

Left: As the neuropathy ascends in the legs, the fingers become involved. The classic Cuirass distribution of involvement of the intercostal nerves is shown. Right: Mononeuritis multiplex with different peripheral nerve distribution involvement. Left peroneal and right ulnar nerve sensory changes is shown.

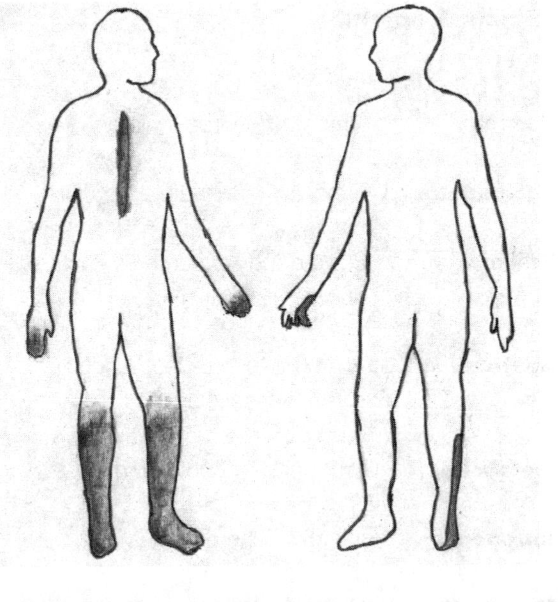

Chronic Axonal PN

Chronic axonal polyneuropathies are the most common of the polyneuropathies. By the nature of it being an axonal injury, severity tends to be related to axon length. Longer axons are affected first, resulting in symptoms which begin in the lower extremities. Sensory symptoms usually precede motor symptoms. Patients typically present with slowly progressive sensory loss and paresthesias. This may take the form of the familiar "stocking and glove" sensory loss; as the ascending sensory loss reaches the mid-calf, the fingertips become affected. When weakness develops, it presents first in the foot dorsiflexors and toe extensors and flexors.

Diabetes is the prototypical chronic axonal PN. However, a range of systemic diseases and metabolic disorders such as nutritional deficiencies, uremia, and malignant diseases—as well as toxins, medications, alcohol abuse with malnutrition, or chemical agents—can result in this pattern of neuropathy. Several varieties of HSMN, especially the axonal forms of Charcot-Marie-Tooth disease (CMT-II), can present with this pattern of neuropathy. A typical phenotype with pes cavus and clawed toes with a positive family history are helpful in directing one toward further genetic work-up for an inherited PN, as with CMT-I.

Figure 4

Skin biopsy demonstrating normal nerve fiber density

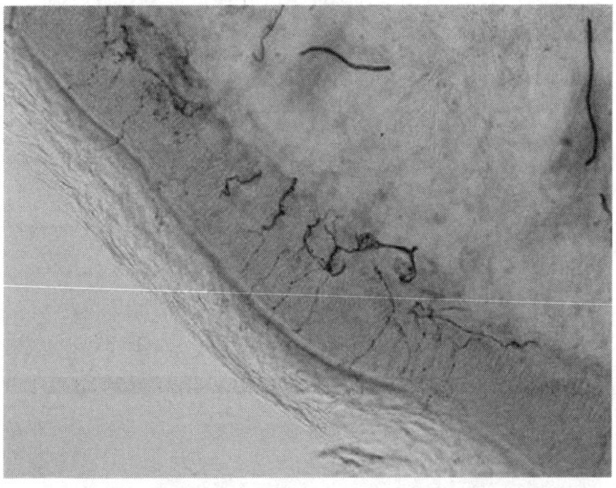

Courtesy of Therapath

Figure 5

Skin biopsy demonstrating decreased nerve fiber density, small fiber neuropathy

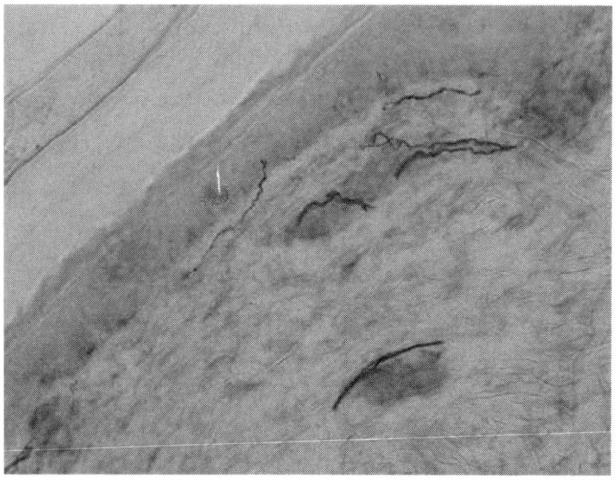

Courtesy of Therapath

Often no clear etiology is found after evaluation for PN. Many of these chronic idiopathic polyneuropathies are mild, predominantly sensory, distal, and symmetrical. Many of these patients have a predominantly small fiber PN that presents with pain and numbness in the feet ("burning feet syndrome"). Physical examination is normal, as are nerve conduction studies. Recently advances in objectifying and proving this diagnosis have been made using skin biopsy. Nerve density in unmyelinated fibers is decreased. The technique is commercially available (Figures 4 and 5).

Table 7

Chemotherapeutic Agents

Vinca alkaloids	inhibit microtubule polymerization; cause sensorimotor & autonomic neuropathy, small fiber
Taxanes	stabilize microtubule polymerization; cause predominantly sensory neuropathy, large and small fiber
Platins	compounds are directly neurotoxic; cause predominantly sensory neuropathy, large fiber

Table 8

Conditions Associated with Mononeuropathies

Vascular	Diabetes, microcirculatory disease
Inflammatory	Synovitis, rheumatoid arthritis
Trauma	Supracondylar humerus fracture, lunate dislocation
Anatomical	Anomalous muscles, vascular plexus, fascial bands
Metabolic	Pregnancy, hypothyroidism
Iatrogenic	Injections, hematomas
Neoplastic	Ganglion, lipoma, sarcoma

6. Specific Mononeuropathies

Mononeuropathies are lesions to specific nerves, most commonly from entrapment by proximity to other structures, trauma, or external compression. A comprehensive review of the nerves and their individual courses and formation from the brachial or lumbosacral plexus is beyond the scope of this review. Major anatomical structures and relationships will be mentioned for clarity of the presentation of specific lesions associated with anatomical compression.

Mononeuropathies caused by trauma or compression can be classified into three categories. Neuropraxia refers to a transient "stunning" of a nerve with short-term nerve conduction disruption. Connective tissue sheaths and axons remain intact so there is no permanent loss of function. Axonotmesis is a more severe nerve injury, with disruption of the axon with maintenance of the nerve connective tissue sheath. Motor, sensory, and autonomic dysfunction results. Recovery is usually complete, as the integrity of the nerve sheath is intact. Neurotmesis is the most serious injury. The nerve axon and its connective tissue sheath are disrupted. Although recovery may occur, it is never complete, due to loss of nerve continuity during regeneration.

Familiarity with a specific peripheral nerve's muscle and sensory innervation make recognizing a patient's pattern of symptoms easy. The weak muscles and the areas of diminished sensation should all conform to a particular peripheral nerve distribution. The pattern of pain may be misleading, as it may radiate beyond the classic distribution of the nerve–such as shoulder pain in carpal tunnel syndrome.

An understanding of the mechanism of nerve injury may aid in diagnosis. Repetitive use of the hands and wrists suggest problems in this area may be due to carpal tunnel syndrome. Recent surgery under anesthesia or positional compression may aid in diagnosing radial or peroneal nerve injuries (Table 7).

Median Nerve

The median nerve forms from the junction of the lateral and medial cords of the brachial plexus. It travels through the arm lateral to the brachial artery; at the level of the antecubital fossa, it courses under the bicipital aponeurosis. It emerges in proximity to the palmaris longus tendon, and enters the carpal tunnel superficial to the flexor tendons. The motor branch emerges distally to innervate the thenar muscles and lateral two lumbricals.

Sensory branches of the median nerve innervate the skin over the thenar eminence. The major palmar branch courses superficial to the carpal tunnel, and so is spared in carpal tunnel syndrome. Sensory branches in the hand supply the lateral 3.5 fingers.

The anterior interosseous nerve is an important branch of the median nerve originating in the antecubital fossa. The nerve lies on the interosseous membrane and innervates the portion of the flexor digitorum profundus muscle controlling the lateral two digits, flexor pollicis longus, and the pronator quadratus.

Two median nerve mononeuropathies discussed are the anterior interosseous syndrome and carpal tunnel syndrome. The anterior interosseous syndrome is most commonly seen with fractures of the forearm, but has also been described as being caused by tendinous bands and aberrant blood supply to the nerve. Symptoms include pain in the proximal forearm. Rarely, the syndrome may be due to an inflammatory neuropathy. On physical examination, the patient cannot form a circle by pinching their thumb and index finger. Also weakness of the flexor pollicis longus and flexor digitorum profundus to the second digit may be elicited. This nerve has no sensory branch, so no sensory involvement is found. Treatment is usually conservative, though surgical exploration is warranted in certain circumstances.

Carpal tunnel syndrome (CTS) is the most common of the mononeuropathies. The carpal tunnel is formed by carpal bones and the transverse carpal ligament. CTS is caused when pressure within the tunnel increases. Commonly this is attributed to tenosynovitis from overuse, but can be associated with pregnancy, carpal bone fractures or dislocations, diabetes, rheumatoid arthritis, hypothyroidism, and amyloidosis.

Symptoms include decreased sensation, paresthesias of digits 1, 2, 3 and half of the fourth, and weakness of the thumb. These may worsen with repetitive use. Nocturnal awakening with tingling or numbness is very common. There may be symptoms of proximal arm or shoulder pain. On examination, a positive Tinel's or Phalen's sign or compression at the wrist can be helpful in making the diagnosis. Thenar muscle wasting is present with advanced cases.

The mainstay of treatment is nonsurgical, including wrist splints, anti-inflammatory medications (including oral prednisone), and steroid injections. If the cause is from repetitive motion, then alteration to the work environment or avocational activity is warranted. Surgical therapy is indicated in refractory cases or those not responsive to nonsurgical measures. All surgical techniques focus on release of the transverse carpal ligament.

The Ulnar Nerve

The ulnar nerve lies in the anterior compartment of the upper extremity posterior to the brachial artery. When it reaches the medial epicondyle, the nerve courses posterior to the medial epicondyle, then enters the anterior antebrachial compartment. It exits the distal forearm just medial to the ulnar artery. The ulnar nerve then travels within Guyon's canal to innervate the hypothenar muscles, two medial lumbrical muscles, the interossei of the hand, and the deep head of the flexor pollicis brevis muscle. The ulnar nerve supplies sensation to the medial one-and-a-half digits.

There are two main mononeuropathies associated with the ulnar nerve—the first at the medial epicondyle and the second at the wrist within Guyon's canal. Cubital tunnel syndrome refers to entrapment of the ulnar nerve posterior to the medial epicondyle. The cubital tunnel is formed by the aponeurosis of the two heads of the flexor carpi ulnaris covered by an overlying retinaculum.

Symptoms of cubital tunnel syndrome include pain or numbness in the forearm within the distribution of the ulnar nerve and paresthesias in the medial one-and-a-half fingers. On examination, atrophy or weakness of intrinsic hand muscles may be present, as well as a positive compression or Tinel's test at the elbow. The thumb and second digit pinch may be weak (Froment's sign). Subluxation of the nerve over the epicondyle may also occur. Nonsurgical treatments include splints or casting, rest, anti-inflammatory medications, and modification of aggravating motions. Surgical treatments focus on releasing the nerve along its course at sites of compression. These options include decompression, medial epicondylectomy, and anterior transposition of the nerve. Transposition of the ulnar nerve may result in worsening of ulnar function if vascular compromise or increasing compression occurs.

The second main ulnar entrapment mononeuropathy is ulnar tunnel syndrome occurring at Guyon's canal. Commonly, injuries of the nerve are caused by blunt trauma, though carpal fractures may be seen as well. Nonsurgical treatment includes rest and modification of activities. Immobilization with a splint and corticosteroid injections are effective. Surgical treatment may include decompression of Guyon's canal.

The Radial Nerve

The radial nerve courses along the posterior humerus in the spiral groove, where it is susceptible to injury. In the arm, it innervates the triceps muscle and sends a branch to the supinator distally. After leaving the posterior arm, it travels anterior to the elbow joint, then divides into the posterior interosseous nerve and the superficial radial nerve. The superficial radial nerve supplies sensation to the lateral half of the posterior hand. The posterior interosseous nerve courses along the interosseous membrane, innervating the muscles of the posterior forearm.

Radial nerve neuropathies are less common compared to the median and ulnar nerve mononeuropathies. The most relevant radial nerve mononeuropathy is in the middle third of the arm due to compression (Saturday night palsy, crutch palsy), or secondary to trauma with fractures of the humerus. This radial neuropathy is characterized by paresis or paralysis of all extensors of the wrist and digits (wrist drop), and the supinator. Very proximal lesions also may affect the triceps and hand supination. Sensory change occurs on the dorsolateral aspect of the hand and the dorsal aspect of the lateral three-and-a-half digits. It is important to remember that MMN may present with features of a radial neuropathy, but there are no sensory symptoms or history of injury.

Medical therapy varies according to the cause of radial nerve neuropathy. The mainstay of treatment is immobilization with functional splints or casting, and anti-inflammatory medications. This is a protective measure while nerve healing occurs. In the event of failure of medical management, surgical exploration may be warranted.

Lower Extremity Mononeuropathies

Lateral femoral cutaneous nerve mononeuropathy is known as meralgia paresthetica. It is a syndrome of paresthesia and pain in the lateral and anterolateral thigh. This nerve arises from the lumbar plexus. It courses out of the pelvis deep to the inguinal ligament to innervate the skin over the lateral thigh.

Entrapment usually occurs at the inguinal ligament. The entrapment may be from intrapelvic causes such as pregnancy or malignancy. Extrapelvic causes such as trauma from seat belts, tight clothes, or obesity are commonly seen as well. Excessive weight loss and malnutrition may also be causative.

Symptoms include anterior and lateral thigh burning, tingling, and/or numbness. Sensory examination often reveals hyperesthesia or hypoesthesia over the lateral thigh. There is no weakness. NCS and EMG are performed to rule out other causes such as radiculopathy.

Treatment is usually conservative, with improvement after modifying compressive forces such as belts or holsters. Weight loss can be beneficial in overweight patients. Injection of local anesthetics or steroids may be helpful. Persistent neurogenic pain may be treated with AEDs, tricyclics, or topical anesthetics. In the event conservative management fails, surgical exploration may be necessary.

Peroneal neuropathy is a common mononeuropathy of the lower extremity. The common peroneal nerve courses around the fibular neck and divides into the superficial and deep peroneal nerves. The superficial peroneal nerve provides innervation to the lateral compartment of the leg and sensation to the dorsum of the foot. The deep peroneal nerve courses through the anterior compartment of the leg, innervating its muscles. The sensory portion of the deep peroneal nerve innervates the web space between the first and second toes.

Most peroneal nerve injuries occur at the region of the fibular head. This is usually due to habitual leg crossing, compression of the nerve against a bed railing in debilitated patients, or in patients under anesthesia unable to move from a compressive force. Trauma from fibular fractures or dislocation and knee injuries, arthroscopy, and arthroplasty are seen as well. Short casts or braces can also result in external compression on the fibular neck region.

Clinically, peroneal nerve lesions usually present as difficulty walking due to weakness of the ankle dorsiflexors. On examination, the patient may have a positive Tinel's sign at the fibular head. Observation of gait and manual muscle testing reveals a foot drop, high stepped gait, and weakness of the ankle and toe dorsiflexors and everters. The pattern of weakness may be variable. Plantar flexion and inversion are spared. Sensory loss in the distribution of the superficial and deep peroneal nerve may help localize the lesion to above or below the fibular head. NCS and EMG are very helpful in determining the anatomical location of the injury and whether the injury involves the sciatic nerve, lumbosacral plexus, or nerve roots.

Treatment should focus on maximizing mobility and function. In addition, the cause of nerve compromise should be corrected to reduce further nerve damage. The use of an ankle-foot orthosis, splints, or orthopedic shoes may provide gait assistance during nerve recovery.

Tarsal tunnel syndrome is entrapment of the tibial nerve or one of its branches, the medial and lateral plantar nerves, within or distal to the tarsal canal. The tarsal tunnel itself is formed by the medial talus, the inferomedial navicular, the sustentaculum tali, and the medial surface of the calcaneus. The fibrous portion of the tunnel is the flexor retinaculum. The most common etiology of tarsal tunnel syndrome is a fracture or dislocation of the talus, calcaneus, or medial malleolus. Another cause is inflammation or tenosynovitis, such as in rheumatoid arthritis, which may also cause a compression neuropathy. We have also seen tibial neuropathy due to extremely tight ski boots.

Clinically, patients present with aching, burning, numbness, and parenthesis involving the plantar surface of the foot, toes, and/or heel. The pain may radiate up to the calf or higher. Symptoms may worsen after standing. EMG is an important test in suspected tarsal tunnel syndrome to rule out other disorders, especially PN. Often tarsal tunnel symptoms are the initial presentation of an undiagnosed peripheral neuropathy.

Treatment is directed toward rectifying the underlying etiology of neural compression. Conservative management is aimed at relieving any external nerve compression. This can include the use of nonsteroidal anti-inflammatory drugs (NSAIDs), podiatric care including orthotics, and physical therapy.

7. Radiculopathy

Cervical radiculopathy refers to impairment in a spinal nerve innervating the upper extremity and causing neurologic dysfunction. This is usually the result of an abnormality in the cervical vertebral column causing spinal nerve compression. In the majority of cases this is due to foraminal encroachment from degenerative arthritis, cervical spondylosis, or osteophyte formation. In approximately 20%, a herniated disc is the cause of the radiculopathy. Disc herniation is more common in younger patients. Most cervical radiculopathies occur in the lower cervical spine, C5 and below.

Relevant Anatomy

The cervical spine is comprised of seven vertebrae. There are eight cervical nerves. One through seven exit superior to the corresponding vertebrae, C8 exits between C7 and T1. C5 innervates the deltoid and biceps muscles; C6 the wrist extensors and abductor and extensors of the thumb; C7 the triceps, wrist flexors, and finger extensors; C8 the finger flexors; and T1 the intrinsic hand muscles. The biceps and brachioradialis reflexes are mediated by the C5-6 roots, and the triceps reflex by the C6-7 roots (mainly C7).

Patients commonly present with numbness and paresthesias in the fingers and lancinating pain radiating down the arm. A careful description by the patient usually points to a specific dermatomal distribution. Unilateral sensory symptoms are typical and there are usually no motor deficits. When patients report weakness it is important to elicit whether there are myelopathic features as well.

Examination of the patient with suspected cervical radiculopathy includes a detailed neurological examination, Spurling's maneuver as well as cervical traction, and examination of the neck. Evidence of weakness, dermatomal sensory change, or asymmetric reflexes can help localize the lesion. Spurling's maneuver and vertical traction may exacerbate or alleviate cervical radiculopathies respectively. Care should be taken in performing any maneuvers in patients with suspected traumatic spine pathology or rheumatoid arthritis, as manipulation may worsen the situation.

MRI is useful in detecting disc herniation or other

causes of spinal nerve injury and should always be obtained in cases of suspected myelopathy. EMG can help differentiate a peripheral nerve disorder from a cervical radiculopathy. In cervical radiculopathy, paraspinal muscle denervation is a helpful finding. Treatment of painful cervical radiculopathy is aimed at reducing nerve irritation and pressure and increasing neck flexibility.

Therapy in the acute phase of injury is conservative, with application of ice or heat, gentle message, and stretching to reduce secondary muscle irritation and spasm. Muscle relaxants and NSAIDs may help with sleep, muscle spasm, inflammation and pain. If there is motor involvement, the degree of pathology may be more significant and require more aggressive early therapy, including cervical traction and neurosurgical consultation. Conservative measures are all that are required in the majority of cases, with resolution of symptoms occurring in 3 to 6 weeks.

Patients with persistent symptoms should be reevaluated to rule out progression. More aggressive treatments may be employed, generally after an MRI. Vertical traction with physical therapy can be useful, although it is not well studied. Cervical epidural corticosteroid injections may be helpful in alleviating persistent radicular pain, and avoid the need for surgery in patients who have not responded to conservative treatment.

Most patients with cervical radiculopathy will improve. Referral to a spine surgeon after failure of conservative management is appropriate.

Lumbosacral Radiculopathy

Low back pain is one of the most common maladies. It is the fifth-leading cause of physician visits and accounts for almost one-third of all workers compensation claims. Most lower back pain is attributable to mechanical or functional soft tissue injury such as muscle strain or ligamentous sprain. True radiculopathic low back pain is present in only about 4% of cases. The nerve roots commonly associated with this in order of descending frequency are S1, L5, and L4. Radiculopathy of L1 to L3 accounts for only 5% of cases. The most common causes of nerve root irritation are herniated disc, foraminal or spinal stenosis, and ligamentous hypertrophy. Other space occupying lesions which cause foraminal compromise are abscesses, cysts, or tumors. These are less common but important considerations in any case where there are symptoms such as fevers, chills, or weight loss. Particular attention to bowel, bladder and sexual dysfunction may suggest a cauda equina syndrome.

The history can be quite varied, but in most radiculopathies the pain is usually brief, sharp and lancinating, often increased by straining, and usually relieved by lying down or finding a characteristic position of comfort. Pain that radiates below the knee is a good predictor of nerve compression, as is a history of weakness and/or numbness. A precise description of radiating pain will help localize a specific nerve root level.

Physical examination is best discussed in terms of individual nerve involvement. Involvement of S1 spinal nerve often results in leg pain that is worse than low back pain. The pain is in the buttock, posterior thigh, calf and heel. Sensation loss over the lateral foot and fifth toe is common, as is weakness of the toe flexors and gastrocnemius. The ankle jerk is often diminished or absent compared to the unaffected extremity.

Involvement of L5 spinal nerve often manifests with worse low back pain than leg pain. Pain is more likely to radiate to the posterior thigh, groin, calf, medial foot and first two digits. Sensory loss is usually found in the hallux and medial foot. Weakness may lead to a foot drop. Reflexes are usually intact.

Involvement of L4 or L3 spinal nerves results in worse pain in the low back than the leg. Pain radiates to the anteromedial thigh and knee with sensory loss in the same area. Weakness of knee extension and hip flexion may be found. The patellar reflex may be decreased or absent.

The straight leg raise (SLR) test, if positive at 60 degrees or less, has good sensitivity for herniated disc, but is not specific. Rectal examination in cases of suspected cauda equina syndrome is essential to evaluate sphincter tone.

Electrodiagnostic studies are helpful when the diagnosis remains unclear, such as a peroneal neuropathy versus radiculopathy. Again, paraspinal muscle denervation is supportive of lumbosacral radiculopathy. They are also helpful in excluding and or differentiating among other causes of sensory and motor disturbances, such as peripheral neuropathy and motor neuron disease. Additionally, they can provide useful prognostic information by quantifying the extent and acuity of axonal involvement in radiculopathies.

MRI with gadolinium is the imaging study of choice in evaluating lumbosacral radiculopathy. Most patients without alarming signs or symptoms will respond to conservative management. In those who fail a reasonable trial in this manner, or have progressive or worrisome features such as significant motor weakness or sensory loss, imaging should be done sooner. Conservative management includes NSAIDs, physical therapy, analgesic medications, epidural steroid injection, transcutaneous electrical nerve stimulation, and chiropractic care. Surgery may be considered with persistent neurological signs and symptoms.

8. Plexopathy

Brachial plexopathy, also known as Parsonage-Turner syndrome, is a disorder involving the brachial plexus and/or individual terminal nerves. It is characterized by the acute onset of unilateral shoulder pain, followed by paralysis and atrophy of the shoulder and scapular muscles. The presentation may vary substantially from case to case. The cause of the disorder is unknown, though thought to be an autoimmune disorder.

The typical history of brachial plexopathy is one of acute onset severe shoulder pain in a person following illness, trauma, immunization or other physiological stressor, such as exercise or childbirth. This pain is localized to the shoulder region in most cases, though it may be bilateral. The pain can mimic orthopedic pain (rotator cuff, bursitis) with exacerbation by movement, and be throbbing and constant, or more like a radicular pain that is lancinating.

Weakness is usually maximal at onset, primarily affecting the muscles of the shoulder girdle. Atrophy can be quite striking. Phrenic nerve involvement with diaphragmatic paralysis may occur rarely.

Physical examination is usually limited in the acute phase by pain. Myalgias are common, and depending on the nerves involved reflexes may be depressed or absent. Sensory changes are not usually prominent but may be detected.

MRI of the cervical spine and brachial plexus will

Table 9

Findings in Motor Neuron Disease

ALS	Most common, UMN LMN findings	EMG diffuse denervation
PLS	Symmetrical, slow progression, UMN findings	EMG no denervation, MRI, PET may be helpful
PMA	Asymmetric, progressive, paraspinal and respiratory involvement	EMG diffuse denervation
Familial ALS	Can be younger, cognitive impairment	EMG denervation SOD 1 testing

help rule out cervical radiculopathy or infiltrative lesion, respectively. Plain films should be done in cases of antecedent trauma to rule out bony fracture or dislocation. EMG studies should be performed at an appropriate time (usually at least 5-7 days after onset) to confirm the diagnosis and to rule out other etiologies.

Conservative management is the rule. Physical therapy to ensure range of motion and prevent complications of shoulder immobility is important. If the disorder is suspected early, an empiric trail of high-dose steroids or IVIG may be tried. Treatment is usually limited by the disorder being diagnosed, far after the onset of symptoms.

Lumbosacral plexopathy is most commonly associated with diabetes. It is known by the eponym Bruns-Garland syndrome (BGS). There is usually the acute onset of hip pain and weakness of the iliopsoas, quadriceps and thigh adductor muscles. Sensory complaints are minimal. The knee reflex is usually absent. NCS and EMG are helpful to confirm the diagnosis and exclude radiculopathy. BGS usually occurs in patients with diabetic PN, systemic symptoms, and poor diabetic control. There have been reports of immunotherapy (corticosteroids and IVIG) helping with recovery. It is important to exercise caution in treating diabetics with steroids.

Lumbosacral plexopathy may also occur as an idiopathic disorder in the elderly or in patients with connective tissue disorders, especially Sjögren syndrome. Immunotherapy may be helpful.

9. Motor Neuron Diseases

Amyotrophic lateral sclerosis (ALS), also called Lou Gehrig disease, is a progressive disorder which usually results in death within three to five years after diagnosis. ALS is one of the motor neuron diseases (MND). These include: primary lateral sclerosis (PLS), which is a pure upper motor neuron (UMN) disorder; progressive muscular atrophy (PMA), which is a pure lower motor neuron (LMN) disorder; and familial ALS (Table 8). ALS is the most common MND, with an overall incidence of 2/100,000 per year. ALS is slightly more common in men than women. ALS is most common in individuals aged 50-70 years, but is seen in patients from their twenties to their eighties. There are reports of ALS clusters. Recently, an association of ALS and military service (specifically those who served in Operation Desert Storm) was published. There are reports of associations with trauma, athletics, thin body stature, dairy products, toxin exposure and pets. The reasons for these associations are not clear.

Clinical Features

ALS usually presents with asymmetrical weakness of a distal extremity, eg, a foot drop or weakness of the hand. ALS is a disorder of both the UMN and LMN. There is no significant sensory deficit or pain. Bowel and bladder function are maintained until late in the course of the illness, where there may be incontinence due to inability to ambulate or move. Cognitive impairment in the form of a frontotemporal dementia can occur. The LMN findings in ALS patients include: atrophy, fasciculations, absent reflexes, weakness and cramps. Fasciculations and atrophy of the tongue are very suggestive of ALS. Electromyographic examination demonstrates this LMN involvement: the recording of denervation (fibrillations and sharp waves), fasciculations, neuropathic motor unit potentials, and decreased voluntary motor recruitment. The UMN findings include: increased tone, increased reflexes, pathological reflexes (Babinski sign, Hoffman sign, palmomental reflex), weakness, and decreased rapid alternating movements. Patients can have emotional lability when there is corticobulbar tract involvement. This can be manifested as laughing or crying when the situation would not normally provoke that emotional response from the patient. Crying is usually more common than laughter. As the disease progresses, significant weight loss occurs as the result of pronounced chewing and swallowing problems, as well as loss of muscle mass. Speech becomes more difficult, and anarthria may ensue. Respiratory insufficiency due to diaphragmatic and accessory muscle weakness is usual.

Differential Diagnosis

The diagnosis is usually not difficult as ALS progresses. Diagnosis can be difficult if only corticobulbar symptoms and signs are present. The EMG is usually not clear in this situation. If the patient's symptoms and signs do not include cranial nerve involvement, MRI scanning of the cervical spinal cord is essential to exclude a cervical myelopathy. Table 9 outlines differential diagnosis and required testing, if indicated.

Diagnostic Testing

Nerve conduction studies (NCS) and EMG are performed to confirm the diagnosis. NCS velocities are usually normal. If there is significant loss of anterior horn cells and muscle atrophy, the compound muscle action potential will be decreased. EMG examination documents widespread active denervation, fasciculations, neuropathic MUPs, and decreased voluntary motor recruitment. These changes should be present in three extremities or the cranial musculature and one extremity. MRI is important to exclude a cervical myelopathy.

Clinical Course

Death usually occurs within 3-5 years after the onset of symptoms. There is progressive weakness, atrophy, and spasticity of the extremities. This results in significant gait impairment and difficulty with activities of daily living such as writing and dressing. In

Table 10

Differential Diagnosis of ALS and Appropriate Testing

Cervical myelopathy	Sensory level, bowel and bladder symptoms, paucity of LMN signs	Cervical MRI
Lyme disease	Rash, arthritis, sensory deficits, specific nerves or roots, serology blood CSF	Lyme serology
HIV	Risk factors, other features of illness, altered immunity	HIV testing
Inclusion body myositis	Significant CK elevation (less common in ALS), flexor weakness UEs, no UMN findings	Muscle biopsy
Multifocal motor neuropathy	Specific nerves, NCS abnormalities, conduction block, no UMN findings	GM1 Ab, NCS SPEP
Myasthenia gravis	Diplopia, ptosis, EMG no significant denervation, repetitive nerve stimulation	AChR Abs

Other testing for less likely diagnoses: Thyroid, if indicated: SOD 1, CIDP lumbar puncture, Hex A, Amyloid for tissue biopsy, Kennedy syndrome

Table 11

Symptomatic Treatment for ALS

Increased salivation	Amitryptline, Botox injections	Can use other antidepressants with anticholinergic effects
Emotional lability	Amitryptline	Can use fluoxetine or other SSRIs
Spasticity	Baclofen, tizanidine	Slowly increase, do not stop abruptly

addition, with cranial nerve involvement there is progressive difficulty with speech, chewing, and swallowing. Bulbar ALS (initial cranial nerve involvement) has a worse prognosis. Cognitive impairment may become manifest as the disease progresses. Emotional liability can occur with corticobulbar involvement. Respiratory insufficiency ensues with CO_2 retention and disordered sleep. Finally, aspiration pneumonia and respiratory failure is the usual cause of death.

Familial ALS

Approximately 10%-20% of ALS cases are familial, with 20% of these cases having a mutation of the superoxide dismutase 1 gene (SOD1). This abnormality can be documented by commercial testing. Familial ALS cases may have an earlier onset of illness and may have more significant cognitive impairment.

Treatment

A multidisciplinary ALS clinic which includes nursing, neurology, pulmonology, speech therapy, occupational therapy (OT), physical therapy (PT), dietetics, and social service is highly desirable. OT and PT can assist with therapy and adaptive devices. Speech therapy can assess and help with communication and swallowing difficulties. Dietetics can follow the patient's nutritional status and help alter the patient's diet when chewing and swallowing become more difficult. Assessment of the need for percutaneous esophageal gastrostomy (PEG) can also be performed. Pulmonary function testing should be done serially. Sleep disturbances and confusion can be a sign of impending respiratory failure. The question of assisted ventilation and PEG placement needs to be discussed with the patient and family early and frankly. Social workers are essential for these discussions and for end-of-life discussions. The social worker and mental health workers support the patient and family in this difficult illness. Medications which may help with symptoms of ALS are outlined in Table 10. There is one medication approved for the treatment of ALS—riluzole, which increases life expectancy by three months. The major side effect is gastrointestinal upset.

10. References

Manuscripts

1. Sindrup SH, Jensen TS. Pharmacologic treatment of pain in polyneuropathy. *Neurology*. 2000; 55:915.

   (A very good review of the rational treatment of polyneuropathy pain.)

2. Shapiro BE, Preston DC. Entrapment and compressive neuropathies. *Med Clin North Am*. 2003 May;87(3):663-96, viii.

   (A nice review article of common entrapment neuropathies and their approach.)

3. Miller JD, Pruitt S, McDonald TJ. Acute brachial plexus neuritis: an uncommon cause of shoulder pain. *Am Fam Physician*. 2000 Nov 1;62(9):2067-72.

   (Inflammatory brachial plexopathies are common in neurology practice. This article is a good review of the clinical presentation and differential diagnosis of this disorder.)

4. England JD, Asbury AK. Peripheral neuropathy. *Lancet*. 2004 Jun 26;363(9427):2151-61.

   (Excellent review on differential diagnosis of peripheral neuropathy.)

5. Berciano J, Combarros O. Hereditary neuropathies. *Curr Opin in Neuro*. 2003;16:613-622.

   (Very good review of the hereditary neuropathies; which are common referrals for the practicing neurologist.)

6. Bayramoglu M. Entrapment neuropathies of the upper extremity. *Neuroanatomy*. 2004; May 24, Volume 3:18-24.

   (A useful review of the common entrapment neuropathies of the upper extremity.)

Textbooks

Aminoff MJ. *Electrodiagnosis in Clinical Neurology*. New York, NY: Churchill Livingstone; 1998.

(This is an excellent review text for NCS/EMG, as well as all clinical neurophysiological testing.)

Web Sites

http://www.neuro.wustl.edu/neuromuscular/

Washington University; St. Louis, Mo. Neuromuscular Disease Center

(The best site for diagnosis and treatment of neuromuscular disorders. Always updated; an excellent work. It is indispensable for the clinician.)

http://www.neuropathy.org/site/

The Neuropathy Association

(Has contacts and information for the patient with neuropathy.)

11. Questions

1-4. A 40-year-old woman is tripping because her feet get caught in the carpet. On examination, she has high arches. Which of the following information would NOT be helpful?

A. If her parents have high arches and curled toes

B. Did the patient receive chemotherapy?

C. Is the patient diabetic?

D. Does the patient live near high tension lines?

If nerve conduction studies are performed on this patient, which findings would be most likely?

A. Incremental response of the median CMAP with high frequency stimulation

B. Decremental response of the ulnar CMAP with low frequency stimulation

C. Normal peroneal F-waves

D. Slowed peroneal nerve conduction velocity

The patient would like a precise diagnosis since she has 2 children and worries if this is hereditary. Which of the following would be LEAST helpful?

A. Examination of the patient's mother and father

B. Genetic testing

C. Examination of the patient's 2 daughters

D. Sural nerve biopsy of the patient's husband

Which of the following would be NOT important for the patient?

A. If she is to receive chemotherapy in the future to let her doctors know she has a peripheral neuropathy

B. Proper fitting shoes and care of her feet

C. Evaluation by physical therapy and podiatry

D. High dose B_6 therapy

5-8. A 56-year-old diabetic accountant began having severe pain in his right hip and thigh 2 weeks ago after playing in a golf tournament. Approximately 5 days later because of the continued severe pain he went to his family practice doctor who suspected a hip bursitis and gave him diclofenac. The pain was not relieved by the diclofenac and yesterday morning the patient became worried when he noticed he had trouble getting out of bed and difficulty climbing upstairs. He returns to his family practice doctor who notes right hip flexor, right thigh adductor, and right knee extensor weakness. The right knee reflex is absent and there is a stocking loss of pin and temperature sensation to the ankles bilaterally. A lumbosacral MRI shows degenerative changes L5 S1. The family practice doctor wants your opinion re surgery. You would probably want to do:

A. A lumbar puncture

B. A sural nerve biopsy

C. Get a stat physical therapy consult

D. Help the surgeon schedule the surgery

E. Perform an EMG/Nerve conduction study

Which of the following would be a LIKELY finding on this patient's NCS?

A. Absent sural nerve conduction

B. A normal H reflex

C. Normal peroneal F-waves

D. Abnormal blink reflexes

Which of the following would be a likely finding on this patient's EMG?

A. Active denervation in the cranial musculature

B. Low amplitude short duration polyphasic motor units in the deltoid

C. Myotonic discharges in the abductor pollicis brevis

D. Myokima in the biceps

E. Active denervation in the right iliopsoas, right vastus lateralis, right thigh adductors

All the following may be helpful for the patient EXCEPT:

A. Better control of the patient's diabetes

B. Pain control with amitriptyline or gabapentin

C. Physical therapy

D. IVIG

E. Mestinon®

9-12. A 49-year-old carpenter noticed that over the last 2 months he keeps dropping his hammer. He also will have cramping in his right arm when holding his power tools for a while. His wife has commented that the muscles in his right arm look smaller. In the past year he has seen his internist for carpal tunnel syndrome and also neck pain. He assumes that his symptoms must be the carpal tunnel syndrome. His wife makes an appointment with the internist because she has noted he is losing weight. The internist is worried because the patient has lost weight, has a smoking history, and there is atrophy and weakness of the intrinsics, deltoid, and biceps muscles on the right.

The patient on examination also has brisk reflexes in the upper extremities and difficulty walking on his heels on the left. These findings:

A. Make brachial neuritis likely

B. Suggest upper and lower motor neuron involvement

C. Localize to the thoracic spine

D. Are consistent with Güillain-Barré Syndrome

E. Suggest Miller Fisher variant

Which of the following would NOT be helpful in evaluation?

A. GM1 antibody level

B. EMG/NCS

C. Cervical MRI

D. Lumbar puncture

E. anti-Yo antibody testing

The patient's EMG most likely would demonstrate:

A. Low amplitude shore duration polyphasic motor unit potentials in the tongue

B. Diver bomber potentials in the APB

C. Full recruitment patterns with minimal effort

D. Electrically silent cramps

E. Active denervation in 3 extremities

As the patient's disease progresses, which of the following would NOT be helpful:

A. IVIG

B. Antidepressants

C. Bi-PAP

D. Baclofen

E. Swallowing evaluation

13-16. A 55-year-old woman who has recently completed a course of treatment radiation therapy and chemotherapy for right-sided breast cancer is complaining of a painful distal neuropathy:

A. A sural nerve biopsy should be the first step

B. At this point, nerve conductions would not be helpful

C. EMG examination of the cranial musculature should be done

D. A complete history of the patient's chemotherapy and medications should be obtained

The patient gives a history of chemotherapy treatment with Taxol®. Which of the following statements is NOT true?

A. Taxenes cause a predominately motor neuropathy

B. If a patient has a pre-existing peripheral neuropathy, chemotherapy usually worsens it

C. Nerve conduction studies can help in documenting and characterizing the patient's peripheral neuropathy

D. Nerve biopsy is usually not indicated in the diagnosis of chemotherapy-induced peripheral neuropathy

The nerve conduction studies and EMG will most likely demonstrate:

A. Low amplitude sensory nerve action potentials

B. Myopathic motor units in the cranial muscles

C. Conduction block

D. Decremental response of the ulnar nerve with 2 Hz stimulation

After one year this patient complains of progressive weakness of her right arm. Which of the following would be least helpful?

A. A serum CK level

B. Nerve conduction and EMG studies

C. Re-evaluation of the patient's breast cancer

D. MRI of the brachial plexus

17-20. A 45-year-old physician complains of 2 days of progressive numbness and weakness of his feet 2 weeks after a stomach virus. On examination he has absent ankle reflexes and weakness of foot dorsiflexion. Which of the following is NOT recommended?

A. CSF studies

B. Nerve conduction studies

C. Assessment of pulmonary function

D. Careful monitoring of his clinical status

E. Immediate high dose IV Solu-Medrol®

Which of the following is associated with Güillain-Barré syndrome?

A. Brisk reflexes

B. Present H reflex

C. CSF pleocytosis

D. Prolonged F-wave latencies

E. Response to Tensilon®

The patient continues to weaken and is having trouble with secretions. You should:

A. Repeat the CSF studies

B. Repeat the NCS

C. Perform repetitive stimulation

D. Transfer the patient to the ICU

E. Do a stat barium swallow study

Care of the patient with Güillian-Barré may include all the following EXCEPT:

A. Prevention measures for deep vein thrombosis

B. Monitor respiratory status

C. IVIG

D. Mestinon

E. Monitor autonomic function

Answers

1. D.
The patient has weakness in dorsiflexion of her feet. The high arches suggest a hereditary peripheral neuropathy. All of these answers except D. may be related to peripheral neuropathy.

2. D.
The slowed peroneal nerve conduction velocities are present in hereditary peripheral neuropathy in, specifically, Charcot-Marie-Tooth I.

3. B.
Family history is important to obtain for the diagnosis of hereditary neuropathy. The husband's history would not be germane.

4. D.
All of the following except B_6 therapy would be important. High dose B_6 therapy may cause severe dorsal root ganglion pathology.

5. E.
An NCS/EMG would help document whether this is a diabetic lumbosacral plexopathy. It is unlikely that L5 S1 root changes would cause proximal lower extremity weakness. An LP may be done later if the diagnosis is not clear.

6. D.
Most patients with diabetic lumbosacral plexopathy have a peripheral neuropathy (absent ankle jerks). Therefore, the H reflex, the electrophysiological equivalent of the ankle jerk, would be absent.

7. C.
With the patient's proximal weakness, active denervation in the right proximal muscles would be likely.

8 E.
All may be helpful including IVIG (recent reports) except Mestinon, which is used for myasthenia gravis.

9. B.
The brisk reflexes with the upper extremity atrophy and weakness suggests upper and lower motor neuron involvement.

10. E.
All would be helpful except E. in ruling out the following: multifocal motor neuropathy, cervical spine disease, and CIDP, and the EMG would confirm the diagnosis of ALS.

11. E
Active denervation in three extremities would help establish the diagnosis of ALS.

12. A.
This patient has ALS. IVIG is not an effective treatment for ALS.

13. D.
This is a patient with breast cancer. It would be important to know if her chemotherapy could cause a peripheral neuropathy.

14. A.
Taxenes cause predominately a sensory neuropathy.

15. A.
Taxenes cause an axonal sensory neuropathy (low amplitude sensory nerve action potentials).

16. A.
Consideration should be given to the spread of the cancer to the brachial plexus or radiation damage to the brachial plexus. Metastatic brain lesions could also be a cause of the patient's weakness.

17. E.
High dose Solu-Medrol is ineffective in the treatment of Güillian-Barré Syndrome. The other strategies are important in the care of the patient.

18. D.
Prolonged F-wave latencies can be an early finding in GBS.

19. D.
Transfer to the ICU is important when a GBS patient has trouble with secretions. Aspiration pneumonia and respiratory failure can lead to mortality in GBS.

20. D.
Mestinon is not usually used in the treatment of GBS. Autonomic failure may be occur in GBS.

Chapter 18: Neuromuscular Junction and Muscle Disease

Elijah Stommel, MD, PhD

Contents

Introduction

There are a myriad of neurological diseases that involve the neuromuscular junction and muscle. The purpose of this review is to educate the reader about some of the important principles and common diseases affecting these anatomical locations. It is not possible to discuss all of these disorders here, but this chapter is intended to stress those common diseases seen in the neuromuscular clinic in adult patients and to give the reader an overall concept of what to expect, how to differentiate and how to treat such illnesses. The diseases covered in these sections are for the most part acquired and do not include congenital muscle or neuromuscular disorders.

1. Myasthenia Gravis

Myasthenia gravis (MG) is a prototypic autoimmune disorder which presents with variable weakness to the extremity, bulbar and ocular muscles. Over half of patients diagnosed with MG present with diplopia and ptosis and as many as an additional 30% of patients will develop such symptoms at some point in the course of their illness. Most patients that present with ocular symptoms will eventually develop more generalized symptoms.

The susceptibility of muscles to fatigue reflects the physiological nature of the disease. Involvement of swallowing and respiratory muscles require immediate attention as such disability can lead to severe compromise to the patient. Ocular MG is more common in older men. Isolated ocular symptoms that persist for over two years are less likely to generalize. Often weakness of extraocular muscles is initially interpreted as blurred vision and later as diplopia that corrects itself with looking through one eye. Although ocular findings of MG may mimic internuclear ophthalmoplegia as in multiple sclerosis, generally fatiguability on sustained gaze and the overall clinical picture make the distinction of this peripheral neuromuscular illness obvious. Photophobia is not uncommon in patients with MG and thought to be related to fatiguability of the constrictor pupillae in response to constant light exposure.

Other cranial nerve abnormalities are common, such as fatiguablility in chewing usually related to eating steak or other tough meat; facial weakness that can give the patient unintended facial expressions; neck weakness; dysarthria and unintelligible speech, especially with prolonged talking and pharyngeal weakness leading to a nasal voice, again especially with extended talking. Aspiration and weight loss are not uncommon as a consequence of swallowing difficulties. Extremity weakness usually involves proximal upper and lower extremities in addition to extensor muscles and typically worsens with sustained effort. The proximal distribution of the weakness can lead to the misdiagnosis of myopathy, especially when other clinical findings are not apparent. Dyspnea on exertion is not uncommon and careful monitoring of pulmonary function is important to avoid respiratory compromise in such patients. Not infrequently it has been noted that patients with MG are often argumentative and disagreeable, often correlating with the length of illness. Although there is no proof and the theory is controversial, it has been postulated that acetylcholine receptor (AChR) antibodies may penetrate the blood-brain barrier and have unexpected central nervous system effects on behavior.

Etiology

MG is caused by autoantibodies that target AChR epitopes in the muscle membrane. Using the Ach-rich solublized membrane of the torpedo fish electric organ, Patrick and Lindstrom were able to demonstrate a disease similar to MG in immunized rabbits. Shortly thereafter, AChR antibodies were discovered in human sera. These antibodies may block the binding of acetylcholine to their receptors and may also degrade the receptors themselves and the surrounding neuromuscular junction through an immune cascade, effectively reducing their number. This interference with receptors causes a reduction in the total membrane depolarization of the muscle fibers, leading to a reduction in the number of muscle fibers that reach the threshold necessary for contraction. Such a reduction in contracting fibers can result in clinical weakness. With each binding of acetylcholine molecules to their postsynaptic receptor, there is a miniature endplate potential (MEPP). The total number of MEEPs determines the total endplate potential, which in turn determines whether or not the muscle fiber depolarizes enough to reach the threshold to cause an action potential ultimately leading to muscle fiber contraction. In acquired MG not only do the antibodies block receptors but they decrease their numbers and density and lead to immune-mediated damage of the postsynaptic membrane through flattening of its convolutions and widening of the synaptic cleft. There is a "safety margin" in normal subjects where despite declining acetylcholine output with sustained activation of the motor nerve there is still depolarization of muscle to threshold because of an excess of postsynaptic receptors. Such a "safety margin" is lost in MG patients.

The immunology of MG is complex. The nicotinic AChR is a transmembrane protein with 5 subunits (alpha, beta, gamma, delta, and epsilon) arranged radially around a central ion channel. Antibodies (mostly of the IgG class) to multiple sites on the extracellular portion of the acteylcholine receptor are generated with MG; however, antibodies directed against the alpha subunit are most prevalent. The binding of antibodies to the various portions of the receptor cause a number of different physiological responses such as a direct blocking of acetylcholine to its binding site, promoting degradation of the receptor through stimulation of the complement system and interfering with ion conduction through the central channel.

Thymic abnormalities have been clearly demonstrated with MG both in experimental models and in the clinical setting. Ten percent of patients with MG have a thymic tumor and 70% have hyperplastic abnormalities that suggest an active immune response. Nearly 20% of patients with MG whose symptoms begin between the ages of 30 and 60 years have thymoma. After the age of 60 the incidence is much lower. These hyperplastic abnormalities of the thymus are within lymphoid tissue where B-cells interact with helper T-cells to produce antibodies. It is clear that both B- and T-cells are involved in MG. The thymus is a crucial organ for immunological self-tolerance, and likely a failure in tolerance leads to the immune-mediated attack on AChR in MG. The tissue of the thymus is a perfect system for promoting MG, containing myoid cells that express the AChR antigen, antigen presenting cells, and immunocompetent T-cells. Although it is still uncertain what role the thymus plays in MG, thymus tissue from patients with MG produces AChR antibodies when implanted into immunodeficient mice. Most thymomas are benign and can be completely removed with surgery. MG tends to be worse in patients with thymoma, demonstrating higher levels of AChR antibodies and more striking abnormalities on EMG. MG can develop long after thymoma removal, and the HLA haplotypes that predominate in patients with thymic hyperplasia are different from those with thymomas.

Diagnostic Tests

The administration of edrophonium (Tensilon®) improves weakness in MG and can be analyzed objectively if there are obvious abnormalities. Some patients who don't respond because of the short half-life of intravenous edrophonium chloride may respond to intramuscular or oral neostigmine because of the longer duration of action. The use of intramuscular neostigmine may be more helpful in infants and where observation may be impaired because of the short half-life of edrophonium. This clinician's own experience is that a therapeutic trial of daily oral pyridostigmine may be more productive where subtle transient responses may be missed with a single dose of edrophonium chloride or neostigmine. The Lancaster Red-Green test is used to evaluate ocular misalignment before and after edrophonium and is positive in 90% of patients with ocular MG.

AChR Antibodies

AChR antibody testing is a useful confirmatory test for MG. Seventy-four percent of patients with acquired generalized MG and 54% with isolated ocular myasthenia have serum positive antibodies for the AChR. The serum antibody concentration varies widely among MG patients with similar disability and should not be used to predict the severity or stage of disease in any individual patients. There is no clear correlation between antibody titres and the severity of disease. False positive results of AchR-binding antibodies concentrations can be seen in patients with a number of autoimmune disorders including systemic lupus erythematosus, inflammatory neuropathy, amyotrophic lateral sclerosis, rheumatoid arthritis taking D-penicillamine, thymoma without myasthenia gravis, and in relatives of patients with myasthenia gravis. What's more, false positive tests can occur in blood drawn within 48 hours of a surgical procedure involving the use of general anesthesia and muscle relaxants.

As a rule, an elevated concentration of AchR-binding antibodies in patients having clinical features consistent with the diagnosis of MG can be confirmatory; however, normal antibody concentrations do not exclude a diagnosis of MG. Another antibody associated with MG is the muscle-specific kinase (MuSK). A recent article showed that 17 of 24 otherwise seronegative patients were found to be MuSK positive. Thymectomy was performed in seven patients with MuSK antibodies and was shown to have no obvious benefit at eight-month follow up. Younger female patients have a higher prevalence of MuSK antibodies, with prominent bulbar symptoms and a high rate of respiratory compromise. Responses to immunomodulatory therapy in this subgroup of MG patients is good, but with a particularly good response to plasma exchange (PE). On electrodiagnostic testing, this subgroup of patients shows less decrement on repetitive stimulation and more myopathic changes on needle EMG. Other antibodies that can be helpful in the setting of MG are the striational antibodies that correlate well with older MG patients and thymoma. False positive results with this antibody are seen with other autoimmune disorders, primary lung cancer, and some paraneoplastic syndromes. Other antibodies are found in a significant percentage of MG patients, including antinuclear (20%-40%), lymphocyte (40%-90%), rheumatoid factor (10%-40%), thyroid (15%-40%), gastric parietal cell (10%-20%), and platelet (5%-50%) antibodies, as well as anti-smooth muscle, mitochondrial, red blood cell, and squamous epithelial antibodies.

Electrodiagnostic Testing

Repetitive nerve stimulation (RS), using the compound motor action potential (CMAP) in affected muscles is a useful study with repeated supramaximal stimulation at a frequency of 1, 2, 3, or 5 Hz. There is the potential for a rate of 1 Hz to allow for replenishment of depleted stores of Ach while a rate of 5 Hz may repair any decrement, producing facilitation. Generally a train of 5 to 10 waveforms are recorded, after 30 to 60 seconds of maximal voluntary contraction, at variable intervals. The objective is to compare the initial CMAP with subsequent CMAPs looking for a decrease or increase in amplitude within each train of impulses.

Generally, the greatest maximal change occurs between the first CMAP and the fourth CMAP. MG patients generally show a decrement in the CMAP amplitude in excess of 10%-15% to the baseline CMAP (Figure 1). Postexercise, waveform size can increase by 10%-50% with improved decrement. This phenomenon is known as postexercise facilitation and is thought to be related to a transient increase in the release of acetylcholine following a short-lived maximal contraction. A reduction of this enhancement occurs over the subsequent 3 to 4 minutes, with reduction of the increment and deterioration of the decrement often below baseline levels known as postactivation exhaustion, as neuromus-

Figure 1

Repetitive stimulation studies in myasthenia gravis

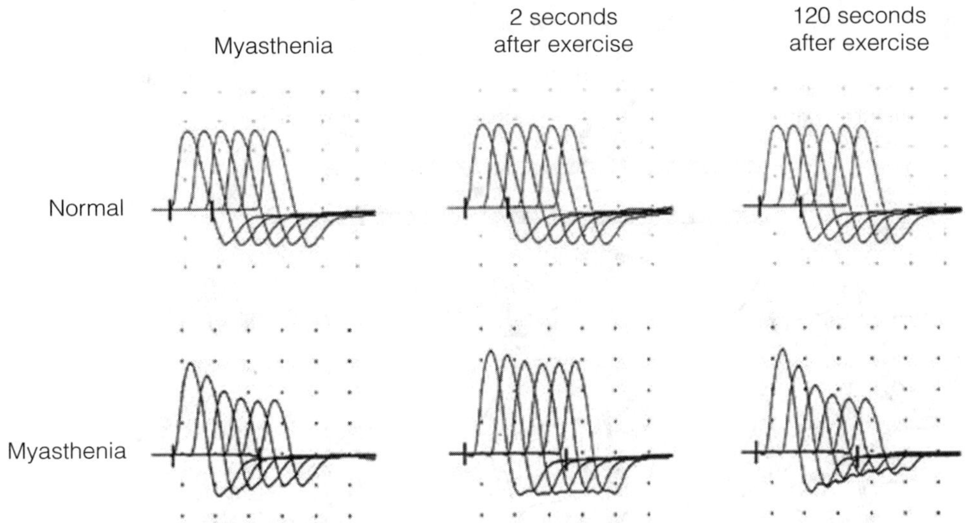

Repetitive stimulation studies in healthy patients and in those with myasthenia gravis. Defective transmission at neuromuscular junctions can be caused either by impaired release of acetylcholine-containing vesicles from the motor terminal (Lambert-Eaton myasthenic syndrome and botulism) or by a reduction in the capacity of postsynaptic skeletal muscle receptors to respond to acetylcholine (myasthenia gravis). These neuromuscular junction abnormalities can be diagnosed by repetitive stimulation studies. In the upper three tracings, responses are shown in a normal individual before exercise, immediately after exercise, and 120 seconds after exercise. Exercise is maximal voluntary contraction of the muscle under study for 30 to 60 seconds. The successive compound motor action potentials (CMAPs) are displayed after six supramaximal stimuli at 2 Hz (cycles/second). Note that the amplitude and configuration of the CMAP does not change in each series. In the lower left tracing, a decrementing response is shown at rest with stimulation at 3 Hz in a patient with myasthenia gravis. A decrement, reflecting abnormal neuromuscular transmission of any cause, is best seen with low rates of stimulation (2 to 5 Hz). A decrementing response is a reproducible decline in the CMAP amplitude (or area) with repetitive stimulation. In this example, there is a 38% decrement in the rested muscle. Immediately after maximal exercise, there is brief improvement in neuromuscular transmission, termed postexercise facilitation. This is reflected in a smaller decrement (in this example, of 13%). For several minutes after maximal exercise, there is a larger decrementing response than is seen in the rested muscle, termed postexercise depression or exhaustion. The decrement in this example is 48% when tested 120 seconds after exercise. These abnormalities with low rates of stimulation are seen in disorders that produce abnormal neuromuscular transmission, including myasthenia gravis, Lambert-Eaton syndrome, and botulism (sensitivity = 5 μV/div; sweep speed = 5 ms/div).

From http://images.md

cular junction and reserve ACh levels are reduced. Generally after 5 minutes, the parameters come back to baseline. RS in appropriate muscles has a sensitivity of approximately 75% in generalized MG and less than 50% in ocular MG. On EMG patients with advanced MG often display short, unstable, small, polyphasic potentials and recruitment is generally either normal or early. RS should not be performed if patients are taking cholinesterase inhibitors (should be discontinued a minimum of 12 hours prior to study), and unless the muscle tested is at normal temperature (amplitude and duration of the MEPP and EPP increase and the duration of the nerve action potential are prolonged

Figure 2

Neurophysiologic testing in myasthenia gravis

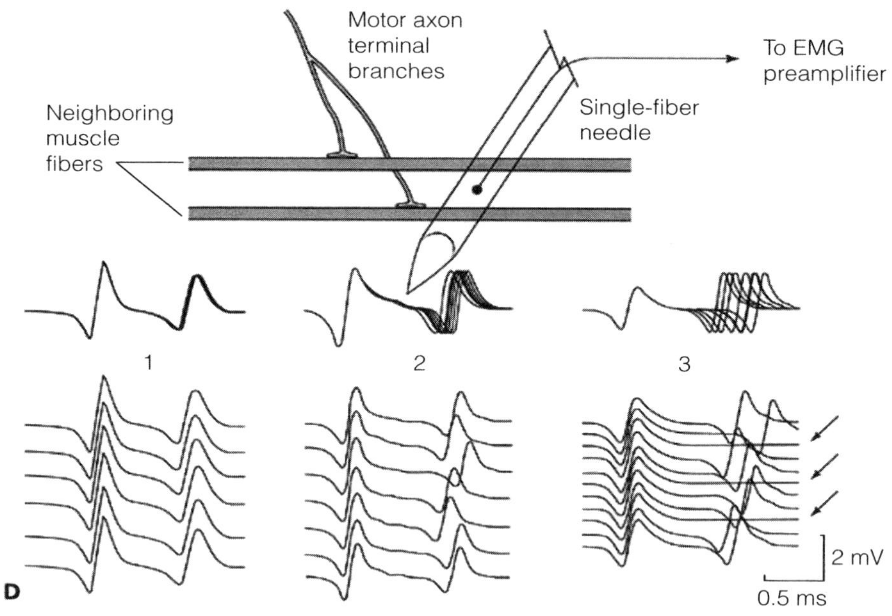

Neurophysiologic testing in myasthenia gravis. A) Repetitive nerve conduction testing in a normal subject demonstrates a constant compound motor action potential (CMAP) amplitude with repetitive nerve stimulation at slow and rapid rates. B) In a patient with symptomatic myasthenia gravis, the amplitude of the compound motor action potential decrements at low rates of 2 to 5 Hz, showing greatest change between the first and second responses. This decrement may correct with administration of intravenous edrophonium (Tensilon, Hoffmann-LaRoche, Nutley, NJ), a short-acting acetylcholinesterase inhibitor. C) Comparison of repetitive nerve stimulation in normal (N) subjects, myasthenia gravis (MG) patients, and Lambert-Eaton myasthenic syndrome (LEMS) patients. The decrementing seen in symptomatic MG can be repaired by 30 seconds of exercise, but increasing decrementation occurs after about 2 minutes. In LEMS, the initial CMAP is of very low amplitude, increasing by greater than 200% after brief, 10-second exercise. After a few minutes, the amplitude again is low. D) Use of a special single fiber needle allows the recording of action potentials from individual muscle fibers. Triggering on one muscle cell action potential, the potential from a neighboring fiber of the same motor unit is also captured and appears time-locked with the first as a pair on the oscilloscope. (1) The first potential is held steady on the screen by the instrument; the second fires with variable timing, a phenomenon called jitter. The jitter is increased in myasthenia gravis (2); and blocking of the second potential occurs when the neuromuscular junction fails (3) (arrows).

From http://images.md

with lowered temperature). False positive results can occur, as when the stimulator slips off the nerve or when the patient withdraws in pain.

Single fiber EMG is another more challenging but helpful technique in establishing a diagnosis of MG (Figure 2). This technique requires a specialized needle to record single muscle fiber discharges. The technique involves the measurement of the variation of the time interval of neuromuscular transmission at individual endplates. This measurement is known as jitter and in MG patients is markedly increased related to the intermittent blocking of neuromuscular transmission and hence the intermittent physiological breakdown of contraction in single muscle fibers. This test is operator dependent and technically difficult but can yield a sensitivity of 95% or greater in generalized MG and 90% or greater in ocular MG, with the testing of appropriate muscles. Single fiber EMG is most useful in MG with mild generalized, ocular, or seronegative MG. Other disorders of the neuromuscular junction can yield positive results with single fiber EMG and hence need to be considered with positive results.

Differential Diagnosis

Because of the ability to narrow down the diagnosis of MG with so many tests, it is hard to misdiagnose the disorder. Nevertheless, in the differential diagnosis, a number of disorders should come to mind.

1. Motor neuron disease such as ALS should be considered although generally easily excluded with electrodiagnostic testing, clinical history and neurological exam.

2. The same can be said for a peripheral neuropathy such as multifocal motorneuropathy or an acquired immune demyelinating polyradiculoneuropathy where electrodiagnostic testing might show conduction block or a decrease in conduction velocity, and the neurological exam would likely be very different.

3. With the C. Miller variant of Guillain-Barré syndrome (GBS), the spinal fluid protein is usually elevated as well. The hallmarks of repetitive stimulation would not be seen as with MG.

4. Botulism should be considered but as mentioned below can usually be excluded by history.

5. A primary myopathy can usually be differentiated by electrodiagnostic testing and neurological exam.

6. LEMS, although relatively rare and a distinctively different neuromuscular disorder (see below) from MG can be differentiated based on the history and largely the electrodiagnostic tests. Antibody testing is also important.

Treatment and Prognosis

One of the first lines of therapy for MG are the anticholinesterase medications, which effectively increase the Ach at the neuromuscular junction. Pyridostigmine (Mestinon®) is generally the most widely used of this class. Dose titration of pyridostigmine is important because of its side effect profile. The onset of action is usually within 30 minutes from ingestion and peak action occurs at approximately two hours. Hence, patients generally require dosing every four to six hours, at least early in the disease. This author likes to start with a dose of 30 mg every 6 hours as a start. Exceeding doses of 120 mg every three hours is generally not helpful. The long-acting form (Mestinon® Timespan®, 180 mg) can be helpful at bedtime for those patients with incapacitating morning weakness. Common side effects include abdominal cramping, diarrhea, increased oral secretions and fasciculations. Weakness is another common side effect thought to be related to excessive depolarization of the postsynaptic membrane or to densensitization.

The majority of patients with MG have thymic abnormalities including hyperplasia in 60%-70% and thymoma in 10%-12%. Imaging of the chest with MRI or CT is standard protocol in MG patients looking for thymoma. Treatment options for thymoma include complete excision or radiation for both relief of MG symptoms and also for prevention of local invasion. Thymectomy is a frequently used intervention for generalized MG in patients from the age of puberty to age of 60 years. It has been established that removing the thymus/thymoma in its entirety is very important, with residual tissue causing ongoing disease. Because of a lack of well-controlled studies, the efficacy and use of thymectomy in the absence of thymoma is controversial at best. A postoperative (thymectomy) worsening of MG is well described and thought to be related to the suppressive effect of the tumor on the immune system. Mestinon or PE have been shown to be helpful in this setting.

Immunosuppressive medications play a key role in the treatment of MG and often offer long-term remission of disease. This article is not detailed enough to give an extensive review of each one. Standard medications for immunosuppressant include corticosteroids, azothiaprine, cyclosporine and mycophenolate. PE and intravenous immunoglobulin (IVIG) are also effective. About

30% of MG patients go into remission with corticosteroids and another 45% have a positive response, with the onset of benefit taking about two to four weeks. The common side effects of steroid use are no different than with other diseases; however, there is a transient worsening of weakness that can occur during the first few weeks of treatment with corticosteroid use in MG. Respiratory weakness or dysphagia in this setting needs to be monitored carefully with the initiation of steroids, generally as an inpatient. Patients are often treated with PE prior to initiation of steroids in this setting. GI prophyalaxis in patients with acid reflux or peptic ulcer should be undertaken. To minimize side effects, an every other day regimen is preferred. Prednisone is generally continued for about a year before tapering is considered. In patients who cannot tolerate daily or every other day corticosteroids, pulsed IV administration of methylprednisolone is another option.

Azathioprine is another option for treatment although it can take six months to a year to benefit. Because of this time lag to efficacy, it is generally not used as a first-line drug of choice. Azathioprine is often used in combination with corticosteroids and a clinical trial did show this combination to be advantageous over corticosteroids alone. Interestingly, the AChR-Ab titres were no different between the two groups. Other immunosuppressive agents that have been used with some success include cyclosporine, mycophenolate and even rituximab, all with their own potential side effects. Cyclosporine, at a dose of 5 mg/kg per day, has been shown to lower AChR-Ab production faster than azathioprine (one to two months) but otherwise does not offer any benefit, and the side effect profile of cyclosporine also makes it a difficult medicine to use.

PE is another useful option in the treatment of MG. The mechanism of action of PE is to directly remove AChR-Ab from the serum, and its ability to do so appears to correlate with a direct reduction in AChR-Ab levels. These effects are seen in days, as early as during the initial treatment; thus, PE is particularly useful in seriously ill patients. The response to PE is transient, usually only lasting a month or so, but can help at the beginning of treatment in patients severely compromised with MG. Repeated exchanges make this treatment poorly tolerated for the long term. It also has the potential to cause a MG crisis. More modern techniques of PE, as with columns using staphylococcus protein A, make the technique more effective. PE may be preferred in patients in myasthenic crisis.

IVIG is effective for MG although the mechanism is not known. It is used in the same clinical situation as PE, useful in the setting of severe, refractory MG and effective in up to 75% of cases. The recommended dose is 0.4 g/kg per day for five days (not to exceed 2 g/kg). It is as effective as PE, but has fewer side effects than PE. IVIG is reported to be effective in nearly 75% of cases. The benefit begins within days and often lasts for one to two months. IVIG has side effects including anaphylaxis, which is associated with an IgA deficiency. Screening for this deficiency is recommended prior to using IVIG.

2. Lambert-Eaton Myasthenic Syndrome (LEMS)

LEMS is a relatively rare disease, but is important to understand as a neurologist because it explains a lot about the pathophysiology of the neuromuscular junction. Smoking is the single biggest risk factor for developing this rare neuromuscular disorder because of the potential for developing small cell lung cancer (SCLC). Although it is rare to see this disorder in the neuromuscular clinic, the prevalence of LEMS with SCLC patients is 1%-3%. LEMS is caused by an autoimmune response against voltage-gated calcium channels (VGCC) on the presynaptic motor nerve terminal. In addition to its association with SCLC, the syndrome has also been associated with other neoplasms including non-SCLC, thyroid cancer, malignant thymoma, small cell carcinoma of the cervix, germinoma, and leukemia. Rarely, LEMS has been seen in children with or without a documented malignancy.

As with other paraneoplastic syndromes, the clinical manifestations of the disorder often precede the identification of the cancer. Generally, the cancer is discovered within the first 2 years after onset of LEMS and, in almost all cases, within 4 years. Approximately one-half of patients with LEMS have a documented neoplasm, but in fact it is more difficult to detect neoplasms that may be affected by an immune response. LEMS in patients with small cell lung cancer generally has a relatively favorable survival outcome, suggesting that the autoimmune response in these patients prevents tumor growth. Such a phenomenon has been documented in other paraneoplastic syndromes. Nonparaneoplastic LEMS exists as well. Patients with paraneoplastic (notably SCCL) as opposed to nonparaneoplastic LEMS may often have other syndromes such as concomitant paraneoplastic cerebellar degeneration, paraneoplastic encephalomyelitis and sensorimotor polyneuropathy.

Diagnosis

The clinical manifestations and electrophysiologic features of LEMS are identical between paraneoplastic and nonparaneoplastic patients. Most LEMS patients have the insidious onset of weakness and fatigue. Early in the disease the neurological exam may only demonstrate subtle abnormalities out of proportion to the patient's symptoms of fatigue and weakness. The pattern of weakness is generally symmetric and proximal, affecting the legs more than the arms. Patients may complain of extremity parasthesias as well as pain. Deep tendon reflexes are generally diminished or absent although they can often be brought out after sustained contraction. A positive edrophonium test is not unusual. Autonomic dysfunction is not unusual, with symptoms such as dry mouth, impotence, blurred vision, constipation, difficulty with micturition, and reduced sweating prevailing. Mild ocular and bulbar symptoms including ptosis, diplopia, dysarthria, or dysphagia often occur usually after patients have developed notable limb weakness. Respiratory failure is distinctly uncommon, but can be inadvertently induced by a number of drugs, including fluorquinolone antibiotics and calcium channel blockers.

Figure 3

Paraneoplastic Lambert-Easton myasthenic syndrome

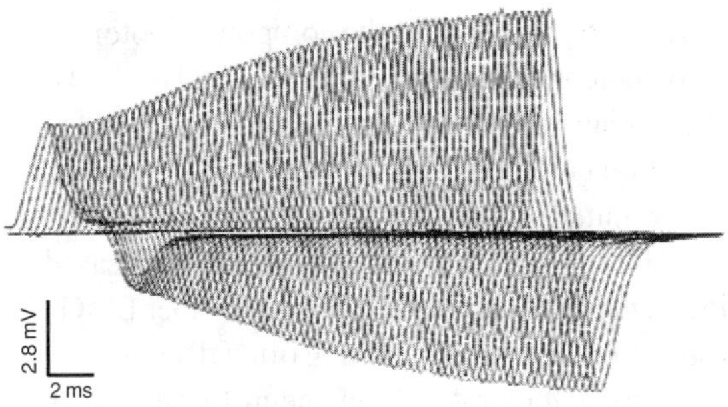

Electromyogram (EMG) in a patient with paraneoplastic Lambert-Eaton myasthenic syndrome (LEMS). This paraneoplastic syndrome produces progressive proximal weakness, and is most often associated with small cell lung cancer. The EMG is characteristic in patients with LEMS. At high frequencies of stimulation, the compound motor action potentials (CMAPs) become progressively larger with time, as seen in this patient with fatigability and a history of smoking. A computed tomography scan showed a nodule within the lung that was a small cell lung cancer on resection.

From http://images.md

Electrodiagnostic Testing

Electrodiagnostic testing remains the best test for LEMS. Common features include a reduced amplitude of muscle action potentials evoked by a supramaximal stimulus (to as little as10% of normal); a decremental response of the compound motor action potential of greater than 7% at 2 Hz to 5 Hz RS; a greater than 100% increase in compound muscle action potentials after several seconds of maximal voluntary contraction (postexercise facilitation) or at 20 Hz to 50 Hz RS (a painful test); increased jitter and impulse blocking on single-fiber EMG testing. The jitter and blocking often decrease at rapid stimulation rates. Many neurologists prefer testing for facilitation after maximal voluntary contraction rather than performing high frequency RS at 20 Hz to 50 Hz, as it is less painful. It is recommended that high frequency RS be reserved in patients where exercise is not possible. One should keep the duration of RS (25-100 stimuli) to a minimum and consider using sedation. In the awake patient who is not extremely weak, a withdrawal reflex can be expected leading to artifact. Often electrophysiological findings can be found in asymptomatic muscles. As a rule of thumb, testing three hand muscles gives a sensitivity exceeding 90%. The distal nerves are generally easier to study. Electrophysiologic tests cannot distinguish between the paraneoplastic and nonparaneoplastic forms of LEMS. Previous studies have demonstrated that serial measurements of stimulation or single-fiber EMG generally reflect the clinical response to treatment.

If a diagnosis of LEMS is determined, an exhaustive search for tumor should be undertaken with chest CT, MR scanning and even FDG-PET scanning if other studies prove unrevealing. Occasionally SCLC is found on bronchoscopy where imaging studies have been negative. In cases where no tumor is discovered, the studies should be repeated at regular intervals. After five years, if no tumor is discovered, it is likely that the patient has a nonparaneoplastic variant of LEMS.

LEMS is a rare syndrome. There are several distinguishing features and findings between LEMS and MG. With the correct diagnostic approach, there is little else that fits the overall clinical picture. It is sometimes missed because it can be masked by other diseases (paraneoplastic and otherwise), can look like mild MG on RS, can be missed by a poor effort on exercise testing, and lastly and likely most commonly, because the physician doesn't think of it.

Pathogenesis

The primary physiological defect in LEMS is a reduction in the quantal release of Ach as a result of decreased presynaptic calcium influx with nerve impulses. LEMS is an autoimmune disease. There is both an increase in other autoimmune disorders in nonpareaneoplastic LEMS patients, an over-representation of the HLA-B8 histocompatibility antigen, and of a number of autoantibodies associated with it. Laboratory experiments using passive transfer experiments (purified IgG from LEMS patients) injected into mice blocks the nerve impulse-evoked release of acetylcholine in a dose-dependent manner, and reproduces the typical electrophysiologic abnormalities of LES and produces histological abnormalities typical of LEMS, as well as inhibiting the calcium influx into cultured SCCL cells and impairing neurotransmitter release from parasympathetic and sympathetic mouse neurons.

Sera from the majority of LEMS patients have serum IgG antibodies against P/Q-type voltage gated calcium channels; however, quantitative titers of these antibodies do not correlate with the severity of the disease nor distinguish between paraneoplastic and nonparaneoplastic disease. Diminishing antibody titres in response to therapy have been demonstrated. It has also been observed that seronegative LEMS patients are less likely to have an associated neoplasm.

Differential Diagnosis (Same as Above for MG)

Probably ALS is most likely confused with this diagnosis, but usually possible to differentiate based on electrodiagnostic testing, clinical exam, clinical history and, if necessary, a muscle biopsy.

Treatment

Successful treatment of LEMS is targeted towards reduction of autoantibodies, which improves neuromuscular transmission. In some cases, the muscle weakness of LEMS will improve with successful cancer treatment. In individuals with the syndrome but without cancer, immunosuppressive drugs such as prednisone and azathioprine are used to reduce the autoimmune response and lessen symptoms. The typical neuromuscular medications can help with LEMS, including pyridostigmine bromide (Mestinon), 3,4-diaminopyridine (DAP), and guanidine. Because muscle weakness may increase with increasing core body temperature, hot weather, use of hot tubs or hot showers, and fever should be avoided. DAP has been shown to be helpful both with and without an associated neoplasm. Sometimes the use of guanidine and pyridostigmine together may allow a lower dose of both drugs, reducing the likelihood of guanidine toxicity. For patients with paraneoplastic LEMS who are receiving or will receive tumor treatment, it is usually reasonable to use pyridostigmine, DAP, or guanidine, and to defer immunotherapy.

The initial avoidance of immunotherapy may be beneficial in patients with known tumor, as treatment for the tumor may obviate such treatment. The use of the immunospressive agents prednisone (60 mg to 80 mg per day) and azathioprine (up to 2.5 mg/kg per day) alone or in combination generally has been shown to be beneficial as immunosuppressive therapy, but a response may take weeks or months. Occasionally cyclosporine has been shown to be beneficial for LEMS in those individuals not responsive to prednisone and azothioprine, but the side effects can be serious. Both plasma exchange and IVIG have been shown to be helpful with sustained effects over several months. A good response to immunosuppressive therapy is more likely to occur in nonparaneoplastic patients. The outcome with LEMS is generally related to the virulence of the associated tumor if one indeed exists.

3. Polymyositis (PM) and Dermatomyositis (DM)

Thirty years ago, Bohan and Peter came up with diagnostic criteria for DM and PM which are still a useful approach to these two disorders. The criteria include: 1) symmetric proximal muscle weakness; 2) typical rash of dermatomyositis; 3) elevated serum muscle enzymes (? what range); 4) EMG showing myopathic changes in affected muscles; and 5) muscle biopsy consistent with typical findings for DM and PM. It should be noted that patients that meet the above criteria may well have some other disorder such as muscular dystrophy, inclusion body myositis, or rhabdomyolysis, to name a few. Both of the inflammatory myopathies, DM and PM, are rare (about 1/100,000), with a 2/1 female predominance and a peak incidence around the fifth decade. DM and PM have similarities, but they are distinct disorders. DM is associated with a higher incidence of malignancy. The pathophysiology of DM is associated with immune complex deposition in blood vessels in contrast to PM, which appears to be associated with T cell-mediated muscle damage, and related to graft-versus-host disease following bone marrow transplantation.

Diagnosis

In most cases the onset of insidious proximal, symmetric muscle weakness is the presenting feature for both these disorders. Dysphagia, nasal regurgitation and aspiration are not uncommon, especially in more elderly patients. Mild myalgias occur in up to half of these patients. Signs of extramuscular organ involvement, such as the lungs or joints, may also point to the diagnosis and serologic tests may provide diagnostic and prognostic information. Continued observation for such involvement is valuable, as indicated by one retrospective study that included 65 patients with an initial diagnosis of "unspecified myositis." Among these patients, 10 (15%) subsequently developed a well-defined disorder with a known association with myositis (eg, systemic lupus, scleroderma, Sjögren syndrome).

Several distinct rashes occur in DM and are frequently the presenting feature. However, the cutaneous manifestations may be transient and may have resolved by the time the patient presents with muscle weakness. Although the rash of DM can be subtle and transient, when present there is a classic Gottron's sign, a symmetric, scaly, erythematous eruption over the extensor surfaces of the metacarpophalangeal and interphalangeal joints of the fingers as well as the extensor aspects of the elbows and knees. An erythematous shawl-like distribution rash can also be seen over the chest and shoulders with additional involvement of the anterior neck and chest forehead, chin or malar region, all of which can be exacerbated by sun exposure. Although rare, a reddish heliotrope rash can also be seen on the upper eyelids, often with associated swelling of the eyelids accompanied by swelling of the eyelid specific for DM (Figure 4). A number of other skin abnormalities have been described. Abnormalities of the fingers and nails include periungual erythema, abnormal nailbed capillary loops, and painful cracking of the skin of the tips and lateral aspects of the fingers. Constitutional symptoms include fever and weight loss. Other findings that can occur include inflammatory polyarthritis, Raynaud's phenomenon, myocarditis and interstitial lung disease.

Both PM and DM have been associated with other connective tissue diseases including systemic lupus erythematosus, rheumatoid arthritis, Sjögren syndrome, Crohn disease and ulcerative colitis. Dermatomyositis sine myositis or amyopathic dermatomyositis are terms that have been used to describe patients with the typical rash and dermatohistologic changes of DM without evidence of myopathy. Many of these patients eventually develop clinical and/or histologic evidence of myositis; in some cases, however, muscle involvement is not seen as long as six years in follow-up.

This author generally only checks creatinine kinase (CK) levels although a variety of muscle enzymes can be checked, including LDH, aldolase, ALT and AST. GGT is generally specific for liver disease.

Figure 4

Dermatomyositis

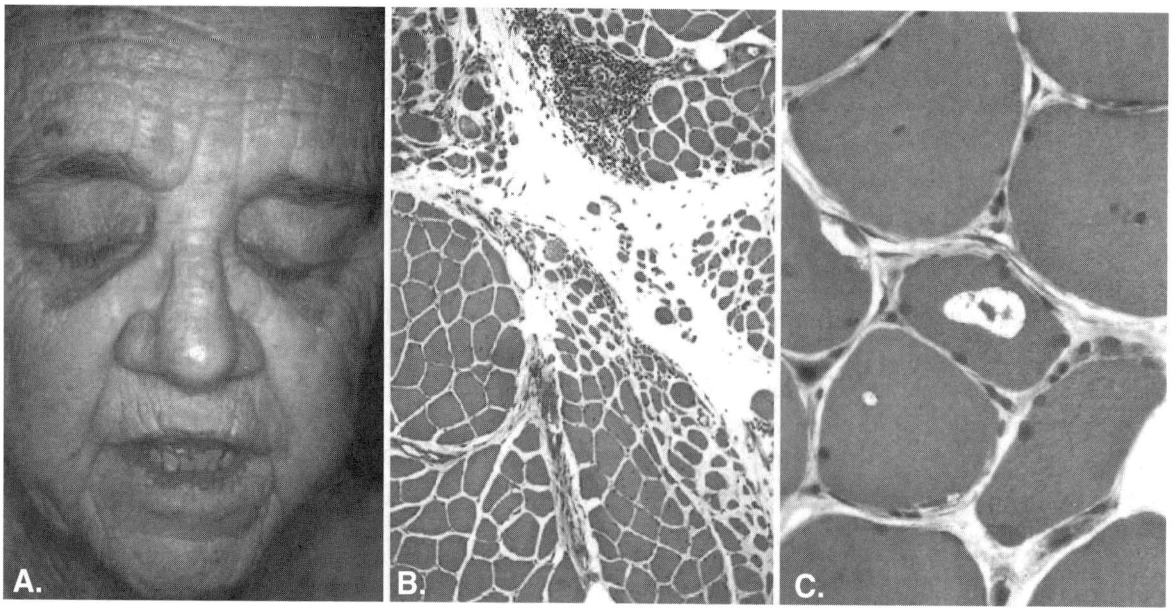

A) Note the rash affecting the eyelids. B) Dermatomyositis. The histologic appearance of muscle shows perifascicular atrophy of muscle fibers and inflammation. C) Inclusion body myositis showing a vacuole within a myocyte.

From Kumar V et al, eds. Robbins and Cotran Pathologic Basis of Disease. *7th ed. 2005; Elsevier:342-1343. Figure 27-14. With permission.*

The trauma of needle EMG is such that it can falsely elevate muscle enzyme levels, hence these levels should be checked prior to EMG. With PM and DM, CK levels can reach 50 times the upper limits of normal, but the degree of elevation does not necessarily correlate well with the degree of weakness. In rare cases the CK and other muscle enzymes can remain normal despite histological evidence of myositis and weakness. If a positive CK-MB is found, a cardiac troponin level should be checked, as the CK-MB fraction can be elevated in DM and PM from inflammation to skeletal muscle and cardiac muscle, and not necessarily from cardiac ischemia. Normal troponin levels effectively exclude a cardiac source. Nonspecific, positive antibody titres are seen with DM and PM, including ANA and anti-ribonucleoprotein; but some are more specific, especially for DM.

EMG is helpful in establishing a diagnosis of myopathy exemplified by active denervation, low amplitude, short duration, polyphasic potentials, high-frequency discharges and early recruitment of motor units, but all such findings are not diagnostic for a specific myopathy. In addition to confirming a diagnosis of myopathy, it can be helpful in finding muscles that are affected to direct a muscle biopsy. Only about 10% of DM and PM have a normal EMG, but caution should be taken in concluding a normal EMG without sampling adequate muscles, including paraspinal muscles.

The only test that can really confirm a diagnosis of PM or DM is a muscle biopsy. Generally the biopsy is obtained from the deltoid or quadriceps, but not a muscle that is so weak that histological findings will be obscured by atrophy, and not in a muscle that has recently been tested with EMG where localized trauma may occur. Nevertheless, a muscle group on the contralateral side of a muscle testing positive by EMG for myopathy may give a higher diagnostic yield. MRI scanning can also be helpful in localizing affected muscles for biopsy purposes, as the muscle will show evidence of inflammation on the correct sequences (Flair, T2). This author performs open biopsies to obtain ample samples of muscle, although percutaneous needle biopsies are performed with moderately successful results. The preparation of the sample and quantity of sample procured is all important in addition to special testing, some of which requires liquid nitrogen freezing for metabolic, biochemical and genetic testing.

The histologic features of both DM and PM include muscle fiber necrosis, degeneration, and regeneration. The histological features of DM reflect a humoral response where the abnormalities are primarily seen in blood vessels, showing both perfascicular and perivascular cellular infiltrates (B-cells and an increased ratio of CD4+ to CD8+ T-cells). Distinct areas of perifascicular atrophy and fibrosis as a result of the inflammation is a hallmark of DM, suggesting areas of microinfarction (Figure 4). Unlike DM, with PM cellular infiltrates are seen to invade (Figure 5) the fascicles themselves. Strictly speaking, you cannot make the diagnosis of PM with histology alone. The abnormalities are generally more diffuse and there are no signs of vasculopathy or immune complex deposition. With PM, cell-mediated immune mechanisms prevail (cytotoxic CD8+ T cells, against an antigen on the muscle fiber cell membranes), as well as an increased expression by muscle fibers of major histocompatibility complex (MHC) antigens. There also appears

Figure 5

Dermatomyositis

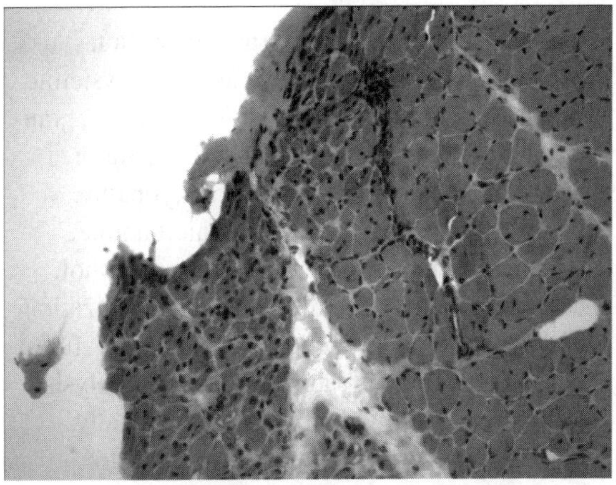

Hematoxylin and eosin staining of a muscle showing the typical appearance of dermatomyositis of perifascicular atrophy and inflammation.

With permission from Brent Harris, MD, PhD, Dartmouth Medical School.

to be a function for cytokines, which may contribute to muscle weakness in the absence of inflammation, as both IL-1 and TNF-alpha are increased in muscle of patients with PM.

In addition to the role of MR in selecting inflammed muscles with PM and DM for biopsy, one can also use it to evaluate the response to treatment. Needless to say it is an expensive means of following patients. MRS has been used in patients to detect abnormalities in DM where muscle strength and CK levels have been normal.

Differential Diagnosis

1. Hereditary neuromuscular diseases. Endomysial inflammation can occur with muscular dystrophies (dysferlinopathies, fascioscapulohumeral dystrophy, Becker's muscular dystrophy), common in patients below the age of 18 years. Disorders of carbohydrate and lipid metabolism are often associated with transient spells of acute, often post-exertional muscle pain with myoglobulinuria. Chronic weakness can develop with repeated spells.

2. Metabolic myopathies, endocrinopathies (hypothyroidism), electrolyte disturbances (periodic paralyses), mitochondriopathies.

3. Systemic medical diseases (malabsorption syndromes, alcoholism, cancer, vasculitis, systemic infections, sarcoidosis, parasitic infections, granulomatous disease, drugs and toxins). Statin drugs are a major drug leading to myopathy. Other common drugs include penicillamine, colchicine and hydroxychloroquine. Alcohol, cocaine, heroin, viral infections, immobilization, and trauma typically present with an acute, fulminant onset with the features of rhabdomyolysis. HIV associated myopathy characteristically demonstrates weakness not only related to cachexia and chronic disease but also can mimic an inflammatory myopathy that is similar to PM. Treatment for HIV with zidovudine can cause a mitochondrial myopathy that can be distinguished on muscle biopsy and goes away with discontinuation of the drug.

4. Neurogenic muscular atrophies or neurogenic conditions. ALS can present with elevated muscle enzymes, but upper motor signs are common and distal motor weakness is more common. EMG shows neurogenic findings.

5. Biochemical muscle diseases (enzyme deficiencies).

6. MG can cause diffuse weakness, but bulbar signs are common, muscle enzymes are normal, EMG shows typical findings and AChR antibodies are usually elevated.

7. Amyloid (both familial and immunoglobulin related) myopathy can show markedly elevated CK levels and typical myopathic potentials on EMG. The classical histological finding of Congo red staining, lack of response to steroid therapy and the systemic involvement (peripheral neuropathy, hepatosplenomegaly, muscle hypertrophy and nephritic syndrome) make the distinction relatively easy.

8. Inclusion body myositis (IBM) is commonly mistaken for PM and ALS (see below). The distribution of weakness with IBM tends to be more distal and commonly involves the finger and wrist flexors in the upper extremities and the tibialis anterior and quadriceps in the lower extremities, all with associated atrophy. Muscle biopsy may be nondiagnostic in 20%-30% of cases lacking the typical inclusion bodies. MRI has proven helpful in making this distinction with the inflammation being more prominent in the fascial planes with PM and being more diffuse with IBM.

9. Hypereosinophilic syndrome demonstrates eosinophilic infiltrates on muscle biopsy and peripheral eosinophilia.

10. Focal myositis: limited form of PM.

11. Familial idiopathic myositis: homozygosity at the HLA-DQA1 locus is a risk factor.

12. PM in the setting of graft-versus-host disease.

PM and DM Therapy

In assessing response to therapy it is recommended that the neurological exam, specifically the motor exam, be followed for PM and DM, as following the CK values may lead to erroneous conclusions. Therapies for PM and DM are essentially the same, but clinical trials have not grouped the two diseases together and hence individual treatments may not mirror each other for both diseases.

Commonly Used Therapies Include:

1. Prednisone (80-100 mg/day times three to four weeks, followed by a taper over 10 weeks to 80 every other day, followed by a very gradual taper to a level that appears to control the disease). The usual side effects of prednisone have to be considered (aseptic necrosis of the hip, diabetes, steroid myopathy, hypertension, osteoporosis). The consideration of another agent needs to be evaluated when prednisone side effects are intolerable, and there is relapsing disease, and progressive disease with respiratory involvement.

2. Azathioprine acts slowly but generally is well tolerated at a dose of 1.5-3 mg/kg. It should not be given with allopurinol and can be toxic to bone marrow and liver.

3. Methotrexate acts faster than azothiaprine, but has the potential to cause pneumonitis. The usual dosing is 7.5 mg weekly times three weeks (2.5 mg every 12 hours) increased by 2.5 mg/week up to 25 mg/week. An interstitial pneumonitis can occur and is difficult to differentiate from polymyositis induced interstitial lung involvement.

4. Cyclophosphamide (0.5-1 gm/m^2/month) may be helpful in patients with interstitial lung disease.

5. Cyclosporine acts faster than azathioprine but its efficacy is limited.

6. Mycophenolate shows promise, but clinical trials are ongoing.

7. PE was found to be ineffective in a double-blind, placebo-controlled study. Rarely, PE may be helpful in combination with an immunosuppressive agent with DM.

8. IVIG shows promise both for DM and PM.

9. Rituximab shows promise in the treatment of DM, but should be considered experimental at this point. There is currently a phase 2 clinical trial underway looking at the efficacy of rituximab for PM and DM.

4. Inclusion Body Myositis

IBM is an adult disease with a predominance of males to females of 3:1. It is a common myopathy in patients over 50 years of age and for unknown reasons is distinctly unusual in patients of African descent. The age of onset in hereditary IBM patients is in the second and third decades, but sometimes later in life. Early clinical manifestations of IBM include weakness of quadriceps and foot extensors, distal hand muscle weakness (especially finger and wrist flexors), and dysphagia. Involvement of distal lower limb musculature is a hallmark of IBM, but proximal musculature is also usually involved. The quadriceps are almost always involved and this may lead to unexpected falls. The weakness is often asymmetric and atrophy is common with advanced disease. Tendon reflexes may be depressed, especially at the knees because of quadriceps atrophy. Subtle facial weakness is common. Barium swallow testing abnormalities are usually found in IBM patients secondary to esophageal muscle dysfunction. Sensory abnormalities are generally not found; however, an underlying axonal sensory neuropathy can be seen on NCVs. Atrophy of involved muscles is the rule.

Despite the fact that IBM is unresponsive to immunomodulating medications, inflammation is seen on histology and as with PM there is an association with autoimmune disorders. There are autosomal dominant and autosomal recessive forms of IBM with distinct patterns of weakness. Histological evidence of inflammation is generally confined to sporadic IBM. The inflammation seen in IBM appears to be similar to that of PM. Endomysial infiltrates are made up of macrophages (30%) and mostly CD8+ cytotoxic T-cells (70%). The major histocompatibility complex class I antigen, which is absent in normal muscle fibers, is powerfully expressed nearby and far from the inflammatory infiltrates. These findings suggest a cytotoxic process similar to that described for polymyositis, involving a T-cell mediated and major histocompatibility complex-I restricted, cytotoxic process.

Although there is no hard evidence to suggest a viral etiology for IBM, there is an association of inflammatory myopathies with retroviruses HIV and HTLV-I. These viruses appear to trigger an autoimmune mechanism that reroutes cytotoxic T-cells to the muscles, without directly infecting the muscle fiber. Overexpression of beta-amyloid precursor protein and mitochondrial abnormalities in sporadic cases have been implicated in IBM as well.

Diagnosis

PM/DM, the distal myopathies with rimmed vacuoles, ALS, and oculopharyngeal muscular dystrophy are all easily confused with IBM (Table 2). The pattern of weakness is distinctly different for IBM and PM. Knee extensor weakness that surpasses hip flexor weakness as well as finger and wrist flexor weakness that surpasses shoulder abductor weakness is consistent with IBM. This pattern of weakness may be more important than the presence of rimmed vacuoles on muscle biopsy in making the diagnosis of IBM, as such patients generally have the same bad response to immunosuppressive therapy as do patients with histologically confirmed IBM. The diagnosis of IBM is confirmed by elevated serum muscle enzymes (2- to 10-fold elevation), electrodiagnostic testing and, most importantly, muscle histology. Occasionally the CK can be normal. Electrodiagnostic testing is useful for ruling out a significant peripheral neuropathy, motor neuron involvement, and confirming a myopathic process, particularly in distal muscles, is indicative of IBM. Neurogenic motor unit potentials (long duration, increased amplitude) can be seen in long-standing IBM as well as PM, which can confound making a proper diagnosis, and are not inconsistent with a long-standing myopathy.

Table 2

Differential Diagnosis of IBM

DM
PM
Distal myopathies with rimmed vacuoles
Oculopharyngeal muscular dystrophy
Welander distal myopathy
Distal myopathy with vacuolar formation

Light microscopic features of IBM reveal rimmed vacuoles, endomysial inflammation, atrophic fibers, hypertrophic large fibers (similar to chronic dystropies, but not in PM), vacuolated or swollen nuclei, and eosinophilic cytoplasmic inclusions. Strictly speaking, you cannot rule out IBM with a muscle biopsy. The swollen or vacuolated nuclei are ubiquitous and appear similar to a primary nucleopathy. There is a high incidence of ragged red fibers present due to abnormal mitochondria. Electron microscopy shows that the eosinophilic inclusions are composed of 12 nm to 18 nm intranuclear and cytoplasmic filaments. The rimmed vacuoles of inclusion-body myositis, which are variably present, have a diameter of 2 m to 25 m (Figure 6). Any individual muscle fiber may contain 1 vacuole or multiple vacuoles located in the subsarcolemmal region or more centrally. The vacuoles are made of cytoplasmic degradation products, such as membranous whorls, myeloid structures, and filaments. The inflammation seen in inclusion-body myositis is a primary endomysial; however, in up to 15% of the cases, the inflammation may be sparse or absent. Amyloid deposition mostly in the subsarcolemmal regions can appear histochemically, similar to those seen in Alzheimer disease. Cytoplasmic filaments stain positive for ubiquitin. Both of these findings are also seen in oculopharyngeal muscular dystrophy, making the association with Alzheimer disease unlikely. Oculopharyngeal muscular dystrophy is an autosomal dominant disorder that differs from IBM by the predominant involvement of ocular, bulbar and pharyngeal muscles. Although oculopharyngeal dystrophy has evidence of inclusions similar to those of IBM, there are also distinct 8.5 nm tubular filaments in the nucleus, not seen in IBM. Welander myopathy, an autosomal dominant distal myopathy, has histologic features of IBM and is considered a hereditary form of IBM.

Figure 6

Polymyositis

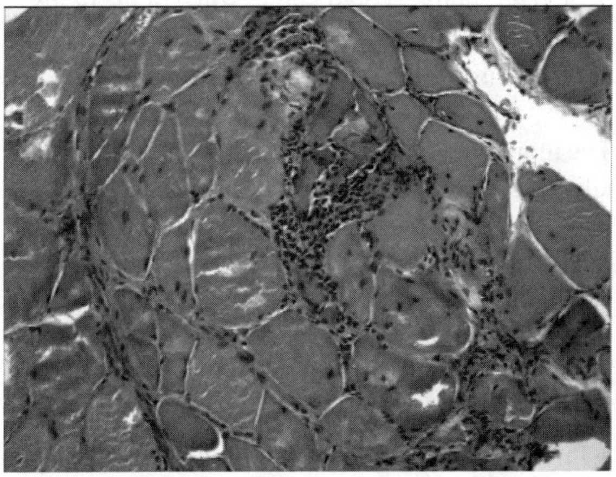

Hematoxylin and eosin stain of skeletal muscle showing typical features of polymyositis. There is focal lymphocytic infiltration, segmental floccular degeneration and degenerating and regenerating muscle fibers.

From Brent Harris, MD, PhD, Dartmouth Medical School. With permission.

Differential Diagnosis

Therapy

IBM has no proven therapeutic protocol. There are potential treatments for IBM, but careful, double-blind, placebo-controlled therapeutic trials have yet to be carried out.

5. Other Neuromuscular/Myopathy Syndromes or Imitators

Sarcoid myopathy sarcoidosis can affect muscle in addition to other organs. Generally involvement of muscle is concurrent with other organ involvement. Often patients with sarcoid myopathy have no symptoms referable to their muscles. Muscle may well be involved in half of patients with sarcoidosis in the absence of muscular symptoms. Generally the muscular involvement is proximal. The presence of palpable nodules in muscle is not uncommon, in addition to a rarer diffuse muscular hypertrophy. Sarcoidosis of muscle occurs more frequently in women (4:1) and appears later in life in women (postmenopausal). Generally the disease is not fuliminant and the CKs are relatively normal. The disease is diagnosed with the usual diagnostic tests for sarcoid including a chest x-ray and skin testing (Kviem-Siltzbach antigen). Prednisone, as with other forms of sarcoidosis, is the standard therapy.

Endocrine Myopathies

Categories of endocrine myopathy include those associated with: 1) adrenal dysfunction (as in Cushing disease or steroid myopathy); 2) thyroid dysfunction (as in myxedema coma or thyrotoxic myopathy); 3) hypothyroid myopathy; 4) parathyroid dysfunction (as in multiple endocrine neoplasia); 5) pituitary axis pathology; and 6) diabetic myopathy, as with ischemic infarction of the femoral muscles. The scope of this chapter does not allow a full discussion.

Myositis Ossificans

This disorder should not be mistaken for calcinosis universalis (the subcutaneous calcifications seen in dermatomyositis). The former is a rare disease associated with skeletal deformities, such as finger and toe deformities, begins early in life (usually second year), and involves bone and subcutaneous tissue as opposed to muscle. Bone deposition is found beneath the skin or within the muscle in the limbs or paraspinal regions, accompanied by localized swelling.

Drug-Induced Myopathies

Drug-induced myopathy usually develops insidiously over days to months after exposure to the inciting agent. Common symptoms include progressive, generalized muscle weakness, and muscle pain (myalgias). As with most other myopathies, the weakness is largely proximal involving both the arms and legs with or without myalgias. Rhabdomyolysis occurs, with more serious cases leading to potential acute renal failure, but reversible when treated promptly. Table 1 shows some of the more common inciting agents, but by no means represents an all-inclusive list.

Table 1

Drugs that Induce Myopathy

Penicillamine
Zidovudine
Chloroquine
Colchicine
Cocaine
Alcohol
Corticosteroids
Hydroxychloroquine
Lipid-lowering agents:
  Fibric acids derivatives (clofibrate, gemfibrozil)
  Certain HMG-CoA reductase inhibitors (lovastatin, fluvastatin, simvastatin)

The majority of causative agents, such as antimalarials, colchicine, corticosteroids, fibric acid derivatives, HMG-CoA reductase inhibitors, and zidovudine usually invoke myopathy in a generalized manner when administered systemically. Indirect myotoxic effects as a result of drug-induced coma (and subsequent ischemic muscle compression, seizures, and rhabdomyolysis) are typical with acute ingestion of alcohol, heroin or cocaine. Penicillamine causes a prototypical drug-induced immune complex-mediated myositis. Diagnostic tools are not really different for drug-induced myopathies as opposed to a myositis (elevation in CK, weakness, EMG findings). Not all drugs will cause an elevation in CK, case in point being a steroid-induced myopathy. A biopsy may be helpful although not usually performed unless there is a strong indication to rule out other muscles diseases where the histology is diagnostic. Histological assessment may determine the presence of vacuoles, inflammation or necrosis, which are characteristic findings of muscle injury associated with drug-induced myopathies. All of these features can also be seen with PM and hence may not be diagnostic. The clinical history is probably as important as anything, as is discontinuation of the suspected drug. Myoglobinuric renal failure is a serious complication of drug-induced myopathies. Treatment is supportive.

Güillain-Barré Syndrome (GBS)

This acquired inflammatory demyelinating polyradiculoneuropathy is generally easily distinguishable from neuromuscular disorders or primary myopathy. The C. Miller variant of GBS is often confused with MG, as the patient may have occular findings. Electrodiagnostic findings (NCVs and EMG) and CSF analysis (looking for a cyto-albuminemic dissociation) help make the distinction. Pupillary involvement can occur with botulism but also with GBS.

Amyotrophic Lateral Sclerosis (ALS)

Atrophy, spasticity, bulbar signs and weakness without sensory complaints are hallmarks of ALS. Not infrequently ALS can be confused with myopathy although findings of upper and lower motor neuron findings is generally not seen with myopathies. In fulminant cases of ALS the CK can often be elevated, but generally no more than 3-4 times the upper limits of normal. Usually an EMG can distinguish between a neuropathic disease such as ALS vs. a myopathy, but if there is any doubt, a biopsy in an affected muscle is reasonable considering the graveness of ALS.

6. Biological Toxins

Botulism

The sources of botulism are through improperly prepared or stored canned foods, and wounds. A variety of distinct types of *C botulinum* exist, but the three most associated with botulism are A, B and E. Types A and B, which are common in the eastern United States, are more related to contaminated, canned foods, whereas E is more commonly associated with contaminated food products. Ingested botulism is more common at high elevations where water boils at a lower temperature, not allowing the high enough temperature to destroy the toxin as with a lower altitude. The majority of wound-related infections are related to type A. Botulism is a high affinity toxin that impairs Ach release, blocking exocytosis from the nerve terminal. Ingestion of the toxin can lead to symptoms within 2 hours to several days, whereas with wound botulism the effects take longer (up to 14 days).

Usually symptoms begin acutely, over 24-48 hours in the bulbar muscles, often associated with blurred vision, difficulty chewing, dysphagia and diplopia. Nausea and vomiting are common with the ingested form of botulism. A more generalized weakness ensues with arm and leg paralysis and respiratory compromise. A flaccid paralysis with areflexia and extraoccular paralysis are common, looking similar to advanced GBS. Pupillary involvement may occur in some cases, but perhaps not as commonly as often reported. The lack of elevation in the CSF protein is one means of differentiating botulism from GBS. The history is often important in making the diagnosis as often multiple people are affected with botulism. Without intervention, respiratory compromise can lead to death with a mortality rate reaching 25%. Electrophysiological abnormalities are similar to LEMS. Small CMAPs and low EPP are found in affected muscles. Post-tetanic facilitation is seen in the majority of cases, but not as notably as with LEMS. A decremental response is less common at slow rates of stimulation, and at high rates of RS mild to moderate facilitation occurs depending on the severity of exposure. NCVs are normal. Needle EMG shows small MUPs and, if far enough out from the exposure, fibrillation potentials. Single-fiber electromyography may be helpful. Gastric and fecal samples should be examined for toxin. Some laboratories are equipped to test for the lethal dose of affected human serum on the lethal dose in mice.

Supportive care is key with special attention to respiratory function. Patients will sometimes respond to acetylcholinsterase inhibitors as with MG and LEMS. Gastric lavage and enemas may help pass the toxins from the gastrointestinal tract. Antitoxins exist for botulism, but the side effects should be weighed against the severity of the case. With intervention, a full recovery may take up to several months, largely a function of the turnover of receptors.

Tick Paralysis

Toxins are contained in the tick saliva. Typically the patient will have an acute ascending paralysis over several days with no sensory symptoms. The toxins have been shown to block axonal sodium channels and also inhibit the release of acetylcholine at presynaptic motor nerve terminals causing total neuromuscular blockade. The tick species responsible for most cases of human tick paralysis in the United States and Canada are *Dermacenter andersonii* (the Rocky Mountain wood tick), and *D variabilis* (the American dog tick). Tick paralysis can be confused for a number of disorders, but usually is mistaken for GBS. Detection and removal of the tick usually results in rapid improvement in the patient's condition in hours to one or two days. A careful search for the tick with a fine-toothed comb can be helpful. Antiserum is generally not recommended nor necessary.

Marine Toxins

Marine toxins such as ciguatera, saxitoxin and tetrodotoxin need to be considered in the differential of acute weakness, but generally these disorders can be determined largely by the presentation and history. Usually more than one person gets sick when eating a tainted meal. PM may be a long-term sequelae of ciguatera exposure.

Black Widow Envenomation

Black widow spiders (Latrodectus) contain latrotoxins which stimulate neuronal calcium channels to result in excessive exocytosis of synaptic vesicles, leading to serious neuromuscular, neurosecretory, and cardiovascular effects. The latrodectus genus is found throughout the world. The black widow is commonly found in fields, woodpiles, and unoccupied dwellings, not necessarily out of sight or mind. Before indoor plumbing, bites were fairly frequent in outhouses, particularly on male genitals. Patients who are unwittingly bitten by a black widow may be worked up for cardiac symptoms because of the chest pain. Abdominal pain, cramping and nausea are also common. Other general neurologically-related symptoms include agitation, hyperhydrosis, anxiety, dyspnea and dysarthria. Angiodema may be experienced in the extremities and eyelids but rarely at the bite site. Acute symptoms increase in severity during the first day after a bite. Most symptoms generally decline after 2-3 days but some mild residua may continue for several weeks after recovery. Death is rare, but may occur in young children or elderly hypertensive individuals. Latrotoxins do not cross the blood-brain barrier, and symptoms derive from somatic and autonomic PNS cholinergic and neuromuscular junction actions. A specific antivenin neutralizes the venom of all Latrodectus species, and should be administered according to package insert. Symptomatic treatment includes the use of analgesics, muscle relaxants, and intravenous calcium gluconate.

7. Critical Illness Myopathy (CIM)

CIM is by definition associated with patients who have been critically ill and should be considered in the differential of any patient with such a history and acute quadriplegia. The disorder goes by other names, including thick filament myopathy, ICU myopathy, and acute corticosteroid myopathy. Risk factors for developing the disorder include a cumulative dose of IV steroids in excess of 1000 mg methylprednisolone; exposure to a neuromuscular blocking agent; a systemic inflammatory response (two or more of the following: temperature >38 degrees C or <36 degrees C; HR >90/min; RR > 20/min or $PaCO_2$<32 torr; WBC >12K, less than 4K or 10% bands); degree of severity of underlying disease; hyperglycemia and other organ failure. Clinical features of CIM include a flaccid quadraparesis, inability to wean from a mechanical ventilator, reduced or normal reflexes, and if testable, normal sensation (lack of signs of polyneuropathy; however, a superimposed critical illness polyneuropathy can be seen). The typical weakness is proximal more than distal or generalized and sometimes the facial muscles can be involved and, rarely, extraocular muscles. The CK is usually elevated with CIM; however, it can be missed in patients where the myopathy remains undiagnosed over a period of weeks in the ICU and hence returns to normal by the time that the patient is suspected of having CIM. Other entities that might mimic CIM include rhabdomyolysis from infection or pharmacologic agents, cachetic myopathy, prolonged neuromuscular blockade (often in the setting of renal or hepatic insufficiency), and inflammatory or underlying inherited metabolic myopathies that may surface in the setting of the ICU.

Electrodiagnostic studies typically show low amplitude motor responses with normal CV and distal latencies. The duration of motor responses may also be prolonged. Sensory values are generally normal unless there is a superimposed critical illness polyneuropathy or preexisting peripheral neuropathy. Typical myopathic features are seen on EMG. Active denervation can occur as early as 1 week after IV corticosteroids. Recruitment should be early unless the patient is so compromised as to not be able to move. Recent research suggests that there is a component of a sodium channelopathy with CIM.

If the patient has not received IV steroids, a muscle biopsy should be done to exclude other disorders that cannot be adequately differentiated by exam, history and electrodiagnostic testing. Histopathology reveals a predominance of type 2 atrophy, necrosis and myofibrillar disorganization, and a

Figure 7

Electron micrographs from the biceps muscle of patient 3

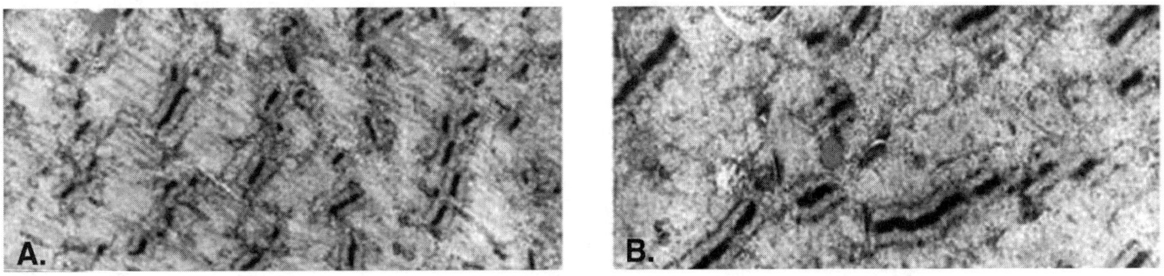

A) Extensive selective loss of thick filaments (original magnification x 24,000)
B) In higher magnification, the marked loss of thick filaments is better appreciated. Thin filaments and Z-discs are well preserved (original magnification x 40,150)

From Sander HW, Golden M, Danon MJ. Quadriplegic areflexic ICU illness: selective thick filament loss and normal nerve histology. Muscle Nerve. *2002 Oct;26(4):499-505. With permission from Wiley Press.*

characteristic loss of myosin out of proportion to other proteins (Figure 7). The pathogenesis appears to involve the overexpression of calpain and other proteolytic enzymes, leading to myosin depletion, as well as the upregulation of apoptotic pathways as a consequence of stress and corticosteroids. Treatment is supportive.

8. Conclusion

This chapter has covered neither all of the syndromes involving the neuromuscular junction syndromes nor all of the acquired myopathies. The intent has been made to focus on those syndromes that are commonly seen and to provide the reader basic concepts about their pathophysiology, clinical features, pathology and treatments. A thorough understanding of this chapter should serve as a basis to understanding these related entities.

9. References

1. Patrick J, Lindstrom, J. Autoimmune response to acetylcholine receptor. *Science*.1973;180(88):871-2.

   (A landmark paper.)

2. Drachman DB. Myasthenia gravis. *N Engl J Med*. 1994;330(25):1797-810.

   (A very good review of myasthenia gravis and still relevant despite being 11 years old.)

3. Hoch W, et al. Auto-antibodies to the receptor tyrosine kinase MuSK in patients with myasthenia gravis without acetylcholine receptor antibodies. *Nat Med*. 2001;7(3):365-8.

4. Vernino S, Lennon VA. Autoantibody profiles and neurological correlations of thymoma. *Clin Cancer Res*. 2004;10(21):7270-5.

5. Sanders DB. Clinical neurophysiology of disorders of the neuromuscular junction. *J Clin Neurophysiol*. 1993;10(2):167-80.

6. Jaretzki A III. Thymectomy for myasthenia gravis: analysis of controversies – patient management. *Neurologist*. 2003;9(2):77-92.

7. Sanders DB, Scoppetta C. The treatment of patients with myasthenia gravis. *Neurol Clin*. 1994;12(2):343-68.

8. Clark WF, et al. Therapeutic plasma exchange: an update from the Canadian Apheresis Group. *Ann Intern Med*. 1999;131(6):453-62.

9. Dalakas MC. Intravenous immunoglobulin in the treatment of autoimmune neuromuscular diseases: present status and practical therapeutic guidelines. *Muscle Nerve*. 1999;22(11):1479-97.

   (A practical paper of clinical interest.)

10. Seute T, et al. Neurologic disorders in 432 consecutive patients with small cell lung carcinoma. *Cancer*. 2004;100(4):801-6.

11. Wirtz PW, et al. The epidemiology of the Lambert-Eaton myasthenic syndrome in the Netherlands. *Neurology*. 2004;63(2):397-8.

12. Maddison P, et al. Favourable prognosis in Lambert-Eaton myasthenic syndrome and small-cell lung carcinoma. *Lancet*. 1999;353(9147):117-8.

13. Nakao YK, et al. Seronegative Lambert-Eaton myasthenic syndrome: study of 110 Japanese patients. *Neurology*. 2002;59(11):1773-5.

14. O'Neill JH, Murray NM, Newsom-Davis J. The Lambert-Eaton myasthenic syndrome. A review of 50 cases. *Brain*. 1988;111 (Pt 3):577-96.

15. Beydoun SR. Delayed diagnosis of Lambert-Eaton myasthenic syndrome in a patient presenting with recurrent refractory respiratory failure. *Muscle Nerve*. 1994;17(6):689-90.

16. Sanders DB. Lambert-Eaton myasthenic syndrome: diagnosis and treatment. *Ann NY Acad Sci*. 2003;998:500-8.

    (A very good recent review.)

17. Tim RW, Massey JM, Sanders DB. Lambert-Eaton myasthenic syndrome: electrodiagnostic findings and response to treatment. *Neurology*. 2000;54(11):2176-8.

18. Wirtz PW, et al. Differences in clinical features between the Lambert-Eaton myasthenic syndrome with and without cancer: an analysis of 227 published cases. *Clin Neurol Neurosurg*. 2002;104(4):359-63.

19. Waterman SA, Lang B, Newsom-Davis J. Effect of Lambert-Eaton myasthenic syndrome antibodies on autonomic neurons in the mouse. *Ann Neurol*. 1997;42(2):147-56.

20. Motomura M, et al. Incidence of serum anti-P/O-type and anti-N-type calcium channel autoantibodies in the Lambert-Eaton myasthenic syndrome. *J Neurol Sci*. 1997;147(1):35-42.

21. Newsom-Davis J. Therapy in myasthenia gravis and Lambert-Eaton myasthenic syndrome. *Semin Neurol*. 2003;23(2):191-8.

(An excellent, recent paper on therapy for these two major neuromuscular diseases.)

22. Bohan A, Peter JB. Polymyositis and dermatomyositis (first of two parts). *N Engl J Med*. 1975; 292(7):344-7.

23. Bohan A, Peter JB. Polymyositis and dermatomyositis (second of two parts). *N Engl J Med*. 1975;292(8):403-7.

24. van der Meulen MF, et al. Polymyositis: an overdiagnosed entity. *Neurology*. 2003;61(3): 316-21.

25. Emslie-Smith AM, Arahata K, Engel AG. Major histocompatibility complex class I antigen expression, immunolocalization of interferon subtypes, and T cell-mediated cytotoxicity in myopathies. *Hum Pathol*. 1989;20(3):224-31.

26. Euwer RL, Sontheimer RD. Amyopathic dermatomyositis: a review. *J Invest Dermatol*. 1993;100(1):124S-127S.

27. Hohlfeld R, Engel AG. The immunobiology of muscle. *Immunol Today*. 1994;15(6):269-74.

28. Dalakas MC, et al. Mitochondrial myopathy caused by long-term zidovudine therapy. *N Engl J Med*. 1990;322(16):1098-105.

29. Spuler S, Emslie-Smith A, Engel AG. Amyloid myopathy: an underdiagnosed entity. *Ann Neurol*. 1998;43(6):719-28.

30. Amato AA, et al. Inclusion body myositis: clinical and pathological boundaries. *Ann Neurol*. 1996;40(4):581-6.

31. Pickering MC, Walport MJ. Eosinophilic myopathic syndromes. *Curr Opin Rheumatol*. 1998;10(6):504-10.

32. Rider LG, et al. Clinical, serologic, and immunogenetic features of familial idiopathic inflammatory myopathy. *Arthritis Rheum*. 1998; 41(4):710-9.

33. Stevens AM, Sullivan KM, Nelson JL. Polymyositis as a manifestation of chronic graft-versus-host disease. *Rheumatology*. (Oxford). 2003; 42(1):34-9.

34. Amato AA, Barohn RJ. Idiopathic inflammatory myopathies. *Neurol Clin*. 1997; 15(3):615-48.

(An excellent, relatively recent review on these disorders.)

35. Lotz BP, et al. Inclusion body myositis. Observations in 40 patients. *Brain*. 1989; 112 (Pt 3):727-47.

36. Arahata K, Engel AG. Monoclonal antibody analysis of mononuclear cells in myopathies. I: Quantitation of subsets according to diagnosis and sites of accumulation and demonstration and counts of muscle fibers invaded by T-cells. *Ann Neurol*. 1984;16(2):193-208.

37. Karpati G, Pouliot Y, Carpenter S. Expression of immunoreactive major histocompatibility complex products in human skeletal muscles. *Ann Neurol*. 1988;23(1):64-72.

38. Dalakas MC. Polymyositis, dermatomyositis and inclusion-body myositis. *N Engl J Med*. 1991;325(21):1487-98.

39. Griggs RC, Askanas V, DiMauro S. Inclusion body myositis and myopathies. *Ann Neurol*. 1995;38:705.

40. Askanas V, Engel WK, Mirabella M. Idiopathic inflammatory myopathies: inclusion body myositis, polymyositis, and dermatomyositis. *Curr Opin Neurol*. 1994;7(5): 448-56.

41. Mendell JR, et al. Amyloid filaments in inclusion body myositis. Novel findings provide insight into nature of filaments. *Arch Neurol.* 1991;48(12):1229-34.

42. Amato AA, Griggs RC. Treatment of idiopathic inflammatory myopathies. *Curr Opin Neurol.* 2003;16(5):569-75.

(A thorough, recent evaluation of treatment options for the inflammatory myopathies.)

43. Douglas AC, Macleod JG, Matthews JD. Symptomatic sarcoidosis of skeletal muscle. *J Neurol Neurosurg Psychiatry.* 1973;36(6): 1034-40.

44. Prendergast CD. Drug-induced rhabdomyolysis: mechanism and management. *Postgrad Med J.* 1993;69:33-66.

45. Stommel EW, Parsonnet J, Jenkyn LR. Polymyositis after ciguatera toxin exposure. *Arch Neurol.* 1991;48(8):874-7.

46. Rich MM, Pinter MJ. Sodium channel inactivation in an animal model of acute quadriplegic myopathy. *Ann Neurol.* 2001;50(1):26-33.

47. Di Giovanni S, et al. Constitutive activation of MAPK cascade in acute quadriplegic myopathy. *Ann Neurol.* 2004;55(2):195-206.

(An interesting paper dealing with the pathophysiology of critical illness myopathy.)

10. Questions

1. A 58-year-old heavy cigarette smoker presents with a several month history of progressive proximal leg>arm weakness and a productive cough. He has noticed a recent dry mouth, constipation and blurred vision. He undergoes a chest x-ray in the process of his diagnostic workup, which reveals a large right upper lobe tumor. A bronchoscopy reveals SCLC. Which of the following would typically be associated with LEMS and are associated with this man's diagnosis?

A. Antibodies to presynaptic calcium channels

B. Elevation in AChR antibodies

C. Postexercise increase in size of CMAP

D. Elevated CSF protein

E. All of the above

2. CK levels are typically increased in MG?

A. True

B. False

3. A 59-year-old man presents to clinic with progressive upper extremity weakness that appears to involve the forearm flexors for the most part. He feels slightly weak in his lower extremities. He denies any dysarthria or dysphagia and still is able to climb stairs.

Which of the following answers regarding IBM are correct and associated with this man's diagnosis of IBM?

A. With IBM, histology shows inflammation and rimmed vacuoles

B. Muscle atrophy is a common feature

C. Forearm flexors frequently involved

D. IBM responds poorly to immunomodulatory therapy

E. All of the above

4. Which of the following treatments is ineffective for PM/DM?

A. Methotrexate

B. Steroids

C. Azathioprine

D. Plasma exchange

5. A 45-year-old male camper cooks and then eats some canned food that he made himself at a height of 10,000 feet in the Colorado Rockies where he lives. Within a few hours the patient starts to develop diffuse weakness, shortness of breath, ptosis and double vision. Luckily the patient was with friends who did not eat the food and were able to get him to medical care. What would be useful ways to differentiate botulism from MG?

A. Autonomic dysfunction

B. Electroneuromyography

C. Antibody studies

D. Clinical history

E. All of the above

6. What are the typical electromyographic findings with MG?

A. A reduction in CMAP amplitude with RS at 2-5 Hz in excess of 10%-15% to the baseline CMAP amplitude

B. Postexercise, waveform size can increase by 10%-50%

C. Increased jitter with SFEMG

D. RS involving appropriate muscles has a sensitivity of approximately 75% in generalized MG

E. All of the above

7. The typical histological features of DM include all of the following except:

A. Perifascicular atrophy

B. Perivascular infiltrates

C. Microinfarction

D. Cellular infiltrates invading the fascicles

8. Typical clinical manifestations of DM include which of the following?

A. Transient rash that can disappear before weakness is noticed

B. Gottron's sign

C. Periungual erythema

D. Eyelid swelling and an associated rash of the eyelids

E. All of the above

9. Which of the following could be confused with PM?

   A. ALS

   B. IBM

   C. Statin-induced myopathy

   D. DM

   E. All of the above

10. Statin-induced myopathy is sometimes difficult to differentiate from PM. True or false?

   A. True

   B. False

11. MRI is helpful in the setting of myopathy for:

   A. Diagnostic purposes

   B. Prognostic purposes

   C. Guiding the site for muscle biopsy

   D. Adding to the radiologist's income

   E. All of the above

12. Which of the following are true regarding botulism?

   A. The symptoms may begin within 2 hours of ingestion of contaminated food

   B. The symptoms usually begin within the bulbar muscles

   C. Ingested toxin is sometimes associated with nausea and vomiting

   D. Recovery from intoxication may take several months

   E. All of the above

13. Which of the following are common with botulism?

   A. Flaccidity

   B. Areflexia

   C. Pupillary paralysis

   D. High CSF protein

   E. Sensory abnormalities

14. Which of the following are common with tick paralysis?

   A. Anti-serum is generally not recommended or necessary

   B. The tick is usually embedded near the hair-line

   C. The paralysis often starts in the legs and rapidly becomes more generalized

   D. Cranial nerve abnormalities are common

   E. All of the above

15. The mode of action of the black widow spider venom is to:

A. Stimulate neuronal calcium channels

B. Block sodium channels

C. Heighten exocytosis at the neuromuscular junction

D. None of the above

16. LEMS is associated with:

A. Bulbar weakness

B. Autonomic dysfunction

C. Sensory complaints

D. Frequent respiratory failure

E. All of the above

17. Common features of the neuromuscular junction disorders include:

A. A failure of the EPP to reach threshold

B. A clinical weakness that is worse with exertion

C. A transient improvement with brief exercise (postexercise facilitation) or AchE-inhibition

D. A variation of the MUP amplitude on needle EMG

E. All of the above

18. The CPK is generally elevated in steroid-induced myopathy?

A. True

B. False

19. Checking the CSF is a useful test for differentiating GBS from botulism.

A. True

B. False

20. A 54-year-old man presents with diffuse weakness, atrophy, spasticity, dysarthria and dysphagia. He has recently noticed rippling in his muscles, which his internist tells him are fasciculations. He is losing weight and goes to a neurologist who performs NCVs/EMG and a complete neurological assessment. He has diffuse, active denervation in all four extremities by electrical testing. He has both upper and power motor neuron findings on neurological exam consistent with ALS.

The patient's CPK comes back 2 times the upper limit of normal. Is this consistent with the patient's diagnosis of ALS?

A. True

B. False

21. A 55-year-old man presents to the neurology clinic with worsening (4 weeks) proximal pain and weakness in his upper and lower extremities over a period of several weeks. He denies any sensory complaints. Cranial nerves are normal. His strength is 4/5 in the proximal muscles of the upper and lower extremities. Reflexes are still present and his sensory exam is intact. He has a waddling gait and has a difficult time getting out of a chair without using his arms to push off his knees. He has no rash and is on no medications.

What might be the first tests that you would want to do in the clinic?

A. CPK level

B. Spinal fluid analysis

C. EMG

D. Genetic testing

22. A 10-year-old female presents to the clinic with worsening ascending weakness and SOB. She has no sensory complaints. An astute neurologist evaluates the patient and finds her to have dysarthria, facial weakness, ophthalmoplegia without papillary involvement, 3/5 weakness in the lower extremities and 4/5 weakness in the upper extremities associated with hypotonia in all extremities. DTRs were absent. She was unable to walk. A subsequent workup reveals normal spinal fluid. NCVs showed low amplitude CMAPs with active denervation on EMG. RS was normal in proximal and distal muscles tested.

Which of the following diagnoses would seem the most likely?

A. Tick paralysis

B. MG

C. GBS

D. DM

23. A 22-year-old female presents with progressive weakness, ptosis, diplopia, dysarthria and dysphagia. She is thought to have myasthenia gravis. Her internist orders an acetylcholine receptor antibody titer to help confirm the diagnosis. Which of the additional tests would not be considered helpful at further confirming the diagnosis?

A. CPK

B. RS testing and single fiber EMG

C. Pulmonary function tests

D. Chest CT

24. A 58-year-old female presents with a 4-week history of progressive weakness and muscle pain that is more proximal than distal. She denies any sensory loss. She has a waddling gait. Her family history is unremarkable for muscle disorders. A CPK is drawn and comes back at 10,000 U/L. She is sent for a right vastus lateralis muscle biopsy after a n EMG of the left quadriceps shows myopathic potentials. The muscle biopsy is read within 24 hours and shows no evidence of inflammation.

Does this result confirm that the patient does not have an inflammatory myopathy?

A. Yes

B. No

25. What other history or tests might you want to know about or order based on the above presentation?

A. Use of cholesterol lowering agents

B. MRI of the leg

C. Repeat EMG

D. Repeat CPK

26. A 25-year-old male went camping with friends. He was sitting in a poorly lighted outhouse when he had a very distinct sting to his genitals. He quickly left the outhouse without seeing any culprit for the sting. Over a period of 2 hours the patient developed chest tightness and pain, agitation, hyperhydrosis, anxiety, dyspnea and dysarthria. Careful inspection in the local emergency room demonstrated an inflamed bite on his right scrotum where he had initially felt the pain.

What would be a likely culprit for the patient's symptoms?

A. Tick bite

B. Snake bite

C. Black widow bite

27. A 60-year-old man is worked-up for progressive proximal weakness associated with pain and cramping that presents over a period of 2 months. He was found to have myopathic potentials proximally in his arms and legs with EMG. CPK was 3000 U/L. A muscle biopsy was performed and showed some necrotic fibers, but no evidence of inflammation. He has been on a statin over the last 4 months.

What would be a good approach to this patient's situation?

A. Assume this is PM and treat accordingly with immunosuppressive agents

B. Assume this is a statin-induced myopathy and discontinue the statin and observe for a month or so

C. Treat for statin-induced myopathy with steroids

D. Repeat the EMG

28. A 57-year-old female had an URI that lasted for a week. About 6 days later she started to develop ascending weakness, ataxia, numbness in her extremities and shortness of breath. She goes to the clinic where she is found to be weak, especially in her legs distally, weak in her face with some mild ophthalmoplegia, and is arreflexic. She has great difficulty ambulating. Which of the following tests would you want to order next?

A. MRI of the brain

B. LP

C. Muscle biopsy

D. NCVs/EMG

E. All of the above

Answers

1. A., C.

2. B.

3. E.

4. D.

5. E.
The temperature of boiling water decreases as the altitude increases. Thus, the temperature at which foods are processed is reduced. The canning pressure for low-acid foods must be increased by 1/2 pound for every 1,000 feet rise in elevation. Overlooking these changes increases the risk of botulism.

6. E.

7. A., B., C.

8. E.

9. E.

10. A.

11. E.

12. E.

13. A., B., C.

14. E.

15. A., C.

16. A., B., C.

17. E.

18. B.

19. A.
An elevated CSF protein would be consistent with GBS.

20. A.
The fulminant loss of motor neurons leads to the death of muscle and can generally elevate the CPK 2-3 times the upper limits of normal.

21. A., C.
The patient is presenting with what would appear to be a rapidly acquired proximal myopathy. The pain and weakness would likely be consistent with a PM. He is on no medications and has no rash consistent DM. Spinal fluid analysis is unlikely to be of any benefit as it does look like he has GBS, and a genetic abnormality would be unlikely to present so quickly and over such a short period of time.

22. A.
This case is most consistent with tick paralysis. Normal CSF would go against a diagnosis of GBS. The normal RS would go against MG as would the presentation, although it could still be possible. The history and exam are not consistent with DM. A careful inspection of the scalp and elsewhere is important to look for a tick. The use of a fine toothcomb can be helpful.

23. A.
A CPK would not be useful in confirming the diagnosis of MG. It is helpful for evaluating myopathies, where it is often increased.

24.
No. The biopsy may well miss an area of inflammation. The use of MRI on the leg can help direct the surgeon to an area of inflammation.

25. B.
The statins frequently are associated with myopathy, but it would be somewhat unusual to cause a CPK level as high as 10,000 U/L. As mentioned above, the use of MRI on the leg can help direct the surgeon to an area of inflammation. A repeat biopsy is likely indicated. A repeat CPK or repeat EMG is not likely to be of any diagnostic value.

26. C.
Black widow bite. The patient's symptoms fit this description well. Over a period of a week the patient's symptoms completely resolved. Careful inspection with a flashlight in the outhouse demonstrated a large spider web and a large black widow spider.

27. B.
The best solution in the setting of recent statin use with no inflammation on the biopsy would be to assume this may be related to the statin and to wait and watch carefully.

28. B., D.

The patient is likely to have GBS with a prodromal infection. Her symptoms as described are neuropathic. The two most helpful confirmatory tests for GBS are CSF analysis looking for a cytoalbuminemic dissociation and NCVs/EMG to look for typical finding of demyelination (temporal dispersion and absent F waves). Axonal involvement portends a worse prognosis and can be looked for with EMG.

Chapter 19: Neuromuscular Disease in Childhood

John Sladky, MD

Contents

1. Introduction

This chapter summarizes the topic of neuromuscular disorders in children. Although there is considerable overlap with some diseases occurring in both children and adults, this chapter will focus predominantly on those which exhibit initial manifestations in childhood. The scope of this text necessitates a minimalist approach to specific arenas. The topic of this chapter alone has spawned entire textbooks. You will note obvious omissions of intriguing entities or those closely related to the focus of discussion. Please accept apology for those topics of particular interest which may have received short shrift.

There are several paradigms which have been employed to provide a conceptual structure for the discussion of neuromuscular diseases. A traditional approach is to begin centrally and progress toward the periphery. There are shortcomings to this strategy, but over decades it has been engrafted into the consciousness of teachers of clinical neuroscience. The paradigm provides an Aristotelian, linear organization to the subject of neuromuscular disease, which allows the student to orient centrifugally along the projection of the lower motor unit. The nature of the disease is characterized by identifying clinical features, which distinguish among different pathological locations along the lower motor unit, ie, motor neuron versus neuromuscular junction. An additional calculus can be brought to bear in the process of investigating neuromuscular disease in children. Unlike the more typical circumstance in adults, where age of onset may not impart additional insight as to the cause of symptoms, many of the neuromuscular disorders encountered in children have a predictable time of life at which they emerge (Table 1). These two approaches can act synergistically in the course of sorting out the nature of the cause of motor dysfunction in children.

Table 1

Typical Age at Presentation of Neuromuscular Disorders in Childhood

This table summarizes the most common pediatric neuromuscular disorders and the typical age at which symptoms become apparent. Some of these entities with a greater degree of clinical heterogeneity appear in more than one column. Those in bold face type represent disorders that most often come to medical attention in their particular age bracket.

Perinatal Period	**Infant/Toddler**	**Preadolescent**
Spinal muscular atrophy	**Spinal muscular atrophy**	Spinal muscular atrophy
Congenital neuropathy	Hereditary sensory-motor neuropathy	**Hereditary sensory** or **sensory-motor neuropathy**
Transient neonatal myasthenia	Guillain-Barré syndrome	Guillain-Barré syndrome
Congenital myasthenic syndromes	**Myasthenia gravis**	**Chronic inflammatory demyelinating polyneuropathy**
Congenital myopathy	Congenital myasthenic syndromes	**Myasthenia gravis**
Congenital muscular dystrophy	**Infant botulism**	Congenital myasthenic syndromes
	Congenital myopathy	Botulism (food or wound)
	Inflammatory myopathy	**Dystrophinopathies**
	Metabolic myopathy	**Limb-girdle dystrophies**
	Mitochondrial myopathy	Myotonic dystrophy
		Inflammatory myopathy
		Metabolic myopathy
		Mitochondrial myopathy

2. Motor Neuron Diseases

Spinal Muscular Atrophies

The predominant reason for parents of children with spinal muscular atrophy (SMA) to seek medical attention is the failure to achieve gross motor milestones. Clinical findings in SMA types I and II also referred to as Werdnig-Hoffman disease are generalized hypotonia, weakness of axial and appendicular muscles with relative sparing of facial and bulbar muscles (early on), and areflexia. Electrodiagnostic testing will document normal sensory nerve conduction with widespread denervation on electromyography. The numerical classification of the SMAs, Types I through III (type III is traditionally termed Kugelberg-Welander disease), is based on age of onset of symptoms, which can often be difficult to precisely ascertain. The first of these phenotypes has a high incidence of mortality by two years of age.

All of the spinal muscular atrophies are caused by homozygous deletions involving exons 7 and 8 in the survival motor neuron gene (SMN1) located on chromosome 5q13. The severity of the disorder is modified by the expression of a second duplicate homologous gene (SMN2). Both SMN genes, found on chromosome 5q, are closely linked, with SMN1 located on the telomeric side of the duplication. Children with severe early onset SMA have typical deletions in SMN1 genes with only one or two residual copies of the SMN2 genes. Those with milder phenotypes have the SMN1 deletions but also possess three or more copies of SMN2. Deletions of both SMN1 and SMN2 genes is probably a lethal permutation since this genotype has not been described in affected humans. Current genotypic diagnosis is based on analysis of the integrity of the SMN1 alleles. Determination of the number of copies of the SMN2 allele adds limited insight to the clinical profile regarding prognosis. Strategies to enhance expression of residual SMN2 alleles may someday provide an avenue to modify disease severity.

Although many issues require attention, the principle management consideration for children with SMA (predominantly infants/toddlers with type 1 SMA) is weakness of respiratory muscles. In the early stages, a proactive stance to prevent or minimize pulmonary infection by avoiding unnecessary exposure and employing a low threshold for antibiotic treatment for upper respiratory infections is prudent. SMAs have been thought to represent degenerative disorders with progressive loss of motor neurons resulting in a relentless decline in strength. The evidence for that explanation for the clinical course of the disease is scant. An equally or even more compelling argument can be made that the disease process compromises the ability of the motor unit to generate increased force to accommodate somatic growth. In the case of gross motor activity, increased skeletal mass imposes a greater load burden with consequent functional decline. Chronic decrements in lung compliance due to repeated episodes of atelectasis and pneumonia result in increased work of breathing, greater difficulty in clearing secretions and, consequently, a vicious cycle leading to respiratory failure. In addition to restrictive lung disease, the course in these children may be further complicated by obstructive airway pathology. Aggressive pulmonary toilette along with broncholytic treatment when necessary can slow the pace of respiratory compromise. In older children, the problem of scoliosis will almost invariably rear its head. Suggested guidelines regarding the timing of surgical intervention in relationship to severity of curvature is a difficult balancing act and is contextually specific for individual patients.

In the later stages of the illness, it is not uncommon for children with SMA to present with acute respiratory failure, often with a precipitating cause such as infection or aspiration, requiring mechanical ventilatory support. Many of these children, primarily in the SMA type 1 category, have a concomitant defect in fatty acid utilization, which may be unmasked during a catabolic state such as infection or fasting, which often coincide. The clinical implication of this underlying metabolic defect in critically ill children is to exacerbate weakness contributing to persistent respiratory failure. Although controlled clinical trials are not available to support this position, it has been my practice to infuse super-normal concentrations of dextrose in maintenance fluids during the acute illness until an adequate nutritional status can be restored.

The prognosis in the SMAs is quite variable. It is clear that age of presentation is related to residual SMN2 gene activity and that early onset and low residual SMN2 number are associated with less favorable outcome. Careful attention to pulmonary complications, however, can certainly affect the course of the illness.

3. Inherited Peripheral Neuropathies

Congenital Neuropathies

Most of the peripheral neuropathies presenting early in life are associated with slowing of sensory and motor nerve conduction velocities with absent or diminished amplitudes of sensory nerve action potentials and compound motor action potentials. They are classified under the category of demyelinating neuropathies, often more accurately as congenital hypomyelinating neuropathies (CHN), since there is rarely evidence of formation of normal myelin sheaths on large caliber axons (Figure 1, see color plates).

Clinical examination typically reveals hypotonia with generalized weakness and absent reflexes. Motor nerve conduction velocities are diminished and may be as slow as 2 m/sec. There is only limited correlation between the magnitude of conduction velocity slowing and the severity of the clinical syndrome. In one series, it was reported that the presence of arthrogryposis multiplex congenita and the absence of onion bulb formations within the endoneurium were phenotypic markers associated with a poor prognosis. This category of peripheral neuropathy is often referred to as Dejerine-Sottas disease. The term brings with it little specificity since the diagnosis includes children with substantial variability in terms of both genotype and phenotype. Homologous gene defects result in different phenotypes, and diverse gene mutations produce similar clinical presentations. Hence, there is considerable genotypic overlap between those neuropathies presenting in infancy and those with a later onset which fall under the rubric of Charcot-Marie-Tooth disease, or hereditary motor and sensory neuropathy.

Hereditary Motor and Sensory Neuropathy

The peroneal muscular atrophy syndrome was originally described in 1886 by Howard Henery Tooth, an English medical student. Later that year, a more detailed description of the disorder was published by the French neurologists Charcot and his pupil Marie. The clinical features common to this group of disorders, for most of the twentieth century referred to as Charcot-Marie-Tooth disease, are quite homogeneous, including progressive loss of strength in a fiber length dependent distribution and, usually to a lesser degree, diminished sensation predominantly involving those modalities related to large caliber myelinated axons, proprioception and vibration. In some cases, sensory impulses are transmitted via small myelinated and unmyelinated axons; touch, temperature and pain are also affected. Myotactic reflexes are diminished or absent at early stages of the disease. In the large majority of cases, the neuropathy is inherited in an autosomal dominant fashion.

The initial subclassification of these disorders came as a result of the work by Dyck and Lambert. Electrophysiological testing permitted distinction between kinships with autosomal dominantly transmitted hereditary motor and sensory neuropathies (HMSN) based on motor nerve conduction velocities in the forearm. Patients with nerve conduction velocity below 40 meters/second were classified as having the demyelinating form of the disease (HMSN Type I), while those with motor conduction velocity of greater than 40 m/sec were classified as the axonal form (HMSN Type II). This classification schema was validated by histopathological characteristics on sural nerve biopsies wherein the predominant pathological features were either of axons showing evidence of demyelination and remyelination or features of axonal degeneration and regeneration. In time, evidence accumulated that subgroups of HMSN were genetically heterogeneous.

Genetic analysis is available to confirm the diagnosis in some HMSN subtypes. The initial mutations identified in autosomal dominantly inherited demyelinating neuropathies were in genes encoding peripheral myelin protein 22 (PMP22) and myelin protein 0 (MPZ). Mutations in the Connexin 32 gene (Cx32) were shown to be responsible for an x-linked pattern of inherited demyelinating neuropathy. Since then, numerous genes have been identified with both axonal and demyelinating subtypes of hereditary sensory-motor neuropathies transmitted in autosomal dominant, recessive, or x-linked modes. There also appear to be instances of spontaneous mutation, although this phenomenon is probably relatively uncommon. To make matters more difficult, mutations in the same gene in different kinships can result in divergent phenotypes with features of either axonal or demyelinating neuropathy. This phenomenon is most likely related to the effect of specific mutations at different sites within the gene resulting in altered protein products with differing pathological effects on the functional integrity of Schwann cell-axonal relationships. In the last few years, enormous strides have been made in identifying genes and specific mutations within those genes responsible for various HMSN categories. The accelerated pace of growth in this field has resulted in review articles shortly becoming outdated.

At present, there is no specific therapy for inherited sensory-motor neuropathies. Interventions such as physical therapy are useful in attempting to maintain range of motion. As that undertaking becomes more difficult or, additionally, to assist in providing greater gait stability, orthotics may be incorporated into the therapeutic armamentarium. The institution of night splints relatively early in the course of the disease is helpful in preserving a more physiological conformation of the foot. Later, the orthotic may assist in preventing falls due to ankle instability or foot drop. Despite the best efforts of patients, therapists and physicians, many patients go on to develop foot deformities typically including pes cavus, hammer toes, and valgus angulation of the fore and hindfoot requiring surgical intervention. Newer orthopedic approaches with early soft tissue interventions may obviate the need for more radical procedures later in the course of the disease.

4. Immune-Mediated Peripheral Neuropathies

Guillain-Barré Syndrome

Guillain-Barré syndrome warrants a more expanded discussion because it is the single most common cause of acute flaccid paralysis in children among countries with widespread immunization programs. A high point on the landscape of diagnostic concerns should be reserved for Guillain-Barré syndrome for three reasons: first, the disease is potentially life threatening; second, it is eminently treatable; and finally, delay in instituting therapy appears to have a deleterious effect on treatment efficacy. The incidence of the disease has been variously estimated to be between 5 and 15/million in children less than eighteen years of age. In most series there is male predominance, with a male:female ratio of approximately 1.2:1. A typical patient might experience ascending weakness beginning in the legs and advancing to involve the arms. The onset of weakness may be associated with moderate-to-severe back and leg pain in up to 75% of patients. The accepted diagnostic criteria are purely clinical, consisting of the subacute or acute onset of progressive weakness involving more than one extremity along with diminished or absent stretch reflexes. Laboratory investigations can serve to reinforce the diagnosis and include the presence of albumino-cytologic dissociation on spinal fluid examination and electrodiagnostic findings indicative of a multifocal, acquired, demyelinating neuropathy.

Roughly two-thirds of GBS patients will identify an antecedent event in the 30 to 60 days prior to the onset of symptoms. These events are diverse in character, ranging from infections, immunizations, trauma, surgery and parturition to animal exposures and insect bites. Upper respiratory tract infection is the single most commonly identified. Over the past few years it has come to be appreciated that campylobacter enteritis may be the commonest antecedent infection, which instigates an immune response resulting in GBS. This is particularly true in developing countries and in areas where the water supply may be contaminated.

The clinical course of GBS conforms to a triphasic model. There is an initial progressive phase which includes the interval from the first appearance of symptoms until the point of maximal clinical severity. This is followed by a plateau phase which lasts until the beginning of a recovery phase which is typically more prolonged than the progressive phase. Review of several series describing the natural history of GBS in both adults and children reveals remarkable consistently with the mean duration of the progressive and plateau phases each lasting approximately 10-11 days. The pace of recovery was much more variable.

The clinical severity at the nadir of the disease in children hospitalized for GBS is also fairly consistent. Approximately 25% of patients retained the ability to ambulate 5 meters without assistance. Forty percent of children were bed or wheelchair bound with roughly 15% requiring mechanical ventilatory support. The prognosis for recovery is, in general, excellent. A large study of children with GBS from western Europe found that after six months all children were ambulatory and, at worst, had minimal functional deficits (Jones, 2000; Korinthenberg et al, 1996). In tertiary care centers with sophisticated life support facilities, the mortality in childhood GBS is virtually zero.

The pathobiology of GBS remains incompletely understood and a comprehensive discussion of this topic is outside the scope of this chapter. It is reasonable to conceptualize the pathogenesis as reflecting a series of discrete processes which ultimately orchestrate an immune mediated attack on the peripheral nervous system. Whether identifiable or not, there must be an event which initiates an autoimmune process. This is followed by breakdown of immune tolerance. The immune system then targets specific epitopes on Schwann cells or axons, or both, within peripheral nerves. Specific immune components, including immunoglobulin, T cells, macrophages and proinflammatory cytokines, must traverse the blood:nerve barrier. This cascade of events ultimately results in a T cell and immunoglobulin orchestrated, macrophage-mediated attack on endoneurial contents.

The specific components of the peripheral nervous system which are injured in this autoimmune process determine the clinical phenotype in the affected child. GBS has been subclassified into several distinct syndromes. The most common in North America and Western Europe is acute inflammatory demyelinating polyradiculoneuropathy (AIDP). This disorder accounts for more than 90% of cases of GBS in these regions. Children with AIDP present with typical ascending paralysis with electrophysiological and histopathological evidence of multi-focal demyelination. A second, much less frequent GBS sub-type is acute motor and sensory axonal neuropathy or AMSAN. In this syndrome the electrophysiology and histopathology are indicative of axonal degeneration rather than demyelination affecting both sensory and motor axonal populations. Fisher syndrome is a clinical diagnosis based on the triad of external ophthalmoplegia, ataxia and areflexia. This syndrome has been estimated to account for approximately 2% of cases of childhood GBS. Acute motor axonal neuropathy (AMAN) is a distinctive syndrome, uncommon in North America and Western Europe. Electrodiagnostic testing reveals normal motor and sensory nerve conduction velocities with preservation of sensory nerve action potential amplitudes. Histopathological studies have demonstrated sparing of sensory axons with axonal degeneration discretely limited to the motor axonal population without features suggestive of demyelination. Although rare in the United States, this disorder may account for up to 40% of cases of GBS in China, South America and elsewhere. There is a significant correlation with campylobacter infection acquired through contaminated local water supplies. In China, where the disorder has been best characterized, this is a disease of children from predominantly rural regions. Other GBS subsyndromes have been reported; however, their incidence is insignificant compared to those described above (Table 2).

There is no evidence-based rationale regarding optimal treatment of children with GBS. Although it would seem counter-intuitive, there is no correlation between institution of (other than supportive) treatment and the long-term outcome of the disease in children. Some have argued on that basis that the risk of therapies, such as plasmapheresis or human intravenous immunoglobulin, are not warranted. There are several case series examining the efficacy of both plasmapheresis and human intravenous immunoglobulin (IVIg) in the treatment of children with GBS. Many have concluded that children treated with either modality may have a more rapid recovery. There have been no randomized con-

Table 2

Guillain-Barré Syndrome Clinical Subtypes

Acute inflammatory demyelinating polyneuropathy
Acute motor and sensory axonal neuropathy
Acute motor axonal neuropathy
Miller Fisher syndrome
Polyneuritis cranialis
Acute dysautonomia

trolled trials of treatment for GBS in children. Data are available from several large randomized trials in adults with GBS using plasmapheresis, IVIg and a combination of both treatment modalities. The eligibility criteria for most of these trials include loss of independent ambulation with one of the end-points being the time to regain the ability to walk 5 meters unaided. Both treatments appear to reduce the time to recover independent walking by about 30%-35%. A study comparing plasmapheresis, IVIg and a combination of both found that the three treatment strategies were equivalent in augmenting the pace of recovery. Meta-analysis of several case series in children with GBS suggests a very similar treatment effect from plasmapheresis or IVIg in children as in adult trials. These observations in childhood GBS are important because the recovery of stable independent ambulation is often the factor which determines when the child can be discharged from the hospital. Reducing the duration of morbidity through therapeutic intervention has obvious implications for both psychological well-being and health care economics.

Several trials in adults have documented an increased incidence of adverse events in the plasmapheresis treated cohorts compared to the patients treated with IVIg. Extrapolating from this experience, it would seem reasonable to choose a therapy based on logistical issues and the adverse event profiles in adult trials. Based on these considerations, many neurologists have concluded that IVIg is the treatment of choice in pediatric GBS. This opinion, however, is based more on belief than on scientific method. Given the quality of currently available data, it is not possible to designate either plasmapheresis or IVIg as the treatment of choice. There is, however, a persuasive rationale to believe that in more severe cases of GBS, treatment is superior to supportive care alone.

Independent of the severity of the acute clinical course of the disease, the long-term prognosis for children with GBS is generally excellent. In their descriptive series, Korinthenberg and Monting found that after six months the majority of children had recovered from their GBS completely or had only mild residua, which did not preclude return to previously undertaken activities of life. These findings are consonant with most other reports describing the outcome of childhood GBS in industrialized nations.

Chronic Inflammatory Demyelinating Neuropathy

Chronic inflammatory demyelinating neuropathy (CIDP) is the great pretender in pediatric neuromuscular clinics. The disorder is reasonably easily identified when it presents acutely, mimicking GBS followed by sequential relapses, or when the symptoms evolve subacutely in a previously well child. In some cases, however, the onset is indolent with slow progression. In this setting CIDP can mimic virtually any inherited neuropathy and should always be kept in mind in a child when no other evidence of neuropathy can be confirmed in the kinship. Because many of the inherited neuropathies are transmitted in a dominant mode, careful family history, and when practical, examination of available family members, may establish a presumptive genetic cause for the disorder. On occasion, electrodiagnostic testing will distinguish hereditary from acquired neuropathies; however, asymmetrical slowing of nerve conduction velocities, conduction block and other features suggestive of an acquired demyelinating neuropathy may not be evident. On occasion, these two entities, HMSN and CIDP, overlap. DNA analysis for common mutations associated with hereditary neuropathies may confirm the diagnosis; however, in the best of hands, it appears that a specific mutation cannot be identified in roughly 25%-30% of cases. In the absence of a detectible mutation, however, it may be necessary to perform a nerve biopsy or undertake a trial of an immunosuppression in order to sort out the question of autoimmune versus inherited disease.

Several immunosuppressant agents have been shown to be effective in the treatment of CIDP. The choice of an optimal treatment in this disorder is personal and idiosyncratic. Corticosteroids are often a first line therapy because they are relatively inexpensive and because the majority of children with CIDP initially respond well to this treatment. If there is an inadequate response or if cumulative side effects occur because of an ongoing high dosage requirement, additional steroid sparing strategies can be employed. Plasmapheresis, IVIg, cyclosporine, azathioprine and cyclophosphamide all have been used with variable success.

5. Disorders of the Neuromuscular Junction

Neonatal Myasthenia Gravis

Neonatal myasthenia gravis may result in transient weakness in the newborn. This syndrome occurs in infants of mothers with active autoimmune myasthenia and, most commonly, will be manifest at birth or within the first days of life. Some infants are born with arthrogryposis multiplex congenita, as a rule in untreated, often minimally affected women with autoimmune myasthenia. Maternal IgG directed against epitopes associated with the postsynaptic acetylcholine receptor is passively transferred across the placenta during late gestation, resulting in receptor blockade with concomitant transient bulbar and somatic weakness. Alternatively, in a poorly controlled myasthenic mother who produces antibodies which cross-react with the fetal AChR, transplacental diffusion of the IgG may result in diminished fetal movement resulting in arthrogryposis. As AChRs mature in these affected fetuses, they are no longer primarily targeted by the antibody, and at birth the infants are minimally weak but movement is restricted by multiple joint contractures.

Congenital Myasthenic Syndromes

Congenital myasthenic syndromes may present in the newborn period or at a later age. Arthrogryposis can be an initial manifestation in these disorders as well as those related to maternal autoimmune MG described above. This finding has been a prominent feature in congenital myasthenia associated with mutations in the rapsyn gene (receptor-associated protein at the synapse). These are typically inherited disorders with either autosomal dominant or recessive modes of transmission. Mutations in genes encoding components of the neuromuscular junction result in defective neuromuscular transmission with variable manifestations ranging from diminished endurance to respiratory failure. The electrochemical defect can be presynaptic, postsynaptic, or at the end plate itself; therefore, symptoms may not respond to anticholinesterase medications. A primary acetylcholine receptor deficiency accounts for most of the nonautoimmune congenital myasthenic syndromes. A striking congenital myasthenic syndrome is caused by a recessively inherited defect in the enzyme choline acetyltransferase, resulting in diminished presynaptic acetylcholine availability.

This disease presents with abrupt onset of bulbar weakness in infancy with acute episodes of apnea (Table 3).

Myasthenia Gravis

Myasthenia gravis, an autoimmune disorder, is characterized by a deficiency of acetylcholine receptors on postsynaptic nerve terminals at neuromuscular junctions. The most common expression of myasthenia gravis (MG) in children is ptosis with variable involvement of other muscles. Conventionally, MG has been said to comprise three clinical syndromes: ocular, bulbar, and generalized myasthenia. Pure ocular MG accounts for about 15%-25% of autoimmune myasthenia in children, depending on the age group and ethnic background. It is often the herald symptom, antedating the appearance of weakness in other muscle groups. Among those children who present with symptoms of ocular MG, roughly 75% will progress to involve bulbar muscles or develop generalized MG. Ptosis with variable degrees of external ophthalmoparesis can develop at any age and evolve to include nearly any combination of striate muscles. Most children who present with ocular symptoms which later generalize do so within the first year. The symptoms typically wax and wane over time and may be exacerbated by intercurrent infection which upregulates activity of the immune system. There is also, typically, fluctuation in the severity of symptoms in proportion to the degree of exertion; hence, the frequently heard complaint that ptosis and other weakness increases during the course of the day. Myasthenia gravis may take a heavy toll on the patient's psychological well being, especially in older age groups. This is because of the marked fluctuations in strength and function in some myasthenic patients. The patient may exhibit normal, or nearly so, functional abilities at one point and within a short period of time become progressively weaker to the point of requiring mechanical ventilatory support.

As stated above, MG is an immune mediated disorder with a predominantly IgG class of antibodies directed toward various epitopes of the post-synaptic acetylcholine receptor (AChR). These antibodies are detectable in 50%-75% of children with generalized MG (seropositive), and cannot be identified in the balance of (seronegative) children with MG. Although the pathogenesis of the disease is thought to be mediated predominantly via anti-AChR antibodies, there is evidence that suggest cellular immune mechanisms also play a role in orchestrating the elimination of postsynaptic receptors. Roughly 25%-50% of younger children will be found to be seronegative. It is difficult to quantitate precisely, but a proportion of these seronegative patients, influenced again by age and ethnic background, have pathogenic autoantibodies to muscle specific tyrosine kinase (MuSK). MuSK is localized on the sarcolemmal surface of the neuromuscular junction. This kinase participates in the agrin-induced clustering of AChRs on the postsynaptic nerve terminal during the ontogenesis of the neuromuscular junction. The role this molecule plays in the mature neuromuscular junction is not precisely understood. It is thought, however, that immune mediated reduction in MuSK results in diminished numbers or inappropriate distribution of AChRs at the post-synaptic nerve terminal. Anti-AChR antibodies and anti-MuSK antibodies appear to be mutually exclusive in that these two antibody species do not coexist in individual patients with myasthenia. The autoimmune mediated attack directed at epitopes from either of these entities results in weakness of variable severity and distribution; however, patients with anti-MuSK mediated MG tend to have greater bulbar involvement and a more treatment resistant course. Myasthenia may occur in concert with other autoimmune processes such as thyroiditis, or lupus. The diagnosis of juvenile myasthenia gravis is based on the clinical history and examination. Other diagnostic modalities in addition to testing for pathogenic antibodies

Table 3

Myasthenic Syndromes in Children

Transient intrauterine paralysis with arthrogryposis
Transient neonatal myasthenia
Congenital myasthenic syndromes
Familial infantile myasthenia with acute apnea
Acquired autoimmune myasthenia gravis

include an edrophonium challenge or electrodiagnostic testing to confirm a post-synaptic defect in neuromuscular transmission. In children with prominent ptosis, a useful bedside maneuver is the application of an ice pack over the ptotic eye for several minutes, which may induce remarkable, transient improvement highly suggestive of myasthenia gravis.

The goal of therapy in myasthenia gravis is to enhance the efficiency of neuromuscular transmission at the synaptic junction. This can be accomplished by increasing the availability of acetylcholine to post-synaptic receptors or by augmenting the sensitivity of the junctional end plate. Acetylcholinesterase inhibitors, pyridostigmine and neostigmine, have been used to ameliorate the symptoms of myasthenia by preventing catabolism of acetylcholine within the synaptic cleft and altering the kinetics of ion channel behavior on the post-synaptic membrane. The therapeutic effect of this category of drug can be highly variable among patients. In general, symptoms of mild-to-moderate severity may respond to anticholinesterase treatment. In the face of impending respiratory failure, it is often wise to discontinue these drugs until the patient can be stabilized with more aggressive management strategies such as plasmapheresis or IVIg administration.

The first-line treatment for myasthenia gravis has classically been pyridostigmine, initially at a dose of 1 mg/kg every four to six hours. This drug alone is often adequate for symptoms of ptosis, but when the disease affects bulbar and somatic muscles, immunosuppression is warranted. Corticosteroids followed by IVIg and plasmapheresis are the initial front line therapies, often in combination. The effect of each of these therapies is mediated by their ability to diminish the level of circulating antibodies directed against postsynaptic AChRs. Chronic daily immunosuppression may require intermittent augmentation with plasmapheresis or IVIg. If these approaches are ineffective, or are complicated by unacceptable side effects, alternate immunosuppressants such as cyclosporine or mycophenylate may prove to be useful. My own bias is to reserve azathioprine and cyclophosphamide for children who are refractory to the aforementioned regimens. Because of the association of myasthenia gravis with thymoma, almost every patient undergoes a CT or MRI examination of the mediastinum to exclude underlying malignancy. Thymic hyperplasia is common; however, a thymoma is almost never uncovered.

Thymectomy can be a useful treatment strategy. One study indicated that the efficacy is time sensitive and is more likely to induce remission if performed within one year of the onset of symptoms. It is most effective for bulbar and generalized myasthenia. It is difficult to imagine undertaking such invasive therapy for isolated ocular myasthenia. In children with bulbar or generalized myasthenia it is reasonable to treat with anticholinesterase medications and immunosuppressants for one year in hope of a spontaneous remission. When the disorder persists beyond that time frame or the child develops an episode of respiratory failure, thymectomy is warranted. Because of the varied clinical course in juvenile myasthenia, it is difficult to distinguish a thymectomy-induced versus spontaneous remission in an individual child.

Infant Botulism

The clinical manifestations of infant botulism are quite stereotypical and consist of constipation, external ophthalmoparesis and feeding difficulties. Generalized weakness and hypo- to areflexia evolve thereafter. The disease results when botulinum spores are ingested, germinate in the GI tract, and slowly elaborate botulinum toxin, which is absorbed and disseminated through systemic circulation, ultimately interrupting neuromuscular transmission. The toxin binds at a presynaptic site on the neuronal membrane. Circulating and externally bound toxin are accessible to antibody directed against epitopes of the toxin. The toxin then traverses the neurolemma, probably by endocytotic mechanisms, and enters the cytoplasm where it binds to acetylcholine release sites and prevents release of acetylcholine vesicles into the synaptic cleft. Once the toxin is internalized, it is inaccessible to circulating antibody and irreversibly blocks acetylcholine release. The course of the disorder typically progresses over a relatively short period after initial presentation. Many of these patients will require mechanical ventilatory support. Autonomic dysfunction may accompany weakness, especially in the more severely affected infants.

The disease can be caused by several *Clostridia botulinum* species, types A through G, which are subclassified based on the characteristics of the elaborated toxin. The vast majority of cases of infant botulism are caused by types A and B. The spores of *C botulinum* are ubiquitously distributed and typically present in soil. The often described exposure to honey is overemphasized, and colonization from honey-containing spores accounts for a minute fraction of cases. *Clostridium botulinum* types A and B have a geographically distinct distribution, with type A predominantly found in states from the Rocky Mountains and west, while type B is located in regions east of the mountain range. Diagnosis of the disease is suspected based on typical clinical findings. The diagnosis may be confirmed based on the electrophysiological characteristics from nerve conduction studies and EMG. The nature and presynaptic localization of neuromuscular blockade in these infants results in a reproducible constellation of findings. Sensory nerve conduction studies are normal, while motor nerve conduction velocities are normal, usually with diminished compound motor action potential amplitude (CMAP). The hallmark features of electrodiagnostic testing are the presence of a decremental response in the CMAP amplitude with low frequency repetitive motor nerve stimulation (2-3 Hz) and a marked increment with higher rates of stimulation (10-50 Hz). EMG reveals mixed features including widespread fibrillation potentials due to chemical denervation of myofibers along with abundant small amplitude, short duration, myopathic appearing motor unit potentials also called brief, short duration action potentials (BSAPs) because of fragmentation of motor units. This latter finding is related to the electrochemical inexcitability of myofibers scattered within the motor unit, resulting in motor unit potentials with reduced amplitude and a polyphasic morphology.

Despite the severity of the clinical syndrome, with adequate supportive care the vast majority of these infants recover fully. The mechanism of recovery from the disease is probably multifactorial. The first step is likely recognition of the toxin by the immune system and elaboration of an antibody response to the toxin. During, and in some cases, after recovery, toxin can still be recovered from the gastrointestinal tract. If there is sufficient binding and internalization of toxin at a particular neuromuscular junction, transmission at that junction is permanently blocked with subsequent degeneration of that nerve terminal. Neuromuscular transmission to that myofiber is reestablished by sprouting of a new axon from the distal nerve fiber and the generation of a new neuromuscular junction.

Treatment of infant botulism is largely supportive. Attention to maintaining respiratory function is critical and physical therapy should be involved early in the course of illness. In addition to supportive treatment, it is also important to avoid agents which can further compromise function at the neuromuscular junction, such as aminoglycosides. In some infants, a relatively small decrement in the efficiency of neuromuscular transmission may have profound functional consequences resulting in respiratory failure. Because feeding difficulties are a nearly ubiquitous feature early in the illness, many infants present with protein-calorie deprivation. Ensuring adequate nutrition, therefore, is critical. Barring unforeseen complications, the prognosis is excellent with a complete, albeit sometimes prolonged recovery. The pace of recuperation can be enhanced by administration of an antibody directed toward botulinum toxin, which has recently become commercially available.

6. Disorders of Muscle

Congenital Muscle Disease

Within the broad spectrum of muscle diseases presenting in infancy, the first branch point in the diagnostic pathway is making a distinction between disorders classified as congenital myopathy or congenital muscular dystrophy. The primary characteristics utilized to distinguish congenital myopathies and congenital muscular dystrophies (CMD) are the presence of myofibrillar necrosis and regeneration, along with endomysial fibrosis and deposition of fat on histopathological examination of muscle biopsy. These features are usually associated with dystrophic disorders. In addition to weakness and hyporeflexia (usually areflexia), these children may have elevated CPK measurements of several times the upper limit of normal.

As a generality, the disorders conforming to a diagnosis of congenital muscular dystrophy carry a less favorable prognosis than congenital myopathy. That having been said, there is considerable variability in the course of these entities, with the consequence that categorical identification provides suboptimal prognostic information to pass along to the parents of these children. Further subclassification of these disorders, based primarily on family history or the histopathological findings in a biopsy specimen, permits design of a rational schema to pursue more specific diagnosis via DNA analysis.

Congenital Myopathies

Congenital myotonic dystrophy (MD) is probably the single most common neuromuscular disorder presenting at birth. Children with congenital myotonic dystrophy are almost exclusively born to mothers with myotonic dystrophy. Because of the marked variability in genotype and phenotype in successive generations, the mother may be unaware of her disorder and her diagnosis may be the byproduct of investigating the cause for weakness in her infant. As is obvious from the above, myotonic dystrophy is a dominantly inherited disorder in which about half of infants of mothers with MD are symptomatic at birth, with gradual improvement in the severity of weakness with maturation. The genetic substrate for the disease is an expansion of a CTG repeat sequence within the 3' untranslated portion of the DM protein kinase gene (DMPK) on chromosome 19. In normal individuals the CTG repeat may range from 5-37 repeats. Individuals affected with MD show greater than 50 repeats. In infants with congenital myotonic dystrophy, the number of CTG repeats may reach up to 2000. The greater the number of repeats, the earlier and more severe the clinical presentation. The CTG sequence is unstable, and with succeeding generations may undergo progressive expansion, providing the molecular explanation for the clinical phenomenon of genetic anticipation in this disorder. Roughly half the progeny of mothers affected with myotonic dystrophy will consequently have a markedly larger repeat sequence than their mother, with an earlier presentation and more severe disease. The majority of patients with myotonic dystrophy associated with a lesser number of repeats present later in life. This variety is discussed in the chapter dealing with neuromuscular disorders in adults.

Other congenital myopathies may present with a similar clinical picture. There are a host of myopathic disorders presenting in infancy, some of which have specific and unique gene defects, while others are genetically heterogeneous. Traditionally, congenital myopathies are classified on the basis of abnormalities of myofibrillar structure on histochemical studies and on electron microscopy. Some congenital myopathies are identified based on abnormal inclusions such as nemaline or rod-body myopathy (Figure 2, color plates), or fingerprint body myopathy, while others have myofibrillar abnormalities like central core disease or mini-core disease. Myotubular myopathy, also known as centronuclear myopathy, is characterized by myofibers which are similar to developing muscle in early gestation in which myofibers have a tubular appearance with centrally located nuclei (Figure 3, color plates).

The prognosis in these disorders is highly variable as there are, in many cases, multiple genotypes with similar phenotypical expressions. Many severely affected children at birth—even those requiring mechanical ventilatory support—may improve over time and survive into adulthood.

Table 4

Examples of Congenital Myopathies with Characteristic Histopathology

Centronuclear myopathy
Nemaline myopathy
Tubular aggregate disease
Fingerprint myopathy
Central core disease
Multi-Minicore disease
Myofibrillar myopathy
Congenital fiber type disproportion

Congenital Muscular Dystrophy

Most of these disorders are inherited in an autosomal recessive fashion. The initial step in classifying these diseases is based on the presence or absence of merosin (alpha-2 chain of laminin 2) on immunocytochemical studies of muscle biopsies or in Western blots. Absence of the protein can be a primary or secondary phenomenon. Congenital muscular dystrophies, therefore, are described as those that are merosin-deficient or are merosin-positive. The proportions of these disorders varies among different ethnic groups, but worldwide, each accounts for about half of CMDs. Cognitive development is normal in most cases of CMD, although some are associated with central nervous system abnormalities including structural abnormalities on MRI and mental retardation. In Japan, the Fukayama type of CMD is the most common form. This disorder is inherited in a recessive mode with a defect in the gene which codes for the protein fukutin. Diminished expression of laminin 2 or β-dystroglycan, which is often abnormal in Fukayama type dystrophy, is thought to be a secondary phenomenon in this disorder. There is typically moderate-to-severe mental retardation with variable structural brain abnormalities including pachygyria/microgyria, and high signal intensity changes in white matter on T2 MRI sequences. Other examples of congenital muscular dystrophy associated with central nervous system and other somatic abnormalities include Walker-Warburg syndrome and muscle-eye-brain disease.

Duchenne/Becker Muscular Dystrophy

These muscular dystrophies are the most frequently encountered entities in the two- to 10-year-old age group. Duchenne muscular dystrophy is also the most clinically stereotypical among neuromuscular diseases affecting males of this age. The Duchenne variety generally presents early in the first decade of life, while the Becker phenotype may not become clinically evident until late adolescence. These boys typically exhibit proximal weakness with variable segmental muscle pseudohypertrophy or atrophy. Most will have an identifiable mutation in the dystrophin gene. Dystrophin itself is a cytoskeletal protein which, among others, is critical in stabilizing the link between the intracellular contractile apparatus, the sarcolemmal membrane, and the extracellular matrix. In the absence of the protein, the sarcolemmal membrane is fragile and susceptible to fenestration during myofibrillar contraction and relaxation. Defects in the sarcolemma result in permeability to extracellular ions and subsequent accumulation of intracellular calcium, which initiates several pathways, ultimately resulting in cell death.

In Duchenne muscular dystrophy a clinical diagnosis is usually not difficult. Several laboratory studies can reinforce the diagnostic impression. A markedly elevated level of creatine phosphokinase (CPK) in serum is often on the order of 15- to 25,000 units in boys between two and five years of age. Electrodiagnostic testing is usually unnecessary and, if performed, is often nonspecific. DNA analysis from peripheral blood samples can be diagnostic with a deletion at Xp21, which can be demonstrated in about two-thirds of these boys with traditional DNA screening. In the absence of an identifiable deletion, full length screening of the coding sequences of the dystrophin gene is now available and will define a mutation in an additional segment of the boys in whom there is no detectable deletion. A small but significant group of boys with presumed dystrophin mutations are not identified by DNA analyses and will require muscle biopsy for confirmation of the diagnosis. When there is no family history to suggest the likely rate of progression of the disease, a muscle sample for immunocytochemical staining or Western blot analysis of the dystrophin protein will distinguish between the Duchenne and Becker variants.

In the current environment, the therapeutic arsenal for Duchenne/Becker muscular dystrophy is limited to corticosteroids. Both prednisone and deflazacort have undergone blinded, controlled trials and have been shown to be superior to no treatment. It is clear from the experience using immunosuppression during the period that myoblast transplantation garnered such enthusiasm that other immunosuppressants also may enhance strength in these affected boys. Absent the need for immunosuppression for the purpose of tissue transplantation, the side effect profile does not justify employing more toxic immuno-modulating agents for amelioration of weakness in these boys. There is experimental evidence from a murine model of DMD that when the pathogenic mutation is a stop codon, aminoglycoside administration may allow bypassing the stop codon with dystrophin assembly in a fraction of myofibers. Studies in humans, however, have yielded disappointing results. Based on recent studies, also in mice, stem cell therapy appears to have the greatest potential to restore dystrophin expression in muscles of boys with DMD. Recently, interest has focused on the protein myostatin, which is a constituent of a regulatory pathway which limits muscle growth. Decreasing the availability of this protein either in animal knockout models, or by administration of immunoglobulin directed against the protein itself, results in enhanced muscle size and strength. One attractive aspect of this possible therapeutic intervention is its nonspecificity and potential applicability to neuromuscular disorders of diverse etiology.

As noted above, a serum CPK which is elevated 50- to 100-fold is nearly pathognomic for dystrophinopathy in this age group although other defects in cytoskeletal proteins can mimic dystrophin deficient muscular dystrophy. A relatively recently described group of such dystrophies are related to mutations in genes encoding the sarcoglycan family of cytoskeletal proteins. These disorders have been nosologically grouped under the acronym SCARMD, or severe childhood autosomal recessive muscular dystrophy. Other muscular dystrophies may also have similar clinical characteristics and fall under the rubric of limb-girdle dystrophies. With the exception of Emery-Dreifuss dystrophy, most are inherited in an autosomal fashion and therefore may affect either sex.

In our contemporaneous state of available therapeutic interventions for muscular dystrophy—and here I want to focus on the Duchenne/Becker varieties—the disease complications, which are almost ubiquitously encountered, appear in this order: joint contractures; progressive weakness with loss of ambulation; scoliosis; respiratory compromise and cardiomyopathy. Muscle, and consequently, joint contractures are inevitable; however, the timing of onset and pace of progression of the processes are highly variable from patient to patient. Achilles tightening results from the toe walking gait pattern, which occurs due to proximal hip-girdle weakness and is among the first of the contractures to emerge. Early incorporation of physical therapy and a daily stretching regimen are useful in, at least, slowing this process. If in spite of aggressive physical therapy, loss of range of motion occurs, and institution of nocturnal orthotics may prove helpful. Instituting orthotics for ambulation is rarely necessary and usually not helpful.

Debate continues—although it seems to be abating—regarding the role of surgery and bracing to maintain ambulation. As a rule, physical therapy can forestall early contractures, and by the time Achilles contractures become the rate, limiting step in interfering with ambulation, the child is wheelchair dependent or confined. Among wheelchair-confined boys, Achilles lengthening and bracing may become necessary to preserve physiological positioning of the feet in the chair. Some neuromuscular clinics advocate using long-leg (foot-ankle-knee-hip) bracing to maintain ambulation in end-stage walkers. The motivation for this strategy is understandable from the psychological perspective; however, it is not the most reliable way to achieve safe, independent mobility. This goal is best realized with a motorized wheelchair. Although there are logistical difficulties associated with these devices, at a time in life when developing increasing social, psychological and physical independence are important developmental processes, a motorized chair allows the child the greatest opportunity to achieve a more independent lifestyle. In a similar vein, late ambulatory children with muscular dystrophy and typical hip-girdle weakness generally fall because of knee joint collapse on foot strike due to quadriceps weakness. When that happens, the initial point of impact with the ground is usually the buttocks. When a child in long-leg braces falls, the initial impact is more often the outstretched arm and torso or the head.

After a period of wheelchair dependency, some boys with DMD will begin to develop scoliosis. The evolution of the curvature deformity can sometimes be slowed with chair positioning, lateral supports, or thoracic braces. It is not clear what factor or factors influence which boys will develop scoliosis and potentially go on to require surgery. Mitigating tactics can be employed early in the course, but once the curve exceeds approximately 35 degrees, progression is almost inevitable. Having reached this juncture, surgical intervention should be considered sooner rather than later.

Pulmonary function studies provide a reliable measurement of respiratory muscle strength and, in some cases, permit prediction of when enhanced vigilance for respiratory complications is necessary. The rationale for obtaining serial pulmonary function studies at some point after the child becomes wheelchair confined is to document the stage of the disease and later to begin to explore and discuss the patient's feelings regarding respiratory support at an appropriate time before such interventions are imminent. Conventionally, it is taught that when the forced vital capacity reaches a value of 25% predicted, there is increased risk of pneumonia. At a level of approximately 15%, nocturnal respiratory insufficiency becomes a tangible concern, frequently manifested as excessive daytime drowsiness. The role for mechanical ventilation in the management of the illness at this stage is individually determined. The question generally must be addressed around the end of the second decade, a time when the patient is capable of playing an essential role in the decision-making process. Whether a patient elects mechanical respiratory support is less dependent on medical issues than individual beliefs, social mores and personal experience. The opportunity to interact with and know other patients using assistive technology often proves to be the most informative and useful in confronting this quality of life decision.

Cardiomyopathy is invariably present in older patients with DMD, fortunately it is infrequently of clinical significance. Because of minimal physical activity, the demand on cardiac output in a wheelchair-confined patient is also limited and usually met even with myocardial disease. Rarely, the progression of cardiomyopathy exceeds the pace of respiratory muscle weakening and may be fatal before frank respiratory failure. Female heterozygotes may rarely develop relatively isolated cardiomyopathy. It is sincerely hoped that the need to consider the aforementioned series of complications from dystrophin deficiency disease will be obviated by effective treatment.

Inflammatory Myopathy

Inflammatory myopathies are relatively rare in childhood. They occur, most commonly, in preadolescent and adolescent age groups. These disorders are conventionally divided into three broad categories: infectious myositis, autoimmune polymyositis, and dermatomyositis. There are a host of viruses with myotrophic properties which can produce focal or generalized muscle inflammation and injury. A not unusual scenario is a child in the mid-first decade of life who, rather acutely, complains of calf pain and is reluctant or unable to walk. In general there will be tenderness to palpation in affected muscles. Serum CPK and muscle transaminases may be elevated. These symptoms usually resolve over several days and further evaluation is rarely necessary. In addition to viral infections, a host of other agents can infect muscle and produce clinical disease. Causative organisms for infectious myositis include a range of bacteria and parasites. In the past, *Trichinella spiralis* was the most common myotrophic parasite and was often asymptomatic. The incidence of trichinosis has dramatically fallen in North America and Europe since the mid-twentieth century.

Autoimmune inflammatory myopathies, for the most part, fall into the category of polymyositis or dermatomyositis. There are rare myopathies associated with other connective tissue disorders, systemic vasculitities or paraneoplastic syndromes. These will not be addressed in this chapter. Although many authors have written that polymyositis is exceedingly rare in childhood, this has not been my experience. Many children present with complaints of fatigue or weakness with or without muscle swelling or tenderness and absent cutaneous abnormalities. Electrodiagnostic testing will confirm a myopathic disorder, frequently without "irritable" features typically associated with muscle inflammation. The serum CPK level may be mildly or massively elevated with variable elevations in the erythrocyte sedimentation rate and other satellite markers for inflammation or other autoimmune disorders. Magnetic resonance imaging of muscle may demonstrate multifocal areas of increased signal intensity on T2 spin echo sequences. The findings on MRI may provide some guidance for choosing a biopsy site. Muscle biopsy may be normal because of the multifocal nature of inflammation. When an active area of inflammation is sampled, typical features include myofibrillar degeneration and regeneration with primary endomysial inflammation, and occasionally perivascular collections of inflammatory cells, without evidence of vasonecrosis.

Dermatomyositis is one of the few disorders in clinical neurology where the nosology accurately reflects the pathology of the disease. Children with this disease may present with muscle pain and weakness or with a painful rash as their primary complaint. The classic syndrome features a malar rash, Gottron papules over extensor surfaces of the fingers, elbows and knees, and subungual flame hemorrhages. As in polymyositis, there may be serological evidence of muscle injury and systemic inflammation. Testing in the electrophysiology laboratory may be similar to polymyositis as well, and muscle MRI may demonstrate evidence of multifocal myoedema. Dermatomyositis is a vasculitic myopathy, so that in addition to the biopsy features seen in polymyositis, these are evidence of frank vasonecrosis indicative of active vasculitis. A hallmark histopathological feature of dermatomyositis is perifascicular myofibrillar atrophy. This is due to the distribution of endomysial blood flow with areas of ischemia most commonly affecting the periphery of the fascicle.

Unlike the situation in adults, where dermatomyositis is commonly a paraneoplastic disease often associated with small cell carcinoma of the lung, neoplasia is almost never a feature of the disease in children. Therapy in both disorders consists of immunosuppression. Again, corticosteroids are probably the first-line therapeutic agents. IVIg and methotrexate are also quite helpful when chronic steroid side effects become unacceptable.

Metabolic Myopathies

Metabolic myopathies account for a small fraction of muscle disease in childhood. The majority fall into three broad categories: glycogen storage disorders, defects in fatty acid oxidation, and mitochondrial cytopathies. It is well recognized that these metabolic disturbances often affect other organ systems and weakness may not be the dominant symptom which brings a child to attention. Some of the more common diagnoses encountered are listed in Table 5.

Glycogen Storage Diseases

A common clinical theme with many of the glycogenoses is the presence of exercise intolerance and muscle cramps; however, some are also associated with progressive weakness. Many of the disorders which present in this fashion may also be associated with episodic myoglobinuria. Four of the more well-recognized glycogen storage disorders are myophosphorylase deficiency (glycogenosis Type V or McArdle disease); phosfructokinase deficiency (glycogenosis Type VII or Tauri disease); alpha-glycosidase deficiency (glycogenosis Type II or Pompe disease); and debrancher

Table 5

Metabolic Myopathies

Myophosphorylase deficiency
Pompe disease
Phosfructokinase deficiency
Debrancher deficiency
Phosphoglycerokinase deficiency
alpha-Glucosidase deficiency
Methylglutaconic aciduria
Acyl co-A-dehydrogenase deficiency (multiple variants)
Mitochondrial disorders

enzyme deficiency (glycogenosis Type III or Forbes disease). The first two of these disorders may share the initial manifestations of exercise intolerance and muscle cramps. Either disease can present at almost any age; however, they are more likely to present in mid-childhood or later at a time when strenuous physical exertion is more likely to occur. Prolonged exercise may result in rhabdomyolysis and pigmenturia. In severe cases this can cause transient or permanent renal failure. The initial appearance of symptoms in older children or adults is more common in alpha-glucosidase deficiency and debrancher deficiency but both may cause hypotonia and weakness in infancy. These later disorders are not typically associated with episodes of rhabdomyolysis. In addition to involvement of striate muscle, both of these diseases typically involve other organ systems.

Disorders of Fatty Acid Metabolism

Carnitine palmitoyltransferase II (CPT II) deficiency is arguably the most often identified disorder of fatty acid oxidation. Like many enzyme deficiency diseases, it is genetically determined and has an autosomal recessive mode of inheritance. The salient clinical feature of the disorder is recurrent rhabdomyolysis. Unlike the glycogenoses, there is usually no exercise intolerance in CPT II deficiency. Affected individuals will generally not experience muscle pain or cramping during vigorous exertion. Rather, after an episode of prolonged exercise, they will develop muscle pain followed by pigmenturia. Often, similar bouts will occur spontaneously or in association with intercurrent infection. Between bouts of rhabdomyolysis, these individuals appear normal and very rarely develop weakness. The most important risk from CPT II deficiency is renal failure induced by myoglobinuria. For unclear reasons, the frequency and severity of episodes of rhabdomyolysis seem to improve with maturation.

Another well recognized category of fatty oxidation disorders are the various species of acyl-CoA dehydrogenase or deficiency, or CAD. The acyl-CoA dehydrogenases participate in the process of mitochondrial B-oxidation and are specific for the length of the associated fatty acid, short chain (4 carbon), medium chain (8 carbon), and long chain (up to 18 carbon) acyl-CoA dehydrogenase. Again, at the risk of oversimplification, children with these disorders most commonly present with an acute encephalopathy, nonketotic hypoglycemia and features suggestive of Reye syndrome. These episodes may be associated with rhabdomyolysis; however, this is usually a less dramatic feature of the diseases. The episodes are often precipitated by prolonged fasting. This often occurs in the setting of intercurrent infection. Over time, slowly progressive weakness may evolve, particularly in SCAD and LCAD. There are many other enzymatic defects which result in impaired fatty acid oxidation and are beyond the scope of this discussion.

Mitochondrial Disease

Disorders of oxidative phosphorylation or mitochondrial cytopathies are a group of disorders which are diverse in molecular etiology and protean in clinical manifestations. The prototypical mitochondrial disorder is the Kearns-Sayre syndrome. The clinical characteristics of this disease include: short stature, external ophthalmoparesis, myopathy, pigmentary retinopathy, and cardiac conduction defects. When followed over the long term, the majority of these patients will develop cardiomyopathy, progressive encephalopathy and blindness. Like many of the classic, phenotypically characterized, mitochondrial disorders such as MERRF (myopathy encephalopathy and ragged red fibers), MELAS (myopathy encephalopathy lactic acidosis and stroke-like episodes), or Leigh syndrome, Kearns-Sayre syndrome is inherited via the maternal transmission of the defective mitochondrial gene. As our understanding of these disorders matures, the role of mutations in nuclear DNA resulting in abnormalities in oxidative phosphorylation has become increasingly evident. In addition to the clinical features enumerated above, mitochondrial cytopathies almost always ultimately demonstrate multi-organ involvement which may include ataxia, deafness, anemia, liver or kidney failure, gastrointestinal hypomotility, autonomic failure and peripheral neuropathy.

There may be considerable variability in the severity of the expression of homologous gene defects in members of the same kinship which is thought to be attributable to at least two independent factors. The first is determined by the basal metabolic requirements of particular cell and tissue types. Those organ systems with the highest energy substrate requirements are likely to be preferentially susceptible to injury due to defective energy production. Inheritance of mitochondrial DNA occurs through the maternal lineage in which the gene may be heterogeneous for mutations, with each cell containing both mutated and normal mitochondrial DNA. Consequently, during the earliest phases of embryonal development, populations of primordial stem cells contain different ratios of abnormal-to-normal mitochondria. This heterogeneous group of embryonic cells is segregated into progenitor cell lines, which develop into tissues with variable burdens of dysfunctional mitochondria. These factors result in a mismatch between the level of basal energy substrate requirements in a particular tissue and the ability of that tissue to generate the required amount of energy. Hence, there are different thresholds for energy failure among different organ systems within individual patients.

The symptoms of early fatiguability, myalgias and episodic rhabdomyolysis are shared by all three categories of metabolic defects described above, along with other entities which may not be associated with known metabolic defects. Measurement of serum lactate, pyruvate and quantitative amino acids, along with determination of quantitative organic acid concentrations in urine, are effective screening tools for many of these disorders. Analysis of acylcarnitine profiles with double mass spectroscopy or screening for specific gene defects is indicated if clinical suspicion suggests the possibility of one of the family of acyl-CoA dehydrogenase defects. Skin biopsy and isolation of cultured fibroblasts may be required to confirm defects of lipid metabolism. In selected patients with suspected defects in oxidative phosphorylation, fresh muscle tissue may be necessary for enzyme determination, oxidative phosphorylation measurements, mitochondrial DNA analysis, and morphological studies. When enzymatic studies are not diagnostic, the presence of ragged red fibers on routine histochemical examination of biopsy material (Figure 4, color plates), or the presence of typical mitochondrial inclusions with electron-microscopy (Figure 5), provide strong circumstantial evidence for a disorder of oxidative phosphorylation.

Figure 5

Mitochondrial myopathy

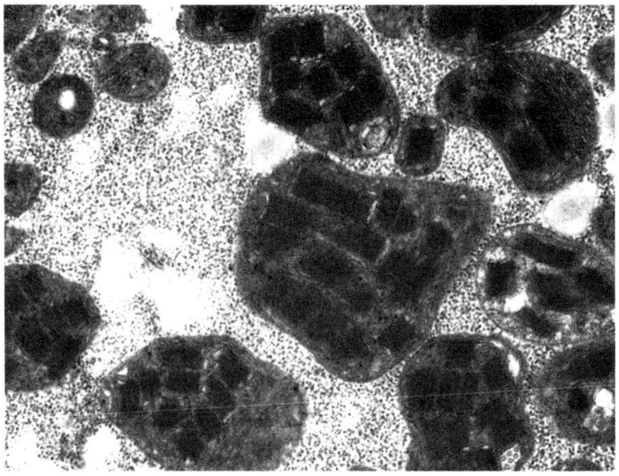

This electronmicrograph illustrates a region proliferation of dystrophic mitochondria. There are prominent intra-mitochondrial inclusions. Multiple types of inclusions may be present. The inclusions presented here are classic paracrystalline arrays.

7. References

1. Afifi AK, Bell WE. Tests for juvenile myasthenia gravis: comparative diagnostic yield and prediction of outcome. *J Child Neurol*. 1993;8 (4):403-11.

   (Guidelines to assist in diagnostic evaluation.)

2. Andrews PI. A treatment algorithm for autoimmune myasthenia gravis in childhood. *Ann NY Acad Sci*. 1998;841:789-802.

   (Useful management strategy for this disorder.)

3. Andrews PI, Massey JM, Sanders DB. Acetylcholine receptor antibodies in juvenile myasthenia gravis. *Neurology*. 1993;43(5):977-82.

   (Provides estimates of the utility of immune diagnostic markers.)

4. Arnon SS. Infant botulism. *Ann Rev Med*. 1980;31:541-60.

   (Dated, but it remains one of the best overviews of this disorder.)

5. Asbury AK, Cornblath DR. Assessment of current diagnostic criteria for Guillain-Barré syndrome. *Ann Neurol*. 1990;27 Suppl:S21-4.

   (This remains the gold standard in terms of diagnostic features in GBS.)

6. Bird TD, Ott J, Giblett ER et al. Genetic linkage evidence for heterogeneity in Charcot-Marie-Tooth neuropathy (HMSN type I). *Ann Neurol*. 1983;14(6):679-84.

   (The first evidence for genotypic heterogeneity in HMSN type I.)

7. Boerkoel CF, Takashima H, Garcia CA et al. Charcot-Marie-Tooth disease and related neuropathies: mutation distribution and genotype-phenotype correlation. *Ann Neurol*. 2002;51 (2):190-201.

   (Another communication which was quickly out of date. However, it provides an excellent conceptual framework on which to add new genotype/phenotype information.)

8. Burke G, Cossins J, Maxwell S et al. Rapsyn mutations in hereditary myasthenia: distinct early- and late-onset phenotypes. *Neurology*. 2003;61(6):826-8.

   (Example of functional consequences of mutations in this protein.)

9. Charnas L, Trapp B, Griffin J. Congenital absence of peripheral myelin: abnormal Schwann cell development causes lethal arthrogryposis multiplex congenita. *Neurology*. 1988;38(6):966-74.

   (Informative monograph on histopathological features in CHN.)

10. Connolly AM. Chronic inflammatory demyelinating polyneuropathy in childhood. *Pediatr Neurol*. 2001;24(3):177-82.

    (Describes the clinical features and response to therapy in childhood CIDP.)

11. Cornblath DR, Sladky JT, Sumner AJ. Clinical electrophysiology of infantile botulism. *Muscle Nerve*. 1983;6(6):448-52.

    (Presents electrophysiological characteristics of presynaptic failure of neuromuscular transmission in infant botulism.)

12. Crawford TO, Sladky JT, Hurko O, Besner-Johnson A, Kelley RI. Abnormal fatty acid metabolism in childhood spinal muscular atrophy. *Annals of Neurology*. 1999;45(3): 337-343.

    (A catabolic state unmasks a defect in fatty acid metabolism in infants with type 1 SMA.)

13. Crawford T. Spinal muscular atrophies. In: H Jones, DeDivo, DC, Darras, BT, eds. *Neuromuscular Disorders of Infancy, Childhood and Adolescence: A Clinician's Approach*. Boston, Mass: Butterworth-Heinemann; 2003.

(An excellent review of the historical, clinical and molecular genetic aspects of SMAs.)

14. Dalakas MC. Basic aspects of neuroimmunology as they relate to immunotherapeutic targets: present and future prospects. *Ann Neurol*. 1995;37 Suppl 1:S2-13.

(Some of the details may be outmoded, but this paper lays out an organizational strategy for assimilating a large amount of complex, ever-expanding information regarding the immuno-biology of autoimmune disorders.)

15. DiMauro S, Lamperti C. Muscle Glycogenoses. *Muscle & Nerve*. 2001; 24:984-999.

(Comprehensive review of muscle involvement in the glycogenoses.)

16. Dyck PJ, Lambert EH. Lower motor and primary sensory neuron diseases with peroneal muscular atrophy. I. Neurologic, genetic, and electrophysiologic findings in hereditary polyneuropathies. *Arch Neurol*. 1968a;18 (6):603-18.

(Seminal work illustrating that electrophysiological measures are segregated discretely within kinships with Charcot-Marie-Tooth disease despite similar phenotypical characteristics.)

17. Dyck PJ, Lambert EH. Lower motor and primary sensory neuron diseases with peroneal muscular atrophy. II. Neurologic, genetic, and electrophysiologic findings in various neuronal degenerations. *Arch Neurol*. 1968b;18 (6):619-25.

(The electrophysiological features reliably distinguished families with different sub-types of the peroneal muscular atrophy syndrome.)

18. Dyck PJ, Swanson CJ, Low PA et al. Prednisone-responsive hereditary motor and sensory neuropathy. *Mayo Clin Proc*. 1982;57 (4):239-46.

(The first report of individuals with HMSN who also had a presumed acquired component responsive to immunosuppression.)

19. Efficiency of plasma exchange in Guillain-Barré syndrome: role of replacement fluids. French Cooperative Group on Plasma Exchange in Guillain-Barré syndrome. *Ann Neurol*. 1987;22(6):753-61.

(The second of the multicenter controlled trials establishing plasmapheresis as an effective therapy for GBS.)

20. Engel AG, Ohno K, Milone M et al. Congenital myasthenic syndromes. New insights from molecular genetic and patch-clamp studies. *Ann NY Acad Sci*. 1998;841:140-56.

(One of many influential papers from this laboratory providing a conceptual framework for understanding congenital myasthenic syndromes to which new information can be added.)

21. Evoli A, Tonali PA, Padua L et al. Clinical correlates with anti-MuSK antibodies in generalized seronegative myasthenia gravis. *Brain*. 2003;126(Pt 10):2304-11.

(Clinical features of autoimmune myasthenia gravis mediated by antibodies directed at this alternative post-synaptic protein.)

22. Fox CK, Keet CA, Strober JB. Recent advances in infant botulism. *Pediatr Neurol*. 2005;32(3):149-54.

(A recent comprehensive review of the disorder.)

23. Gabreels-Festen A. Dejerine-Sottas syndrome grown to maturity: overview of genetic and morphological heterogeneity and follow-up of 25 patients. *J Anat*. 2002;200(4):341-56.

(Excellent summary of aspects, including correlative histopathology for neuropathies in the CHN spectrum.)

24. Gabreels-Festen AA, Gabreels FJ, Hoogendijk JE et al. Chronic inflammatory demyelinating polyneuropathy or hereditary motor and sensory neuropathy? Diagnostic value of morphological criteria. *Acta Neuropathol*. (Berl) 1993;86(6):630-5.

(Ancillary features which can help in making the sometimes subtle distinction between HMSN and CIDP when genotypical markers are not informative.)

25. Griffin JW, Li CY, Ho TW et al. Guillain-Barré syndrome in northern China. The spectrum of neuropathological changes in clinically defined cases. *Brain*. 1995;118(Pt 3):577-95.

(Follow-up of the work described earlier by McKhann et al.)

26. Hughes RA, Hadden RD, Gregson NA et al. Pathogenesis of Guillain-Barré syndrome. *J Neuroimmunol*. 1999;100(1-2):74-97.

(Although six years old, a virtually undated and superb review of the pathobiology of GBS.)

27. Hughes RA, Rees JH. Clinical and epidemiologic features of Guillain-Barré syndrome. *J Infect Dis*. 1997;176 Suppl 2:S92-8.

(An exploration of the possible nature of that elusive "antecedent event.")

28. Iannaccone ST, Russman BS, Browne RH et al. Prospective analysis of strength in spinal muscular atrophy. DCN/Spinal Muscular Atrophy Group. *J Child Neurol*. 2000;15 (2):97-101.

(Characterization of quantitative measures of the course of the disease.)

29. Jones HR, Jr. Guillain-Barré syndrome: perspectives with infants and children. *Semin Pediatr Neurol*. 2000;7(2):91-102.

(A perspective from an author with a great depth of personal experience.)

30. Juel VC, Massey JM. Autoimmune myasthenia gravis: recommendations for treatment and immunologic modulation. *Curr Treat Options Neurol*. 2005;7(1):3-14.

(This provides a useful algorithm for the design of treatment regimens for children with MG.)

31. Korinthenberg R. Chronic inflammatory demyelinating Polyradiculoneuropathy in children and their response to treatment. *Neuropediatrics*. 1999;30(4):190-6.

(This manuscript is widely referred to regarding CIDP in children.)

32. Korinthenberg R, Monting JS. Natural history and treatment effects in Guillain-Barré syndrome: a multicentre study. *Arch Dis Child*. 1996;74(4):281-7.

(The most extensive series to date to examine the long-term outcome in childhood GBS.)

33. McKhann GM, Cornblath DR, Griffin JW et al. Acute motor axonal neuropathy: a frequent cause of acute flaccid paralysis in China. *Ann Neurol*. 1993;33(4):333-42.

(The original description of this fascinating disease among children in rural China.)

34. Muntoni F, Torelli S, Ferlini A. Dystrophin and mutations: one gene, several proteins, multiple phenotypes. *Lancet Neurology*. 2003; 2:731-740.

(More in-depth exploration into genotype/phenotype correlations than was possible in this chapter.)

35. Ohno K, Tsujino A, Brengman JM et al. Choline acetyltransferase mutations cause myasthenic syndrome associated with episodic apnea in humans. *Proc Natl Acad Sci USA*. 2001;98 (4):2017-22.

(A clinically and genotypically distinct form of a congenital myasthenic syndrome.)

36. Ouvrier RA, McLeod JG, Pollard JD, eds. *Peripheral Neuropathy in Childhood*. 2nd ed. London: Mac Keith Press; 1999. (Procopis PG, ed. *The International Review of Child Neurology Series*).

(Although there are three, this monograph has the special characteristics of a single author text.)

37. Pachman L. Juvenile dermatomyositis and other inflammatory myopathies. In: H Jones, DeVivo D, Darras B, eds. *Neuromuscular Disorders of Infancy, Childhood and Adolescence: A Clinician's Approach*. Boston, Mass: Butterworth-Heinemann; 2003:901.

(A definitive review of inflammatory myopathies in children.)

38. Paradiso G, Tripoli J, Galicchio S et al. Epidemiological, clinical, and electrodiagnostic findings in childhood Guillain-Barré syndrome: a reappraisal. *Ann Neurol*. 1999;46 (5):701-7.

(Important insight into the different spectra of childhood GBS in South and North America.)

39. Pickett J, Berg B, Chaplin E et al. Syndrome of botulism in infancy: clinical and electrophysiologic study. *N Engl J Med*. 1976;295 (14):770-2.

(The initial report describing the stereotypical clinical features of the illness and linking the pathophysiology of the disease to clostridial toxico-infection.)

40. Plasmapheresis and acute Guillain-Barré syndrome. The Guillain-Barré syndrome Study Group. *Neurology*. 1985;35(8):1096-104.

(The first definitive demonstration of an effective treatment for GBS.)

41. Randomized trial of plasma exchange, intravenous immunoglobulin, and combined treatments in Guillain-Barré syndrome. Plasma Exchange/Sandoglobulin Guillain-Barré Syndrome Trial Group. *Lancet*. 1997;349 (9047):225-30.

(Showed that treatment with plasmapheresis and IVIg were equally efficacious and equivalent to the combination.)

42. Research criteria for diagnosis of chronic inflammatory demyelinating polyneuropathy (CIDP). Report from an Ad Hoc Subcommittee of the American Academy of Neurology AIDS Task Force. *Neurology*. 1991;41 (5):617-8.

(Perhaps overly stringent for application in the clinic, nevertheless provides a diagnostic benchmark.)

43. Rodriguez M, Gomez MR, Howard FM, Jr. et al. Myasthenia gravis in children: long-term follow-up. *Ann Neurol*. 1983;13(5):504-10.

(Remains the best data available on thymectomy for the treatment of MG in children.)

44. Sladky JT. Guillain-Barré syndrome in childhood. *J Child Neurology*. 2004;191-200.

(A recent concise review on Guillain-Barré syndrome.)

45. Sumner CJ, Huynh TN, Markowitz JA et al. Valproic acid increases SMN levels in spinal muscular atrophy patient cells. *Ann Neurol.* 2003;54 (5):647-54.

(An example of a potential therapeutic strategy for this currently untreatable disease.)

46. Swoboda KJ, Prior TW, Scott CB et al. Natural history of denervation in SMA: relation to age, SMN2 copy number, and function. *Ann Neurol.* 2005;57(5):704-12.

(A description of the genotype-phenotype correlation in SMA.)

47. Tein I. Lipid Storage Muscular Disorders. In: Jones, HR, DiVivo DC, Darras BT, eds. *Neuromuscular Disorders of Infancy, Childhood and Adolescence*. Boston, Mass: Butterworth-Heinemann; 2003.

(A comprehensive review of lipid storage disorders in childhood.)

48. Wilmshurst JM, Pollard JD, Nicholson G et al. Peripheral neuropathies of infancy. *Dev Med Child Neurol*. 2003;45(6):408-14.

(A relatively extensive series from this experienced group.)

49. Zeviani M, Di Donato S. Mitochondrial disorders. *Brain*. 2004;127:2153-2172.

(A comprehensive review of the relatively current status of our understanding of this group of disorders.)

8. Questions

1. You are asked to evaluate a three-year-old girl for delayed acquisition of motor skills. Her language and cognitive development have been normal. There is no family history of similar conditions. On examination she has intact cranial nerves. You find diffuse weakness, proximal more than distal and lower more than upper extremities. Sensation appears to be normal. She is areflexic. Electrodiagnostic testing is consistent with motor neuron disease. DNA analysis reveals homozygous deletions of exons 7 and 8 of the SMN gene on chromosome 5q, diagnostic for spinal muscular atrophy (SMA).

Children with SMA usually come to medical attention due to:

A. Difficulties with feeding

B. Problems with chronic constipation

C. Failure to attain motor milestones

D. Regression of motor skills

2. One week later you're seeing a six-month-old boy with hypotonia and failure to attain motor milestones. The family history is negative for neurological disorders. Cranial nerve examination discloses tongue fasciculations. He has axial and appendicular weakness with a paradoxical respiratory pattern. Sensation appears intact. Deep tendon reflexes are absent. His electrodiagnostic testing also is consistent with motor neuron disease. He too has a homozygous deletion of exons 7 and 8 of the SMN1 gene.

The severity of the clinical expression of spinal muscular atrophy is related to:

A. The size of the deletion at the locus on chromosome 5q

B. The distance of the deletion from the telomere of chromosome 5

C. The number of residual copies of the SMN2 gene

D. None of the above

3. A previously healthy seven-year-old boy comes to the emergency room complaining of leg weakness and back pain, which has progressed over the prior 48 hours. Cognitive function and cranial nerve examinations are normal. He exhibits distal>proximal weakness of the lower extremities while arm strength appears normal. There is a mild decrement in vibratory and proprioceptive sensations below the knees bilaterally. Reflexes are absent throughout with normal plantar reflexes. Based on these clinical features the attending physician tells his parents that the probable diagnosis is Guillain-Barré syndrome.

The diagnosis of Guillain-Barré syndrome is confirmed by:

A. A clinical presentation of ascending paralysis and areflexia

B. The presence of albumino-cytologic dissociation on CSF examination

C. Evidence of asymmetrical slowing of motor nerve conduction velocities and the presence of conduction block on nerve conduction studies

D. All of the above

4. The patient described above is admitted to the hospital for further evaluation and treatment. Ancillary studies confirm the diagnosis of Guillain-Barré syndrome. Therapy is initiated.

Treatment of children with acute Guillain-Barré syndrome:

A. Minimizes long-term disability

B. Is most effective during the progressive phase of the disease

C. Should begin with IVIg, based on controlled trials in adults

D. Is directed at eliminating pathogenic antibodies targeting myelin-related epitopes

5. A four-month-old girl is brought to the emergency room by her parents. She has been intermittently constipated for the prior two weeks. Over the course of the past two days she has become hypotonic with generalized weakness and inability to suck, and choking on her feeds. On examination she appears somnolent. She has dilated, poorly reactive pupils, external ophthalmoparesis with facial and bulbar weakness. There is generalized weakness of the extremities more severe proximally. She withdraws to painful stimuli. Tendon reflexes are absent. Based on the constellation of clinical features, infant botulism is thought to be the most likely diagnosis. Because of concerns regarding airway compromise, she is intubated and transferred to the intensive care unit. Electrodiagnostic testing confirms a pre-synaptic defect in neuromuscular transmission consistent with infant botulism.

Infant botulism:

A. Is often caused by ingestion of clostridium botulinum spores in honey

B. Should be treated with gentamycin to eradicate the bacterium from the affected infant's gastrointestinal tract

C. Should be treated with antibody to the toxin elaborated by the bacterium

D. Is more common east of the Rocky Mountains

6. A 30-month-old boy is evaluated for delayed motor development. He was noted shortly after birth to be hypotonic with diminished spontaneous movements and a poor suck. The acquisition of motor skills was delayed in that he sat at 9 months and walked at 20 months. Cognitive development is age appropriate. There is no family history of neuromuscular disease. At the time of evaluation he is hypotonic with symmetrical proximal weakness. Deep tendon reflexes are normal. Additionally he has bilateral ptosis and restricted extraocular motility. There is bilateral facial weakness. Routing sensory and motor nerve conduction studies are normal, as is needle EMG. Repetitive nerve stimulation at 3 Hz elicits a 47% decrement in the amplitude of the compound motor action potential consistent with a post-synaptic defect in neuromuscular transmission. Anti-acetylcholine receptor and MUSK antibodies are not detected. The presumed diagnosis is a congenital myasthenic syndrome.

   Congenital myasthenic syndromes:

   A. Respond well to treatment with anticholinesterases

   B. Are more commonly due to defects in the post-synaptic acetylcholine receptor

   C. Resolve as anti-AChR antibody titers diminish with age

   D. Are transmitted with a recessive pattern of inheritance

7. The patient is a 9-year-old girl who was born at term without perinatal complications. Early development was normal. She was in her usual state of good health until three months prior to evaluation when her parents noted intermittent left eyelid ptosis. Over the month prior to evaluation she noted increasing fatigue and complained of occasional diplopia. There is no family history of neuromuscular disease; however, her 15-year-old sister is said to have lupus. On examination she has mild bilateral ptosis, worse on the left, and restricted ocular abduction bilaterally. Pupils are normally reactive. Facial movement is normal and she has no apparent bulbar weakness. She has mild symmetrical weakness of shoulder girdle muscles. Distal muscles in the arms appear to have normal power. Lower extremities have normal strength to formal testing; however, when asked to perform serial deep knee bends, she can only do five. Sensation, cerebellar function and tendon reflexes are normal. Electrodiagnostic studies reveal a decremental response in the compound motor amplitude of the trapezius. Repetitive simulation of the median nerve recording over abductor pollicis brevis is normal. Needle EMG is also normal. Serological testing reveals an elevated anti-acetylcholine receptor antibody titer.

   Myasthenia gravis in children:

   A. Is caused predominantly by antibodies directed against acetylcholine receptor or muscle specific kinase epitopes

   B. Often occurs in infants born to mothers with poorly controlled myasthenia

   C. Is frequently associated with thymoma

   D. Responds poorly to immunosuppressants

8. You are asked to see a 10-year-old boy because of an increasing clumsiness for the past year. He is the product of an uncomplicated gestation and delivery with normal subsequent neurological development. He is currently an otherwise healthy straight-A student in the fourth grade. The general medical examination is remarkable for highly arched feet and mild Achilles contractures bilaterally. Cranial nerve examination is normal. Muscle strength is normal with the exception of tibialis anterior and peroneus longus and brevis, which are mildly weak. Vibratory sensation and proprioception are mildly diminished below the ankles. Cerebellar exam is normal. Deep tendon reflexes are unelicitable throughout. Electrophysiological

testing demonstrates absent sural and posterior sensory nerve action potentials (SNAPs) bilaterally. Median and ulnar SNAP amplitudes are markedly diminished with mild slowed conduction velocities. Motor nerve conductions are markedly slowed with disproportionately prolonged distal latencies and absent F-waves. There is prominent conduction block and or dispersion of proximally-evoked compound motor action potentials. EMG revealed evidence of chronic partial denervation in a fiber length dependent pattern of severity. These features were thought to be indicative of chronic inflammatory demyelinating polyneuropathy.

CIDP in children:

A. May mimic HMSN

B. May mimic GBS

C. Usually responds to treatment with corticosteroids

D. May be distinguished from HMSN with sural nerve biopsy

E. All of the above

9. The patient is a four-year-old boy who is referred for evaluation of weakness. He is the product of a normal gestation and delivery with an uncomplicated perinatal period. Early milestones were acquired in a normal fashion. Since he began walking at 15 months of age his parents have noted that he runs more slowly and has decreased endurance compared to other children his age. He has a maternal uncle who is said to have died from muscular dystrophy. There is no other pertinent family history. He has otherwise been in good health. On examination he has prominent calves, a mildly hyperlordotic gate, and uses a modified Gower's maneuver to rise from sitting on the floor. Preliminary testing is remarkable for a serum CPK of 23,00 IU.

Which of the following are true about Duchenne muscular dystrophy?

A. It can be ruled out based on the absence of an out of frame deletion in the dystrophin gene

B. The severity of the disease correlates with the size of the deletion

C. Pulmonary function tests are predictive of the risk for respiratory complications

D. Will often require Achilles tendon lengthening to maintain ambulation

10. The patient is a seven-year-old girl who is being evaluated for episodic inability to walk. Over the past 18 months she had three episodes associated with relatively mild intercurrent infections during which she complains of fatigue and feels so unsteady that she is unable to walk. These episodes have lasted from 3 to 9 days. She was the product of a normal gestation and delivery without perinatal complications. Neurological development has been normal. She has been healthy and is a good student. She has a maternal uncle who has similar episodes albeit much less frequently. Her general examination is normal. Her neurological examination is remarkable for mild bilateral ptosis, restricted extraocular motility to all fields, and areflexia at the ankles. Serological studies document an elevated lactic acid level. Lactate is also elevated in her urine. The presumptive diagnosis is a disorder of oxidative phosphorylation.

The following are true about mitochondrial disorders in children:

A. They are most often inherited via mutations in maternal mitochondrial DNA

B. Often present with recurrent hemiparesis

C. Are frequently asymptomatic

D. Are best diagnosed based on histopathological features in muscle biopsy specimens

Answers

1. C.

2. C.

3. D.

4. C.

5. B.

6. A.

7. B.

8. E.

9. C.

10. C.

Color Plates

Figure 1

Congenital hypomyelinating neuropathy

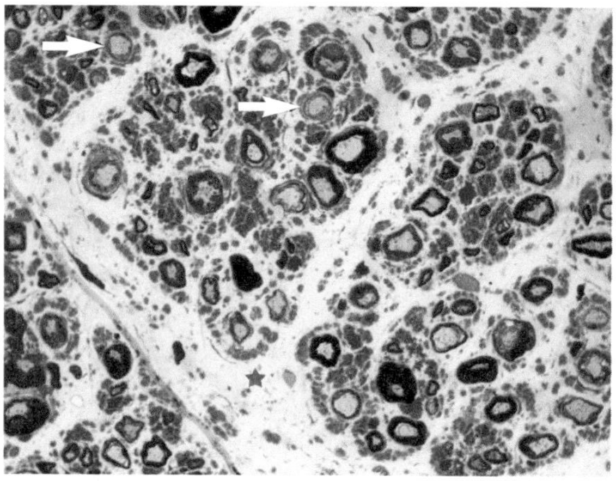

Note massive endoneurial edema (red star) indicative of endoneurial denervation. None of the large caliber axons exhibit normal compact myelin. Several axons of a diameter which should undergo myelination have no myelin sheath (arrows).

Figure 2

Nemaline myopathy

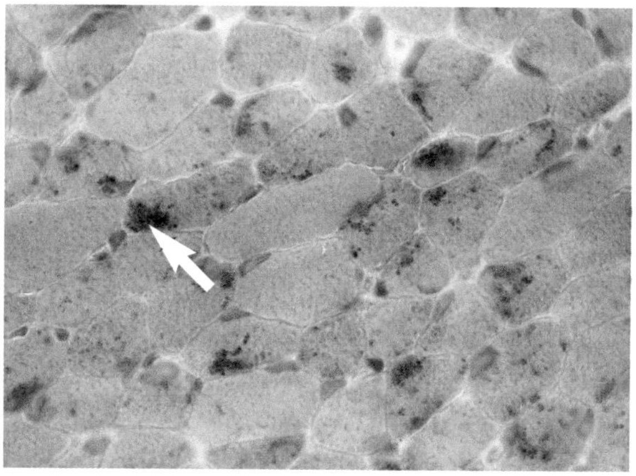

Note nemaline or rod bodies accumulating within several myofibers in this field.

Figure 3

Centronuclear myopathy

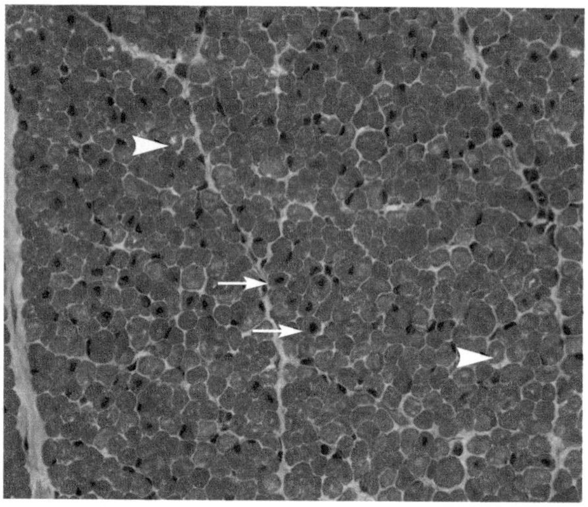

The majority of the myonuclei within the plane of section are centrally located as apposed to the normal peripheral, subsarcolemmal location (arrows). There is typically a halo around the central nucleus which, when the cross section does not include the nucleus, results in an apparent hole in the center of the myofiber (arrowheads).

Figure 4

Mitochondrial myopathy

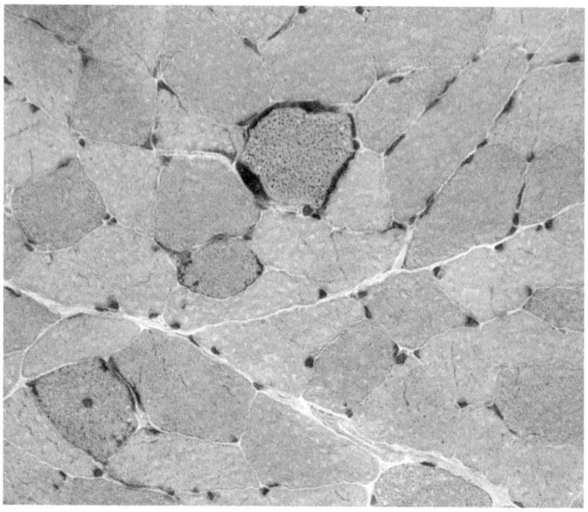

Note nemaline or rod bodies accumulating within several myofibers in this field.

Chapter 20: Spinal Cord Disorders

Rand Swenson, MD

Contents

1. Introduction

Disorders of the spinal cord are common and may appear either as an isolated finding or in concert with other central neurologic or systemic problems. Every category of medical condition can affect the spinal cord, complicating differential diagnosis in patients with evidence of spinal cord dysfunction. The focus of the chapter will be on conditions that preferentially or exclusively affect the spinal cord, although we will briefly consider conditions that can damage the spinal cord while preferentially affecting other parts of the nervous system.

2. Myelopathy

Myelopathy is a generic term indicating damage to the spinal cord from any cause. It is often possible to determine that there is myelopathy present even when it is more challenging to determine the cause.

The syndrome of myelopathy incorporates some combination of symptoms resulting from damage to the tracts of the spinal cord (descending and ascending, Figure 1), possibly accompanied by evidence of damage to local structures of the cord such as the gray matter or nerve roots. Long tract damage represents a particular challenge, since it is often challenging to determine the precise level of the lesion. Theoretically, the level of long tract damage can be determined by identifying the upper limit of preserved tract function (ie, *spinal level*). In practice, this can be difficult and the true level of damage is usually some distance above this "spinal level."

The "long tract signs" usually include motor signs of corticospinal involvement (that is, upper motor neuron signs) or signs of sensory tract damage (ie, dorsal columns or spinothalamic tract), or both.

On the motor side, the characteristic findings of upper motor neuron involvement include spastic weakness of muscles along with hyperreflexia (potentially including clonus or pathological spread of reflexes). Acute damage to the spinal cord can result in a variable duration (often up to several days) of flaccid paralysis, termed *spinal shock*.

On the sensory side, loss of dorsal columns sensations (such as vibration sense, joint position sense or well-localized touch sensation) or evidence of spinothalamic tract damage (loss of pain and/or temperature sense) should be sought. If sensory deficits are found, some attempt should be made to determine the upper limit of this involvement (usually by testing trunk sensations). This is substantially easier to do for spinothalamic tract involvement than for dorsal columns. Of course, when sensory deficits are identified is also important to consider whether these might be due to peripheral nerve, nerve root or intracranial damage before concluding that it is to the result of myelopathy. Bilateral involvement, particularly with a sensory level over the trunk, would probably represent myelopathy, while loss of sensation in a restricted area of a limb (particularly if there are sharp borders to the sensory loss) would probably be peripheral. Also, it is important to determine if there are other signs pointing toward myelopathy.

In addition to damage to sensory and motor tracts in the spinal cord, there may be evidence of damage to descending autonomic control pathways. Symptoms may result from loss of control over sympathetic nervous system responses or from loss of descending control of the urinary bladder.

Damage to descending sympathetic nervous system control pathways may present as inadequate response to being upright (orthostasis) but also may result in mass reflexes with overactivity of the sympathetic nervous system. On occasion this can result in dangerous elevations of blood pressure (usually in response to some stimulus below the level of the spinal cord damage).

Descending pathways participate in bladder control by inhibiting reflex activity of the urinary bladder. Urinary urgency is the most common finding with partial interruption of these descending pathways and is most evident with slowly progressive conditions. Rapidly progressive spinal cord damage or lesions involving the sacral spinal cord (conus medullaris) can produce a flaccid bladder, particularly in the acute phase.

While damage to spinal cord tracts produces symptoms below the level of lesion, damage to the gray matter of the spinal cord or to the nerve roots produces symptoms at the level of damage. This makes symptoms of gray matter or nerve root damage particularly useful in localizing the level of the disease process. Injury to gray matter usually affects the anterior horn cells (lower motor neurons). Lower motor neuron damage is characterized by: 1) flaccid weakness of muscles that are innervated at that par-

Figure 1

Location of ascending and descending tracts of the spinal cord

Ascending tracts on the right and descending on the left.

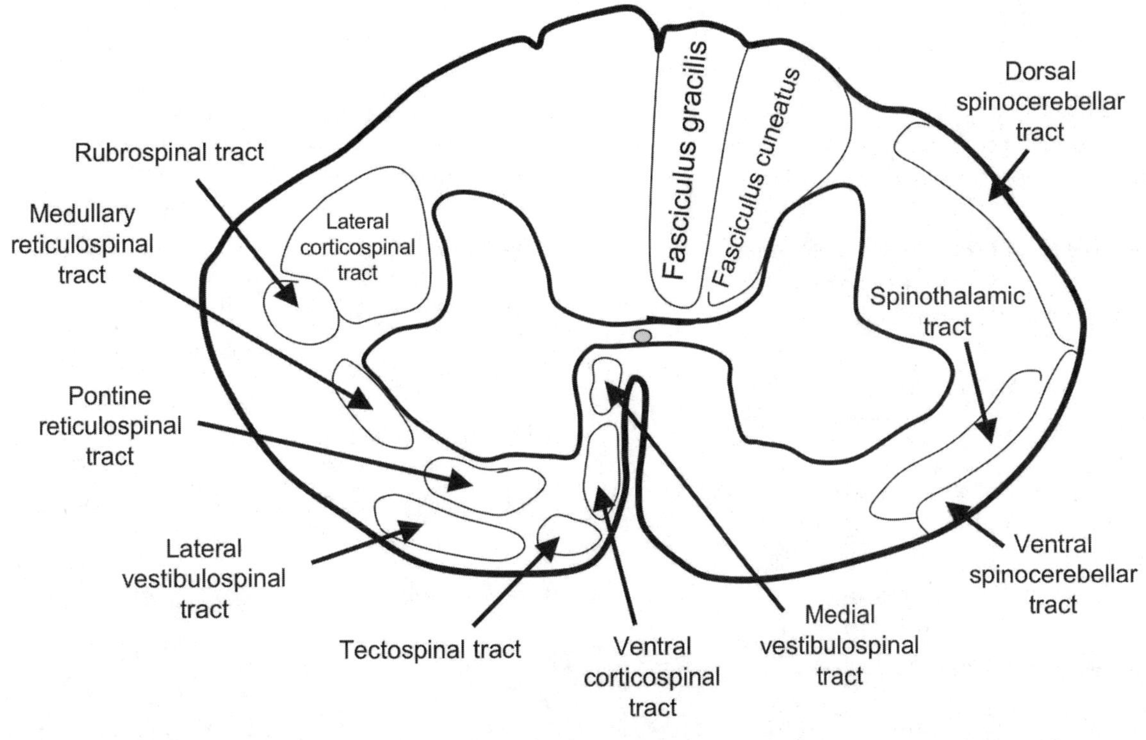

ticular spinal level; 2) atrophy; 3) decrease in the reflexes mediated at that level; and, often, 4) fasciculations. Injury to gray matter can, at times, also produce neuropathic pain. Nerve root damage (radiculopathy) often occurs at the level of spinal cord damage particularly when the spinal cord is affected by conditions arising outside of the cord. This is recognized by radicular pain, and weakness or loss of local reflexes. When present, findings of lower motor neuron damage or radiculopathy are excellent localizers of the site of damage and can give important guidance to the most appropriate areas for imaging.

When myelopathy begins before skeletal maturity, scoliosis and pes cavus are common (both of which may be associated with other neurologic abnormalities as well). Most idiopathic adolescent scoliosis has a convexity toward the patient's right in the thoracic region. A scoliosis with convexity to the left raises questions about possible underlying neurologic abnormality, particularly myelopathy.

Table 1

Red and Yellow Flags in Patients with Back Pain

Red Flags Consideration should be given to additional testing because of a higher than acceptable possibility that there is something serious causing the patient's symptoms.	**Yellow Flags** A sign or symptom that is rarely seen in uncomplicated back pain; suggests closer observation or more testing.
Significant trauma	Bilateral sciatica or neurological deficits
Immunosuppressive or anticoagulant use	Perianal paresthesia
New pain in patient greater than 55 years	Bladder dysfunction
Prior cancer or recent infection	Multiple nerve root involvements
Fever with new back pain	Pulsatile abdominal mass
ESR >20	Colicky pain, or writhing with pain
IV drug abuse	Lack of a story consistent with mechanical low back pain
Back pain that is worse with rest	Lack of improvement with conservative treatment
Deteriorating neurologic function	

3. Back Pain

Back pain is among the most common of complaints in humans and rarely results from a serious underlying neurologic disorder. For this reason, it is often difficult to determine when and if to image the region and, if so, at which location. Back pain that is associated with signs and symptoms of myelopathy is a red flag requiring further investigation. Additionally, when localized back pain is present in the myelopathic patient, the pain is the best predictor of the level of involvement.

There are several other red flags and yellow flags that should prompt additional thought prior to determining that the back pain represents benign disease. These red and yellow flags consist of symptoms and circumstances that are relatively rare in patients that have uncomplicated, benign back pain. Attention to these red and yellow flags appear in Table 1 and can help identify individuals with higher than anticipated prior probability of disease.

4. Extramedullary Spinal Cord Compression

The syndrome of extramedullary spinal cord compression is important to recognize since it often results from conditions that can cause rapid and permanent deterioration. There are many such conditions, with major categories listed in Table 2. The syndrome may begin with lateralized symptoms, with evolution to bilateral involvement. Damage to nerve roots (radiculopathy) may develop since the compressive lesion (particularly if acute) can distort the course of a nerve root. The most important conditions producing extramedullary spinal cord compression are neoplastic, traumatic, infectious (epidural abscess) and hemorrhagic (epidural hematoma).

Neoplastic spinal cord compression usually results from metastasis to the spine, although direct metastasis to the epidural space can also occur. Epidural metastasis is more difficult to diagnosis since regular x-rays will not show the lesion. Other extramedullary neoplasms, including primary tumors of the spine (such as multiple myeloma), or primary tumors of the meninges (meningioma), or nerve sheaths (neurofibroma or schwannoma), can compress the cord.

Epidural abscesses are almost always painful and they elevate the ESR (sometimes without fever or elevated WBC count). These usually occur in immunocompromised individuals (including diabetic patients), often without a very obvious infection elsewhere. Epidural abscess can result in rapid deterioration in neurologic status if untreated and the outcome is far from assured even with aggressive treatment.

Trauma can compromise the spinal canal and thereby the spinal cord by displacement of various bony or discal elements. Additionally, trauma may result in epidural hematoma that can also distort the cord. These hematomas may also occur spontaneously in anticoagulated patients or following spinal procedures that violate the epidural space.

Table 2

Conditions That Can Cause Extramedullary and Intramedullary Spinal Cord Compression

Etiology	Intramedullary	Extramedullary
Neoplastic	Glioma Ependymoma Hemangioblastoma Metastasis (rare)	Extradural Metastatic Primary bone (rare: myeloma, etc.) Entradural Neurofibroma Meningioma Drop metastasis Lymphoma Carcinomatous meningitis
Radiation	Radiation myelopathy	
Traumatic	Traumatic myelopathy with or without hematoma	Fracture/dislocation Traumatic hematoma
Degenerative	Motor neuron disease	Spondylotic myelopathy OPLL
Genetic	Spinocerebellar ataxias Friedreich ataxia	
Infectious	Bacterial (uncommon) Granuloma: brucellosis, turberculosis, etc. Spirochetal Syphilis Lyme Fungal (rare) Parasitic Toxoplasma Schistosomiasis Echinococcus Viral HIV Cytomegalovirus Epstein-Barr Other Herpes virus (VZ, HSV-2) Enterovirus (including Polio) HTLV-1	Epidural abcess (bacterial usually, may be fungal) With osteomyelitis/discitis Without osteomyelitis/discitis

(continued)

Table 2 *(continued)*

Conditions That Can Cause Extramedullary and Intramedullary Spinal Cord Compression

Etiology	Intramedullary	Extramedullary
Vascular/hemorrhagic	Arteriovenous malformation Dural arteriovenous fistula Infarction (anterior spinal a.) Microangiopathy	Epidural hematoma
Inflammatory	Multiple sclerosis Devic disease ADEM	
Vascular/hemorrhagic	Arteriovenous malformation Dural arteriovenous fistula Infarction (anterior spinal a.) Microangiopathy	Epidural hematoma
Inflammatory	Multiple sclerosis Devic disease ADEM Transverse myelitis Vasculitis (lupus, etc.) Sarcoid Celiac; Whipple	
Toxic/metabolic	Subacute combined degeneration (PLS) Other deficiency (copper, Vitamin E) Cuban epidemic neuropathy Drugs of abuse (especially nitrous oxide and heroin) Medications (especially intrathecal methotrexate or amphotericin B) Poisons (including strychnine, cycad seeds)	Epidural lipomatosis
Congenital/Developmental	Syrinx	Congenital spinal stenosis Tethered cord

Early recognition of extramedullary spinal cord compression is important since this generally leads to early imaging which is usually necessary for definitive diagnosis and treatment. In cases where there is a high index of suspicion for spinal cord trauma or metastatic disease (especially if imaging is expected to be delayed) high dose steroids may be used empirically (see below).

5. Intramedullary Disease of the Spinal Cord

Intramedullary spinal cord disease has a wider differential than extramedullary compression (Table 2). Intramedullary causes of myelopathy are unlikely to result in radicular involvement and are rarely painful (unless accompanied by meningeal inflammation, as in some infectious causes). A full range of diseases must be considered in the differential: neoplastic, traumatic, degenerative, infectious, hemorrhagic, vascular, inflammatory, toxic/metabolic, and congenital. Expansile intramedullary lesions can produce suspended sensory losses, involving loss of pain and temperature sensation in the upper body while sparing sensations in the lower portion of the body (due to involvement of crossing fibers of the spinothalamic system). Certain lesions preferentially affect the white matter of the spinal cord (such as inflammatory, demyelinative lesions). These disorders of white matter produce signs and symptoms of damage to long tracts. Other conditions attack the gray matter and may damage neurons, such as the anterior horn cells, producing amyotrophy, often accompanied by fasciculations.

6. Etiologic Differential Diagnosis of Myelopathy

The following sections will consider the potential causes of myelopathy by etiology. Virtually all categories of disease can affect the spinal cord, adding to the challenge of differentially diagnosing myelopathy (Table 2). Specifically, we will discuss neoplastic, traumatic, degenerative, infectious, hemorrhagic, vascular, inflammatory, toxic/metabolic, and congenital causes of myelopathy.

Neoplastic

Neoplasms can be located in the extradural or intradural regions. Intradural conditions can be further categorized into extramedullary or intramedullary. Both the extradural and the intradural/extramedullary neoplasms often damage nerve roots in addition to affecting the spinal cord. Certain primary neoplasms have a particular tendency to involve each of these specific locations. Therefore, the location of a tumor can be a guide to the type of further workup and management. Most extradural tumors are metastatic. However, primary tumors of bone, such as multiple myeloma, can affect the spine and produce extramedullary spinal cord compression (EMSCC) by promoting fracture or by extending into the epidural space. Intradural/extramedullary tumors either derive from tissues in the region (meningiomas or nerve sheath tumors), or result from metastasis via cerebrospinal pathways (lymphoma or drop metastasis from intracranial tumors, such as medulloblastomas, ependymomas or, rarely, malignant gliomas). Intramedullary spinal cord tumors include gliomas, ependymomas and hemangioblastomas, although metastatic tumors can (rarely) go directly to the spinal cord.

Neoplastic EMSCC represents one of the most feared complications of metastatic cancer. Many neoplasms metastasize to the spine including, particularly, lung, breast, prostate, renal and lymphoma. While most involve bone (increasing the likelihood of detection by plain radiographs or bone scans) some only involve the epidural space adjacent to the spinal cord. These can be particularly challenging to diagnose.

Most neoplastic EMSCC occurs in the thoracic region due to the high frequency of metastasis to that region of the spine. The most common symptom is pain, which occurs in about 95% of patients, often before other symptoms. While back pain itself is not a very strong predictor of metastatic cancer (because of the large number of individuals with benign back pain), new back pain or highly localized back pain, especially in the patient with a history of cancer, requires strong consideration for imaging. About 70% of patients with malignant EMSCC have point tenderness to pressure or percussion.

About 80% of patients with EMSCC complain of weakness, 55% have paresthesias or numbness, and 40% have bowel and bladder problems. Examination reveals weakness in about 85%, a sensory level in about 70%, abnormal reflexes in 65%, Babinski response in 50%, and decreased rectal tone in 60%.

The reason that it is critical to recognize this process early is that outcome generally depends on the patient's neurologic status at the time of institution of therapy. Steroids and radiation have been the gold standard treatment, although more radical surgical approaches to decompression have been gaining favor in patients who have a better prognosis from their underlying disease. Typically, treatment will stabilize the patient's clinical status, although improvement is uncertain. Therefore, starting treatment prior to major dysfunction improves outcome.

Tumors that are intradural but extramedullary include meningiomas, tumors of the nerve sheaths (schwannomas or neurofibromas) and "drop metastasis" (usually from ependymomas, medulloblastomas or, occasionally, gliomas). Management varies depending on the particular neoplasm, with the benign tumors being treated surgically (when they become symptomatic) and the more malignant ones being treated by radiation and/or intrathecal chemotherapy. Certain tumors can invade the spinal meninges (carcinomatous meningitis), producing a picture that suggests polyradiculopathy with or without evidence of myelopathy. This type of tumor metastasis, while rare, has a very poor prognosis, although some tumors may be more responsive to treatment in the short run than others (lymphoma, for example).

Intramedullary spinal cord tumors are rare but most often are gliomas, ependymomas or hemangioblastomas. Furthermore, there are rare intramedullary metastases. The symptoms of intramedullary neoplasms would include myelopathy, but are much less likely to be accompanied by pain or radiculopathy. They may be associated with a "suspended" sensory loss of pinprick sense due to damage to crossing spinothalamic tract fibers.

In addition to the direct effects of neoplasms, paraneoplastic syndromes may affect the spinal cord. These often accompany other signs of paraneoplastic involvement of the CNS, but it is important to note that the symptoms of the paraneoplastic syndrome can occur as an initial manifestation of cancer. Paraneoplastic myelopathy appears in two main forms, a rapidly progressive necrotic myelopathy, usually accompanying lung cancers or lymphomas, or a chronic paraneoplastic involvement of white matter. This latter condition typically involves the dorsal and lateral columns and is most common with breast and ovarian cancers or Hodgkin disease. While there is promise of effective treatment of these conditions via immune modulation, this remains uncertain.

Radiation

Radiation myelitis is a potential complication of radiation therapy. The treatment of tumors of the respiratory system (including nasopharynx) and upper gastrointestinal tract presents particular risks if the nervous system is included in the field. Radiation myelitis typically develops after a latent period of over 6 months (although this can be shorter if the radiation dose is high). It can develop many years after treatment. The condition usually affects the lateral and ventral columns of the spinal cord, producing spastic weakness of the legs, often with a loss of temperature sense. Symptoms are usually slowly progressive and are thought to result from demyelination due to damage of small blood vessels. Sensitivity to this complication appears to be higher in patients who are also treated with chemotherapy.

Unfortunately, there are no definitive tests for radiation myelitis. MRI scans may show some cord swelling initially with increased T2 signal and, later, atrophy. CSF often shows nonspecific elevation of protein and, possibly, a few lymphocytes. Again, however, this is completely nonspecific and diagnosis is based on history and ruling out alternative causes.

Traumatic

Trauma is a common cause of myelopathy. This may be rapid, often associated with a fracture, fracture-dislocation, or large, acute disc herniation, or may be subtler, due to repeated traumas associated with congenital or acquired spinal stenosis. This latter situation usually is due to spondylotic changes in discs and joints, although it can also result from conditions such as ossification of the posterior longitudinal ligament (OPLL). Osteoporosis, in addition to being a cause of back pain, can cause compression fractures. In most cases these compression fractures do not compromise the posterior part of the vertebral body and therefore do not damage the spinal cord. However, in some cases they may be unstable and also involve the posterior body in a pattern akin to a "burst fracture."

Acute traumatic myelopathy is treated with a protocol of high-dose intravenous methylprednisolone based on one study showing marginally better outcomes. This is quite controversial, but is most often used since it is the only treatment that is known to have any favorable effect on prognosis. While unstable spinal fractures, including burst fractures, typically require some surgical intervention, more stable fractures are managed nonoperatively. The goals are to prevent further damage to neural tissue, to decrease pain, and to facilitate further care of the patient with spinal cord injury.

Cervical spondylotic myelopathy (CSM) is an acquired condition that can have the additional substrate of congenital stenosis (either as an isolated condition or part of a systemic disorder, as with achondroplasia). It usually affects the mid-to-lower cervical spine and is associated with thickening and buckling of the ligmentum flavum, bulging of the intervertebral disc, hypertrophy of facets and development of posterior osteophytes, all of which contribute to narrowing of the vertebral canal. Ossification of the posterior longitudinal ligament (OPLL) is an idiopathic condition that occurs with higher frequency in Asians. This contributes to development of the myelopathy and is more likely to be progressive, with a much higher incidence of requiring surgery than the average case of spondylotic myelopathy.

The pathology of chronic, low-grade compression usually includes demyelination that is most evident in the lateral and dorsal columns of the spinal cord (producing upper motor neuron symptoms and loss of proprioceptive and epicritic functions in the legs). It can also damage anterior horn cells, producing amyotrophy in the upper limbs. Experimental studies on animals suggest that it is due to mild but repeated ischemia, the result of impairment of blood flow by compression. This has not been confirmed in humans.

CSM must, of course, be distinguished from other conditions damaging the cord. This is particularly true of demyelinating conditions and motor neuron disease. Rheumatoid arthritis can result in thickening of spinal ligaments with a loosening of these ligaments (especially in the upper cervical region) that can produce a chronic movement and position-associated cord compression. While symptoms may have acute onset after trauma or extreme head position, there can also be chronic myelopathic findings.

The treatment of spondylotic myelopathy is controversial. About 30%-50% of patients will show some improvement with immobilization in a collar. The condition can be stable over many years but it can also be slowly progressive, or even have some episodic exacerbations. Fortunately, it rarely progresses to complete debility after its initial recognition unless trauma intervenes. Surgical treatment should be considered early for those who have

Figure 2

A myelomere of the spinal cord, and one of its two associated spinal nerves

In A: A, anterior median fissure; P, posterior median sulcus. B shows the arterial supply to the cord.

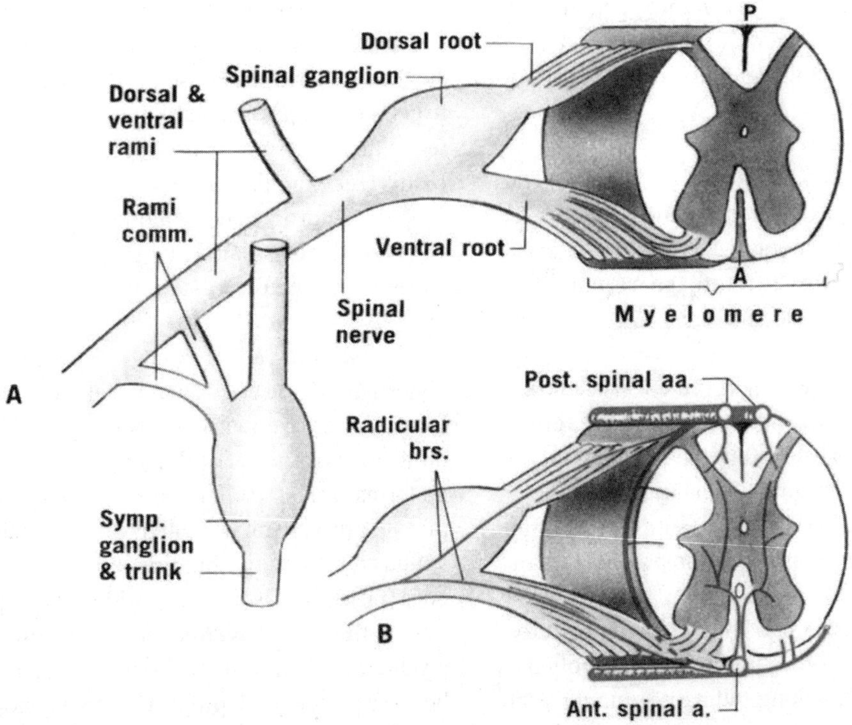

severe underlying pathology (or OPLL) or that show signs of continuing to deteriorate despite conservative measures.

Vascular and Hemorrhagic

Just as cerebrovascular disease encompasses a range of pathophysiologies, there are several types of vascular conditions that affect the spinal cord. These may be extradural (including epidural hematoma) or intramedullary (hemorrhage or ischemia). Additionally, abnormalities of blood vessels (arteriovenous fistulas or malformations) can contribute to myelopathy.

Epidural hematoma is characterized by pain and myelopathy (or cauda equina compression, depending on the level). The pain may be only in the back or have the additional component of radiculopathic pain. Epidural hematomas arise from one of several conditions. They may be a complication of a spinal procedure (including, rarely, lumbar puncture), or they can result from a bleeding dyscrasia (including anticoagulation). Trauma is a common cause of epidural hematoma but they also can develop spontaneously from an extradural vascular malformation. If the neurologic symptoms are not severe, patients can often be closely monitored and managed conservatively, especially if the hematoma resulted from a reversible condition, such as anticoagulation.

Intramedullary hematoma is usually traumatic. The extent of hemorrhage does correspond (loosely) with clinical outcome in trauma. However, evacuation of an intrameduallry hemorrhage has not been shown to improve clinical outcome.

The blood supply of the spinal cord consists of a single anterior spinal artery that arises from the vertebral arteries superiorly and runs the length of the spinal cord in the anterior median fissure of the spinal cord (Figure 2). This artery supplies the anterior two-thirds of the spinal cord (in practical terms, everything but the dorsal columns). The two posterior spinal arteries are small and run on the posterolateral aspect of the cord. They basically supply the dorsal columns. These longitudinally-running arteries are not robust enough to supply the lower reaches of the spinal cord without periodic contribution from radicular arteries. The radicular arteries appear every 4 to 6 segments along the spinal cord and follow the nerve roots to reach the spinal cord, replenishing the flow in the longitudinal arteries. There is one very large radicular artery that usually arises from one of the lower thoracic segmental arteries, the arteria magna (of Adamkiewicz). If flow in this artery is disrupted, the lower portion of the spinal cord often infarcts. Atherosclerosis and instrumentation of the upper lumbar aorta are the most common causes of spinal cord infarction, although other causes of vascular occlusion such as arterial dissection or embolus can produce it.

Anterior spinal artery syndrome is due to disruption of blood flow in that artery. This most commonly results from occlusion of one of the main radicular arteries, although pressure on the central part of the spinal cord can directly occlude the anterior spinal artery. Since this artery supplies the anterior two-thirds of the spinal cord, infarction is usually recognized by the acute onset of paraplegia with preservation of dorsal column sensation.

Microangiopathy of the spinal cord can result from vasculitis, occlusion by microemboli, hyperviscosity (due to abnormal proteins or blood cells) or due to obstruction by foreign bodies in the arterial circulation (such as gas bubbles with decompression sickness). All of these conditions are rare and are usually only one of several manifestations of systemic disease. Some causes of inflammatory vasculitis (for example, connective tissue disorders like Sjögren syndrome and systemic lupus erythmatosis) can produce an isolated myelopathy that may be extremely difficult to diagnose.

The spinal cord can be damaged by the presence of abnormal blood vessels that usually either take the form of arteriovenous malformations (AVMs) or of dural arteriovenous fistulas (A-V fistulas). These abnormal vascular channels can damage the cord by putting pressure on normal tissue, by impairing venous return, or by shunting blood away from the cord (producing ischemia). Additionally, particularly in the case of AVMs, they may hemorrhage, producing acute damage. These vascular lesions can be challenging to identify. Although abnormal vascular channels can usually be seen on MRI scans, occasionally they are quite difficult to distinguish from CSF flow artifacts. Angiography requires the identification of the correct radicular feeding artery, which may arise at some distance from the malformation.

Dural arteriovenous fistulas are acquired conditions of uncertain etiology that are most common in middle-aged men. These typically result in venous congestion, producing edema of the spinal cord along with ischemia. Dural A-V fistulas produce symptoms by compression of neural structures or by producing low-pressure shunts that divert blood from normal capillary beds, producing ischemia.

Successful treatment of the AVM or A-V fistula requires identification of the feeding arteries. Depending on the location, surgical or endovascular treatment may be attempted, although the relatively high potential for injury to the spinal cord must be considered in decision making.

Degenerative

There are many disorders of the spinal cord that have been classified as degenerative. As more is learned about some of these conditions, metabolic or genetic causes are identified and we will consider these conditions with their appropriate etiologic groupings. Degenerative conditions can be classified as those involving gray matter or white matter or a combination of both.

Motor neuron disease is a prototypical degenerative condition of the spinal cord. This family of conditions involves non-inflammatory degeneration of anterior horn cells (lower motor neurons), descending tracts (upper motor neurons), or both. Most cases occur sporadically, although there are familial clusters of the disease associated with genetic lack of intraneuronal cytoprotective mechanisms. There are also cases that relate to toxic exposures (cycad neurotoxins in ALS-Parkinson disease complex of Guam, for example) that have led to theories of causation relating to possible toxic exposure.

Motor neuron disease is seen most commonly in middle age and above. The prototypical condition, amyotrophic lateral sclerosis (ALS), has symptoms that include progressive damage to lower motor neurons (flaccid paresis with atrophy) and upper motor neurons (spastic paresis with hyperreflexia and Babinski sign). It spares the pathways involved in bladder control. The condition may involve mostly brain stem muscles (bulbar palsy), sparing the eye muscles. In rare cases, the condition may only produce upper motor neuron signs ("primary lateral sclerosis"), although this diagnosis is controversial and should be used with great caution. Death in motor neuron disease usually results from failure of respiration and protective reflexes, as well as the general effects of debility.

There are variants of motor neuron disease. Some of these develop in infancy and childhood (spinal muscular atrophies). These go by a variety of names (Werdnig-Hoffmann disease, with the later-developing Wohlfart-Kugelberg-Welander type being the most common). These conditions are hereditary and are due to deficiencies in survival factors in motor neurons. More recently, many adult forms of progressive spinal muscular atrophy (some of which can be segmental and rather indolent) have been found to be due to lack of survival of motor neuron (SMN) protein, or the complex in which this protein participates. This has further reinforced enthusiasm for the possibility of a unifying cause of motor neuron disease. However, this has remained elusive.

Genetic

There are a growing number of genetic disorders that have myelopathy as a feature. Any condition that mainly affects the development of central nervous system myelin will have a component of myelopathy. This includes the early-life leukodystrophies, such as adrenoleukodystrophy and metachromatic leukodystrophy. These conditions are mostly recognized by their relatively early onset and progressive nature, while specific biological markers are used for definitive diagnosis. Of course, leukodystrophies affect many brain systems and their symptoms are usually dominated by involvement of the optic nerve, cortical white matter or cerebellar connections. These conditions will not be further considered in this chapter.

Spinocerebellar ataxias (degenerations) are a large and growing family of hereditary conditions that present with ataxia in late childhood through adulthood. Many of these disorders show pathology in spinal tracts as well as in the cerebellum. The best known of these are the autosomal dominant SCAs, where specific genes and, for many, gene products are known. This list is growing, and there are also autosomal recessive SCAs to add to the list. Despite the fact that may of these conditions do produce spinal cord pathology, for most of them this represents a minor and inconsistent part of their clinical presentation. However, for SCA-1 the myelopathic symptoms can be very prominent and this diagnosis enters into the differential of a slowly progressive myelopathy with severe ataxic symptoms.

Friedreich ataxia is an autosomal recessive condition that usually begins in late childhood, but whose onset can be delayed until early adulthood. Several spinal cord pathways are progressively damaged, including the dorsal columns and the lateral columns (upper motor neurons). After a reasonably normal early childhood, progressive clumsiness of gait and skeletal deformity (such as scoliosis) is noted, typically with progression to a wheelchair after about 10 years of symptoms. The gene product was found in 1996 to be a mitochondrial protein, frataxin. This leads to iron deposition in mitochondria and cell damage, and patients die from cardiomyopathy, typically 30-40 years after onset of symptoms.

Infectious

There are a large number of infectious conditions that affect the spinal cord or spinal cord tracts. Some of these involve tissues around the spinal cord (epidural abscess and meningitis) and some directly infect the cord (myelitis). Additionally, there may be postinfectious spinal cord involvement.

Epidural abscess is important to diagnose as early as possible, since this is treatable and can result in precipitous damage to the spinal cord. The epidural abscesses may result from extension of an infection of the spine (osteomyelitis) or intervertebral disc (discitis). The abscess can also develop *de novo* in the epidural space. Risk factors for epidural abscess include recent invasive procedure, infection elsewhere, or immunosuppression (including diabetes). The clinical presentation almost always involves back pain (often worse at night and not relieved by lying down), along with elevated ESR. Nerve roots may be involved (radiculitis). Remarkably, many of these patients do not have fever and some do not have elevated white blood cell counts. The source of infection may not be identified and, when it is, it can be a small abscess or dental infection. The organisms are usually staphylococci although anaerobes may also be present. One reason that this is so important to recognize as early as possible is that once neurologic signs and symptoms of myelopathy begin to develop, there can be very precipitous destruction of the cord (probably by damage of microcirculation, with subsequent infarction).

Tuberculosis can result in a somewhat more slowly evolving epidural abscess that is usually associated with adjacent spinal tuberculous osteomyelitis (Pott disease). Patients are typically somewhat immunocompromised, but do not necessarily have apparent pulmonary disease.

Meningitis (discussed in the section on infectious diseases) can damage the spinal cord and nerve roots. This damage usually corresponds to the severity of the inflammation and an associated inflammatory vasculitis can further compromise the cord.

Intramedullary infections run the gamut from bacterial and fungal infections to parasitic infections and infections with viruses. Additionally, the symptoms may result from direct action of the organism or as a postinfectious, presumably immune-mediated phenomenon.

Bacterial infections of the spinal cord are uncommon. Granulomas can result from hematogenous spread of tuberculosis or brucellosis. Additionally, infections of adjacent structures can invade the spinal cord, resulting in abscess formation.

Spirocheteal diseases such a neurosyphilis and Lyme disease can produce myelopathy. *Treponema pallidum*, the causative agent for syphilis, can affect the spinal cord either by producing a meningomyelitis or tabes dorsalis, which was once the most common spinal cord infection. Syphilitic meningomyelitis usually produces a slowly progressive spastic weakness (sometimes mimicking spondylotic myelopathy). While the characteristic symptoms of tabes dorsalis are sensory, tabes dorsalis is also slowly progressive and is due to infection of sensory neurons of the dorsal root ganglion (which is why it is often associated with shooting pains and diminished reflexes). The dorsal columns degenerate because these tracts arise from large neurons of the dorsal root ganglia. Loss of normal sensation often results in injury to skin, bones and joints (Charçot joints).

Myelopathy in lyme disease is reported, although it is quite rare. It appears in three main types: acute transverse myelitis; as part of a meningomyelitis; or as a chronic myelopathy. Fungal infections of the spinal cord are not common and, when they occur, usually exist as an extension of fungal meningitis or from adjacent epidural or spinal infections. *Cryptococcus*, *Blastomycetes*, *Aspergillus* and *Coccidioides* are all potential pathogens and are more likely in patients who are immunosuppressed. These infections can produce symptoms by extrinsic compression from fungal abscesses, by directly invading the spinal cord, or by producing a vasculitis.

Parasitic myelopathy is rare in the developed world, with the occasional exception of invasion of the spinal cord by *Toxoplasma gondii* in patients with AIDS. In Asia, South America and Africa, infections with schistosomes (via contact with contaminated water that contains infected snails) can infect the cord. The dog tapeworm (*Echinococcus granulosis*) or the pork tapeworm (*Taenia solium*) can cause cysts in the spinal cord or infect the adjacent spine with potential abscess. Pork tapeworms are most common in Latin America and they most often produce cysts in the brain.

Viral infections of the spinal cord are more common than bacterial, fungal or parasitic infections. Immunocompromised individuals are at particular risk and these infections are a feared complication of HIV/AIDS. Vacuolar myelopathy is a condition associated with infection by the HIV virus. The pathology of vacuolar myelopathy probably results from activation of inflammatory cells with high concentrations of inflammatory cytokines. Only a small percentage of patients show actual presence of the virus in the site of lesions. There is some recent evidence that there is disturbance of vitamin B_{12} metabolic pathways, and this may explain the predilection for dorsal and lateral columns of the cord (as with subacute combined degeneration see below). This condition usually presents as subacute myelopathy with paraparesis with or without sensory loss. Occasionally, it can be quite asymmetrical. The bladder is usually involved and incontinence of urine and stool is common. This must be distinguished from cytomegalovirus infection, which can be treated by antiviral agents.

Other herpes viruses (including varicella zoster and herpes simplex type 2) are known to produce myelopathy in rare cases. In some cases this occurs during the appearance of classic viral radiculitis, with the virus extending centrally from the dorsal root ganglion. In other cases (including the Epstein-Barr virus and cytomegalovirus), classic transverse myelitis can occur during primary infection. In the case of the herpes viruses, specific antiviral agents should be employed for treatment.

Enteroviruses can produce myelopathy. The prototypical infection in the group is with poliovirus. When this virus attacks the nervous system, it usually produces meningitis, which may or may not progress to involvement of lower motor neurons. If it does damage anterior horn neurons, it produces flaccid paresis with no sensory involvement. The lack of sensory loss with poliomyelitis is an important distinguishing feature between polio and Güillain-Barré syndrome.

Tropical spastic paraparesis is the result of infection with HTLV-1 virus. This retrovirus is transmitted sexually, parenterally and vertically (mother to infant). The condition is characterized by a chronic and progressive spastic paraparesis along with a spastic bladder. While it is endemic to Asia, it has been a growing concern in other portions of the world, especially Africa and the Caribbean. The pool of individuals infected with the virus is also increasing in the United States, although only about 1:250 will go on to develop symptoms of myelopathy. There is no definitive treatment for this condition although many small trials of antiviral and anti-inflammatory treatments have been attempted.

Transverse myelitis is a syndrome characterized by acutely evolving myelopathy. This syndrome has several causes, and these are not always easy to distinguish at the outset. Although transverse myelitis is often a monophasic, demyelinative illness that follows an infection, it may be the first manifestation of multiple sclerosis or Devic disease (neuromyelitis optica), and a search for other white matter lesions and serology for neuromyelitis optica would be appropriate (see below). The syndrome can also develop as a paraneoplastic process or in cases of rheumatologic disease (such as SLE, Sjögren syndrome and mixed connective tissue disease) and granulomatous disease (such as sarcoidosis). Many cases are post-infectious and, in these cases, infection is usually viral or with mycoplasma. Typically, symptoms begin 4 days to 3 weeks after the infection, though they can be coincident. In some instances transverse myelitis may be due to direct spinal cord infection. These cases are more likely to have pain (due to inflammation of the meninges) and are more likely to have significant numbers of white cells in the spinal fluid (postinfectious causes often have elevated protein and some lymphocytes). In cases of suspected infection with the herpes virus group, PCR may help determine whether specific antiviral agents would be indicated. The presence of pain and fever as well as a high and mixed white count in CSF are all clues to suggest acute infectious transverse myelitis. With more intensive investigation, a cause is often identified. However there are still cases of "idiopathic" transverse myelitis.

Treatment is supportive, unless there is a specific virus present for which antiviral therapy may be effective (such as for herpes viruses). The prognosis of transverse myelitis correlates with the length of the affected spinal cord and with the concentration of inflammatory markers in the spinal fluid.

Due to the rapid onset of symptoms in transverse myelitis, usually reaching a peak in 4-21 days, it is common that there is flaccid paraplegia and an atonic urinary bladder with urinary retention. However, as symptoms persist, spasticity (of limbs as well as bladder) usually develops. In the great majority of cases it is necessary to rule out epidural spinal cord compression (from tumor, abscess or hematoma) since these will require different treatment.

Congenital/Developmental Disease

The most common congenital abnormality of the spinal cord is spina bifida. This may exist as an isolated defect in the posterior connective tissue of the spine (spina bifida occulta), which is of no neurological significance, or there may be a meningeal cyst (meningocele) that can contain the spinal cord (meningomyelocele). In the latter case, there are almost always neurological sequellae that depend on the particular level of the lesion. In rare cases, the spinal cord itself may fail to close and can be exposed (rachishisis). This is incompatible with neurologic function of the lower part of the cord and is often associated with other neurologic abnormalities.

Tethered cord can develop as a result of congenital abnormalities of the lower spine (such as a lipoma of the filum terminale), or may be acquired as a result of scarring from infection or from early spinal procedures (such as repair of a meningocele). The usual findings are progressive gait abnormality with a variable mix of signs of myelopathy (spasticity, hyper-reflexia, Babinski sign, spastic bladder), and radiculopathy (radiating pain, diminished reflexes, atonic bladder). Imaging to determine the precise location of the conus medullaris (normally at the L1 level) is the best initial test. This may also show an abnormality that may or may not be amenable to surgical treatment.

A syrinx is a cystic dilation of the central canal of the spinal cord, often associated with abnormality at the foramen magnum (such as Chiari malformation) or with other cord lesions (such as intramedullary tumors). It is attractive to suppose that the lesion is obstructing the free passage of fluid through the central canal, resulting in pressure dilation of the syrinx. This is particularly true since correction of a Chiari malformation (when one exists) may produce some degree of resolution of neurologic symptoms. Also, shunting of large syrinx cavities (usually into the subarachnoid space, though sometimes into the peritoneal cavity) may also be helpful. However, this theory remains unproven.

The classic picture of a syrinx results from damage to the anterior white commissure since this is immediately adjacent to the central canal. This commissure is the location of decussation of fibers conveying pain and temperature sensations from the several spinal segments below the lesion. Therefore, a loss of pain and temperature sense extending for several dermatomal segments below the level of lesion would be expected, while touch sensation would be preserved. The patient may unknowingly injure him- or herself, especially with hot items. This has been termed a *suspended sensory loss or vest-like sensory loss*, because the lower part of the body is spared.

This classic presentation for syringomyelia is not all that common. Damage to anterior horn cells (amyotrophy) or even of dorsal horn with neuropathic pain are also potential presentations. In this era of MRI scans, benign syrinxes are increasingly identified and some have been shown to resolve over time. Whenever a syrinx is identified, it is critical to consider whether it is secondary to another condition. In addition to being associated with Chiari malformation, it may result from trauma or intramedullary tumor. When it is associated with Chiari malformation, it may resolve following treatment directed at the Chiari malformation.

Inflammatory Disease

Several inflammatory conditions produce myelopathy. The prototypical inflammatory disease of the spinal cord is multiple sclerosis. The spinal cord is a frequent target of MS and myelopathy may be the initial presentation. Sensory or motor tracts can be involved, as can descending control pathways for the bladder, resulting in a spastic bladder (with urge incontinence) or bladder dysynergia. MS should not involve anterior horn cells, and the finding of amyotrophy points to alternative diagnoses.

MS only very rarely results in radicular pain, so symptoms suggestive of radiculopathy would also point to the need for further investigation.

Acute disseminated encephalomyelitis (ADEM) is an acute demyelinating disorder of the central nervous system. It is a monphasic illness with multiple inflammatory white matter lesions that often include the spinal cord. By analogy with animal studies, this appears to be a T-cell mediated immune response to myelin basic protein that may be triggered by infection or inoculation. CSF can be normal, or it may show inflammatory markers. While the inflammatory markers are not distinct from those in MS, there is more likely to be a substantially elevated lymphocyte count and there is a lower frequency of oligoclonal bands. As in MS, the CSF can be completely normal. While the initial attack can be quite severe, patients usually show good to excellent recovery over time. There is no distinctive biomarker that will distinguish the condition from a first episode of MS, and these patients are often treated as a first exacerbation (with immune modifying therapy). It is still controversial how many of these patients will go on to develop classic MS.

There is an acute demyelinative myelopathy called *neuromyelitis optica* (NMO, Devic), which is more common in Asia, especially Japan. Although at one time it was considered to be a variant of MS, it is now thought to be a separate condition. NMO is characterized by the acute onset of optic neuritis and myelopathy affecting the long tracts of the spinal cord. The condition follows any one of several courses. It may be fulminant and fatal, it can be monophasic (often with significant recovery), it may follow relapsing-remitting course (usually with progressive disability), or it can be progressive. Bilateral optic neuritis should raise suspicion of this condition (although this is still more common in MS). Additional features that would suggest NMO rather than MS include pain at onset, bilateral cord involvement and high cell count in CSF, although none of these definitively indicate NMO. Most cases have a serum autoantibody (NMO-IgG), which appears to target the aquaphorin-4 channel. This fixes complement and triggers inflammation. The finding of the antibody is highly specific for NMO.

The prognosis of NMO is very guarded. Patients with progressive or relapsing NMO have been tried on a variety of immune modulating treatments (including plasmapheresis, IVIg, and some of the agents that have been effective in MS). However, despite some positive case reports and small series, the effects of treatment remain uncertain.

NMO must be distinguished from other causes of white matter disease including ADEM, rheumatologic conditions (such as Sjögren syndrome, mixed connective tissue disorder, antiphospholipid antibody syndrome and SLE), since treatment would differ in these conditions. It should also be distinguished from viral infection (described above).

There are several other systemic inflammatory conditions that can present with inflammatory spinal cord lesions. These conditions enter into the differential diagnosis of MS, but they arc usually recognized by their involvement of other organ systems or other parts of the nervous system. In the relatively rare case where the spinal cord is the only site of lesion, diagnosis can be extremely difficult. Both celiac disease and Whipple disease, which are classically inflammatory disorders of the gastrointestinal tract, can produce myelopathy. Often there are other foci of central nervous system disease. Neurosarcoid is an idiopathic condition characterized by multifocal granulomatous disease. In some cases central nervous system manifestations can occur without other systemic disease and biopsy may be the only definitive test. Treatment of these other inflammatory myelopathies is quite different from the management of MS and therefore they should be considered in the differential.

Toxic/Metabolic Disease

The prototypical nutritional deficiency affecting the spinal cord is subacute combined degeneration (*posterolateral sclerosis*). This may or may not be associated with pernicious anemia (it appears that different metabolic pathways are involved in nervous system and hematopoetic effects of vitamin B12). Deficiency usually results from poor absorption of the vitamin rather than actual dietary insufficiency. Spinal cord involvement is usually symmetrical and symptoms begin with paresthesias in the legs, often extending onto the trunk. Later, ataxia, weakness of the legs and finally spasticity develop. This progression can evolve over weeks to months and may be quite rapid in some patients. Diagnosis can be complicated by a polyneuropathy which may be ascribed a role in some of the early paresthesias. It has a proclivity for affecting the cortical descending tracts, producing spastic, upper motor neuron weakness. It also affects the dorsal columns, producing loss of epicritic sensations, including joint position and vibratory sense and impairing two-point discrimination.

Direct vitamin B_{12} assay has been the most common test for deficiency. However, there are many documented cases of deficiency with normal B_{12} levels and without anemia. This has led some authors to recommend measures of methylmalonic acid and homocystine, since B_{12} is a cofactor in metabolism of these compounds. However, it is not clear that this metabolic pathway is the one that is responsible for symptoms and therefore it is not entirely clear that these are the most direct tests of deficiency. Nonetheless, recognition of B_{12} deficiency is important since the nervous system symptoms are largely reversible if identified early, especially in the first few weeks.

Other nutritional deficiencies producing myelopathy have been reported from time to time. For example, it has recently been reported that copper deficiency can produce a syndrome virtually identical to the subacute combined degeneration of B_{12} deficiency. Also, severe vitamin E deficiency has been shown to produce a myeloneuropathy. Fortunately, most of these deficiencies are quite rare and the clinical picture is often dominated by other symptoms of the deficiency.

Cuban epidemic neuropathy was a condition identified in the early 1990s in an isolated part of the island. It was determined to be due to nutritional deficiency, and was characterized by optic neuropathy, sensory and autonomic peripheral neuropathy, neural deafness, and myelopathy.

Various toxins have been associated with myelopathy. These roughly fall into the categories of drugs of abuse, medications, poisons and environmental toxins. Chronic abusers of nitrous oxide frequently develop myelopathy, probably on the basis of ischemia of the cord. Heroin abusers may also develop the condition, possibly due to injection of an adulterant. Certain medications that are administered intrathecally are known to potentially produce myelopathy. These include intrathecal methotrexate or amphotericin B and the effect may also be by damage to blood vessels.

Strychnine is a poison used primarily to kill rodents. It binds to glycine receptors (the primary inhibitory transmitter in the spinal cord), blocking the receptors. Therefore, poisoning results in overactivity of neurons, causing spasm and failure of normal functions. There is little actual tissue destruction. On the other hand, chronic intake of a toxin from cycad seeds has been shown to result in the ALS-Parkinson-dementia complex of Guam (see above). This has led to concerns that toxins may contribute to other neurodegenerative disorders.

7. Cauda Equina and Neurogenic Claudication

Cauda equina lesions are not, technically, related to spinal cord disease. However, they often coexist with myelopathies and may present symptoms that have to be distinguished from myelopathy. The cauda equina consists of lumbosacral nerve roots arising from the lower portion of the spinal cord that pass caudally to reach the intervertebral foramina. These roots can be damaged by space-occupying lesions below the end of the spinal cord, which is around the L1-2 level. It is critical to identify these lesions early (bilateral sciatica, loss of sensations in the buttocks, or loss of rectal tone are important signs).

A special case is lumbar spinal stenosis, which may result in the syndrome of neurogenic claudication. This syndrome occurs with narrowing of the vertebral canal either congenitally or due to degenerative arthritis accompanied by some intervertebral disc bulging. Most often there is a combination of some congenital narrowing along with the degenerative changes.

Relatively light pressure on the cauda equina nerve roots results in impairment of circulation, with blockage first of venous flow and, later, of arterial. The effect of this compression is magnified when there are several levels of compression (as there often are) since this impairs flow into a segment of nerve root from both sides, producing an ischemic segment. This compression is worst when the individual stands and particularly when extending the spine (since this further narrows the vertebral canal and also causes some additional disc bulging). Therefore, patients have symptoms that worsen as they stand, but that are fairly promptly relieved by forward flexion. Riding a bicycle is usually quite comfortable even though walking may be progressively limited. Walking uphill (due to a natural forward lean into a hill) is often easier than walking downhill.

The most common symptoms of neurogenic claudication are heaviness and fatigue of the legs, often accompanied by an aching discomfort in the calves while standing or walking. There may be some paresthesias, especially in the L5 dermatome. The lower extremity symptoms are usually bilateral, while vascular claudication is more often unilateral. Although there is no definitive diagnostic test (imaging may show narrowing that is inconclusive in terms of clinical significance), the diagnosis is usually based on all of the elements of the syndrome, including provocative and relieving factors.

8. Conclusion

In summary, while the recognition of myelopathy is usually quite easy (based on a combination of signs and symptoms of damage to long tracts as well as to gray matter and nerve roots), the etiology is often unclear. It is important to be systematic, considering the potential etiologic entities, including: neoplastic; traumatic; degenerative; infectious; hemorrhagic; inflammatory; toxic/metabolic; and vascular. Although the investigations may be extensive, the reward for proper diagnosis is often identification of a treatable condition that would produce severe deficits if left to follow its natural course.

9. References

1. Swenson RS. The evaluation of low back pain: A reasonable approach. *Neurologic Clinics of NA*. 1999;17:43-63.

   (This is a discussion of the differential diagnosis of low back pain and the red and yellow flags useful in its assessment.)

2. Loblaw DA, Perry J, Chambers A, Laperriere NJ. Systematic review of the diagnosis and management of malignant extradural spinal cord compression: the Cancer Care Ontario Practice Guidelines Initiative's Neuro-Oncology Disease Site Group. *J Clin Oncol*. 2005;23:2028-37.

   (This is a recent, state-of-the-art review of the evaluation and management of epidural spinal cord compression.)

3. Bluman EM, Palumbo MA, Lucas PR. Spinal epidural abscess in adults. *J Am Acad Orthop Surg*. 2004;12:155-63.

   (This is a recent discussion on the spectrum of evaluation and management of epidural abscess.)

4. Bataller L, Dalmau J. Paraneoplastic neurologic syndromes: approaches to diagnosis and treatment. *Semin Neurol*. 2003;23:215-24.

   (This is an excellent review of paraneoplastic disease of the spinal cord.)

5. Behin A, Delattre JY. Complications of radiation therapy on the brain and spinal cord. *Semin Neurol*. 2004;24:405-17.

   (This article reviews the literature on radiation myelopathy.)

6. Sekhon LH, Fehlings MG. Epidemiology, demographics, and pathophysiology of acute spinal cord injury. *Spine*. 2001;26(24 Suppl):S2-12.

   (This is a review of the literature on spinal cord injury.)

7. Bracken MB. Steroids for acute spinal cord injury. *Cochrane Database Syst Rev*. 2002;(3):CD001046.

   (This review takes a critical look at the evidence for a weak effect of steroids on the outcome of spinal cord injury.)

8. Schmidt MH, Quinones-Hinojosa A, Rosenberg WS. Cervical myelopathy associated with degenerative spine disease and ossification of the posterior longitudinal ligament. *Semin Neurol*. 2002;22:143-48.

   (This article reviews the pathophysiology and treatment of spondylotic myelopathy.)

9. Caragine LP Jr, Halbach VV, Ng PP, Dowd CF. Vascular myelopathies-vascular malformations of the spinal cord: presentation and endovascular surgical management. *Semin Neurol*. 2002;22:123-32.

   (This review article describes the evaluation and management of vascular malformations of the spinal cord.)

10. Schols L, Bauer P, Schmidt T, Schulte T, Riess O. Autosomal dominant cerebellar ataxias: clinical features, genetics, and pathogenesis. *Lancet Neurol*. 2004;3:291-304.

    (This is a well-written recent review of the state of the art in understanding of inherited ataxias.)

11. Voncken M, Ioannou P, Delatycki MB. Friedreich ataxia-update on pathogenesis and possible therapies. *Neurogenetics*. 2004;5:1-8.

    (This review focuses on mechanisms of pathology of Friedreich ataxia.)

12. Berger JR, Sabet A. Infectious myelopathies. *Semin Neurol*. 2002;22(2):133-42.

    (This is an excellent review of infectious diseases of the spinal cord.)

13. Kaplin A, Krishnan C, Deshpande D, Pardo C, Kerr D. Diagnosis and management of acute myelopathies. *The Neurologist*. 2005;11:2-18.

(This article summarizes the evaluation and management of transverse myelitis.)

14. Yamada S, Won DJ, Siddiqi J, Yamada SM. Tethered cord syndrome: overview of diagnosis and treatment. *Neurol Res*. 2004;26: 719-21.

(This is an excellent review of the pathophysiology and clinical aspects of tethered cord syndrome.)

15. Levine DN. The pathogenesis of syringomyelia associated with lesions at the foramen magnum: a critical review of existing theories and proposal of a new hypothesis. *J Neurol Sci*. 2004;220:3-21.

(An interesting discussion of the state of current understanding of syringomyelia.)

16. Binder DK, Schmidt MH, Weinstein PR. Lumbar spinal stenosis. *Semin Neurol*. 2002;22:157-66.

(This review article considers the presentation, evaluation and treatment of lumbar spinal stenosis.)

10. Questions

1. Which of the following is least likely to indicate myelopathy?

A. Pinprick sensory level on the trunk

B. Hyperreflexia in the lower extremity with normal upper extremity reflexes

C. Stocking distribution of paresthesia

D. Atrophy and fasciculations in both hands

E. Urge incontinence of urine

2. Most back pain is due to:

A. Musculoskeletal causes

B. Neoplastic causes

C. Infectious causes

D. Inflammatory causes

E. Vascular causes

3. A 45-year-old diabetic woman presents with three days of severe mid-thoracic back pain. The back pain awakened her from sleep. She tried to get out of bed and fell to the floor. She was incontinent of urine. In considering the possibility of epidural abscess, which of the following is true?

A. The erythrocyte sedimentation rate is almost always elevated

B. There is almost always a high fever

C. A normal white blood cell count rules out epidural abscess

D. There is an obvious focus of infection elsewhere in the body in almost all cases

E. There are obvious signs of meningial infection in virtually all cases

4. A 52-year-old woman had a history of adenocarcinoma of the breast treated five years ago with lumpectomy and radiation to the left breast and axilla. She had two weeks of new, gradually increasing upper thoracic back pain. Regarding the possibility of malignant extramedullary spinal cord compression (EMSCC):

A. EMSCC usually results from primary tumors of the spine

B. Back pain is the most common early symptom

C. This is always associated with direct metastasis to vertebrae

D. Back pain is highly predictive of EMSCC

E. Myelopathy is very slowly progressive

5. Which of the following is NOT correct regarding intramedullary spinal cord tumors:

A. They are usually not painful

B. Findings of myelopathy may be the first signs or symptoms

C. Ependymomas may be intramedullary

D. Most of them are metastatic

E. There may be a "suspended" sensory loss

6. Which of the following is the most likely location for a meningioma?

A. Extradural/extramedullary

B. Intradural/extramedullary

C. Intradural/intramedullary

D. Extradural/intramedullary

7. Which of the following symptoms would be the most helpful in distinguishing an intradural/extramedullary lesion from an intramedullary lesion?

A. Spasticity in the legs

B. Spastic bladder

C. Sensory level on the trunk

D. Radicular pain

E. Upgoing toes

8. A 28-year-old man with a history of Hodgkin disease treated 18 months ago with chemotherapy and radiation presented with one month of dysesthesias in both lower limbs and more recent difficulty "tripping over things." Exam showed decreased pin and temperature sense in both lower limbs with no clear sensory level. There was spastic weakness of both lower extremities with upgoing toes and hyperactive reflexes at the knees and ankles, bilaterally. Which of the following is false concerning the possibility of radiation myelitis?

A. It usually involves the ventral and lateral columns of the spinal cord

B. It is easily distinguished from other forms of myelopathy by conventional MRI scans

C. It rarely develops before six months from the time of treatment

D. In most cases the symptoms are slowly progressive

E. Cerebrospinal fluid findings are non-specific

9. A 72-year-old man presented with slowly progressive ataxia. He was found to have spasticity in both lower extremities with hyperactive lower extremity reflexes and bilateral upgoing toes. He also had loss of vibratory and position sense of both great toes. You correctly think of possible spondylotic myelopathy. Concerning this diagnosis:

A. It usually develops in the upper cervical region

B. It is usually acute in onset

C. It can stabilize for many years

D. It is always associated with ossification of the posterior longitudinal ligament

E. It is a surgical emergency

10. Which of the following is not a known risk factor for epidural hematoma?

A. Sickle cell anemia

B. Anticoagulation

C. Trauma

D. Spinal procedures

E. Extradural vascular malformation

11. A 62-year-old man undergoes surgery for an abdominal aortic aneurysm. In the recovery room he is noted to be unable to move his lower limbs and could not feel pinprick over his lower limbs. In considering possible anterior spinal artery syndrome, this condition usually spares:

A. Temperature sense in the buttocks

B. Bladder control

C. Strength of the legs

D. Conscious proprioception in the legs

E. Pin sensitivity

12. Which of the following is the most likely candidate for dural A-V fistula?

A. 5-year-old boy

B. 14-year-old girl

C. 50-year-old man

D. 80-year-old woman

E. 22-year-old man

13. A 57-year-old woman presented with several months of gradually increasing clumsiness of gait and weakness of the arms (left greater than right). Diffuse fasciculations were visible in the muscles of both shoulders and upper limbs and atrophy was most evident in intrinsic muscles of the left hand. Which finding would call the diagnosis of amyotrophic lateral sclerosis into question?

A. Urinary urge incontinence

B. Fasciculations in intercostal muscles

C. Spasticity in the legs

D. Bilateral upgoing toes

E. Atrophy of shoulder girdle muscles

14. A 14-year-old boy was brought in by his mother because his gait appeared to be worsening. His early development was normal and his 2 other siblings were normal. He appeared otherwise healthy except for a scoliosis and very high arches in the feet. In considering the possibility of Friedreich ataxia, all the following are correct EXCEPT:

A. Children are usually normal in early childhood

B. It is autosomal dominant

C. The abnormal gene product is known

D. The problem is with mitochondrial functions

E. Dorsal and lateral columns are usually affected

15. Which of the following is most likely to indicate that acute paraplegia is due to acute traumatic myelopathy rather than traumatic cauda equina syndrome:

A. Lower extremity radiculopathic pain

B. Urinary incontinence

C. Flaccid weakness

D. Sensory level at the umbilicus

E. Loss of pin sensitivity in the buttocks

16. The primary area of infection in tabes dorsalis is:

A. Lumbosacral dorsal root ganglia

B. Thoracic gray matter

C. Cervical white matter

D. Central canal

E. Peripheral ends of nerves to feet

17. A 32-year-old man with HIV/AIDS, currently on antiretroviral therapy was tripping and falling when he would walk in the park near his house. In considering the diagnosis of vacuolar myelopathy:

A. It is always symmetrical

B. It is easily distinguished from cytomegalovirus myelopathy

C. It often produces incontinence, including of stool

D. It presents acutely, with deterioration in hours to days

E. HIV virus can always be identified from the lesions

18. HTLV-1:

A. Produces a myelopathy that is more rapidly progressive than that associated with HIV

B. Is not found in Europe or North America

C. Invariably produces myelopathy in infected individuals

D. Is caused by a retrovirus

E. Spares bladder function

19. Concerning syringomyelia, all of the following are true, EXCEPT:

A. It is often associated with other congenital abnormalities or structural cord lesions

B. It can present with a picture of amyotrophy of intrinsic hand muscles

C. It typically abolishes sensitivity in a saddle distribution early in it course

D. It often results in unrecognized injury

E. It may be associated with intraspinal neoplasms

20. Neuromyelitis optica:

A. Is simply a first onset of multiple sclerosis targeting specific parts of the nervous system

B. Is almost always a benign and self-limited condition

C. Is more likely to be painful at the onset than multiple sclerosis

D. Usually has fewer white cells in the spinal fluid than multiple sclerosis

E. Always affects the spinal cord before damaging the optic nerves

21. There are several rheumatologic conditions that can produce myelopathy. Many of these appear to have their effect by producing a vasculitis. Which of the following is least likely to be associated with a vasculitis of the cord?

A. Rheumatoid arthritis

B. Mixed connective tissue disorder

C. Systemic lupus erythematosis

D. Sjögren syndrome

22. A 68-year-old woman had bariatric surgery 10 years ago. She noted that she was having increased difficulty with gait. You consider the possibility of subacute combined degeneration. This condition:

A. Always shows low serum vitamin B_{12} levels

B. Almost always starts with sensory symptoms

C. Almost always has an associated anemia

D. Almost always is irreversible

E. Almost always affects bladder function

23. A 75-year-old woman comes to clinic with a principal complaint of bilateral lower extremity pain with walking. She has to sit down after about two blocks due to aching and "heaviness." Her legs feel much better after a few minutes of sitting. She has had normal vascular studies of her lower extremities. Which of the following is most suggestive of symptomatic lumbar spinal stenosis?

A. Symptoms that are worse when pushing a cart than walking on the level

B. Symptoms that are brought on by walking but completely relieved by standing in one place

C. Greater lower extremity symptoms walking downhill than uphill

D. Symptoms provoked by walking that are restricted to one leg

E. Associated loss of bowel control

Answers

1. C.
All the listed symptoms are common in myelopathy with the exception of stocking distribution of paresthesia. This is much more common in peripheral neuropathies. The pinprick's sensory level on the trunk suggests damage to spinothalamic tract, while hyperreflexia in the lower extremities suggests damage to upper motor neurons. Atrophy with prominent fasciculations suggests a process damaging anterior horn cells, and urge incontinence of urine indicates damage to descending bladder control tracts.

2. A.
The vast majority of back pain is musculoskeletal in origin. Unfortunately, rare cases of more severe conditions must be considered. Using red and yellow flags to try to detect patients requiring further investigation may be a fruitful approach to selecting patients for further investigation.

3. A.
Epidural abscess may be very difficult to diagnose in patients. Typically there is some level of immunosuppression (including, possibly, diabetes mellitus). Despite the infectious nature of the condition, white blood cell count may be normal and fever is typically low-grade or absent. The remote infection may be occult and may consist of dental abscesses or infections in other relatively hidden sites. It is rare that meninges are involved sufficiently to produce meningeal signs and it would be very rare that the infection spreads to the subarachnoid space. However, damage to the spinal cord can occur quite rapidly.

4. B.
Malignant extramedullary spinal cord compression is a feared complication of metastatic cancer. Back pain is the most common early symptom, though the significance of the pain may not be recognized. While the metastasis is often to the vertebrae (and may be visible on x-rays) it may also be to the epidural space. The myelopathy may progress very rapidly once the cord begins to be affected. Fortunately, even in patients with cancer, most back pain is not due to metastasis. Nonetheless, a high index of suspicion must be maintained in this group.

5. D.
Intramedullary spinal cord tumors are rare. They are usually primary tumors of the cord, such as ependymomas or gliomas. They are usually not painful and usually result in a myelopathy that may include a suspended sensory loss, indicating damage to crossing spinothalamic tract fibers.

6. B.
Meningiomas appear as intradural, extramedullary space occupying lesions. Some nerve root sheath tumors appear in the same location and should be considered in the differential of intradural extramedullary masses.

7. D.
Extramedullary masses are much more likely to damage nerve roots, thereby producing radicular pain, than are intramedullary masses. Intramedullary masses are typically painless. Otherwise, symptoms of myelopathy may be the same in both extramedullary and intramedullary space occupying lesions.

8. B.
Radiation myelitis typically occurs as a delayed complication of radiation therapy (usually greater than six months). This condition may be quite challenging to diagnose since symptoms are similar to other slowly progressive myelopathies. Cerebrospinal fluid findings do not help much, other than ruling out infectious causes.

9. C.
Spondylotic myelopathy is a condition that typically develops due to degenerative changes in the cervical spine, though it may be contributed to by congenital stenosis as well as conditions such as ossification of the posterior longitudinal ligament. He is usually insidious and can stabilize for many years. Surgical treatment is somewhat controversial, unless there is clear evidence of progression or symptoms are severe.

10. A.
Sickle cell anemia is not a known risk factor for epidural hematoma. Anticoagulation and other bleeding dyscrasias are risk factors. Epidural hematoma can also be due to trauma or spinal procedures (including lumbar puncture). Extradural vascular malformations also can contribute on rare occasions.

11. D.
Anterior spinal artery syndrome typically involves the anterior two-thirds of the spinal cord. This usually spares the dorsal columns, with preserved vibratory sense, joint position sense, and well-localized touch. Spinothalamic tract and upper motor neurons are usually involved and produce the predominant symptoms below the level of damage.

12. C.
Dural arteriovenous fistulas typically become symptomatic in middle-aged men.

13. A.
Amyotrophic lateral sclerosis does not affect bladder control. It typically damages upper and lower motor neurons with signs of spasticity, increased reflexes and upgoing toes in the lower extremities and fasciculations and atrophy in regions of lower motor neurons involvement. The condition spares sensory tracts and those that control the bladder and bowel.

14. B.
Friedreich ataxia is an autosomal recessive condition. The abnormal gene product is known and mitochondrial functions are affected. The symptoms are typically due to abnormality in the dorsal and lateral columns of the spinal cord, and cerebellar signs are also prominent. Early development is typically normal before slowly progressive symptoms begin. Patients usually die in their middle ages due to cardiomyopathy.

15. D.
Acute traumatic myelopathy and cauda equina syndrome share many similarities. However, sensory level at the umbilicus would indicate damage at the T10 level or above. This is well above the level of the cauda equina. Although chronic spinal cord injury would be expected to produce spasticity, acute injury to the cord often produces spinal cord shock with decreased reflexes and flaccidity. Loss of pin sensitivity in the buttock region could be due to either a myelopathy or cauda equina syndrome and radiculopathy in the lower extremities is more likely the result of cauda equina syndrome nerve root involvement.

16. A.
The primary site of infection in tabes dorsalis is the sensory neurons in the dorsal root ganglia. Damage to the larger of these neurons will result in degeneration of the dorsal columns, from whence the condition receives its name. However, small sensory neurons can also be damaged, producing loss of pain and temperature sense as the condition progresses. This is often associated with lancinating, neuropathic pain.

17. C.
Vacuolar myelopathy is a relatively common condition with HIV/AIDS, though autopsy studies have indicated it can be subclinical. This condition does not appear to be the direct result of viral infection, but rather to activation of inflammatory mediators that are the cause of the damage. Incontinence is common, and the myelopathic symptoms may be quite asymmetrical. Deterioration is typically of a subacute nature, and the condition may be difficult to distinguish from other, more treatable causes of myelopathy immunocompromised individuals.

18. D.

Tropical spastic paraparesis results from viral infection with the HTLV-1 virus. The condition is characterized by a chronic and progressive spastic weakness along with neurogenic bladder. Actually most individuals infected with the virus are asymptomatic. Despite its name, it can be found in all parts of the world.

19. C.

Syringomyelia is a condition characterized by cystic dilatation of the central canal of the spinal cord. The classic clinical picture is one of suspended sensory loss with loss of sensitivity to pain and temperature around the level of the cystic cavity, with sparing of sensations below. The "saddle" distribution is the last to be affected. Patients may injure themselves without being aware due to loss of pain and temperature sense. The condition may damage other elements of the spinal cord including anterior motor neurons. A search for congenital abnormalities, such as Chiari malformation, may provide a target for treatment. Syrinx cavities may also be seen due to other cord abnormalities such as neoplasms, presumably by blocking spinal fluid pathways.

20. C.

Neuromyelitis optica is a condition that was once thought to be closely associated with multiple sclerosis. The condition now appears to be an immune attack on the spinal cord and optic nerves by other mechanisms, since specific antibodies can usually be detected in the blood. This condition may be quite severe and recurrent and there are no definitive treatments. It usually has a higher white cell count than seen with multiple sclerosis and painful bilateral optic neuritis is often the earliest symptom.

21. A.

The vasculitis associated with rheumatoid arthritis is not associated with damage to the spinal cord (although instability of the cervical spine due to this condition can produce a traumatic myelopathy). Other rheumatologic conditions, including systemic lupus erythmatosis, Sjögren syndrome, and mixed connective tissue disorder are more likely to do this, though myelopathy is a rare presentation of any of these conditions.

22. B.

Subacute combined degeneration results from deficiency of vitamin B_{12}, even though vitamin B_{12} levels in the blood may be within normal limits. It's not clear exactly what metabolic pathway is most responsible for the myelopathy, however. Surrogate markers, including methylmalonic acid and homocysteine, have been recommended. This condition may not have an associated anemia, especially in the face of adequate folate levels. In the developed world this is usually the result of poor absorption, rather than insufficient intake. Early on, the symptoms are quite reversible, though permanent damage may occur as the condition progresses. This progression may be rapid in some cases though it is usually subacute. Typically, bladder function is spared at the outset, with damage being most evident in sensory tracts of the dorsal columns and, later, in upper motor neurons of the lateral column.

23. C.

Neurogenic claudication has some important distinctions from vascular claudication. Typically, symptoms are relieved, promptly when sitting down or flexing the spine, and patients are able to walk better while leaning forward. Patients naturally lean forward while pushing something or while walking uphill (so these are comfortable actions). Standing erect, even in one place, does not relieve the symptoms, while bending forward (such as by sitting) does. Symptoms of neurogenic claudication are more likely to be bilateral than are symptoms of vascular claudication. Neurogenic claudication does not affect bladder or bowel control (which may suggest cauda equina syndrome).

Chapter 21: Epilepsy in Adults

Vijay M. Thadani, MD

Contents

1. Introduction

The word epilepsy is derived from a Greek word meaning "to seize." Many primitive cultures shared the belief that during an epileptic seizure the victim was seized by an external and possibly divine force. Thus, we are quite unhistorical if we speak of a patient "seizing;" rather, he is "seized." In Western thought, the earliest view that epilepsy is a natural disease of the brain, as opposed to a supernatural one, comes from the Greek school of medicine that traces its origin to Hippocrates. This view was maintained and amplified in the Roman era by Galen and his school. The religious and magical view, however, remained powerful until at least the 18th century ACE, and is perhaps not yet extinct today.

While the followers of Hippocrates and Galen and their successors in orthodox medicine may have been more rational in their view of epilepsy than the supernaturalists, it made little practical difference in therapy until the middle of the 19th century. It is even arguable that prayer was more beneficial than some of the natural therapies, which included cauterization of the skull, castration, and the drinking of blood.

An improvement in the understanding of epilepsy began in the 18th and 19th centuries. Tissot (c. 1770) described childhood absence epilepsy and Esquirol (c. 1815) distinguished between grand mal seizures (convulsions) and minor seizures, which he described as petit mal. Reynolds (c. 1861) distinguished between petit mal epilepsy and epilepsy with generalized convulsions, and also between idiopathic epilepsy and seizures due to other causes. The distinction between focal and generalized seizures was not, however, clearly established. Hughlings Jackson (c. 1874), who was far ahead of his time in recognizing seizures to be a consequence of abnormal cortical discharge, believed all seizures to be of focal origin, differing only in location and extent. Gowers (c. 1881) attempted a classification in which epilepsies due to focal cerebral lesions were separated from those caused by non-specific brain abnormalities.

The modern classification of seizures and epilepsies depends on an understanding of their electrophysiological basis. All seizures result from an abnormal electrical discharge in the brain, which may be due to a variety of cerebral irritants. Epilepsy is the habitual occurrence of seizures, often in a pattern that constitutes a syndrome, and can have a variety of causes, even though the resultant seizures may be clinically and electrically very similar.

2. Pathophysiology of Seizures and Epilepsy

Cellular Excitability

Normal neuronal activity requires the maintenance of a resting membrane potential, which is periodically disturbed by depolarization. When the depolarization reaches a critical level, an action potential is generated by ion exchange and current flow across the cell membrane. In some parts of the central nervous system, neuronal firing is regulated by intrinsic ionic membrane mechanisms which cause cyclical depolarization and resultant action potentials. Elsewhere, the action potential depends on synaptic transmission producing depolarization.

Epileptic seizures happen when there is excessive excitability of neuronal populations, resulting in repetitive massed action potentials. For a seizure to occur, abnormal excitation, as well as abnormal synchronization of populations of neurons must be present.

Electrical Properties of Single Neurons

The resting membrane potential of the nerve cell is negative inside, and this is maintained by the active extrusion of sodium. Chemical or electrical events that open channels for sodium permit depolarization of the cell and, at a critical level of depolarization there is an all-or-none action potential which is dependent on the opening of voltage-dependent sodium channels. During and immediately after an action potential, sodium channels become refractory, and potassium channels open; and this transiently hyperpolarizes the cell until the normal resting membrane potential is restored. The opening of calcium channels can result in prolonged depolarization of neuronal membranes, and this is associated with repetitive action potentials. Events causing the opening of sodium and calcium channels thus tend to depolarize the membrane and are excitatory, while those that open potassium and chloride channels tend to hyperpolarize the cell membrane and are inhibitory.

Role of Neurotransmitters

In the central nervous system, glutamate is probably the main excitatory neurotransmitter, and when it binds to one of its several receptor subtypes, there is an opening of sodium channels and depolarization of the postsynaptic neuron. When it causes a critical level of depolarization, this excitatory postsynaptic potential (EPSP) results in the all-or-none firing of an action potential in the postsynaptic neuron. The binding of gamma-amino-butyric acid (GABA) to its receptor opens a chloride channel, and the resulting inhibitory postsynaptic potential (IPSP) hyperpolarizes the cell and makes the firing of an action potential less likely. The occurrence and cessation of seizures thus depends on a balance between excitation and inhibition.

Thalamic Synchronization

Thalamic projections to the cerebral cortex act as synchronizers of cerebral electrical activity. EPSP-IPSP complexes typically last for 100 msec and project to the posterior cortical areas where they are responsible for the 10 cps posterior-dominant alpha rhythm. Faster EPSP-IPSP complexes in the frontal part of the thalamus project to anterior cortical structures, and are responsible for the faster beta rhythms. Abnormal thalamic oscillations with consequent entrainment of the neocortex at a frequency of 3 cps are probably responsible for the absence seizures seen in various forms of primary generalized epilepsy, but cortical abnormalities may also play a role. Abnormal activation of T-type calcium channels in the thalamus has been implicated in this type of seizure activity. Not only abnormal excitation, but abnormal inhibition is of critical importance, since it is the breakdown of inhibition that probably results in the conversion of the petit mal (absence) seizure to the generalized tonic-clonic convulsive seizure.

Epileptic Foci

Partial seizures are, by definition, the result of abnormal electrical activity in one region of the brain with varying degrees of spread. Epileptic foci arise from a variety of injuries and irritations to the brain, and many experimental models are based on artificially-induced injury. For example, in the penicillin-induced epileptic focus, microelectrode recordings show that there are paroxysmal depolarizations, as well as prolonged hyperpolarizations. These presumably depend on calcium and sodium, as well as potassium currents. There is evidence for abnormal and decreased dendrite branching, as well as a reduced number of inhibitory synapses. There is also evidence for redistribution of calcium channels.

Intracellular recording shows focal bursts of neuronal firing, which are reflected as abnormal spikes on the EEG. These bursts are presumably prevented, for the most part, from becoming seizures by the presence of a hyperpolarized inhibitory zone which surrounds the epileptic focus. The breakdown of this inhibition, which happens for unclear reasons, periodically results in the propagation of the interictal spike to surrounding regions. The end result is a focal seizure or secondarily generalized seizure.

Another model for focal epilepsy is kindling in animals, where weak electrical stimulation delivered repeatedly over time to one part of the brain causes a spontaneously firing epileptic focus to develop. Kindled foci show both enhanced excitation and inhibition. These are probably both necessary for the abnormal synchronized firing of neurons that leads to epileptic seizures.

In human epilepsy, temporal lobe seizures are frequently associated with a characteristic pattern of hippocampal sclerosis. Loss of hilar neurons may prevent the activation of inhibitory neurons that would normally inhibit granular neurons of the dentate gyrus. It has been hypothesized that disinhibited granule cells develop synchronous and autonomous firing patterns that then spread to the rest of the hippocampus and the temporal lobe.

Developmental Aspects of Epilepsy

Epilepsy is fundamentally a disorder of cortical and subcortical neurons. Thus, developmental abnormalities of the cerebral cortex are frequently associated with epilepsy. In normal development of the cerebral cortex, neuroblasts migrate toward the surface along radially oriented glial fibers. The organization of the six-layered neocortex requires a precisely orchestrated migration of neurons, with the migration of deep layers preceding that of the more superficial ones. Thus, the neurons destined for the more superficial cortical layers have to migrate through the ones that are already in place in deeper layers. This occurs over several weeks, and errors in this process lead to a variety of developmental abnormalities, some of which are highly epileptogenic. Similarly, disorders of morphogenetic movement that result in the formation of abnormal gyri and sulci can also be associated with epilepsy.

Lissencephaly

Several types exist, some of which are genetically determined. There is a failure of normal layering to occur, and the brain has a smooth appearance. Macro- and microgyria are variations on the same theme. Epilepsy and mental retardation are common in such patients.

Heterotopias

These are probably focal defects of neural migration resulting in abnormally placed neurons, often in subcortical locations. They are highly epileptogenic. The cells themselves, neurons and glia, are often atypical in morphology. One common glial variety is the "Taylor type" balloon cell.

Microdysgenesis

Minor distortions of cerebral architecture, including the abnormal positioning of single neurons or clusters of neurons, are probably a cause of epilepsy. Such anomalies often cannot be seen in imaging studies. They are found often in brain tissue that has been resected for the treatment of epilepsy. Such minor dysgenesis is found not only in neocortex, but in the hippocampus as well.

Cortical Dysgenesis and Neoplasia

Abnormal clusters of neurons and glia often show neoplastic properties as well as being causes of epilepsy. One such tumor is the ganglioglioma which is a low-grade malignancy containing both an astrocytic and a neuronal component. Tuberous sclerosis is associated with subcortical heterotopias, and a variety of other disorders of cerebral architecture. Malignant degeneration is possible. Hypothalamic hamartomas are of special interest because of the association with gelastic seizures (seizures accompanied by laughter). Removal of the lesion is often curative.

Specific Etiologies of Epilepsy and Seizures

Genetic Causes of Epilepsy

Some of the primary generalized epilepsies, and more rarely the focal epilepsies, show a dominant pattern of inheritance, but the genetic and biochemical defects have not been well characterized. A number of syndromes where the specific defects are known are discussed below.

Vascular Causes of Epilepsy

Strokes are a common cause of epilepsy, particularly in the elderly. Approximately 10% of patients with cortical infarctions will subsequently develop epilepsy. This can often be quite refractory. Presumably, the scar from the stroke becomes an irritative epileptic focus. Lacunar infarctions, since they involve primarily the white matter, are less likely to be epileptogenic. Strokes *in utero* occur for unclear reasons and often result in the formation of porencephalic cysts. These are a fairly common cause of epilepsy in childhood, and are often associated with the infantile hemiplegia syndrome.

Vascular malformations also cause epilepsy. The decomposition products of blood, particularly iron, are quite epileptogenic, so if an aneurysm or arteriovenous malformation bleeds, and the patient survives, epilepsy frequently develops. Abnormal cortical architecture around vascular malformations may also contribute to epileptogenesis. Cavernous hemangiomas, although they do not bleed catastrophically, may by repeated leaks create epileptic foci with hemosiderin staining of surrounding brain tissue. Some hemangiomas are familial, particularly when there are multiple lesions.

Infectious Causes of Epilepsy

Bacterial infections, such as meningitis, are associated with seizures in the acute phase and may, by cerebral scarring, cause chronic epilepsy. Bacterial meningitis is also associated with the subsequent development of hippocampal sclerosis and temporal lobe epilepsy. Tuberculosis, Lyme disease, and syphilis are other bacterial disorders associated with epilepsy.

Among parasites, echinococcus, malaria, and toxoplasmosis represent major problems, but worldwide, cysticercosis is the most common parasitic cause of epilepsy.

Viral meningitis is not usually associated with seizures or epilepsy, but encephalitis may produce acute seizures, as well as chronic epilepsy. Herpes encephalitis has a predilection for the temporal lobes and is associated both with amnesia and epileptic seizures. MRI shows localization abnormalities in the temporal region. In recent years, HIV infection has been associated with epilepsy. In about half the cases, HIV appears to be directly responsible, while in others it predisposes toward other diseases that cause seizures, such as CNS toxoplasmosis.

Traumatic Epilepsy

Head trauma is a major cause of epilepsy. The likelihood of developing epilepsy after a significant head trauma is directly proportional to the severity of the injury. Bleeding and focal neurological deficits are added risk factors. Early use of phenytoin reduces the likelihood of acute seizures, but does not affect the subsequent development of epilepsy.

Autoimmune Causes of Epilepsy

A variety of autoimmune disorders has been associated with epilepsy. Lupus is a multi-system autoimmune inflammatory disorder which can involve the brain as well. Lupus cerebritis is frequently a cause of encephalopathy as well as epilepsy. Seizures may be focal or secondarily generalized. It is necessary to treat both the epilepsy and the underlying immune disorder. Neurosarcoidosis is another autoimmune inflammatory cause of epilepsy. Here too it is necessary to treat the autoimmune disorder with steroids and/or immunosuppressive drugs, and at the same time, to treat the epilepsy with antiepileptic medications.

Vasculitis may be more than one disorder and has a variety of manifestations. The most focal extracerebral form is temporal arteritis, which is treated with steroids, but widespread systemic vasculitis is not uncommon. This may also involve the intracranial vessels, or more rarely, involvement is limited to the intracranial vessels. When the intracranial vasculature is involved, strokes and seizures are frequent.

Immune suppression with cyclophosphamide is the key to therapy.

Rasmussen's encephalitis is a chronic focal parenchymal and vascular inflammation limited to one hemisphere. It has been associated with a variety of viral syndromes, but the active disease, at least in some cases, involves an antibody to a glutamate receptor. Focal seizures are often uncontrollable, but plasmapheresis may help. Hemispherectomy is often necessary.

Metabolic Factors

Acute or chronic metabolic derangements are rarely causes of epilepsy, but are frequently associated with lowering of the seizure threshold and the occurrence of isolated (or even repeated) seizures.

Electrolyte imbalance. Changes in the levels of various electrolytes, particularly if they occur over a short period of time, can precipitate seizures. Hyponatremia and hypocalcemia are particularly likely to cause seizures, while hypercalcemia is more associated with encephalopathy. Over-rapid correction of abnormalities, particularly correction of hyponatremia, must be avoided since it can precipitate irreversible myelinolysis. The seizures associated with electrolyte imbalances are usually generalized tonic-clonic seizures.

Hyperglycemia and hypoglycemia are also associated with seizures. Hypoglycemia is particularly associated with convulsive seizures, but either hypo- or hyperglycemia can produce focal seizures in patients who have an underlying brain injury.

Hepatic and renal failure. Patients with uremia or hepatic encephalopathy are at increased risk for seizures. The exact mechanisms are uncertain. Characteristic EEG abnormalities with triphasic waves are commonly seen. Control of seizures is rarely achieved without an improvement in the underlying metabolic disorders. Dialysis is helpful in controlling seizures associated with renal failure. Anticonvulsant drugs must be administered with caution because of altered clearance.

Toxic substances. Lead poisoning in children and lithium poisoning in all age groups are associated with seizures and epilepsy. Other heavy metals may act similarly. Intoxication with organic solvents is an occasional cause of seizures, but long-term epileptogenic consequences are less certain. A variety of drugs, including tricyclic antidepressants and neuroleptics, lower the seizure threshold somewhat, but not usually enough to preclude their use in patients with epilepsy. Among the drugs of abuse, cocaine can cause acute strokes, as well as seizures, and has also been associated with persistent abnormalities of EEG and the development of epilepsy. It is used as an epileptogenic agent in a variety of experimental models. Amphetamines also lower the seizure threshold, but opiates and cannabis probably do not.

Alcohol is a special case. In and of itself, it is not a cause of seizures or epilepsy. However, falling levels of alcohol are associated with alcohol withdrawal seizures. These usually occur 24-48 hours after the cessation of heavy drinking. Alcohol withdrawal seizures are generalized tonic-clonic convulsions. Benzodiazepines or phenobarbital are prophylactic and therapeutic, while drugs such as Dilantin® and Tegretol® probably are not. Alcohol withdrawal may also lower the seizure threshold in a person with focal brain disease, and thus act as a trigger for focal and secondarily generalized seizures. Such seizures are best treated with benzodiazepines, in combination with conventional antiepileptic medications.

Neoplastic Causes of Epilepsy

Both extra-axial lesions such as meningiomas, as well as intra-axial ones such as astrocytomas, can be causes of epilepsy. It is not uncommon for such lesions to present as epilepsy without associated neurological signs. The seizures are usually focal with or without secondary generalization. There is some evidence that primary intra-axial brain neoplasms which present as epilepsy are smaller and more superficial than those which present with mass effect and neurological deficits. The epileptogenic ones may also have a better prognosis.

Metastatic cancers are also frequent causes of epilepsy, while carcinomatous meningitis is a less common cause.

3. Classification of Seizures and Epilepsy

The classification of seizures and the classification of epilepsies are related but separate topics, because the types of epilepsy are not always well correlated with the types of seizures that a patient suffers.

Classification of Seizures

Primary Generalized Seizures

These are defined as seizures in which the clinical manifestations and electroencephalographic (EEG) patterns suggest bilateral and diffuse cerebral involvement at the time of onset.

Tonic-clonic seizures. These are the prototypical convulsive seizures. They are characterized by sudden stiffening, crying out, loss of consciousness, and varying degrees of tonic (stiffening) and clonic (jerking) muscular activity. Tongue biting and incontinence are common. Postictally, the patient is lethargic. The EEG shows a mixture of polyspike and spike and wave activity, and during the postictal phase may be diffusely slow.

Absence (petit mal) seizures. These are brief seizures lasting for a few seconds. They are characterized by sudden loss of contact and staring into space. Minor automatisms may be seen. Recovery is rapid. These are classified as generalized seizures because of the EEG abnormality, which is a characteristic generalized 3 Hz spike and wave discharge.

Myoclonic seizures. These are characterized by sudden bilateral single or repetitive muscle jerks. All extremities may be affected. Brief seizures are not associated with loss of consciousness, but they often lead into generalized convulsive seizures in which consciousness is lost. The EEG shows generalized irregular polyspike and spike-wave complexes.

Tonic seizures. These are quite uncommon and are characterized by sustained muscle contraction. The ictal EEG shows prolonged fast sharp spike activity, and the rigid axial musculature often results in severe falls.

Atonic seizures. These seizures are characterized by a sudden loss of tone in various muscle groups and frequently result in falls. The EEG may show a variety of generalized abnormalities.

Partial Seizures

Partial (focal) seizures are characterized by clinical and EEG abnormalities that suggest initial involvement of only one cerebral region or hemisphere. By definition, in simple partial seizures, consciousness is always preserved; whereas in complex partial seizures, it is altered or lost. Partial seizures can become secondarily generalized when a focal electrical discharge spreads to both hemispheres. Often focal motor or focal sensory signs and symptoms are evident for many seconds before generalization, but sometimes a brief subjective aura or brief focal motor activity is the only indication of a focal onset. In contrast, primary generalized seizures, in which the abnormal electrical discharge begins diffusely, almost never have an aura. In some cases, however, secondary generalization is so rapid that it cannot be distinguished from a primary generalized seizure.

The symptomatology of partial seizures depends substantially on where in the brain they begin. For example, focal seizures beginning in the occipital lobe are often accompanied by visual phenomena. Certain patterns of symptomatology give rise to epilepsy syndromes which we will consider below.

Classification of Epilepsies

The present system of classification distinguishes first between epilepsies with generalized seizures (generalized epilepsies) and those with focal or partial seizures (localization-related, focal or partial epilepsies). A second major distinction in the modern classification of epilepsy separates idiopathic epilepsies from those that are symptomatic. In idiopathic epilepsy, no underlying cause is found, and usually the patient is asymptomatic except for seizures. A hereditary predisposition often exists, and different syndromes are defined by age of onset, clinical characteristics of the seizures, and typical EEG abnormalities. In symptomatic epilepsy, the seizures are believed to be secondary to an underlying brain disease. This may be a congenital malformation, inborn error of metabolism, trauma, anoxic injury, tumor, or any of the known causes of epilepsy.

The distinction between idiopathic and symptomatic epilepsies cannot be sustained indefinitely. As the genetic basis of the idiopathic epilepsies is elucidated at a molecular level, subtle biochemical defects will doubtless become apparent. Once such defects are recognized, the distinction will not be between idiopathic epilepsies and symptomatic ones, but between those that have a biochemical basis (with grossly normal brain structure) and those that are caused by structural lesions.

A brief review of the epilepsies will be considered here. The pediatric epilepsy syndromes are discussed in more detail in the chapter on pediatric epilepsy.

Generalized Epilepsy

Generalized epilepsies are, by definition, those with primary generalized seizures. These seizures involve the whole brain diffusely, and the EEG shows a diffuse bilateral onset.

Generalized epilepsies are divided into the idiopathic and the symptomatic. Some common syndromes are described below.

Idiopathic Generalized Epilepsies

Benign familial neonatal seizures. This is a relatively rare disorder. It is dominantly inherited and produces frequent tonic and clonic seizures with autonomic changes during the first week of life. Imaging studies are normal. Seizures are characterized by clonus or apnea. EEG abnormalities are nonspecific. The prognosis is good. This syndrome is due to potassium channel mutations (KCNW2, KCNQ3).

Benign familial neonatal-infantile seizures. There are several overlapping syndromes here with focal and generalized seizures occurring in the first 6 months of life. The prognosis is usually good, but adults are occasionally affected. Imaging studies are normal, and EEG often shows focal abnormalities. Sodium channel mutations (SCN2A) have been implicated.

Childhood and juvenile absence epilepsy (petit mal, pyknolepsy). These are related syndromes with dominant or polygenic transmission. They are characterized by a normal MRI and 3 Hz spike-wave abnormality on the EEG. Seizures are brief, typically lasting 10 to 30 seconds, and are characterized by sudden loss of contact and staring into space. Minor automatisms are occasionally seen. These automatisms can cause absence seizures to be confused with temporal lobe seizures (see below), but the EEG is diagnostic. Patients with petit mal epilepsy usually outgrow it, but may also develop generalized tonic-clonic seizures in later life. Different genes are involved in different families, but GABA receptor (GABRG2) mutations have been found in some families with febrile seizures and petit mal.

Juvenile myoclonic epilepsy. This epilepsy manifests itself in adolescence and is characterized by a mixed seizure pattern, including absence, myoclonic and generalized tonic-clonic seizures. The EEG shows generalized irregular polyspike and spike-wave complexes. In some families, this epilepsy has been mapped to chromosome 6, but the biochemical defect remains unknown. In other lineages, GABA receptors (GABRA1) and calcium channels (CACN4) are probably abnormal.

Other idiopathic generalized epilepsies. A number of patients have epilepsy with primary generalized seizures but not any other syndromic features. These probably represent a heterogeneous group of as yet uncharacterized epilepsies. In some families, sodium channel mutations (SCN1A, 2B, 1B) have been found and many of these patients have a prior history of febrile seizures. This has been described as the generalized epilepsy with febrile seizures plus (GEFS+) syndrome.

Symptomatic Generalized Epilepsies

This is a very broad category and includes a variety of brain diseases in which seizures are a prominent feature.

Infantile spasms (West syndrome). This is devastating infantile epilepsy. It is characterized by spasms (these may be flexor, extensor, or a mixture), developmental plateauing or regression, and a diffusely abnormal EEG with high amplitude sharp and slow waves (hypsarrhythmia).

A variety of causes can lead to this syndrome, including intrauterine infection, inborn errors of metabolism, structural brain abnormalities, or hypoxia at birth. Often, however, there is no obvious etiology. As adults, such patients have a variety of seizure types.

Lennox-Gastaut syndrome. This syndrome appears between the ages of 1 and 10 years, sometimes de novo and sometimes following infantile spasms. There is no single etiology. These patients have a diffusely abnormal EEG which becomes more abnormal in sleep. Multiple seizure types are common, and most patients are at least moderately retarded. These patients may have a mixture of absence, myoclonic, generalized tonic-clonic, as well as partial seizures. Not surprisingly, studies of brain metabolism show both diffuse and focal abnormalities.

Diseases with seizures as a prominent symptom. Many congenital malformations, errors of metabolism and storage diseases have seizures as a major manifestation. Among diseases with obvious structural abnormalities, lissencephaly and tuberous sclerosis may produce West syndrome and Lennox-Gastaut syndrome. Hyperglycinemia has been associated with myoclonic encephalopathy in infancy, and phenylketonuria, if untreated, can be a cause of West syndrome. Disorders of mitochondrial metabolism can produce seizures, mental retardation, and stroke-like episodes. A variety of storage diseases with known enzymatic defects, such as Tay-Sachs disease, can present with myoclonus that develops into focal and generalized epilepsy. Such disorders are often progressive. Ceroid lipofuscinosis, Lafora body disease, and other similar disorders, all feature mental retardation, cognitive decline, myoclonus and generalized seizures.

Focal Epilepsy

While focal epilepsies may occasionally be idiopathic, with no evidence of structural brain disease or other cerebral dysfunction, most focal epilepsies arise from structural lesions, including congenital disorders of brain architecture, tumors, trauma, infection, and stroke. The nature of the lesion seems less important in defining the syndrome than its location.

Temporal lobe epilepsy. The seizures of temporal lobe epilepsy are the archetypal complex partial (psychomotor) seizures, although complex partial seizures may have extratemporal origin. Typically a seizure of temporal lobe origin begins with an aura. Auras with a gastric sensation, emotional content, déjà vu, and visual disturbances are common, but other sensory and autonomic symptoms may also be present. The seizure itself often begins with oral automatisms such as lip smacking and swallowing. Consciousness is often not initially impaired but becomes so as the seizure spreads. More complex automatisms such as walking, drinking, and undressing may occur later in the seizure. Ictal violence is very rare, but postictal confusion and agitation is quite frequent. Some temporal lobe seizures become secondarily generalized and end in tonic-clonic convulsions. Automatisms may be unilateral or bilateral, as may dystonia. These can sometimes be correlated with lateralized EEG abnormalities during the seizures.

Temporal lobe epilepsy is usually due to an acquired structural lesion such as a tumor or mesial temporal sclerosis. Mesial temporal (hippocampal) sclerosis is one of the common causes of temporal lobe epilepsy. The pathogenesis of the lesion itself is uncertain. There is an association with prolonged febrile convulsions in childhood, and in animal models such seizures can cause permanent hippocampal damage. However, human pathological specimens often show ectopic neurons, which raises the possibility that the damaged hippocampus was developmentally defective to begin with. Serial MRI scans may be one way in which this question can be addressed. Meanwhile, it is clear that seizures associated with the MRI finding of mesial temporal sclerosis are often medically refractory but very amenable to surgical treatment. In addition, there are some families with LGI1 mutations where temporal lobe epilepsy with auditory symptoms is dominantly inherited. MRI in such patients shows minor structural abnormalities.

Occipital lobe epilepsy. Seizures originating in the occipital lobes are characterized by an aura or onset that includes elementary visual hallucinations, flashing lights, and often loss in vision. Contralateral head deviation and rapid forced eye movements are also common. When seizure spread is from the occipital lobe into the temporal lobe, the seizure may develop into something resembling a temporal lobe seizure, as described above. If the pattern of seizure spread is above the Sylvian fissure, focal sensory and motor phenomena are more likely. In adults, occipital lobe epilepsy is usually acquired from structural lesions. In contrast, children can have idiopathic forms which overlap with some of the generalized epilepsies of children.

Frontal lobe epilepsy. Frontal lobe seizures can produce a very wide range of epileptic phenomena. This includes simple and complex partial seizures, asymmetric motor seizures, and generalized tonic-clonic convulsions. Supplementary motor areas (SMA) seizures are quite characteristic. Contraversive head and eye deviation is typical, with posturing of the contralateral arm so that it is externally rotated and flexed at the elbow. Speech arrest or forced vocalization may occur, as well as elaborate coordinated or dystonic movements. Consciousness is often preserved, or lost only briefly.

Complex partial seizures of frontal lobe origin also share certain features which enable one to define a frontal lobe seizure syndrome. Such seizures often occur in clusters and are usually brief. They often come out of sleep. They begin and end abruptly, and postictal confusion is rare. The associated automatisms are complex and often appear to be semipurposeful. Sexual automatisms, forced vocalization and bizarre behavior patterns occur, which are hard to distinguish from nonepileptic psychogenic seizures.

Frontal lobe epilepsy, like the other lobar epilepsies, usually arises from structural lesions. There is, however, at least one genetic form without a structural brain lesion. Autosomal dominant nocturnal frontal lobe epilepsy was initially thought to be a sleep disorder, but is now recognized as an epilepsy caused by a mutation in a nicotinic acetylcholine receptor (CHRNA2,4). Bizarre behavioral events occur out of sleep and usually respond well to treatment with Tegretol®.

Parietal lobe epilepsy. Parietal lobe epilepsy appears to be a rarer phenomenon than the other focal epilepsy syndromes described above. Somatosensory auras and pain are characteristic findings, but need not be present. Patterns of electrical spread from the parietal lobe are variable, and such seizures can evolve into patterns indistinguishable from the other lobar epilepsies.

Reflex epilepsies. This is a heterogeneous group of disorders. Most are inherited, though the specific genes have not been identified. They are characterized by seizures resulting from specific stimuli. Among the stimuli that cause seizures in individuals and families are reading, hot water, visual scanning, flashing lights, and specific sounds. Imaging studies in such individuals are usually normal, though startle epilepsy has been associated with large porencephalic cysts. EEG abnormalities are usually regional or focal and show varying degrees of spread.

4. Diagnosis of Epilepsy

History

The history is critical in making a diagnosis of epilepsy. It is essential to obtain history, not only from the patient, but from parents, relatives and friends who have witnessed the seizures. More often than not, a patient does not know what happens during a seizure. Clinical features of the seizure often assist in localization of the seizure focus or identification of the epilepsy syndrome. Early medical history, particularly that pertaining to birth injury, febrile convulsions, or childhood meningitis, is best obtained from parents.

Physical Examination

The physical examination is often unhelpful by virtue of being normal. Nevertheless, useful information can be obtained. Café-au-lait spots are associated with neurofibromatosis, while hypomelanotic spots and adenoma sebaceum are seen in tuberous sclerosis. Subtle lateralized findings on the neurological examination are often contralateral to the seizure focus, while mild diffuse cognitive impairments may be a consequence of underlying brain disease, epilepsy, or the side effects of antiepileptic medications. Physical examination is also helpful with regard to the differential diagnosis, since heart murmurs, carotid bruits, and orthostatic hypotension may point to disorders other than epilepsy.

EEG

Routine EEG

As described in the chapter on clinical neurophysiology, EEG is useful for diagnosing what type of epilepsy a patient has. For example, the regular 3 Hz spike-wave discharge is very strongly suggestive of primary generalized epilepsy with petit mal seizures, while lateralized temporal spikes during drowsiness and sleep are suggestive of temporal lobe epilepsy. Generalized slowing with sharp activity is suggestive of a diffuse encephalopathy associated with seizures, and focal slowing alone is often seen following stroke or head injury, or in the presence of a brain tumor.

A normal EEG does not, however, rule out a diagnosis of epilepsy. More than half of all routine outpatient EEGs done in patients with a well-established diagnosis of epilepsy are normal.

Special EEG Techniques

Long-term video and EEG monitoring. Video and EEG monitoring is usually carried out in specialized epilepsy units over a period of several days. Anticonvulsant medications are gradually withdrawn and this not only brings out interictal EEG abnormalities, but often precipitates occurrence of the patient's habitual seizures. Ictal EEG gives valuable lateralizing and localizing information with regard to the seizure focus that is not obtained from interictal recording. Long-term video-EEG monitoring gives a definite diagnosis in 80%-90% of patients who submit to it. This includes patients with non-epileptic psychogenic seizures.

Intracranial EEG. Intracranial EEG is a powerful tool that can localize seizures in cases where the scalp EEG is quite unrevealing. A variety of techniques have been developed, including intraparenchymal depth electrodes, subdural strip electrodes, and subdural grids. Usually, the clinical features of the seizures, as well as the interictal and ictal scalp EEG recordings, give clues as to the rough lateralization and localization of the seizure focus. Then intracranial electrodes are placed, and often exquisitely focal regions of seizure onset can be identified.

The placement of subdural grids also allows functional mapping to be done. Instead of only recording spontaneous interictal and ictal seizure activity, it is possible to stimulate the contacts of the grid in adjacent pair-wise combinations to functionally map the brain. It is particularly necessary to map sensory and motor cortex, as well as the language areas. Focal resection to cure epilepsy is then tailored to avoid critically important regions.

Imaging Studies

Radiographs

Radiographs have largely been superseded by more modern imaging techniques. However, depressed skull fractures, which can be a cause of focal seizures, Paget disease, and the typical calcifications of tuberous sclerosis, are often well appreciated on plain films.

Cerebral Angiography

Cerebral angiography, now usually practiced with digital subtraction techniques, remains an essential tool for the characterization of vascular lesions that are often a cause of epilepsy. Arteriovenous malformations (AVM), with or without evidence of rupture, frequently cause epilepsy; and angiography is essential for anatomic delineation prior to surgery, as well as for presurgical embolization procedures.

Cavernous hemangiomas, which are often epileptogenic, are not well seen on conventional angiography because of their low flow state, and are best defined by MRI.

CT Scan

Widespread availability, and the ease with which images can be obtained, has made CT scanning with and without contrast material the most common initial imaging study in the evaluation of epilepsy. A variety of epileptogenic lesions are easily demonstrated, including tumors, arteriovenous malformations, and old infarctions. In the context of trauma, CT scanning is probably superior to all other modalities in the demonstration of acute bleeding. CT angiography is faster than the corresponding MRI study and may have higher resolution.

There are, however, drawbacks to CT scanning. Dye allergy may necessitate noncontrast scanning only, which can miss tumors and vascular lesions. In the temporal lobes, even with contrast, significant epileptogenic lesions are missed on CT scan, which are easily appreciated on MRI.

Magnetic Resonance Imaging (MRI)

MRI has revolutionized the evaluation of epilepsy. The presence of a structural lesion does not establish a diagnosis of epilepsy, but once this has been established on clinical grounds, the presence of an appropriate lesion is confirmatory, and often influences treatment. Every patient with even a possibility of focal seizure onset should have an MRI scan.

Mesial temporal (hippocampal) sclerosis is a good example of the utility of MRI. With the possible exception of tumors, mesial temporal sclerosis (MTS) is the most common cause of temporal lobe epilepsy. The lesion is completely invisible on CT scan. It is easily seen on MRI, and patients who have this lesion, while often refractory to medications, are excellent candidates for epilepsy surgery. Neuronal migration disorders and minor structural abnormalities are also best seen on MRI.

Positron Emission Tomography (PET)

PET scans produce metabolic maps of the brain. The most commonly used tracer is 18F-fluorodeoxyglucose (FDG). This provides a measure of regional glucose metabolism. Many studies have shown that in the interictal period, epileptic foci have decreased metabolism and blood flow compared to the surrounding regions, and compared to the contralateral nonepileptic region. Intracranial electrode studies have demonstrated that the zone of hypometabolism correlates well with the zone of seizure onset, and is a very useful guide to resective epilepsy surgery. This is particularly true for the temporal lobes. Recent advances in PET scanning include the use of benzodiazepine receptor ligands, and it appears that regions of seizure onset are markedly deficient in benzodiazepine receptors.

Ictal PET scanning is difficult logistically, since the isotope has a short half-life and has to be continuously available, so that it can be injected at the moment of seizure onset. Ictal scans, when obtained, often show hyper-metabolism in the region of seizure onset, and are complementary to interictal ones in guiding surgery.

Single Photon Emission Computer Tomography (SPECT)

SPECT scanning uses radioactive isotopes whose distribution in the brain is proportional to blood flow and presumably to cerebral metabolism. In the evaluation of epilepsy, the most commonly used isotope is 99m technetium. Regions of hypoperfusion correlate with the epileptic focus, similar to PET scans, but the sensitivity is quite low.

Ictal SPECT is a far more promising technique. Because the isotope is relatively long-lived, an onsite cyclotron is not needed as it is for PET. Also, once injected, the isotope localizes rapidly in the brain, with regional absorption proportional to blood flow, and is then stable for an hour or more. It is thus possible to inject the isotope at the time of seizure onset while the patient is undergoing video and EEG monitoring, and then to scan the patient later at one's convenience. Regions of seizure onset show hyperperfusion relative to the rest of the brain, provided the injection is done within a few seconds of the first clinical signs and symptoms.

Magnetic Resonance Spectroscopy (MRS)
MRS is still a research technique in the evaluation of epilepsy, but holds great promise. PET and SPECT scans, as noted above, are very useful for delineating regions of abnormal brain metabolism, but tell one little at the biochemical level. MRS of selected brain regions can give precise information regarding molecular composition and the ratios of molecules involved in energy transfer. In the temporal lobes, this correlates with the structural finding of mesial temporal sclerosis, as well as with the decreased blood flow and metabolism seen with SPECT and PET scans. N-acetyl aspartate (NAA) is a neuronal compound, and is reduced in gliotic scans that are often epileptogenic. Choline and creatine are found in glia, and the NAA/choline and creatine ratio is a biomarker for normal and abnormal brain tissues.

With MRS, SPECT, and PET, major structural lesions can make the metabolic picture uninterpretable, and for localizing the epileptogenic region, these techniques work best in combination with anatomical and electrical studies.

5. Differential Diagnosis of Epilepsy

General Considerations

By no means is every episode of loss of consciousness epileptic. A variety of ordinary medical, as well as psychiatric disorders can masquerade as epilepsy. Breath-holding spells in infants, hyperventilation in adolescents, syncope and cardiac arrhythmias in older individuals, migraine, transient ischemic attacks, narcolepsy, and dystonias can all masquerade as epilepsy. Psychogenic nonepileptic seizures (NES) are also frequently mistaken for epilepsy. It is often impossible to sort out these different possibilities by history, examination, and response to treatment alone; and long-term video/EEG monitoring with recording of the actual spells is often essential for making a diagnosis.

Infantile Syncope

This is associated with loss of consciousness and sometimes with minor seizure activity. There is a cyanotic as well as a pallid form. It may or may not be associated with breath holding. The EEG shows nonspecific slowing, and the convulsive activity is presumably due to cerebral hypoperfusion. Other infantile spells that can be confused with epilepsy include benign myoclonus in sleep, and Sandifer syndrome (reflux).

Hyperventilation

Anxiety and stress are the underlying causes of hyperventilation and a variety of symptoms, including lightheadedness, blurred vision, and loss of consciousness can occur. Parasthesias and muscle spasms are common. Hyperventilation can occasionally cause epileptic convulsions in patients with primary generalized epilepsy. Hyperventilation is also associated with panic attacks, which can sometimes mimic epileptic auras.

Adult Syncope

The direct cause of syncope, with or without convulsion, is cerebral ischemia. This can result from abnormal cardiac and cerebral reflexes (vasovagal or vasodepressor syncope), and can also be induced by stimuli such as carotid massage, paroxysmal coughing, and voiding. Cardiac arrhythmias, such as sick sinus syndrome, are a somewhat less common cause of syncope. Orthostatic hypotension, often resulting from hypovolemia or side effects of medications, is a frequent cause of syncope in the elderly.

Transient Ischemic Attacks (TIAs)

These can be stereotypical with focal neurological symptoms, and may therefore be confused with focal epilepsy. Sudden falls, with little or no loss of consciousness, particularly in the elderly, are often due to posterior circulation ischemia, and are rarely epileptic. Strokes can, of course, result in the formation of scar tissue, which then secondarily becomes a cause of true epilepsy.

Transient global amnesia is a syndrome of sudden memory loss lasting from minutes to hours. It is occasionally confused with postictal amnesia. Most investigators believe that it is an ischemic phenomenon, although some EEG abnormalities have been described.

Sleep Disorders

Narcolepsy is characterized by sudden attacks of irresistible sleepiness in the daytime. This, and a characteristic syndrome of cataplexy (sudden loss of muscle tone), sleep paralysis, and hypnagogic hallucinations, is occasionally confused with epilepsy.

Night terrors in children, when the patient awakens screaming, and somnambulism, are problems of non-REM sleep. Disagreeable dreams occur in REM sleep. Polysomnography and video EEG may be required to make a definite diagnosis. Some of these disorders respond to anticonvulsant therapy and may represent frontal lobe epilepsy masquerading as a sleep disorder.

Migraine

A variety of focal neurological symptoms and signs can be seen during migraine, including scotomata, hemisensory parasthesias, and impairment of consciousness. The gradual onset and remission of these symptoms, and the usual association with headaches, serves to distinguish them from epilepsy.

Movement Disorders

Movement disorders that masquerade as epilepsy are rare. Some paroxysmal dyskinesias can look like focal or generalized motor seizures, but the EEG is always normal. Also, dystonic postures can continue unchanged or occur repetitively for minutes or even hours, which is distinctly unusual for epileptic seizures. Paroxysmal movements are sometimes seen in multiple sclerosis, and often respond to anti-epileptic drugs. It is doubtful whether these are truly epileptic seizures.

6. Medical Treatment of Epilepsy

General Principles

Unless there is a clear cause for recurrent seizures, for example, a brain tumor, most neurologists will not treat a first seizure, since only about half of these will recur. Recurrent seizures are usually treated unless they are so minor as to be not incapacitating. For initial treatment, therapy with a single drug (monotherapy) is always preferable, since one does not then have to worry about pharmacokinetic and pharmacodynamic drug interactions. The choice of drugs depends partly on the nature of the epilepsy, and partly on the individual patient's response. The monitoring of anticonvulsant blood levels is important, since both efficacy and side effects, for most antiepileptic drugs, depend on blood levels. Realistically, about 75% of patients can have their seizures controlled on one or more antiepileptic medications without significant side effects. The remaining 25% will either have uncontrollable seizures, or will suffer significant side effects from the currently available medications. Many of these patients who are medically refractory are good candidates for epilepsy surgery (see below).

Mechanisms of Action of Antiepileptic Drugs

Normal brain function is characterized by a fine balance between excitatory (depolarizing) or inhibitory (hyperpolarizing) forces. Excessive excitation or reduced inhibition can result in the paroxysmal excessive discharge of neurons that characterize a seizure. Thus, seizures occur when the threshold for firing of the neuronal membrane is reduced beyond the capability of intrinsic membrane threshold-stabilizing mechanisms to prevent firing.

Antiepileptic drugs typically work by influencing this excitatory-inhibitory balance in the brain. Approaches used to reduce excitability include increasing the inactivation gate of the sodium channel, thus reducing number of action potentials during membrane depolarization or blocking calcium channels to reduce neurotransmitter release. The older antiepileptic drugs, carbamazepine and phenytoin, work through blocking of Na^+ channels. Enhancing inhibition by modulating the gamma-amino-butyric acid (GABA) receptor is another well-established mechanism. Phenobarbital and the barbiturates work by modulating Cl-flow through the GABA receptor. Excitation can be reduced by blocking glutamate release or binding to the receptor.

T-calcium currents are one of three different voltage-dependent calcium currents (L, N, T) known to exist in the human brain. T-calcium currents are small, rapidly inactivated currents that act as pacemakers for normal rhythmic brain activity, especially in the thalamus. T-calcium currents also appear to have an important role in pacing the three-per-second spike-wave activity of absence seizures (but not other seizure types). Drugs inhibiting T-calcium currents specifically inhibit absence seizures.

Table 1 provides a summary of the mechanisms of action of the antiepileptic drugs.

Old Antiepileptic Drugs

Just about any substance that can be ingested, and many that should not, have at one time or another been used as antiepileptic agents. Most of the drugs in current use were discovered by accident or by trial and error; we are only now starting to synthesize compounds on the basis of their likely antiepileptic effects at the molecular level. It is reasonable, therefore, to discuss medications from an historical and chronological point of view. A summary of the old antiepileptic drugs is included in Table 2.

Bromide

Potassium bromide was used more or less accidentally for the treatment of catamenial epilepsy in 1867. It was found to be effective against this type of epilepsy, particularly for those patients with generalized tonic-clonic seizures. Bromide augments $GABA_A$ receptor mediated inhibition by increasing the sensitivity of the $GABA_A$ receptors to GABA and increasing $GABA_A$ receptor currents owing to the threefold increase in permeability of bromide over chloride. Side effects include sedation and an acneiform rash. Today, it has been almost completely superseded.

Table 1

Major Mechanisms of Action of the New Antiepileptic Drugs

Target / Mechanism	Effect	Antiepileptic Drugs Using This Mechanism
Na^+ channel	↓ Action potential frequency	Lamotrigine Oxcarbazepine Topiramate Zonisamide
Ca^{2+} channel T-type L-type N-type	 ↓ Thalamocortical oscillations ↓ Cortical excitation ↓ Neurotransmitter release	Gabapentin (L) Lamotrigine (N) Levetiracetam (N) Topiramate (L) Zonisamide (L/T)
GABAergic transmission ↑ $GABA_A$ receptor activation ↑ GABA synthesis/release ↓ GABA reuptake	↑ Inhibition	Tiagabine (↓ uptake) Vigabatrin (↓ metabolism of GABA)
Glutamatergic transmission inhibits glutamate receptors ↓ glutamate synthesis/release	↑ Excitation	Gabapentin (↓ release) Lamotrigine (↓ release) Topiramate (blocks AMPA and KA)

Phenobarbital (Luminal®)

Barbiturates were introduced as antiepileptic drugs as 1912. They are still regarded as highly effective and safe, although, owing to their sedating effect, they are no longer first line drugs in economically advanced countries. Phenobarbital and primidone (Mysoline®) are the two most commonly used barbiturates, and they are effective against focal seizures with or without secondary generalization, as well as against the generalized convulsive seizures, with diffuse onset, that are seen in the various forms of generalized epilepsy. The parenteral form of phenobarbital is very useful for rapid seizure control. Barbiturates are not as effective against atypical generalized seizures such as tonic and atonic seizures, and not at all effective against absence seizures. Because phenobarbital is inexpensive as well as effective, it remains the drug of choice in many poorer countries.

Mechanism of action. The mechanism of barbiturate drugs probably includes binding to the $GABA_A$ receptor and hyperpolarizing the cells via increased chloride transport.

Pharmacokinetics. Phenobarbital is absorbed slowly (over 6 to 18 hours) but completely from the small intestine. The drug is 40%-60% protein-bound. Approximately one-third of an administered dose of phenobarbital is excreted unchanged in the urine, and two-thirds is excreted as metabolites created by hepatic biotransformation. Phenobarbital exhibits linear pharmacokinetics with an elimination half-life of approximately four days in adults (40-136 hours). Phenobarbital steady-state plasma concentration is attained 14 to 20 days after initiating therapy or changing dosing rate. The phenobarbital plasma concentration is increased after the addition of valproic acid. As an enzyme inducer, phenobarbital may lower the plasma concentrations

Table 2

Summary of the Old Antiepileptic Drugs

Antiepileptic Drug	Indications	Maintenance Dosage (mg/day)	Half-life (hours)	Therapeutic Range (mg/mL)	Common Side Effects	Serious Idiosyncratic Side Effects
Carbamazepine	Adjunctive for partial seizures. Adjunctive for primary generalized seizures. Monotherapy for partial seizures. Monotherapy for primary generalized seizures.	600-1200	14-27	8-12	Ataxia Blurred vision Nausea	Rash Blood dyscrasias Hepatoxicity Hyponatremia
Ethosuximide	Monotherapy for absence seizures.	500-1500	20-60	40-100	Gastrointestinal distress Dizziness	
Phenobarbital	Adjunctive for partial seizures. Adjunctive for primary generalized seizures. Monotherapy for partial seizures. Monotherapy for primary generalized seizures.	90-120	40-136	15-45	Lethargy Irritability	Rash
Phenytoin	Adjunctive therapy for partial seizures. Adjunctive therapy for primary generalized seizures. Monotherapy for partial seizures. Monotherapy for primary generalized seizures.	200-400	12-36 (nonlinear kinetic)	10-20	Gingival hypertrophy Hirsutism	Rash
Valproate	Monotherapy and adjunctive for complex partial seizures. Monotherapy and adjunctive for simple and complex absence seizures.	1000-3000	6-15	80-150	Gastrointestinal distress Hair loss Tremor Weight gain	Hepatotoxicity Pancreatitis Blood dyscrasias

of many drugs including the antiepileptic drugs carbamazepine, valproic acid, lamotrigine, tiagabine, and zonisamide. In addition, phenobarbital can reduce levels of warfarin, theophylline, and cimetidine.

Adverse side effects. Dose-related toxicity includes sedation, irritability, hyperactivity, slowed thinking, and ataxia. These behavioral changes limit the usefulness of the drug. Rash is a common idiosyncratic toxicity, and agranulocytosis, aplastic anemia, and hepatitis are very rare idiosyncratic reactions. Long-term toxicity includes folic acid, vitamin K, and vitamin D deficiency.

Phenytoin (Dilantin)

Merritt and Putnam discovered phenytoin and related hydantoin drugs by screening compounds for their ability to prevent electroconvulsive seizures in cats. Phenytoin was marketed in 1938, and is effective against the same spectrum of seizures as phenobarbital. The parenteral form of phenytoin, which is very useful for rapid seizure control, has been largely replaced by a pro-drug fosphenytoin, which is easier to use and less likely to cause hypotension. The lack of sedation is a distinct advantage of phenytoin over phenobarbital.

Mechanism of action. Phenytoin probably has more than one mechanism of action, but the most significant of these is its effect on voltage-gated sodium channels. By blocking sodium channels, it prevents abnormal neuronal firing and seizure spread.

Pharmacokinetics. Approximately 85% of an orally administered phenytoin is absorbed slowly over a period of 24 hours. Phenytoin is 69%-96% protein-bound and is biotransformed by the liver. Phenytoin has concentration-dependent (nonlinear) pharmacokinetics that makes it difficult to predict blood level following a change in dosage. If the patient's blood level is near the therapeutic range (10-20mcg/mL), increases or decreases in dose must be done cautiously. Due to the nonlinear kinetics, a small increase in dose can result in a large increase in blood concentration.

Adverse side effects. The side effects include gingival hyperplasia, hirsutism, coarsening of features, and liver function abnormalities. Osteoporosis, particularly in older men and women, is another problem. Calcium supplements and vitamin D are recommended for patients on long-term therapy with phenytoin.

Ethosuximide (Zarontin®)

Available since 1960, ethosuximide is a drug with a narrow spectrum of action having efficacy only in absence seizures. The drug is not used frequently in adults but is commonly used in children.

Mechanism of action. The drug inhibits calcium currents through the T-type Ca^{++} channel of thalamic neurons.

Pharmacokinetics. Ethosuximide is readily and almost completely absorbed in the alimentary tract. Little or no binding to serum proteins occurs. The drug is transformed in the liver to either a ketone or an alcohol metabolite, which is then excreted with or without glucuronide conjugation. The half-life is 20-60 hours. No significant drug interactions occur.

Adverse side effects. Gastrointestinal complaints are common and include stomach irritation, anorexia, nausea, and vomiting. Dose-related toxicity includes drowsiness, dizziness, and headache. Idiosyncratic toxicity includes rash and leukopenia and, very rarely, pancytopenia, agranulocytosis, aplastic anemia, psychosis, and systemic lupus erythematosus (SLE).

Benzodiazepines

Diazepam (Valium®) became available in 1968. Its mechanism, like that of other benzodiazepines, involves binding to the $GABA_A$ receptor at a site different from phenobarbital, with resultant hyperpolarization of the cell. Intravenous diazepam or lorazepam (Ativan®) are the drugs of choice for the rapid termination of status epilepticus, but tolerance develops rapidly to all benzodiazepine drugs if they are used for the chronic treatment of epilepsy. Clonazepam (Klonopin®) has some limited utility in the treatment of atypical generalized seizures, such as refractory absence, atonic and tonic seizures.

Carbamazepine (Tegretol, Carbatrol®)

Carbamazepine became available in 1974, and is chemically related to the tricyclic antidepressants. It has the same spectrum of activity as phenytoin and phenobarbital, and is an effective drug for complex partial and secondarily generalized seizures. Carbamazepine is also useful for the treatment of trigeminal neuralgia, bipolar disorder, and painful peripheral neuropathy.

Mechanism of action. Its mechanism of action is believed to be similar to that of phenytoin in blocking voltage-gated sodium channels. It also, however, binds to the adenosine receptor as an agonist compound. This may contribute to its role as an antiepileptic medication.

Pharmacokinetics. Approximately 75%-85% of an orally administered dose is absorbed after oral administration. Carbamazepine is 70%-80% protein-bound and is metabolized by the liver into many metabolites, some of which (especially carbamazepine epoxide) possess antiepileptic activity. Carbamazepine biotransformation exhibits time-dependent pharmacokinetics (self-induction), which means that the plasma concentration may fall unexpectedly during the first two months of administration when self-induction occurs. The half-life is 14-27 hours.

Drug interactions are common. Adding carbamazepine may increase the plasma concentration of phenytoin and lower the plasma concentrations of felbamate, lamotrigine, oral contraceptives, theophylline, valproic acid, and zonisamide. Propoxyphene, erythromycin, chloramphenicol, isoniazid, verapamil, and cimetidine may elevate the carbamazepine plasma concentration, whereas phenobarbital, phenytoin, felbamate, and primidone may lower the carbamazepine plasma concentration. Adding lamotrigine or oxcarbazepine to carbamazepine may enhance the side effects of carbamazepine.

Adverse side effects. Side effects are rare, but include sedation, suppression of bone marrow, hyponatremia, and liver toxicity. Some patients with idiopathic generalized epilepsy get worse on carbamazepine.

Common dose-related toxicity includes diplopia or blurred vision, dizziness, drowsiness, ataxia, and headache. At high plasma concentrations, tremor, dystonia, chorea, depression, irritability, psychosis, convulsions, water retention (inappropriate antidiuretic hormone-like syndrome), congestive heart failure, and cardiac arrhythmias may occur. Idiosyncratic reactions such as rash are common. Rarely, anemia, agranulocytosis, leukopenia, thrombocytopenia, hypersensitivity syndrome (dermatitis, eosinophilia, lymphadenopathy, splenomegaly), and cholestatic and hepatocellular jaundice can occur.

Valproate Sodium, Valproic Acid, Divalproex Sodium (Depakote®)

Valproate became available in 1978. It has a very broad spectrum of activity, including generalized convulsive seizures, tonic, atonic, and myoclonic generalized seizures, absence seizures, and focal seizures with or without secondary generalization. It is a very effective drug for the idiopathic generalized epilepsies. It is also useful for migraine and bipolar disorder.

Parenteral valproate (Depacon®) is useful for those who cannot take it orally, but its role in the rapid control of seizures is still unclear.

Mechanisms of action. Valproate has multiple modes of action. Blocking of sodium channels and increasing endogenous levels of GABA in the brain are only two of the many mechanisms that have been suggested.

Pharmacokinetics. Valproate is rapidly and completely absorbed after oral administration, with a slight delay in absorption when it is taken after meals. The drug is approximately 90% protein-bound. Protein binding varies with drug plasma concentration, and the free fraction increases with increasing plasma concentration. Primary metabolism is by hepatic hydroxylation and conjugation with glucuronide. Valproate also appears in the bowel and undergoes enterohepatic circulation. Beta and omega oxidation may also take place. Excretion as glucuronide in the urine follows, with minor amounts lost in feces and expired air. The half-life is short, 6-15 hours. Valproate raises the plasma concentration of lamotrigine and phenobarbital. Phenytoin, phenobarbital, and carbamazepine lower the plasma concentration of valproic acid. Felbamate increases the plasma concentration of valproate.

Adverse side effects. Some gastrointestinal distress occurs with valproic acid but is rare with the divalproex sodium preparation. Dose-related toxicities include tremor, elevated plasma transaminase, and hyperammonemia. Weight gain and hair loss can occur but it is not clear if these are dose-related. Idiosyncratic toxicity includes hepatic failure, thrombocytopenia, pancreatitis, stupor and coma. The risk of hepatic fatality is greatest in children younger than two years and in persons taking valproic acid in combination with other antiepileptic drugs. Long-term toxicities are weight gain, hair loss, and platelet dysfunction.

ACTH and Prednisone

Steroids are rarely useful in epilepsy, but infantile spasms (West syndrome) sometimes respond dramatically to short courses of ACTH or prednisone. The mechanism of action is uncertain.

New Antiepileptic Drugs

In the past ten years, several new antiepileptic drugs have become available. A number of patients who are refractory to currently used medications, or cannot tolerate them, do significantly better with one of the newer ones. The new drugs appear to have side effect profiles that are somewhat more benign than those of older drugs, and their effectiveness, overall, appears similar to that of conventional therapy. A major advantage of most of the new drugs is that they are not stimulators of the hepatic cytochrome P450 enzyme system, and so have far fewer pharmacokinetic interactions with other drugs. Conventional antiepileptic drugs such as Dilantin, Tegretol and barbiturates can, by stimulating the liver, lower the levels and effectiveness of a wide range of medications, including birth control pills, coumadin, theophylline, antidepressants, and antihypertensives. Chemotherapy may also be less effective.

While some of the new drugs were found by accident or by trial and error, others are "designer drugs" which were selected and tested on the basis of their ability to influence the known neurophysiological mechanisms of epilepsy. A summary of the new antiepileptic drugs is included in Table 3.

Felbamate (Felbatol®)

In 1993, felbamate became the first in a series of new antiepileptic drugs introduced, and quickly became widely used in both children and adults. Felbamate, which is an analog of the tranquilizer meprobamate (Miltown®), is a highly effective antiepileptic drug for all seizure types except absence. The drug is approved by the FDA as monotherapy or adjunctive therapy for adult patients with partial seizures with or without secondary generalization and adjunctive therapy for partial or generalized seizures in children with Lennox-Gastaut syndrome. While it remains a highly efficacious antiepileptic drug, the molecule is associated with a significant risk of aplastic anemia and hepatotoxicity. It is now used only in patients with severe epilepsy that do not respond to other antiepileptic drugs.

Mechanisms of action. Felbamate has multiple modes of action including potentiating Cl- current flow through the GABA receptor, inhibition of Na+ channels, and inhibition of N-methyl-D-aspartate receptors. The drug is broad spectrum and has been shown to be effective in both partial and generalized seizures.

Pharmacokinetics. Felbamate is well-absorbed orally and is about 25% protein-bound. Metabolism is mainly in the liver with hydroxylation and glucoronidation. Excretion of the glucoronide and unchanged drug (about 50%) is through the kidney. The half-life of felbamate in monotherapy is 16-22 hours. Felbamate inhibits the metabolism of phenytoin and valproate, with concomitant increases in level. Carbamazepine levels fall with co-adminis-

Table 3

Summary of the New Antiepileptic Drugs

Antiepileptic Drug	Indications	Maintenance Dosage (mg/day)	Half-life (hours)	Therapeutic Range (mcg/mL)	Common Side Effects	Serious Idiosyncratic Side Effects
Felbamate (Felbatol®)	Adjunctive for partial seizures. Adjunctive for partial and generalized seizures associated with Lennox-Gastaut.	2400-3600	13-24	Not established	Anorexia Insomnia Somnolence	Blood dyscrasias (aplastic anemia) Hepatoxicity
Gabapentin (Neurontin®)	Adjunctive for partial seizures.	900-3600	5-7	Not established	Lethargy Irritability Dizziness Weight gain	None
Lamotrigine (Lamictal®)	Adjunctive for partial seizures. Adjunctive for the generalized seizures of Lennox-Gastaut. Indicated for conversion to monotherapy in adults with partial seizures receiving treatment with carbamazepine, phenytoin, phenobarbital, primidone, or valproate as the single AED.	Highly dependent upon other drugs used; if on enzyme inducers, 200-400; if on valproate, 100-200	7-60; (Highly dependent on concomitant antiepileptic drugs)	Not established (Maintain <20 g/mL)	Lethargy Irritability Insomnia	Rash
Levetiracetam (Keppra®)	Adjunctive for partial seizures	2000-3000	4-8	Not established	Irritability Lethargy	None
Oxcarbazepine (Trileptal®)	Adjunctive for partial seizures Monotherapy for partial seizures	1200-2400	7-12	Not established	Lethargy Confusion	Rash Hyponatremia
Pregabalin (Lyrica®)	Adjunctive for partial seizures	150-600 mg	6-7	Not established	Lethargy Dizziness	None
Tiagabine (Gabitril®)	Adjunctive for partial seizures	32-56; dosage dependent upon other drugs used; if on enzyme inducers, use higher dose range	4-9	Not established	Lethargy Confusion Mental dullness Difficulties with concentration	Induction of spike-wave status epilepticus
Topiramate (Topamax®)	Adjunctive for partial seizures. Adjunctive for primary generalized tonic-clonic seizures. Adjunctive for seizures associated with Lennox-Gastaut syndrome. Monotherapy for partial seizures and primary generalized tonic-clonic seizures.	100-400	12-20	Not established	Irritability Hyperactivity Mental dullness Weight loss	Glaucoma
Zonisamide (Zonegran®)	Adjunctive for partial seizures in adults (≥16 years)	300-400	20-50	Not established	Dizziness Anorexia Tiredness Renal stones	Hyperthermia Oligohidrosis Rash

tration of felbamate, but carbamazepine epoxide (an active metabolite) levels rise, so the net effect is uncertain. Enzyme-inducing drugs such as phenytoin and carbamazepine lower the blood levels of felbamate.

Adverse side effects. Common adverse effects include anorexia, insomnia, nausea, ataxia, and emesis. However, after the drug was released it was found to result in fatal aplastic anemia and hepatic failure. The overall risk of aplastic anemia for patients taking felbamate is estimated to be 1:5000, 100 times greater than the risk in the normal population; and the risk of fatal outcome is approximately 1:10,000. No felbamate-associated aplastic anemia was reported in children younger than 13 years. Risk factors associated with aplastic anemia include a history of blood dyscrasia, a history of substantial toxicity to other antiepileptic drugs, serologic or clinical evidence of an autoimmune disorder, and a history of treatment with felbamate for less than a year.

Gabapentin (Neurontin®)

While released as an antiepileptic drug, gabapentin is now prescribed more often for conditions such as pain and migraine than epilepsy. The widespread prescribing of gabapentin for conditions other than epilepsy is related to its ease of use as much as to its efficacy in these conditions. The drug has no pharmacokinetic interactions and no serious side effects. Despite the emphasis on non-epileptic conditions, the drug still has a valuable role in the treatment of epilepsy. It is clearly effective for focal and secondarily generalized seizures, but may exacerbate idiopathic generalized epilepsy.

In the United States, gabapentin is indicated as adjunctive therapy for children (>12 years) and adults with partial seizures (with or without secondary generalization).

Mechanisms of action. Despite its structural relationship to GABA, gabapentin is not an agonist at the $GABA_A$ receptor. The drug inhibits glutamate release, affects L-type Ca2, channels, and is a weak inhibitor of GABA transaminase. It probably increases levels of endogenous GABA in the brain.

Pharmacokinetics. Gabapentin has a bioavailability of approximately 60% at low doses. At higher doses bioavailability decreases, because gabapentin is absorbed through the saturable L-amino-acid transport system in the proximal small intestine. Gabapentin is not appreciably metabolized in humans and is eliminated by renal excretion as unchanged gabapentin. The gabapentin elimination half-life is 5-7 hours. There are no drug interactions.

Adverse side effects. Gabapentin is well tolerated and no unique side effects have been detected. A minority of patients experience one or more of the following side effects: fatigue, dizziness, or ataxia. Myoclonus may begin or be exacerbated by gabapentin. Weight gain and pedal edema have been reported in some patients. Behavioral changes consisting of aggression, hyperactivity, and oppositional behavior may be seen in children taking gabapentin, although usually it is an exacerbation of the child's underlying behavior. No laboratory abnormalities have been attributed to gabapentin and routine blood studies are not required.

Lamotrigine (Lamictal®)

Lamotrigine is a broad-spectrum antiepileptic drug that has a number of attractive features for childhood and adult use. However, there is a risk of rash and the drug must be used with care. It is indicated as adjunctive therapy for adults with partial seizures and generalized seizures in children with Lennox-Gastaut syndrome. There are indications the drug is useful in absence seizures, and for other idiopathic generalized forms of epilepsy.

Mechanisms of action. The drug works by prolonging the inactivation of voltage-sensitive Na+ channels and inhibits glutamine and glutamate release.

Pharmacokinetics. Lamotrigine is rapidly and completely absorbed after oral administration. Lamotrigine undergoes hepatic metabolism and is excreted primarily as the 2-N-glucuronide metabolite. The elimination half-life of lamotrigine is highly dependent upon whether the drug is taken with other drugs. In children also taking carbamazepine, phenytoin, or phenobarbital, the elimination half-life is 7-15 hours. Co-administration with valproate (divalproex sodium, valproic acid) increases the elimination half-life of lamotrigine to 40-60 hours or more, and doubles the serum concentration. The half-life of lamotrigine in children on no other medications is approximately 20 hours. Lamotrigine does not affect the plasma concentration of carbamazepine, phenobarbital, phenytoin, primidone, or valproate.

Adverse side effects. Lamotrigine is generally well tolerated. The drug is not associated with behavioral or cognitive side effects. With high doses, particularly when used as adjunctive therapy, dizziness, diplopia, headache, ataxia, tremor, and nausea may occur. The incidence of rash associated with hospitalization among adults treated with lamotrigine is 0.3% and the incidence among children is 1.0%. The incidence of cases reported as possible Stevens-Johnson syndrome is 0.1% for adult patients and 0.5% for pediatric patients. The risk of rash is higher in children who are taking valproate, presumably because it decreases the metabolism of lamotrigine. Most rashes occur during the first 6 weeks of therapy. The risk of rash is reduced by slow upward titration of dose. No hematological or hepatic disturbances have been reported and routine laboratory studies are not required.

Levetiracetam (Keppra®)

Drug screening for antiepileptic drugs has relied, to a major degree, on anticonvulsant efficacy against single acute seizures induced by maximal electrical or chemical stimulation in rodents. The most widely used models have been maximal electroshock seizure threshold and the pentylenetetrazol seizure test. All established antiepileptic drugs have demonstrated activity in at least one of these two models. Levetiracetam is noteworthy since it is devoid of anticonvulsant activity in the acute maximal electroshock seizure and pentylenetetrazol models, despite offering potent protection against seizures in other models, including kindling. It is approved as adjunctive therapy for partial and secondarily seizures in adults and children (≥4 years). It is also useful in idiopathic and symptomatic generalized epilepsy.

Keppra is favored by surgeons, intensivists and oncologists. It has equivalent parenteral and oral dosing, and does not induce liver enzymes. Such induction can make chemotherapy less effective.

Mechanisms of action. The mechanism of action of levetiracetam is not entirely clear. However, the drug does block N-type Ca2+ channels, and reverses inhibition, by the negative allosteric modulators zinc and beta-carbolines, of neuronal GABA- and glycine-gated currents. In addition, it binds to a synaptic vesicle protein, SV2. How this binding would affect seizures is not clear.

Pharmacokinetics. Levetiracetam is rapidly and almost completely absorbed after oral administration. The absorption and elimination of levetiracetam are linear. Levetiracetam is not extensively metabolized in humans; the majority of the drug is excreted unchanged in the urine. The major metabolic pathway of levetiracetam is enzymatic hydrolysis of the acetamide group. Levetiracetam produces no inhibition of cytochrome P450 isoforms, epoxide hydrolase, or UDP-glucuronide enzymes. There are no reports of drug interactions between levetiracetam and antiepileptic drugs or other drugs. The metabolites have no known pharmacological activity and are excreted in the urine. The elimination half-life is 4-8 hours in children. The pharmacodynamic effects of levetiracetam are longer than would be predicted by half-life and the drug can be given twice daily.

Adverse effects. There are no reports of serious toxicity with levetiracetam. The drug is well tolerated in children. In children, headache, anorexia, somnolence, and mild infection (otitis media, pharyngitis, and gastroenteritis) have been reported. The central nervous system side effects usually occur early in treatment and can be reduced by slow drug initiation and/or dose reduction. Levetiracetam has caused irritability and aggressiveness. Reversible treatment-emergent psychosis has been associated with levetiracetam therapy. No hematological or hepatic disturbances have been reported and routine laboratory studies are not recommended.

Oxcarbazepine (Trileptal®)

Oxcarbazepine is a derivative of carbamazepine, and is an efficacious antiepileptic drug in the treatment of partial and secondarily generalized seizures. Its role in the treatment of generalized epilepsy is less certain. Oxcarbazepine appears to have fewer side effects than carbamazepine and may be effective in patients who have not responded to carbamazepine. The opposite is also true. Oxcarbazepine is indicated for use as monotherapy or adjunctive therapy in the treatment of partial seizures (simple, complex, secondarily generalized) in adults and children, including newly diagnosed patients. The drug is also indicated for adjunctive therapy for partial seizures in children (≥4 years of age).

Mechanisms of action. The drug works primarily through blockade of voltage-sensitive Na+ channels.

Pharmacokinetics. The antiepileptic activity of oxcarbazepine is exerted primarily by its 10-monohydroxy metabolite (MHD). The parent drug has no antiepileptic activity. Following oral administration, oxcarbazepine is completely absorbed and extensively metabolized to its active MHD metabolite. Maximum plasma concentration of MHD occurs 45 hours after administration. MHD has an elimination half-life of 7-12 hours in adults and children over 8 years of age. In children, the clearance of MHD is greater and the elimination half-life of MHD is shorter than in young adults. MHD is further metabolized via glucuronide formation. Approximately 80% of an administered dose of oxcarbazepine is excreted as MHD or MHD glucuronide. Oxcarbazepine, unlike carbamazepine, does not exhibit autoinduction of its own metabolism.

Carbamazepine, phenobarbital, phenytoin, and valproic acid may decrease MHD plasma concentration. Oxcarbazepine may increase plasma concentrations of phenytoin and phenobarbital and decrease plasma concentrations of carbamazepine and carbamazepine epoxide.

Adverse effects. The most commonly observed adverse events associated with use of oxcarbazepine are headache, somnolence, dizziness, nausea, and fatigue. The reported rate of skin rash with oxcarbazepine is approximately a third of that seen with carbamazepine, phenobarbital, and phenytoin. Cross reactivity occurs; approximately 25%-30% of patients who have skin rash with carbamazepine will have a skin rash with oxcarbazepine. A multiorgan hypersensitivity disorder characterized by rash, lymphadenopathy, abnormal liver functions, eosinophilia, and arthralgias has been reported. Cases of Stevens-Johnson syndrome and systemic lupus erythematosus have been reported. The risks of aplastic anemia and hepatitis with oxcarbazepine have not been established. Minor drops in counts of red blood cells, granulocytes, leukocytes, or platelets may occur. Oxcarbazepine is rarely associated with hyponatremia (125 mmol per L or less) in children. Routine monitoring of blood counts or hepatic function is not necessary.

Pregabalin (Lyrica®)

Pregabalin is the most recently added approved antiepileptic drug. It is approved for adjunctive therapy in adults with partial and secondarily generalized seizures. Its role in the treatment of idiopathic and symptomatic generalized epilepsies is unclear. Because of its structural similarity to gabapentin, there is concern it could make generalized forms of epilepsy worse.

Mechanism of action. Pregabalin is a 3-substituted analogue of gamma-amino butyric acid (GABA). It binds to calcium channels, modulates calcium influx, and also influences GABAergic neurotransmission.

Pharmacokinetics. Pregabalin is well absorbed after oral administration, is eliminated largely by renal excretion, and has an elimination half-life of about 6 hours. Following oral administration of pregabalin capsules under fasting conditions, peak plasma concentrations occur within 1.5 hours. Pregabalin oral bioavailability is ≥90% and is independent of dose. There are no drug interactions.

Adverse effects. Pregabalin is well tolerated by the majority of patients. Somnolence, ataxia, and dizziness may occur in some patients. Mild weight gain has been observed in some patients. In a small study of recreational users of sedative/hypnotic drugs, including alcohol, pregabalin received subjective ratings of "good drug effect," "high," and "liking" to a degree that was similar to diazepam. In controlled clinical studies in over 5,500 patients, 4% of pregabalin treated patients and 1% of placebo treated patients overall reported euphoria as an adverse event, though in some patient populations studied this reporting rate was higher and ranged from 1%-12%. In clinical studies, following abrupt or rapid discontinuation of pregabalin, some patients reported symptoms including insomnia, nausea, headache or diarrhea. For this reason, pregabalin is a Schedule V controlled substance.

Tiagabine (Gabitril®)

Tiagabine was released with considerable interest since it was a "designer drug" with a single mechanism of action. It is indicated as adjunctive therapy for persons 12 years and older with partial and secondarily generalized seizures. It is uncertain whether it is effective in generalized forms of epilepsy, but the same concerns that exist for gabapentin and pregabalin probably apply to tiagabine also.

Mechanisms of action. Tiagabine enhances GABAergic activity by inhibiting neuronal and astrocytic GABA reuptake.

Pharmacokinetics. Tiagabine is absorbed well, with food altering the rate but not the extent of absorption. The drug is metabolized by ring oxidation to 5-oxo-tiagabine, an inactive compound, and by glucuronidation. The elimination half-life of tiagabine is 7-9 hours in patients on monotherapy and 4-7 hours in patients receiving hepatic enzyme-inducing drugs (carbamazepine, phenytoin, primidone, and phenobarbital). After multiple dosing, steady-state plasma concentration is reached within two days. No clear relationship exists between tiagabine plasma concentration and clinical efficacy.

Carbamazepine, phenytoin, phenobarbital, and primidone decrease tiagabine plasma concentration. Valproate significantly reduces tiagabine protein binding *in vitro*. Tiagabine has no effect on steady-state plasma concentrations of carbamazepine or phenytoin and probably has no effect on steady-state plasma concentrations of phenobarbital or primidone. Tiagabine may cause a mild decrease in valproate plasma concentrations.

Adverse side effects. The most common CNS side effects seen with use of tiagabine in children include asthenia, dizziness, and somnolence. Rarely, children will have episodes in which they will have momentary loss of muscle tone and stumble or fall. These episodes need to be distinguished from atonic seizures. The most concerning adverse event is the worsening of seizures with tiagabine. Nonconvulsive status epilepticus has been reported on several occasions. Unfortunately, it has not been possible to predict which patients are at risk for an exacerbation of seizures. No laboratory abnormalities have been attributed to tiagabine and routine blood studies are not necessary.

Topiramate (Topamax®)

Topiramate is a broad spectrum antiepileptic drug with several mechanisms of action. It is approved as initial monotherapy in patients 10 years of age and older with partial-onset or primary generalized tonic-clonic seizures. Effectiveness was demonstrated in a controlled trial in patients with epilepsy that had no more than two seizures in the three months prior to enrollment. Safety and effectiveness in patients who were converted to monotherapy from a previous regimen of other anticonvulsant drugs has not been established in controlled trials, but is generally believed to be feasible.

Topiramate is also approved as adjunctive therapy for patients ≥2 years of age with primary generalized tonic-clonic seizures, partial-onset seizures, or seizures associated with Lennox-Gastaut syndrome.

Mechanism of action. Topiramate is a fructopyranose compound that has multiple mechanisms of action. It inhibits voltage-gated Na+ channels, blocks glutamate transmission via the seizure threshold, but opiates and cannabis probably do not.

Alcohol is a special case. In and of itself, it is not a cause of seizures or epilepsy. However, falling levels of alcohol are associated with alcohol withdrawal seizures. These usually occur 24-48 hours after the cessation of heavy drinking. Alcohol withdrawal seizures are generalized tonic-clonic convulsions. Benzodiazepines or phenobarbital are prophylactic and therapeutic, while drugs such as Dilantin® and Tegretol® probably are not. Alcohol withdrawal may also lower the seizure threshold in a person with focal brain disease, and thus act as a trigger for focal and secondarily generalized seizures. Such seizures are best treated with benzodiazepines, in combination with conventional antiepileptic medications.

Neoplastic Causes of Epilepsy

Both extra-axial lesions such as meningiomas, as well as intra-axial ones such as astrocytomas, can be causes of epilepsy. It is not uncommon for such lesions to present as epilepsy without associated neurological signs. The seizures are usually focal with or without secondary generalization. There is some evidence that primary intra-axial brain neoplasms which present as epilepsy are smaller and more superficial than those which present with mass effect and neurological deficits. The epileptogenic ones may also have a better prognosis.

Metastatic cancers are also frequent causes of epilepsy, while carcinomatous meningitis is a less common cause.

7. Epilepsy Surgery

Evaluation for Surgery

After several medication trials, about 25% of patients with epilepsy will be refractory. It is estimated that more than half of these may benefit from surgery. Evaluation for surgery requires a multidisciplinary approach. A combination of structural and functional imaging is necessary to define the region of abnormal brain tissue. This has to be correlated with electrographic abnormalities, and long-term video/EEG monitoring is essential. Both interictal and ictal EEG abnormalities are useful in localizing the region of seizure onset. Usually when a structural lesion is apparent, scalp EEG is sufficient, but when ambiguity exists, particularly in nonlesional epilepsy, intracranial EEG recording is invaluable. A combination of intraparenchymal depth electrodes, subdural strip electrodes, and subdural grids is often used to precisely localize the seizure focus. Clinical features of the seizures need to be correlated with the imaging and electrographic findings.

Neuropsychological assessment is an important part of presurgical evaluation. A battery of neuropsychometric tests can lateralize and localize deficits of cerebral functioning, and these can be correlated with seizure foci identified using techniques described above. The intra-arterial amytal procedure (Wada test) is useful for determining cerebral dominance. After a routine angiogram, sodium amytal is injected into one, and subsequently the other carotid artery. A hemiparesis rapidly develops, and if it is accompanied by aphasia, this permits identification of the language-dominant hemisphere. Also, during the time of hemiparesis, it is presumed that one entire hemisphere's function is temporarily suppressed, and memory testing permits assessment of each hemisphere's memory capability independently. Since the hippocampus is an essential structure for the coding of memory, it is essential when hippocampectomy is contemplated for seizure control to know that the contralateral hippocampus and temporal lobe are capable of supporting memory. Lateralized memory failure also predicts the side of seizure onset.

When resection is contemplated near the motor cortex or the speech areas, functional cortical mapping by stimulation of a subdural grid is essential for localizing regions of brain that must be spared.

Types of Surgery

A focal resection is the most common, as well as the most effective form of epilepsy surgery. When a lesion can be identified, complete removal of the lesion with a narrow margin almost always gives complete control of the seizures. How much additional structurally normal brain, which nevertheless shows electrical epileptiform abnormalities (the epileptogenic zone), should be resected remains controversial. Temporal lobectomy is another highly successful operation. Rates of cure and significant improvement approach 90 percent. When the pathology is mesial temporal sclerosis, selective hippocampectomy is less invasive and probably just as successful.

Multilobar resections are feasible on the basis of careful functional mapping and precise definition of the epileptogenic zone. The extreme case is hemispherectomy, where the entire hemisphere is deemed to be epileptogenic. Rasmussen syndrome, a progressive inflammatory disorder with focal and secondarily generalized seizures, is best treated with hemispherectomy.

When, for whatever reason, localization is not possible, or the seizure focus is nonresectable because of its proximity to essential brain tissue, corpus callosotomy is a reasonable alternative. This procedure involves division of the anterior two-thirds of the corpus callosum, and subsequently the posterior one-third may also be divided. Callosotomy often prevents secondary generalization of focal seizures, and is very effective in preventing seizures that cause drop attacks. Such patients do, however, continue to have focal seizures. Transient disturbances of language, as well as disturbances of coordination in one side of the body, are not uncommon postoperative complications.

Multiple subpial transections are another palliative procedure. This technique permits surgery in regions of cortex that involve essential functions and cannot be resected. The procedure disrupts lateral cortical connections and prevents seizure spread, but leaves intact the columnar cortical architecture that is essential for cortical functioning.

Cerebral Stimulation

Intracranial Stimulation

Electrical stimulation of the cerebellum was attempted over 40 years ago as a treatment for epilepsy. Anecdotal success was reported, but the procedure is probably futile. More recently, stimulation of the thalamus and subthalamic nucleus has shown promising results, but no patients have become seizure free. Deep brain stimulation probably disrupts cortical-reticular networks that propagate seizures, but the mechanism of action is unknown. Chronic stimulation of epileptogenic cortical structures such as the hippocampus has also been attempted with encouraging preliminary results.

Vagus Nerve Stimulation

A variety of animal studies have shown that intermittent stimulation of the vagus nerve has a desynchronizing effect on the EEG, and can also acutely stop seizures. In human studies, patients with refractory partial and secondarily generalized seizures have experienced reductions in seizure frequency of about 50 percent. Few patients become seizure free, though the benefit appears to increase over time. The role of vagus nerve stimulation in idiopathic generalized epilepsy is as yet unclear. Side effects are relatively benign and include hoarseness, cough and sleep apnea. Cardiac arrhythmia has not been a problem. Although there are no direct comparisons, the device appears more effective than any single new drug in patients with refractory epilepsy.

Outcome and Psychosocial Factors in Relation to Epilepsy Surgery

The outcome of epilepsy surgery, even when it is narrowly defined as seizure control, is quite variable. The classification of Engel, ranging from class I (seizure free) to class IV (no improvement), has gained general acceptance. Temporal lobectomy for mass lesions or hippocampal sclerosis appears to be the most successful procedure with 60%-70% of patients becoming seizure free. Outside of the temporal lobes, complete success rates are closer to 50 percent. Only about 20% of patients show no improvement, and about 5% are worse. Recently, more complex measures of outcome are being employed, and some of these may be applicable to medical therapy as well. Quality of life, as measured on a variety of scales, appears to be significantly improved following epilepsy surgery, particularly when patients become seizure free. In refractory temporal lobe epilepsy, surgery is clearly superior to medical therapy. Fewer role limitations and higher social function are commonly seen. Improvement in employment status is also significant.

Psychometric tests have shown variable results, but the overall trend appears to be towards improvement, particularly when the surgery is in the non-dominant hemisphere, and the patient becomes seizure free. Conversely, dominant hemisphere resections and surgical failure are associated with deterioration of cognitive function. Depression and psychosis have occasionally followed epilepsy surgery, but it is uncertain whether these are directly caused by surgery, or whether surgery is only a precipitant in a population that already has a marked increase in the incidence and prevalence of such problems.

8. Psychiatric and Psychosocial Problems in Epilepsy

It is estimated that about 30% of patients with epilepsy have significant psychiatric problems. Most are depressed, but less than 5% appear to be psychotic. Anxiety is another major problem. The treatment of these problems is no different than for nonepileptic patients, although antipsychotic as well as antidepressant drugs may lower the seizure threshold. In most cases such drugs are not contraindicated. Certain antiepileptic drugs, particularly barbiturates, are associated with depression. In contrast, Tegretol, Depakote and Lamictal are mood stabilizers. A high rate of suicide is seen among patients with epilepsy, and careful observation is indicated.

Chronic schizophreniform psychosis sometimes accompanies epilepsy. It remains uncertain whether the epilepsy is responsible for the psychosis, or whether such patients have two separate disorders. There is also some evidence to support the interesting idea that improved control of seizures and normalization of the EEG ("forced normalization") is sometimes associated with a worsening of psychosis. Conversely, a flurry of seizures is sometimes associated with acute psychosis. This usually improves over several days, and responds like other forms of psychosis to treatment with neuroleptics.

Personality disorders are not uncommon in epilepsy. Chronic illness in and of itself is associated with personality disorders, but temporal lobe epilepsy, in particular, has been associated with a constellation of personality characteristics, including hypergraphia, hyper-religiosity, and hypo- or hypersexuality. The vast majority of patients with epilepsy do not show such abnormalities.

Learning disabilities are common among children with epilepsy, and it is unclear to what extent the epilepsy is directly responsible. More diffuse brain damage, as well as psychosocial factors, may be contributory. Federal legislation, particularly the Americans with Disabilities Act, prohibits discrimination against patients with epilepsy and other physical or mental handicaps. In certain circumstances, employers may be obliged to provide modified work conditions that enable patients with epilepsy to work.

Patients with uncontrolled epilepsy are prohibited everywhere from driving. In most jurisdictions, freedom from seizures for at least three months is required before a driver's license can be obtained or re-obtained. However, the number of patients with epilepsy who actually have accidents while driving due to seizures is quite small.

9. Conclusion

Epilepsy is a group of disorders with the unifying feature that abnormal electrical activity in the brain is associated with disordered consciousness. The problem is a chronic one, and affects all aspects of a patient's life. Recent advances in both medical and surgical epilepsy give us the hope of being able to control seizures in most patients. Control of seizures is not, however, an end in itself. Improvement of the patient's quality of life requires attention to a variety of psychosocial problems that often exist along with the seizures.

10. References

1. Bernardo LS. Prevention of epilepsy after head trauma: do we need new drugs or a new approach? *Epilepsia*. 2003;44 (Suppl 10): 27-33.

   (One of the last works of a subtle thinker. Old drugs are not good enough.)

2. Cendes F. Febrile seizures and mesial temporal sclerosis. *Curr Opinion Neurology*. 2004;17:161-164.

   (An interesting review of a controversial topic. One does not necessarily cause the other.)

3. Engel J Jr, Pedley TA, eds. *Epilepsy: A Comprehensive Textbook*. Philadelphia, Pa: Lippincott Williams & Wilkins; 1998.

   (Everything you ever wanted to know about epilepsy but were afraid to ask.)

4. French J, Kanner AM, Bautista J. Efficacy and tolerability of the new antiepileptic drugs. I. Treatment of new onset epilepsy. *Neurology*. 2004;62:1252-1260.

   (Up-to-date review of new anti-epileptic drugs.)

5. Fried I, Kim JH, Spencer DD. Limbic and neocortical gliomas associated with intractable seizures: a distinct clinicopathological group. *Neurosurgery*. 1994;34:851-824.

   (A fascinating paper which shows that epilepsy-producing tumors have a better-than-expected prognosis if resected.)

6. Hirsch LJ, Hauser WA. Can sudden unexplained death in epilepsy be prevented? *Lancet*. 2004;Dec 18:364(9452):2157-2158.

   (Stopping seizures is not the only goal in treating epilepsy.)

7. Karceski S, Morrell M, Carpenter D. The expert consensus guidelines series. Treatment of Epilepsy. *Epilepsy Behav*. 2001;2:A1-A50.

   ("Evidence-based" guidelines are not the only way to solve a problem.)

8. Kwan P, Brodie MJ. Early identification of refractory epilepsy. *N Engl J Med*. 200;342:314-319.

   (A modern classic. Solid data and logical reasoning really clarify the prognosis of epilepsy.)

9. Mattson RH, Cramer JA, Collins JF, et al. A comparison of carbamazepine, phenobarbital, phenytoin, and primidone in partial and secondarily generalized tonic-clonic seizures. *N Engl J Med*. 1985;313; 145-151.

   (One of two papers that showed the world how to do antiepileptic drug trials and come up with really useful and meaningful comparative data.)

10. Mattson RH, Cramer JA. Comparison of valproate with carbamazepine for the treatment of complex partial seizures and secondarily generalized tonic-clonic seizures in adults. *N Engl J Med*. 1992;327:765-771.

    (One of two papers that showed the world how to do antiepileptic drug trials and come up with really useful and meaningful comparative data.)

11. Morrell MJ. Reproductive and metabolic disorders in women with epilepsy. *Epilepsia*. 2003;44 (Suppl 4); 11-20.

    (Highlights some less well-recognized aspects of the disease as well as problems caused by the drugs used to treat it.)

12. Noebels JL. The biology of epilepsy genes. *Ann Rev Neurosci*. 2003;26:599-625.

    (An up-to-date review of what will be an increasingly important topic.)

13. Rowe CC, Berkovic SF, Sia STB, Austin M, McKay WJ, Kalnins RM, Bladin PF. Localization of epileptic foci with postictal single photo emission computed tomography. *Ann Neurol.* 1989;26:660-668.

(This paper represented a major advance in imaging epileptic foci.)

14. Sloviter RS. The functional organization of the hippocampal dentate gyrus and its relevance to the pathogenesis of temporal lobe epilepsy. *Ann Neurol.* 1994;35:640-654.

(An interesting hypothesis about epileptogenesis at the cellular level. True or not, it stimulates thought and further experiments.)

15. Thadani VM, Siegel A, Lewis P, Siegel AM, Jobst BC, Gilbert, KL, Darcey TM, Roberts DW, Williamson PD. Validation of ictal single photon emission computed tomography with depth encephalography and epilepsy surgery. *Neurosurg Rev.* 2004 ;27:27-33.

(Summary of Dartmouth's ictal SPECT series.)

16. Theodore WH, Katz D, Kufts C, Patronas N, Smothers P, Bromfield E. Pathology of temporal lobe foci: correlation of CT, MRI and PET. *Neurology.* 1990;40:797-803.

(An important comparison of structural and functional imaging in epilepsy.)

17. Treiman DM, Meyers PD, Walton NY, et al. A comparison of four treatments for generalized convulsive status epilepticus. *N Engl J Med.* 1998;339:792-798.

(The best comparative trial of how to treat status epilepticus.)

18. Wiebe S, Blume WT, Girvin JP, et al. A randomized, controlled trial of surgery for temporal-lobe epilepsy. *N Engl J Med.* 2001;345:311-318.

(For one epilepsy syndrome, surgery really is superior to medical management, both with regard to seizure outcome and overall quality of life.)

19. Williamson PD, Spencer DD, Spencer SS, Novelly RA, Mattson RH. Complex partial seizures of frontal lobe origin. *Ann Neurol.* 1985; 18:497-504.

(Shrewd observation combined with a deep knowledge of what was observed led to identification of a new syndrome.)

21. Wyllie E, ed. *The Treatment of Epilepsy*. 3rd ed. Philadelphia, Pa: Lippincott Williams & Wilkins; 2001.

(Another comprehensive text. Well written but not as exhaustive as Engel and Pedley.)

11. Questions

1. A man develops severe abdominal pain and tenderness and absent bowel sounds after being started on valproate. The clinical problem is most likely associated with:

   A. Valproate level of 115

   B. Prothrombin time and partial thromboplastin time two times normal

   C. Amylase level three times normal

   D. Ammonia level two times normal

   E. Aspartate transaminase level three times normal

2. Complex partial seizures are always:

   A. Associated with visible changes on scalp electroencephalogram

   B. Accompanied by jerking of more than one extremity

   C. Caused by structural brain lesions

   D. Associated with changes in behavior or consciousness

   E. Originating in the temporal lobes

3. Early myoclonic encephalopathy is associated with all of the following except:

   A. Electroencephalogram with burst-suppression activity

   B. Variable partial seizures

   C. Normal development in later life

   D. Onset before 3 months of age

   E. Fragmentary myoclonus

4. Common epileptic auras include all of the following except:

   A. Gastric sensation

   B. Feeling of fear

   C. Unusual taste or smell

   D. Desire to commit violence

   E. Indescribable feeling

5. The following statements about the NMDA-type glutamate receptor are true except:

   A. The binding of glutamate usually has an excitatory effect

   B. Receptor-blocking drugs are potential anticonvulsants

   C. A glycine binding site is associated with it

   D. Barbiturate drugs bind to it

   E. It is associated with Na+ and Ca++ ion channels

6. The $GABA_A$ receptor binds all of the following except:

   A. Phenytoin

   B. Barbiturates

   C. Benzodiazepines

   D. GABA

   E. Topiramate

7. Which of the following statements is (are) true of valproate?

A. It is one of the most effective drugs for idiopathic generalized epilepsy with convulsive seizures

B. It is effective in the treatment of absence seizures and complex partial seizures with or without secondary generalization

C. Side effects include gastrointestinal upset, weight gain, hair loss, thrombocytopenia, and menstrual irregularities

D. A. and C.

E. A., B. and C.

8. Corpus callosotomy for the treatment of epilepsy may:

A. Prevent secondary generalization of focal onset epilepsy

B. Prevent falls from atonic seizures

C. Reduce the severity of some complex partial seizures

D. Make a hemiparesis worse

E. All of the above

9. Mental functions that may be preserved during a complex partial seizure include:

A. Visual perception

B. Auditory perception

C. Verbal responsiveness

D. Behavioral responsiveness

E. All of the above

10. Sudden falls are associated with all of the following seizure types except:

A. Atonic seizures

B. Tonic seizures

C. Myoclonic seizures

D. Gelastic seizures

E. Tonic-clonic seizures

11. Which of the following antiepileptic drugs is unlikely to cause an exacerbation of porphyria?

A. Phenytoin

B. Phenobarbital

C. Carbamazepine

D. Gabapentin

E. Primidone

12. In focal epilepsy one might expect to see:

A. Interictal focal hypometabolism on PET scan

B. Interictal focal hypoperfusion or normal perfusion on SPECT scan

C. Ictal focal hyperperfusion on SPECT scan

D. Decreased numbers of benzodiazepine (GABA) receptors binding labeled ligand on interictal PET scan

E. All of the above

13. A 50-year-old man has a history of complex partial seizures. These have been refractory to several medications, and he is taking Keppra 1000 mg bid. His exam is normal, MRI is normal, and video-EEG recording shows seizures with maximal electrographic change in the left temporal region. An intracarotid Amytal study (Wada test) shows that the right hemisphere does not support memory functions. Which treatment option is contraindicated?

A. Vagus nerve stimulation

B. Cerebral stimulation

C. Left temporal lobectomy

D. An experimental drug trial

E. Addition of phenobarbital to his medical regimen

14. A 65-year-old man who is taking coumadin for atrial fibrillation suffers a cardioembolic stroke and develops epilepsy. He also suffers from depression, and nephrolithiasis. He is quite thin. Among the drugs listed below, the best choice is likely to be:

A. Phenytoin

B. Carbamazepine

C. Phenobarbital

D. Lamotrigine

E. Topiramate

15. A 60-year-old woman who smokes and has COPD develops bronchitis. She has a history of seizures that have been well controlled on Tegretol with a level of 10mg/L. Her PCP treats her with Zithromax®, codeine, a prednisone taper and inhaled terbutaline and inhaled ipratropium. She then develops ataxia, nystagmus and confusion. The likely culprit is:

A. Codeine

B. Zithromax

C. Ipratropium

D. Prednisone

E. Terbutaline

16. A 25-year-old woman with history of petit mal (absence) seizures in childhood and convulsive seizures as an adult has done well on valproate. When she decides to become pregnant it would be logical to convert her to:

A. Lamotrigine

B. Phenobarbital

C. Carbamazepine

D. Ethosuximide

E. Pregabalin

17. A 40-year-old man with complex partial and secondarily generalized seizures has done well on Dilantin 300 mg daily with a blood level of 13 mg/L. After his insurance refuses to pay for the brand name drug, he switches to generic phenytoin and has a breakthrough seizure with a measured drug level of 7. At a dose of 400 mg daily, his level is 11 and he has another seizure. His dose of phenytoin is further increased to 500 mg daily and this results in ataxia, nausea and nystagmus. His phenytoin level is now 22. The relevant pharmacological principle is:

A. Displacement of bound drug from protein

B. First-order kinetics

C. Saturation of the renal transporter of conjugated phenytoin metabolites

D. Induction of hepatic enzymes

E. Zero-order kinetics

18. A 28-year-old woman is being evaluated for epilepsy surgery. Her seizures involve frequent and sudden arousals from sleep, and dystonic posturing that is more prominent of the right. Her exam and MRI scan and interictal EEG are normal, and ictal EEG shows artifacts only. Interictal and ictal SPECT scans are obtained. These will most likely show:

A. Ictal hyperperfusion of the left frontal lobe.

B. Interictal hypoperfusion of the left frontal lobe.

C. Ictal hyperperfusion of both frontal lobes.

D. Interictal hypoperfusion of the right temporal lobe.

E. Ictal hyperperfusion of the right frontal lobe.

19. A patient with end-stage renal disease is placed on dialysis and suffers a seizure. He is loaded with Dilantin and the level is noted to be low in spite of adequate maintenance dosing. Seizure control is good. An increase in the maintenance dose of Dilantin to achieve a "therapeutic" blood level results in ataxia and nausea. This has happened because:

A. Dialysis dementia makes patients susceptible to side effects of phenytoin.

B. Dilantin is being dialyzed away, and large doses are producing fluctuating levels which result in toxic symptoms.

C. Protein binding of Dilantin is reduced in dialysis patients, while the percentage of free Dilantin is relatively high.

D. Hepatic metabolism of Dilantin is increased in dialysis patients, and active metabolites are producing toxicity.

E. The patient is confused and has taken more Dilantin than was recommended.

20. A 25-year-old man with a family history of relatives with nocturnal spells is noted to have sudden arousals at night, with dystonia, thrashing in bed, and brief confusion. This is probably a case of:

A. Hereditary Lewy body dementia with REM sleep behavior disorder.

B. A nicotinic acetylcholine receptor mutation.

C. A GABA receptor mutation.

D. A sodium channel mutation.

E. A potassium channel mutation.

21. An 18-year-old woman has episodes of suddenly falling to the ground when she laughs at a joke. She also describes some vivid dreams, and is sometimes unable to move as she awakens from sleep. She is often sleepy in the daytime. It is likely she is suffering from:

A. Atonic epileptic seizures.

B. Psychogenic non-epileptic seizures.

C. Cataplexy with narcolepsy and sleep paralysis.

D. Gelastic epilepsy with hypothalamic hamartoma.

E. Complex partial seizures of frontal lobe origin with disturbed sleep patterns.

22. A 55-year-old man has had medically refractory complex partial seizures, 2-3/month, for much of his life. He is not interested in brain surgery, and is offered a vagus nerve stimulator. The most accurate advice statement is:

A. He will not be able to have an MRI of the brain afterwards.

B. There is a 50% chance that he will have a 50% reduction in seizure frequency.

C. There is a 50% chance that he will be seizure free.

D. He will probably have throat pain.

E. Homeland Security will arrest him when the device sets off an alarm at the airport.

Answers

1. C.

Pancreatitis is a complication of treatment with valproate. An elevated valproate level of 115 could produce nausea, vomiting, or diarrhea, but would be unlikely to present as an acute abdomen. Valproate does not usually affect the prothrombin time and partial thromboplastin time. Thrombocytopenia is a common side effect but is usually not clinically significant. Children, more commonly than adults, can have elevations of ammonia; other liver function tests can also be abnormal. Abnormal liver function tests are sometimes associated with encephalopathy but not usually an acute abdomen.

2. D.

Complex partial seizures are by definition associated with changes in behavior or consciousness. They can originate in any lobe of the brain. Sometimes there is no obvious structural lesion, only an electrical abnormality. They are not always associated with motor activity. Complex partial seizures, particularly of frontal lobe origin, may not produce changes in the scalp electroencephalogram. An intracranial electroencephalogram recording is sometimes necessary.

3. C.

Patients with early myoclonic encephalopathy usually do very poorly. They commonly develop multiple seizure types and are often severely retarded. There may be some benign variants of this condition.

4. D.

All the other choices are quite common epileptic auras. A desire to commit violence is almost unheard of as a true epileptic aura. Directed violence during or after a seizure is also extremely rare. Nondirected, random striking out during the period of ictal or postictal confusion is somewhat more common.

5. D.

Barbiturate drugs bind to the $GABA_A$ receptor and exert an anticonvulsant effect by hyperpolarizing the cell. The $GABA_A$ receptor is associated with a chloride ion channel, and the inward passage of chloride ions hyperpolarizes the cell and makes firing less likely. The other statements are all true of the NMDA-type glutamate receptor. The binding of glutamate depolarizes the cell and makes firing more likely. There is inward passage of sodium and calcium ions. The binding of glycine at an accessory site is necessary for glutamate-mediated depolarization.

6. A.

GABA is the endogenous substrate for the $GABA_A$ receptor. Barbiturates and benzodiazepines exert their anticonvulsant effects by binding to the $GABA_A$ receptor and producing hyperpolarization of the cell. Topiramate mimics the action of GABA at the $GABA_A$ receptor. Phenytoin exerts its anticonvulsant effect by blocking the transmission of sodium ions through the voltage-gated sodium channel.

7. E.

This answer is self-explanatory.

8. E.

Cutting the major connecting pathway between the two hemispheres can prevent secondary generalization of focal seizures. Falls often occur when seizures spread from one side of the brain to the other, so anything that prevents seizure spread is likely to reduce falling. Impairment of consciousness in complex partial seizures is also associated with spread to both sides of the brain, so consciousness is less likely to be impaired if seizure spread is inhibited. Callosotomy may make a hemiparesis worse because the damaged hemisphere is then deprived of input from the undamaged hemisphere.

9. E.

Complex partial seizures can impair any or all of the listed alternatives; however, any of the alternatives may be preserved. The only requirement for a complex partial seizure is that consciousness should in some way be altered.

10. D.

Atonic, tonic, tonic-clonic, and myoclonic seizures can all produce sudden falls because of alterations in muscle tone. Gelastic seizures are associated with inappropriate laughter and do not usually produce falls.

11. D.

Seizures associated with porphyria can be exacerbated by phenytoin, phenobarbital, primidone, or carbamazepine, all of which exacerbate the underlying disease. Gabapentin, because it has no hepatic metabolism, does not exacerbate porphyria and can be used to treat seizures associated with porphyria.

12. E.

Glucose metabolism is often reduced in and around a seizure focus, and this can be detected by PET scan using FDG-glucose. Perfusion is sometimes decreased interictally, but interictal SPECT scan is not a very sensitive or specific test. Ictally, perfusion is often increased, and this can be detected with SPECT, provided the isotope is injected within seconds, or at most within minutes, of seizure onset. Recent research with PET scans suggests that the binding of radio-labeled flumazenil (a measure of the number of GABA receptors) is decreased in the vicinity of a seizure focus.

13. C.

A left temporal lobectomy in these circumstances is likely to produce a severe anterograde amnesia. The other options are all reasonable.

14. D.

Phenytoin, carbamazepine and phenobarbital interfere with coumadin metabolism. Phenobarbital can produce depression. Topiramate is associated with kidney stones and weight loss. Lamotrigine is therefore the best choice. The only drawbacks are that it cannot be loaded rapidly and carries a relatively high risk of rash.

15. B.

Zithromax and other macrolide antibiotics increase blood levels of carbamazepine by inhibition of the cytochrome P-450 enzyme system. The patient is probably suffering from Tegretol toxicity. The other medications are probably harmless in this situation.

16. A.

Lamotrigine is effective against petit mal and grand mal seizures in idiopathic generalized epilepsy. It has a good track record in pregnancy. Phenobarbital and carbamazepine are not effective against petit mal seizures. Ethosuximide is not effective against grand mal seizures. Pregabalin may not be effective against either seizure type and is an unknown quantity in pregnancy.

17. E.

Phenytoin metabolism shows zero order kinetics at high doses because of saturation of the metabolizing hepatic enzyme.

Thus a relatively small increase in the dose, in the 400-600 mg range in adults, may produce a dramatic increase in the blood level, and consequent toxic side effects. The other pharmacological principles exist, and are in principle true, but do not apply here.

18. A.

The epileptic syndrome is suggestive of frontal lobe epilepsy, and the greater dystonia on the right suggests a contralateral (left-sided) electrographic seizure focus. In the interictal state seizure foci are hypoperfused, and become hyperperfused seconds after seizure onset. Ictal SPECT is more sensitive than interictal SPECT. So we are most likely to see left frontal hyperperfusion on the ictal SPECT study.

19. C.

A. is true, but probably irrelevant early in the course of dialysis. If E. were true, levels of Dilantin would fluctuate randomly. B. is unlikely because Dilantin is not dialyzed and levels do not usually fluctuate. C. is false because hepatic metabolism of Dilantin is not increased in dialysis patients, and hepatic metabolites of Dilantin are mostly inactive. C. is the correct answer, and it is important to measure free as well as total Dilantin levels in patients with any type of metabolic derangement.

20. B.

This is probably a case of autosomal dominant frontal lobe epilepsy.

21. C.

Atonic seizures are not usually induced by emotion. Gelastic seizures are not caused by laughter, but laughter is part of the seizure. Drop attacks can be psychogenic, but it seems unlikely in this case, which clearly fits into a syndromic pattern. Complex partial seizures can be atonic, and can disturb sleep to produce daytime somnolence, but are not usually associated with sleep paralysis or emotional triggers.

22. B.

Throat pain is rare in patients with vagus nerve stimulators. MRI of the brain is feasible, but body MRI may cause heating of wires and is not recommended. Almost no one becomes seizure free with VNS, but 50% seizure reductions are quite common. No one can predict what Homeland Security will do, but metal detectors at airports have not been a major issue. Close contact with any sort of microwave radiation is contraindicated.

Chapter 22: Epilepsy in Children

Carl E. Stafstrom, MD, PhD

Contents

1. Introduction

Definitions and Epidemiology

This chapter reviews the diagnosis and treatment of childhood epilepsy. For further information, the reader is referred to the comprehensive textbooks and other sources listed in the References.

A *seizure* is a paroxysmal alteration of neurologic function caused by the excessive, hypersynchronous discharge of neurons in the brain. *Epileptic seizure* is used to distinguish a seizure caused by abnormal neuronal firing from a nonepileptic event such as a pseudoseizure. *Epilepsy* is a chronic condition of recurrent, unprovoked seizures. Epilepsy is not a single disease but rather a sign of underlying brain dysfunction. Seizures provoked by a reversible insult (eg, fever or hypoglycemia) do not fall under the definition of epilepsy because they are a short-lived, secondary condition rather than a chronic state.

An *epilepsy syndrome* refers to a group of clinical characteristics that consistently occur together, with similar seizure type, age of onset, electroencephalogram (EEG) findings, triggering factors, genetics, natural history, prognosis, and response to antiepileptic drugs (AEDs). The nonspecific term "seizure disorder" should not be used.

Epilepsy is one of the most common neurologic conditions, with an incidence of approximately 50 new cases per year per 100,000 population. Approximately 1% of the population suffers from epilepsy, one-third of which is refractory (ie, not controlled by several anticonvulsant medications or other therapies). Approximately 75% of epilepsy begins during childhood.

Classification of Seizures and Epilepsies

The International League Against Epilepsy (ILAE) has developed separate classifications of epileptic seizures and epilepsies (epilepsy syndromes), as detailed in the chapter on epilepsy in adults. Epileptic seizures are classified according to: clinical seizure phenotype, ictal EEG pattern, and interictal EEG pattern. The first step is to categorize a seizure as partial (focal) or generalized using clinical criteria. Partial seizures originate in one part of the brain and begin with focal clinical signs. Generalized seizures begin simultaneously in both hemispheres, without focal clinical features such as eye deviation or one-sided tonic-clonic movements. The second step is to further classify a seizure as generalized or partial according to its interictal and ictal EEG features, if available. After classification based on a reliable history and EEG, the physician can formulate an appropriate diagnostic evaluation and treatment plan.

Epilepsies and epilepsy syndromes are classified according to: 1.) their onset (generalized or localization-related); and 2.) whether a cause is known (symptomatic) or not known (idiopathic). An updated classification system is being developed that takes into account ictal phenomenology, seizure type, syndrome diagnosis (if present), etiology, and degree of functional impairment. New classification schemes will evolve as knowledge about epilepsy pathophysiology and genetics emerges.

2. Pathophysiology and Genetics

The developing brain is very prone to seizures, for several physiological reasons (Table 1). A seizure may result when there is distortion of the normal balance between excitation and inhibition in the brain. This balance can be upset by genetic or acquired factors. Genetic pathologies leading to epilepsy can occur anywhere from the circuit level (eg, abnormal synaptic connectivity in cortical dysplasia); to the receptor level (eg, abnormal gamma-amino-butyric acid ((GABA)) receptor subunits in Angelman syndrome); to abnormal ionic channel function (eg, potassium channel mutations in benign familial neonatal convulsions). Similarly, acquired cerebral insults can alter circuit function (eg, structural alterations of hippocampal circuitry following prolonged febrile seizures or head trauma). Even in the normal developing brain, excitatory synaptic function develops prior to inhibitory synaptic function, favoring enhanced excitation and seizure generation. In addition, perhaps paradoxically, early in life GABA can act as an excitatory neurotransmitter rather than an inhibitory one, due to a reversed chloride ion gradient and immature pattern of chloride transport by membrane pumps. These observations partly explain why the very young brain is especially susceptible to seizures. Fortunately, seizures seem to cause less structural damage in the developing brain than in the adult brain.

There has been a recent explosion of information about the genetic basis of epilepsy syndromes, some of which is summarized in Table 2. Both monogenic and polygenic mutations can lead to epilepsy. It is clear that mutations proteins governing a wide variety of physiological functions can lead to the state of hyperexcitability that underlies epilepsy. As these syndromes become better elucidated, there is hope that syndrome-specific therapies can be designed.

3. Diagnostic Evaluation

History and Examination

The history and neurologic examination are the cornerstones of neurologic diagnosis, with laboratory studies properly used to augment or confirm the diagnosis (Table 3). Historical features include the clinical context in which the seizure occurred, features of the seizure itself, duration, and postictal signs. It is important to determine whether an epilepsy syndrome is present, to guide the nature and extent of the evaluation, treatment, and prognosis. If there is uncertainty about the diagnosis, it is usually better to withhold treatment and wait for another attack than to embark on an extensive work-up and initiation of AEDs.

The extent of diagnostic evaluation is determined by the clinical context. In a child who presents in status epilepticus, in coma, or with a fever, there is an urgency to determine the acute cause of the seizures, such as infection, brain injury, or metabolic disturbance. In a child who has recovered completely by the time of evaluation, the work-up is less urgent.

Table 1

Factors Predisposing the Developing Brain to Hyperexcitability and Seizures

Early development of excitatory synapses and neurotransmitters
Delayed development of inhibitory synapses and neurotransmitters
Early development of sodium and calcium channels
Later development of potassium channels
Exuberant axonal branching pattern early in life (more excitatory synapses)
Paradoxical depolarizing action of GABA early in development
Delayed glial clearance of extracellular potassium after neuronal firing

GABA, gamma-aminobutyric acid

Electroencephalography (EEG)

An EEG is a recording of the brain's electrical activity. It can detect abnormal electrical activity such as focal spikes or sharp waves (consistent with partial epilepsy) or diffuse bilateral spike-waves (consistent with generalized epilepsy). A routine EEG should be obtained on any child with a suspected seizure, preferably during both wakefulness and sleep and with hyperventilation and photic stimulation. Simultaneous video-EEG monitoring can increase the diagnostic yield or differentiate an epileptic seizure from a nonepileptic event. The EEG can be normal in a child with epilepsy, especially in partial-onset seizures of frontal or temporal lobe origin. In such cases, intracranial EEG monitoring may be necessary to detect the seizure focus. However, the diagnosis of epilepsy is based on clinical information, and the EEG should be regarded as confirmatory, not diagnostic. While we ordinarily should "treat the child, not the EEG," certain exceptions exist in which electrographic abnormalities themselves portend clinical impairment. These include absence epilepsy, the syndrome of continuous spike-wave discharges of slow wave sleep, and hypsarrhythmia in infantile spasms (West syndrome) (each syndrome is detailed in section 4).

Neuroimaging

Computed tomography (CT) and magnetic resonance imaging (MRI) scans are important adjuncts to the clinical examination and EEG in the evaluation of a child with seizures. Neuroimaging techniques are especially sensitive for CNS structural lesions. MRI is more likely to show an abnormality in a child with partial seizures, abnormal neurologic findings, or focal discharges on the EEG. A child with focal neurologic findings on examination requires urgent neuroimaging.

MRI is more sensitive than CT and is therefore preferred, especially for the detection of cortical malformation, dysgenesis, or hippocampal sclerosis. Quantitative, computer-assisted volume analysis of the temporal lobes may allow detection of asymme-

Table 2

Epilepsy Genetics in Selected Syndromes

Syndrome	Chromosomes	Genes
Autosomal dominant nocturnal frontal lobe epilepsy (ADNFLE)	20q13, 1p21	Acetylcholine receptors
Benign familial neonatal convulsions (BFNC)	20q13, 8q24	Potassium channels
Generalized epilepsy with febrile seizures plus (GEFS+)	19q13, 2q24, 5q34	Sodium channels $GABA_A$ receptors
Severe myoclonic epilepsy of infancy (SMEI)	2q24, 5q31	Sodium receptors
Juvenile myoclonic epilepsy	5q34, 2q22-23	$GABA_A$ receptors Calcium channels
Childhood absence epilepsy	5q34, 19p	$GABA_A$ receptors Calcium channels

GABA, gamma-aminobutyric acid

Table 3

Suggested Laboratory Evaluation of a Child With Seizures

Seizure Type/Syndrome	Test	Comments
Simple partial	MRI	Rule out structural lesion
Complex partial	MRI	Rule out structural lesion
Generalized tonic-clonic	MRI	Rule out structural lesion
Absence	None required	
Infantile spasms and other refractory epilepsies and epileptic encephalopathies	Skin examination including Wood's lamp	Hypopigmented lesions (tuberous sclerosis complex)
	MRI	Rule out congenital malformation, neuronal migration disorder
	Serum/urine amino/organic acids; serum biotinidase	Screen for inborn error of metabolism
	Serum ammonia	Screen for urea cycle defect
	Serum lactate/pyruvate	Screen for mitochondrial disorder
	Pyroxidine infusion	Rule out vitamin B_6-dependent seizures
	Ophthalmologic examination	Chorioretinitis might indicate congenital infection. Chorioretinal lacunes might indicate Aicardi syndrome.
	Lumbar puncture	Rule out neurotransmitter disorder

tries that are not readily apparent on visual analysis of the scan. CT is valuable in the acute setting to detect hemorrhage, calcification, tumors and other lesions that require immediate attention.

Several new imaging techniques are available to aid in the assessment of epilepsy. MRI abnormalities can be correlated directly with EEG activity. MR spectroscopy measures the concentrations of a variety of neurochemicals in different brain regions and can sometimes help to localize a seizure focus. Positron emission tomography (PET) images the brain's regional utilization of glucose, with asymmetries suggesting areas of interictal or ictal abnormality. Single photon emission computed tomography (SPECT) compares local blood flow discrepancies, information that is most useful when recorded during a seizure. Magnetoencephalography (MEG) assesses the brain's dynamic electromagnetic fields and can localize areas of abnormal function. These new modalities are used mainly in epilepsy centers for presurgical evaluations.

Metabolic Evaluation

The type of seizure and syndrome dictates the extent of the metabolic work-up. For example, a child with infantile spasms or Lennox-Gastaut syndrome is more likely to have a metabolic or degenerative disorder than one presenting with simple partial seizures. In metabolic disorders, seizures typically accompany other abnormal findings, such as developmental delay. In neonatal seizures, a metabolic evaluation is mandatory (see section 4). Table 3 outlines some of the metabolic and genetic tests useful for the evaluation of various seizure types and syndromes.

4. Differential Diagnosis

Seizure Types

Partial Seizures

As discussed in the chapter on adult epilepsy, seizures are classified according to their onset as partial or generalized. Partial (focal) seizures are those in which the first clinical and EEG changes indicate activation of neurons limited to part of one cerebral hemisphere. Partial seizures are further classified as to whether or not consciousness is impaired during the attack. When consciousness is not impaired, the seizure is termed simple partial. When consciousness is impaired, that is, the child is unable to respond normally to exogenous stimuli by virtue of altered awareness or responsiveness, the seizure is classified as complex partial. The clinical manifestations of partial seizures are determined by the cortical area involved. For example, a simple partial seizure arising from the occipital lobe presents with visual phenomena; from the precentral gyrus, with motor activity; and from the postcentral gyrus, with sensory symptoms. Seizures arising from the temporal lobe are usually associated with an altered state of consciousness and are therefore complex partial seizures. Partial complex seizures can secondarily generalize, that is, spread from the focus to both sides of the brain.

Generalized Seizures

Generalized seizures, on the other hand, begin in both cerebral hemispheres simultaneously, with alteration of responsiveness and sometimes other clinical signs. There are several types of generalized seizure. Absence seizures (formerly called petit mal) involve sudden staring with unresponsiveness to external verbal stimuli, and often eye blinking or head nodding. Note that "absence" refers to both a seizure type and an epilepsy syndrome (see below).

Generalized tonic-clonic seizures (formerly called grand mal), consist of bilaterally symmetric convulsive movements of all limbs, with impairment of consciousness. Some children have prodromal symptoms, such as headache, insomnia, irritability, or a change in mood hours or even days before a seizure. Prodromal symptoms are to be distinguished from an aura, which generally precedes the GTC by seconds or minutes. The aura is a partial seizure, whereas a prodrome is not associated with epileptiform discharges. The aura is useful in distinguishing between a GTC seizure that begins focally from one that does not secondarily generalize. Auras vary considerably from patient to patient and may encompass any of the manifestations of simple partial seizures including focal motor, sensory, autonomic, or psychic symptoms. Occasionally, a seizure is clonic or tonic without the other component.

Atonic seizures consist of sudden loss of tone in the axial musculature, causing the individual to fall or slump to the ground. Atonic seizures are often associated with other seizure types in the same person, and are often seen in epilepsies such as Lennox-Gastaut syndrome. A patient with atonic seizures often has significant neurologic impairment and may need to wear a protective helmet due to the high risk of head injury.

Myoclonic seizures consist of sudden, brief ("lightning-like") movements that are not associated with any obvious disturbance of consciousness. These brief involuntary muscle contractions may affect one or several muscles; therefore, myoclonic seizures can be generalized or partial. Myoclonus can be associated with a lesion at any level of the neuraxis, including cortex, cerebellum, brainstem, or spinal cord. Myoclonic seizures have numerous causes. Myoclonic movements may be normal phenomena such as hypnogogic jerks or sleep starts. Conversely, myoclonus can be associated with virtually any severe insult to the brain, including toxic, metabolic, infectious, traumatic, or degenerative insults. Likewise, the pathophysiology of myoclonus varies; some myoclonus is nonepileptic and classified as a movement disorder, whereas other myoclonus has an epileptic basis.

Epilepsy Syndromes in Children

These examples of childhood epilepsy syndromes were selected based on their importance or frequency, and are categorized according to the 1989 ILAE classification scheme.

Generalized Epilepsy Syndromes

Idiopathic Generalized Epilepsy Syndromes

Benign familial neonatal convulsions. Benign familial neonatal convulsions (BFNC) is a neonatal epilepsy syndrome in which seizures begin in the first week of life. The seizure type is focal clonic or focal tonic (although it is currently classified as a generalized epilepsy), often accompanied by apnea. The seizures occur in sleep and are usually brief, lasting 1 to 2 minutes, but may occur as many as 20 to 30 times per day. They usually stop after a few days or weeks. Ictal EEG recordings show initial generalized voltage attenuation, followed by bilateral spikes and sharp waves. Except for seizures, the infants are normal, and evaluation fails to detect an etiology of the seizures. The key to the diagnosis is a positive family history of newborn or infantile seizures with benign outcome. However, even with a positive family history, other more ominous causes of seizures should be ruled out before concluding that the seizures are inherited.

Infants can be treated with phenobarbital until seizures remit. The prognosis of BFNC is good, although about 10%-15% of affected infants continue to have seizures beyond the neonatal period, even into adulthood.

BFNC is a familial disorder that has been linked to at least two chromosomal loci. The identified genes (KCNQ2 on chromosome 20q and KCNQ3 on chromosome 8q) code for voltage-gated potassium channel subunits that appear to regulate the "M-current," a muscarine-activated neuronal current that turns off potassium channels. The M-current ordinarily stabilizes resting membrane potential, so its dysfunction causes increased neuronal excitability and seizures. It is not known why seizures in BFNC affect neonates primarily, since the genetic defect is presumably present throughout life.

Generalized epilepsy with febrile seizures plus. Generalized epilepsy with febrile seizures plus (GEFS+) is a recently described disorder in which children have febrile seizures beyond the age at which febrile seizures usually stop (age 5 years). In addition, these children may develop additional afebrile seizure types, including generalized tonic-clonic, absence, myoclonic, and atonic. Therefore, this syndrome is not the same as simple febrile seizures, and represents a genetic predisposition to epilepsy. GEFS+ is transmitted in an autosomal dominant pattern with high penetrance. In different families, genetic defects have been identified in neuronal sodium channels and GABA receptors. There may be a spectrum of disorders, with different phenotypes, caused by sodium channel dysfunction. For example, the same sodium channel mutation has been identified in severe myoclonic epilepsy of infancy (Dravet syndrome). In GEFS+, the outcome is variable: seizures resolve in some children, whereas in others, epilepsy persists.

Childhood absence epilepsy. Absence seizures can be part of several epilepsy syndromes, including childhood absence epilepsy (CAE), juvenile absence epilepsy, and juvenile myoclonic epilepsy (JME). CAE is characterized by typical absence seizures with an onset between 4 and 10 years of age. In CAE, absence seizures consist of staring with altered alertness, sometimes with motor phenomena such as blinking or head nodding. Because absence seizures are brief and nonconvulsive, they can be easily missed or misdiagnosed. Their recognition and treatment is important because frequent absence seizures can cause a decline in school performance, or may result in injury.

Clinical Characteristics

The hallmark of a typical absence spell is the suppression of mental function, usually to the point of complete abolition of awareness, responsiveness, and memory. The seizures start abruptly and generally last from 5 to 15 seconds. Ongoing activity is suddenly interrupted, the facial expression changes, and the child stares off. When the seizure ends, the child immediately resumes his or her previous conversation or activity. The child may be momentarily confused afterwards, but there is no prolonged postictal state.

The frequency of absence seizures varies considerably, from a few per day to hundreds per day. Stress and fatigue can increase their frequency. Most children with typical absence seizures have a normal neurologic examination and intelligence, although school performance may be impaired if seizures are frequent. GTC seizures eventually occur in 10%-20% of patients with CAE.

Electroencephalography

Children with CAE have a normal EEG background. The ictal EEG pattern of an absence seizure consists of the sudden onset of generalized symmetric spike or multiple spike- and slow-wave complexes at a frequency of 3 Hz. For practical purposes, generalized spike-wave activity lasting longer than 1 second or so can be considered a seizure. Hyperventilation is a potent activator of absence seizures, and this simple test can be used in the clinic to diagnose absence seizures and assess treatment effectiveness. Failure to induce an absence attack with several trials of hyperventilation of 3- to 5-minutes duration in an untreated patient would make the diagnosis of absence seizures unlikely.

Atypical Absence Seizures

Atypical absence seizures involve an altered state of awareness or staring, with an onset and cessation that is not as abrupt as a typical absence seizure. Atypical absences are often accompanied by automatisms, clonic movements, autonomic components, and changes in tone. Atypical absence seizures are usually longer than typical absences, sometimes lasting several minutes. Unlike the usual 3 Hz spike-wave discharges that occur in typical absence seizures, slower spike-wave discharges occurring at 1.5 to 2.5 Hz are more characteristic of atypical absence seizures. The interictal EEG is usually abnormal in children with atypical absences, many of whom have Lennox-Gastaut syndrome (see below).

Etiology

The differential diagnosis of staring spells includes absence seizures, complex partial seizures, and inattention. The pathophysiology of absence seizures involves altered function of thalamo-cortical circuits. CAE has a genetic basis, although a single gene mutation has not yet been found. Some families with CAE have been identified with GABA receptor loss-of-function mutations. EEG studies of families with CAE have shown age-related increased incidences of spike-wave abnormalities among asymptomatic siblings. Therefore, the EEG abnormality is a marker for genetic susceptibility to absence epilepsy, although the seizures will not manifest in everyone with the EEG trait. The EEG abnormality is the expression of an autosomal dominant gene with the unusual characteristic of having a very low penetrance at birth that rises to nearly complete penetrance during childhood before decreasing again.

Evaluation

In a child with typical absence seizures, a classic 3 Hz spike-wave ictal EEG, a normal interictal EEG, and a normal neurologic examination, no further diagnostic studies are necessary. If there is an abnormal developmental history, neurologic deficits, or focality on the EEG, a brain MRI scan is recommended. Because absence seizures are brief and subtle, their frequency is often underestimated. Each follow-up evaluation should include a trial of hyperventilation. Activation of a seizure by hyperventilation indicates that the seizures are not under optimal control, regardless of the history supplied by the parent or other observer.

Treatment

Ethosuximide and VPA are equally effective in the treatment of absence seizures. A child with CAE has a better than 70% chance of achieving seizure control on either drug. Ethosuximide is usually tried first, because of concerns about adverse reactions with VPA. VPA should be considered the drug of choice in a child who has both absence and GTC seizures. The combination of ethosuximide and VPA sometimes works better than either drug alone, though signs of toxicity must be closely monitored. Lamotrigine is also effective in CAE.

Prognosis

The prognosis of CAE is good, with most children outgrowing the absence seizures during adolescence. However, at least 15% of children with CAE have persistent seizures or evolve into JME. A general guideline is to withdraw AEDs slowly after the child has been seizure free for 2 years and no longer has generalized spike-wave discharges on the EEG (including a hyperventilation trial). Spike-wave discharges on the routine EEG indicates a high recurrence risk if the medication is withdrawn.

Juvenile myoclonic epilepsy. Myoclonic seizures in children may occur as a component of an epilepsy syndrome known as juvenile myoclonic epilepsy (JME). JME typically begins in adolescence, and 15% of JME cases evolve from CAE. The myoclonic seizures in JME involve jerks of the neck, shoulders, or arms, occurring singly or repetitively. The myoclonic jerks may cause the patient to drop objects, which may be attributed to nervousness or clumsiness. The myoclonic seizures most often occur shortly after awakening from sleep. They are exacerbated by fatigue, sleep deprivation, and alcohol use.

GTC seizures also occur in as many as 90% of patients with JME and the syndrome often presents with GTC seizures. GTC seizures also occur soon after awakening. Sometimes a series of myoclonic seizures culminates in a GTC seizure. Up to 35% of patients with JME also have absence seizures.

The neurologic examination and intelligence are usually normal in JME. Multifactorial inheritance is presumed. Studies have linked the syndrome to chromosome 6p, a locus that appears to be dominantly inherited, but a responsible gene has not yet been identified.

The interictal EEG in JME shows characteristic bursts of fast (3.5 Hz to 6 Hz) spike-wave complexes. This pattern contrasts with the 3-Hz spike-wave complexes seen in childhood absence epilepsy and the slow (1.5 Hz to 2.5 Hz) spike-wave complexes of Lennox-Gastaut syndrome. Photic stimulation may activate the epileptiform discharges in JME. If the diagnosis is suspected and the awake EEG is normal, a sleep-deprived EEG should be obtained.

VPA is the treatment of choice for JME, though other broad spectrum AEDs (eg, lamotrigine, topiramate, methsuximide) may also be effective. The seizures in JME often respond quite promptly to VPA, but long-term treatment is required. Patients rarely tolerate drug withdrawal and seizures only rarely remit spontaneously. JME is considered relatively benign because most children continue to exhibit normal neurologic function.

Cryptogenic or Symptomatic Generalized Epilepsy Syndromes

Infantile spasms. Infantile spasms (IS) is an epilepsy syndrome characterized by seizures known as epileptic spasms, an interictal EEG pattern called hypsarrhythmia, and mental retardation. This triad is known as West syndrome. IS is an age-specific disorder beginning primarily in the first year of life; the peak age of onset is between 4 and 6 months.

Clinical Manifestations

The epileptic spasms of IS vary considerably and the diagnosis is often delayed due to their subtle features. The duration of a spasm is intermediate between myoclonic jerks (which are briefer) and tonic seizures (which are more sustained). Some seizures are characterized by brief head nods, whereas others consist of forceful flexion or extension of the trunk and limbs. The epileptic spasms may be predominantly flexor, extensor, or mixed flexor-extensor in type.

The seizures characteristically occur in clusters of a few to tens of individual spasms. The number of clusters per day varies from a few to 50 or more. Spasms typically occur during sleep transitions, especially upon awakening.

Differential Diagnosis

Several disorders may be confused with infantile spasms. IS are often misdiagnosed as colic or other nonepileptic phenomena. In benign myoclonus of early infancy, infants have clusters of tonic or myoclonic movements, but unlike infants with IS, these children are normal neurologically and developmentally and have normal EEGs. The movements stop by 18 months of age. Benign neonatal sleep myoclonus consists of erratic myoclonic jerks only when the child is asleep. The jerks are usually quicker than IS. The myoclonus occurs during non-REM sleep and stops upon awakening. Neurologic function and EEG are normal, and treatment is unnecessary.

Electroencephalography

The interictal EEG in children with IS is called hypsarrhythmia, which consists of a disorganized, "chaotic" pattern of very high voltage slow waves and spikes in multiple cortical areas. Variants include hypsarrhythmia that is more prominent over one hemisphere or the presence of a focus of spike activity. The classic ictal EEG pattern is generalized slow wave followed by background voltage attenuation in all channels ("electrodecremental response"), usually accompanied by a clinical spasm.

Etiology

IS cases are conventionally classified into those in which there is no identified preceding neurologic disorder or etiology (cryptogenic) and those in which there is a preexisting pathologic event or disorder (symptomatic). With modern neuroimaging and other diagnostic advances, the proportion of cryptogenic cases is decreasing: only about 10%-15% of cases are currently considered cryptogenic.

Several specific conditions are associated with IS. Common etiologies include hypoxic-ischemic encephalopathy, neonatal intracranial hemorrhage, meningitis or encephalitis, congenital infection, developmental anomaly of the CNS, and metabolic disease. Tuberous sclerosis complex (TSC) is associated with an especially high incidence of infantile spasms (up to 50% of TSC patients). A causal relationship between vaccination and IS has not been proven.

Evaluation

An infant who presents with IS requires a thorough evaluation, including a developmental assessment, neurologic examination, and laboratory studies. The neurodevelopmental status at the time of diagnosis is an important indicator of prognosis. Every child with the possible diagnosis should have an EEG and neuroimaging. A normal EEG (including sleep) would suggest that the child has benign myoclonus of early infancy rather than IS, although in some affected children, hypsarrhythmia develops after spasm onset. An MRI scan is recommended, which may uncover brain anomalies such as agenesis of the corpus callosum or cortical dysplasia.

In children in whom an etiology cannot be definitely established, an infusion of 50 to 100 mg pyridoxine intravenously during EEG monitoring may be useful. Infants with pyridoxine dependency should have an improvement in the seizures and EEG within minutes. Infants with frequent vomiting, lethargy, failure to thrive, peculiar odors, and unexplained neurologic findings should have urine amino and organic acid screening, serum ammonia and liver function tests. Because most children will be placed on adrenocorticotropic hormone (ACTH), electrolytes, calcium, phosphorous, glucose, and urine analysis should be obtained. Examination of the spinal fluid, including CSF glycine, is indicated if there is concern about an active infection or a metabolic disorder.

Treatment

ACTH and corticosteroids are the primary drugs used to treat IS. Vigabatrin appears to be promising for children with TSC. The anticonvulsant mechanism of ACTH is not known; it may work via the hypothalamic-pituitary axis or directly on neuronal membrane excitability.

The effects of ACTH on long-term outcome are controversial. Several authors have found no developmental differences as a function of treatment. For infants with preexisting brain damage, it is unlikely that any form of therapy will greatly influence the long-range mental and motor outcome. An important question is whether treatment of cryptogenic IS in children that were normal before the onset of seizures alters outcome. Long-term studies on infants with cryptogenic IS who received either ACTH, oral steroids, or other AEDs, show that those who received ACTH had a lower incidence of seizures and better psychomotor development.

There is no consensus about the optimal dosage regimen or ACTH treatment duration. A commonly used protocol suggests a starting dose of nonsynthetic ACTH gel of 40 international units (IU) per day given intramuscularly. The response to ACTH can be dramatic, with cessation of seizures and EEG improvement within a few days. The ACTH is given for 1 month following the cessation of seizures. At that time a taper is begun, decreasing by 10 units a week. If the seizures do not completely resolve by 2 weeks, the dosage should be increased by 10 IU increments each week until the seizures cease or a daily dose of 80 IU is reached. If at that point the seizures still persist, VPA, topiramate, or a benzodiazepine can be tried. If relapse occurs during the taper or after ACTH discontinuation, the ACTH can be restarted at the dosage that originally stopped the spasms.

Adverse ACTH side effects include cushingoid obesity, growth retardation, acne, and irritability. More serious side effects include infection, hypertension, cardiomyopathy, osteoporosis, gastrointestinal bleeding, and electrolyte disturbances. Monitoring should include twice weekly blood pressure and stool guaiac checks and weekly serum electrolytes. If the child develops hypertension or hypokalemic alkalosis, a reduction in dosage is recommended. Some children require salt restriction or antihypertensives. Fever should be investigated promptly, as infections are more likely during steroid-induced immunosuppression.

Vigabatrin, a selective inhibitor of GABA-transaminase, has been shown to exert a favorable effect on IS, especially in children with TSC. Vigabatrin is not approved for use in the United States. There have been some reports of vigabatrin-induced visual field defects. Other therapies that might be beneficial in the treatment of IS are topiramate and the ketogenic diet.

Infants with IS that have a consistent focal onset may benefit from resective surgery. A structural lesion such as focal dysgenesis may correlate with the focal EEG and clinical features. Some infants with cryptogenic infantile spasms and normal MRI scans have deficits of cerebral metabolism (detected by PET). When this area of cortical hypometabolism is removed under the guidance of intraoperative corticography, the seizures may be reduced or eliminated.

Prognosis

As an epileptic encephalopathy, the prognosis of IS is poor. Many affected children have psychomotor retardation and persistent seizures. With age, the seizures often change from spasms to mixed seizures of the types seen in the Lennox-Gastaut syndrome. About two-thirds of affected children are mentally retarded and motor impairment such as cerebral palsy is common. Because a large number of children have neurologic impairment before the onset of the spasms, it is not surprising that the outcome is so poor. Prognosis is directly related to etiology, with crytpogenic cases having a significantly better prognosis than symptomatic ones.

Lennox-Gastaut syndrome. The Lennox-Gastaut syndrome (LGS) is a generalized epilepsy syndrome in which children have frequent, medically intractable seizures (up to hundreds per day). LGS has the following characteristics: 1.) a slow spike-wave EEG pattern (less than 3 Hz); 2.) mental retardation; and 3.) multiple seizure types. Most children with LGS also have motor impairments.

Clinical Characteristics

LGS begins between the ages of 1 and 6 years. Seizure types include tonic, GTC, atypical absence, atonic, or myoclonic. Tonic seizures consist of periods of sustained muscle contractions accompanied by altered consciousness. These are especially frequent during sleep. Atonic (astatic) seizures, or drop attacks, occur without warning. If standing, the child will quickly fall to the floor. Head or facial injuries often occur, and these children often need to wear protective head gear. The loss of tone may affect the head only; such head drops can occur singly or in a series of head nods. Consciousness is momentarily impaired, but the child regains alertness promptly.

Atypical absences occur frequently in children with LGS. These have a gradual onset and cessation, and may involve clonic components, automatisms, autonomic changes, and myoclonic jerks. Atypical absences may be prolonged, during which the child has a dull appearance, with confusion, drooling, and behavioral arrest. It is often difficult to tell when one seizure ends and the next one begins, because alertness and activity level do not improve between the absences. GTC seizures also occur in children with LGS, usually at night or during sleep transitions.

Electroencephalography

The characteristic EEG finding in LGS is generalized slow spike-wave discharges, at a frequency of 1.5 Hz to 2.5 Hz. These discharges occur in long runs during wakefulness and are even more frequent in sleep.

Etiology

LGS is usually diagnosed in a child who is already neurologically or mentally handicapped. The etiology may not be known specifically (cryptogenic) or can result from a definable etiology, such as hypoxic brain injury, a cerebral dysgenesis, or a neurocutaneous disorder. The etiologies of LGS overlap those of IS. The majority of children with symptomatic LGS have a static encephalopathy; though rarely, children with degenerative disorders such as neuronal ceroid lipofuscinosis present with LGS.

Evaluation

In the absence of an obvious medical condition, the child needs to be thoroughly evaluated, with the specific evaluation guided by the history and physical examination. In view of the devastating nature of the syndrome, every effort should be made to rule out a treatable disorder. Abnormalities on neuroimaging are common, especially cortical or subcortical atrophy.

Treatment

Many affected children are notoriously refractory to AEDs. Because the syndrome is heterogeneous, there is some variability in how the children will respond to an AED. Drug therapy should be individualized to address the types and frequency of seizures in each child. Children with LGS may benefit from VPA, clonazepam, lamotrigine, or topiramate, or some combination of these. Felbamate is reserved for particularly refractory cases. Because of the intractable nature of the seizures, there is a tendency to place the children on numerous AEDs. This polypharmaceutical approach usually results in drug toxicity with somnolence, fatigue, nausea, ataxia, and rarely, optimal seizure control.

Prognosis

Children with LGS have a poor neurologic prognosis. Over time, the atonic, myoclonic, and atypical absence seizures may decrease, but GTC seizures increase and partial seizures emerge. In addition to debilitating seizures, intellectual impairment hinders children with LGS from leading independent lives. Some children have a progressive deterioration in mental function despite vigorous attempts to control their seizures.

Localization-Related Epilepsy Syndromes

Idiopathic Localization-Related Epilepsy Syndromes

Rolandic epilepsy (benign childhood epilepsy with centrotemporal spikes). Rolandic epilepsy (RE) is a common, distinctive epilepsy syndrome of childhood characterized by seizures arising from the lower central sulcus of Rolando. The EEG pattern is characteristic, consisting of spikes in one or both midtemporal-central regions. The evaluation and prognosis of a child with RE differs considerably from other, less benign focal epilepsies.

Clinical Characteristics

Seizures typically begin between the ages of 5 and 11 years and usually remit spontaneously in early adolescence. Children have a normal neurologic examination and normal intellectual function. The classic presentation is a nocturnal seizure with clonic movements of the mouth and face, salivation, and garbled or arrested speech, but consciousness is maintained. Motor phenomena during RE attacks are usually restricted to one side of the body, typically the face, but sometimes affect the arm or leg. This simple partial seizure may secondarily generalize. There is little or no postictal state. Seizures of RE are distinguishable from partial complex seizures because they lack automatisms, auras, hallucinations, and affective symptoms.

Electroencephalography

The classic interictal EEG shows a normal background with superimposed high-amplitude spikes-wave complexes, which occur singly or in brief runs over the midtemporal and central (rolandic) regions. Rolandic spikes are not diagnostic of epilepsy and may occur in children without a seizure history.

Genetics

RE has a strong familial occurrence. The EEG trait, but not the clinical syndrome, is inherited as autosomal dominant with age-dependency and incomplete penetrance. About half of first-degree relatives demonstrate the EEG abnormality between the ages of 5 and 15 years. Before 5 and after 15 years of age, penetrance is low, with few patients exhibiting the EEG abnormality. Only about 12% of children who inherit the EEG abnormality develop seizures.

Evaluation
If the child has a clinical history and EEG characteristic of RE, plus a normal neurologic examination, further workup is not necessary. If the neurologic examination is abnormal or the EEG demonstrates any atypical features, a brain MRI is warranted.

Treatment and Prognosis
Since the seizures of RE are benign and often infrequent, many clinicians do not treat the first or even the second seizure. The seizures are usually controlled with a single AED, such as carbamazepine (usually the first choice), phenytoin, or VPA. The efficacy of the newer AEDs in RE is not known. In Europe, sulthiame has proven effective in clinical trials.

Treatment is recommended for 1 to 2 years before the AED is tapered. Resolution of the EEG abnormalities is a favorable sign. Children usually outgrow both seizures and EEG abnormalities around adolescence. Long-term prognosis is usually excellent, although caution is advised if atypical clinical or electrographic features are present.

Benign childhood epilepsy with occipital paroxysms. Benign childhood epilepsy with occipital paroxysms (BCEOP) resembles RE in that focal seizures occur in neurologically normal children, who tend to outgrow their epilepsy before adulthood. The syndromes differ in the localization of the epileptiform discharges and the phenomenology of the seizures. In BCEOP, the peak age of seizures onset is between 5 and 9 years. The seizures consist of elementary visual phenomena such as hallucinations, illusions, blindness, or phosphenes, though any seizure type may occur. Progression to a hemiclonic seizure is not unusual. A seizure is often followed by a migraine headache. Interictal occipital rhythmic spikes are maximal upon eye closure. A genetic etiology is assumed.

Panayiotopoulos syndrome is a subtype of BCEOP, seen in slightly younger children (3 to 7 years old). Nocturnal seizures predominate, accompanied by eye deviation and vomiting, but description of visual phenomena may be minimal. This syndrome also remits by adolescence. Both BCEOP and Panayiotopoulos syndrome are commonly associated with migraine, and these disorders may share a similar pathogenetic mechanism.

Symptomatic Localization-Related Epilepsy Syndromes
Symptomatic localization-related epilepsy syndromes are those that arise in a particular region of brain, due to an acquired or congenital lesion. Etiologies include tumors, scars (eg, hippocampal sclerosis), cortical dysplasias, porencephalic cysts (resulting from perinatal infarction), and vascular malformations. The seizure features are related to the region of brain affected; usually, the seizure will begin as simple partial or complex partial and then generalize secondarily. The EEG will show focal spikes, sharp waves, or slowing, related to the area of brain involved.

These syndromes are sometimes divided into those originating in the neocortex or mesial temporal structures. In children, a neocortical localization is more common, while in adults, the mesial temporal lobe is a frequent epileptogenic site. Neocortical etiologies in children may include low-grade neoplasms and the wide spectrum of migrational abnormalities and developmental dysplasias. Symptoms and EEG findings are related to brain region affected.

Some important childhood localization-related epilepsy syndromes involve an entire hemisphere. Rasmussen encephalitis is a focal encephalitis that affects only one hemisphere, and results in progressive hemiparesis, intractable epilepsy (partial seizures that may progress to epilepsia partialis continua), and cognitive decline. The etiology of Rasmussen encephalitis is unknown but it might have an autoimmune basis, with antibodies to certain glutamate receptor subunits. The unilateral pathology may be due to focal breakdown of the blood-brain barrier. Neuroimaging shows progressive unilateral cortical atrophy. Another hemispheric syndrome, Sturge-Weber syndrome (encephalotrigeminal angiomatosis), consists of a hemispheric vascular malformation, leading to intractable epilepsy and hemiparesis. The degree of cerebral involvement is reflected by the degree of facial angiomatosis. Some authorities feel that early surgery (hemispherectomy) affords a better prognosis in the hemispheric localization-related epilepsy syndromes.

Indeterminate Epilepsy Syndromes

Neonatal Seizures

Neonatal seizures are classified as "indeterminate" because the typical seizure types in newborns do not conform to the ILAE scheme. Seizures may be the first and only sign of CNS dysfunction in a newborn, so their recognition is extremely important. Despite advances in obstetrics and perinatal care, many infants with neonatal seizures have a poor neurologic outcome.

Clinical characteristics. Seizures in the neonatal period (first 30 days of life) differ considerably from those seen in older children and adults. Due to immature myelination and cortical organization, the neonatal brain is unable to sustain generalized epileptiform discharges, so GTC seizures rarely, if ever, occur in neonates, and absence seizures never do.

Neonatal seizures are classified clinically into four types, based on behavioral manifestations: subtle, generalized tonic, focal or multifocal clonic, and myoclonic. Subtle seizures may include repetitive oral-buccal-lingual movements such as sucking, pedaling movements of the legs or arms, eye deviation, nystagmus, or apnea. Subtle seizures are often associated with severe CNS insults. Neonatal tonic seizures resemble decerebrate or opisthotonic posturing with intermittent tonic extension of the arms and legs; they are usually associated with severe brain lesions and most often occur in preterm infants. Clonic seizures consist of rhythmic jerking of groups of muscles in a focal or multifocal pattern. In multifocal clonic seizures, movements may migrate from one part of the body to another. Focal seizures may be seen with localized brain malformations or insults, such as a perinatal stroke, as well as in disorders that diffusely affect the brain, such as asphyxia, metabolic derangement, or infection. Myoclonic seizures are similar to those seen in older children, with rapid isolated jerks, focally or bilaterally.

Simultaneous video-EEG monitoring can differentiate behaviors with EEG correlates ("epileptic seizures") from behaviors that do not have associated EEG changes. Focal clonic seizures have the highest correlation with EEG ictal abnormalities. Many behaviors considered to be subtle seizures on clinical grounds (for example, chewing or pedaling movements) are not associated with EEG abnormalities, suggesting that these behaviors are not epileptic in nature. Subtle seizures may represent "brainstem release" phenomena or epileptic seizures originating from deep subcortical structures not recordable on surface EEG. In either case, subtle seizures often reflect severe CNS dysfunction. Apnea alone is rarely the sole manifestation of a neonatal seizure. Myoclonic and tonic events are variable in their relationship to EEG abnormalities.

Neonatal jitteriness needs to be distinguished from neonatal seizures. Jitteriness is an intermittent involuntary movement of the limbs that may mimic a seizure. The movements resemble a coarse tremor of the limbs and are not accompanied by eye deviation. The movements can be spontaneous or evoked by limb movement, and can be suppressed by passive flexion of an involved extremity. Jitteriness often appears in the context of other CNS excitation, such as irritability and excessive startle. It is often seen in infants of substance-abusing mothers and in hypoxic-ischemic encephalopathy. The etiologies of seizures and jitteriness overlap, but in jitteriness the EEG does not show epileptiform abnormalities.

Electroencephalography. The neonatal EEG is usually not specific for a particular etiology, but it may supply clues about the severity and time course of a CNS insult. The EEG may support the clinical diagnosis of seizures in infants with atypical or minimal behavioral manifestations if the recording includes the episode in question. The EEG may also document seizure discharges that are not accompanied by overt clinical manifestations ("uncoupling" of electrographic and clinical seizures, or "electroclinical dissociation"). In infants who are paralyzed and dependent on respiratory support, the EEG may be the only objective means for assessing cerebral function and determining the presence of seizure activity. For prognostic purposes, EEG background patterns and sleep-wake cycles are especially important.

Etiology. Establishing the etiology of a neonatal seizure is critical because the cause determines the therapy and is highly correlated with outcome. Major causes of neonatal seizures include hypoxic-ischemia (H-I), hypocalcemia, hypoglycemia, hyponatremia, intracranial hemorrhage, infection, congenital malformations, genetic factors, inherited metabolic disorders, and drug withdrawal. H-I is the most common cause of neonatal seizures. Most asphyxia occurs before delivery (20% of cases), during delivery (35%), or a combination of antepartum and intrapartum (35%); only 10% of cases result from postnatal causes. Timing of the seizure is related to etiology. Seizures due to H-I usually occur in the first day of life, those caused by metabolic derangements begin in the first few days, while those secondary to cortical malformations do not appear until several weeks of life or later.

Treatment. After ventilation and adequate glucose levels are ensured, initial goals are to establish the underlying cause and institute appropriate therapy. Metabolic derangements should be corrected and antibiotics given when appropriate. The decision to treat an infant with recurrent seizures is based on the seizure duration and frequency, associated autonomic dysfunction, etiology, and EEG abnormalities. If seizures are brief and not associated with autonomic instability, treatment may be deferred or a short-acting benzodiazepine used. Conversely, neonates with frequent seizures, especially if they interfere with ventilation, require prompt and vigorous treatment.

Phenobarbital is the primary drug used to treat neonatal seizures, despite its limited effectiveness. The initial loading dose is 20 mg/kg intravenously with a maintenance dosage of 5 to 6 mg/kg per day, given once or twice daily. Most infants require serum levels between 10 and 40 mg/dL to suppress seizures, but the dose is often pushed higher before resorting to polytherapy. Serum levels above 40 mg/dL may result in lethargy.

If phenobarbital is ineffective, a second drug is added (usually fosphenytoin). As in older children, phenytoin follows nonlinear kinetics in the newborn period. The drug is usually administered in two boluses of 10 mg/kg intravenously, which results in a blood level of 15 to 20 mg/dL. Phenytoin is poorly absorbed from the gastrointestinal tract of newborns, and it is often difficult to maintain therapeutic levels using the oral route; 8 mg/kg per day or higher is sometimes required to obtain a therapeutic level. Commonly, phenobarbital or phenytoin will suppress clinical seizures but the baby continues to have electrographic seizures ("uncoupling"). In such cases, the physician must decide, in the context of the clinical situation, how far to push medications to suppress electrographic seizures.

Diazepam and lorazepam are commonly used to treat neonatal seizures. A diazepam dose of 0.2 to 0.5 mg/kg intravenously is recommended for the acute management of neonatal seizures. Due to its short distribution phase, diazepam is not an optimal maintenance AED.

There is little information about the efficacy of the newer AEDs in neonatal seizures. In general, AEDs should be weaned once seizures stop and medical abnormalities are corrected, preferably before the infant is discharged from the nursery.

Neonatal Epilepsy Syndromes

Most neonatal seizures are reactions of the brain to a neurologic insult. However, several neonatal epilepsy syndromes have been defined. The syndrome of benign familial neonatal convulsions was discussed above.

Early myoclonic encephalopathy (EME) is characterized by sporadic and erratic fragmentary myoclonus, usually in combination with other seizure types. The EEG shows burst suppression. A variety of etiologies has been associated with EME, including metabolic diseases, cerebral dysgenesis, and H-I insults. The prognosis is very poor. Most infants die within a year or survive with severe neurologic sequelae.

Ohtahara syndrome, or early infantile epileptic encephalopathy (EIEE), begins in early infancy, with severe, frequent tonic seizures and burst suppression on the EEG. Affected infants have severe developmental deficits. EIEE may evolve into West syndrome. As with EME, a host of etiologies has been described in EIEE, but cerebral dysgenesis is the most common association.

Landau-Kleffner Syndrome

Landau-Kleffner syndrome (LKS; acquired epileptic aphasia) is a rare epilepsy in which a child loses previously acquired language abilities and has seizures or epileptiform abnormalities on EEG. In its pure form, LKS occurs in previously normal children with normal language development, who gradually lose the ability to understand spoken language and produce speech. Recently, some authors have expanded the syndrome to include behavioral and cognitive deterioration, including symptoms seen in autistic spectrum disorders. Regression of social and language skills is frequently seen in children with autism, with or without accompanying seizures, so the differentiation of autism and LKS can be difficult. In LKS, compared to autism, social skills are better preserved. The pathophysiology of LKS is unknown. Imaging studies are generally negative although recent PET studies have shown bitemporal abnormalities, supporting the hypothesis that language-related brain regions are dysfunctional in LKS.

EEG abnormalities in LKS may include generalized, focal, or multifocal spikes, spike-waves or sharp waves. If focal, the discharges commonly involve one or both temporal or temporoparietal (perisylvian) regions. The hypothesis has arisen that the epileptiform discharges interfere with language production, although it is possible that both the language dysfunction and EEG abnormalities are independent consequences of the same underlying brain pathology. Successful treatment of the seizures or even the EEG discharges is not usually accompanied by language or behavioral improvement. The outcome is quite variable; some children recover completely, usually in adolescence, while others have persistent aphasia in adulthood.

Evaluation should include hearing assessment, an overnight EEG and a MRI scan of brain. The seizures usually respond readily to AEDs (eg, VPA, benzodiazepines), while the language impairment does not. Attempts to treat children with steroids or subpial resection have been controversial.

Electrical Status Epilepticus of Sleep (ESES; Continuous Spike-Wave Discharges During Slow-Wave Sleep or CSWDS)

ESES is an electrographic diagnosis and CSWDS is considered the electroclinical syndrome. Children have normal language development prior to the onset of seizures, which are usually partial complex in type, followed by language and cognitive or behavioral deterioration. The cognitive changes may range from inattention to psychosis. The EEG shows a fairly normal background during wakefulness and rapid eye movement (REM) sleep, but more than 85% of the slow wave sleep (non-REM) record consists of generalized spike-wave discharges (although focal spikes or fragmentary generalized spike-wave can be seen during wakefulness). These discharges are often slow (1.5 Hz to 2 Hz) and have a frontocentral predominance. The cognitive and behavioral deterioration is often less dramatic than in children with LKS, and ESES remits during adolescence. Similar treatment options are used in ESES and LKS. Carbamazepine may worsen the syndrome. The outcome of ESES is quite variable; some children eventually regain normal language function.

Special Syndromes (Situation Related)

Febrile Seizures

Febrile seizures occur in children from about 6 months to 5 years of age. Although the exact pathophysiology is unknown, febrile seizures represent an age-dependent response of the developing brain to fever. There is a genetic association, with febrile seizures occurring 2 to 3 times more frequently in affected families than in the general population. Overall, febrile seizures occur in 2%-5% of children in the susceptible age range. Seizures with fever before or after those ages suggest another cause.

Clinical characteristics. The two main types of febrile seizures are: 1.) simple, and 2.) complex or complicated. (The term "complicated" is preferred, to avoid confusion with afebrile complex partial seizures.) Simple febrile seizures are brief (less than 15 minutes in duration), generalized, and do not recur within 24 hours of the first one. Simple febrile seizures usually occur in normal children without neurologic deficits. Complicated febrile seizures are either prolonged (longer than 15 minutes), the seizures have focal components (eg, the seizure begins on one side of the body or there is lateralized eye deviation), or another seizure occurs within 24 hours of the first one. As discussed below, simple and complicated febrile seizures differ in their prognosis and in the risk for development of epilepsy.

Differential diagnosis and evaluation. In a child presenting with fever and seizure, there are three possibilities: febrile seizure, seizure secondary to meningitis or intracranial infection, or underlying epilepsy unmasked by the fever. If the seizure was brief, the child promptly returns to baseline mental status, and a source of fever is identified (eg, otitis media or gastroenteritis). A simple febrile seizure is the most likely cause and an extensive evaluation is not necessary. On the other hand, if there is a concern about persistent lethargy or diminished responsiveness, a lumbar puncture should be performed to rule out meningitis or encephalitis. In a complicated febrile seizure, especially if there is focality to the seizure, a neuroimaging study should be performed to rule out an intracranial injury, stroke, mass, or dysplasia. A head CT scan will rule out an acute bleed, but an MRI scan is preferred to evaluate for cortical malformations and dysplasia. In a simple febrile seizure, an EEG will usually be unrevealing, whereas in a complicated febrile seizure, an EEG is useful to evaluate for focal spikes or slowing.

Treatment. Simple febrile seizures do not require treatment, nor do most complicated febrile seizures. For a child with prolonged febrile seizures, the family can be provided with diazepam rectal gel for emergency use. For children with frequent febrile seizures, intermittent oral diazepam can be given for the duration of the fever only, at a dose of 0.3 mg/kg every 8 hours. Only in exceptional circumstances would prophylactic medication be prescribed, and usually only if there is concern about epilepsy rather than febrile seizures. Only phenobarbital and valproic acid have been shown to be effective in preventing febrile seizures.

Prognosis. A child who has had a single simple febrile seizure has about a 33% chance of another febrile seizure with a subsequent febrile illness (50% chance if the first febrile seizure occurs at less than 12 months of age). If a child has had two simple febrile seizures, there is about a 50% chance of a third febrile seizure. The recurrence risk for additional febrile seizures is greatest if a child has had a first febrile seizure under 12 months of age or there is a family history of febrile seizures.

The most concerning risk is not for recurrent febrile seizures, but rather for the development of afebrile seizures (ie, epilepsy). A significant proportion of adults with temporal lobe epilepsy (due to mesial temporal sclerosis) had a prolonged febrile seizure as a child. After a simple febrile seizure, the risk for epilepsy later in life is only slightly higher than for the general population, about 2%. The risk of developing epilepsy after febrile seizures is greatest if the child has preexisting neurologic impairment such as developmental delay or cerebral palsy, if there is a family history of epilepsy, or if the febrile seizure was complicated in type. Depending on the specific complicated febrile seizure feature (prolonged, focal, recurrent), the risk for epilepsy varies from 6.5%-9.3%; if all three features are present, the risk for epilepsy is 49%.

Status Epilepticus

Status epilepticus (SE) is defined as more than 30 minutes of continuous seizure activity, or multiple shorter seizures over the same time period without full recovery of consciousness between seizures. There is unequivocal clinical and experimental evidence that SE can lead to brain damage and therefore must be stopped as quickly as possible.

Clinical features. Any seizure type can progress into SE. SE is usually classified as convulsive and nonconvulsive. In convulsive status, the seizure type is usually GTC, accompanied by significant autonomic manifestations including tachycardia, respiratory compromise, and hypersecretion. If the seizure continues, the patient may develop fever, hypotension, acidosis, and respiratory depression. Nonconvulsive status refers to SE with absence or partial seizures. Nonconvulsive SE can present as a continuous or fluctuating state of confusion and incomplete responsiveness. In addition, partial status may involve motor function (epilepsia partialis continua), sensory symptoms, or focal impairment of function (eg, aphasia) not associated with altered consciousness.

Etiology. The etiologies of SE are as varied as those of epilepsy in general. Most SE is symptomatic; some cases are idiopathic. In children, nonspecific febrile illness, hypoxic-ischemic encephalopathy, and CNS infection account for the majority of cases of symptomatic SE. In patients already being treated for epilepsy, SE can be precipitated by abrupt withdrawal of anticonvulsant medications (particularly barbiturates and benzodiazepines), sleep deprivation, or intercurrent infection.

Treatment. In practical terms, any child seizing upon arrival at the emergency department or found seizing in the community should be treated for SE. Failure to treat SE quickly may result in neurologic sequelae or even death. A protocol for the treatment of SE is found in Table 4. Systemic abnormalities such as hyperpyrexia, hypoglycemia, hypotension, and hypoxia may occur during SE and exacerbate the cerebral damage. Therefore, it is critical to achieve systemic metabolic stability as well as stop the seizures. As the SE is being treated, the search for precipitating causes should proceed.

Initial therapy aims to provide the basics of life support, such as maintaining adequate cardiac output and cerebral perfusion and preventing injury as a result of the violent motor activity. Because cerebral hypoxia can be both a cause and consequence of status epilepticus, immediate needs are to assess cardiorespiratory function and insert an oral airway. Oxygen should be administered and endotracheal intubation may be necessary. Once the airway is secure, intravenous access should be obtained. Blood should then be sent for laboratory studies (Table 4), glucose given by bolus injection, and maintenance fluids started. Blood pressure must be monitored, especially during AED administration. Body temperature should be monitored continuously as it may rise quickly during SE and necessitate a cooling blanket or ice packs.

Once systemic conditions are addressed, AEDs should be given. Table 5 lists the doses and other data about the five most commonly used drugs in children with SE. Each drug is efficacious, and there is no proscribed order of administration. The usual protocol is to administer a fast acting benzodiazepine (one or more times) to stop the SE, then to load with a longer acting agent such as fosphenytoin or phenobarbital. For SE refractory to these agents, more drastic measures may need to be undertaken, such as a midazolam drip or pentobarbital coma.

Table 4

Emergency Treatment of Status Epilepticus

1. Place patient in safe position
2. Assess cardiorespiratory function
3. Insert oral airway and administer oxygen
4. Insert intravenous catheter
5. Draw venous blood for measurement of AED levels CBC, BUN, electrolytes, glucose, and ammonia
6. Draw arterial blood gas
7. Give 50% glucose solution (1-2 mL/kg)
8. Start maintenance fluids unless there is evidence of fluid overload, concern about increased intracranial pressure, or dehydration
9. Give diazepam or lorazepam (Table 5)
10. If seizures stop, a longer-acting AED (phenobarbital or phenytoin/fosphenytoin) should be considered
11. If status continues, give phenobarbital or phenytoin/fosphenytoin (Table 5)
12. If status continues, intubate child and admit to intensive care unit. Give propofol bolus then maintenance drip. Alternatively, use a midazolam bolus and maintenance drip (Table 5).
13. If status continues, consider general anethesia

Prognosis. The outcome of SE is improving with earlier and more effective medical management. The SE-related mortality rate in children is less than 5 percent. Fewer than 10% of children with SE develop new neurologic deficits, and most of those patients have preexisting neurologic impairment. The consensus is that the etiology of SE, rather than the seizure itself, is the main determinant of neurologic outcome. Risk factors for neurologic sequelae from SE include age of onset under 6 years, a remote symptomatic cause, and partial seizures.

Nonepileptic Disorders That Mimic Seizures

Numerous nonepileptic paroxysmal alterations of motor activity or behavior mimic seizures by history or clinical presentation. A few of the more common disorders are described here. From a therapeutic point of view, it is important to distinguish epileptic from nonepileptic behaviors, because some nonepileptic phenomena respond to medications other than AEDs and others require no specific treatment other than reassurance or avoidance of the circumstances that precipitate the spell.

Benign Paroxysmal Vertigo

Benign paroxysmal vertigo (BPV) manifests as sudden, brief overwhelming sensations of vertigo that cause a child to stagger, lose balance, and sometimes fall to the ground. The child appears distressed and frightened and may become pale, diaphoretic, and nauseous, but consciousness is maintained. Episodes last from a few minutes to several hours and recur every few months to several times per week. BPV is considered a migraine variant. It usually affects preschool-age children and resolves by 7 years of age, although most affected children go on to develop more typical migraine symptoms later in life. In contrast to other causes of vertigo, in BPV there is no tinnitus, hearing impairment, or other brainstem dysfunction except for occasional nystagmus. The diagnosis is aided by a normal EEG and neurologic examination and supported by a family history of migraine. The lack of rhythmic movements or altered consciousness further differentiates BPV from epilepsy. The attacks typically fail to respond to anticonvulsant or antimigraine medications, and the best treatment is to reassure the parents of the benign nature of the spells.

Table 5

Commonly Used Antiepileptic Drugs for the Treatment of Status Epilepticus

Property	Diazepam	Lorazepam	Fosphenytoin	Phenobarbital	Midazolam
Dose	0.2-0.4 mg/kg (maximum dose 20 mg)	0.05-0.1 mh/kg	15-20 mg/kg	15-20 mh/kg	Bolus: 0.1-0.3 mg/kg Drip: 0.75-10 mcg/kg/min
Time to stop seizure	3-10 min	1-20 minutes	5-30 minutes	10-30 minutes	15 minutes
Half-life	50 hours	15 hours	10-15 hours	80-100 hours	1.7-4.0 hours
Duration of action	Minutes	Hours	12-24 hours	Days	30-80 minutes
Side effects	Hypotension Apnea Somnolence	Hypotension Apnea Somnolence	Cardiac arrhythmias Hypotension	Hypotension Apnea Somnolence	Hypotension Apnea Somnolence

Breath-holding Spells

Despite their name, breath-holding spells (BHSs) are involuntary reflex responses with a benign prognosis. They are age related and are typically outgrown by school age. Two types of BHSs occur: cyanotic (also called cyanotic infantile syncope) and pallid (also called pallid infantile syncope or reflex anoxic seizures).

Cyanotic BHSs, the more common type, are precipitated by upset, anger, or frustration. The hallmark is crying, during which the child will stop breathing (usually in expiration), become cyanotic, then lose consciousness. At that point the child may become rigid, limp or even shake, raising the concern about a seizure. The unconsciousness lasts from seconds to a minute. The pathogenesis of cyanotic BHS is complex, probably involving an interaction between hyperventilation, Valsalva maneuver, expiratory apnea, and intrinsic pulmonary mechanics.

Pallid BHSs are similar to cyanotic BHSs in some respects but are more likely to be provoked by fright or a mild unpleasant stimulus (such as mild trauma). There will be a gasp but little or no cry, followed by loss of consciousness, pallor, bradycardia, diaphoresis, and limpness. Pallid BHSs result from vasovagally mediated cardiac inhibition, causing diminished cerebral blood flow.

Neither type of BHS is associated with an increased predisposition to epilepsy, although seizure activity can occur at the end of a cyanotic or pallid BHS. These so-called "seizures" manifest as tonic stiffening of the extremities, sometimes followed by brief clonic jerking. Such seizures are not epileptic in nature and instead represent a response of the brain to acute, mild hypoxia. These seizures terminate spontaneously and do not require anticonvulsant treatment. Notably, in a BHS, cyanosis occurs before the seizure, whereas in an epileptic seizure, cyanosis usually occurs during or after the seizure.

Evaluation with an EEG is usually not needed. An electrocardiogram can rule out prolonged QT syndrome, which can mimic epilepsy. In addition, anemia can worsen BHS and should be excluded. Management of BHS consists mainly of parental reassurance that the spells will be outgrown, usually by school age, and that the BHS will not lead to future epilepsy or brain damage. Some children with the pallid type develop syncope later in life.

Syncope

Syncope (fainting), seen commonly in older children and adolescents, can often be differentiated from an epileptic seizure by history. Attacks may be preceded by warning (presyncopal) signs such as lightheadedness, blurred vision, pallor, nausea, or diaphoresis. These warning signs are followed by a loss of consciousness and a slow slump to the ground, as opposed to the more violent fall seen with a myoclonic or atonic seizure. Late in a syncopal spell, there may be a brief tonic or clonic seizure secondary to cerebral hypoperfusion and hypoxia; these are not epileptic seizures. Consciousness is regained rapidly, compared to a more prolonged epileptic postictal state. A child may be tired after syncope but is not ordinarily confused for more than a few seconds. Seizure is further differentiated from syncope in that a seizure is not associated with cold, clammy skin.

Syncope is caused by transiently diminished cerebral blood flow, due to an irregular heart rate (an arrhythmia causing decreased cardiac output), decreased venous return (orthostasis or Valsalva), a vasovagal mechanism (fright, pain, emotional upset), or, rarely, cough- or micturition-induced reflex syncope. Vasovagal attacks often occur in a hot, stuffy environment. Orthostasis is most commonly precipitated by rising from a sitting or recumbent position. A child who has an arrhythmia or who faints from any position other than standing requires a cardiac evaluation. Orthostatic blood pressures should be documented. The EEG is usually normal. The key to treatment is the avoidance of precipitating factors as much as possible.

Pseudoseizures

Pseudoseizures (psychogenic seizures; nonepileptic seizures) are paroxysmal changes in motor activity or behavior that resemble epileptic seizures clinically but have no EEG correlate. The diagnosis of pseudoseizure should be considered in any child with seizures refractory to anticonvulsants or with consistently normal EEGs. A history of strong emotional overlay or psychiatric disturbance in the child or family may suggest pseudoseizures. Clinically, it may be very difficult to differentiate between epileptic seizures and pseudoseizures, and simultaneous video-EEG monitoring can be helpful. Diagnosis relies on prolonged monitoring and careful correlation of clinical and electrographic findings. To complicate the diagnostic evaluation, pseudoseizures and epileptic seizures may coexist in the same child.

Pseudoseizures can be disabling and often reflect major underlying psychopathology. As with many psychosomatic illnesses, pseudoseizures can arise because of unresolved psychological conflicts and anxiety that are converted into a physical symptom. In children with pseudoseizures, one must be suspicious of physical or sexual abuse. Many children with pseudoseizures have witnessed a real seizure, either first-hand or in the media.

Pseudoseizures present with a variety of clinical forms. Many resemble generalized tonic-clonic seizures, although the two sides of the body are more likely to jerk out of phase with each other. Pseudoseizures can also simulate complex partial, atonic, myoclonic, and even absence seizures. Sometimes the behavioral manifestations of the spell are a clue to its nonepileptic nature. For example, GTC activity in the setting of preserved consciousness favors a nonepileptic event. However, caution is warranted, as some behaviors previously thought to be pseudoseizures are actually epileptic events generated by brain areas distant from scalp EEG electrodes. For example, seizures arising from the frontal lobe may give rise to behavioral ictal manifestations that were formerly thought to be characteristic of pseudoseizures. Seizures originating in the supplementary area (SMA) of the frontal lobe involve bilateral motor activity with preserved consciousness. Compared with pseudoseizures, SMA seizures are briefer, more stereotyped, frequently occur during sleep, and initially manifest with arm abduction (fencer's pose). Seizures originating in the orbitofrontal region are now recognized to include nonspecific screaming, affective changes such as intense fear, bilateral nonrhythmic leg or arm movements, and even sexual automatisms such as pelvic thrusting. Such behaviors were previously considered to be the sine qua non of pseudoseizures. These observations underscore the difficulty of differentiating between epileptic seizures and pseudoseizures on clinical grounds.

A child with pseudoseizures must be approached with a great deal of sensitivity. It is usually best to avoid confronting the child directly with the diagnosis, and one's suspicions should be discussed with the family in a supportive fashion. Therapy should involve both the child and family and might include psychotherapy and stress management strategies. Patients are best co-managed with a psychiatrist experienced with this disorder. Family members should be assured that the symptom (pseudoseizure) is real but does not involve epileptic neuronal discharges, and that therapy is designed to address the underlying psychological cause of the symptom. The main therapeutic goal is to teach the child alternative coping skills, so that anxiety or psychological stress does not need to manifest in such a maladaptive fashion.

Several methods have been described to induce or terminate a pseudoseizure, but interpretation of such procedures is difficult. Provocative methods should be used with extreme caution if at all, ideally with concurrent EEG monitoring. Serum levels of prolactin, cortisol, and other substances have been reported to correlate with an epileptic seizure, but are not routinely recommended in children for diagnosing pseudoseizures. The outcome of pseudoseizures in children varies but is generally more favorable than in adults.

Episodic Dyscontrol

Episodic dyscontrol (rage attacks) are episodes of aggression that are out of proportion to the precipitating event and the social context. They are common in school-aged children and adolescents. The attacks appear suddenly and explosively and consist of uncontrolled behaviors such as hitting, kicking, and biting. After an attack, the child may be completely or partially amnestic for the event or show signs of remorse. Fatigue may follow an episode, but not usually the prolonged postictal confusional state that follows an epileptic seizure. In episodic dyscontrol, motor activity is usually directed at a specific object or person, motor activity is random rather than rhythmic, and the child recalls the attack or its trigger afterwards. Rage attacks often occur in children who are mildly impaired neurologically, including those with such conditions as autism, attention deficit disorder or following traumatic injury to the temporal or frontal lobe. Children who experience rage attacks sometimes respond to propanolol, carbamazepine, or selective serotonin reuptake inhibitors.

Night Terrors
Night terrors (pavor nocturnas) is a common parasomnia that is often confused with seizures. Night terrors occur in children from about 18 months to 8 years of age, with a peak around 4-5 years of age. They occur in the early stages of sleep (non-REM, stages 3 and 4). The child will awaken with inconsolable, frantic screaming, sweating and other signs of sympathetic activation, and flailing of all extremities in a nonrhythmic fashion for several minutes, then fall back to sleep without memory of the episode in the morning. There is often a family history of night terrors. The diagnosis is based on clinical history; video-EEG recording is rarely needed. The main differential diagnosis is nightmares (which occur during REM sleep) and nocturnal epileptic seizures such as frontal lobe seizures. The only treatment is reassurance.

5. Treatment

General Principles

The primary mode of treatment in children with epilepsy is pharmacologic although epilepsy surgery, vagus nerve stimulation, and ketogenic diet therapy are useful in selected cases. In the past decade, several new AEDs have been introduced, along with improved formulations and modes of administration. For children, compliance and effectiveness are enhanced by several available formulations of AEDs (eg, chewable tablets, sprinkles, suspension, extended-release preparations), as well as a variety of delivery routes (oral, sublingual, intravenous, rectal).

The goal in the pharmacologic treatment of epilepsy is to reduce or eliminate seizures while minimizing the adverse effects of treatment. Drug treatment is only one component of the overall management strategy. Psychological, educational, and social complications of epilepsy and its treatment must also be considered. Failure to address these quality of life issues will result in treatment program failure, regardless of whether seizures are controlled.

Medical treatment should always begin with a single AED. Monotherapy controls approximately 60% of newly diagnosed epilepsy. Even in children with multiple seizure types, a single drug is started and increased to high therapeutic serum levels or until toxicity ensues. If, at that time, seizures are not controlled, a second drug can be initiated while the first one is either continued or tapered. If more than one AED is used simultaneously, it is never certain which one is controlling seizures or causing toxicity. Addition of a second AED will control seizures in only another 10% of patients, and the side effects of multiple medications are cumulative. "Rational polytherapy," that is, using more than one AED with complementary mechanisms of action, is sometimes effective.

Therapeutic ranges—the plasma concentrations for which optimal seizure control is likely to occur without side effects—have been established for most AEDs. However, these levels are only approximate, and individual patients may have complete control with levels below the therapeutic range, while others may tolerate and require levels outside the usual therapeutic range. Conversely, some children develop intolerable side effects at serum levels within the therapeutic range. Trough levels are preferable for most AEDs.

Certain drugs are more effective in specific seizure types and syndromes (Tables 6 and 7). A summary of some important properties of the commonly used AEDs in children is found in Table 8. Further details about AEDs can be found in the References.

Starting AEDs

Many factors need to be considered when deciding whether to start AED therapy, and each child must be evaluated individually. Potential benefits of treatment (prevention of further seizures and development of epilepsy) must be weighed against potential adverse effects (cognitive/behavioral changes, toxicity, cost, stigma, etc.). The decision of whether or not to begin an AED is related strongly to the epilepsy syndrome. For example, absence seizures that affect a child's attention span and school performance warrant treatment, whereas in a child with a single nocturnal seizure and an interictal EEG showing classic rolandic spikes, immediate treatment may not be required. The approach to a first unprovoked (nonsyndromic) seizure is more controversial. Less than half of children with a first unprovoked seizure will have another seizure in the initial two years, the period of greatest recurrence risk. Children with prior neurologic impairment are at the greatest risk for recurrence. Therapy does not seem to change the recurrence rate, and the EEG is a good predictor of recurrence. In view of the risk of adverse effects encountered with AEDs, in most children it is reasonable to wait for a second seizure before subjecting the child to years of drug therapy.

Withdrawing AEDs

The decision of when to withdraw AEDs is also based on age-specific risks and benefits, psychosocial considerations, and syndrome diagnosis. Traditionally, the practice has been to taper AEDs in children who remain seizure free for two years, although shorter times may be sufficient in certain syndromes. A history of focal seizures, especially with a persistently abnormal EEG, is the main risk factor for seizure recurrence after AED taper in children who are well-controlled for more than two years. Children with absence epilepsy or benign rolandic epilepsy will likely outgrow their seizures, whereas those with juvenile myoclonic epilepsy or a structural lesion are less likely to remit.

Summary of Antiepileptic Therapy

From the plethora of treatment options discussed above, it is clear that the physician has a wide range of options available to treat the child with epilepsy. Of course, if the seizures are due to a systemic derangement (eg, hypocalcemia or hypoglycemia), the primary etiology can be corrected without AED therapy. Once the decision to treat with an AED is made, the choice of agent will depend on the child's age, lifestyle, syndrome, and concurrent medical conditions and treatments, as well as the side effect profile of the AED and its cost, potential toxicity, kinetics, and drug interactions. Therefore, the decision is not always straightforward and must be tailored individually to the patient. While the newer AEDs claim to have fewer idiosyncratic reactions, the full spectrum of drug interactions and side effects will not become clear until these newer AEDs have been used more extensively. For traditional AEDs, we have a better appreciation of the range of adverse reactions and side effects, but their efficacy is often not optimal. Finally, for refractory epilepsy, the complexities of multiple concurrent AEDs must be dealt with, and consideration given to alternative epilepsy treatments such as the ketogenic diet, vagus nerve stimulation, and epilepsy surgery.

Table 6

Antiepileptic Drugs for the Treatment of Childhood Seizures

Seizure Type	Antiepileptic Drugs	
Partial Seizures	**First Choice**	**Second Choice**
Simple or complex	Carbamazepine Phenytoin Valproic acid Oxcarbazepine	Lamotrigine Topiramate Tiagabine Levitiracetam Zonisamide Gabapentin Phenobarbital Primidone Benzodiazepines
Generalized Seizures	**First Choice**	**Second Choice**
Absence	Ethosuximide Valproic acid	Lamotrigine Acetazolamide Clonazepam
Generalized tonic-clonic	Carbamazepine Phenytoin Valproic acid Oxcarbazepine	Lamotrigine Topiramate Tiagabine Gabapentin Phenobarbital Primidone Benzodiazepines
Myoclonic	Valproic acid	Lamotrigine Clonazepam Levetiracetam
Clonic	Valproic acid	Lamotrigine Phenobarbital
Tonic	Valproic acid	Carbamazepine Phenytoin Lamotrigine Phenobarbital
Atonic	Valproic acid	Lamotrigine Clonazepam

6. Prognosis

The outcome of childhood epilepsy is strongly dependent upon the epilepsy syndrome and several other factors, including preexisting neurologic impairment, age of seizure onset, duration of epilepsy, and ease with which seizures come under control. When discussing outcome, seizures themselves are only one aspect to consider. Children with epilepsy often have significant psychological, social, and educational challenges that, in many cases, outweigh the burden of the actual seizures. In addition, seizure control (ie, with AEDs) must be distinguished from seizure remission.

Prognosis related to individual syndromes was discussed above. Generally, the idiopathic benign epilepsies of childhood (eg, rolandic epilepsy) have a favorable prognosis, with seizure remission and continued normal neurologic function. Generalized epilepsy syndromes such as childhood absence epilepsy and GEFS+ have an intermediate prognosis in that seizures resolve in some cases but persist in others. Some epilepsy syndromes are considered catastrophic in that seizures persist, become refractory to medical treatment, and are accompanied by severe cognitive impairment (eg, infantile spasms, Lennox-Gastaut syndrome). The question of whether the occurrence of a seizure increases the likelihood that a subsequent seizure will occur, has not yet been answered definitively in either human studies or animal experiments.

Finally, some children with epilepsy die unexpectedly, without an obvious cause determined either historically or by postmortem examination. Sudden unexplained death in epilepsy (SUDEP) has been seen in both adults and children. Definitive risk factors have not been established, but children with severe, intractable generalized epilepsies on multiple AEDs appear to be at greater risk.

Table 7

Antiepileptic Drugs for the Treatment of Childhood Epilepsy Syndromes

	First Choice	Second Choice
Childhood absence epilepsy	Ethosuximide Valproic acid	Lamotrigine Acetazolamide Clonazepam
Rolandic epilepsy	Carbamazepine Phenytoin Valproic acid	Gabapentin Lamotrigine Topiramate
Infantile spasms	Adrenocorticotrophic hormone Vigabatrin	Topiramate Lamotrigine Valproic acid Pyridoxine (vitamin B_6)
Lennox-Gastaut syndrome	Valproic acid	Lamotrigine Topiramate Felbamate*

** Consider only in children refractory to several AEDs.*

Table 8

Summary of Commonly Used Antiepileptic Drugs in Children

AED (Trade names)	Starting Dosage	Typical Maintenance Dosage	Half-life (Hours)	Therapeutic Range (mg/L)	Common Side Effects	Serious Idiosyncratic Side Effects
Phenobarbital	<1 yr; 4-6 mg/kg/day >1 yr: 3-4 mg/kg/day Teenagers, adults: 3 mg/kg/day	Same as starting dosage	40-70	15-40	Irritability Hyperactivity Lethargy	Rash Hepatic failure Agranulocytosis Stevens-Jobs syndrome
Primidone (Mysoline®)	1-2 mg/kg	10-25 mg/kg/day once a day at bedtime	5-8	5-12	Irritability Hyperactivity Lethargy Nausea	Rash Agranulocytosis
Phenytoin (Dilantin®)	5 mg/kg/day (may need higher dose in children <5 years)	Same as starting dosage	5-34	10-20	Lethargy Dizziness Ataxia Gingival hyperplasia Hirsutism	Rash Hepatic failure Lymphadenopathy Pancreatitis Agranulocytosis Stevens-Jobs syndrome
Carbamazepine (Tegretol®, Tegretol XR® Carbatrol®)	5-10 mg/kg/day	10-30 mg/kg/day	8-25	6-12	Diplopia Lethargy Blurred vision Ataxia	Rash Hepatic failure Pancreatitis Leukopenia Aplastic anemia Hyponatremia
Valproic acid (Depakote®, Depakene®, Depacon®)	15 mg/kg/day	15-60 mg/kg/day	4-14	50-100	Lethargy Weight gain (or rarely weight loss) Hair loss Tremor	Rash Hepatic failure Pancreatitis Thrombocytopenia Anemia Agranuloctosis Stevens-Jobs syndrome Polycystic ovary syndrome

(continued)

Table 8

Summary of Commonly Used Antiepileptic Drugs in Children ***(continued)***

AED (Trade names)	Starting Dosage	Typical Maintenance Dosage	Half-life (Hours)	Therapeutic Range (mg/L)	Common Side Effects	Serious Idiosyncratic Side Effects
Ethosuximide (Zarontin®)	10 mg/kg/day	15-40 mg/kg/day	25-40	40-100	Gastric distress Hiccups Lethargy	Rash Leukopenia Pancytopenia Systemic lupus erythramatosus
Gabapentin (Neurontin®)	10 mg/kg/day increase in 5 mg/kg increments	20-100 mg/kg/day; optimal dose not established	5-8	2-12 Usefulness not established	Lethargy Dizziness Ataxia Agitation Weight gain Headache	Rash
Lamotrigine (Lamictal®)	Add-on therapy: If on valproate: Weeks 1-2: 0.2 mg.kg.day Weeks 3-4: 0.5 mg/kg/day If on other AEDs: Weeks 1-2: 2 mg/kg/day Weeks 3-4: 5 mg/kg/day	Add on therapy: If on valproate: 1-5 mg/kg/day If on other AEDs: 5-15 mg/kg/day	On monotherapy: 25 On valproate: 30-70	4-20	Lethargy Dizziness Ataxia	Rash Stevens-Jobs syndrome
Topiramate (Topamax®)	0.5-1 mg/kg/day	5-9 mg/kg/day	12-24	4-10	Somnolence Dizziness Ataxia Headache Nausea Fatigue Weight loss Acidosis	Rash Glaucoma

(continued)

Table 8

Summary of Commonly Used Antiepileptic Drugs in Children *(continued)*

AED (Trade names)	Starting Dosage	Typical Maintenance Dosage	Half-life (Hours)	Therapeutic Range (mg/L)	Common Side Effects	Serious Idiosyncratic Side Effects
Tiagabine (Gabatril®)	0.1 mg/kg/day	0.6-1 mg/kg/day	3-9	0.1-0.3	Somnolence Dizziness Ataxia Nausea	Rash
Zonisamide (Zonegram®)	1-2 mg/kg/day	4-8 mg/kg/day	30	20-40	Somnolence Dizziness Ataxia	Rash
Levitiracetam (Keppra®)	10 mg/kg/day	40-60 mg/kg/day	6-8	5-40	Somnolence Dizziness Ataxia	Rash
Oxcarbazepine (Trileptal®)	8-10 mg/kg/day	20-45 mg/kg/day	9 (of active metabolite monohydroxy-carbazepine)	4-12 (MHD* 12-30)	Somnolence Dizziness Ataxia Headache Nausea	Rash Hyponatremia
Felbamate (Felbatol®)	15 mg/kg/day	15-45 mg/kg/day	16	30-80	Insomnia Nausea	Aplastic anemia Hepatic failure

** MHD (10-monohydroxy-carbazepine) is the active metabolite of oxcarbazepine.*

7. References

1. Arzimanoglou A, Guerrini R, Aicardi J. *Aicardi's Epilepsy in Children*. 3rd ed. Philadelphia, PA: Lippincott Williams & Wilkins; 2004.

   (This is a recently updated edition of Aicardi's classic textbook on pediatric epilepsy. With more than 4,000 references, it covers all aspects of epilepsy diagnosis, common and rare syndromes, and a general approach to epilepsy management.)

2. Baram TZ, Shinnar S. *Febrile Seizures*. San Diego, Calif: Academic Press; 2002.

   (Comprehensive monograph that covers all aspects of febrile seizures including epidemiology, risk factors, clinical features, neurobiology, treatment, and prognosis.)

3. Crunelli V, Leresche N. Childhood absence epilepsy: genes, channels, neurons, and networks. *Nature Rev Neurosci*.2002;3:371-382.

   (This review describes the neuronal networks underlying absence epilepsy and animal mutants with absence seizures that could shed some light on the pathophysiological basis of this common epilepsy.)

4. Engel J Jr. A proposed diagnostic scheme for people with epileptic seizures and epilepsy: report of the ILAE task force on classification and terminology. *Epilepsia*. 2001;42:796-803.

   (This article presents the revised classification scheme of epilepsies and epilepsy syndromes. Several new aspects are taken into account, including the ictal features, seizure type, etiology, and degree of functional impairment.)

5. Fukuyama Y. West syndrome and other infantile epileptic encephalopathies. *Brain Dev*. (special issue) 2001;23(7):441-777.

   (Special issue of *Brain & Development* that contains articles on all aspects of infantile spasms, including pathophysiology, epidemiology, diagnosis, EEG, and treatment.)

6. Hirtz D, et al. Practice parameter: Treatment of the child with a first unprovoked seizure. *Neurology*. 2003;60:166-175.

   (Consensus by expert subcommittees of the American Academy of Neurology and the Child Neurology Society, presenting detailed recommendations and rationale as to when to treat a first unprovoked seizure in a child.)

7. Levy RH et al, eds. *Antiepileptic Drugs*. 5th ed. Philadelphia, Pa: Lippincott, Williams & Wilkins; 2002.

   (The "bible" of AEDs, now in its 5th edition, provides detailed information about all AEDs, old and new.)

8. Mitchell WG. Status epilepticus and acute serial seizures in children. *J Child Neurol*. 2002;17(Suppl. 1):S36-S43.

   (A superb overview of the risk factors, consequences, and treatment protocol of status epilepticus in children.)

9. Nordli DR Jr. Diagnostic difficulty in infants and children. *J Child Neurol*. 2002;17(Suppl. 1):S28-S35.

   (The author discusses some of the difficulties in classifying seizures and epileptic syndromes in young children, as well as an orderly approach to epilepsy classification at very young ages.)

10. Obeid M, Mikati MA. Expanding spectrum of paroxysmal events in children: potential mimickers of epilepsy. *Pediatr Neurol*. 2007;37:309-316.

    (An overview of clinical spells that are often misidentified as seizures.)

11. Rho JM, Stafstrom CE. Neurophysiology of epilepsy. In: Swaiman KF, Ashwal S, Ferreiro DM (eds.), *Pediatric Neurology: Principles and Practice*. 4th ed., Philadelphia: Mosby Elsevier, 2006, pp. 991-1007.

(The pathophysiology of seizures and epilepsy is covered in depth, with a focus on developmental mechanisms.)

12. Scheffer IE, SF Berkovic. The genetics of human epilepsy. *Trends Pharmacol Sci*. 2003;24:428-433.

(Excellent update of epilepsy genetics by internationally recognized authorities that have made pivotal advances in this rapidly evolving field.)

13. Silverstein FS, Jensen FE. Neonatal seizures. *Ann Neurol*. 2007; 62:112-120.

(A timely review covering the clinical aspects of neonatal seizures with a discussion of pathophysiological factors that can lead to hyperexcitability in the developing brain.)

14. Stephenson JBP. *Fits and Faints*. Oxford: MacKeith Press; 1990.

(A classic monograph that explores the pathophysiology and clinical manifestations of anoxic seizures and related spells.)

15. Wheless JW, Constantinou JEC. Lennox-Gastaut syndrome. *Pediatr Neurol*. 1997;17: 203-211.

(An extremely well-written overview of LGS, packed with helpful hints about patient management.)

8. Questions

1. In defining an epilepsy syndrome, which of the following features are considered?

A. Age of onset

B. Etiology

C. EEG findings

D. Prognosis

E. All of the above

2. Which of the following is NOT considered an epilepsy syndrome?

A. Rolandic epilepsy (benign childhood epilepsy with centrotemporal spikes)

B. Childhood absence epilepsy

C. Hypoglycemia

D. Lennox-Gastaut syndrome

E. Juvenile myoclonic epilepsy

3. Most epilepsy begins in childhood. Possible pathophysiological explanations include all of the following EXCEPT:

A. Earlier development of excitatory synapses

B. Depolarizing action of GABA early in life

C. Consistently lower serum calcium levels in children compared to adults

D. Earlier development of sodium and calcium channels

E. Prolific dendritic arborizations early in life with widespread excitatory synaptic connections

4. A 7-year-old girl presents with her first unprovoked, afebrile seizure. Which of the following would be the most useful initial study?

A. Serum cortisol

B. Serum prolactin

C. MRI scan

D. EEG

E. Blood cultures

5. A 5-year old boy has his first afebrile complex partial seizure, with unresponsiveness and left-hand tonic-clonic movements for 2 minutes. His examination is normal except for mild developmental delays and clumsy fine motor function of the left side. You decide to order an MRI scan of brain as opposed to a head CT scan because MRI is better for detection of:

A. Subtle cortical dysplasia

B. Hemorrhage

C. Calcium

D. Glucose metabolism

E. Cerebral blood flow

6. A 7-year-old child has a seizure consisting of focal right hand clonic activity. This simple partial seizure is distinguishable from a complex partial seizure in that a simple partial seizure:

A. Lasts longer

B. Shows more distinctive EEG changes

C. Rarely has observable clinical features

D. Is not accompanied by alteration of awareness or consciousness

E. Never has an aura

7. A 10-year-old girl with complex partial seizures could have a seizure focus in the:

A. Temporal lobe only

B. Frontal lobe only

C. Occipital lobe only

D. All of the above

E. None of the above

8. An 8-year-old boy presents with several 10-second long staring spells per day, accompanied by unresponsiveness. The EEG will most likely show:

A. 3 Hz spike-wave

B. 6 Hz spike-wave

C. Multifocal sharp waves

D. Focal spikes

E. All of the above

9. You diagnose childhood absence epilepsy in the above child. Which antiepileptic drug would be your best initial choice?

A. Carbamazepine

B. Valproic acid

C. Ethosuximide

D. A or B

E. B or C

10. Benign familial neonatal convulsions is a neonatal epilepsy syndrome with dysfunction of which ion channel(s)?

A. Sodium

B. Calcium

C. Chloride

D. Potassium

E. A and B

11. Seizures in generalized epilepsy with febrile seizures plus (GEFS+):

A. Do not appear until adolescence

B. Occur in response to fever at any age

C. Present as febrile seizures before age 5 years and as afebrile seizures after age 5 years

D. First occur in the neonatal period

E. None of the above

12. A 15-year-old girl is diagnosed with juvenile myoclonic epilepsy (JME). In counseling the family, you mention that all of the following are characteristics of JME EXCEPT:

A. Myoclonic seizures

B. Generalized tonic-clonic seizures

C. Bursts of 4 Hz to 6 Hz spike-wave on EEG

D. Probable need for lifelong AED treatment

E. All of the above are characteristic of JME

13. A 6-month-old girl with tuberous sclerosis complex presents with flexor spasms in clusters most noticeable shortly after she awakens from sleep. In this syndrome, you would expect all of the following EXCEPT:

A. Ictal EEG showing hypsarrhythmia

B. Interictal EEG showing hypsarrhythmia

C. Spasms should respond to vigabatrin or ACTH treatment

D. Prognosis will be poorer because she has a symptomatic etiology

E. Even if spasms respond to treatment, other seizure types will probably emerge

14. A 4-year-old boy has Lennox-Gastaut syndrome. He would be expected to exhibit all of the following EXCEPT:

A. Multiple seizure types

B. EEG showing slow spike-waves

C. Difficult to control seizures

D. A poor prognosis for seizure control and intellectual development

E. All of the above

15. A 9-year-old healthy, normally developing boy develops episodes of unilateral facial contortion and twitching accompanied by speech arrest. His alertness is maintained and there are no convulsive movements of his limbs. In counseling the family, you mention that children with this epilepsy syndrome:

A. Rarely outgrow their seizures

B. Often outgrow their seizures by adolescence

C. Should be treated with phenobarbital until adolescence

D. Usually have prior neurologic impairment or developmental delay

E. Should never be treated since the outcome is benign

16. A 2-week-old infant develops episodes of rhythmic, synchronous clonic movements of both arms and legs. Neonatal seizures are especially concerning because:

A. They usually persist throughout life despite treatment

B. They always cause brain damage

C. They usually reflect an underlying brain injury or CNS dysfunction

D. No anticonvulsant is effective

E. They cannot be detected reliably on EEG

17. A 2-day-old boy has an EEG to evaluate seizures. Which type of neonatal seizure has the most consistent ictal EEG correlate?

A. Focal clonic

B. Generalized tonic

C. Subtle

D. Absence

E. Benign neonatal sleep myoclonus

18. A previously healthy, normally developing 2-year-old girl presents to the emergency room with a fever of 103 degrees Fahrenheit. Earlier that day, she had a 1-minute episode of unresponsiveness accompanied by stiffness of all extremities followed by generalized hypotonia for 2 minutes, after which she regained full alertness and baseline function. On examination, she has bilateral otitis media and a normal neurologic examination. Children with this diagnosis:

A. Should always be treated prophylactically because these seizures are associated with brain damage

B. Should always be treated prophylactically because these seizures are inevitably associated with intellectual decline

C. Should always be treated prophylactically because prolonged febrile seizures have been associated with mesial temporal sclerosis later in life

D. Can be treated intermittently with oral diazepam, which has been shown to reduce the occurrence of additional febrile seizures in the same illness

E. Can be subdivided into simple and complicated types, which have the same prognosis

19. A 13-year-old boy with which of the following diagnoses should be treated with an AED?

A. Breath-holding spells

B. Syncope

C. Rage attacks

D. Parasomnias

E. None of the above

20. A 4-year-old girl with Lennox-Gastaut syndrome is failing AED monotherapy and you are considering adding a second AED. In general, which of the following statements is NOT true regarding antiepileptic drug treatment of childhood epilepsy?

A. Monotherapy is preferred

B. Polytherapy increases the chance of toxic medication-related side effects

C. In polytherapy, one drug may affect the other drug's metabolism

D. The pharmacokinetics of AED metabolism are different in children and adults

E. It is preferable to start a "newer" AED first, because of fewer adverse effects

Answers

1. E.
An epilepsy syndrome is characterized by a consistent set of clinical features that include seizure type, age of onset, EEG findings, etiology, natural history, treatment response, and prognosis.

2. C.
Seizures caused by hypoglycemia are considered reactive in nature. Once the hypoglycemia is corrected, there is no reason to expect seizures to recur. Each of the other options is an epilepsy syndrome.

3. C.
Processes mediating excitation typically develop prior to their inhibitory counterparts. Therefore, excitatory synapses, depolarizing GABA action, early development of sodium and calcium channels, and excitatory synaptic connections all favor increased cellular and network excitability in the developing brain. Hypocalcemia can cause seizures, but baseline serum calcium levels are similar in children and adults.

4. D.
An EEG is the first test of choice in this situation. Serum prolactin and cortisol levels have been reported to accompany epileptic seizures (as opposed to pseudoseizures), but they are actually quite unreliable as indicators of epileptic seizure activity. A brain MRI scan may be indicated, but not emergently. Blood cultures are reasonable if the child is febrile.

5. A.
In this non-emergent scenario, cortical dysplasia is among the more likely etiologies. MRI is superior to CT for determination of this structural abnormality. In an emergency situation, a head CT scan can detect blood. Both MRI and CT can detect calcium, but may be easier to see on CT. Glucose metabolism is demonstrated by a PET scan and cerebral blood flow by a SPECT scan; neither of those is indicated in this setting.

6. D.
The primary feature that distinguishes a simple partial seizure from a complex partial seizure is preservation of awareness. Seizure duration and EEG features do not differentiate the two types. Both seizure types have observable clinical features, and an aura is actually considered to be a simple partial seizure.

7. D.
Any lobe of the brain can support a complex partial seizure.

8. A.
This boy most likely has childhood absence epilepsy with an EEG pattern of 3 Hz spike-waves during an absence seizure. Less likely, he could have complex partial seizures and have an EEG with focal or multifocal paroxysmal disturbances; complex partial seizures are typically longer than absence seizures and occur less frequently.

9. E. (B or C would also be acceptable)
Ethosuximide is usually the first AED prescribed for a child with absence epilepsy, unless the child also has GTC seizures, in which case VPA would be preferable. Some physicians choose VPA first; the choice is also determined by considering the child's age and concern about side effects. Carbamazepine can exacerbate absence seizures.

10. D.
BFNC is caused by an inherited mutation in neuronal potassium channels. In all neonatal seizures, specific causes should be ruled out before concluding that the cause is genetic.

11. C.
GEFS+ presents as febrile seizures that either do not cease at the expected age (around 5 years) or evolve into afebrile seizures of a variety of types after the febrile seizures stop. Choice B is incorrect because fever-induced seizures are not seen in GEFS+ in adulthood. Choice D is incorrect because the syndrome cannot be diagnosed with certainty until after age 5 years.

12. E.
All of the statements are true about JME, which typically responds to treatment (eg, VPA), but lifelong treatment is usually necessary to avert recurrent seizures.

13. A.
In infantile spasms, the ictal EEG shows electrodecrement while the interictal EEG shows hypsarrhythmia. Infantile spasms in children with tuberous sclerosis may respond to vigabatrin or ACTH, but these children typically develop multifocal seizures at older ages. Prognosis is poorer in symptomatic compared to cryptogenic infantile spasms.

14. E.
All of the statements characterize Lennox-Gastaut syndrome. Children with LGS typically have multiple seizure types that are refractory to several AEDs.

15. B.
Children with rolandic epilepsy typically outgrow their seizures by adolescence, hence the common use of the term "benign" in referring to this syndrome. The decision to treat is tailored to the child's particular circumstances, including time of day during which seizures occur (if nocturnal only, AED may not be necessary); frequency of seizures (the first seizure is often not treated); and age (younger age at presentation suggests a longer period of seizure susceptibility). Carbamazepine is the usual AED chosen.

16. C.
Neonatal seizures are usually a marker of CNS insult or dysfunction. Their prognosis is related to the etiology so they may cease when the pathology is reversed. Neonatal seizures can often be detected on EEG, with EEG correlation related to seizure type (focal clonic seizures are most highly correlated). The typically chosen medications (phenobarbital, phenytoin, benzodiazepines) have limited effectiveness. Hopefully, mechanism-specific treatments for neonatal seizures will be developed.

17. A.
Video-EEG studies have shown that focal clonic seizures are most highly correlated with EEG discharges. Generalized tonic seizures and subtle seizures, such as those involving bicycling or chewing movements, are less tightly correlated with EEG changes and might represent brainstem release phenomena rather than epileptic seizures.

18. D.
Simple febrile seizures are not associated with brain damage or cognitive impairment and are ordinarily not treated prophylactically. Prolonged febrile seizures have been associated with subsequent mesial temporal sclerosis, but preventative treatment is not indicated. Simple and complicated febrile seizures have different prognoses; most children with either febrile seizure type do well, but there is a higher chance of subsequent afebrile seizures in children with complicated febrile seizures.

19. E.
Breath-holding spells are seen in preschool aged children and are not treated with AEDs. Likewise, syncope, episodic dyscontrol (rage attacks), and sleep-related disorders (parasomnias) are not treated with AEDs, because of their non-epileptic etiologies. Of note, children with rage attacks occasionally improve on AEDs by a mechanism thought to involve an overall decrease in neuronal membrane excitability, but this disorder is not considered to be epileptic in nature.

20. E.
Accumulating clinical experience is showing that the "newer" AEDs have side effects, perhaps little different than the older generation of AEDs. It is certainly preferable to treat a child with a single agent, to reduce the chance of adverse effects. Keep in mind that drugs can interact and induce adverse side effects by altering each other's metabolism. Children and adults metabolize drugs differently in terms of volume of distribution, pharmacokinetics and, to some extent, side effect profile. Occasionally, as in children with LGS, polytherapy is necessary and the choice of drugs is aimed at the predominant seizure types.

Chapter 23: Electrophysiology

Barbara C. Jobst, MD
Gregory L. Holmes, MD

Contents

1. Introduction

Signaling via electrical action potentials is the basis for neuronal functioning and a fundamental principle of the nervous system. Although only compounded electrical potentials can be recorded on the surface of the head, electrophysiology is one of the fundamental diagnostic tools for the neurologist.

Berger, in 1929, was the first to record "brain waves" in the form of an electroencephalogram (EEG). Other electrophysiologic diagnostic tools, like evoked potentials, followed thereafter. Despite advances in MRI and neuroimaging, electrophysiology remains fundamental in the evaluation of neurological disorders and more specialized applications like intraoperative monitoring and polysomnography have become indispensable to the neurologist.

2. EEG

Methods and Procedure

EEG represents a limited sampling of electrical activity on the surface of the brain. Only the electrical currents in the radially oriented apical dentrites of the neocortical pyramidal neurons can be measured. Most pyramidal cell currents are excitatory and inhibitory postsynaptic potentials (EPSPs and IPSPs) in the dentrites, but "intrinsic" membrane oscillations arising from voltage-dependent ion-channels also contribute to the EEG signal.

To record EEG electrodes made out of silver chloride, gold or platinum are applied in a standardized way using the 10/20 international system on the scalp of the patient (Figure 1). Electrodes are named by their location (F = frontal, P = parietal, O = occipital, T = temporal, C = central) and an associated number. Odd numbers are assigned to the left hemisphere, even numbers are assigned to the right hemisphere (Hughes, 1994). Midline electrodes are designated by "Z" (Fz, Cz, Pz, and Oz).

The electrodes are wired to the electroencephalograph via amplifiers. Amplifiers enhance the signal as brain activity is only microvolts (μV) in amplitude. Amplifiers filter environmental noise (com-

Figure 1

Placement of electrodes in the international 10/20 system system

Standard longitudinal bipolar montage is demonstrated by the arrows connecting the electrodes.

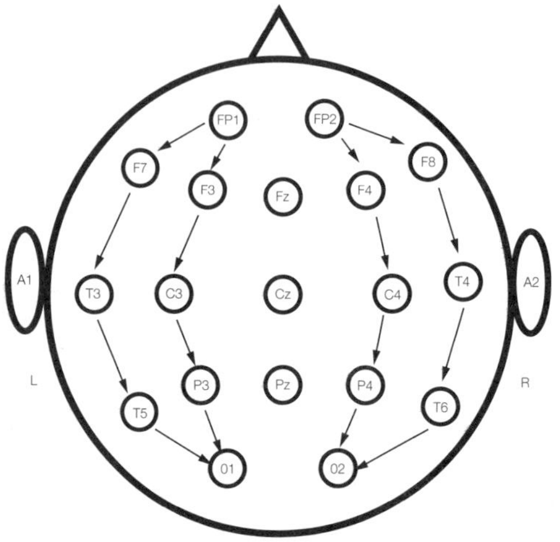

mon mode rejection). Low frequency (high pass) and high frequency (low pass) filters are then applied to exclude frequencies outside the range of interest. The usual bandwidths examined in the human EEG are between 0.3 Hz to 70 Hz.

Electroencephalographs record the voltage difference between two electrodes (Figure 2). Various electrode configurations, termed montages, are used to identify abnormalities. Referential montages involve the difference between an active electrode on the scalp and an inactive electrode, for example, an electrode on the ear or chin. However, it is important to keep in mind that an inactive electrode placed anywhere on the body will detect some electrical activity and is not truly inactive. Nevertheless, judicious use of an inactive electrode allows comparison of EEG signals of interest with electrical activity outside the field of interest. Bipolar montages record the voltage difference between two active scalp electrodes. In referential recording, an abnormality is localized by identifying the channels where the abnormalities are of highest amplitude. In a bipolar recording, a phase reversal of an abnormal signal indicates the localization of the origin of an abnormality. By convention, signals with an upward deflection are considered negative and signals with a downward deflection are considered positive.

Figure 2

Example of a differential amplifier

The EEG signal is the difference between the inputs, termed grids (G1 and G2). If G1 and G2 are recording identical voltages the output will be a flat line.

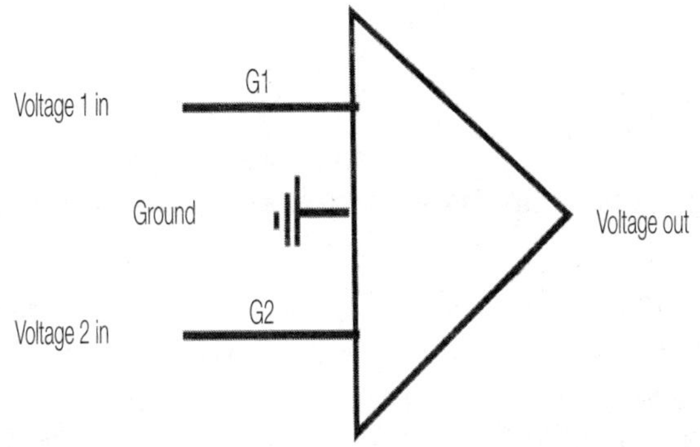

Although analogue electroencephalographs remain available, most machines now use digital technology. The advantages of digital machines are enormous. A digital apparatus allows the reader to change electrode montage, sensitivity, "paper" speed, and filters at will after the recording. Regardless of the recording method, calibration is required in every EEG recording to ensure that the amplifier and filter settings are identical in each channel. Impedance checks of all electrodes are necessary in digital and analog recording in order not to contaminate physiologic signal by environmental noise.

Usually 16 to 18 channels of scalp EEG are recorded. EKG is recorded to recognize EKG and pulse artifacts. In addition, electrodes are placed near the outer canthi of both eyes to detect eye movements to aid the reader in differentiating eye movements from cerebral electrical activity.

A routine EEG should include referential and bipolar montages. The EEG should be recorded with the patient awake and asleep. Age and state (awake or asleep) need to be known to the interpreter. Epileptiform activity is enhanced with sleep. Provocation maneuvers like eye opening and closing, hyperventilation, and photic stimulation should be performed. The recording should be at least 20 minutes long in adults and 1 hour long in neonates. Repeat EEG recordings or prolonged EEG recordings increase the yield for detecting abnormalities. An EEG report should be produced that includes an introduction, description and interpretation

Normal EEG

For definitions of basic EEG rhythms, see Table 1.

During wakefulness, with the eyes closed, the background rhythm should be most prominent in the occipital leads and represent an alpha rhythm. The normal amplitude should vary between 15-50 μV. Frontally faster frequencies in the beta range are normal. Eye opening results in blockage of the alpha rhythm with only beta frequencies present (Figure 3).

Drowsiness results in amplitude attenuation and replacement of the background rhythm with a mixture of theta, alpha and beta frequencies. With sleep stage II, sleep spindles, vertex waves and K-complexes appear (Figure 4). These waveforms are most prominent centrally. With sleep stages III and IV, there is an increase in delta slowing and disappearance of spindles and vertex waves. REM sleep is characterized by a low voltage mixture of alpha and beta frequencies, as well as frequent eye movements.

Normal Variants

Apart from the above described rhythms, there are normal variants that have no pathologic significance and can be difficult to distinguish from abnormal rhythms (Table 2). For example, EEGs that only contain beta frequencies are considered a normal variant. Predominant beta frequencies may also be the result of medication effect and are frequently associated with benzodiazepines or barbiturate intake. For other normal variants see Table 2.

Artifacts

Artifacts, especially movement artifacts, or muscle artifacts, can obscure the recording due to tension in the temporal muscles (Figure 5 and Table 3). It is essential for the electroencephalographer to recognize artifacts and distinguish those from physiological brain abnormalities. As a general rule, abnormal activity generated in the brain usually has a broader field and should be apparent in more than one electrode.

Activation Procedures

Hyperventilation, sleep deprivation and photic stimulation are activation procedures that can elicit abnormal activity on EEG, especially epileptiform activity. During hyperventilation the patient is asked to breathe deeply and rapidly for three minutes. The resulting hypocapnia is responsible for slowing of the background rhythm, which is considered within normal limits during hyperventilation (Figure 6). Slowing is more prominent in the frontal regions in adults and adolescents and occipital region in children. Slowing during hyperventilation is more extensive in children than adults and is exacerbated by fasting. Slowing should subside one minute after cessation of hyperventilation. The appearance of epileptiform activity in the form of spikes, sharp waves or spike-and-wave discharges is abnormal. Hyperventilation is most useful in typical absence epilepsy of childhood. The vast majority of

Table 1

Basic EEG Elements and Stages of Sleep

Alpha-rhythm	8-12 Hz
Beta-rhythm	13-40 Hz
Theta-rhythm	4-7.5 Hz
Delta-rhythm	1-3 Hz
Spike	Sharp element <70 ms duration
Sharp wave	Sharp element 71-200 ms duration
Spike wave complex	Spike followed by a slow wave
Polyspike	Several spikes in a row
Sleep spindle	14 Hz rhythmic activity
Vertex wave	Central sharp wave
K-complex	High amplitude sharp wave followed by sleep spindle
Drowsiness (Sleep stage I)	Alpha attenuation, increase in theta
Sleep stage II	Vertex waves, sleep spindles, K complexes; High amplitude (>70 µV <2 Hz) delta activity <20%
Sleep stage III	High amplitude (>70 µV <2 Hz) delta 20%-50%
Sleep stage IV	High amplitude (>70 µV <2 Hz) delta >50%
REM sleep	Saw tooth waves and mixed frequencies

Figure 3

Normal EEG with well-developed alpha background with the eyes closed

Note the attenuation of the alpha at the beginning of the recording with eyes opened.

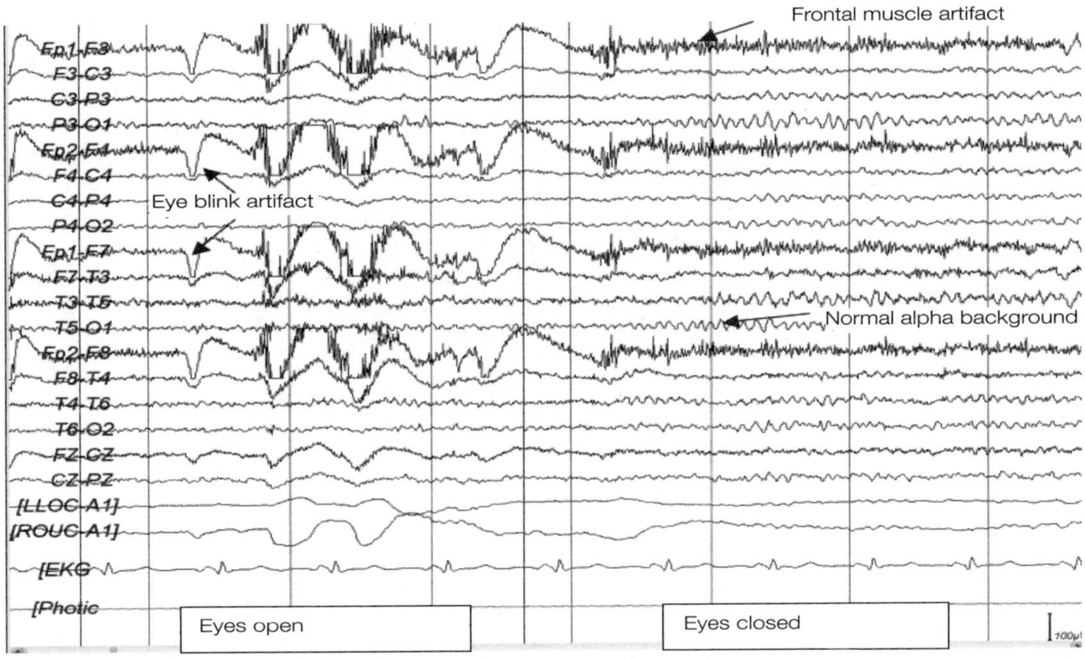

Figure 4

Normal stage II sleep in a 12-year-old boy with vertex waves and sleep spindles in a transverse montage

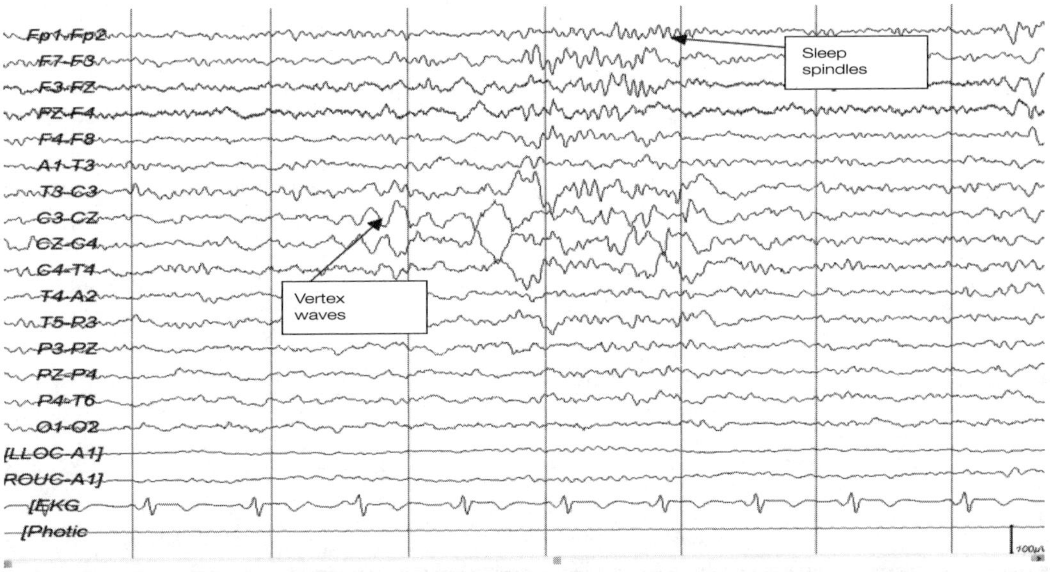

Table 2

Normal EEG Variants

Normal Variant	Description and Location	Occurs in
Rhythmic temporal theta burst of drowsiness (RTTD) = psychomotor variant	Notched temporal rhythm	Adolescents and young adults
Alpha variant (slow and fast)	Harmonic relationship to alpha rhythm *Slow alpha variant:* half the frequency of alpha *Fast alpha variant:* double the frequency of alpha rhythm	Adults
Frontal arousal rhythms	7-20 Hz over frontal regions lasting up to 20 seconds	Children, during arousal
Subclinical rhythmic electrographic theta discharges in adults (SREDA)	High voltage monophasic sharp component, followed by one second lower amplitude rhythms, followed by 5-7 Hz sinusoidal theta. Bilateral, posterior temporal 40-80 sec long	>50 years old during drowsiness or hyperventilation
Midline theta rhythms	5-7 Hz over vertex	
Fourteen and 6 Hertz positive bursts	Resembles sleep spindles with sharp positive phase; posterior temporal asynchronous	Children and adolescents
Small sharp spikes = benign epileptiform transients of sleep	Small spikes <50 μV unilateral	Drowsiness and light sleep
Six Hertz spike and wave = phantom spike wave	Bilateral synchronous 6 Hz spike and wave	Drowsiness and relaxed wakefulness
Wicket spikes	Temporal arc-like waves that look like a "wicket"	30 years old Drowsiness and light sleep
Posterior slow waves of youth = youth waves	Posterior theta activity	Children and adolescents
Positive occipital slow transients of sleep = POSTS	Positive repetitive sharp waves occipitally, bilateral synchronous	15-35 y/o during sleep
Lambda waves	Positive repetitive sharp waves occipitally	Occur with scanning eye movements, more common in children
Mu (μ) rhythm	Rhythmic arc-like activity of alpha frequency centrally	Young adults, disappears with hand movement

Figure 5

Muscle artifact primarily over the temporal regions (Fp1-F7, F7-T3, Fp2-F8, F8-T4)

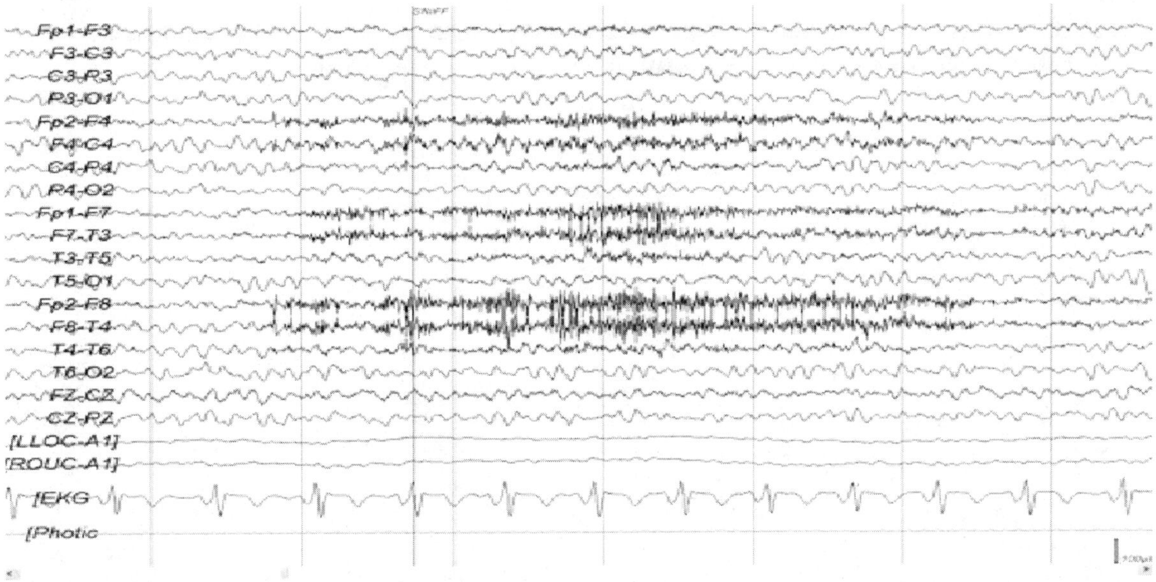

Table 3

Common EEG Artifacts

Artifact	Characteristics
Muscle/EMG	High frequency artifact often artifact temporal
Movement artifact	High amplitude irregular activity often in all channels
60 cycle artifact	Sinusoidal artifact of 60 Hz
Electrode pop	Localizes to only one electrode
Eye movement artifact Eye blinks	Retina is negative, cornea is positive. Upward movement of eyeball creates positive potential in frontal leads and "out of phase activity" in eye channels
Sweating/perspiration	High amplitude slow potentials <1 Hz
EKG artifact	Synchronized with EKG
Pulse artifact	Time locked to EKG
IV-drip artifact	Electrostatic periodic artifact
Digital artifact	Due to sampling
In infants:	
Hiccups	Periodic movement artifact
Sucking	High amplitude sharp activity bitemporal
Padding	Rhythmic artifact that follows frequency of padding

Figure 6

Normal diffuse slowing during hyperventilation in an 8-year-old boy

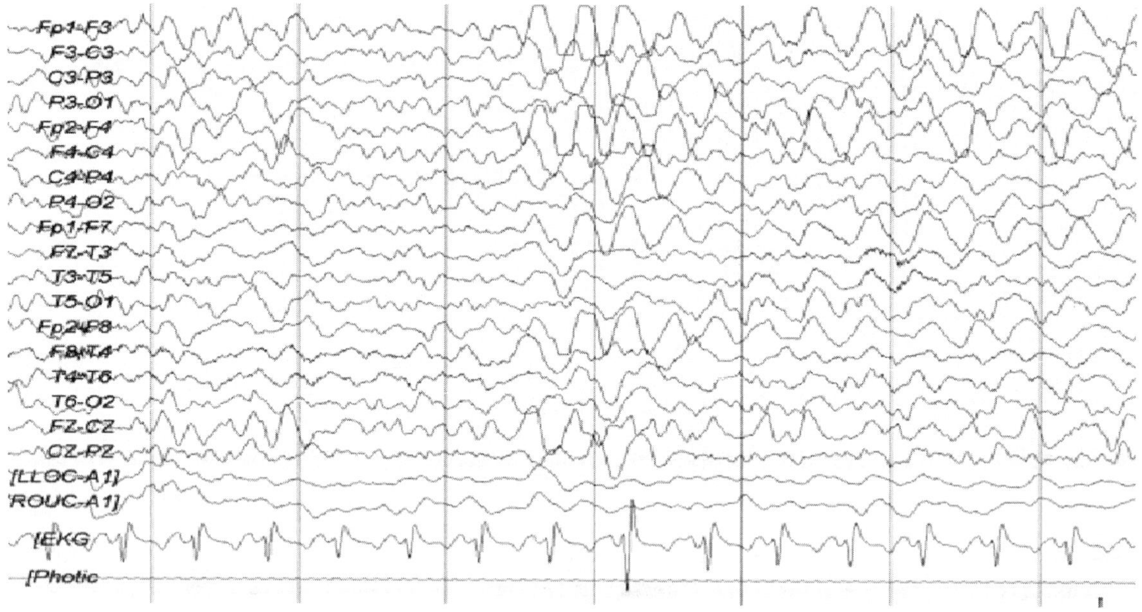

children with untreated absence epilepsy will have an absence seizure during hyperventilation with typical 2.5-3.5 Hz generalized spike-and-wave discharges (Figure 7). Hyperventilation is contraindicated in patients with a previous stroke or severe cardiac or pulmonary disease.

During photic stimulation, a stroboscopic light is flashed at increasing frequencies between 1 and 30 Hz. This may activate epileptiform activity. Photic stimulation can result in no change of the background rhythm, photic driving, a photomyogenic response or a photoconvulsive (also termed photoparoxysmal) response. With photic driving the occipital activity of the EEG follows the frequency of the photic stimulus. These so-called driving responses are visual evoked potentials and usually have no pathological significance when present bilaterally. A variety of storage diseases will result in high amplitude spikes or sharp waves with photic stimulation at low frequencies. Some patients with migraine headaches will drive at high frequencies or at harmonics of the photic stimulation, eg, a 24 Hz driving response with a 12 Hz photic stimulation.

A photomyogenic response is time-locked muscle artifact to the stimulation. This activity is seen in the frontal region of the head. The abnormal activity immediately ceases at the end of the stimulus. A photoparoxysmal or photoconvulsive response consists of spikes, sharp waves, and spike-and-wave activity occurring during the photic stimulation. This abnormal activity usually extends beyond the occipital electrodes and frequently persists beyond the end of the photic stimulation (Figure 8). Not all patients with a photoconvulsive response have epilepsy. However, if the EEG changes are widespread and last longer than the photic stimulation, the likelihood of epilepsy is high. Photosensitivity is most commonly associated with generalized seizures but can also occur in patients with partial seizures.

EEG of Childhood

Electrical brain activity matures during infancy and childhood. Therefore neonatal and childhood EEG defers substantially from adult recordings. In very premature neonates (< 30 weeks conceptional age),

Figure 7

Generalized 3 Hz spike wave discharge in a 11-year-old with typical childhood absence epilepsy

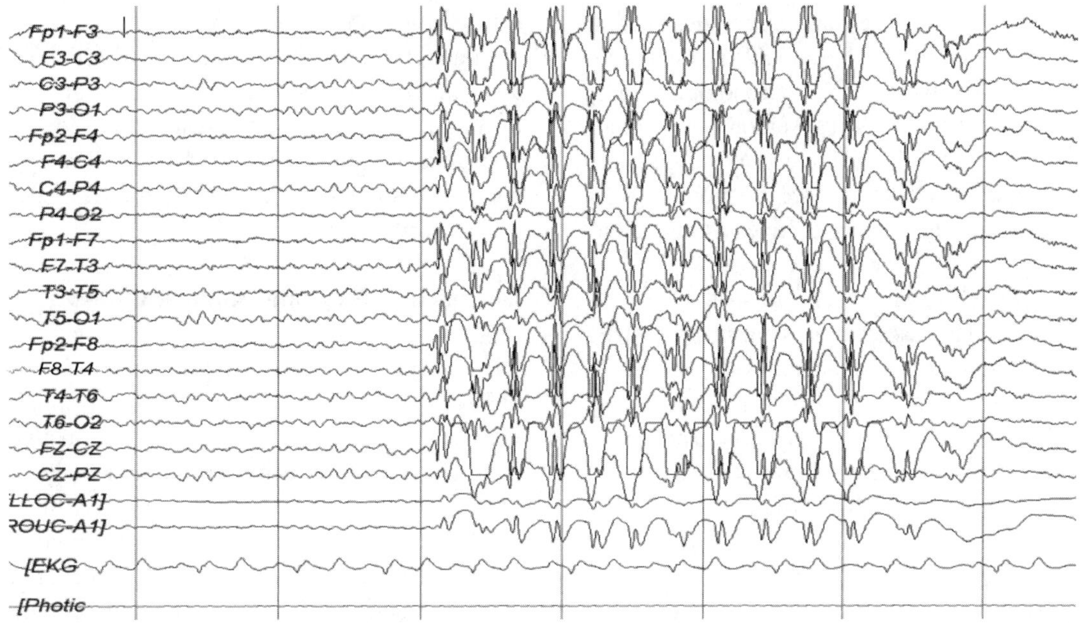

Figure 8

Photoconvulsive response in 14-year-old girl with generalized tonic-clonic seizures

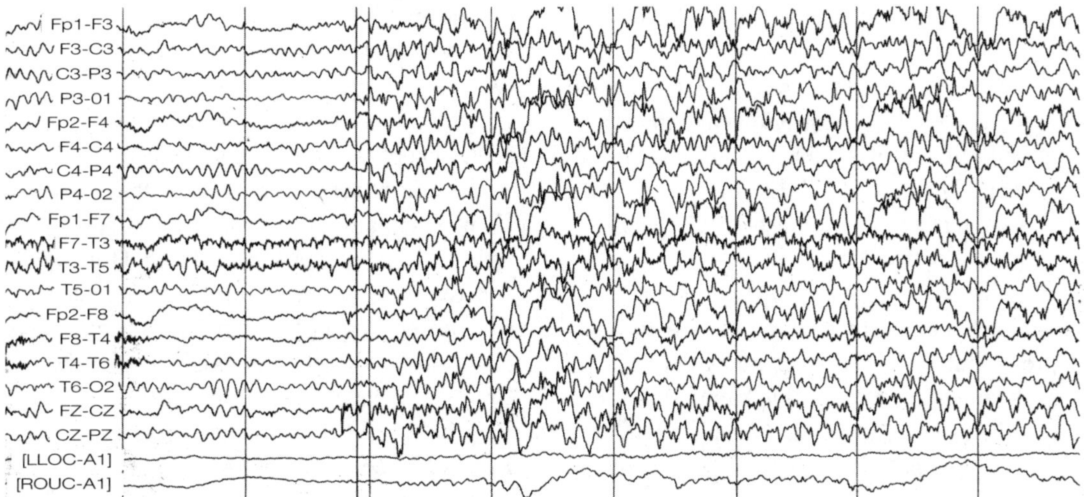

a modified montage with fewer electrodes is used due to head size. In addition, respirations and EMG are monitored.

Maturation of electrical brain activity is related far more with gestational age than chronological age. The electroencephalographer should know the conceptional age (gestational age + chronological age). Between 29 and 36 weeks of gestation there is rapid evolution of brain activity (Table 4). It is important to know whether a neonatal record is continuous or discontinuous and whether it is reactive to stimulation.

At full term (36-40 weeks gestational age) the record can still be discontinuous during quiet sleep, but interburst intervals should not be longer than 2-4 seconds (*tracé alternant* pattern). Slow wave sleep in the delta range may gradually develop at full term. During wakefulness, continuous activity constitutes the predominant background rhythm in a full-term infant, which is a mixture of low-to-medium amplitude mixed frequencies. This continuous activity is observed during wakefulness (eyes open) and active sleep (eyes closed). Delta brushes, which are high amplitude delta waves superimposed with spindle-like activity, are present until 44 weeks of gestation.

At the age of 3-4 months the background activity should be more organized and in the frequency range of 3-4 Hz. Slow wave sleep should be clearly present. Vertex waves appear between 4-6 months. Sleep spindles may already appear at the age of 1-2 months but are initially asynchronous. Well-defined sleep spindles should be present by 6 months of age. At 12 months of age the waking background frequency should increase to 6-7 Hz. An 8 Hz background rhythm is usually established at 3 years of age.

Hypnagogic hypersynchrony is a pattern that is most prominent in childhood after the age of 12 months. It consists of bilateral high amplitude rhythmic theta waves at the onset of sleep. It may be mistaken for epileptiform activity. However, hypnagogic hypersynchrony does not exhibit embedded spikes or sharp waves.

Abnormal EEG

Abnormalities on EEG can be diffuse, regional, or focal. Diffuse abnormalities are usually seen in all channels and indicate some sort of an encephalopathy. Regional abnormalities involve lesser brain volumes and can be bilateral or lateralized. Focal abnormalities are restricted to discrete regions of the brain and may indicate a structural abnormality. Sharp waves, spikes, spike-and-wave discharges and paroxysmal rhythmic activity is classified as epileptiform activity.

Diffuse and Regional Abnormalities

Diffuse irregular generalized slowing in the theta or delta range indicating diffuse cerebral dysfunction. Is is frequntly referred to as an encephalopathic pattern. There are multiple etiologies (Table 5). Diffuse slowing can be intermittent or continuous. Diffuse intermittent slowing indicates a mild encephalopathy. Diffuse continuous slowing indicates a moderate to severe encephalopathy. Diffuse intermittent rhythmic slow activity predominantly over the frontal regions (FIRDA = frontal intermittent rhythmic delta activity) is frequently noted in adults with an encephalopathy. In children, occipital diffuse intermittent rhythmic activity is more frequent (OIRDA = occipital intermittent rhythmic delta activity). FIRDA is also associated with subfrontal or diencephalic lesions and obstructive hydrocephalus. Rarely, OIRDA can be associated with typical absence epilepsy.

Periodic patterns are typical for more severe and acute encephalopathies. Those consist of sharp waves or triphasic waves that occur in a periodic fashion. Triphasic waves are large positive sharp waves >70 μV that are preceded and followed by a negative wave of lower amplitude. Triphasic waves were initially described in hepatic encephalopathy but occur also in other types of encephalopathy, Creutzfeldt-Jacob disease or SSPE.

Focal Abnormalities

Focal slowing can be rhythmic or arrhythmic (polymorphic), intermittent or continuous. Continuous focal slowing usually indicates a structural lesion. Continuous focal polymorphic delta activity is asso-

Table 4

Neonatal EEG

Gestational Age	Wakefulness	Active Sleep (eyes closed like REM)	Quiet Sleep
<29 weeks	Discontinuous, monorhythmic occipital delta, bursts of rhythmic occipital and temporal theta, bursts 90% synchronized	No state organization	No state organization
30-32 weeks	Monorhythmic delta, posterior delta brushes, marginally reactive	More continuous, increased body movements	Trace discontinue (<25 μV during suppression) IBI 5-8 sec; 70% synchronous bursts; Differentiation between quiet and active sleep possible
33-34 weeks	Reactive, delta brushes, sharp waves temporal and central, monorhythmic delta decreases	Delta brushes	Trace discontinue IBI 5-6 sec 80% synchronous bursts
35-36 weeks	Activity moyenne, anterior slow dysrhythmia; Encoches pointues frontales (frontal sharp waves)	Delta brushes	Trace alternans (>25 μV during suppression) IBI 4-6 sec 85% synchronous bursts
37-40 weeks	Activity moyenne, sharp waves decrease	25% indeterminate sleep; delta brushes disappear	Trace alternans IBI <4 sec, 100% synchronous bursts; continuous slow wave sleep appears
41-44 weeks	Activity moyenne	50% of record active sleep	Trace alternans, continuous slow wave sleep

IBI = interburst interval

Table 5

Encephalopathies

Metabolic	Uremic, hepatic electrolyte imbalance, hypo- / hyperglycemic
Anoxic	
Endocrine	Thyroid, calcium, adrenal
Nutritional	B_1, B_{12}
Infectious and Inflammatory	Meningitis, encephalitis, Creutzfeldt-Jacobs, AIDS, autoimmune
Hypertensive	
Epileptic	Progressive and myoclonic epilepsies
Hereditary and Neurodegenerative	Leukodystrophies, inborn errors of metabolism

ciated with tumor, stroke, abscess, or hematoma. It can also occur in encephalitis and other inflammatory diseases. Focal slowing intermixed with epileptiform activity suggests epilepsy (Figure 9). Voltage of delta activity usually ranges between 100-150 μV.

Focal attenuation of beta frequencies can also indicate structural lesions like subdural hematomas, stroke, tumor or abscess. A breach rhythm is focal high amplitude intermixed theta and alpha frequencies (6-11 Hz) intermixed with sharp components. It is the result of a skull defect and by itself does not have pathological significance.

Epileptiform Abnormalities

Spikes, spike-and-waves, sharp waves, polyspikes (multiple spikes), polyspike-and-waves discharges and paroxysmal rhythmic activity are considered epileptiform discharges. Epileptiform abnormalities are highly correlated with seizures and epilepsy but the association is not exclusive. Epileptiform activity can also be noted in healthy individuals and the diagnosis of epileptic seizures and epilepsy should not be made on the basis of the EEG alone. The exception to this rule is in cases where electrical seizures with behavioral changes are actually recorded during the EEG. For example, it is relatively easy to record an absence seizure with hyperventilation or photic stimulation in an untreated child with absence epilepsy. The clinical context should always be taken into consideration when interpreting an EEG.

Diffuse focal slowing and FIRDA can also be associated with epilepsy but is not specific. Temporal intermittent rhythmic delta activity is associated with temporal lobe epilepsy. Focal slowing can be seen in the postictal EEG.

PLEDs are periodic lateralized epileptiform discharges that most often have a frequency of 1 Hz (Figure 10). They were thought to be pathognomonic for Herpes encephalitis but they also occur with stroke, epilepsy and Creutzfeldt-Jacob disease. Generalized periodic epileptiform discharges are similar to PLEDS, but epileptiform activity occurs in all leads. Generalized periodic epileptiform discharges are associated with status epilepticus. A normal interictal EEG does not rule out epilepsy.

Many patients with epilepsy have a single normal interictal EEG. Repeated EEGs may increase the yield of discovering an abnormality in 80%-90% of individuals with epilepsy. In patients with a single seizure, the probability of recording epileptiform activity on interictal EEG is highest within 24 hours of the seizure. If an ictal EEG is normal, an epileptic disorder is unlikely, but patients with frontal lobes seizures may have no discernible changes on EEG, even during the seizure.

Figure 9

Focal delta slowing over the left temporal region with intermixed sharp waves in a 28-year-old patient with seizures

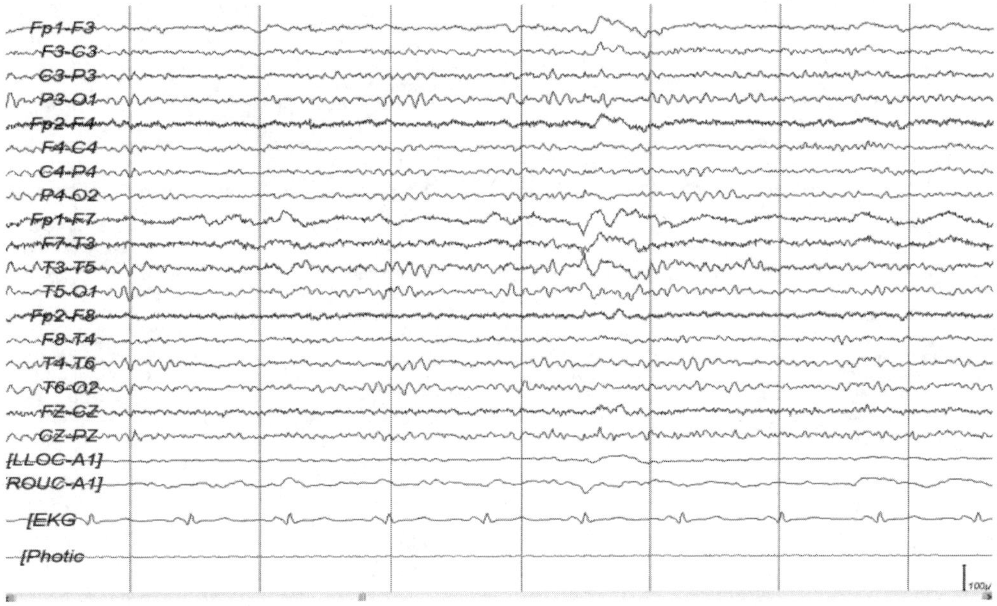

Figure 10

Periodic lateralizing epileptiform discharges over the right fronto-central region (PLEDS)

59-year-old patient with a structural lesion in the right central area due to toxoplasmosis in the setting of immunosuppression in Wegener disease.

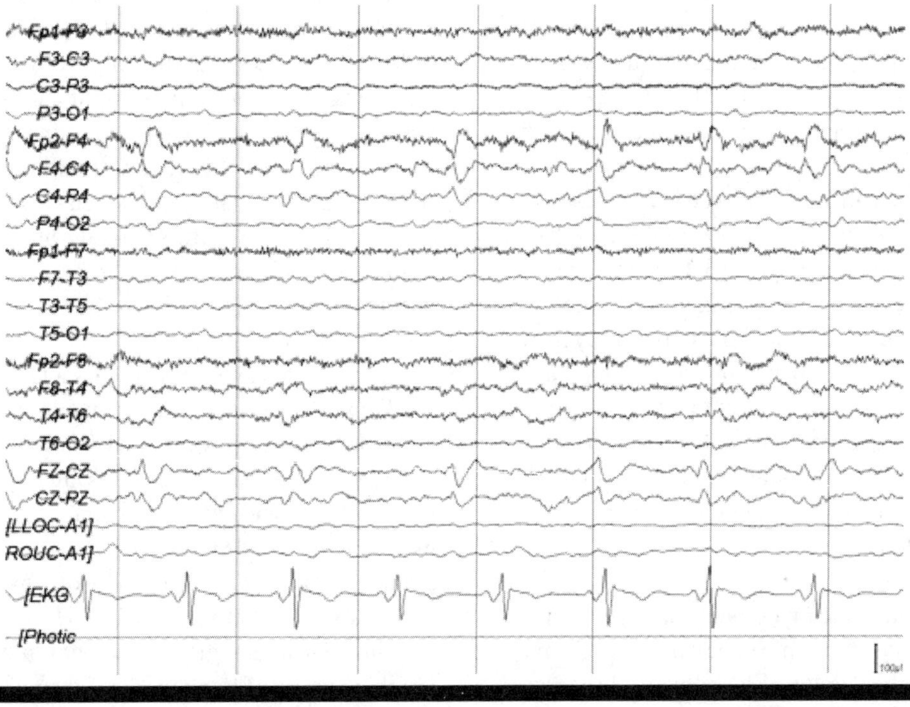

Figure 11

Generalized isolated spike-wave discharges

13-year-old girl with a history of tonic-clonic seizures and absence seizures due to idiopathic primary generalized epilepsy.

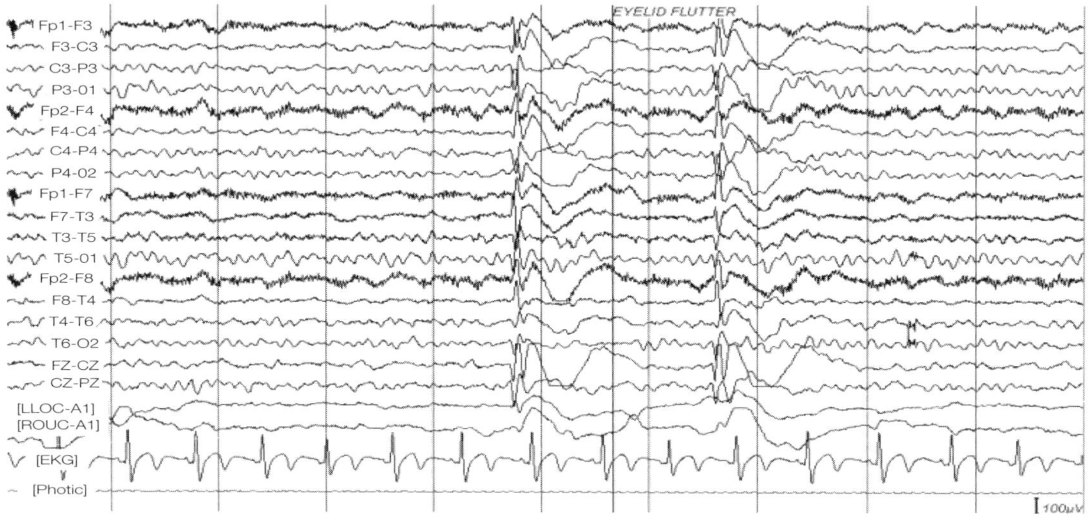

Seizures and Epilepsy

Epilepsy syndromes are divided into primarily generalized and focal (partial) epilepsies. Primary generalized epilepsies are characterized by generalized EEG changes involving all channels on ictal recordings (Figures 7 and 11). In focal or partial epilepsy syndromes, epileptiform activity originates in circumscribed areas of the cortex (Figure 12) and seizures may secondarily spread to the entire cortex.

Primary Generalized Epilepsy Syndromes
Childhood and juvenile absence epilepsy is characterized by paroxysmal typical 3Hz generalized spike-and-wave discharges (Figure 7). Spike-and-wave discharges are frequently activated by hyperventilation (Table 6). Brief episodes of spike-and-wave discharges already seem to interfere with awareness. Absences are usually no longer than 12 seconds. OIRDA (occipital intermittent rhythmic delta activity) is seen frequently in children with absence epilepsy.

The EEG in juvenile myoclonic epilepsy is characterized by less stereotypic generalized spike-and-wave discharges. Polyspike-and-wave discharges are frequent, with the frequency of the spike-wave discharges varying from 3.5 to 6 Hz. Photosensitivity is more commonly seen than activation by hyperventilation (Table 6).

West syndrome is characterized by infantile spasms, hypsarrhythmia and developmental delay. Hypsarrythmia is an EEG pattern of highly disorganized, chaotic delta waves of high amplitude (>300 V), which is continuous (Figure 13). Infantile spasms show an electrodecremental response on EEG. A frontally predominant generalized slow wave transient is followed by diffuse voltage attenuation. Some patients with West syndrome have a partial onset to their seizures.

Lennox-Gastaut syndrome is characterized by the triad of multiple seizure types, mental retardation and slow spike-and-wave discharges on EEG. The slow spike-and-wave discharges are large complexes of biphasic or triphasic sharp waves followed by a high amplitude negative slow wave. Those complexes appear at a frequency of 1.5-2.5 Hz. Paroxysmal fast activity of 15-20 Hz most prominent in the frontal region is another typical electrographic feature of Lennox-Gastaut syndrome.

Figure 12

Focal epileptiform activity over the right temporal region in form of sharp wave discharges

34-year-old man with intractable temporal lobe epilepsy and typical complex partial seizures.

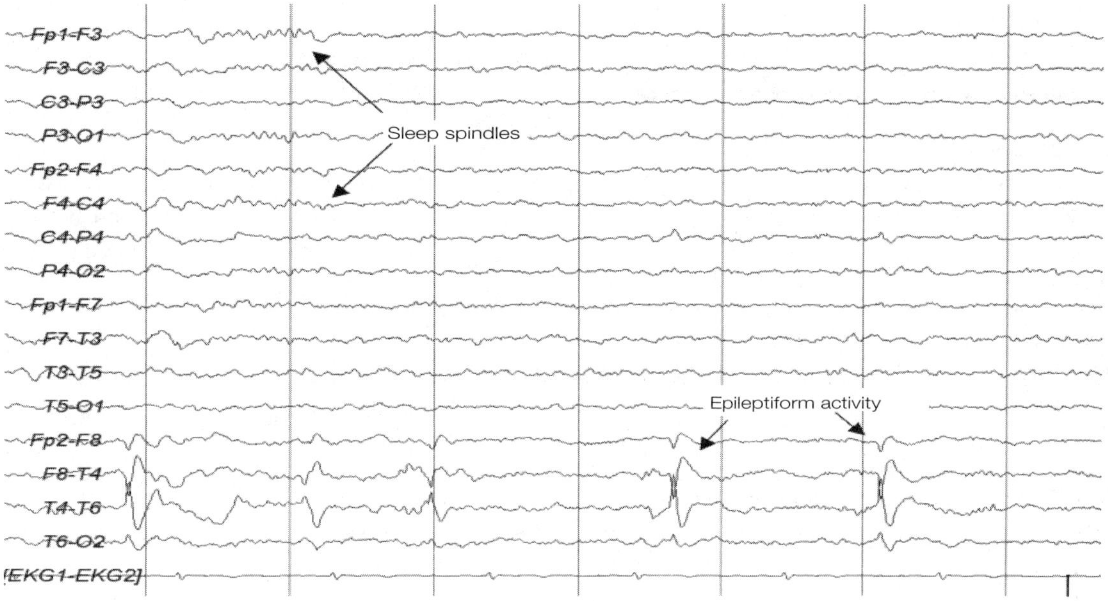

Figure 13

Hypsarrhythmia pattern in a 8-month-old infant

Note high amplitude chaotic disorganized delta waves with intermixed spikes.

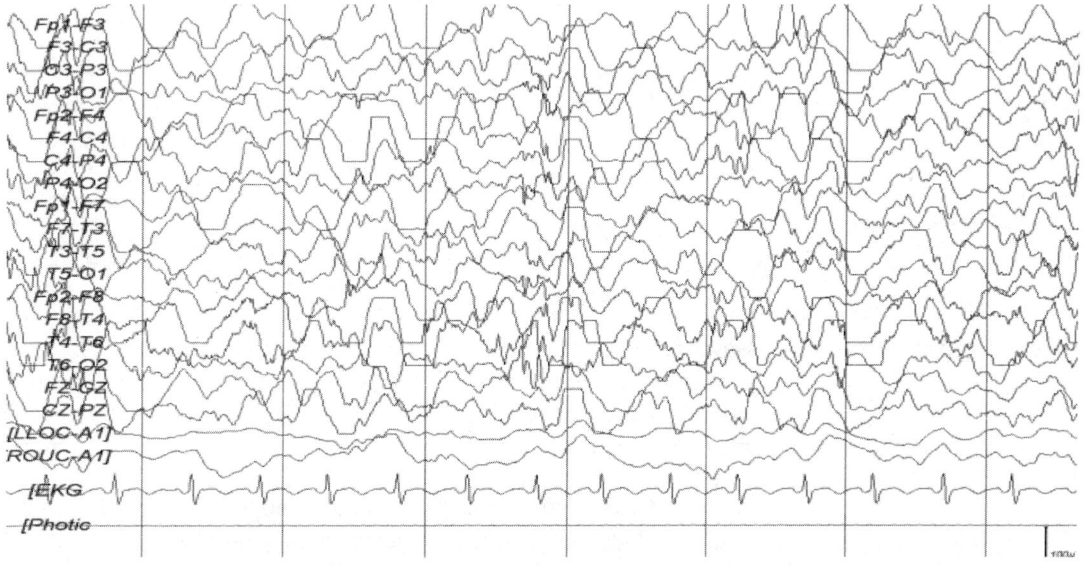

Table 6

EEG of Certain Epilepsy Syndromes During Various Stages and Activation Procedures

Hyperventilation	Photic Stimulation	Awake	Non-REM Sleep	REM
Absence epilepsy				
85% activation OIRDA	20% activation	Organized 3 Hz SW burst	Increased SW bursts, fragmented non-REM sleep polyspikes	Like awake state, but decreased SW
Benign epilepsy with centro-temporal spikes				
No effect	No effect	Poss. unilateral centro-temporal spikes	Marked increase in spiking, mainly in stage III and IV	Rare spikes
Childhood epilepsy with occipital paroxysms				
No effect	No effect	Fixation off sensitivity (increased spiking with eye closure, blocked with eye-opening)	Increased spiking	Inhibits spikes
Juvenile myoclonic epilepsy				
Some activation	Significant activation	Eye closure activates generalized SW and polyspike wave	Suppresses SW discharges	Less SW than in awake, but more than in NREM
West syndrome				
		64% hypsarrhythmia	99% hypsarrhythmia in stage II, III	Hypsarrhythmia disappears
Lennox-Gastaut syndrome				
Activates slow spike wave	No effect	Slow-spike wave 1.5-2.5 Hz	15-20 Hz frontal paroxysmal fast and increased slow spike wave	Reduced or absent slow spike wave
Landau-Kleffner syndrome				
		Focal epileptiform discharges	Activation with increased discharges	Like awake
Continuous spike and wave of slow wave sleep				
		3-5 Hz intermittent SW	>85% generalized SW	SW disappear <5%
Temporal lobe epilepsy				
		Lateralized temporal epileptiform activity	Bilateral independent temporal epileptiform activity	

OIRDA = occipital intermittent rhythmic delta activity; SW = spike wave

Figure 14

Example of rapid spikes in a 9-year-old patient with tonic seizures

The child has Lennox-Gastaut syndrome.

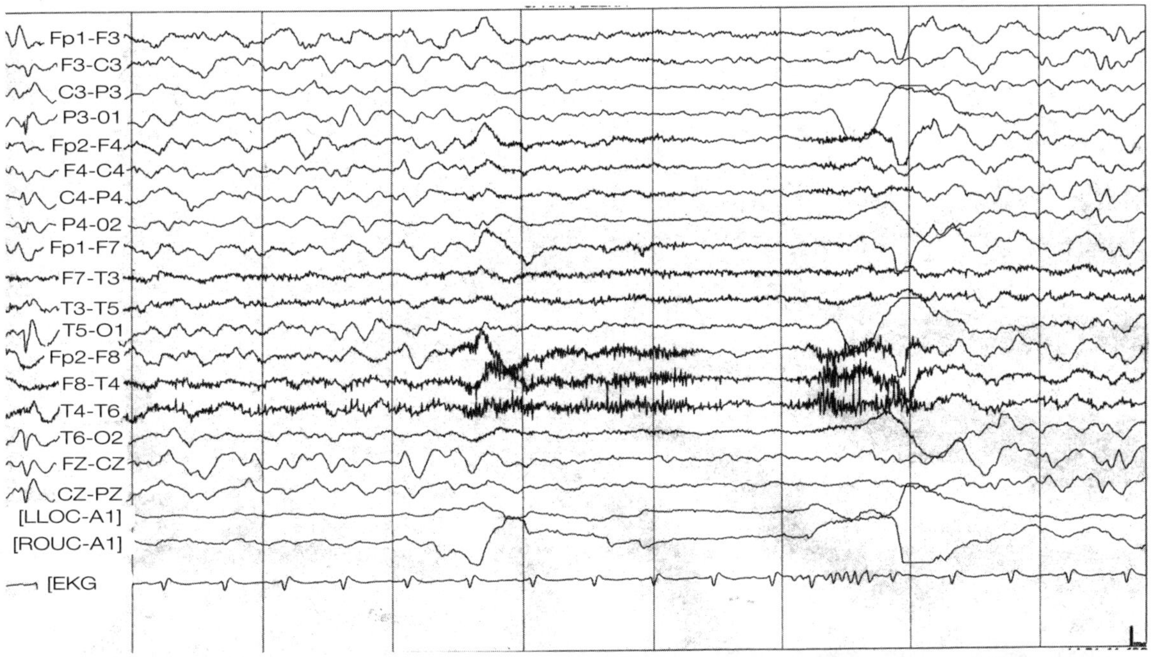

Paroxysmal fast activity is activated by sleep (Table 6). Focal and multifocal epileptiform discharges are seen in addition to slow spike-and-wave complexes and paroxysmal fast activity. Slowing of the background is the norm and usually correlates with cognitive impairment.

Tonic, atonic, atypical absence seizures, and myoclonic seizures are common, in addition to generalized tonic-clonic seizures and focal seizures. The ictal EEG, during tonic seizures, consists of paroxysmal fast activity (Figure 14) and the EEG of atypical absences consists of diffuse, bisynchronous, high amplitude 1-2.5 Hz spike-and-wave activity, which can be difficult to distinguish from interictal activity (Figure 15). Other ictal patterns like rhythmic theta activity or 7 Hz spike-and-wave are also possible.

Focal or Localization Related Epilepsies

Temporal lobe epilepsy can either originate in the mesial structures (hippocampus, amygdala and parahippocampal gyrus) or in the lateral temporal neocortex. Mesial temporal and lateral neocortical temporal lobe seizure can be difficult to distinguish based on clinical and EEG criteria. Anterior temporal sharp waves with intermittent temporal slowing are typical interictal findings (Figure 9). Temporal epileptiform activity can be bitemporal and occur synchronously or independently over both hemispheres (Table 6). The interictal neocortical temporal sharp waves typically have a broader field than mesial ones. Ictal EEG consists of lateralized temporal rhythmic theta build-up over the involved temporal lobe (Figure 16).

Ictal and interictal EEG in frontal, parietal and occipital lobe epilepsy can be quite variable. Interictal epileptiform activity in the form of spikes or sharp waves may localize to the epileptogenic region. Frontal lobe epilepsy is recognized as having minimal ictal and interictal EEG changes, especially if seizures originate on the medial surface of the brain, eg, the supplementary motor area seizures.

Figure 15

Slow spike-wave discharges in a child with Lennox-Gastaut syndrome

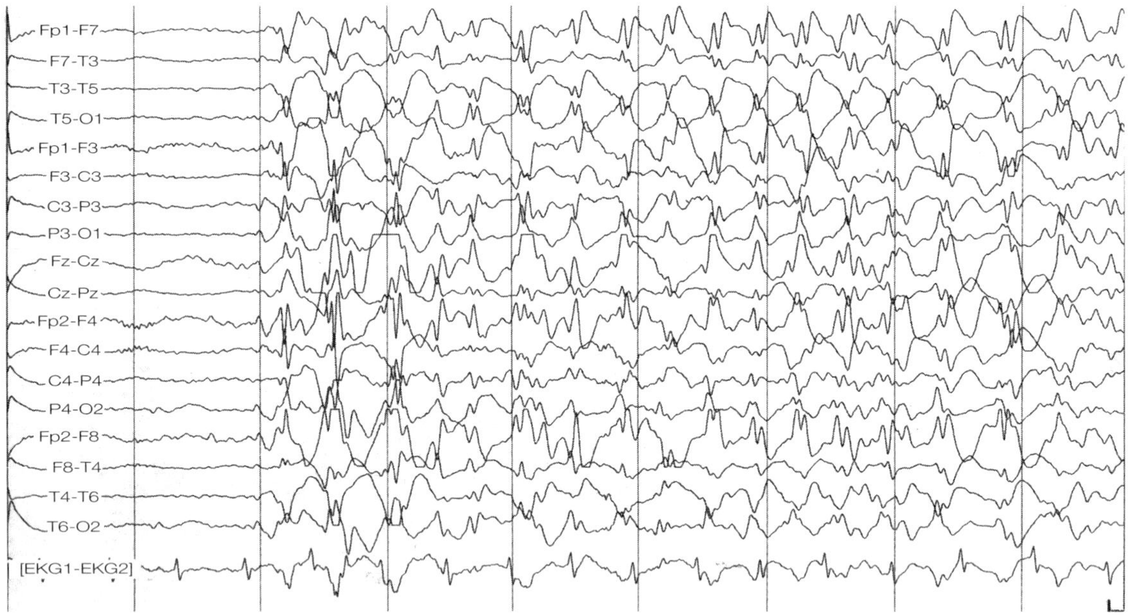

Figure 16

Temporal lobe focal seizure with rhythmic sharp theta build-up (arrow)

33-year-old patient with a history of a perinatal middle cerebral artery infarction and subsequent intractable localization related epilepsy.

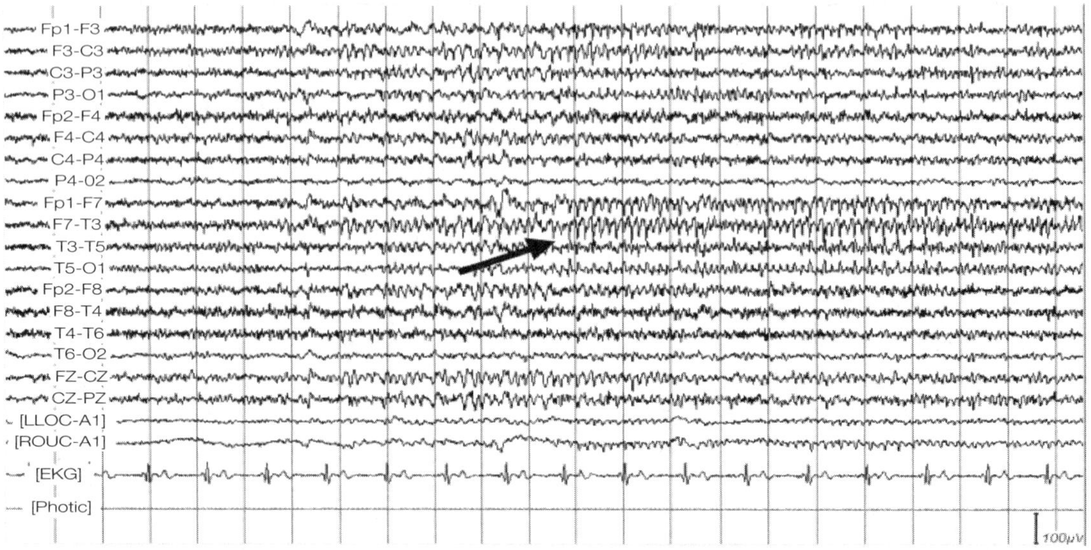

Figure 17A,B

Central-temporal spikes using bipolar montage in an 8-year-old boy with BECTS

A) Bipolar montage. Note the phase reversal across C3-P3 and T3-T5 (arrows). This demonstrates a maximum negative field in the central and mid-temporal region.

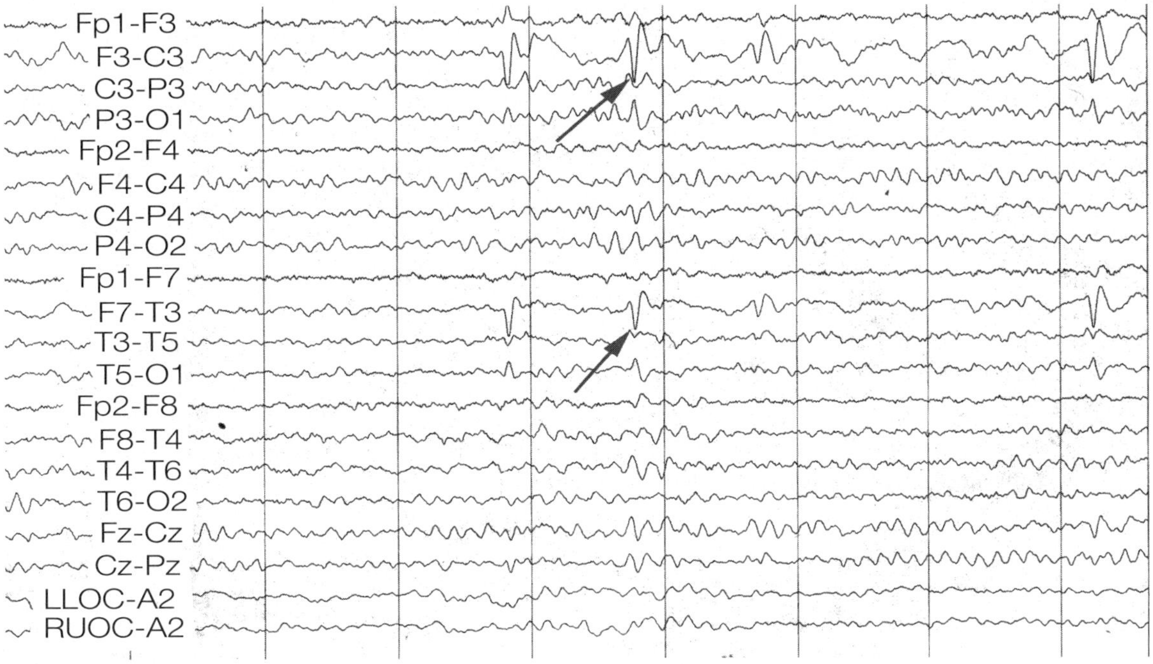

B) Referential montage. Note the phase reversal with the waveform in Fp2 and F4 going downward, indicating positivity (top arrow) with C4 going upward, indication positivity (lower arrow). This represents a horizontal dipole, common in BECTS.

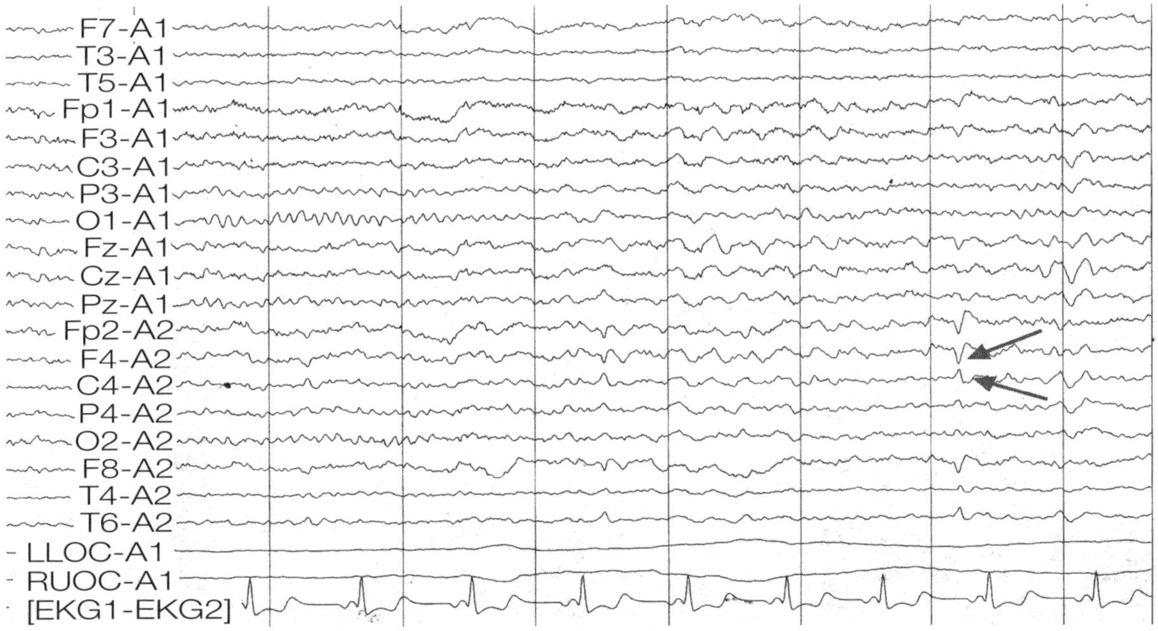

Benign epilepsy of childhood with centro-temporal spikes (BECTS), previously termed benign rolandic epilepsy, is characterized by interictal mid-temporal and central spikes and sharp waves. The maximal voltage of the epileptiform activity is in the C3-C4 or T3-T4 region (Figure 17 A and B). Rolandic spikes often are characterized by a horizontal dipole which can be readily seen when a referential montage is used. Sharp waves and spikes are dramatically increased during slow wave sleep (Table 6). Centro-temporal spikes are also seen in other neurological diseases like perinatal hypoxia, Rett syndrome, fragile X-syndrome, cortical dysplasias, tumor and agenesis of the corpus callosum.

Childhood epilepsy with occipital paroxysms is characterized by interictal diphasic sharp waves or spikes of high amplitude in the occipital region (Figure 18). Epileptiform activity disappears with eye opening and promptly returns after eye closure (Table 6).

Landau-Kleffner syndrome (LKS) and continuous spike-and-waves of slow sleep (CSWS) are related syndromes. The ictal aphasia in LKS is attributed to high-voltage multifocal spikes and spike-and-wave epileptiform activity in the language dominant temporal region. Epileptiform activity is activated by non-REM sleep and may become generalized similar to CSWS (Table 6). In CSWS, generalized spike-and-wave discharges are the predominant pattern throughout NREM sleep and occupy more than 85% of the NREM record (Figure 19). This EEG pattern is called electrical status epilepticus of sleep (ESES). During wakefulness, spike-and-wave discharges are present but markedly decreased as compared to the sleep record.

Status Epilepticus

Status epilepticus can be convulsive or nonconvulsive. In convulsive status epilepticus, seizures with associated EEG change, occur initially discretely followed by a period of continuous rhythmic discharges (Figure 20). This is followed by periods of attenuation and finally GPEDs (generalized periodic epileptiform discharges) are seen in a severely attenuated background.

Figure 18

Left occipital spikes (arrow) in a patient with childhood epilepsy with occipital paroxysms

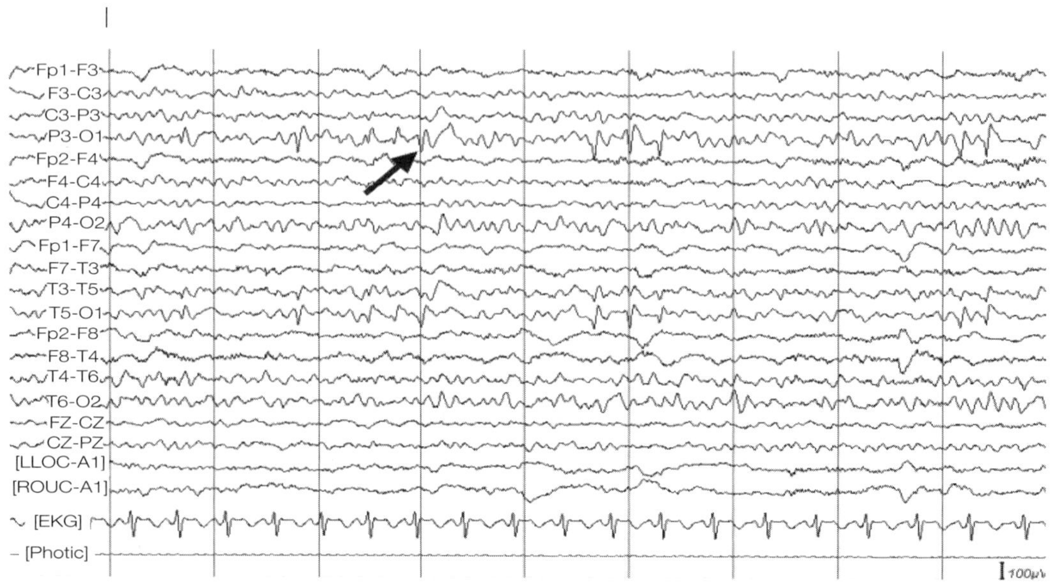

Figure 19

Electrical status epilepticus of sleep

EEG shows almost continuous spike-wave discharges which occupied over 85% of slow wave sleep.

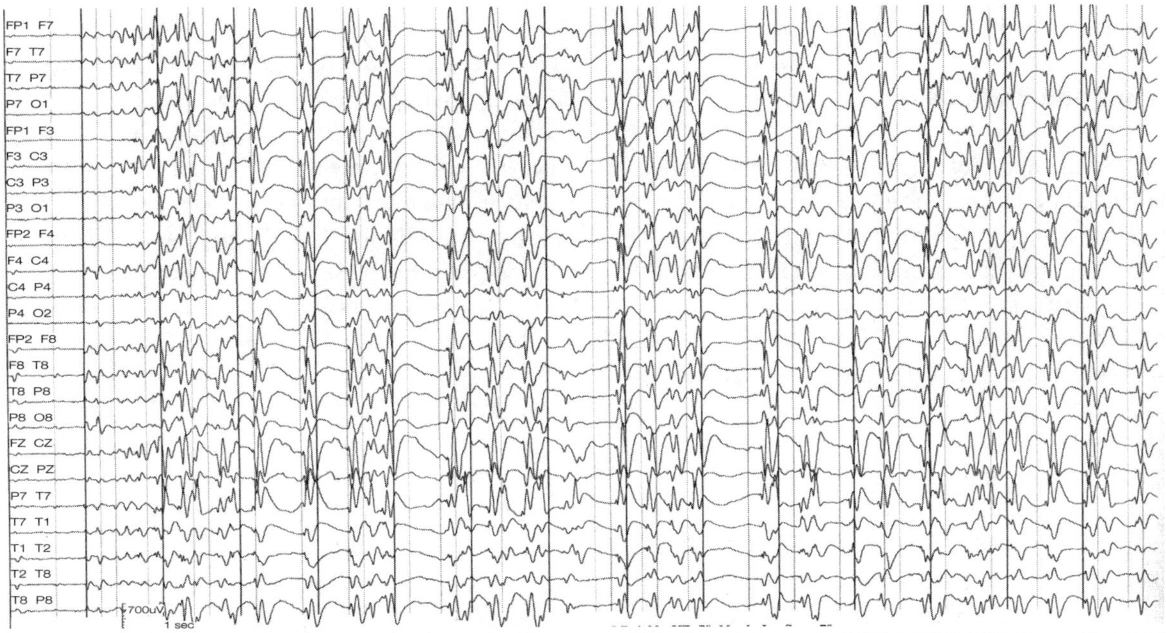

Figure 20

Rhythmic generalized epileptiform delta activity

70-year-old woman with status epilepticus in the setting of alcohol abuse and uremia.

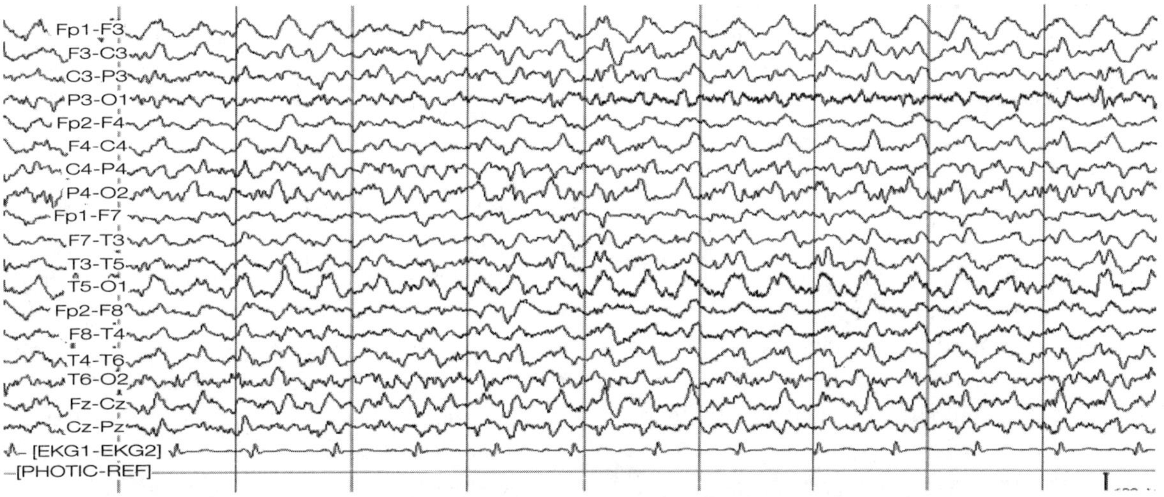

Absence status and complex partial status epilepticus are variations of nonconvulsive status epilepticus. During absence status, generalized spike-and-wave discharges at the frequency of the underlying epilepsy syndrome are present. Continuous bilateral sharp-slow activity is the hallmark of complex partial status epilepticus.

Coma and Brain Death

EEG is an important diagnostic tool for the evaluation of coma and can be helpful to determine the prognosis of a patient in coma. EEG is useful to determine the depth of coma. Stimulation with alerting or painful stimuli can contribute important information. A reactive EEG, one that changes with stimulation, carries a better prognosis than a nonreactive, monotonous recording.

Intermittent rhythmic delta activity or patterns of generalized high voltage delta activity alternating with lower voltage irregular potentials (alternating pattern) with preserved reactivity indicate less severe coma. High voltage nonreactive delta activity is associated with an unfavorable prognosis.

Burst suppression patterns and periodic patterns are associated with a poor prognosis. Bursts of irregular high amplitude theta and delta waves, with or without intermixed spikes or sharp waves, alternate with episodes of suppression in burst suppression patterns. Burst suppression can occur with severe anoxic encephalopathy or hypothermia. Acute drug intoxication as well as anesthetic agents are reversible causes of burst suppression patterns. In severe progressive anoxic injury, burst suppression precedes electrocerebral inactivity. Electrocerebral inactivity is defined as no electrical brain activity exceeding 2 μV, and if sustained it indicates brain death.

A slow, nonreactive, low voltage (<20 μV) EEG in coma indicates cortical damage. This has to be distinguished from normal low voltage variants in awake patients. Alpha coma refers to an EEG that indicates diffuse monorhythmic alpha activity in all leads. This is different from the awake state, in which there are faster mixed frequencies over the frontal regions. Alpha coma is seen in anoxic encephalopathy and pontomesencephalic lesions and is thought to be a poor prognostic sign. If in a comatose patient the EEG contains features that are usually seen in sleep stage II, it is termed spindle coma. Spindle coma is associated with high mesencephalic lesions and generally carries a better prognosis.

The EEG can be a confirmatory test to determine brain death, but the recording has to be modified as compared to routine EEG testing. At least 30 minutes of recording are required, montages should include double spacing of electrodes and sensitivity should be 2 μV/mm. Stimuli should be applied and the EEG recording used for brain death should occur at least 8 hours after the onset of the coma (Table 7).

Somatosensory evoked potentials (SSEPs) are another confirmatory test to diagnose brain death. Clear loss of cortical potentials confirms brain death, but recording of SSEPs in the intensive care unit can be challenging due to electrical noise contamination in the environment.

Special EEG Procedures

As longer recordings increase the yield of detecting epileptiform activity, 24-hour ambulatory EEG monitoring is frequently performed. This can be helpful, as ictal events are more likely to be captured. It is frequently utilized if absence epilepsy is suspected.

Video/EEG monitoring is utilized to determine seizure frequency and type and to distinguish between epileptic and non-epileptic seizures. It is also essential for the evaluation of epilepsy surgery candidates. The patient is admitted to a specialized inpatient EEG monitoring unit. Antiepileptic medications are often tapered and seizures are captured on video with simultaneous EEG monitoring. If epilepsy surgery is pursued, the procedure may be extended and intracranial subdural strip/grid electrodes or depth electrodes may be implanted to identify the region of seizure onset in intractable epilepsy. In a functional mapping procedure, those electrodes can be electrically stimulated. By functional mapping, information can be obtained whether eloquent cortex is covered by the stimulated electrodes (eg, the primary motor cortex or the

Table 7

Procedure to Determine Brain Death

Prerequisites to Determine Brain Death

A. Cause known and irreversible
B. No confounding medical condition
C. Normal metabolics: normal electrolytes, acid base status, endocrine function
D. No drugs or poison
E. Temperature >32° C

Exam

1. Coma
2. No motor response
3. Pupils nonreactive
4. Corneal reflexes absent
5. Caloric testing: no response 1 minute after irrigation, wait 5 minutes in between sides
6. Gag reflex absent
7. No response to suction
8. No sucking/rooting reflex
9. No respiratory drive as per apnea test

Confirmatory Tests

1. Angiography: no filling
2. EEG: 16 electrodes, Impedance <10 KΩ, 10 cm between electrodes, sensitivity: 2 μV/mm, 30 minute recording, 1-30 Hz filters, nonreactive rhythm
3. Transcranial doppler: lack of diastolic flow, reverberating flow and small systolic peaks
4. SPECT: 30 minutes, 60 minutes and 2 hours after injection: hollow skull
5. SSEP: absent responses

Procedure to Determine Brain Death

Age	*Time between exams*	*Number of confirmatory tests needed*
<2 mo	46 h	2
<1 year	24h	1
<18 years	12 h	Optional
Adult	Optional 6h	Optional

Apnea Test

Temp >36.5 BP >90 positive fluid balance or euvolemia necessary

1. Preoxygenate 100% O_2 for 10 min pO_2 >200
2. Start pulse ox / disconnect ventilator
3. 100% O_2 6 L/min per cannula
4. Observe respiratory movements
5. After 8 min get ABG and reconnect
6. If desaturation or hypotensive stop earlier and get ABG.

Positive if pCO_2 >60 mm Hg or 20 mm Hg above baseline

language areas) and whether resection of those brain regions is safe. Intracranial EEG is also used in the operating room to identify epileptogenic tissue (electrocorticography), but due to anesthesia effects, the use of electrocorticography is limited.

3. Evoked Potentials

Evoked potential use has declined with the advent of MRI scanning. However, there remains a role for evoked potentials in assessing neurological lesions and monitoring neurological function during surgery. The three types of evoked potentials that continue to be used are auditory, visual, and somatosensory. Each will be briefly reviewed.

Brainstem Auditory Evoked Potentials

The short latency brainstem auditory evoked potential (BAEP), also commonly known as the auditory brainstem response (ABR), or brainstem auditory evoked response (BAER), is the auditory system's electrical response to an acoustic stimulus. By definition, the short latency auditory evoked potential occurs within the first 10-15 msec following an acoustic stimulation. The response is generated by the auditory nerve, brainstem, and possibly subcortical structures, and can be obtained at almost any

Figure 21

Anatomy of the brainstem auditory evoked potentials

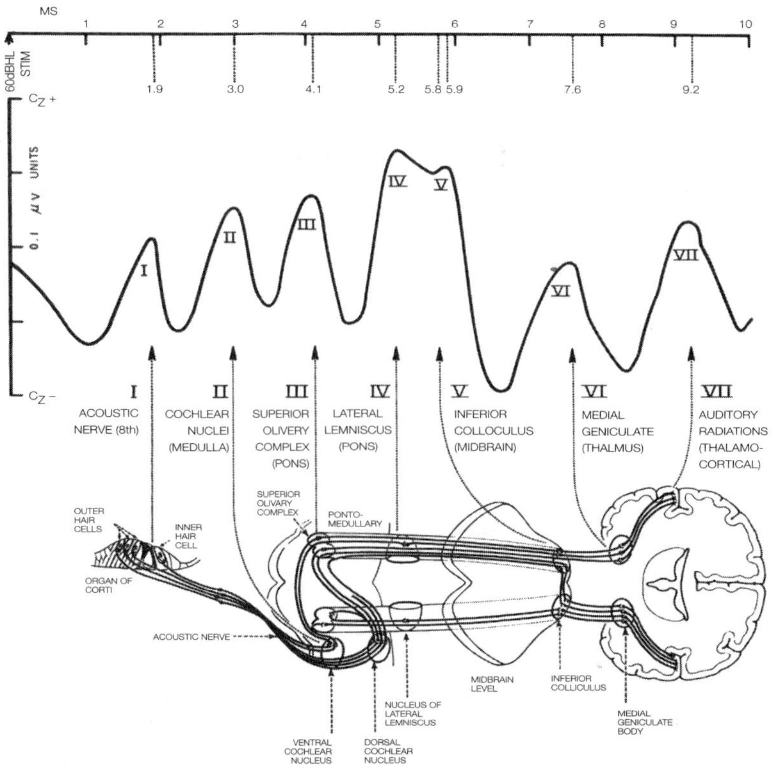

age. These features make the BAEP a very useful test in the evaluation of the peripheral and central brainstem auditory systems at any age. The technique is useful in the evaluation of the peripheral auditory system in patients with hearing and language disorders. BAEPs are also useful in the evaluation of patients with brainstem lesions such as tumors and neurodegenerative diseases. BAEP has also become useful in the operating room to monitor brainstem neurophysiologic function during neurosurgical procedures involving the posterior fossa.

Anatomical Localization of Waveforms

There are five waveforms of clinical interest, recorded most commonly from the scalp (Figure 21). Wave I is generated by the distal eighth nerve near the cochlea. Wave II is attributed to the extramedullary, intracranial eighth nerve or the cochlear nucleus in the lateral medulla. The superior olivary complex and nuclei of the trapezoid body in the lower pons are the generators for wave III. Waves VI and V are generated in the region of the lateral lemniscus and inferior colliculus, which are in the upper pons and lower midbrain. The last two waveforms, waves VI and VII, are more variable and less helpful clinically. It is suggested that their origins are from the medial geniculate body of the thalamus and the auditory radiations respectively.

Clinical Utility

The clinical utility of BAEPs is in both assessment of the peripheral hearing apparatus and the brainstem auditory system. In children, BAEPs are extremely useful and in some cases the only way to test hearing. Normal values are defined as the mean plus 2.5 or 3 standard deviations above the mean.

Abnormalities

In evaluating the BAEPs, the most important feature is the latencies of the various waveforms. Amplitudes of the waveforms are not a very reliable indicator of abnormality due to the large amount of variability. By using modern technology, it is relatively easy to measure the latencies. When evoked potentials were introduced it was recommended that each laboratory develop their own normative data; this is no longer necessary since this information is now available in numerous sources.

The primary generator of wave I is the distal eighth nerve near the cochlea. Therefore, wave I is affected by pathology of the peripheral auditory apparatus, at or distal to this part of the nerve. This includes not only the nerve but the spiral ganglion, middle ear, and external auditory canal. When all waveforms are clearly seen but there is a prolongation of waves I, III and V absolute latencies with normal interpeak latencies (IPLs), a peripheral hearing defect is present with normal central conduction from the peripheral eighth nerve to the midbrain. A shorter than normal I-V IPL with prolongation of all absolute latencies has also been described in high-frequency hearing loss. This is most likely because of a differential response of the cochlea (apical versus basal) due to the hearing loss, therefore changing the absolute latency of wave I to a greater extent. If wave I is absent with a normal III-V IPL, this is also

Figure 22

Normal BAEPs in 16-year-old girl with tinnitus

The first two channels are with left ear stimulation (ipsilateral and contralateral) and the second two traces are with right ear stimulation. The stimulation frequency was 11.1 Hz at 85 dB.

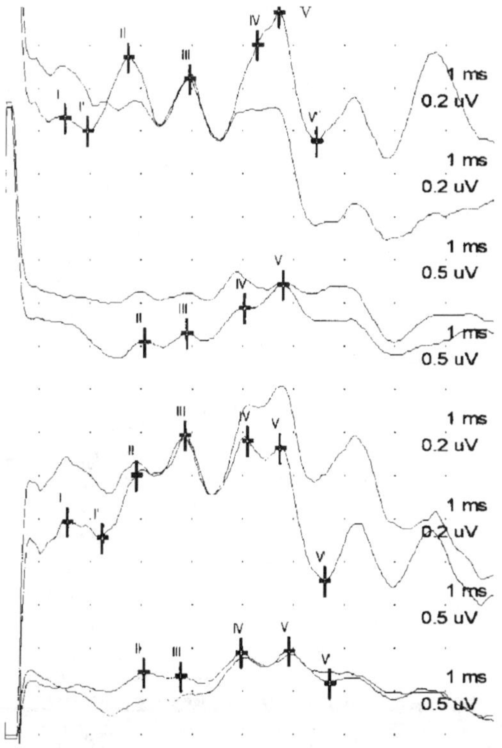

typically due to a peripheral deficit. The conduction of the click stimulus is normal from the lower pons to the midbrain, but the conduction from the peripheral eighth nerve to the lower pons cannot be determined. Complete absence of responses from one or both ears is rare. If this occurs and is not due to technical difficulties, it suggests a severe high frequency hearing loss most commonly, or desynchronization of the conducting pathways, which may take place in multiple sclerosis. In this situation the conduction of the click stimulus from the peripheral eighth nerve through the brainstem cannot be accurately measured. Figure 22 is an example of a normal BAEP.

Figure 23

BAEPs in a one-year-old child with cerebral dysgenesis and a small brainstem on MRI scan

The first two channels are with left ear stimulation (ipsilateral and contralateral) and the second two traces are with right ear stimulation. The stimulation frequency was 11.1 Hz at 85 dB. The absolute latencies of wave I = 2.48 msec. left, 2.54 msec. right; wave III = 4.69 msec. left, 4.58 msec. right; and wave V = 7.36 msec. left, 6.60 msec. right, were all above normal. The I-III interpeak latency was normal bilaterally but the II-V interpeak latency was prolonged.

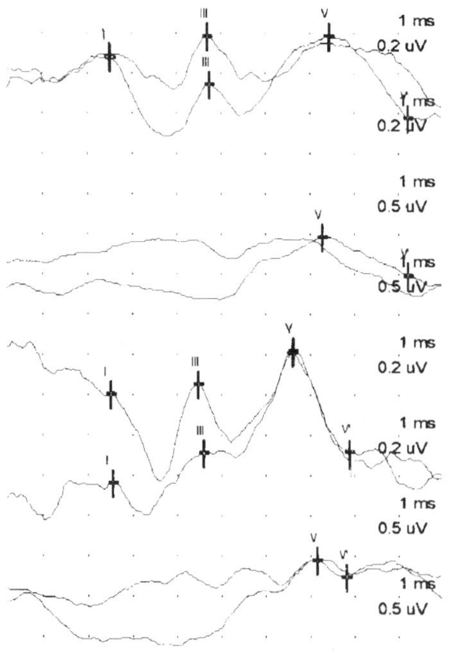

When the I-III IPL is abnormally prolonged, a conduction conduction defect in the brainstem auditory sysytem between the distal eighth nerve and the lower pons is suggested. When an abnormal increase in the III-V IPL occurs, a conduction defect in the brainstem auditory system between the lower pons and midbrain is likely. Figure 23 is an example of an abnormal BAEP.

With monaural stimulation, the responses from each ear should always be compared. If the latencies from both ears are normal, but there is an abnormal asymmetry between the sides, this also suggests a conduction defect from the ear with the relative prolongation.

Audiological Testing

The BAEP can be helpful in assessing the peripheral auditory system by determining hearing thresholds and the type of hearing defect. The latency-intensity study (LIS) or wave V recognition threshold is useful in conjunction with the BAEP, especially in children at risk for hearing impairment.

The latency-intensity study is performed monaurally by decreasing the click stimulus intensity and measuring wave V. The rate of stimulation can be increased to 40/sec or more to allow a quicker performance without significantly attenuating wave V. With decreasing intensities, the latencies of waves I, III, and V increase while the absolute amplitudes decrease, eventually disappearing. Wave I is usually the first waveform to disappear, followed by wave III. Wave V is the last wave to disappear and is therefore a good indicator of peripheral auditory activity. The intensity at which wave V disappears is the threshold of hearing. The use of a 30 dBnHL cutoff level in the screening of infants and young children seems to be a sensitive predictor of a child at high risk for hearing loss. Failure to obtain wave V with stimulation intensities above 30 dB suggests a hearing loss. The severity of the impairment can be determined by increasing the intensity of the click until a wave V is recognized.

Figure 24

Latency-intensity curve in a conductive hearing loss

The curve is shifted to the right as compared to a normal latency-intensity study.

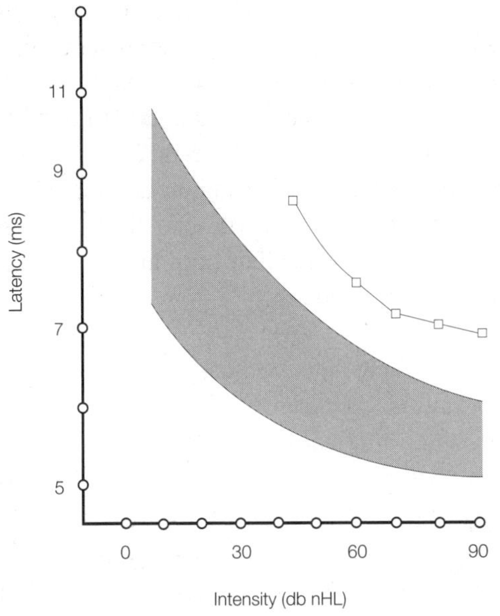

Figure 25

Latency-intensity curve in a cochlear or sensorineural hearing loss

At high intensities the curve is normal, but rapidly shifts to the right with a decrease in the stimulus intensity.

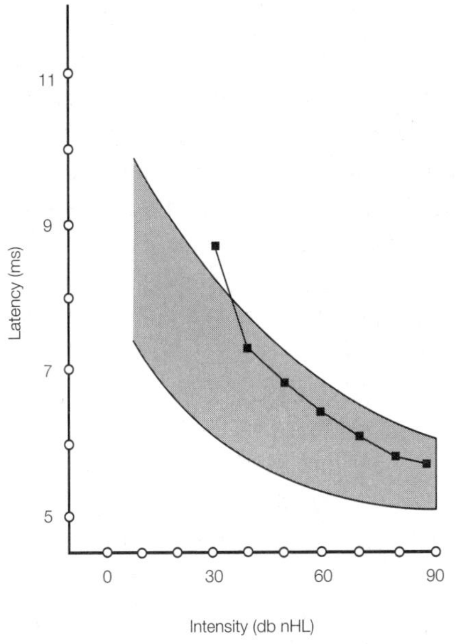

A normal LIS does not necessarily indicate normal hearing. Since the click is a mixed frequency stimulus, if there is at least some part of the frequency range intact, the LIS may be normal. In addition, if wave V is poorly formed in the routine BAEP, the LIS will be difficult, if not impossible to perform.

There are two types of abnormality seen on the latency intensity study. A conductive hearing loss interferes with the effectiveness of transmission of the stimulus to the cochlea. This can delay all waves and causes a shift of the latency intensity curve to the right (Figure 24), with the shift corresponding to the amount of hearing deficit. The second pattern is seen with a cochlear or sensorineural hearing loss. The latency of wave V is normal at high intensities and rapidly increases or disappears with a decrease in the stimulus intensity (Figure 25). Use of the latency intensity study and brainstem auditory evoked potentials can help the clinician determine where the hearing loss is, possible etiologies, and more appropriate treatments.

Neurological Testing

BAEPs are valuable not only in assessing hearing but as part of a neurological evaluation. BAEPs are particularly helpful when a degenerative or demyelinating disease is suspected. BAEPs can complement MRI in the diagnosis of brainstem or posterior fossa tumors. Evaluation and prognosis in encephalopathies and coma using BAEPs can also be useful. Brainstem responses can also be monitored intraoperatively during neurosurgical procedures.

In white matter diseases, the pathologic lesion is either due to demyelination or formation of abnormal myelin and BAEPs are often abnormal, with prolonged latencies of waveforms. As the disease progresses, there is a disappearance of waves II-V. For example, there are prolonged absolute and interpeak latencies in children with metachromatic leukodystrophy. Adrenoleukodystrophy frequently results in abnormal BAEPs. The degree of the BAEP abnormality appears to be related to the severity and stage of the condition. The test can be useful in individuals at risk, since asymptomatic patients may have abnormalities on testing.

The BAEPs are very helpful in the neurological workup in patients with multiple sclerosis. BAEPs can identify silent lesions in the brainstem, thus helping to solidify a diagnosis in equivocal cases. When used in conjunction with the clinical history and neurological examination, the BAEPs can strongly suggest multiple sclerosis. BAEPs can also be used to follow the progression of the disorder and response to therapy.

Visual Evoked Potentials

The visual evoked potential (VEP) is an objective physiological measurement of the electrical activation of the visual pathways of the brain, and has become a valuable tool in vision research and clinical medicine. The VEP is elicited by discreet visual stimulation of the eye, with subsequent recording of the electrical potentials from the scalp produced by the passage of neural impulses from the eye to the occipital lobe. Lesions anywhere along this pathway may interfere with the VEP.

Anatomy of Visual Pathways

Receptor cells of the retina are arranged in a single layer of cells which are shaped like rods and cones. Cones respond to bright light and are responsible for color and form vision, while the rods respond mainly to low-level light and movement. Rods and cones contain disk-like layers of receptor pigment protein which absorb photon energy from the incident light relative to the color sensitivity of the specific protein. This energy absorption causes a summation potential to be generated, which accumulates at the cell body. This summated potential propagates along a neural network consisting of a hierarchy of connections to the ganglion cells. Bipolar cells modulate and process the input from receptor cells on their way to the ganglion cell. These impulses are modulated in turn by intermediate horizontal and amacrine cells. A nerve action potential is generated at the ganglion cell. The ganglion cells have a one-to-one relationship to the nerve fibers in the optic nerve. Axons travel across the retina to the optic nerve and continue on to the next synapse at the lateral geniculate.

The axons of the ganglion cells travel back toward the brain in a manner which is topographic with the retina. As the axons approach the optic chiasm, the medial fibers cross to the contralateral hemisphere while the more lateral remain ipsilateral. Some fibers cross early while others actually initially follow the tract, reverse direction, and cross to the contralateral side. As the axonal fibers assemble into the optic tracts, some fibers descend into the brainstem. Some of these mediate pupillary constriction to light and eye blinking.

The lateral geniculate is organized topographically, and organizes input from each eye separately into layers which alternate in a predictable manner. The first two layers consist of large cells (magnocellular) which respond to low contrast, while the other four layers consist of smaller cells (parvocellular) which respond to high contrast. The lateral geniculate is the first synapse for axons which are coming from the geniculate cells of the retina. The lateral geniculate receives feedback fibers from the occipital lobe and brainstem structures and has cells which respond differently to monocular or binocular stimulation.

Myelinated axons extend from the cell bodies of the lateral geniculate and cross through the posterior aspects of the corona radiata as they travel to the visual cortex. The occipital cortex consists of six well-defined cortical layers. The occipital cortex is separated into columns. The columns are structured to represent line orientation; the stripes represent binocular integration, and the entire array is oriented in a topographic distribution relative to the retina. The fibers of the optic radiations arrive consistently at layer four. It is this layer which has the myelinated fibers of the radiations, and appears as the Line of Genari.

Recording Techniques

VEPs can be evaluated using several techniques depending on the clinical situation:

Strobe flash technique. The most commonly used method for the acquisition of visual evoked potentials in infants and young children is the strobe flash. This technique involves the use of a tungsten filament or xenon gas strobe flash, the same type typically used for EEG photic stimulation studies. The light source is placed in front of the infant's head and is flashed sequentially with the computer sweep. In most settings the infant is placed on its back and is studied during natural or sedated sleep. The strobe is placed one meter away from the bridge of the infant's nose. The rate of stimulation is usually about two per second although some authors recommend a rate of 1 to 1.5 per second. The technique is well established and is available in nearly every neurophysiology laboratory. There are a number of sources of normative data.

Light emitting diode (LED) goggle technique. Another technique for visual stimulation involves the use of light emitting diodes (LEDs). These LED elements can be placed in goggles and arrayed in a pattern on a grid. The goggles are placed over the child's eyes and are taped gently in place for the duration of the examination. The stimulus parameters can be precisely defined as a square wave onset offset curve which provides an effective nervous system stimulus. The intensity and pattern of the LED array can be standardized easily and the red color obviates the variability produced by the red filter effect of the eyelid. The use of the goggles allows for stimulation of each eye separately. An alternating grid pattern of LEDs can provide a pattern-shift method of stimulation, rather than an onset-offset method, so that luminance can remain the same. The LED array can be linked to a computer so that various parameters can be changed systematically throughout a recording sequence.

Pattern reversal technique. The pattern reversal method for VEP stimulation is the most common used in adults. The pattern is produced on a computer monitor screen and most commonly uses a checkerboard pattern reversal. The most effective method for studying central vision is to keep luminance constant, and to stimulate only those aspects of the retina which respond to edge detection and orientation of receptor fields. This can be accomplished by the pattern reversal technique. In the most popular method, a checkerboard pattern is presented to the central vision with an equal number of dark and light squares. With reversal, the black squares turn white, and the white turn black. There is no resultant luminance change, but the retinal receptor units experience linear orientation effects as well as edge detection. This produces specific ganglion cell stimulation in an efficient manner. Experience has shown that this method produces the most consistent, reproducible, and clinically useful VEP waveforms.

Neurological Conditions

There are a host of conditions where VEPs can be useful since they provide information about neural structures from the eye to occipital cortex. The test is useful in evaluating patients with structural, degenerative, and metabolic disorders. VEPs have probably been most widely used in demyelinating and dysmyelinating diseases. Conduction along the white matter tracts of the brain is by saltatory conduction. This provides a highly efficient means of signal transmission which depends on the thick lipid coating of myelin and the intermediate nodes. A variety of disorders may occur which disrupts this signal transmission. The thick lipid coating of myelin may be stripped away. This occurs in multiple sclerosis as well as other disorders such as post-viral processes or in autoimmune hypersensitivity reactions to vaccines. The demyelination in these processes produces delays in the VEP latencies and may also result in a dispersion pattern. This is caused by a mixture of signals being transmitted by demyelinated axons in different stages of disruption including a few remaining normal axons. The signal traveling such a pathway will arrive at different times and may result in a very broad waveform or in a waveform with two or more peaks. The VEP amplitudes usually are normal or near normal, but the waveform components are markedly delayed in latency. Figure 26 demonstrates the VEP from a patient with a normal right eye (A) and a left eye with optic neuritis (B).

Dysmyelination can occur due to defects in the formation of the myelin structure during development, or due to a defective repair process caused by a deficiency in key structural components. Adrenoleukodystrophy and metachromatic leukodystrophy are good examples of this type of disorder. Krabbe disease and hyperglycinemia can

Figures 26A and B

Eighteen-year-old child with left optic neuritis

A. Normal right eye stimulation. P100 = 103 msec. B. Abnormal optic nerve on left. P100 = 114 msec. Filter setting 1.0 Hz LF, 100 Hz HF, rate 1.9 stimuli per second, summed 150 sweeps

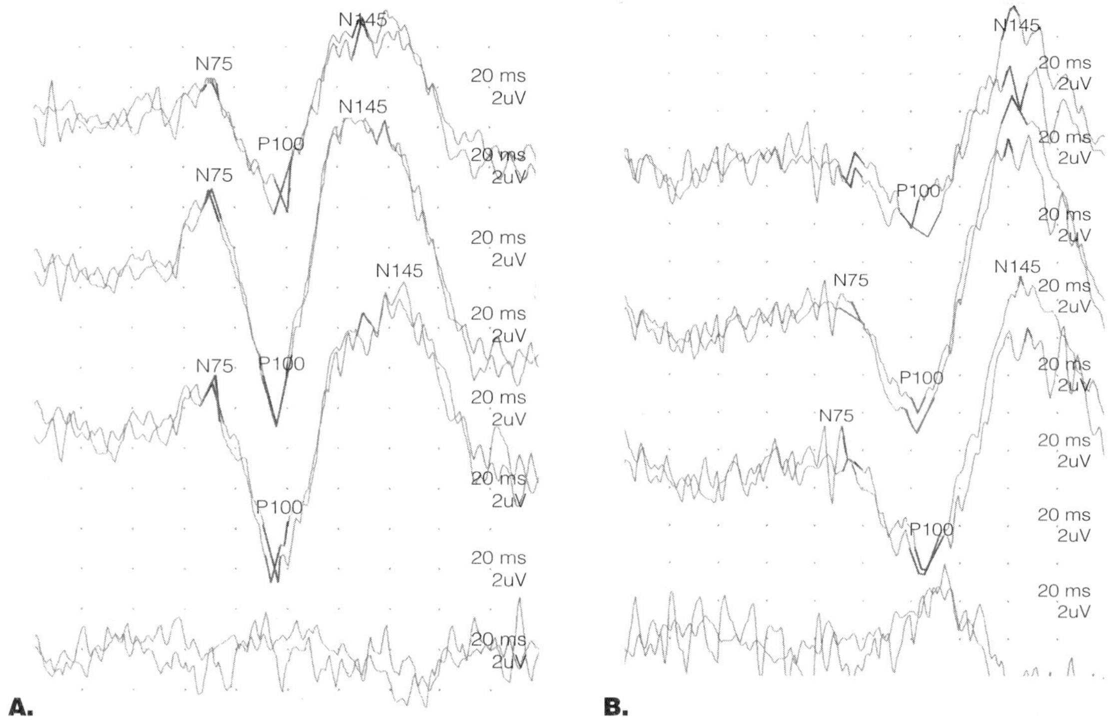

also result in profound dysmyelination and the VEPs in these disorders are usually severely disrupted. It is not clear to what extent the VEP can monitor the progression of these disorders, but it does offer an objective tool for measuring the effects of myelin deterioration. VEPs and other evoked potentials have been used to monitor clinical improvement in recent cases of leukodystrophies which have been treated with bone marrow transplantation.

The speed and efficiency of conduction of an electrical signal depends on the quality of the myelin sheath, the resting membrane potential, and intrinsic properties of the intermediate nodes. Each of these components is critical to the conduction of a VEP signal. A defect of any one or combination of these components will disrupt or delay the VEP signal.

A delayed or disrupted VEP waveform in a patient with an unusual degenerative process should suggest a defect in myelination.

A delayed or disrupted VEP waveform in a patient with an unusual degenerative process should suggest a defect in myelination.

Somatosensory Evoked Potentials

Somatosensory evoked potentials (SSEPs) provide the means to monitor portions of the peripheral and central nervous system. Both median nerve (MN-SSEP) and posterior tibial nerve (PTN-SSEP) are routinely used.

Anatomical Localization of Waveforms

Evoked potentials recorded from the body's surface are either near field or far field in nature. That is, the generator source is close or distant to the site of recording. The generators may be in grey matter or white matter. White matter generates compound action potentials which are propagated through fiber tracts. The latencies of the propagated action potentials increase as a function of the distance from the point of stimulation, and hence, are dependent on recording electrode position. These are recorded only in relative close proximity to the fiber tract itself, and thus are termed near field potentials. Near field potentials have a specific distribution (topographic specificity), latencies which vary according to recording electrode placement, amplitudes >1V, and generally negative polarity. Far field EPs may be recorded at long distances from the point of propagation and are generated when a traveling impulse (signal) passes through a certain anatomical site or fixed point along the nerve. Far field potentials have a diffuse distribution, fixed latencies, amplitudes <1 V, and polarity that reflects volume-conducted positivity.

Table 8

Presumed Generators of MN-SSEP

(Notations in parenthesis are designations for children [1-8 years]).

Component	Origin
P9 (P7)	FFP of brachial plexus
N9	Brachial plexus
P11 (P8)	FFP of dorsal root entry zone
P13-P14 (P9)	Brainstem lemniscal pathways composite of cervical dorsal horn synaptic activity and brainstem lemniscal pathways
N20 (N16)	Subcortical region and sensory cortex
P23 (P20)	Sensory cortex

Potentials are labeled according to the polarity and mean latency of a component derived from a sample of the normal population. As expected, latencies change with body growth and nervous system maturation.

Table 9

Presumed Generators of PTN-SSEPs

(Notations in parenthesis are designations for children [1-8 years]).

Component	Origin
N8 (N5)	Tibial nerve action potential
N19 (N11)	Cauda equine
N22 (N14)	Lumbar cord grey matter
N29 (N20)	Gracile nucleus
P37 (P28)	Mesial sensory cortex
N45 (N41)	Cortex (association?)

Figure 27

Normal median nerve SSEP in a 2-year-old boy

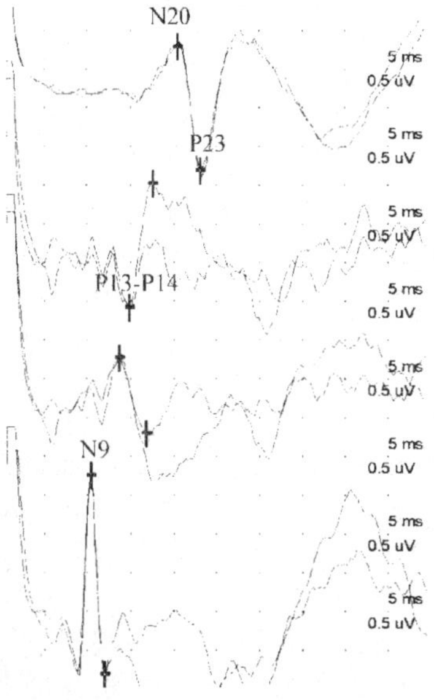

The presumed generators of MN-SSEPs and PTN SSEPs are summarized in Tables 8 and 9.

Median Nerve SSEPs

When SSEPs are recorded from the scalp with a non-cephalic reference (shoulder), three (and sometimes four) positive potentials are obtained: P9, P11, and P13, regardless of recording site. Since they have fixed latencies, these are far field potentials. Two later components are also recorded, the N20 (also called N19) and P23. The P9 is the far field potential of the N9 which arises from the distal portion of the brachial plexus. Because the N11 has a shorter refractory period than the subsequent N13, it is believed to be generated presynaptically from the dorsal root entry zone. The P13 component arises in structures caudal to the thalamus, probably in the brainstem lemniscal pathways. The N20 generator source is not precisely understood. Some have suggested that it is thalamic in origin, while others have supported a thalamocortical or cortical source. Figure 27 is an example of a normal median nerve SSEP.

Posterior Tibial Nerve SSEPs

Designations for EP component of PTN-SSEPs are less consistent than for MN-SSEPs. Following posterior tibial nerve stimulation, electrodes over the popliteal fossa record the electronegative peripheral nerve action potential N8. Electrodes over the lower spine record two electronegative potentials, the N19 and N22. The N19 represents the afferent volley in the cauda equina. The N22 is a stationary potential and probably reflects post-synaptic activity of internuncial neurons in the grey matter of the spinal cord. Electrodes over the cervical spine record another later stationary potential, N27. This component may reflect post-synaptic activity in the gracile nucleus. The P37 is the first major localized scalp recorded component. The P37 waveforms reflect the ipsilaterally oriented cortical surface electropositivity. The electronegative end of the dipole may be recorded contralaterally. There is a great deal of inter-subject variability in the topography of the P37 in adults, and especially, children. This is probably related to known anatomic differences in the location of primary sensory area for the leg. When the leg area is located at the superior edge of the interhemispheric fissure, the cortical generator for P37 is vertically oriented and its amplitude is maximal close to the vertex. When the leg area is located more deeply in the fissure, the cortical generator is more horizontally turned and the P37 projects ipsilaterally. Figure 28 is an example of a normal tibial nerve SSEP.

Figure 28

Normal tibial nerve SSEP in a 34-year-old woman

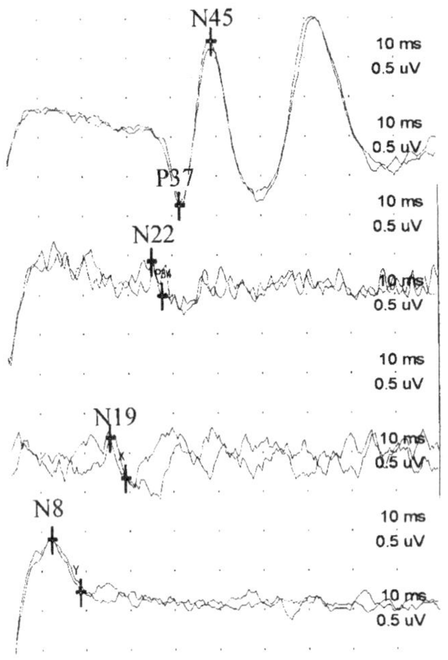

Neurological Disorders

Clinical occasions when somatosensory evoked potentials (SSEPs) are useful occur frequently. It is not necessary to have sensory loss in order to have abnormal SSEPs. There is, however, a good correlation between spinal cord/brainstem lesions involving dorsal column/lemniscal structures and proprioception abnormalities in the adult: If position sense is impaired more than modestly, then the SSEP is likely to be abnormal. Additionally, there may be abnormalities of the SSEP even in the face of a normal sensory exam. This, of course, is what leads to its utility in conditions such as multiple sclerosis.

Abnormalities may consist of prolonged latencies (compared to normal control data), absence of obligatory potentials, or prolongation of interpeak intervals or central conduction times or slowing of "conduction velocities." Decreased amplitude by itself is not a criterion for abnormality.

4. Intraoperative Monitoring

Several electrophysiologic procedures are utilized in the operating room to prevent neurologic disability due to surgery. The most frequently employed methods are EEG/SSEP monitoring during carotid endarterectomies and motor and sensory evoked potentials during spinal procedures.

During carotid endarterectomies, EEG monitoring is performed to screen for cerebral ischemia. If there is unilateral loss of beta frequencies and unilateral increase in delta or theta slowing, ischemia is suspected and shunting during the procedure should be considered. Median or ulnar SSEPs are additionally utilized to monitor for ischemia. Ischemia should be suspected if there is unilateral loss of amplitude or increased latency of cortical components.

During spinal procedures, SSEPs monitoring mainly of the lower extremities has traditionally been used to monitor spinal cord function. Motor evoked potentials specifically monitor loss of motor

Figure 29

Motor and somatosensory evoked potentials during spinal surgery

Motor evoked potentials require only one stimulus. Somatosensory evoked potentials require averaging.

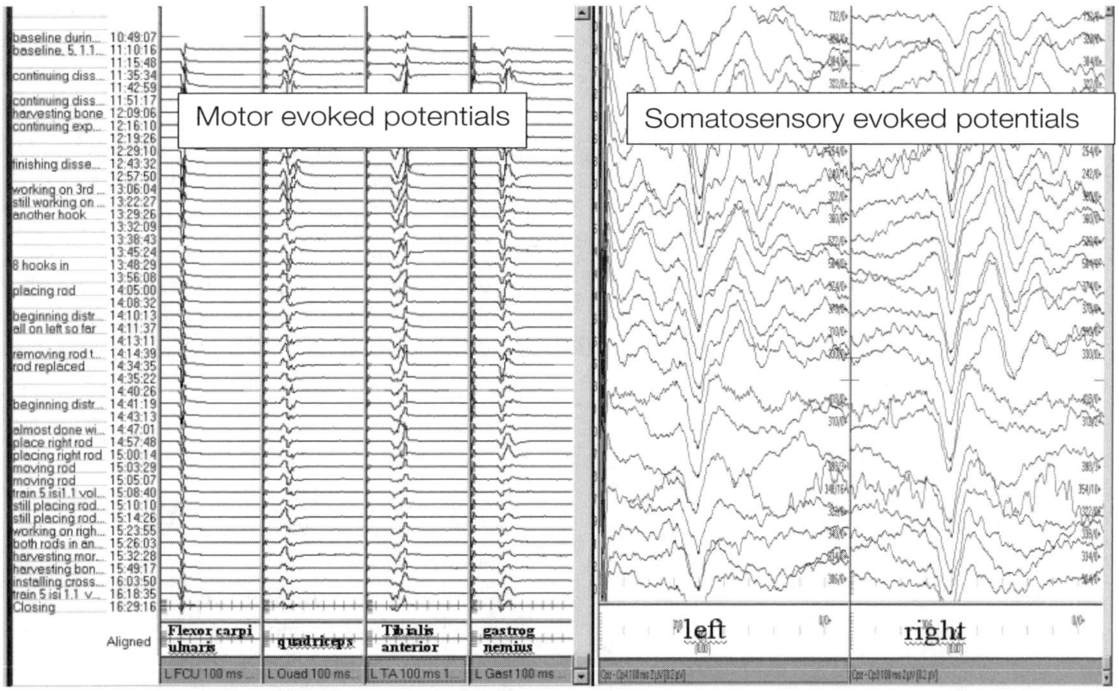

function (Figure 29). Motor evoked potentials in the operating room are elicited by transcranial electrical stimulation of the motor cortex with high currents and recording from upper or lower extremity muscles. To perform motor evoked potentials, anesthesia has to be modified to total intravenous anesthesia to preserve cortical excitability. If there is complete loss of motor evoked potentials during a procedure, this predicts subsequent motor paralysis. In the case of loss of motor evoked potentials, instrumentation that leads to spinal cord compromise can be removed during the surgical procedure and permanent damage can be prevented. SSEPs mainly monitor posterior column function. If there is an amplitude decrease of more than 50% or a latency increase of more than 10% of the cortical potentials, neurological compromise is suspected.

In posterior fossa and brainstem procedures, brainstem monitoring can be performed intraoperatively. Brainstem auditory evoked potentials monitor brainstem and cranial nerve VIII function. EMG monitoring of muscles supplied by cranial nerves can detect injury to other cranial nerves. Monitoring of CN VII during surgery for acoustic schwannomas has decreased morbidity. All other cranial nerves can be monitored in a similar fashion.

5. Magnetoencephalography

Magnetoencephalography (MEG) entails the extracranial detection of brain magnetic fields by use of biomagnetometry. Electric currents which produce the voltages on the scalp that serve as the basis for EEG also produce magnetic fields. MEG records the magnetic flux associated with electrical currents in activated sets of neurons. MEG allows analysis of brain activity in real time, but unlike evoked (electrical) potentials the sources of this activity can be accurately estimated, as they are not distorted by differences in conductivity between the brain, skull and scalp. Deduction of the sources from the measured magnetic field distribution is simple, and both spatial and temporal aspects of the activity can be determined with remarkable accuracy (0.1 to 1 cm and 1 msec respectively). Several algorithms for source modeling of the MEG data have been proposed.

The biomagnetic fields detected by MEG are quite small compared to the earth's magnetic field; at times the neuronal noise may be as much as 10,000 times the neuronal magnetic field being monitored. Detection of the small magnetic field requires both a magnetically shielded room and the use of instrumentation involving superconducting technology.

Repetitive application of a given stimulus results in repeated evocation of the same electrical currents and magnetic fields. MEG consists of: 1.) recording magnetic flux on the head surface associated with electrical currents in activated neuronal aggregates, 2.) estimating the location of neuronal aggregates, referred to as activity sources or event-related fields, and 3.) projecting the event-related fields onto an MRI of the brain to identify and envision the activated brain regions. In most laboratories, recordings are made with multichannel neuromagnetometers consisting of over 100 magnetometers arranged to cover the entire head.

MEG can be performed after somatosensory, auditory or visual stimuli and the corresponding evoked potential is detected and mapped onto a MRI, allowing noninvasive determination of eloquent primary sensory cortices. With recurring presentations of stimuli, these signals can be recorded as event-related fields (ERF) on the head surface. Event related fields, similar to evoked potentials, are waveforms that represent temporal variations in brain activity time-locked to the presentation of stimuli. Some of the waveforms are noted to occur consistently across different experimental conditions, and are known as components. There are two basic components: 1.) early, extending up to 150-200 ms following stimulus onset; and 2.) late, lasting several hundred milliseconds after stimulus onset. Activation of the primary sensory cortex results in early components of the ERF waveforms. Late components have been shown to reflect activation of the association cortex. It is by estimation of the regions that contribute to systematic variations in late portions of the ERF waveform that delineation of the outline of the brain circuits responsible for cognitive and linguistic function can be accomplished. ERFs can be reliably elicited by experimentally controlled events, such as the presentation of auditory, visual, or tactile stimuli, as well as during engagement in cognitive tasks.

MEG is used for: 1.) localization of the epileptic zone in lesional and nonlesional epilepsy surgery patients; 2.) functional mapping of eloquent cortex and demonstrating the relationship of these areas to the brain lesion or epileptogenic area; and 3.) assessment of normal and abnormal language development and the impact of treatment strategies.

6. References

1. Anonymous. Guidelines for writing EEG reports. *Journal of Clinical Neurophysiology.* 1994;11(1):37-39.

   (Lists guidelines for writing a report.)

2. Anonymous. Minimum technical standards for EEG recording in suspected cerebral death. *Journal of Clinical Neurophysiology.* 1994;11(1):10-13.

   (Lists guidelines for the technical standard of recordings for brain death, which are different for standard EEG recordings.)

3. Anonymous. A proposal for standard montages to be used in clinical EEG. *Journal of Clinical Neurophysiology.* 1994;11(1):30-36.

   (Overview of minimal necessary montages in EEG recording.)

4. Clancy RR, Berquist AGC, et al. Neonatal electroencephalography. In: Ebersole JS, Pedley TA, eds. *Current Practice of Electroencephalography.* Philadelphia, Pa: Lippincott, Williams and Wilkins; 2003:160-234.

   (Excellent brief overview of neonatal EEG.)

5. Dalby MA. Epilepsy and 3 per second spike and wave rhythms: A clinical, electroencephalographic and prognostic analysis of 346 patients. *Acta Neurol Scand.* 1969;Suppl 40:3.

   (Early study about the implications and prognosis of 3/sec spike wave discharges.)

6. Hughes J. *EEG in Clinical Practice.* Newton, Mass: Butterworth-Heinemann; 1994.

   (Brief, easy to understand book about the essentials of EEG recordings.)

7. Jayakar P, Chiappa KH. Clinical correlations of photoparoxysmal responses. *Electroencephalogr Clin Neurophysiol.* 1990;75(3):251-4.

(Study that examines the significance of the photoparoxysmal response and the time relation to the stimulus.)

8. King MA, Newton MR, et al. Epileptology of the first-seizure presentation: a clinical, electroencephalographic, and magnetic resonance imaging study of 300 consecutive patients. *Lancet*. 1998; 352(9133):1007-11.

(Study that examines the possibility of epilepsy after a first seizure.)

9. Pedley TA, Mendiratta A, et al. Seizures and epilepsy. In: Ebersol JS, Pedley TA, eds. *Current Practice of Clinical Encephalography.* Philadelphia, Pa: Lippincott, Williams and Wilkins; 2003:506-587.

(Excellent overview about the EEG features of epilepsy.)

10. Treiman DM, Walton NY, et al. A progressive sequence of electroencephalographic changes during generalized convulsive status epilepticus. *Epilepsy Res*. 1990;5(1):49-60.

(Describes the evolution of EEG patterns in status epilepticus.)

11. Westmoreland BF. Epileptiform electroen cephalographic patterns. *Mayo Clin Proc*. 1996;71(5):501-11.

(Describes normal variants that appear epileptiform.)

7. Questions

1. To use EEG as a confirmatory test for brain death:

A. The test should be 30 min long

B. It should be recorded with a higher sensitivity as usual (2 μV/mm)

C. Only electrocerebral inactivity confirms brain death

D. Larger spaced distances between electrodes should be recorded

E. All of the above

An EEG as a confirmatory test for brain death requires a minimum recording for 30 min at a higher sensitivity. Electrodes should be spaced further apart to possibly record smaller potentials as larger distances between electrodes will capture smaller electrical potentials. 16 channels should be recorded and impendances should measure less than 10 kOhms. Use of sedative drugs, hypothermia below 32 degrees Celsius, endocrine and metabolic abnormalities as well as hypotension needs to be excluded before a patient can be assessed for brain death. Only complete electrocerebral inactivity confirms brain death.

2. In a normal EEG of a 3-year-old child:

A. Hypnagogic hypersynchrony may occur

B. There is continuous delta slowing

C. No sleep spindles or vertex waves should be present

D. There is epileptiform activity

E. Photic stimulation results in increased slowing

At three years old, the background rhythm should be in the fast theta (7 Hz) or slow alpha range (8 Hz-10 Hz). Delta slowing would definitely be abnormal in an awake child, but is seen during normal slow wave sleep. Sleep spindles are normal sleep patterns in sleep stage II. Sleep spindles occur at the age of 1-2 months and are initially asymmetric. Vertex waves occur at the age of 4-6 months. Hypnagogic hypersynchrony is a normal pattern of drowsiness in children between 3 month to 13 years and consists of monomorphic high amplitude theta waves most prominent over the vertex.

3. Hyperventilation:

A. Causes hypercapnia

B. Often activates generalized spike wave discharges in absence epilepsy

C. Should not be performed in patients with severe cardiovascular disease

D. B. and C.

E. A., B. and C.

Hyperventilation causes hypocapnia which is responsible for background slowing on EEG. In absence epilepsy hyperventilation often activated the EEG and typical 3 Hz spike-and-wave discharges are noted. Hyperventilation can also be utilized as a clinical test in the office. It is easy to perform and often results in a clinical absence (cessation of breathing, blank llod on face, non-responsive to verbal commands) in a child with typical absence epilepsy. In patients with severe cardiovascular disease, hyperventilation should be used with caution due to cardiovascular risk.

4. Alpha coma:

A. Is associated with a good prognosis

B. Is associated with anoxic brain injury

C. Shows frontal beta activity on most recordings

D. Is considered a reactive pattern

E. Is the same as spindle coma

Alpha coma is characterized by uniform alpha activity over all head regions. In a normal awake EEG alpha activity is only observed over the posterior head regions and beta activity is noted over the frontal head regions. Alpha coma is often associated with anoxic brain injury and has a poor prognosis. The pattern is non-reactive to any type of stimulus. Spindle coma is characterized by typical features of stage II sleep with prominent spindle like activity in a comatose patient and carries a better prognosis than alpha coma.

5. A 15-year-old boy with mental retardation and tonic, atonic and atypical absence seizures has most likely:

A. Generalized slow spike wave complexes on EEG

B. Paroxysmal fast activity on EEG

C. Landau-Kleffner syndrome

D. A. and B.

E. A., B. and C.

Multiple seizure types and mental retardation are typical for Lennox-Gastaut syndrome. The typical EEG pattern consists of generalized slow spike-and-wave complexes at 1.5-2.5 Hz. Paroxysmal fast activity during sleep is the second defining EEG pattern for Lennox-Gastaut syndrome. Landau-

Kleffner syndrome is an epileptic aphasia, which renders children unable to speak due to continuous seizure activity over the temporal language areas and is characterized by temporo-parietal spikes.

6. A 26-year-old man has his first witnessed generalized tonic clonic convulsion. No metabolic or infectious causes could explain the seizure. EEG and MRI are normal.

A. It is unlikely that he has epilepsy as EEG and MRI are normal

B. The likelihood that he has another seizure is more than 80%

C. He has juvenile myoclonic epilepsy

D. A repeat EEG would increase the likelihood to identify epileptiform activity

E. He should be admitted for video/EEG monitoring to clarify the diagnosis

The patient had his first unprovoked seizure. There is an approximately 30% chance that the patient has a recurrent seizure or epilepsy. Juvenile myoclonic epilepsy is a primary generalized seizures disorder with typical myoclonic jerking in the morning and generalized convulsions. On EEG it is characterized by frequent spike-and-wave and polyspike-and-wave discharges between 4-6 Hz, especially during photic stimulation. It typically begins in the teenage years. The patient could still have juvenile myoclonic epilepsy, but the diagnosis cannot be established with a negative EEG. Another EEG in the patient above would increase the possibility of recording epileptiform activity. Video/EEG monitoring would not be appropriate for the evaluation of a single seizure.

7. While recording an EEG:

A. Checking of impedances is unnecessary with digital recording

B. Low and high pass filters should be checked

C. Hyperventilation and photic stimulation should be performed

D. B. and C.

E. A., B. and C.

Impedance measurements determine the resistance between electrodes and scalp and should be performed in digital recordings. Filters are usually set at 1 Hz for the high pass filter and 70 Hz for the low pass filter. Hyperventilation and photic stimulation should be performed with every EEG unless there is a clear contraindication.

8. Hypsarrythmia:

A. Is the EEG pattern of infantile spasm

B. Is of high voltage

C. Represents chaotic delta activity

D. A. and B.

E. A., B. and C.

Hypsarrhythmia is the typical EEG patterns associated with West syndrome. West syndrome consists of infantile spasms and usually manifests at the age of 3-12 months. Hypsarrhythia is high amplitude (> 300 microV), disorganized slow EEG activity in the delta range (Figure 13).

9. A nine-year-old boy who has focal facial twitching with motor aphasia without loss of consciousness will likely have which of the following:

A. An EEG with centro-temporal spikes

B. Enhanced epileptiform activity during sleep

C. A good prognosis

D. A. and B.

E. All of the above

This is a typical story for a child with Benign Epilepsy with Centro-Temporal Spikes. The epileptiform activity typically increases during sleep.

10. Loss of motor evoked potentials during surgery for scoliosis:

A. Is always due to anesthesia effects

B. Is only significant if there is also loss of SSEPs

C. May indicate spinal cord injury

D. Should be ignored

E. Should prompt more instrumentation of the spinal column

Loss of motor evoked potentials can indicate damage to the motor pathways of the spinal cord and can occur without the loss of SSEPs, resulting in a pure motor deficit. Anesthesia with volatile agents, eg, sevoflurane or paralytic agents, can abolish motor evoked potentials, but this should only be assumed if other sources like instrumention by the surgeon have been excluded. Loss of motor evoked potentials should never be ignored and if there is loss of motor evoked potentials due to instrumentation, it may necessitate removal of already placed spinal instrumentation.

11. When all waveforms are clearly seen on BAEPs, but there is a prolongation of waves I, III and V absolute latencies with normal IPLs, which of the following is likely:

A. A peripheral hearing defect

B. A lesion of the superior colliculus

C. A lesion of the dorsal tegmental region

D. A lesion in the dominant auditory cortex

Wave I is thought to be generated at the level of the acoustic nerve, wave III originates in the superior olivary nucleus of the lower pons, and wave V is thought to correlate with the inferior colliculus in the dorsal tegmental region. The superior colliculus is part of the visual system. If all waves are delayed with normal interpeak latencies the lesion is located distal to the acoustic nerve or the acoustic nerve itself and indicates a peripheral hearing defect.

12. When the I-III interpeak latency of BAEPs is abnormally prolonged, which of the following is true:

A. There is a conduction defect in the mid-medulla

B. There is a lesion of the inferior colliculus

C. There is a lesion in the brainstem auditory system between the distal eighth nerve and the lower pons

D. There is a lesion of the cochlea

Prolongation of the interpeak latency between wave I and III would indicate a lesion between the distal eight nerve and the lower pons (Figure 21). A lesion in the cochlea would result in prolonged latencies in waves I-V with normal interpeak latencies. The cochlear nuclei (generator of wave III) are located in the lateral medulla. A lesion in the inferior colliculus would result in a prolonged wave V and subsequently prolonged interpeak latency III-V.

13. In the BAEP, Wave III is generated by:

A. The distal eighth nerve

B. The extramedullary, intracranial eighth nerve or the cochlear nucleus in the lateral medulla

C. The superior olivary complex and nuclei of the trapezoid body in the lower pons

D. The inferior colliculus

Wave III is generated in the superior olivary complex and the trapezoid body in the lower pons (Figure 21).

14. Magnetoencephalography measures:

A. Ionic fluxes

B. Radial electrical signals

C. Synaptic activity

D. Magnetic signals

Magnetencephalography measures magnetic fields on the scalp. EEG measures radial electrical signals. Ionic fluxes and synaptic activity are difficult to measure *in vivo* in humans.

15. Optic neuritis results in which of the following in the VEP:

A. A shortening of the I-II IPL of the VEP

B. A delay of the P100 of the VEP

C. A decrease in amplitude of the P50

D. A reduced amplitude of the P75

Waveforms are only numbered with Roman numerals in brainstem evoked potentials. Delay of the P100 peak is the typical sign of optic neuritis and indicates conduction delay in the optic nerves. Amplitude measurements in evoked potentials are less significant than latency differences.

16. The first major localized scalp recorded component of posterior-tibial SSEPs is the:

A. P37

B. N20

C. P40

D. N40

Peaks in somatosensory evoked potentials are termed by their polarity (by convention positive=P=down or negative=N=up) and the normal value of a particular peak. P 37 is the first positive peak in somatosensory evoked potentials of the lower extremity and should occur around 37 ms. N20 is the first negative peak of somatosensory evoked potentials of the upper extremities.

17. A common feature of spikes in benign epilepsy with centro-temporal spikes is:

A. Phase reversal at F8

B. Phase reversal at Fp1

C. Vertical dipole

D. Horizontal dipole

The typical EEG feature of benign epilepsy with centro-temporal spikes (BCTS) is the horizontal dipole. Spikes are typically seen in the centro-temporal region. In a referential montage if there is a polarity reversal from the frontal to the centro-temporal region, this is indicative of a horizontal dipole.

18. In continuous spike and waves of slow wave sleep (electrical status epilepticus of sleep), what percentage of the slow wave sleep record is occupied by spike-wave:

A. 20%

B. 40%

C. 85%

D. 65%

Greater than 85% spike wave activity of the non-REM sleep record are indicative of continuous spike-and-waves of slow wave sleep. During wakefulness spikes are markedly decreased. The disease occurs in children aged 1-13-years-old. Neuropsychological impairment is common, although the disease often spontaneously remits. It is related to Landau-Kleffner syndrome.

19. The Landau-Kleffner syndrome is characterized by:

A. Low voltage record

B. High amplitude slowing in the occipital regions

C. Temporal or parietal spikes

D. Frontal spikes

Acquired epileptic aphasia (Landau-Kleffner syndrome) is a rare syndrome characterized by language regression and epileptiform discharges involving the temporal or parietal regions of the brain. In this disorder children develop an abrupt or gradual loss of language ability and verbal auditory agnosia, with onset during the first decade of life. This interruption in communication skills is generally closely preceded, accompanied, or followed by the onset of seizures or an abnormal EEG, or both.

20. A photoparoxysmal response:

A. Is diagnostic for epilepsy

B. Is a normal variant

C. Is associated with nocturnal seizures

D. Is common in Landau-Kleffner syndrome

E. None of the above

A photoparoxysmal response is the occurrence of epileptiform activity with photic stimulation during an EEG. This pattern can occur in patients without a history of seizures. About 70% of patients with a photoparoxysmal response have epilepsy and 4% of patient with epilepsy have a photoparoxysmal response. It is not specific for a particular type of epilepsy.

21. A 46-year-old woman experiences her first tonic clonic convulsion after sleep deprivation while on vacation in Germany. An MRI is performed, which is normal, and an EEG is performed as shown below.

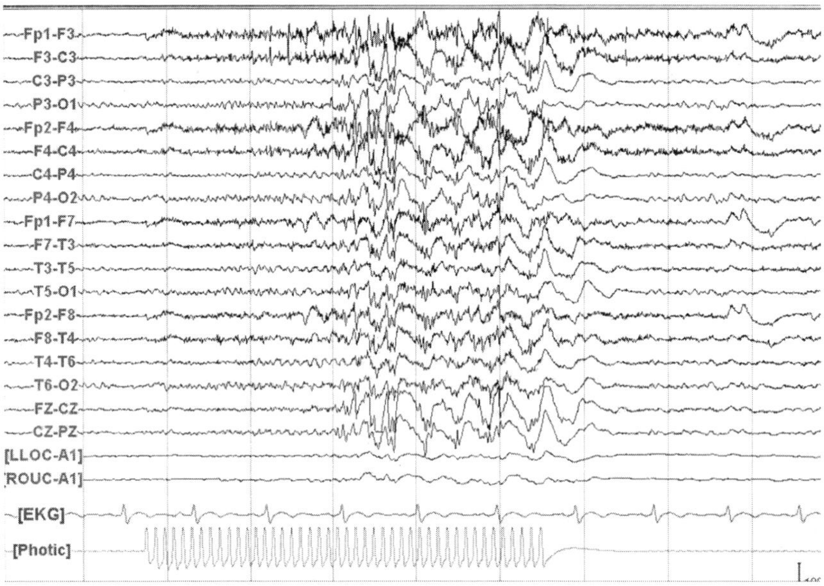

A. The patient very likely has epilepsy and antiepileptic treatment should be considered.

B. The EEG shows photic driving which is considered normal.

C. As the patient never had a seizure before and the seizure was induced by sleep deprivations the likelihood that she will have another seizure is negligible if she maintains good sleep hygiene.

D. The EEG is typical for a localization related (focal) seizure disorder.

E. The EEG does not show epileptiform activity.

The EEG shows a typical photoconvulsive response that outlasts the duration of the photic stimulus (last channel). There are irregular generalized spike wave complexes that are definitely epileptiform. As the patient had a clinical seizure it is likely that the patient suffers from epilepsy. The EEG abnormalities are seen in all channels which suggests a primary generalized epilepsy and not a localization related epilepsy. As the patient already had one clinical seizure and has definite epileptiform abnormalities, it is very likely that she will have recurrent seizures and treatment should be considered. Avoiding sleep deprivation alone may not be sufficient.

22. A 7-year-old boy is seen because of episodes of nighttime drooling and facial twitching. He was born normally and is doing well in school. The neurological exam is normal. His EEG is as below.

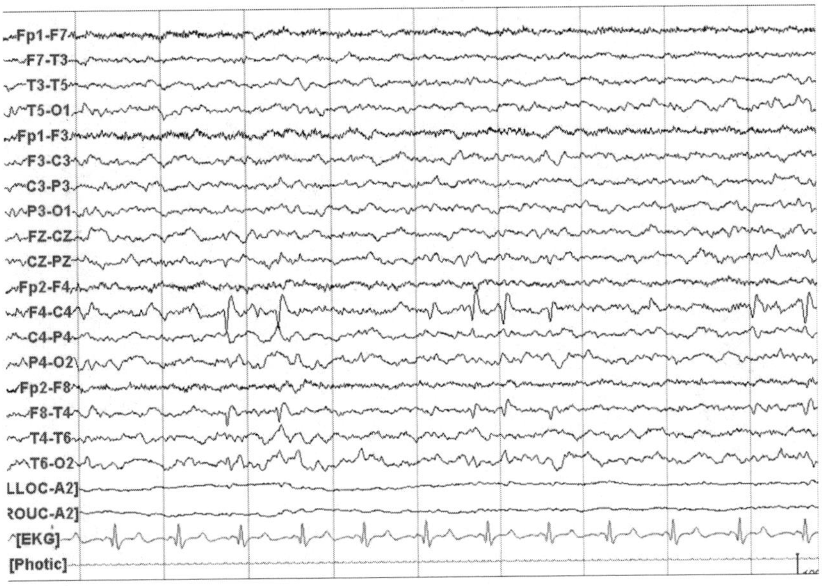

A. The EEG is normal.

B. The patient has typical absence epilepsy.

C. There are centro-temporal spikes that are compatible with a diagnosis of benign epilepsy of childhood with centro-temporal spikes.

D. The EEG background is abnormally slow for a seven-year-old.

E. The patient has Landau-Kleffner syndrome.

The EEG shows centro-temporal spikes with a horizontal dipole as typically seen in benign epilepsy of childhood with centro-temporal spikes. The EEG is recorded during light sleep and therefore the overall background is slower than during the awake states. Centro-temporal spikes are more frequent during drowsiness and sleep. Laundau-Kleffer syndrome is an epileptic syndrome that results in aphasia due to continuous seizure activity in the temporal regions. Patients have severely impaired language and neuropsychological deficits.

23. An 8-year-old previously healthy boy lost consciousness in physical education class. An EEG was obtained as shown below.

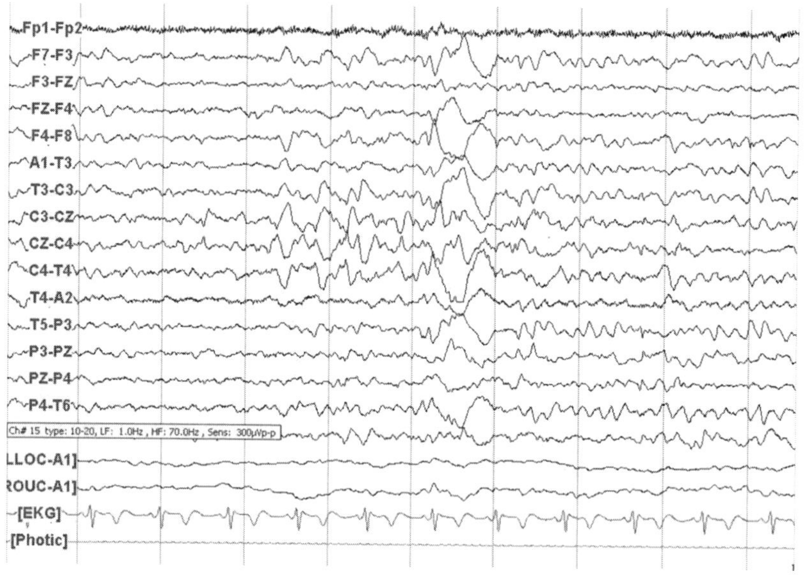

A. The patient is very likely to have epilepsy as he has epileptiform activity on his EEG.

B. The EEG is obtained during sleep.

C. A cardiac evaluation should be considered to assess the etiology of his loss of consciousness.

D. B. and C.

E. All of the above

The EEG shows a normal sleep pattern of sleep stage II with vertex waves over Cz and K-complexes. Most sleep patterns are symmetric and most prominent over the vertex. No epileptiform activity is noted. A cardiac evaluation is indicated to assess other reasons for his loss of consciousness besides epilepsy.

24. A 79-year-old lady is admitted to the ICU with severe generalized spasms. Two weeks earlier she suffered from an injury to her calf from a tree branch while accidentally stepping on it. The patient is suspected to have tetanus. An EEG is obtained as below.

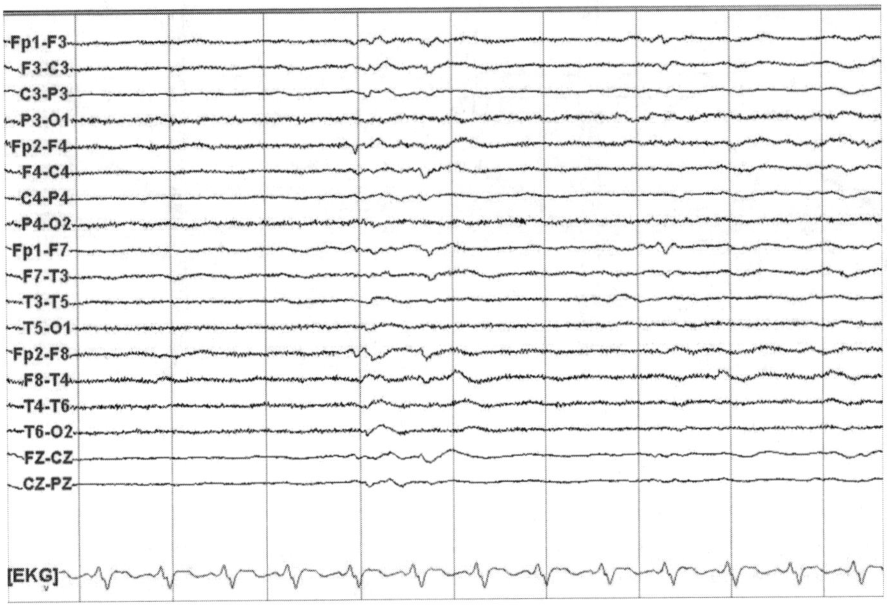

A. The EEG is normal.

B. The patient does not have tetanus but frequent generalized seizure due to epileptiform activity on EEG.

C. The EEG shows burst suppression pattern.

D. The prognosis is good.

E. The patient is brain dead.

The EEG shows a low amplitude burst suppression pattern that usually carries a poor prognosis. Burst suppression can also be seen with sedation due to anesthetics like propofol or benzodiazepines. Burst suppression due to medications is reversible. The EEG above is of low amplitude and also the burst of activity is of low amplitude. As long as there is some cortical activity like intermittent bursts the patient does not meet the criteria for brain death. This particular patient with the above EEG died of the tetanus infection.

25. In a 16-year-old patient with severe congenital scolosis, intraoperative monitoring is performed. Transcranial motor evoked potentials and sensory evoked potentials are performed. Sensory and motor evoked potentials are reproducible and well formed at baseline. During distraction and correction of the spinal axis, motor evoked potentials disappear as shown below (arrows). Median arterial pressure is 50 mmHg.

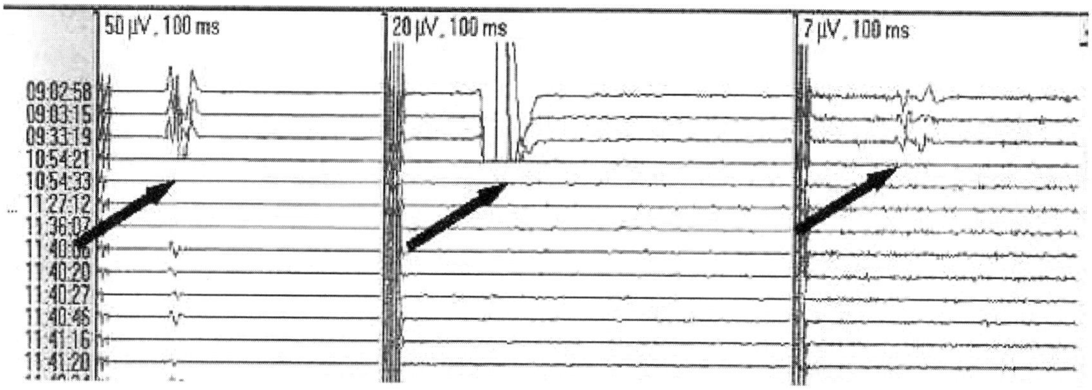

A. The loss of potentials could be due to anesthesiology giving a paralytic agent like succinylcholine.

B. The loss of motor potentials could be due to spinal cord ischemia during distraction and the instrumentation may need to be removed.

C. The blood pressure should be raised.

D. A. and C.

E. All of the above.

The clear loss of motor potentials could be due to an paralytic agent (as actually occurred in this case), or could be due to spinal cord ischemia as a result of instrumentation by the surgeons. It would be important to know whether sensory evoked potentials were lost in addition to the motor evoked potentials. If there is suspicion that spinal cord ischemia occurred as a consequence of instrumentation, instrumentation should be removed. Raising the blood pressure could improve perfusion if spinal ischemia occurred. During instrumentation, mean arterial pressure should be kept above 70 to assure sufficient perfusion pressure during distraction regardless of intraoperative monitoring findings. Intraoperative monitoring has reduced the necessity to wake up the patient during the spine surgery to assess motor function.

26. You are asked to see a 2-day-old infant who was born at term with hypoxic-ischemic encephalopathy due to placenta previa and excessive bleeding at the time of delivery. The infant has had some episodes of chewing and cycling movements of the legs which have not decreased with phenobarbital therapy. An EEG was obtained which demonstrated an invariant pattern shown below:

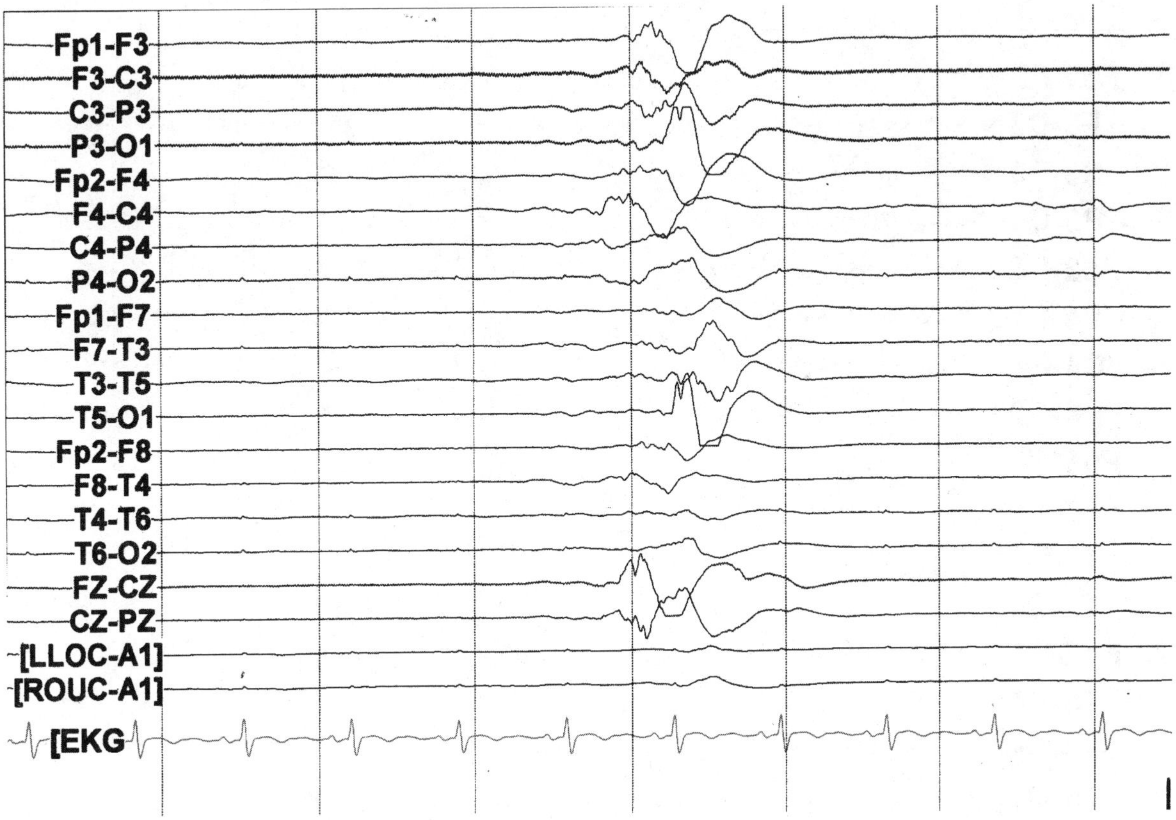

The EEG shows:

A. Tracé discontinu

B. Tracé alternant

C. Normal quiet sleep

D. Burst suppression

The EEG shows severe depression of the background activity interrupted by bursts of higher amplitude polymorphic activity. Since the child was born at term, this would not be a tracé discontinu pattern. The activity in between the bursts is too low to be tracé alternant. This is an example of burst suppression, a severely abnormal EEG pattern.

27. A three-year-old girl is seen in the neurology clinic because of recurrent myoclonic jerks. At age 13 months, she had a 60-minute febrile seizure that involved clonic jerks of the left side of her body. The parents are concerned that she has slowed in her development. The following EEG was obtained. Based on the history and EEG, which disorder do you need to consider?

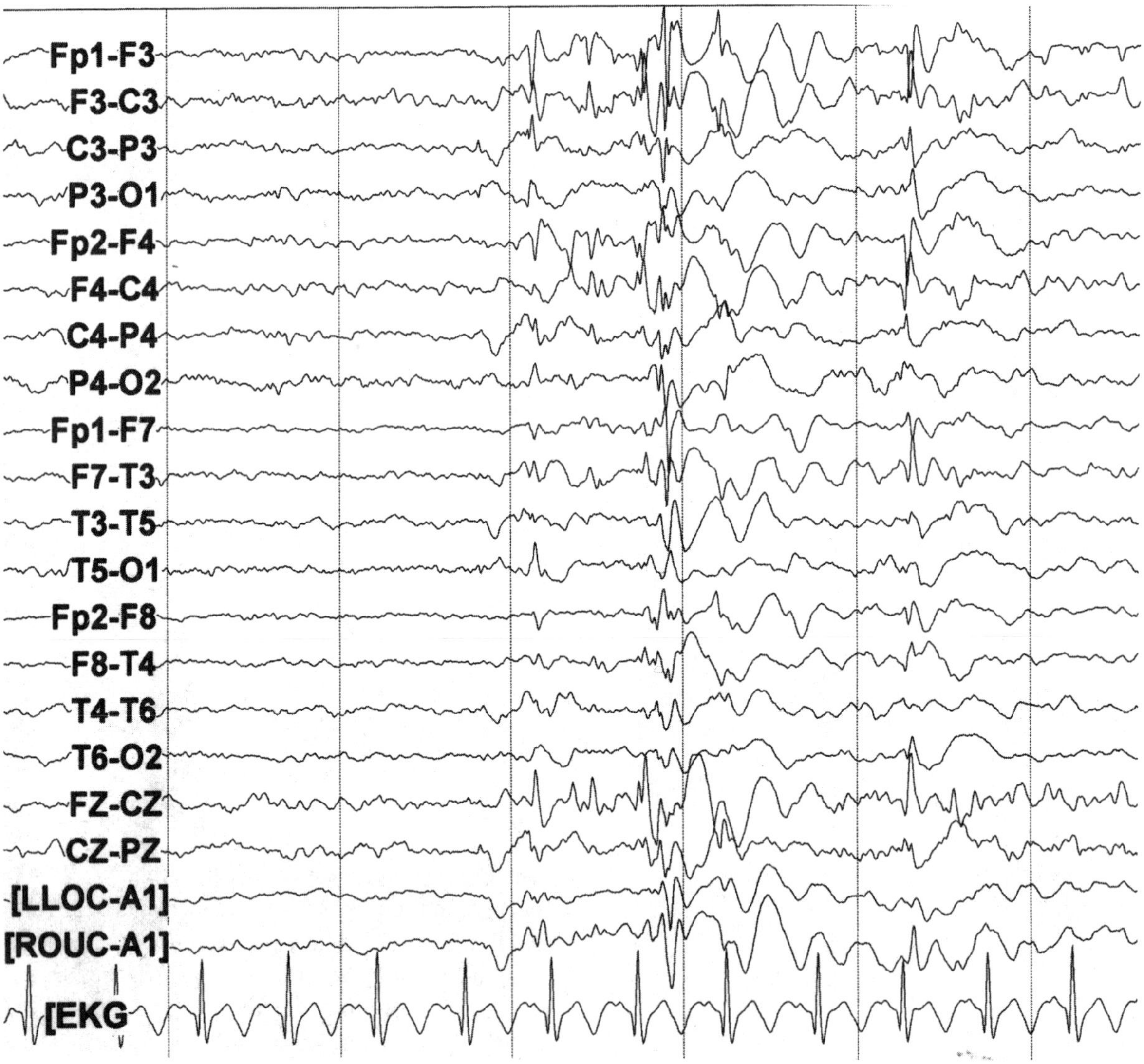

A. Landau-Kleffner syndrome

B. Benign Epilepsy with Centro-Temporal Spikes

C. Dravet syndrome (Severe Myoclonic Epilepsy of Early Childhood)

D. ESES

The prolonged febrile seizure with focal features followed by myoclonic jerks and developmental slowing is suggestive of Dravet syndrome. The generalized spike-wave activity would be consistent, but not diagnostic of the condition. The disorder can be diagnosed by genetic testing.

28. A term infant is transferred from a community hospital because of right arm jerking. The pregnancy and delivery were uneventful. An MRI and EEG were obtained and are shown below. Based on these findings, the etiology of the seizures is most likely:

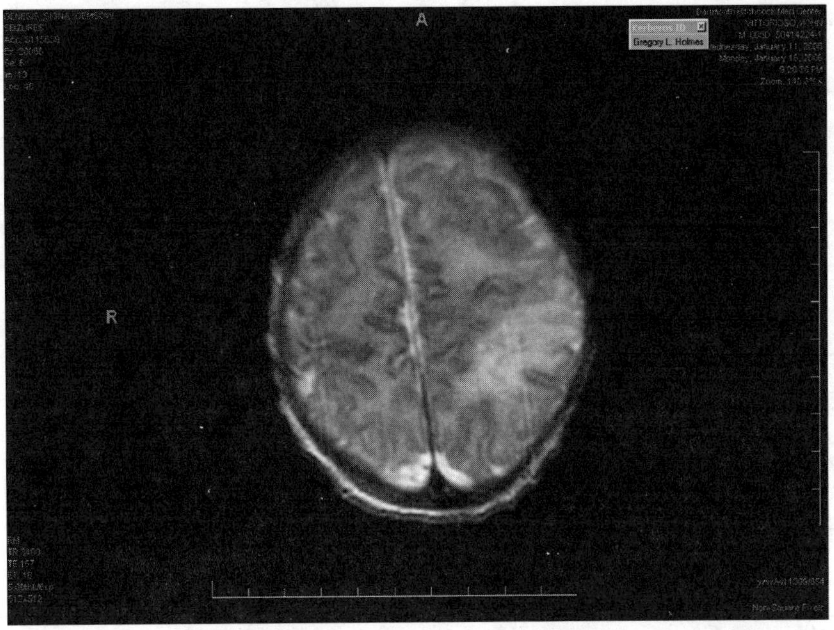

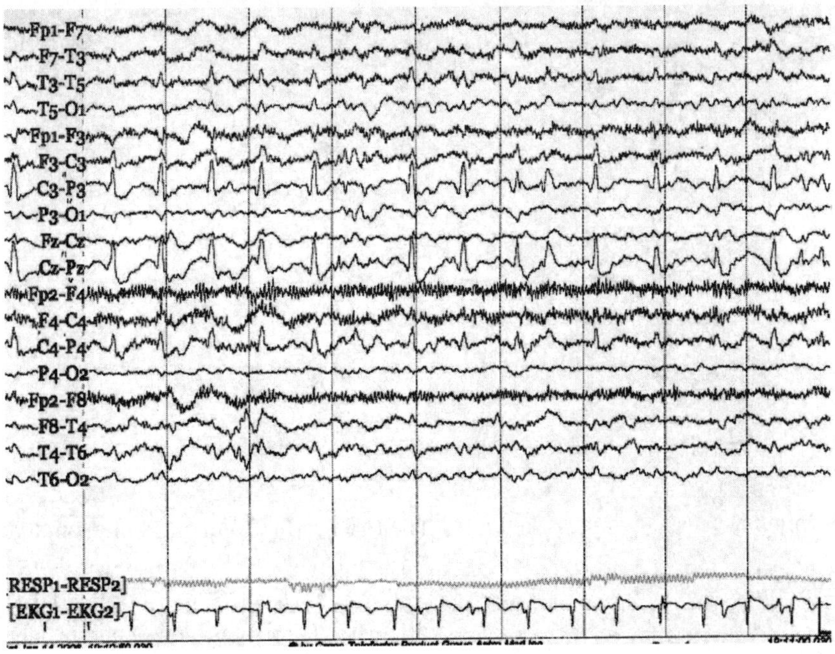

A. Cortical dysplasia

B. Left middle cerebral artery stroke

C. Benign familial neonatal seizures

D. Non-ketotic hyperglycinemia

The MRI shows a signal abnormality in the left hemisphere and is likely a stroke. The EEG shows a focal discharge occurring in the same area.

29. A 12-year-old boy is referred to you for possible night terrors. The following EEG was obtained. Which of the following diagnoses should be considered?

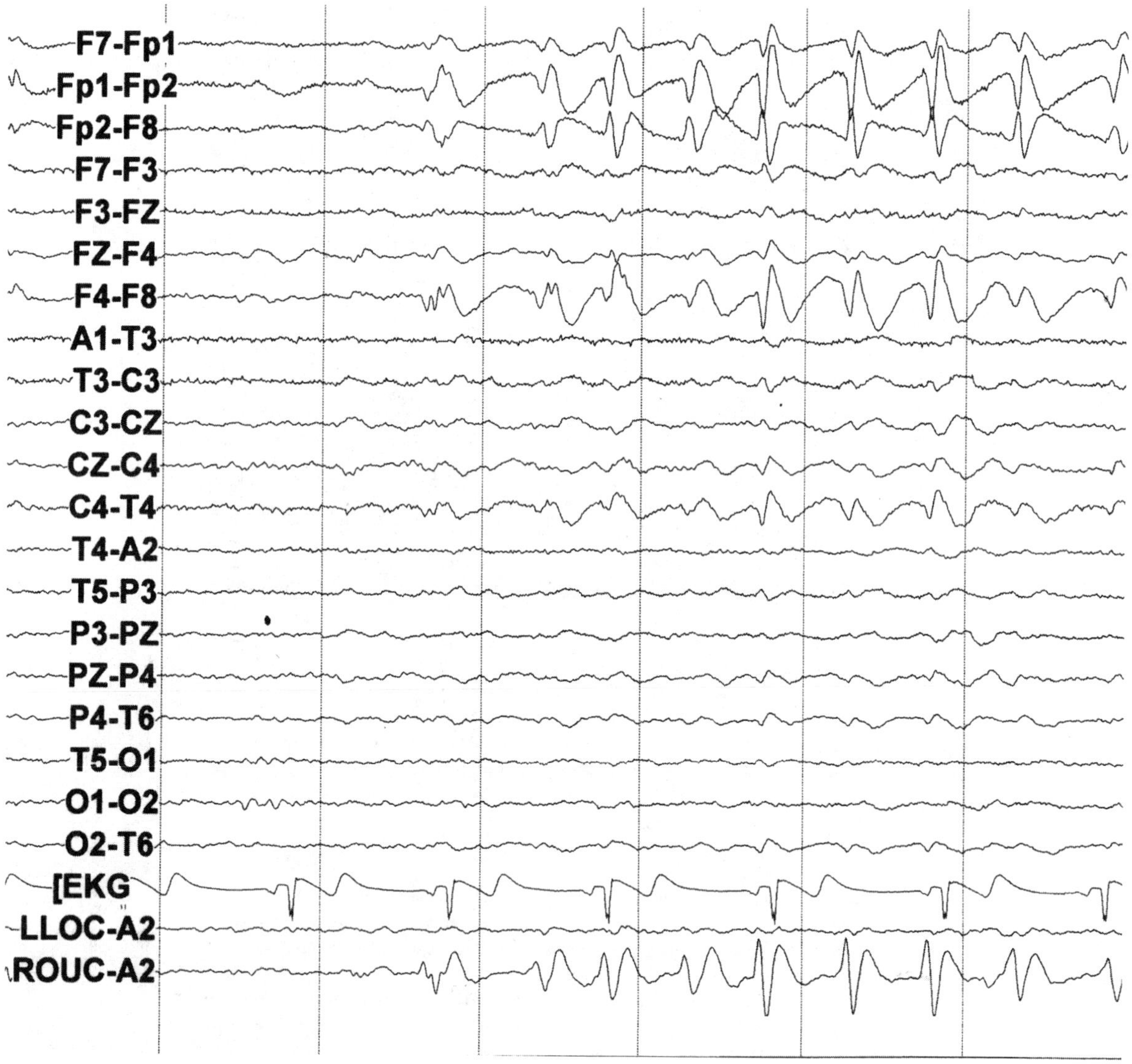

A. Frontal lobe epilepsy

B. Temporal lobe epilepsy

C. Night terrors

D. Parietal lobe epilepsy

The EEG shows frequent right frontal lobe spikes. Night terrors in a 12-year-old would be unusual, but could occur. The frequent frontal lobe spikes would suggest the patient is having nocturnal frontal lobe seizures.

30. You are asked to see a 17-year-old woman who had a generalized tonic-clonic seizure upon awakening. Upon further questioning, you learn she also has episodes of bilateral arm jerking, particularly in the morning. The EEG demonstrated here in conjunction with the clinical history suggests the diagnosis of:

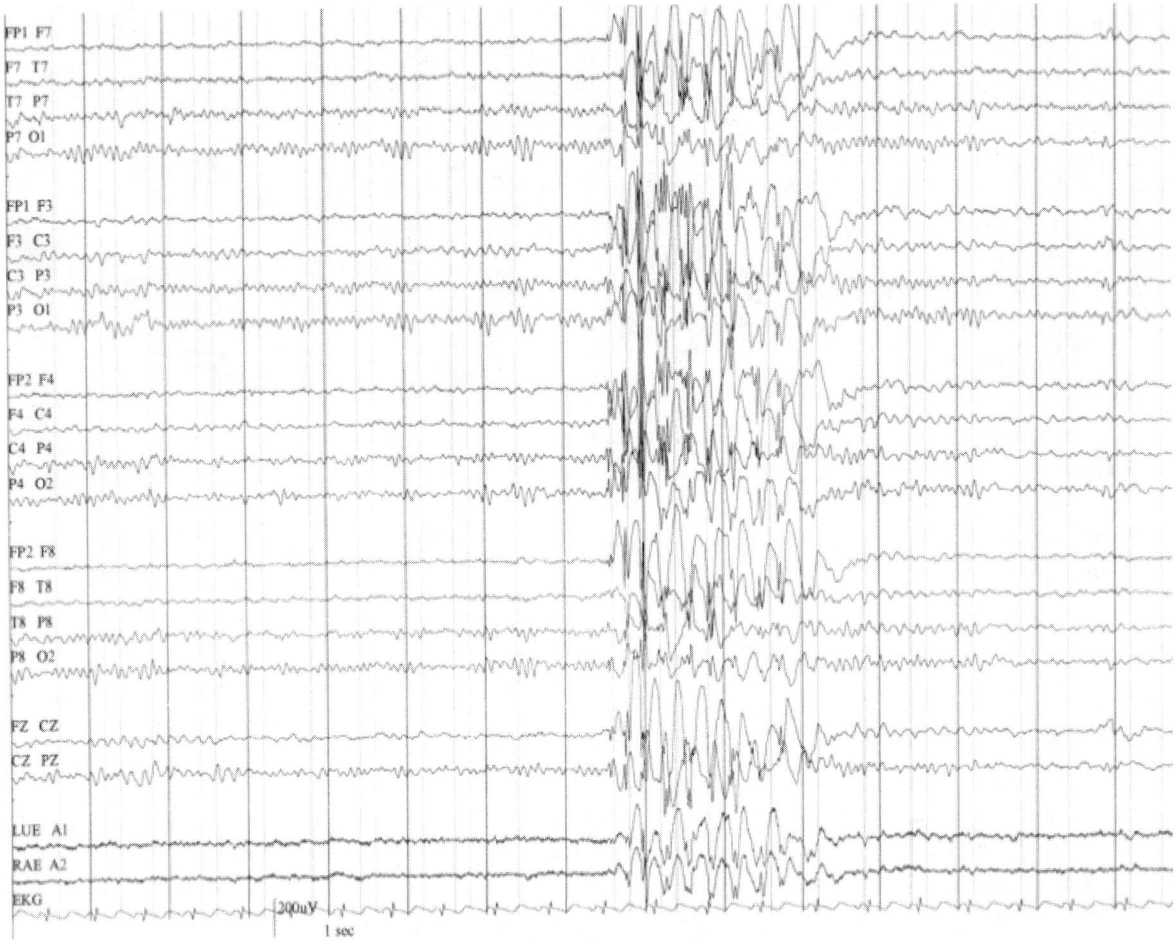

A. Juvenile myoclonic epilepsy

B. Juvenile absence epilepsy

C. Landau-Kleffner syndrome

D. Dravet syndrome

The history is highly suggestive of juvenile myoclonic epilepsy. The EEG, which demonstrates generalized rapid spike-and-wave discharges would be compatible with the diagnosis of juvenile myoclonic epilepsy.

Answers

1. E.
2. A.
3. D.
4. B.
5. E.
6. D.
7. D.
8. E.
9. E.
10. C.
11. A.
12. C.
13. C.
14. D.
15. B.
16. A.
17. D.
18. C.
19. C .
20. E.
21. A.
22. C.
23. D.
24. C.
25. E.
26. D.
27. D.
28. B.
29. A.
30. A.

Chapter 24: Neurological Pain

Morris Levin, MD
Zahid H. Bajwa, MD

Contents

1. Introduction: Understanding and Treating Pain

Despite enormous advances in our knowledge about the physiology, pathophysiology and treatment of pain over the last 50 years, many patients with pain disorders still suffer, leaving their well-meaning clinicians perplexed and frustrated. It isn't uncommon in such situations for the clinician to unconsciously "blame" the patient, if only as a means to release the frustration brought on by the feeling of clinical inadequacy. Many of these difficult to treat syndromes have their bases in the function and dysfunction of the peripheral, central, and autonomic branches of the nervous system, which should therefore fall within the realm of neurology.

Much of what we know today about the complexity of pain is based on seminal work by Melzack and Wall in the 1960s on the gate control theory, which proposed that rather than a straightforward afferent path beginning in the pain receptor, the perception of pain is the result of a number of interactions between different neurons. Their concepts have been revised several times over the years, and have led to innovative therapies including the TENS unit as well as the spinal cord stimulator, and they provided the impetus for widespread basic and clinical research into the study of pain. More recently Clifford Woolf and others have emphasized that there are several mechanisms underlying the production and maintenance of pain, and that successful treatment must be etiology-driven.

Research aimed at understanding pain, from work on the molecular biology of nociceptive pathways and their regulation and processing, to the psychosocial factors that influence the human experience of pain, has led to the development and application of improved treatment strategies for acute, recurrent and chronic persistent pain, both cancer or non-cancer related.

The purpose of this chapter is to provide the neurologist: 1.) a review of the anatomy and physiology of pain; 2.) a synopsis of the current understanding of the pathophysiology of neuropathic pain illnesses and modulation of pain in the CNS; and 3) an overview of representative neurologic pain syndromes and their current clinical management strategies, using evidence-based treatment protocols wherever possible. An exhaustive review of pain-producing conditions will not be attempted. Headache disorders will not be discussed more than briefly, as there is a separate chapter on headaches in this volume.

2. Pain Anatomy and Physiology

The sensation of pain (nociception) begins in the periphery through the activation of pain receptors (nociceptors) that are the terminal endings of primary thinly myelinated or unmyelinated afferent nerve fibers. These are bipolar neurons whose bodies lie in the dorsal root ganglion and whose proximal axons enter the spinal cord via the dorsal ramus, pass through the dorsal root entry zone (DREZ) and synapse in the dorsal horn (DH). Subtypes of nociceptors are further categorized by the kind of stimulation to which they respond as well as the nature or pattern (frequency and intensity) of their response.

Myelinated nociceptors are relatively faster conducting A-delta fibers. These are generally stimulus-specific (pressure, pinching). Some have low thresholds and respond readily to heat. Others are high threshold mechanoreceptors. The rate of discharge of both types of nociceptors is directly proportional to the intensity and/or frequency of the stimulus.

Unmyelinated C fibers, however, constitute the majority of peripheral nociceptors. Most (80%) are polymodal, responding to thermal, mechanical, and chemical stimuli, the remaining 20% being responsive only to chemical stimuli except at times when they are sensitized to mechanical stimulation in the presence of inflammation. These are slow-conducting primary afferents with receptive fields smaller than those of A-delta nociceptors.

Most nociceptors become more sensitive (lowered threshold) to more than the usual stimuli in the presence of tissue damage, even without direct damage to the nociceptor, as a result of high levels of pain producing factors including histamine, bradykinin, serotonin, and prostaglandins. In addition, pain afferent nerve endings release CGRP and substance P in these situations, which further promotes nociceptor activation.

There is growing evidence that itch is mediated not so much by low-level stimulation of nociceptors in general, but by histamine sensitive pruriceptors constituting about 5% of all C-fiber nociceptors. There are likely other peripheral chemical mediators of itch, and the central pathways may be separate from those of pain, with a "scratch reflex" resulting from cortical stimulation of multiple cortical sites instead of the better understood nocifensive withdrawal reflex.

Nociceptors vary not only in their threshold of activation, but in their rate of firing too. This provides an important, if elementary, form of encoding sensory data prior to entering the dorsal horn of the spinal cord where further processing can occur. In the spinal cord, 2nd order neurons, with which primary afferents synapse, vary in terms of the type of stimulus or region of the body they subserve. Some respond to a continuum of stimuli such as warmth through the noxious range of high temperatures ("wide dynamic range"—WDR); others are specific for noxious stimuli (nociceptor specific—NS).

Each of these nociceptors and the 2nd order neurons they excite contributes to the qualitative and quantitative experience of pain. A-delta fibers are responsible for the near immediate detection of sharp pain; while delayed pain, usually characterized as dull or aching, is mediated by C fibers.

First-order neurons have their cell bodies mostly in the dorsal root ganglion (DRG), or in the case of the face and anterior head, the trigeminal ganglion. (Note that there is some sensory input to the CNS via the ventral horn.) In the case of visceral afferents, the fibers travel with sympathetic and parasympathetic fibers. The central processes of these primary nociceptor afferents first access the spinal cord through Lissauer's tract where they may ascend or descend one or two spinal levels prior to synapsing with second-order neurons in the dorsal horn. Gray matter in the dorsal horn is histologically divided into 10 layers, numbered from superficial to deep, otherwise collectively named Rexed's laminae, of which the first two most superficial layers (I, the marginal zone and II, the substantia gelatinosa) are the primary targets for the terminals of the nociceptive primary afferents described above. Levels III and IV may play an inhibitory role. Second order axons emerge largely out of laminae I, II, V, VII, and VIII; lamina V cells contain WDR neurons that receive input from both nociceptive and non-nociceptive afferents. Because of this, there is a greater degree of convergence in lamina V than elsewhere in the dorsal horn. It is believed that the deeper layers receive input from muscles and viscera. Interneurons within the dorsal horn of the spinal

Table 1

The Two Major Nociceptive Pathways

Medial / affective	
Polymodal receptors	
C axons (unmyelinated)	
Slow – "second pain"	
Burning, non-localized pain	
Wide dynamic range (WDR) DH neuron	
DH neuron–Large field	
Spinoreticular tracts	
Medial thalamic nuclei	
Multiple cortical projections	
Lateral / discriminative	
Mechano-, thermo- receptors	
A delta (small, myelinated)	
Fast–"first pain"	
Sharp, localized pain	
DH neuron nociceptive only	
DH neuron–Small field	
Spinothalamic tract	
Lateral thalamic nuclei	
Postcentral gyrus projections	

cord provide "cross-talk" between the various layers or laminae, further modulating ascending impulses. The spinal cord is therefore more than a sensory relay center.

Second order nociceptive neurons give rise to axons, which cross the midline of the spinal cord in the anterior commissure and ascend in afferent nociceptive tracts, most prominently the spinothalamic tract (or, in the case of the face and head, trigeminothalamic tract). The spinothalamic tract is located within the anterolateral quadrant of the spinal cord, and ascends through the brainstem and into the ventral posterior lateral nucleus of the thalamus, where further modulation occurs (and perhaps a crude sense of awareness), and from where distribution of nociceptive information to cortical and subcortical regions occurs. The spinothalamic tract ultimately gives rise to two distinct pathways: 1.) the lateral pathway, projecting to the somatosensory cortex and subserving the sensory-discriminative aspect of pain; and 2.) the paramedian pathways, which project to widespread cortical areas, including the frontal lobes, and in particular, the cingulate gyrus. The former system is faster, as it is subserved by myelinated A delta fibers as primary nociceptors. The latter system processes affective-motivational aspects of pain and is subserved by C fibers (Table 1). Several other ascending tracts (ie, the spinohypothalamic, spinoreticular, and the spinopontoamygdala tracts) are likely involved in additional facets of nociception such as sleep perturbation and arousal, as well as emotional aspects of pain.

Pain from the face and head is carried by cranial nerves V, VII, IX, X, and from the posterior division of the upper cervical nerves (C2 and C3). The cranial primary afferents synapse in the trigeminal system's three sensory nuclei, but the nociception pathway primarily involves the spinal trigeminal nucleus (STN). The trigeminothalamic tract ascend to the ventral posterior medial nucleus of the thalamus, and other targets.

The activity of the spinal cord second-order nociceptive cells can be heightened by several factors. First, with repeated stimulation, they become more active in certain situations (see below in "Central Sensitization"). This process is thought to be mediated by the NMDA receptor complex. Secondly, when receptors are damaged and dorsal horn neurons become "deafferented," they become hyperactive. This denervation hypersensitivity is a widespread phenomenon in the nervous system.

The activity of spinal cord second order neurons can be reduced by several mechanisms as well, in particular: 1.) a peripheral process known as "gating"; and 2.) a central mechanism – the descending antinociceptive system. In the "gating" mechanism, presynaptic inhibition from incoming non-nociceptive afferents occurs at the level of the first synapse. This is the result of primarily A beta fibers and is termed the gating mechanism because these non-nociceptive afferent activity can "close the gate" on nociceptive activity (Figure 1). Clinical examples of pain treatments that employ the gating mechanism are massage, transcutaneous nerve stimulation, and heat/cold therapy.

Figure 1

The gate control mechanism in pain modulation

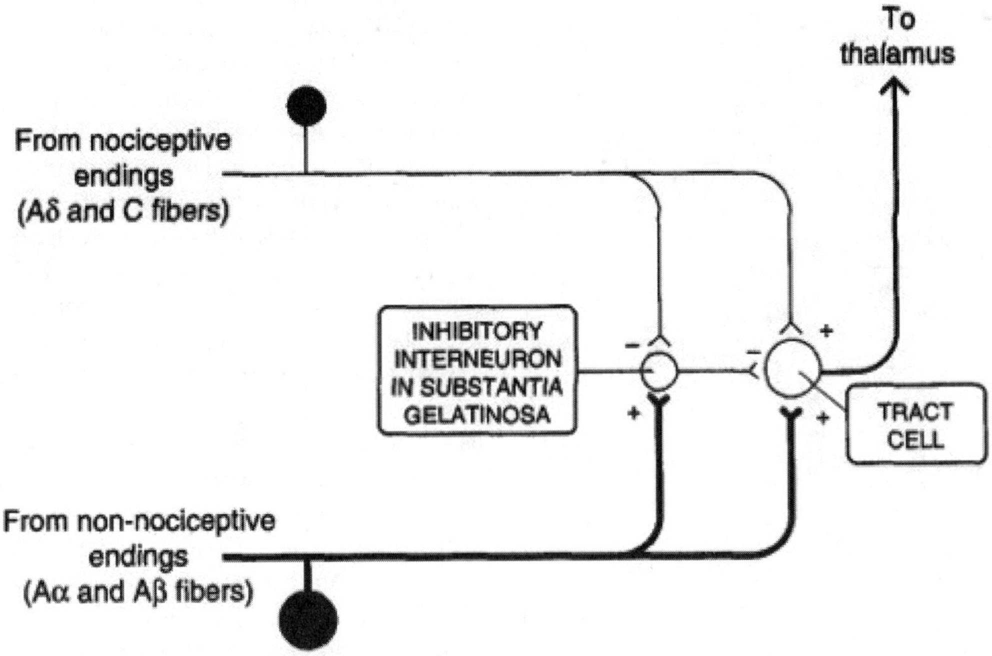

Simple illustration of the gate control theory of pain. Non-nociceptive sensory fibers stimulate the inhibitory interneurons, whereas nociceptive afferents inhibit them. An increase in non-nociceptive input will reduce the rate of firing of the spinothalamic tract neurons.

paininstruct.uwo.caanatomy

Inhibition of pain transmission also results from descending inhibition of the second-order neuron. Inhibitory presynaptic opiate receptors are found on the first-order axon. Other opiate receptors are found throughout the neuroaxis, including the brain stem. These respond to the "descending antinociceptive system," (aka, "the endogenous opioid system") which originates in a number of higher centers, including the cortex, thalamus, and brain stem (Figure 2). The midbrain periaqueductal gray region (PAG) is crucial in this system, which also includes the serotonergic nucleus raphe magnus of the medulla, the noradrenergic locus ceruleus in the pons, and an area referred to as the rostral ventromedial medulla (RVM). This system sends fibers through the dorsolateral funiculus to laminae I and V in the dorsal horn of the spinal cord which inhibit transmission at the first synapse in the nociceptive system. Activation of this system is but one of several mechanisms explaining the analgesic properties of certain classes of medication, including antidepressants, migraine prophylactics, and opioids. Of note, it is a system that remains immature at birth, making the newborn hyperalgesic relative to children and adults. The ascending systems are anatomically in place by the 20-24th week of gestation, possibly affording conscious perception of pain at the cortical level. A cruder, thalamic-based awareness is likely in place and possibly functioning a few weeks earlier.

Figure 2

The descending antinociceptive system

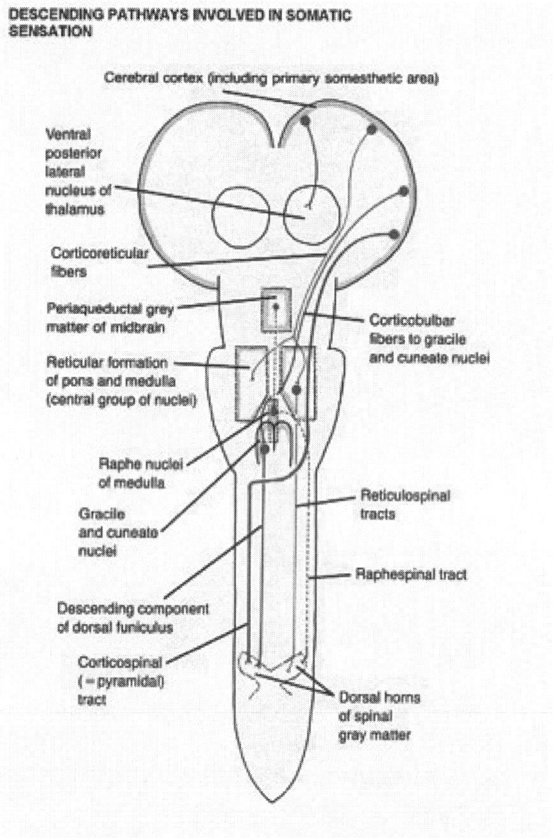

instruct.uwo.caanatomy

3. The Pathophysiology of Pain and Classification of Pain Types

Acute nociceptive pain is a vital, protective mechanism that permits us to live in an environment with potential for physical harm or injury. Its importance is perhaps most spectacularly highlighted by the rare and devastating congenital absence of nociceptors in which babies and children are prone to continuous and potentially life-affecting injuries, often resulting in death at a very young age. A far more common, if less spectacular, condition is the diminution of nociception and general sensation in the distal extremities of diabetics, which also leads to injury. These "negative" symptoms are significantly worsened by the accompaniment of "positive" phenomena like lancinating paresthesiae and dysesthesiae amidst a near constantly present background of burning and aching discomfort. Pain may be an unpleasant and disruptive experience necessary for survival, but when it persists without apparent value it induces a state of suffering that can eliminate hope, destroy self-esteem, and radically alter the quality of the patient's life and, by extension, that of his or her family's. Few have said it more succinctly than Victor Frankl who, following his liberation from a concentration camp in World War II, stated, "It is not suffering that diminishes man, but suffering without meaning."

In the 1980s, the International Society for the Study of Pain (IASP) established a committee to attempt the arduous task of defining and classifying the different types of chronic pain. By 1994, the IASP settled on a definition of pain still in use today: "Pain is an unpleasant sensory and emotional experience associated with actual or potential tissue damage, or described in terms of such damage." The IASP Task Force on the Taxonomy of Pain also devised a scheme coding pain disorders along five axis: the region and systems involved; temporal characteristics; degree of intensity; time since onset; and etiology. This is expanded upon below.

Normal pain signaling is sometimes referred to as eudynia. The pain is generally proportionate to the type and degree of injury and personifies acute forms of pain with which most of us are familiar. In contrast, the experience of chronic persistent pain following tissue healing serves no such physiologic role and becomes a disease state in its own right; it is then referred to by some as maldynia. Most commonly, the cut-off period separating chronic from acute pain is somewhere between 4-12 weeks, although most clinicians are aware of the limitations of such arbitrary cut-offs. The difference in definitions between acute and chronic pain with respect to a definite time line is more than semantics; it can result in serious consequences if used as the basis for making decisions about allocation of therapeutic resources to patients. Clearly, some conditions are best treated aggressively before they are defined as chronic. For example, neuropathic pain following presumed or demonstrable injury to a peripheral nerve may be a harbinger of serious and sometimes untreatable conditions such as the complex regional pain syndromes (CRPS), types 1 and 2, formerly referred to as reflex sympathetic dystrophy (RSD) and causalgia, respectively. Early treatment may significantly improve outcome, while delay may render them progressive and intractable. The transition from a state of acute to chronic pain is therefore best viewed as a continuum along which the earlier the pain mechanism is defined, the better is the chance of developing a successful pain management plan. Continuing this line of logic, mechanism-based diagnoses help to direct timely and appropriate care. Failure to miss a window of opportunity for treatment simply because an arbitrary duration of pain has not been reached may lead to an irreversible and intractable condition analogous to ignoring a precancerous lesion until it becomes a lethal and incurable cancer.

The broadly defined major categories of pain include *Nociceptive* pain and *Neuropathic* pain. Nociceptive pain is the conscious perception of noxious sensory input resulting from direct stimulation of nociceptors by tissue damage or other stimulus. Nociceptive pain is proportional to the degree of tissue damage. While often acute, it can be a major component of chronically painful conditions such as discogenic spine pain. Nociceptive pain is further subdivided into somatic and visceral pain. *Somatic pain* arises from damage to the body wall and skeletal tissues. It is well localized, may be sharp or dull, and varies in description and experience. Examples of acute somatic pain are skeletal fractures or torn hamstring muscles. Osteoarthritis might cause chronic somatic pain. *Visceral pain* is mediated by stretch receptors with thinly myelinated or unmyelinated afferents located in the walls of the viscera, and probably by autonomic afferent fibers as well. Visceral nociceptors can be activated by ischemia, inflammatory cytokines, or traction. The pain may be experienced as a deep and often poorly localized or diffuse sensation that may be referred rather than felt at the source. Knowledge of common referral patterns becomes important in developing a reasonable differential diagnosis. The intensity of pain ranges from mild to extremely intense. It is usually dull and cramping in quality. (Examples include the pain of appendicitis, cholecystitis, the passing of kidney stones, menstrual cramps, mesentery ischemia, and pleurisy.)

Neuropathic pain results from abnormal neural activity or the central processing of such, and is secondary to disease or injury at any level of the nervous system, central, peripheral or both. It is often disproportionate to the amount of injury and can persist with or without ongoing disease (ie, diabetic painful peripheral neuropathy, postherpetic and trigeminal neuralgias, and postamputation phantom pain). It can be spontaneous or evoked, and may manifest as *allodynia* and *hyperalgesia*. Allodynia is the perception of pain in response to a normally non-noxious stimulus. Hyperalgesia is a heightened response to a normally minimally painful stimulus. The pain sensations in neuropathic pain are often unfamiliar or bizarre to the point where normal descriptors are unsatisfactory, although "boring, burning, crushing, shooting and electrical" are commonly used terms. Neuropathic pain is further divided into *peripheral neuropathic pain*, where the neural defect is presumed to be in the 1st order neuron (primary nociceptor) and *central neuropathic pain*, where the dysfunction is at the level of the spinal cord or above. Examples of peripheral neuropathic pain are carpal tunnel syndrome and the pain of spinal radiculopathy. Examples of central neuropathic pain are pain due to midline spinal cord lesions like syringomyelia, and the post-thalamic stroke syndrome (aka "central pain syndrome" or Dejerine-Roussy syndrome).

Sympathetically mediated pain is a type of neuropathic pain which usually arises from a peripheral nerve lesion following the development of structural changes in somatic nerve membranes, rendering them hyper-responsive to normal autonomic output. Contrary to popular belief, this oversensitized pain response is not due to excessive autonomic output.

Central pain should not be confused with central sensitization of pain, a neuropathic pain process by which acute peripheral neuropathic (visceral or somatic) pain becomes chronically persistent due to CNS-mediated sensory misprocessing. This is thought to occur, in part, via CNS changes wrought by dysfunction of secondary neurons in the dorsal horn of the spinal cord during and/or following repetitive and longstanding peripheral input from initially but persistently activated C-fibers. Constant and severe bombardment of WDR neurons by C-fiber input sensitizes them to the point where normally "ignored" or subthreshold sensory input from other non-noxious pathways or nerves (AB neurons for example) becomes "important" enough for them to inappropriately activate pain pathways even when the input is non-noxious or nonpainful. These sensitized cells and neural circuits can be homosynaptic or heterosynaptic. The former, also referred to as wind-up, is a specific type of central sensitization involving only those synapses directly potentiated by activity-dependent neural input. It is a hyperresponsiveness that stops as the stimulus comes to an end. The latter, on the other hand, is also a process of neural activity-dependent potentiation and sensitization, but dorsal horn synapses not directly involving change as well. This plasticity persists beyond the term of the stimulus. Glutamate, substance P, and calcitonin gene-related peptide (CGRP) release is involved in disinhibiting NMDA receptors and calcium-activated cation channels that causes a progressive increase in action potential output from dorsal horn cells. Pain thresholds are thereby lowered and the area of perceived pain increases as the fields of dorsal horn cell receptivity increases.

Central sensitization is one of the postulated mechanisms by which neuropathic pain and other chronically painful disorders, such as the fibromyalgia syndrome (FMS), becomes persistent or develops in the first place. In the case of FMS, the inciting repetitive pain signals may come from skeletal sources such as injured spinal facet joints or intervertebral discs.

4. The History and Physical Examination in Pain Disorders

The emphasis on various aspects of the history and physical examination and the diagnostic work-up of patients in chronic pain depends upon the patients' presenting complaint(s). However, certain "routines" are followed regardless of the presentation.

History

As with any medical work-up, the physician begins with a thorough history of the present illness. Specific questions focus the evaluation (see Table 2).

When and how did the pain begin?

A good starting point is to ask the patient to describe how the pain began. Was there a precipitating event, such as an injury or a painful procedure, or did the pain begin spontaneously? Did the current level of pain arise rapidly and acutely, or in a more gradual fashion?

With trauma, it is important to get the details of the injury. With a motor vehicle accident (MVA), for example, it may be important to know how and under what conditions the vehicles collided, what restraint systems were used, the speed and angle of collision, the degree of damage to the vehicles, and so on. In addition, it is important to determine the disposition of the patient following the trauma. Was there loss of consciousness? Did he or she go to an emergency unit and, if so, what did the work-up reveal? Was the patient admitted to the hospital? What treatment did the patient receive? Find out if the injury was work related and, if so, whether the patient is collecting worker's compensation or disability insurance/payments, or if he or she is currently in litigation or plans to be. Answers to these questions may have prognostic relevance by helping the physician determine if the degree of pain is commensurate with the degree of injury; mild trauma associated with a very dramatic clinical presentation of pain might suggest embellishment of symptoms for secondary gain. Nonetheless, it is a common error to assume such at first glance, especially where difficult to image or impossible to objectively measure pain is concerned. This is often the case with fibromyalgia, neuropathic pain, or post-traumatic headaches. Observation of body language, facial expression and consistency of information over time becomes exceedingly important in such cases. Furthermore, one's own behavior can affect the patient's presentation. If one portrays a lack of empathy or distrust in asking pertinent questions, the patient might consciously or unconsciously feel a need to "convince" the examiner of the veracity of the clinical complaint. Doing so by exaggeration could lead to the examiner erroneously concluding malingering by the patient, a common mistake. Physicians must also keep in mind that the response to pain varies not only from one individual to another, but between cultures and gender.

How is the pain described?

Allow the patient to verbalize the painful symptoms. What is the location of the pain? Is it focal, like a frontal headache, or does it exist in various locations that are discrete or contiguous, as might be seen in cases of lumbar radiculopathy or widespread musculoskeletal pain? Does the pain seem to have a point of emanation and if so, does it radiate? Is it associated with other sensations or the loss of sensation? Is it positional— brought on or exacerbated by specific activities? Regarding the "depth" of the pain, is it superficial and easy to localize, as in somatic pain, or does it seem to come from deep within the body over a more generalized region, the way visceral pain presents? Might the localization of pain be due to a common referral pattern involving another area of the body?

It is important to allow the patient to describe the pain using his or her own words. Studies evaluating the adjectives people use reveal two broad categories of descriptors that fall into either sensory or affective groups. In the former, words such as sharp, dull and cramping were noted to communicate a definite sensation in a particular part or region of the body, as opposed to descriptive terms such as dreadful, vicious and cruel, which connote a more emotional component of the patient's pain experience. Uncovering and assisting the patient in coping with negative feelings can be an important part of therapy and devising the treatment plan in general. Help from a mental health professional knowledgeable about pain management might be required.

What is the intensity of pain?

Although there is no quantitative biochemical or neurophysiologic test for pain, tools have been

Table 2

Key Points Defining the Pattern of Pain and Factors That Affect Resolution/Chronicity

1. Location of pain
2. Character of pain
3. How and when the pain started
4. Is it continuous or intermittent?
5. Exacerbating and relieving factors
6. Effects of certain positions and activities on pain
7. Effects of stress on the pain experience
8. Effects of alcohol and other substances on pain
9. Is there an associated sleep disturbance?
10. Is there an associated mood disturbance?
11. Effect of pain on work and school
12. Effect of pain on quality of life including social, sexual and family interactions
13. Effect of pain treatment on cognitive, social, and sexual function
14. Motivation: Issues of secondary gain
15. Is a lawsuit involved?
16. Whom, if anyone, does the patient blame for his or her pain?

Goodwin J, Bajwa ZH. Evaluating the patient in chronic pain. In: Mintzer B, ed. Practical Pain Management. *New York, NY: McGraw Hill; 2001.*

devised to assess pain intensity. The verbal numerical scale, rating pain from zero for "no pain," to 10 for "the worst imaginable pain," is easily implemented and recorded during frequent assessments. Similarly, a visual analog scale may be used, with or without intensity descriptors. These instruments are useful for tracking pain intensity, but are unidimensional and therefore do not reflect the complexity of the pain experience. A visual or verbal analog pain score for one patient may not mean the same thing to another, but it is reliable on repeated use in the same patient, allowing serial assessments by different clinicians over the course of treatment. Pain scores should be recorded, like vital signs, with intervention performed when the score exceeds an acceptable level, although that considered acceptable to one person may not be so to another.

More sophisticated testing is also available, such as the McGill Pain Questionnaire (MPQ), which is frequently used in pain management centers. The patient chooses among 16 groups of descriptor's words that characterize the sensory, affective, and evaluative qualities of the pain. A pain intensity scale, a questionnaire on the use of analgesics, and prior pain experience, and a human figure drawing on which the patient indicates his pain location are also included in the MPQ. The disadvantage of the MPQ is that it is not self-administered, and takes up to 20 minutes to complete.

What improves the pain?

Questioning patients about factors that improve their pain, as well as its temporal characteristics, may prove helpful in deriving the mechanism of pain and directing treatment. Does it exhibit a periodicity, and how long does it last? Determine what types of therapy the patient has tried and what benefit, if any, they experienced. Inquire specifically about surgery, interventional procedures (diagnostic or therapeutic), medication use and side effects, physical therapy, chiropractic or osteopathic manipulation, and behavioral and complementary medicine.

Is there anything of importance in the past medical history?

Discovering comorbid medical conditions that may be associated with pain symptoms, such as diabetic neuropathy, AIDS, osteoarthritis and peripheral vascular disease is crucial not only diagnostically, but in making treatment decisions as well. The psychological history is of particular importance, especially with regards to depression, anxiety, and post-traumatic stress disorder. The presence of coexisting psychopathology may add complexity to the treatment of chronic pain, particularly where drug and alcohol addiction or depression are concerned, but should not lead the physician away from seeking a primary physical diagnosis.

How does the pain impact the patient's life?

It is important to know how the symptoms have impacted the patient's life at home, with friends, and at work. Does the patient have a social support structure in place, and has he or she been able to adapt to the impairment or disability, and the psychological stress that comes with chronic pain? What activities is the patient able or unable to perform as compared to a time prior to the onset of pain? Is the pain preventing the patient from caring for a child, working, or performing basic activities of daily living? Patients with severe and/or long-standing persistent pain are vulnerable to psychological dysfunction such as depression, anxiety, and other mood and sleep disorders. The physician must determine whether progress can be made in the absence of therapy directed toward the psychosocial component of the pain syndrome.

What previous evaluations have occurred?

Much of the work-up may have already been done, obviating the need for additional tests, and reviewing past results can save a lot of time, energy and costs for patients. However, it is important to avoid establishing a diagnostic bias based on chart review prior to meeting with the patient, since inaccuracies may be propagated through the chart over time.

The Physical Examination

The physical examination of patients with chronic pain begins by observing them as they move from the waiting area into the examination room. Do they stand up straight away, or do they push off with their arms, twisting into a stooped standing posture? Observation of gait can be illuminating. Is it antalgic or due to weakness or ataxia? Do they compensate for a bad leg or back by altering their gait, and is this motion placing other structures at risk for strain or injury? Observe pain behaviors throughout the examination, such as facial grimacing, verbalization of pain, and affect. Is affect congruent with apparent mood or topic of conversation? Pain behavior may represent severe discomfort with walking or moving through certain positions; however, it can also be a telltale sign of malingering or simply an attempt by the patient to convey (in an exaggerated way) that he or she has been suffering. And as previously stated, a patient with a long course of chronic pain may feel that the physician needs convincing that the problem is worthy of his or her time. Embellishment is neither unusual nor an indication that the pain is minimal or does not exist.

Note general appearance, dress, and hygiene. Note splinting and compensatory movements that patients in pain will use to protect a painful region of the body. Is this activity consistent throughout the examination? Although time limits may require a history-based physical examination, ideally a full physical examination should be performed regardless of the patient's complaint, including a complete or at least detailed/focused neurologic examination.

General Approach to Facial Pain

The diagnosis and management of patients with facial pain can prove daunting even to experienced clinicians. The causes are myriad, and misdiagnosis and mismanagement are common. As with other painful conditions, pain felt in the face does not necessarily originate in facial structures; pain may be local in origin or referred. A thorough medical history, including that of trauma and surgical and dental procedures, may provide valuable clues. Is there depression or other psychiatric signs or symptoms? What therapies have been tried and with what outcomes? A thorough physical and neurological examination is ideal and important for the reasons stated earlier.

Neuralgia, whether of the face or elsewhere, is defined as paroxysmal pain in the distribution of a nerve. The pain is typically maximal at onset and may be described as lancinating, "electric shocks," stabbing, or jabbing. There may be an occasional but intense, brief or sustained pain or frequently repetitive pains. It or they can last a fraction of a second, or persist far longer. There may be a refractory period after the severe pain during which such pain will not occur. Interictal aching pain may be present. Some neuralgic conditions have trigger zones (areas which, when stimulated, provoke an attack) or other triggers. Careful history taking may reveal other types of pain, such as continuous aching, burning, or throbbing. Inquiries must be made about all sensations that occur, as some patients mention only the severe ones. Response to treatment may provide a clue to diagnosis, but it can also prove misleading; "diagnostic blocks" in the setting of facial pain do not necessarily define the site from which the pain arises because of the overlap in innervation of cranial structures by cranial nerves V, VII, IX, X—all of which converge on the spinal trigeminal nucleus and the tractus solitarius.

Of particular importance in the evaluation of headache and facial pain are signs of raised intracranial pressure (ICP). Papilledema is the obvious clinical sign to look for, although about 5% of those with raised ICP may not develop it. Cranial nerve dysfunction, including pupillary abnormalities, must be ruled in or out. The head and neck also require careful attention. Are there myofascial trigger points that might be a source of referred pain or the result of an underlying skeletal problem? Is there evidence of dental or sinus pathology? Auscultation for bruits and palpation of the carotid artery are sometimes informative.

The need for imaging studies depends upon the history and physical examination findings, differential diagnosis, and type of films already obtained (and when). Magnetic resonance imaging is the most useful study for identifying mass lesions within the cranium as it is for demyelinating CNS disorders, although for a very recent bleed, CT scanning is the imaging modality of choice.

Trigeminal Neuralgia

Trigeminal neuralgia is one of the better understood, and fairly common causes, of facial pain. It tends to occur in paroxysms and is maximal at or near onset. It has been described as "electric shock-like" or "stabbing." The V2 and/or V3 branches of the 5th cranial nerve are involved far more frequently than is V1 (the lower jaw or mandibular region). Unlike some facial pain syndromes, trigeminal neuralgia typically does not awaken patients at night. The pain usually lasts from one to several seconds, but may occur repetitively. A refractory period of several minutes during which a paroxysm cannot be provoked is common. Occasionally the pain is bilateral, but is usually not on both sides simultaneously. There may also be a coexisting continuous, deep, dull pain. Facial muscle spasms can be seen with severe pain. This finding gave rise to the older term for this disorder, tic douloureux. If there is sensory loss by examination in the distribution of pain, a painful trigeminal neuropathy caused by a mass lesion in Meckel's cave should be suspected and a head MRI ordered immediately.

Many cases of TN may be caused by compression of the trigeminal nerve root, by an aberrant loop of an artery or vein, usually within a few millimeters of entry into the pons (the root entry zone). Other causes of nerve compression include vestibular schwannomas (acoustic neuromas), meningiomas, epidermoid or other cysts, and rarely, a saccular aneurysm or arteriovenous malformation. MS plaques near trigeminal nerve nuclei, or other structural lesions of the brainstem near the origin of the nerve root, can also lead to TN.

Table 3

Pharmacological Treatment of Trigeminal Neuralgia

Medication	Dose Range
Acute	
Phenytoin, IV	IV 250-1000 mg (no more than 50 mg/min)
Lidocaine , IV	IV 100 to 300 mg over one half hour
Chronic	
Carbamazepine	400 to 1200 mg/day
Gabapentin	900 to 2400 mg/day
Lamotrigine	200 to 400 mg/day
Oxcarbazepine	600 to 1200 mg/day
Pregabalin	150-300 mg/day
Valproate	600 to 1200 mg/day
Baclofen	30 to 80 mg/day
Topiramate	200 to 400 mg/day
Tizanidine	6 to 18 mg/day
Tiagabine	12 to 56 mg/day
Pimozide	4 to 12 mg/day
Clonazepam	2 to 8 mg/day

Goodwin J, Bajwa ZH. Evaluating the patient in chronic pain. In: Mintzer B, ed. Practical Pain Management. *New York, NY: McGraw Hill; 2001*

The mechanism by which compression of the nerve leads to symptoms is likely due to demyelination in a circumscribed region around the area of compression. Precisely how demyelination results in the symptoms of TN is not entirely clear, although demyelinative lesions may cause excessive firing of the nerve via accumulation of protein channels in large numbers at the site of demyelination (or within the cell bodies themselves, protein channels usually only found in the nodes of Ranvier). Ephaptic crosstalk between fibers mediating light touch and those involved in pain generation could account for the precipitation of painful attacks by light tactile stimulation of facial trigger zones. Here, one neuron directly excites another by electrical coupling. Another and distinct mechanism is crossed after discharge, where impulses from one neuron results in release of depolarizing substances that excites local neurons that would otherwise be at a subthreshold level for depolarization, and to which the first is not directly coupled. Furthermore, alteration of afferent or descending input may disinhibit pain pathways in the spinal trigeminal nucleus. Evidence for a role of central pain mechanisms includes the presence of refractory periods after a triggered episode, trains of painful sensations after a single stimulus, and latency from the time of stimulation to the onset of pain.

Pharmacologic therapy is the initial treatment of TN not caused by a structural lesion. Surgery or other invasive interventions are reserved for patients whose pain is refractory to medical therapy. About 70%-80% of patients do well with medical therapy. A variety of medications have been studied in the treatment of TN (Table 3). Carbamazepine is believed to be the most effective, although a variety of antiepileptic drugs are gathering support in the literature. The drug is highly effective, and side effects are generally manageable, particular if low doses are initially prescribed with gradual titration. Baclofen, phenytoin, valproate, pimozide, and clonazepam have utility as well, alone or in various combinations. Misoprostol (15-methyl-PGE1 analogue) appears to be effective in TN due to MS. Newer antiepileptic drugs such as gabapentin, pregabalin, lamotrigine, and topiramate have been reported useful, although there is less clinical experience with these agents. Oxcarbazepine, a keto derivative of carbamazepine, has also been reported as successful in treating TN.

Although there are no randomized and placebo controlled studies available regarding the efficacy of opioids in TN, they have been used very effectively in patients with acute exacerbations of TN pain lasting for days to weeks, and also initially while carbamazepine levels are slowly titrated to effect.

Spontaneous and permanent remission of TN has been reported. More often, it tends to wax and wane. Periodic attempts to gradually withdraw therapeutic medications are warranted in patients achieving relief of pain with oral medications.

Interventional Procedures for the Treatment of TN

Microvascular decompression involves the removal or separation of vascular structures from the nerve root, often an ectatic superior cerebellar artery. Long-term follow-up suggests 60%-70% of patients have good outcomes

Percutaneous radiofrequency rhizotomy creates a lesion in the Gasserian ganglion of the trigeminal nerve by application of heat. The lesion is thought to selectively destroy pain impulses carried by unmyelinated or thinly myelinated fibers. The ganglion is approached in Meckel's cave through the foramen ovale. The lesioning is performed in cycles of 45 to 90 seconds at 60 to 90 degrees Celsius. Percutaneous rhizotomy is less invasive than microvascular decompression, is associated with a low rate of morbidity and mortality, and has a higher initial success rate, but a recurrence rate of 25%-50% within 2 to 3 years. Creation of large lesions are more effective in preventing recurrence, but are associated with a higher likelihood of facial numbness and dysesthesia.

Retrogasserian glycerol rhizolysis involves the injection of 0.1 to 0.4 mL of glycerol into the trigeminal cistern. A tingling or burning sensation is felt on the face, and pain relief is usually immediate (although it sometimes requires up to seven days). Sensory loss can occur but is not necessary for pain relief; however, long-term relief may be greater in patients who experience some sensory loss. Pain recurrence is common after glycerol rhizolysis, with recurrence rates by six years as high as 92 percent.

Balloon compression is performed using a Fogarty catheter to compress the gasserian ganglion. The balloon is inflated with 0.5 to 1.0 ml of contrast dye for 1 to 6 minutes. This produces immediate pain relief but there may be persistent discomfort from dysesthesias.

Gamma knife therapy produces lesions with focused gamma radiation. Radiation is aimed at the proximal trigeminal root, since irradiation of the Gasserian ganglion itself produced poor results. The doses used are 70 to 90 Gy. The beams of gamma radiation appear to cause axonal degeneration and necrosis.

Linear accelerator radiosurgery provide a means for a noninvasive, outpatient treatment of TN, without patient sedation. Linear accelerator radiosurgery is similar to gamma knife radiosurgery but with a different source of radiation. A case series of 22 patients refractory to medical therapy, and that either declined or were unsuitable to undergo a surgical procedure, found radiosurgery by this technique to be safe and effective. Twenty-five of 32 patients in another series reported good to excellent results with a median time to pain relief of six weeks. Further study of this technique is warranted.

Peripheral neurectomy can be performed on branches of the trigeminal nerve, including the supraorbital, infraorbital, alveolar, and lingual nerves. Neurectomy is accomplished by incision, alcohol injection, radiofrequency lesioning, or cryotherapy. Cryotherapy involves freezing of the nerve using special probes, in theory to selectively destroy pain fibers.

Postherpetic Neuralgia

An acute outbreak of herpes zoster (shingles) may cause facial pain, especially affecting the V1 branch of the 5th cranial nerve. Postherpetic neuralgia (PHN) is variably defined as pain persisting after the rash has healed. On occasion there is no preceding rash. While PHN most often represents a continuance of pain that was never alleviated following an acute episode of herpes zoster, it has been reported to begin in patients months to years after complete resolution of the initial event. The pain of PHN is usually described as aching, burning, and/or lancinating, and sometimes associated with severe itch. More than 90% of patients with PHN also have allodynia (pain evoked by normally nonpainful stimuli such as light touch), and/or dysesthesias (unpleasant sensations to normally non-noxious stimuli, which often persist for several seconds). Areas of anesthesia as well as deficits in thermal, tactile, pinprick, and vibration sensation may be evident within the affected dermatomes; the contralateral, uninvolved side being normal on neurologic examination.

The major risk factors for PHN are older age, a suppressed immune system, very severe acute onset of pain, and greater severity of rash. Patients under age 40 rarely develop PHN unless immune suppressed; and 75% of patients afflicted with it are over the age of 70.

Treatment of acute herpes zoster with acyclovir, valacyclovir, famciclovir, steroids, pain medications, and even sympathetic nerve blocks may shorten the duration of rash and alleviate the immediate pain, although none has been clearly proven to prevent the occurrence of PHN. PHN may respond to a number of therapies such as antidepressants, analgesic drugs, capsaicin, topical anesthetics, anticonvulsants, intrathecal corticosteroids, NMDA receptor antagonists, cryotherapy and surgery. A systematic review of the literature concluded that the treatments shown to be more effective than placebo for PHN include tricyclic antidepressants (TCAs), topical capsaicin (0.075%), gabapentin, and controlled-release oxycodone, although the long-term benefits are uncertain, and side effects are common. Intrathecal methylprednisolone is of benefit in patients refractory to the above measures.

Opioids and TCAs appear to provide the most benefit. The latter is generally the first medication class of choice because of similar efficacy to opioids without the complication of physical dependency or the risk of addiction. However, opioids can be used if TCAs are unsuccessful. These drugs can also be administered simultaneously since TCAs may not be immediately effective. Frequently, the improvement in sleep associated with these medications results in a significant decrease in overall suffering (but if restless legs syndrome or periodic leg movements of sleep is present, TCAs are likely to worsen them and interfere with sleep). Aggressive titration often produces a discernible analgesic effect within the first week of therapeutic dosing. Anticonvulsant therapy with gabapentin or pregabalin is a reasonable alternative to treatment with TCAs, or may be added to TCA or opioid therapy. Other anticonvulsants appear to be effective as well. Topical capsaicin may provide relief, although it is often poorly tolerated. Topical lidocaine as a compounded cream (with or without TCAs and/or gabapentin used orally or topically), or in the form of commercially available 5% Lidoderm® patches, may provide short-term relief as well. Intravenous lidocaine may be effective in patients that do not respond to the aforementioned treatments. Intrathecal corticosteroid injections might also be considered for patients who continue to have intractable pain despite the measures recommended above. These injections do not work for trigeminal nerve-related pain.

Glossopharyngeal Neuralgia

Glossopharyngeal neuralgia is defined as paroxysmal pain in areas innervated by cranial nerve IX (and on occasion, a contribution by CN X). Demyelination can occur at the root of either cranial nerve—or rarely, where syncope coexists via asystole or bradycardia, input from CN IX into the tractus solitarius impacts the function of the dorsal motor nucleus of CN X. There are numerous similarities of this condition to trigeminal neuralgia, with which it occasionally coexists, although glossopharyngeal neuralgia is much less common, as well as more resistant to medical therapy. It is characterized by paroxysmal, severe, unilateral pain involving the ear, larynx, tonsil, or posterior tongue. It is almost never bilateral. Typical triggers include chewing, swallowing, coughing, speaking, yawning, certain tastes, or touching the neck or external auditory canal.

The pain typically radiates upward from the oropharynx toward the ear. The duration of the severe paroxysms lasts seconds to minutes, but there may also be a low grade, persistent and dull background pain. Several dozen attacks can occur per day, sometimes awakening the patient from sleep. Some episodes may also be associated with strenuous coughing and/or hoarseness. Like trigeminal neuralgia, glossopharyngeal neuralgia can occur in a pattern of episodes lasting weeks to months, alternating with longer periods of remission.

As with TN, there are idiopathic and secondary forms of GN. Secondary causes include demyelinating lesions, cerebellopontine angle tumor, peritonsillar abscess, carotid aneurysm, and Eagle syndrome (in which the glossopharyngeal nerve is compressed laterally against an ossified stylohyoid ligament or elongated styloid process). Vascular compression of CN IX can occur at the nerve root entry zone by the vertebral artery or posterior inferior cerebellar artery. The differential diagnosis of glossopharyngeal neuralgia includes "geniculate neuralgia" (nervus intermedius neuralgia of Hunt). The overlap of clinical features between the two conditions fosters suspicion that they may actually be variations of the same condition.

The evaluation of a patient suspected of suffering from glossopharyngeal neuralgia includes a careful history, especially inquiring about the presence of triggers and nocturnal awakening. MRI/MRA are indicated in virtually all patients to rule out a mass lesion or vascular pathology; plain skull films may reveal an ossified stylohyoid ligament (consistent with Eagle syndrome).

Medical therapy of glossopharyngeal neuralgia is essentially the same as for trigeminal neuralgia. In addition, application of local anesthetics to the oropharynx may prove both diagnostic and therapeutic. Surgical treatment is considered for patients for whom medical therapy failed (more common than with TN, up to 50%). Therapeutic procedures include intracranial sectioning of CN IX plus the upper three to four rootlets of CN X at the jugular foramen, or vascular decompression. The latter is a relatively safe procedure with good short- and long-term outcomes.

Superior Laryngeal Neuralgia

The superior laryngeal nerve is a branch of the vagus nerve that runs adjacent to the carotid bifurcation and innervates the cricothyroid muscle of the larynx. The nerve may be involved by local disease of the carotid artery or injured by carotid endarterectomy. Clinically, the patient suffers from paroxysmal pain radiating from the throat to the ear or eye, similar to that of glossopharyngeal neuralgia. The episodes last seconds to minutes and may occur spontaneously or can be triggered by coughing, swallowing, or speaking. During severe paroxysms the patient can temporarily be rendered mute. On examination, hoarseness of speech and a trigger point superolateral to the thyroid cartilage may be noted. Local blockade of the nerve is diagnostic, and some patients respond to carbamazepine and/or other drugs used for neuralgias. Neurectomy in selected refractory cases may be curative.

Cluster-Tic Syndrome

The cluster-tic syndrome is characterized by two types of pain. One component resembles the pain of trigeminal neuralgia and is paroxysmal, short lasting, and severe. The second component is more like a cluster headache, with autonomic phenomena (lacrimation, tearing). Pain may be provoked by stimulating trigger points or by moving the neck. The two pain manifestations are often time-locked with brief lancinating facial pain leading into an ipsilateral cluster headache. Cluster-tic syndrome can affect patients between 20 and 70 years of age. It may exist in chronic or episodic forms. Medical therapy usually consists of a combination of drugs used to treat trigeminal neuralgia and cluster headache, but is often unsuccessful. It has been reported that if surgery (microvascular decompression or trigeminal rhizotomy) relieves the neuralgia, the cluster-like pain may be lessened and then become more responsive to medical therapy.

Post-Traumatic Facial Pain

Facial pain can occur after trauma, including bullet wounds or other head injuries, and surgery. Facial pain may occur after maxillofacial surgery, orbital enucleations, sinus surgery, and dental procedures. In all cases of post-traumatic facial pain, a careful search must be conducted for underlying pathology, especially dental problems. Some patients manifest constant burning pain, occasionally with tingling and stabbing but without the trophic changes, edema, and redness characteristic of complex regional pain syndrome.

Treatment of post-traumatic facial pain can be extremely difficult. Blockade of the stellate ganglion may be effective in patients who complain of significant burning pain. Brief lancinating pains may respond to agents useful for neuralgias. Amitriptyline or other TCAs, for example, can reduce pain, improve sleep, and lessen associated depression and anxiety. Other agents useful for treating migraine headaches have been employed empirically for symptomatic benefit. Post-traumatic facial pain generally resolves spontaneously within several years.

Atypical Facial Pain

The International Headache Society's definition of atypical facial pain is "persistent facial pain that does not have the characteristics of the cranial neuralgias and is not associated with physical signs or a demonstrable organic cause." Idiopathic facial pain is another term that has been used to describe this condition, which is often ascribed to an underlying psychological disorder. Although such chronic facial pain is frequently associated with psychiatric disorders, particularly depression, this is no different from other chronic pain disorders in which psychiatric co-morbidity is common.

Idiopathic or atypical facial pain is usually a continuous dull ache with intermittent severe episodes, primarily affecting areas of the face other than joints and muscles of mastication. Pain may be bilateral, last for several years, and is unresponsive to analgesics. Patients frequently attribute their pain to an antecedent event such as a dental procedure or minor facial trauma. Some patients also complain of other symptoms such as headache, neck and backache, dermatitis, pruritus, irritable bowel, or dysfunctional uterine bleeding. The neurologic examination is, by definition, normal. It is likely that an equal number of men and women are affected by chronic facial pain, but many more women seek help for it.

In some cases, serious underlying pathology may not declare itself initially, but nasopharyngeal carcinoma and other cancers are eventually implicated. Only when a neurologic deficit appears (eg, cranial nerve palsies) may the real diagnosis become evident. Other reported causes include lung cancer (secondary to referred pain, presumably via CN X), and occult dental pathology (eg, infected cavities of maxillary and mandibular bones at the sites of previous extractions).

All patients presenting with idiopathic facial pain require a careful history and physical examination, including dental consultation, to rule out occult pathology. An MRI of the head, with attention to the base of the brain may also be indicated. A chest x-ray is warranted in smokers to rule out lung cancer. Serial examinations may be required for an occult process to declare itself.

The treatment of idiopathic facial pain is challenging and often requires a multidisciplinary approach. Mainstays of treatment include counseling and antidepressant medication. The efficacy of tricyclic antidepressants has been demonstrated in controlled trials and appears to be independent of the antidepressant effect. Fluoxetine has also been found effective in nondepressed patients with chronic facial pain. Behavioral interventions, such as biofeedback and cognitive behavioral therapy, may also provide some relief. In general, as with all chronic pain syndromes, effective patient-clinician communication facilitates the treatment process.

Burning Mouth Syndrome

Burning mouth syndrome (BMS) is defined as burning pain in one or several oral structures. Affected patients often present with multiple oral complaints, including burning, dryness and taste alterations. Burning mouth complaints are reported more often in women, especially after menopause. Typically, patients awaken without pain but note increasing symptoms through the day and into the evening.

Usually, no obvious etiology is found, but several possibilities exist that can be divided into local and systemic causes. A careful history and oral cavity examination assist in diagnosing the cause of BMS, which locally may include allergy, denture irritation, oral habits, infection (eg, oral candidiasis), and reflux esophagitis. Systemic causes include vitamin and mineral deficiency, diabetes mellitus, and chemotherapy.

Treatment is always aimed at the cause in BMS, when one is evident. In the majority of cases, however, there is no known etiology. In the absence of any local or systemic pathology, treatment is similar to that of other neuropathic conditions. Studies generally support the use of low doses of clonazepam, chlordiazepoxide, and tricyclic antidepressants. Evidence also supports the use of a low dose of gabapentin, and some patients have responded to capsaicin.

Table 4

Waddell's Signs of "Non-organic" Causes of Back Pain

- Superficial tenderness–tenderness of the skin on light palpation.
- Nonanatomic tenderness – tenderness in multiple anatomic distributions
- Axial loading test – production of pain when pressing lightly down on the top of the patient's head
- Pain with simulated rotation (rotating the shoulders and pelvis together)
- Distracted straight leg raising test–if a patient complains of pain on straight leg raising, but not if the examiner extends the knee when the patient is distracted
- Regional sensory change – stocking sensory loss in one limb
- Regional weakness with intermittent resistance
- Overreaction – exaggerated painful response to a stimulus, that is not reproduced when the same stimulus is given later

6. Spinal Radicular Pain

Low back pain is one of the most common reasons for physician office visits. In fact, 4 out of 5 people will have significant low back pain at some point in their lives. Radiculopathy pain is often seen by neurologists, and is also discussed in the "Peripheral Neuropathy" chapter in this volume.

Radicular pain is caused by irritation of the root(s) of spinal nerves. The most common causes in the lumbar region are disk herniation and spondylosis. Cervical radicular pain is caused by irritation of a cervical spinal nerve root, most often caused by disk herniation and foraminal stenosis. The two major factors involved in the radicular pain are compression and inflammation. Thoracic radicular pain is much less common and is generally due to diabetes mellitus or degenerative disk disease.

During the physical examination, the clinician should not overlook low-grade fever, which may signal the presence of an underlying infection such as diskitis or an epidural abscess. Inspection of the skin can help to rule in or out disorders such as psoriasis, neurofibromatosis, and herpes zoster. Examination of the abdomen is important to rule in or out an intra-abdominal process presenting with low back pain or thoracic pain (eg, aortic aneurysm). The neurologic examination should include gait assessment, motor and sensory testing, and the evaluation of reflexes and related phenomena such as the presence or absence of Spurling's sign (axial compression of the spine and rotation to the side of symptoms reproduces/worsening cervical radiculopathy symptoms); L'hermitte's sign (flexion of the neck produces electric shock-like sensations that extend down the spine and at times into the limbs; and Babinski reflex and Hoffman reflex (flicking the terminal phalanx of the third or fourth finger leads to flexion of the terminal phalanx of the thumb).

Waddell's signs (see Table 4) are supposed to help discover malingering or "non-organicity" of pain. Generally it is considered significant if more than two of these signs are present, and that a patient's surgical outcome is statistically less likely to be successful compared to someone with similar physical pathology, but for whom the examination lacks these signs. *It is important to remember that the presence of Waddell's signs does not rule in psychopathology or malingering as probable causes of pain, just as their absence does not rule them out.* If factitious disorder or malingering are suspected, thorough evaluation by a mental health professional, *knowledgeable about pain and its management*, should be sought in order to clarify psychosocial factors.

7. Other Pain Syndromes

Complex Regional Pain Syndrome

Complex regional pain syndrome (CRPS) type I and type II were previously referred to as reflex sympathetic dystrophy (RSD) or causalgia, respectively, depending on whether or not there was demonstrable motor nerve injury (causalgia). The clinical signs and symptoms are very similar, if not identical. They include sensory changes such as allodynia and hyperpathia, hyperalgesia, and hypoalgesia, changes in blood flow, distal limb edema, abnormalities of skin temperature, texture and hair distribution, sweating, tremors, weakness, reactive muscular spasm, localized pain referring trigger points, and dystonia. Before making the diagnosis of CRPS, it is important to exclude other causes of neuropathic pain as diagnostic, such as painful peripheral neuropathies, as well as other medical conditions like infectious, inflammatory and vasospastic disorders. It is not, however, a simple diagnosis of exclusion any more than is fibromyalgia; and neither should it be used inappropriately as a "waste-basket diagnosis." Psychiatric disorders and very common but less clinically severe maladaptive behaviors ("pain" or "illness" behavior) need to be fully addressed as well, usually so more from a therapeutic perspective than a diagnostic one. Even where there is no psychopathology, behavioral intervention can positively impact the outcome when combined with more physical modalities of treatment. The diagnostic criteria for CRPS are defined by the International Association for the Study of Pain (AISP) as outlined in Table 5.

The injury can be as minimal as an immunization shot or as severe as complex fractures. The incidence tends to be higher among women (60%)—the mean age ranging between 36 and 42—although it is seen in children and teenagers as well. The course is different in children, being more easily treated and more likely to spontaneously resolve. The lower extremities tend to be more frequently affected than is the case in adults, where the upper extremities predominate. In children, the female-to-male ratio is 5:1, and Caucasians are the most likely to develop this syndrome even when statistical bias has been taken into account. The reasons for these differences are unclear. The symptoms are generally disproportionate to the trauma, and they are not defined by a dermatomal spread. The pain is felt deep in the distal part of the affected limb.

CRPS is a neurologic disorder affecting the central and peripheral nervous systems. However, the pathogenesis is not completely clear. There are statistical associations between certain Class I and II HLA antigens in patients with poor clinical outcome. The current treatment guidelines focus on pain management, physical rehabilitation and cognitive-behavioral therapy. Pharmacologic therapies include TCAs, gabapentin, steroids, terazosin, phenoxybenzamine, clonidine, ketamine and opioids. Interventional regional anesthetic procedures can be used to provide pain relief in patients with or without sympathetically maintained pain (SMP), depending on the specific needs of the patient. In the past SMP was essential to diagnose CRPS. Today we know that SMP is not present in all the cases of CRPS. Spinal cord stimulation can be used, as can intrathecal pain pumps, when other therapies have failed. Some patients, especially teenagers and younger children, may need to be hospitalized for a few days with an indwelling epidural catheter providing analgesia to facilitate the physical therapist's use of a passive range of motion device, neuromuscular reeducation and desensitization, and the teaching of activity pacing. Individual counseling and the teaching of relaxation techniques and new coping skills and/or family therapy might be started at the same time.

A significant reduction in pain and a much improved level of function, both physically and psychosocially, are the general goals of management. Spinal cord stimulation and intrathecal pain pumps are useful for some patients with CRPS. Some extreme cases may require palliative surgery. Early rehabilitation therapy is crucial for CRPS using stress loading and isometric techniques as mentioned above, although high-dose pain medication is usually needed just to be able to participate.

Central Pain Syndromes

Central pain is defined as "pain associated with lesions of the central nervous system" and can be classified anatomically as spinal cord-related pain or brain-related central pain.

The most common cause of spinal cord pain is trauma from motor vehicle accidents. Other causes include spine surgery, inflammation, neoplasm, vascular diseases and congenital disease. With brain

Table 5

International Association for the Study of Pain (IASP) Criteria for CRPS I and CRPS II

CRPS I

1. The presence of an initiating noxious event, or a cause of immobilization.
2. Continuing pain, allodynia or hyperalgesia, with which the pain is disproportionate to any inciting event.
3. Evidence at some time of edema, changes in skin blood flow, or abnormal sudomotor activity in the region of the pain.
4. This diagnosis is excluded by the existence of conditions that would otherwise account for the degree of pain and dysfunction.

CRPS II

1. The presence of continuing pain, allodynia or hyperalgesia after a nerve injury, not necessarily limited to the distribution of the injured nerve.
2. Evidence at some time of edema, changes in skin blood flow, or abnormal sudomotor activity in the region of the pain.
3. This diagnosis is excluded by the existence of conditions that would otherwise account for the degree of pain and dysfunction.

Table 6

Selected Pain Treatment Options in Palliative Care

Non-opioid analgesics	
Acetaminophen	500-1000 mg po q4-6h
Naproxen sodium	220-550 mg po q8h
Ketorolac	30-60 mg IM/IV
Opioids – initial analgesic doses	
Levorphanol (8x)*	2-4 mg po q6h; 1-2 mg IV q6-8h
Hydromorphone (4x)	4-8 mg po q3h; 1-2 mg IV q3h
Methadone (1.5x)	20 mg po q6-8h; 10 mg IV q6-8h
Morphine (1x)	20-60 mg po q3-4h; 10 mg IV q3-4h
Oxycodone (1x)	5-10 mg po q3-4h
Hydrocodone (1x)	5-10 mg po q3-4h
Meperidine (0.1x)	100 mg IM q2-3h

**relative strength in parentheses – eg, levorphanol is 8x more potent than morphine per mg*

related central pain, approximately 90% of the cases have a vascular etiology. Thalamic and cortical sensory misprocessing has been identified as sources of central pain. Characteristic symptoms include muscle pains or cramps; dysesthesias; hyperthermia due to CNS disinhibition; allodynia; shooting pain; circulatory pain (pins and needles); and peristaltic or visceral pain.

Central pain remains one of the most difficult to treat syndromes for physicians. Lidocaine IV is the most effective therapy for central pain; however, the need to administer the drug intravenously limits its use. The oral analogue of lidocaine, mexilitine, has not proven as effective. Other medications that can be used include amitriptyline 50 to 100 mg/day, lamotrigine, gabapentin, pregabalin, topiramate and opioids. It is also important to treat muscle spasticity; significant increase in muscle tone due to poorly controlled spasticity can lead to significant pain. Medications that can be used include baclofen, tizanidine and benzodiazepines, all of which may also have some anti-pain properties as well.

Thalamic pain is described as unilateral facial and/or body pain and dysesthesia attributed to a lesion in or near the thalamus. It is typically a moderate to severe, burning or aching pain to the contralateral side of the face, trunk and/or limbs of the affected side. Pain can present with hemiplegia, hyperesthesia, allodynia, or hyperalgesia (significantly heightened sensitivity to painful stimuli). MRI or CT scan usually demonstrates a lesion in the thalamic region. Treatment options are varied, including tricyclic antidepressants, antiepileptics or other membrane-stabilizing agents, and opioids alone or in combination (rational polypharmacy). Other options include stimulation-produced analgesia, such as acupuncture, TENS (transcutaneous nerve stimulation), and deep brain stimulation.

Cancer Pain

Pain in cancer patients can be caused by direct effects of the tumor (eg, invasion of bone by tumor, distention of sensate tissues, or direct nerve compression) or by complications of treatment (eg, radiation fibrosis, chemotherapy-induced neuropathy, postoperative surgical pain). In addition, the possibility that pain is unrelated to either the malignancy or its treatment must be considered. In pediatric neoplastic disease, pain is more likely the result of interventions and treatment as opposed to the situation in adults where the pain most often results from the direct effects of the neoplasms themselves.

Any physician involved in the field of pain management needs to recognize the development and progression of cancer-related pain whether due to pharmacologic tolerance, a change in the mechanism of pain due to cancer spread or changing pressure from mass lesions, deconditioning, or anxiety and depression. They should be able to initiate treatment for the more common causes with opioid and non-opioid analgesics (see Table 6). Initially, treatment should include non-opioid with or without adjuvant medications. (Adjuvant medications include antidepressants, antiepileptics, corticosteroids, sedatives, and antinauseants.) With persisting or increasing pain, opioid agents should be added along with addition of other adjuvant medication choices. Clonidine and alpha-2 receptor agonist seems to add analgesic benefit as well in many patients. Calcitonin and biophosphonates are useful in bone pain, as is palliative radiation therapy. Topical analgesics can be useful (lidocaine), and treating uncomfortable systemic dysfunction such as constipation, muscle spasm and nausea is of course essential.

Effective pain relief without intolerable side effects is occasionally difficult to obtain with the use of conventional analgesics, even with escalating doses of opioids. In these circumstances, consultation with a specialist in pain management may be necessary. In terminal cases, more aggressive surgery can be contemplated, including neurolysis, dorsal root ganlionectomy, and a number of spinal cord procedures such as dorsal root entry zone (DREZ) lesioning, cordotomy, and tractotomy. Deep brain stimulation (generally thalamic) is also an option.

It is always important to remember that uncontrolled pain, the adverse effects of opioids and other analgesics, and the fear of pain itself can contribute to depression, which may precipitate suicidal thoughts or requests for aid in dying. Pain also adds to the discomfort experienced by those caring for the dying patient, and managing it well reduces much of the distress to family and friends of the patient, not to mention the patient him or herself. Taking care of the patient's family's emotional needs as well as those of the patient is a central theme in palliative hospice care. A very useful resource for patients with cancer related pain (and their families) is the subpage of the National Institute of Cancer web site: www.cancer.gov/cancertopics/paincontrol.

8. Conclusion

Acute and chronic pain can occur via a number of different mechanisms. The experience of pain is based on physical, psychological and social factors, all of which can be modulated in order to reduce the pain patient's suffering. It is essential for the clinician to understand types of pain (nociceptive vs. neuropathic) and their contributing factors in order to optimize patient care.

9. References

Allen G, Galer BS, Schwartz L. Epidemiology of complex regional pain syndrome: a retrospective chart review of 134 patients. *Pain*.1999;80:539-44

(The main difference between Complex Regional Pain Syndrome type I and type II is the presence of initiating noxious event. The symptoms are generally disproportionate to the trauma, and they are not defined by a dermatomal spread.)

Ashkenazi A, Levin M. Three common neuralgias: how to manage trigeminal, occipital, and postherpetic pain. *Postgraduate Medicine*. 2004;116(3):16-32.

(A summary of the pathologic mechanisms of pain in these common neuralgias with individually tailored pharmacologic and surgical approaches to their treatment.)

Attal N, Caude V, Brasseur L, et al. Intravenous lidocaine in central pain: a double-blind, placebo-controlled, psychophysical study. *Neurology*. 2000;54:564-574.

(IV lidocaine may be the most effective treatment for central pain. Other medications can be used but they are not as effective, and some others like opioids are controversial.)

Butler S. Disuse and CRPS. In: Harden RN, Baron R, Janig W, eds. *Complex Regional Pain Syndrome*. Seattle, Wash: IASP Press; 2001:141-50.

(Early rehabilitation therapy using stress loading and isometric techniques are an essential part of the treatment for CRPS.)

Bruyn GW. Superior laryngeal neuralgia. *Cephalalgia*. 1983;3:235.

(Injury of the superior laryngeal nerve is a common complication after carotid surgery. Local blockade of the nerve is a diagnostic tool to differentiate this neuralgia from glossopharyngeal neuralgia.)

Campbell FG, Graham JG, Zilkha KJ. Clinical trial of carbazepine (Tegretol) in trigeminal neuralgia. *J Neurol Neurosurg Psychiatr*.1966;29:265.

(Carbamazepine is the first-line therapy for trigeminal neuralgia. But due to the side effects it can be combined with other drugs. It should be prescribed initially at a low dose and gradually titrated depending on the patient response and side effects.)

Jaeger B, Singer E, Kroening R. Reflex sympathetic dystrophy of the face. Report of two cases and a review of the literature. *Arch Neurol*.1986;43:693.

(Early and aggressive treatment of complex regional pain syndrome is essential to improve patient outcome. Treatment delay may lead to fast progression of the disease.)

Jannetta PJ. Microsurgical management of trigeminal neuralgia. *Arch Neurol*.1985;42:800.

(Interventional procedures for the treatment of trigeminal neuralgia include microvascular decompression, percutaneous radiofrequency rhizotomy, retrogasserian glycerol rhizolysis, balloon compression, linear accelerator radiosurgery, and peripheral neurectomy. The success rate of each of this procedures varies, and the patient should consider different modalities.)

Kost RG, Straus SE. Postherpetic neuralgia – pathogenesis, treatment, and prevention. *N Engl J Med*. 1996;335:32.

(Most patients with postherpetic neuralgia are older than 70 years. Patients under age of 40 generally will be immune suppressed.)

Levin KH, Covington EC, Devereaux MW, et al. Neck and low back pain. *Continuum* (NY). 2001;7:1-205.

(The most common cause of radicular low back pain and radicular cervical pain is due to nerve root irritation by disc herniation. Physical and neurologic examination should include gait assessment, motor and sensory testing, and evaluation of reflexes.)

Levin M. Changing the face of pain management: mechanism-based treatment most likely to succeed. *Postgraduate Med*. 2004;116(3):45-8.

(Mechanism-based pain treatment is discussed along with an overview of pain mechanisms.)

Love S, Coakham HB. Trigeminal neuralgia: pathology and pathogenesis. *Brain*. 2001;124:2347.

(The most common cause of trigeminal neuralgia is due to compression of the trigeminal nerve root within the entry into the pons or the root entry zone.)

McQuay HJ, Tramer M, Nye BA, et al. A systematic review of antidepressants in neuropathic pain. *Pain*. 1996;68:217.

Melzack R, Wall PD. Pain mechanisms: A new theory. *Science*. 150:171-9, 1965.

(Their famous article proposing the Gating Theory of Pain modulation.)

Melzack R. The McGill pain questionnaire: Major properties and scoring methods. *Pain*. 1975; 1:277.

(The McGill Pain Questionnaire (MPQ) is the standard pain questionnaire used in most pain management centers in the USA. The disadvantage of this questionnaire is that it takes up to 20 minutes to complete and is not self-administered.)

Mersky H. Classification of chronic pain: Description of chronic pain syndromes and definition of pain terms. *Pain*. 1986;S1(3).

(Classification of different types of chronic types of pain by the IASP.)

Revill SI, Robinson JO, Rosen M, Hogg MI. The reliability of a linear analogue for evaluating pain. *Anaesthesia*. 1976;31:1191.

(Pain scores are only reliable if used repeatedly in the same patient, and different patients have different pain scores depending on different factors such as sex, cultural background and lifestyles.)

Schott GD. Triggering of delayed-onset postherpetic neuralgia. *Lancet*. 1998;351:419.

(Postherpetic neuralgia can begin months to years after the first episode; however, in most cases the pain continues from an acute episode of herpes zoster.)

Woolf CJ, Mannion RJ. Neuropathic pain: aetiology, symptoms, mechanisms, and management. *Lancet*. 1999;353:1959.

(A mechanism-based approach to the treatment of neuropathic pain.)

10. Questions

1. The "affective" pain system contains:

A. A delta fibers

B. C fibers

C. 2nd order neurons with small receptive fields

D. Lateral thalamic nuclei

2. A 62-year-old female with hoarseness comes to your office complaining of episodes of sharp pain that radiates from her throat to her eye. Usually, the episodes last 20 to 40 seconds and are triggered when she coughs. During her last visit you injected 4 cc of a long-acting local anesthetic around the trachea using the hyoid bone as a landmark. Today she tells you that after that injection she did not have any episodes of pain for 24 hrs. The most likely diagnosis is:

A. Glossopharyngeal neuralgia

B. Geniculate neuralgia

C. Superior laryngeal neuralgia

D. Carotodynia

3. During a routine phlebotomy, a 31-year-old woman experiences immediate shooting pain in the radial side of her hand. Afterwards, pain persisted in her distal forearm and hand. Over the course of the next several months pain continued, and both color changes and edema were noted in the affected limb. In this patient, one can differentiate CRPS type I from CRPS type II based upon:

A. Time of onset of symptoms

B. Intensity of pain and time of onset

C. Etiology

D. Type of symptoms

4. Which of the following cranial nerves does not contain afferent nociceptive nerves?

A. II

B. VII

C. IX

D. X

5. Hyperalgesia is defined as:

A. Spontaneous pain in an area or region

B. Pain initiated by dysfunction in the nervous system

C. Pain caused by a stimulus that does not normally produce pain

D. Increased pain response to stimulus that is normally painful

6. Allodynia is defined as:

A. Spontaneous pain in an area or region

B. Pain initiated by dysfunction in the nervous system

C. Pain caused by a stimulus that does not normally produce pain

D. Increased response to stimulus that is normally painful

7. A neurology consult is sought for a 64-year-old female patient with a chief complaint of pain in the distribution of the trigeminal nerve for the past 2 weeks. She has no other medical condition except for high blood pressure, for which she takes furosemide once per day. The appropriate treatment would be:

A. Administer fentanyl patch

B. Initiate therapy with IV lidocaine

C. Obtain neurologic workup for multiple sclerosis

D. Initiate therapy with carbamazepine

8. Which of the following is not associated with complex regional pain syndrome?

A. Hyperesthesia

B. Dermatomal distribution of pain

C. Tremors

D. Allodynia

9. The mechanism of the transcutaneous electrical nerve stimulator (TENS) in relieving pain is:

A. Direct electrical inhibition of type A and C fibers

B. Activation of inhibitory neurons

C. Hyperpolarization of spinothalamic tract neurons

D. Depletion of neurotransmitters in nociceptors

10. Types of peripheral neuropathic pain include all but:

A. Diabetic neuropathy

B. Trigeminal neuralgia

C. Dejerine-Roussy syndrome

D. Cervical radiculopathy pain

11. A 32-year-old woman patient has had a history of right-sided headaches and facial pain for the last month. The facial pain generally precedes longer-lasting (1 hour) ipsilateral supraorbital pain of the headaches, and facial pain is variable; however, every time she has the facial pain, her "eye gets really wet like I am crying," and she develops nasal congestion. The most likely diagnosis is:

A. Cluster-tic syndrome

B. SUNCT syndrome

C. Thalamic pain

D. Complex regional pain syndrome

12. A seamstress pricks her index finger while sewing and immediately jerks it away. The type of nerve fibers that initially conducts the afferent pain signal to the CNS will be:

A. Unmyelinated A-delta fibers

B. Myelinated A-delta fibers

C. Unmyelinated C fibers

D. Myelinated C fibers

13. The descending antinociceptive system includes cells in the following nuclei except:

A. Red nucleus

B. Locus ceruleus

C. Nucleus raphe magnus

D. Rostral ventromedial medulla

14. A 74-year-old diabetic hypertensive man had a stroke 2 months ago with residual right-sided numbness in the face and trunk. For the past several weeks he has been complaining of right-sided burning and aching facial pain. The most likely diagnosis is:

A. Complex regional pain syndrome

B. Trigeminal neuralgia

C. SUNCT syndrome

D. Central thalamic pain

15. Which of the following would be most effective in reducing the previous patient's pain?

A. IV lidocaine

B. IV amitriptyline

C. IV gabapentin

D. IV lamotrigine

16. Central sensitization is generally a phenomenon that occurs at the level of the:

A. 1st order nociceptor

B. 2nd order nociceptor

C. Thalamus

D. Cortex

17. A 52-year-old man with R upper lobe lung cancer begins to have pain in his distal R upper extremity. Exam and radiological work-up reveals no neoplastic involvement of the arm. He is most likely to be suffering from:

A. Referred pain

B. Central neuropathic pain

C. Peripheral neuropathic pain

D. Nociceptive pain

18. A 40-year-old mechanic complains of disabling back pain since a twisting injury at work. You decide to investigate possible malingering with Waddell's sign testing. Which of the following is not one of Waddell's signs?

A. Hoover's test

B. Superficial tenderness

C. Axial loading test

D. Distracted straight leg raising test

19. A 68-year-old healthy woman developed "shingles" on her forehead several weeks ago. The scabs have healed but she continues to complain of burning and lancinating pain in the region of the outbreak. Which would be least likely to be effective for her syndrome?

A. Tricyclic antidepressants

B. Sertraline

C. Gabapentin

D. Topical lidocaine patches

20. A 56-year-old man with pancreatic cancer is experiencing moderate to severe pain. Which of the following would be a reasonable starting dose?

A. Levorphanol 20 mg po q6h

B. Hydromorphone 4-8 mg po q 8h

C. Morphine 10 mg IV q3-4h

D. Oxycodone 50 mg po q3-4h

Answers

1. B
The medial or affective nociceptive system begins with C fibers (so is slower), has 2nd order neurons with wide fields, and includes more medial thalamic nuclei.

2. C.
The superior laryngeal nerve (SLN) is a branch of the vagus nerve which provides sensory innervation to the base of the tongue and epiglottis, and motor innervation to the cricothyroid muscle. Clinically, patients with superior laryngeal neuralgia suffer from paroxysmal pain radiating from the throat to the ear or eye, similar to glossopharyngeal neuralgia. The episodes last seconds to minutes and may occur spontaneously or be triggered by coughing, swallowing, or speaking. However, the indication that she was without pain for 24 hrs after blocking the SLN guided the diagnosis to superior laryngeal neuralgia. One of the different approaches to block this nerve is to insert a needle at the level of the thyrohyoid membrane just inferior to the hyoid bone.

3. C.
Complex regional pain syndrome is one of the most challenging pain syndromes to treat and diagnose. Prompt diagnosis and initiation of treatment is crucial. The presence of nerve injury is essential to diagnose CRPS type 2 as defined by the guidelines of the International Association for the Study of Pain (IASP). (International Association for the Study of Pain diagnostic criteria for CRPS I and CRPS II.) In this patient, the lancinating pain initially experienced suggests a median nerve injury.

4. A.
Pain from the face and head is carried by cranial nerves V, VII, IX, X, and from the posterior division of the upper cervical nerves (C2 and C3).

5. D.
Hyperalgesia is exaggerated pain caused by a normally minimally painful stimulus.

6. C.
Allodynia is pain caused by a stimulus that does not normally provoke pain.

7. D.
A response to carbamazepine is considered diagnostic for TN by some experts. The current literature favors it as first-line therapy.

8. B.
One of the most puzzling things about the pain distribution of CRPS is that it is not a dermatomal distribution type of pain.

9. B.
TENS is a low-intensity, mixed frequency electrical stimulation that is thought to produce analgesia either via the gating theory (ie, stimulating A delta fibers which act to inhibit the A delta and C fiber mediated nociceptive pathway), or by leading to the release of endorphins.

10. C.
Neuropathic pain is termed peripheral if the dysfunction lies in the primary afferent neuron. Dejerine-Roussy syndrome is due to a thalamic lesion, generally a stroke.

11. A.
The cluster-tic syndrome is characterized by three types of pain. One component resembles the pain of trigeminal neuralgia and is paroxysmal, short lasting, and severe. The second component is more like a cluster headache, although of variable length, with autonomic phenomena (lacrimation, tearing). The pain of SUNCT (short unilateral neuralgiform pain with conjunctival inflammation and tearing) is similar but very brief and not followed by headaches.

12. B.
Myelinated nociceptors are relatively fast conducting A-delta fibers. Some respond readily to heat, the mechanothermal receptors (MTRs); others are high threshold mechanoreceptors (HTMs). The discharge intensity is linearly related to the degree of the stimulus.

13. A.
The midbrain periaqueductal gray region (PAG) is crucial in the descending antinociceptive system, which also includes the serotonergic nucleus raphe magnus of the medulla, the noradrenergic locus ceruleus in the pons, and the rostral ventromedial medulla (RVM).

14. D.
Central thalamic pain can present with unilateral facial pain and dysesthesia, and is attributed to a lesion in the region of the thalamus. It is typically a moderate to severe burning or aching pain to the contralateral side of the face. Accompanying symptoms may involve the trunk and limb of the affected side, and pain can present with hemiplegia, hyperesthesia, allodynia, or hyperpathia.

15. A.
One of the most effective treatments for central pain is IV lidocaine. It is difficult to use for chronic pain for obvious reasons, but the oral form, mexiletine, may be tried.

16. B.
The 2nd order neuron in the dorsal horn becomes hyperactive in central sensitization as a result of continued stimulation.

17. C.
This patient most likely has neoplastic involvement of the R brachial plexus, a peripheral neuropathic pain syndrome.

18. A.
Hoover's test (designed to show lack of effort in ileopsoas strength testing), like Waddell's tests, is a sign of factitious disorder or malingering. It is not one of Waddell's signs of non-organic spinal pain, however.

19. B.
All of the following are recommended as first line treatments for post-herpetic neuralgia: tricyclic antidepressants, gabapentin, pregabalin, opioids, and topical lidocaine patches.

20. C.
Levorphanol and oxycodone doses are too high for a starting dose. The timing for hydromorphone is too infrequent.

Chapter 25: Inflammatory Demyelinating Disorders of the Central Nervous System

Peter N. Riskind, MD, PhD

Contents

Introduction

Multiple sclerosis (MS) and its variants (neuromyelitis optica, acute disseminated encephalitis) typically affect young and otherwise healthy individuals during their peak childbearing- and career-developing years. The episodic, unpredictable nature of many symptoms and variable but often severe disability further add to the devastating effects of these illnesses. They share many characteristics, such as a presumed autoimmune etiology, CNS inflammation, and loss of both oligodendroglial cells and nerve fibers. At present, it is unclear whether they are completely distinct illnesses or part of a spectrum of a single illness.

1. Multiple Sclerosis

In Western countries, MS is a common inflammatory demyelinating disorder. Indeed, it is the most important neurologic cause of disability in young adults in this country.

Epidemiology

Current estimates suggest that about 400,000 individuals are affected with MS in the United States. The age of onset ranges from childhood up to the sixth decade of life, with peak incidence in the third decade. MS prevalence is highest from 40-59 years of age.

Women are affected more often than men, with an average female-to-male ratio of 2.6:1. In younger patients the female-to-male ratio approaches 4:1, whereas it is nearer to 1:1 in middle-aged onset patients.[19] Some studies suggest that the incidence and prevalence of MS is rising in women in comparison to men. Life expectancy is reduced by about seven years, mainly due to infectious complications of immobility.

Risk Factors

The risk of MS varies widely among different ethnic groups, and in different geographic locations. This phenomenon is thought to reflect genetic as well as environmental factors.

The strongest evidence in support of a genetic basis of MS risk comes from studies on twins and other family members.[27] Identical twins of an affected individual have a risk of MS of 35%, whereas fraternal twins or other sibs have a risk of 4% (which is 20-50 times the overall risk of individuals in this country). The observation that 65% of twins are *discordant* for MS implies that environmental factors have a profound effect upon MS risk.

The clearest linkage of MS with any allele has been the association with HLA-DR2, although recent evidence also suggests linkage to the Interleukin2 and Interleukin7 receptors. It is likely that a large number of alleles help to confer either enhanced susceptibility or protection against acquiring MS, and the resultant combination of those alleles in any individual contributes a sum risk of the disease.

MS is most common in Caucasians, particularly individuals of northern European descent.[31] In contrast, MS is relatively uncommon among Asians or black Africans residing in their regions of origin. In general, African Americans and Asian Americans have a higher risk of MS than individuals remaining in their countries of origin.

MS has an unusual geographic distribution, with lowest overall risk observed in locations near to the equator, and higher risk in either Northern or Southern hemisphere locations that are distant from the equator. This pattern is now thought to result from settlement patterns of different ethnic groups (eg, more Swedish immigrants immigrated to northern parts of the US), and also from important environmental factors that vary with latitude. Individuals emigrating from a high-risk area to a low-risk area (or vice versa) before the age of 15 acquire the risk associated with their new home, whereas immigration after age 15 does not affect subsequent risk.

The recent observation that total sun exposure during childhood and early adulthood substantially affects MS risk suggests one potential explanation.[30] Presumably, sun exposure has a beneficial effect, through induction of vitamin D production (which is immunosuppressive). Indeed, analysis of blood samples obtained at entry into the US armed forces suggests that low vitamin D levels are associated with an increased risk of subsequently developing MS, whereas high vitamin D levels may be protective.

Another proposed mechanism has been geographic differences in either endemic infections or in the age at which individuals might be infected with viruses. For example, delayed initial exposure to infections might promote autoimmunity, or early exposure might have a preventive effect upon MS risk. This issue remains unresolved. A recent study indicates no difference in age of exposure to six common childhood infections in individuals with or without MS, but another study has reported that a higher infant sibling exposure during the first six years of life was associated with a reduced MS risk.

The clearest association of an infection with MS is with the Epstein-Barr virus (EBV). In developing countries EBV infection commonly occurs in infants and young children, causing a relatively nonspecific viral syndrome. However, in the United States and other developed countries, EBV often affects teenagers and young adults, causing "mononucleosis". A history of mononucleosis has been reported to occur more than five times as often in adults that subsequently developed MS than in controls. More importantly, EBV antibody titers measured in more than 3 million members of the United States military were higher in individuals that subsequently developed MS. Indeed, rises in viral titers were found up to five years before MS onset. Premorbid viral titers were identical in controls and in MS patients before 20 years of age, but rose several fold in MS patients at age 25 or higher, independent of age of MS onset. Finally, the rise of EBV titers occurred in individuals that were already EBV-positive, suggesting that they may have been exposed to another strain of EBV or other infection, triggering a second rise of viral titers.

Other candidate infectious factors have also been proposed, with some evidence supporting a role of human herpes virus-6 and *Chlamydia pneumoniae*.

Although associated with a reduced *risk* of MS, both male gender and African-American ethnicity are associated with an increased *severity* of MS.

Late-onset MS (eg, in middle age or later) is associated with both a higher likelihood of primary progressive disease and a shorter latency to develop secondary progressive disease.

Clinical Classification

The clinical classification of MS rests upon two key phenomena, the *flare* and *progression*.

An MS *flare* (attack, exacerbation) is characterized by a relatively rapid development of neurologic symptoms and signs, followed by partial or complete recovery. Most research studies have required at least 24 or 48 hours duration of the neurologic episode in order to qualify as a flare. As flares may be polyphasic, an interval of 30 days stability or improvement is conventionally required before any new events are considered a separate flare. Typical flares evolve over hours to weeks, but in some cases neurologic symptoms and signs may appear suddenly and with maximal severity ("stroke-like onset"). Flares may be followed by incomplete recovery.

The interval between recognized flares is termed *remission*, although imaging and immunological studies suggest that the disease is not actually quiescent. Nonetheless, the term "remission" implies that there is no progressive clinical deterioration or flare activity. Remissions are of extremely variable duration, ranging from months to decades. MS *progression* is a slow, insidious and often initially unrecognized loss of neurologic function occurring over months to years, with or without a previous history of flares.

Current classification of MS rests principally upon whether the illness begins with a flare versus onset of progressive disability in the absence of any history of preceding flare.[15] Flare-onset MS represents about 85% of cases. The initial flare often involves a single part of the CNS, and is termed a *clinically isolated syndrome*. Historically, MS has not been diagnosed until a second episode is recognized, as many patients do not have further episodes. Individuals having at least two flares, but with clinical stability between flares, are diagnosed with relapsing remitting MS. Two subtypes are recognized, relapsing remitting MS with complete recovery, and *relapsing remitting MS* with incomplete recovery. After varying intervals of relapsing remitting disease, the majority of MS patients ultimately develop progression between or in addition to flares. This marks the beginning of *secondary progressive MS*. The precise point of transition from relapsing remitting disease is usually impossible to determine.

About 10% of patients experience progressive disability from onset, without any flares. This pattern is termed *primary progressive MS*. Progressive myelopathy or cerebellar dysfunction are two common presentations of this form of MS. About 5% of MS patients develop progression from onset (like primary progressive MS) but there are superimposed flares (like secondary progressive MS). This pattern is termed *progressive relapsing MS*. This nosology has replaced an older terminology that grouped all progressive forms into a single category, *chronic progressive MS*.

Natural History

Flares are considered to result from acute focal or multifocal inflammation within the CNS, causing acute demyelination as well as elaboration of free radicals and other substances that likely induce local conduction block. Flares correlate reasonably well with acute inflammatory changes on MRI (see below). The occurrence of a clinical flare is determined not only by having an active lesion, but also by the location of the lesion within the CNS. That is, when lesions are located in "clinically-eloquent" areas (those that cause noticeable symptoms and signs) they are clinically detectible, whereas active lesions in "silent" parts of the CNS may not be recognized. Such "silent" active lesions may be appreciated on serial MRI at a rate up to ten times the number of clinical flares. It remains unclear whether most flares are "spontaneous" or whether they are triggered by environmental factors as a rule. There is convincing evidence that up to one-third of flares are triggered by nonspecific viral infections. Claims that MS flares result from physical trauma (eg, motor vehicle accidents) are unsupported. However, severe stress (bereavement) appears to increase the risk of a first MS episode. Another well established influence upon MS flares is the biphasic effect of pregnancy and delivery[5] (see below). Flares should be distinguished from a separate phenomenon, the *pseudo-exacerbation*, in which old symptoms and signs reappear in the context of infection, severe fatigue, or elevated body temperature. In this case the duration of symptoms is much briefer than in most flares and resolves quickly with control of the triggering stimulus.

Recovery from the initial flare is often excellent. The duration of subsequent clinical remission is quite variable, but the highest risk of a second episode is within the next two years. Importantly, frequent inflammatory events may be appreciated on serial MRI scans during "remission", occurring at a ratio of up to 10 times the frequency of clinical flares. Thus, one cannot assume that clinical stability is equivalent to actual disease remission. The frequency of flares is quite variable, but averages about 0.5 per year in most studies of patients with early relapsing remitting disease.

Table 1

Patterns of Demyelination

I	II	III	IV
T lymphocytes + macrophages	T lymphocytes + macrophages	T lymphocytes + macrophages	T lymphocytes + macrophages
no complement	extensive complement	no complement	no complement
perivenous	perivenous	not perivenous	not perivenous
sharp margins	sharp margins	indistinct margins	sharp margins
oligodendrocyte loss in the active lesion border	oligodendrocyte loss in the active lesion border	apoptotic oligodendrocytes and loss of MAG	oligodendrocyte loss in the peri-plaque white matter
oligodendrocyte reappearance in the inactive center	oligodendrocyte reappearance in the inactive center	few oligodendrocytes in the inactive center	few oligodendrocytes in the inactive center
shadow plaques present	shadow plaques present	shadow plaques absent	shadow plaques absent

The frequency of flares and new lesions on MRI imaging are highest early in the disease, when the "inflammatory" component of MS predominates clinically. Clinical variables that suggest earlier onset of disability include a progressive course, frequent relapses in the first two years (especially within the first year), male gender, polysymptomatic onset, and predominant motor or cerebellar involvement.[6,23] Of these variables, development of a progressive course is the strongest predictor of future disability.

Progression of disability is an insidious worsening over months to years. Indeed, progression is typically so slow that it is only recognized long after onset. Although progression may plateau, by definition there is no recovery of disability. The major mechanism underlying progression is thought to be axonal transaction. In contrast to flares, progression correlates best with brain atrophy.

Recently a retrospective population-based study has suggested that progression of disability may be slower than was previously thought.[23] Median times from MS diagnosis to Expanded Disability Status Scores (EDSS) of 3 (mild disability) and 6 (requiring a cane) were 17 and 24 years, respectively. Although the flare rate in the first two years is related to subsequent disability, neither the total number of flares nor the overall flare frequency before the onset of progression are related to time to use of a cane, becoming bed-bound, or death.[6] Indeed, several large studies indicate that most of the variability between patients in the time to disability milestones is contained within the time from disease onset to EDSS 3-4 and/or onset of progressive disability.[23] Once progression has begun, the rate of deterioration is much less variable and is essentially identical for primary progressive as well as secondary progressive forms.

A recent study suggests that the presence of antimyelin antibodies (anti-myelin oligodendrocyte glycoprotein and anti-myelin basic protein antibodies) in patients with CIS strongly predicts a shorter latency to the second relapse and a diagnosis of clinically definite MS.[2] These results should *not* be interpreted as demonstrating a "blood test for MS". Importantly, *all* patients in this study had typical white-matter lesions on brain MRI and oligoclonal bands in the CSF, and had a high probability of ultimately developing clinically definite MS. The presence of one or more anti-myelin antibody is likely a marker of a relatively more acute form of the illness, one that may ultimately be associated with increased disability.

Pregnancy

Many patients with MS are women of childbearing age, and the effect of pregnancy upon MS has accordingly been an issue of particular concern. A large, multicenter prospective study has provided the best assessment of the effects of pregnancy.[5] MS relapse rates were found to decline significantly during pregnancy, particularly during the third trimester. Relapses during that phase of pregnancy averaged 0.2 per person per year (normalized) as compared to 0.7 relapses per person per year during the year before pregnancy. During the initial three months following delivery there is a significantly increased risk of flares, averaging 1.2 flares per woman per year. The net effect of pregnancy upon total flares and disability was negligible. Importantly, neither epidural anesthesia nor breastfeeding increased relapse rates or worsened disability.

Typical Clinically Isolated Syndromes

Optic Neuritis (ON)

ON is characterized by the triad of loss of visual acuity, dyschromatopsia (color desaturation) and ipsilateral eye pain.[33] Pain or visual loss may be absent in some cases, whereas dyschromatopsia is virtually always present. The optic disc is normal in appearance in the majority of cases ("retrobulbar" ON), but disc blurring, hyperemia or peripapillary hemorrhages may be present (papillitis). ON may involve the optic chiasm ("chiasmitis") or both optic nerves during a single attack. Indeed, recent studies suggest that subtle involvement of the "uninvolved" eye often accompanies clinically unilateral ON. Central scotoma, loss of contrast sensitivity, phosphenes (brief light flashes triggered by eye movement or noise) and visual obscurations in bright light may also accompany ON.

Visual loss is usually maximal within one week and begins to improve within the first month. In general, the prognosis for significant visual recovery is quite good. The best predictor of ultimate recovery is baseline visual acuity. However, even in patients with severe visual loss at baseline, more than 80% had recovered to 20/40 by 6 months.

Eye pain typically improves early in the course (within 72 hours) and generally does not persist beyond 7 days.

A relative afferent papillary defect is typically seen in the affected eye during ON, and may persist indefinitely, even with full recovery of visual acuity.

Partial

Transverse Myelitis (TM)

Patients with partial TM typically develop progressive "numbness" (tingling and or loss of sensation) beginning in one or both feet and ascending over days to weeks to involve more of the lower extremities and perhaps the torso. In some cases ascending weakness or "heaviness" of one or both legs may occur in addition to or instead of sensory symptoms, and neurogenic bladder symptoms (frequency, urgency, retention) are common. As the sensory motor symptoms evolve, patients may experience significant gait ataxia. Although the usual sensory level is "at the waist," in most instances the demyelinative focus is situated in the cervical spinal cord rather than in thoracic segments. Partial TM may be accompanied by an "electric" sensation radiating down the spine and/or into the limbs, triggered by neck flexion (Lhermitte phenomenon).

Brainstem Demyelination

Brainstem demyelination may elicit a wide variety of symptoms, including diplopia, dysarthia, dysphagia, ataxia, positional vertigo, nausea and vomiting, and limb ataxia. Helpful diagnostic signs include bilateral ophthalmoplegia and facial myokymia. The progressive course of symptoms over days to weeks also helps to distinguish demyelination from vascular etiologies.

Paroxysmal Phenomena

Paroxysmal phenomena are rapid-onset, brief (10-30 seconds) and often frequent (up to 50 or more per day) neurologic syndromes that occur chiefly in individuals with MS. They include paroxysmal dystonia or hemidystonia ("tonic spasms"), dysarthria-ataxia, akinesia, paresthesiae, pain and other syndromes. In some cases these are the presenting symptom of MS. They may occur in bouts lasting for weeks, then resolve, suggesting that they share some features of a flare. They are thought to occur as a consequence of ephaptic transmission (cross-talk between adjacent demyelinated nerve fibers). Trigeminal neuralgia and glossopharyngeal neuralgia, characterized by repeated severe "electric" pains in their respective distributions, are probably due to the same mechanism.

Pathophysiology of MS

The pathogenesis of MS has not been definitively established, but the prevailing view is that the disease begins with peripheral activation of T lymphocytes that are capable of recognizing some element of myelin. Molecular mimicry, whereby viral or other infection triggers cross-reactivity to self-antigens, is one possible mechanism of generating such T lymphocytes. The activated T lymphocytes gain entry into the CNS via adhesion molecules and their respective ligands that are upregulated on their cell surfaces and on endothelial cells, respectively. Upon entering the CNS, the activated T lymphocytes encounter myelin antigens presented by dendritic cells and with appropriate MHC complex, resulting in an immunologic cascade.[8,20] The results of this immune response are complex, but include cell-mediated damage (resembling delayed hypersensitivity), antibody and complement-mediated damage, and toxic effects of free radical generation. An early effect of this immunological inflammatory response is increased permeability of the blood-brain barrier.

Although myelin is held to be the principal target of the immune response, there are indirect as well as direct neurotoxic effects of the resulting inflammation, resulting in transection of axonal processes, especially within and near the focus of demyelination (the *plaque*) but also in normal appearing white matter.[29]

For many years the prevailing understanding of MS has been that it is principally mediated by the TH1 subtype of CD4+ lymphocytes that secrete gamma-interferon, tumor necrosis factor-alpha (TNF-alpha), TNF-beta and interleukin-2 (IL-2). These "damaging" T lymphocytes are opposed by cells having the TH2 phenotype, which activate B cells and secrete Il-4, IL-5, transforming growth factor-beta (TGF-beta) and IL-10. As a result, one goal of therapy has been to shift T lymphocytes from a TH1 phenotype into a TH2 phenotype. This is largely the result of animal studies utilizing the model of *experimental autoimmune encephalomyelitis (EAE).* Importantly, studies in rodents indicated that EAE could be passively transmitted to healthy animals by selectively injecting CD4+ lymphocytes from affected animals, but other lymphocyte subtypes could not passively confer disease. More recently the potential importance of B-cells as well as other immune cells has been increasingly recognized.

Pathology

Multiple sclerosis refers to the appearance of multiple "scarred" foci (plaques) that are visible within the white matter in the brain and/or spinal cord at autopsy. Microscopic examination of chronic lesions typically reveals a sharply demarcated region of reduced cellularity, loss or reduction of oligodendrocytes and myelin-staining, and relative preservation of axons.[8] Active lesions contain macrophages with phagocytosed myelin, T cells (CD4+ and CD8+), B cells, and plasma cells, as well as microglia.

Immunopathologic Subtypes

MS has long been known to have marked clinical variability between patients, both in terms of disease course and severity as well as in response to specific therapies. One possible explanation for this variability has been that MS is really a syndrome resulting from multiple distinct pathophysiologic etiologies.

This hypothesis has received significant support from evidence that MS lesions can be categorized into four different immunopathologic subtypes.[16] More importantly, evidence suggests that all lesions in any individual patient belong to a single subtype. The pathologic subtypes are shown in Table 1-1. Type I and Type II appear consistent with autoimmune mechanisms, whereas Type III and IV are much more suggestive of dystrophic or degenerative mechanisms. Type I and Type II lesions represent about 20% and 53% of cases, respectively. Pathologically they are similar to the pattern seen with EAE. In contrast, Type III, representing about 25% of cases, resembles a chronic viral infection or ischemic change. Type IV, representing about 2% of cases, resembles an oligodendroglial dystrophy.

These data are based principally on pathologic samples from brain biopsies, and to a lesser extent on autopsy material. One caveat is that the biopsied lesions were primarily large ("tumefactive") lesions that resembled brain tumors, and were therefore atypical. Moreover, the validity of this classification scheme has been challenged by Prineas, with the contention that the different subtypes merely reflect evolutionary stages of plaque development.

Diagnosis of MS

Although multiple consensus criteria for diagnosing MS have been proposed, they all rest upon the principal that MS involves multiple separate lesions within the CNS white matter, separated in time (or for progressive forms, progressing over at least 6 months), and, importantly, not explained by any other illness. Laboratory evidence (evoked responses, cerebrospinal fluid, serological studies, MRI or other imaging) is considered and may have significant influence on the diagnosis. The diagnosis must ultimately be made by a neurologist, based upon the clinical evidence. A key point is that none of the laboratories studies (including MRI imaging and cerebrospinal fluid analysis) is sufficient by itself to determine the diagnosis.

Currently the most widely accepted criteria for the diagnosis are the McDonald criteria (Tables 1-1, 1-2 and 1-3). The most important change from previous criteria is that MRI evidence of new lesions or active inflammation contributes to the diagnosis.

Differential Diagnosis

Differential diagnosis of MS is substantially affected by clinical aspects of the particular syndrome under consideration, including severity of disability, patient age, relapsing versus progressive time course, multifocal versus monofocal illness, and the specific region of the neuraxis affected (eg, myelopathy, optic neuritis or cerebellar syndrome).

Table 1-1

McDonald Criteria: Diagnosis of MS

Relapsing-Remitting or Secondary Progressive MS

Clinical Features	Additional Required
Two or more attacks, with objective evidence of two lesions	Nothing
Two or more attacks, with objective evidence of one lesion	MRI evidence of dissemination in space, ***Or*** Two or more MRI lesions consistent with MS plus positive CSF
One attack, with objective evidence of two or more lesions	MRI evidence of dissemination in time
One attack, with objective evidence of one lesion	MRI evidence of dissemination in space ***And*** MRI evidence of dissemination in time ***Or*** Two or more MRI lesions consistent with MS plus positive CSF ***And*** MRI evidence of dissemination in time

Table 1-2

McDonald Criteria

Dissemination in Space

At least three of the following:
- One Gd-enhancing lesion or nine T2-hyperintense lesions
- At least one infratentorial lesion
- At least one juxtacortical lesion
- At least three periventricular lesions

Dissemination in Time

Gd-enhancing lesion done at least three months after the clinical attack, in a different location from the initial attack

Or

A new T2 hyperintense lesion, compared to an MRI done at least 30 days after the clinical attack

One of the key issues to be determined is whether the neurologic illness is part of a systemic illness. This distinction may be difficult at times, as MS flares may occur in the context of a viral syndrome causing myalgias, diarrhea, fever or other systemic problems. Moreover, it is not unusual for MS patients to experience joint pains or subjective joint swelling (without objective swelling), which might suggest a collagen vascular syndrome. Conversely, collagen-vascular syndromes may initially present with purely CNS involvement and only manifest other systemic features 5 or more years later.

For unclear reasons, MS patients often have functional signs and symptoms in addition to those that are clearly "neurologic". This phenomenon seems particularly evident early in the illness and around the time of diagnosis. Thus, it is essential that neurologists refrain from labeling patients as "hysterical" without carefully considering all of the evidence that might support a "neurologic" diagnosis such as MS.

Table 2 lists some findings that should alert the neurologist to strongly consider alternative diagnoses. Tables 3-1 and 3-2 list illnesses that should be part of the differential diagnosis, and clues to their diagnosis.

Table 1-3

McDonald Criteria: Diagnosis of MS

Clincial Feature Required	Additional
Insidious progression, suggestive of MS for one year, determined prospectively or retrospectively	Two out of the three following: 9 brain lesions ***Or*** 4 brain lesions + prolonged visual evoked potentials ***Or*** 2 or more focal spinal cord lesions ***Or*** Positive spinal fluid (2 or more oligoclonal bands OR increased IgG) ed IgG Index

Laboratory Investigations

The rationale for obtaining blood studies in patients with suspected MS is to determine whether a systemic illness might explain the neurologic syndrome in question. A reasonable minimum panel of blood studies for all MS patients includes an RPR, ESR, Lyme titer, B12 level, blood sugar, and ANA. Additional screening tests might include angiotensin converting enzyme, HTLV-1 and -2, anticardiolipin antibody, lupus anticoagulant, TSH, anti-Ro and -La, and serum protein electrophoresis, depending upon the history and examination.

Low levels of antinuclear antibodies are frequently detected in MS patients. Similarly, low- or moderately-elevated antiphospholipid antibody titers, mildly-elevated angiotensin converting enzyme levels, and borderline- or mildly-low B12 levels may be seen in otherwise typical MS patients. These findings may or may not signify an alternative diagnosis to that of MS, and must be interpreted within the overall clinical context. On the other hand, some laboratory findings in themselves suggest an alternative diagnosis (eg, positive dsDNA).

Evoked Potentials (EPs)

The role of EP has been substantially supplanted by MRI, which is both more sensitive and more specific. However, in selected cases EP may be very helpful in making the diagnosis. For example, demonstration of an occult lesion in the spinal cord or visual pathways may help establish dispersion of lesions in space, even in the context of normal MRI. A corollary of this principle is that EP ordinarily do not add useful information when the pathway in question is obviously clinically affected. EP abnormalities are detectible in 85% of patients with clinically definite MS. Visual and somatosensory EP have higher sensitivity and are generally more helpful than brainstem auditory EP.

Cerebrospinal Fluid (CSF)

CSF in MS patients invariably has normal glucose levels and, in the great majority of cases, normal or minimally elevated protein. A mild lymphocytic pleocytosis (up to 20 cells/mm^3) is often seen, but polymorphonuclear cells, WBC pleocytosis in excess of 50/mm^3, or a total protein greater than 0.8 g/L strongly suggest consideration of alternative diagnoses.

CSF abnormalities reflecting an intrathecal immune response are found in the great majority of MS patients. However, variations in laboratory techniques and parameters analyzed have led to considerable differences in sensitivity and specificity of CSF testing in MS. Criteria for "positive" CSF (supporting a diagnosis of MS) include either two or more oligoclonal bands or an elevated intrathecal production of IgG (usually the IgG index). The presence of a single oligoclonal band (OCB) is of unclear significance. Some patients with one OCB go on to develop more bands over time and meet criteria for MS, whereas others may ultimately be diagnosed with systemic autoimmune illness or other conditions. Most studies indicate that OCB is present in 85%-95%, and elevated IgG index in 70%-90% of patients with clinically definite MS. These abnormalities may be absent in otherwise typical MS, especially in early or mild forms of the disease or in primary progressive MS. OCB may be seen in a host of other illnesses, including infections, lymphoma, systemic autoimmune illness, and in apparently healthy individuals. CSF analysis is not necessary in assessment of patients with typical clinical and MRI findings of MS. However, it may be quite helpful in patients with atypical clinical or MRI features, particularly when the results are incompatible with MS.

Once OCB have developed they are quite stable over time. CSF WBC counts do not correlate well with clinical flares. Thus, there is little to be gained by routinely repeating CSF analyses during suspected flares.

MRI

MS lesions are hyperintense on T2-weighted images (T2), proton density images (PD), and fluid-attenuated inversion recovery (FLAIR) images. An

Table 2

Factors Suggesting Against a Diagnosis of MS

Clinical
"Primary progressive" pattern with onset at less than 40 years of age
Onset at less than ten or greater than seventy years of age
Peripheral neuropathy not otherwise explained by coexisting disease (eg, diabetes)
Consistent association of flares with high fever, rash, joint redness and swelling, or other features that suggest a systemic illness
"Atypical" response to high-dose corticosteroids: No objective response to treatment of a flare early in the course of the disease Immediate recurrence of deficit upon completion of therapy, especially with recurring evidence of steroid-dependence
Absence of any recovery following optic neuritis or transverse myelitis
Excessively strong family history (eg, all sibs and multiple aunts and uncles with MS)
Completely normal neurologic examination, inconsistent with complaints of profound weakness, imbalance or severe sensory loss
Laboratory
Erythrocyte sedimentation rate greater than 80 (unless explained by infection)
Cerebrospinal fluid protein level > 1 g/L or CSF/serum glucose <0.4
Cerebrospinal fluid wbc > 50×10^6
MRI
Extremely bright lesions on diffusion-weighted images (suggesting infarcts)
Marked involvement of basal ganglia
Pronounced, disproportionate involvement of gray matter

identical pattern of hyperintensity is seen in other lesions with increased water content, including foci of gliosis, edema, inflammation, Wallerian degeneration or tumors. Most MS lesions are isointense on T1-weighted images (T1), but in the context of acute inflammation or edema, or with loss of axons and tissue matrix, they may be hypointense on T1.

FLAIR images are particularly useful for detection of cortical or juxtacortical lesions, whereas T2 images are preferable for posterior fossa lesions, and short tau inversion recovery sequences (STIR) may be most sensitive for spinal cord lesions.

Gadolinium enhancement reflects the loss of integrity of the blood-brain barrier that occurs within and near a focus of acute inflammation. This is typically a transient phenomenon in MS lesions,

Table 3-1

Differential Diagnosis of MS

Multiple Sclerosis Mimics	Discriminating Features
Systemic lupus	Positive anti-dsDNA or anti-Smith antibodies, high ESR, protracted seizures, peripheral neuropathy, pronounced steroid dependence, evolution of systemic features
Antiphospholipid syndrome	History of fetal loss or thrombosis, high-positive antiphospholipid antibody or anticardilipin levels
Primary Sjögren syndrome	Sicca syndrome, positive anti-Ro and -La antibodies, positive parotid or minor salivary gland biopsy, peripheral neuropathy, evolution of systemic features
Sarcoidosis	Meningeal enhancement, hilar adeonopathy, pulmonary involvement, prominent hypothalamic-pituitary involvement, pronounced steroid dependence, other systemic features, high angiotensin converting enzyme levels (moderate levels may be seen in MS), biopsy
Isolated CNS vasculitis	Persistent headache, night sweats, seizures, extremely bright lesions on diffusion-weighted MRI, vascular beading on cerebral angiography (MRA is insensitive), positive biopsy of meninges or lesion, steroid dependence
Polyarteritis nodosa	Peripheral neuropathy (abnormal sural nerve biopsy), steroid dependence or unresponsiveness other systemic involvement
Behçet disease	Prominent involvement of basal ganglia, large diffuse brainstem lesions, mucocutaneous ulcerations
Tropical spastic paraparesis	HTLV-1 or HTLV-2 antibodies

lasting three weeks on average. Thus enhancement is a very useful marker for recent disease activity. Several types of enhancement are observed in MS patients, including homogenous enhancement, ring enhancement, and incomplete ring enhancement. Ring-enhancing lesions may be more "damaging" than homogenously enhancing lesions and incomplete ring enhancement may have more specificity for MS than other forms. Interestingly, patterns of enhancement seem to be consistent within individual patients.

The number, location, orientation, size and contrast-enhancement of lesions are all important features when considering the diagnosis of MS. MS lesions are usually ovoid, and range in diameter from a few mm to several cm. The majority of lesions involve only white matter, but gray matter lesions are now known to occur in 4%-5% of total lesions.

Typical locations for MS lesions include the juxtacortical white matter, corpus callosum, periventricular white matter adjacent to the posterior horns of

Table 3-2

Differential Diagnosis of MS

Multiple Sclerosis Mimics	Discriminating Features
Lyme disease	Painful radiculitis, bilateral facial nerve involvement, peripheral neuropathy, other systemic features, serum and CSF antibodies to *B burgdorferi*, polymerase chain reaction + for *B burgorferi*
Adrenoleukodystrophy (including female heterozygotes)	Peripheral neuropathy, adrenal insufficiency, elevated very long-chain fatty acids
CADASIL	"Stroke-like" onset, lack of response to corticosteroids, extremely bright lesions on diffusion-weighted MRI, bilateral anterior temporal involvement on MRI, skin biopsy with Notch3 immunostaining, Notch3 genetic mutations
Neurosyphilis	Seizures, stroke, Argyll Robertson pupils, loss of pain sensation, lancinating pains, positive CSF VDRL
AIDS	Peripheral neuropathy, positive HIV antibody, other systemic features
B_{12} deficiency	Peripheral neuropathy, symmetrical spinal cord involvement, elevated methylmalonic acid or homo cysteine levels (with normal folate levels); low B_{12} (borderline reduction of B_{12} is not rare in MS)
Copper-deficiency myelopathy	Peripheral neuropathy, low copper and ceruloplasmin
Leber hereditary optic neuropathy (or "LHON +" syndrome)	Family history consistent with maternal transmission, simultaneous or sequential bilateral loss of central vision, marked stimulus-induced myoclonus
Spinocerebellar degenerations	Peripheral neuropathy, molecular genetic testing

the lateral ventricles, and the middle cerebellar peduncle. Cervical spinal cord lesions are seen more often than thoracic lesions. Spinal cord lesions typically involve a relatively short length of the cord, corresponding to one or two vertebral bodies.

Several investigators have proposed MRI criteria for establishing a diagnosis of MS. The criteria of Barkhof were reported to have an accuracy of 80% in predicting clinically definite MS in patients presenting with clinically isolated syndromes. These criteria have largely been incorporated into the McDonald Commission proposed diagnostic criteria. However, the typical MRI features of MS can also be seen in other neurologic diseases, and in rare MS patients, MRI imaging may be normal. Thus, it is essential not to rely exclusively upon MRI imaging when considering the diagnosis.

Although MRI imaging has had a dramatic impact upon our understanding of MS and on the design of clinical trials, the limitations of conventional MRI imaging have also become all too obvious. For example, the number and volume of T2 lesions correlate poorly with clinical disability. Moreover, under some circumstances, drug treatments that effectively reduce the number of new T2 lesions fail to affect disability (eg, in secondary progressive MS). Chronic T1 hypodensities ("black holes"), which represent foci of more severe tissue loss, have a somewhat better, but still modest correlation with disability. Perhaps the most useful measure from conventional MRI is assessment of brain *atrophy*.[26] Brain atrophy apparently occurs progressively in many, if not all, MS patients. It may be seen very early in the disease, and correlates fairly well with measures of disability, disease course, and cognitive loss. Importantly, brain atrophy early in the course of the disease is a significant predictive factor for later disability. Cervical spinal cord atrophy may also occur, and has a significant correlation with disability, especially with measures of ambulation. Brain atrophy has been assessed by a variety of computerized software programs measuring different outcomes (eg, the "brain parenchymal fraction", third ventricular width, etc.). In clinical practice, atrophy is appreciated by enlargement of the ventricles beyond that expected for age, and by evidence of cortical tissue loss. It is clear that informal assessments of this sort grossly underestimate the frequency and severity of brain atrophy in MS patients.

Newer MRI techniques, such as magnetization transfer imaging (MTI) and magnetic resonance spectroscopy (MRS) are currently employed in MS research studies and are likely to enter routine clinical practice in the near future. MTI exploits differences in signal intensities generated by protons in free water versus those bound to macromolecules. The magnetization transfer ratio (MTR) is a quantitative measurement thought to reflect damage to the tissue matrix (axons, myelin, etc). MTR is reduced in MS lesions and in whole-brain measurements of patients with MS. It is particularly useful in quantitatively assessing tissue loss within either normal appearing white matter or in MS plaques. MRS is another quantitative technique that relies upon the relationship of N-acetyl aspartate (NAA) to neuronal number (and probably also to neuronal "health"). MRS measurement of the ratio of NAA to creatine correlate well with clinical disability, further supporting the hypothesis that progressive disability is largely due to loss of axons over time.

MRI lesions consistent with MS are seen in 26%-70% of patients presenting with clinically isolated syndromes, suggesting that such patients often have preexisting (but heretofore occult) chronic demyelinative disease (eg, MS), or that they have experienced multifocal demyelination in association with the presenting episode.[4,7] The presence of MRI lesions at disease onset strongly suggests that clinically definite MS will ultimately develop. The overall rate of clinically definite MS after optic neuritis is 30% at five years and 38% at ten years.[21] However, normal baseline MRI was associated with a five-year MS risk of 16% and ten-year risk of 22%. In contrast, at five years, clinically definite MS had been diagnosed in 51% of patients with three or more brain lesions at baseline, and in 56% of patients with at least one lesion by ten years. Another study indicates that patients with clinically isolated syndromes had a high risk of developing clinically definite MS by ten years (>80%) when one or more lesions were present on baseline MRI.[3] Moreover, the baseline lesion volume strongly correlates with both new lesion accumulation and disability at five years.

Treatment

Management of Acute Flares

High-dose intravenous corticosteroids are now considered standard-of-care for severe, disabling MS flares. Although many different regimens have been employed, there is little evidence to support any particular "recipe" over others. Indeed, recent evidence suggests that high-dose oral corticosteroid therapy may be equivalent to similar bioequivalent doses delivered intravenously. A standard, widely used schedule of therapy is five days of intravenous methylprednisolone, 1000 mg daily.

There is no consensus about treating minor MS flares with high-dose corticosteroids. For example, such treatment had no effect upon the long-term outcome of clinically isolated optic neuritis. However, preliminary evidence suggests that corticosteroid therapy may have tissue-sparing effects or benefit long-term outcomes; therefore, some clinicians elect to treat mild episodes.

Disease Modifying Treatments

Until only a few years ago, MS was held to be an inexorably progressive illness, with minimal treatment options. Flares were treated with corticosteroids or ACTH in order to minimize the duration of the attack; oral immunosuppressive agents such as azathioprine were sometimes used, and aggressive treatment with chemotherapeutic agents (eg, cyclophosphamide) was at best controversial for very aggressive forms of the illness.

Until only a few years ago, MS was held to be an inexorably progressive illness, with minimal treatment options. Flares were treated with corticosteroids or ACTH in order to minimize the duration of the attack; oral immunosuppressive agents such as azathioprine were sometimes used, and aggressive treatment with chemotherapeutic agents (eg, cyclophosphamide) was at best controversial for very aggressive forms of the illness.

This situation changed dramatically with the introduction of Betaseron® (interferon beta 1b) in 1993, as the first FDA-approved prophylactic drug for MS.[9] The Betaseron pivotal trial convincingly demonstrated that prophylactic treatment could reduce the frequency of MS flares. A second unique contribution of this trial was the compelling evidence that MRI outcomes were extremely useful markers of disease activity and treatment effectiveness.

In subsequent years three other injectable drugs for MS prophylaxis have been FDA-approved, comprising with Betaseron a new category termed the "ABCR" drugs (Avonex®, Betaseron, Copaxone®, Rebif®).[10,12,25]

Beta-Interferons

Three of the four ABCR drugs (Betaseron, Avonex, Rebif) bear marked structural and functional similarities and exert their actions by mimicking endogenous interferon-beta. Interferon-beta has a variety of immunomodulatory actions on the immune system, including antigen-nonspecific suppression of T-cell proliferation and inhibition of interferon-gamma induced upregulation of MHC class II expression, as well as multiple effects that reduce T-cell migration across the endothelium into the CNS.

Because of its actions on the blood-brain barrier, interferon-beta has a pronounced inhibitory effect upon development of new gadolinium-enhancing lesions. Interferon therapy also appears to induce a clinical benefit somewhat more quickly than does Copaxone (glatiramir acetate).

Betaseron (interferon 1b) differs from human interferon-beta because of one amino acid substitution and is not glycosylated, whereas Avonex (interferon 1a) and Rebif (also interferon 1a) are structurally identical to human interferon-beta. The major differences between each of these drugs are the dose per injection, and the route and frequency of administration (see Table 4).

The Betaseron pivotal trial was done at a time when flare-frequency was thought to be the most robust outcome measure for MS. Accordingly, assessment of disability was only a secondary priority, and effectiveness of Betaseron in retarding progression of disability could not be convincingly demonstrated. This situation was remedied several years later, when the Avonex pivotal trial was designed having disability (EDSS) as the preeminent outcome measure. Avonex treatment was indeed shown to attenuate progression of disability and was subsequently approved by the FDA for that indication.

The ideal dose/frequency of interferon-beta treatments has been quite controversial. A comparison of Avonex 30 mcg once weekly (the standard dose) versus Avonex 60 mcg once weekly showed no advantage of increasing the dose. On the other hand, two head-to-head trials of Avonex 30 mcg weekly versus Rebif (given 3 times per week), or Betaseron (given every other day), supported a benefit of "high dose, high frequency" treatment. Indeed, Rebif received FDA approval in 2002 on the basis of demonstrated superiority over Avonex over a 48-week head-to-head comparison trial in patients with RR MS.[22] Unfortunately, neither of these comparison trials could be double-blinded (the patients knew their own treatments) and both studies were too short to unequivocally demonstrate long-term superiority of Rebif or Betaseron versus Avonex. A reasonable conclusion is that treatment efficacy may be enhanced by giving interferon-beta more than once per week. Importantly, high-dose, high-frequency interferon treatment substantially increases the risk of *neutralizing antibodies (Nabs)*. Recent studies confirm that high-titer Nabs reduce or prevent the benefits of treatment.[13] In such cases, the Nabs generally developed within the first two years of therapy, but did not attenuate treatment benefit until the third year.

The beta-interferon drugs for MS are moderately effective, providing an overall reduction of the flare frequency in RR MS patients of about one-third. Avonex and Rebif also significantly delayed disability, as measured by the likelihood of progressing one point on the EDSS. It appears that individual patients may differ substantially in their responsiveness to treatment with interferon-beta or glatiramer (Copaxone), perhaps because of different underlying pathophysiologies or innate differences in immune function. Thus, "failure" of treatment with one agent does not necessarily mean that another agent from a different drug class cannot be effective.

Importantly, the effectiveness of treatment is substantially affected by the timing of treatment with respect to the duration of illness. Treatment is clearly much less effective, and is likely completely ineffective, when it is initiated in the secondary progressive phase of illness. This is especially true when flares have either ceased or have become quite infrequent. On the other hand, the effectiveness of treatment appears to be substantially enhanced when it is initiated very early in the illness, even before the second demyelinative episode. This was determined by studying clinically isolated syndrome patients at high risk of developing clinically definite MS on the basis of at least three typical lesions on brain MRI.[11] In such patients, Avonex treatment substantially reduced new MRI lesions and delayed the next demyelinative flare.

Side effects of interferon-beta include both *systemic* symptoms (eg, "flu-like" symptoms, fever, transient exacerbation of previous neurologic symptoms, migraines, hepatotoxicity, leukopenia, depression, seizures) and *local* symptoms (injection-site reactions).

Flu-like symptoms occur in most patients, but usually resolve with a few weeks of initiating treatment. Initiation of treatment with a low dose and slow upward titration of the dose may be very helpful in increasing tolerability of the treatment. In addition, many of the side effects of interferon-beta may be attenuated by pretreatment with either an NSAID or acetaminophen.

Injection site reactions commonly include redness and swelling, but rarely, necrotizing ulcers and disfiguring lipodystrophy may also occur. An advantage of intramuscularly administered beta-interferon (Avonex) is that local site reactions are much less common than with the subcutaneously administered drugs.

Glatiramer Acetate (GA, Copaxone, Copolymer I)

GA is a random polymer of glutamic acid, lysine, alanine and tyrosine, the four most prevalent amino acids in myelin basic protein. Its principal mechanisms of action in MS are still unclear. The major postulated mechanisms include tolerance induction of myelin basic protein-reactive T-cells (eg, acting as an altered peptide ligand), or induction of a shift from a TH1 phenotype to a TH2 (anti-inflammatory) phenotype in myelin-reactive T-cells.

GA significantly reduced the frequency of flares by 29% in a two-year pivotal trial of patients with RR MS,[12] but did not reach the predetermined endpoint for significantly attenuating disability. However, recent head-to-head comparison trials with Betaseron and Rebif suggest that GA has very similar clinical efficacy, and latency to clinical effect as interferons.

GA is administered as a daily SC injection. Side effects notably include injection site reactions, hives (especially during initiation of the drug), and infrequent acute systemic reactions (tachycardia, sweating, dyspnea, chest pressure) that last for 10 to 20 minutes. Flu-like symptoms, leucopenia, depression and hepatic injury are much less likely to occur with GA than with interferon-beta.

Mitoxantrone (Novantrone®)

Mitoxantrone is a immunosuppressive agent used for treatment of hairy cell leukemia and other neoplastic disorders. It is FDA-approved for treatment of aggressive relapsingremitting, secondary progressive and progressive-relapsing forms of MS, based on evidence that it delays progression of disability in such patients. However, treatment is limited to a total dose of 140 mg/m^2 (about three years of standard therapy) because of concerns regarding severe cardiomyopathy. In addition, mitoxantrone has been associated with an increased risk of acute myeloblastic leukemia.

Natalizumab (Tysabri®)

Natalizumab is a monoclonal antibody to alpha-4 integrin, a selective adhesion molecule expressed on the surface of leukocytes (except for granulocytes). Given intravenously once per month, natalizumab is remarkably well tolerated and effective. Over a two-year study relapse rate was reduced by

Table 4

The "ABCR" Drugs for Multiple Sclerosis

Drug	**Class**	**Dose**	**Route**	**Frequency**
Betaseron	Interferon beta 1β	250 mcg	s.c.	Alternate days
Avonex	Interferon beta 1α	30 mcg	i.m.	Weekly
Rebif	Interferon beta 1α	44 mcg	s.c.	3/week
Glatiramer (Copaxone)	Random polymer	20 mg	s.c.	Daily

67% and disability progression was reduced by 42% compared to placebo controls. Natalizumab was withdrawn from the market within months of its FDA-approval, because of the unexpected development of progressive multifocal leukoencephalopathy (PML) in three patients. All three affected patients had taken natalizumab in combination with other immunomodulatory agents (two with Avonex). After an intensive safety investigation, the FDA reapproved natalizumab as monotherapy in June, 2006. Thus far there have been no further reports of PML in patients treated with natalizumab.

2. Marburg Variant ("Malignant MS")

The Marburg variant is a rare variant of MS that is pathologically identical to typical MS but is much more severe. It is a monophasic illness leading to death or profound disability within weeks or months from onset. MRI is characterized by extensive areas of T2 hyperintensity in the cerebral hemispheres or brainstem.

3. Balo's Concentric Sclerosis

This is a rare, usually severe variant of MS, clinically similar to Marburg variant. It is distinguished by concentric rings of normal-appearing myelin alternating with demyelination, visible on MRI or upon pathologic evaluation. Most reported patients have been young persons of Chinese or Japanese origin.

4. Neuromyelitis Optica (NMO, Devic Disease, Devic Syndrome)

NMO is a syndrome of severe inflammation and demyelination, usually confined to the spinal cord and optic nerves, having multiple features that are distinct from MS. Recently a sensitive and specific serum marker for NMO has been developed (NMO-Ig), based upon the presence of antibodies that bind to the aquaporin-4 water channel.[14]

Clinical Features

The initial descriptions of NMO were of a fulminant, monophasic illness in which bilateral optic neuritis and severe transverse myelitis, the index events, occurred within an eight-week period. A key feature of the diagnosis was that other CNS structures were spared. More recently both of these criteria have been revised. Two different forms of NMO are now recognized, a monophasic form and a relapsing variant.[32] In addition, MRI lesions outside of the spinal cord and optic nerves are now known to occur in a minority of patients with NMO.

The monophasic form of NMO is characterized by a short interval between the index events (median five days), moderate recovery and absence of subsequent flares. The relapsing form has a longer interval between index events (median 166 days) and milder index event severity, but subsequent flares cause severe incremental disability.[32]

Epidemiology

NMO is an uncommon disease in Western countries, but there are no data regarding its incidence and prevalence. A recent serologic study suggests that the "optic-spinal" form of MS, commonly diagnosed in Japan, may be identical to NMO.

The monophasic form of NMO has a younger age of onset (mean age 29) and lower male:female ratio (approximately 1:1) than the relapsing form (mean onset age 41; male: female ratio approximately 4:1). The relapsing form is associated with other systemic autoimmune disorders (eg, Sjögren syndrome or lupus) in one-third of cases, whereas there is little association of the monophasic form with autoimmune disorders.

Laboratory Features

The most useful laboratory data for distinguishing NMO from MS are the serum NMO-Ig evaluation and cerebrospinal indices. Oligoclonal bands are uncommon in NMO, and some reports suggest that they may resolve following the initial flares. CSF pleocytosis of >50 WBC/mm^3 may be seen in up to 35% of patients. Polymorphonuclear cells are detected in 50% of patients with CSF pleocytosis. The CSF protein may be substantially higher than typical MS.

MRI

The key MRI feature of NMO is a T2 hyperintense confluent spinal cord lesion that extends longitudinally >3 vertebral body lengths. The spinal cord lesions commonly enhance with gadolinium, and there may be focal cord swelling at the site of the lesion.

Otherwise typical "MS lesions" may be seen on brain MRI in less than 10% of patients that otherwise meet criteria for NMO.

Diagnostic Criteria

Multiple sets of diagnostic criteria have been published, but the recent development of a sensitive and specific serologic test has profoundly altered the diagnosis of NMO. Recent proposed criteria from Wingerchuk et al include two *absolute* criteria, optic neuritis and acute myelitis, and two major *supportive* criteria, MRI evidence of a contiguous spinal cord lesion extending > 3 vertebral body lengths and NMO-Ig immunopositivity. The best single "rule-in" criterion was NMO-Ig (93% specific), whereas absence of a spinal cord lesion extending > 3 vertebral body lengths was associated with 97% sensitivity to "rule-out" the diagnosis. Recent studies suggest that the sensitivity of the NMO-Ig serologic test is approximately 60%.

Pathology

NMO generally results in more inflammatory, necrotizing changes within the spinal cord and optic nerves and involves gray matter more than MS. The entire cross-sectional area of the spinal cord may be involved at some levels, and cavitation of the cord is often seen. Hyalinized, thickened blood vessels are seen in the vicinity of lesions.

Microscopically, there is a profound loss of oligodendrocytes within lesions, and pronounced macrophage infiltration with large numbers of perivascular granulocytes and eosinophils. Clinical evidence of a strong humoral immune contribution is supported by perivascular deposition of immunoglobulins and complement C9neo antigen.[17]

Prognosis

Although the index events are typically more severe in the monophasic than in the relapsing form, the long-term prognosis is much better with monophasic NMO. In most cases, individuals with monophasic NMO recover ambulatory ability and avoid complete blindness. In contrast, more than 50% of relapsing NMO patients are unable to ambulate without assistance or develop severe visual loss in one eye within five years. The five-year survival of the monophasic form of NMO is 90%, whereas the relapsing form has a five-year survival rate of only 68%.[32] Deaths in the relapsing form were due to respiratory failure associated with acute cervical myelitis.

Predictors of a relapsing course include longer interval between index events, female sex, milder motor deficit with the index event, and older age of onset.

Treatment

There are no data from large controlled treatment trials in NMO. There is little evidence that interferon-beta or glatiramer are effective, leading most experts to use immunosuppressive agents, especially regimens targeting humoral immune responses. Treatment approaches have included corticosteroids (alone or in combination with other immunosuppressants), IVIG or plasma exchange. A recent preliminary study suggests that the B-cell depleting agent, Rituximab, may be effective.

5. Acute Disseminated Encephalomyelitis (ADEM)

ADEM is an acute, multifocal, monophasic illness involving brain and spinal cord, often with more pronounced alteration of sensorium and meningeal signs than are seen in typical MS. ADEM is generally considered a "postinfectious" syndrome. It was initially linked to infection with measles, smallpox or varicella, or to immunizations against a variety of organisms. In Western countries it occurs most commonly following nonspecific upper respiratory infections or without any clear-cut provocative infection.

Clinical Features

Onset of systemic symptoms (fever, malaise) and meningeal symptoms (headache, nausea and vomiting) usually begins 4-21 days after infection or immunization. Neurologic symptoms (paraparesis, hemiparesis, aphasia, sensory loss, ataxia, rarely bilateral optic neuritis) then develop rapidly, reaching a peak of severity within several days. There is substantial overlap with the features of MS flares, though the marked acuity of the neurologic syndrome in ADEM, as well as loss of consciousness, meningismus and fever differ from typical MS.

Follow-up evaluations, either clinical or MRI studies, eventually determine whether the illness is monophasic (eg, ADEM) or relapsing (eg, MS). In some cases, relapses within the first month of illness are considered consistent with ADEM.

Epidemiology

The incidence and prevalence of ADEM are unknown. It is seen most commonly in prepubertal children, but also occurs in young or even middle-aged adults. There is little or no sex difference in children with ADEM, but adults appear to have a female-predominant pattern similar to MS.

Pathology

As in MS, there are patchy foci of perivenous demyelination, primarily within the white matter. During the acute phase of illness, lesions contain an inflammatory infiltrate of both lymphocytes and macrophages. Local vascular changes, including hyperemia, vessel wall inflammation, and hemorrhage may also be seen. These features, as well as the association with infections, have suggested that ADEM may be quite similar to the experimental animal model of inflammatory CNS demyelination, experimental autoimmune encephalomyelitis.

Laboratory Findings

The CSF findings are usually those of a hyper-acute inflammatory illness, with raised intracranial pressure, increased protein, and pleocytosis (up to 1000 WBC/mm^3), possibly including polymorphonuclear cells. However, CSF may be normal in some patients. Oligoclonal bands and increased intrathecal synthesis of IgG may be seen, and do not help to distinguish ADEM from MS.

MRI

The MRI findings in ADEM are very similar to those in MS, and most investigators are in agreement that MRI outcomes cannot distinguish the two during initial presentation. Simultaneous enhancement of all lesions (which would suggest a "monophasic" process) occurs in both MS and ADEM, and is not a reliable discriminator between them. However, T2 hyperintense lesions within the thalamus, basal ganglia or cortex are more suggestive of ADEM.

Prognosis

ADEM in children is associated with a high mortality rate (10%-30%) and complete recovery in only 50% of patients. In contrast, a recent series of adult patients suggests a more favorable outcome. All patients were treated with corticosteroids or immunosuppressive drugs. Only one of 40 patients died and one patient was unimproved, whereas 31 patients had significantly improved from their peak disability and seven patients had fully recovered.

Treatment

There are no large controlled treatment trials for ADEM, but case reports and small series suggest that high-dose intravenous corticosteroids, intravenous immunoglobulin or plasma exchange may be effective. Immunosuppressive agents such as cyclophosphamide may be helpful in some cases.

6. Hemorrhagic Leukoencephalitis

Hemorrhagic leukoencephalitis is a rare, hyperacute form of ADEM, with even more severe morbidity and risk of mortality. It is often difficult to clinically distinguish from ADEM. On MRI, lesions tend to be larger than in ADEM, and in contrast to ADEM, involvement of the basal ganglia is generally not seen. Cerebrospinal fluid is typically under increased pressure, and is notable for substantial RBC as well as a neutrophilic pleocytosis.

7. References

1. Ascherio A, Munger KL, Lennette ET, et al. Epstein-Barr virus antibodies and risk of multiple sclerosis. *JAMA*. 2001;286:3083-3088.

2. Berger T, Rubner P, Schautzer F, et al. Antimyelin antibodies as a predictor of clinically definite multiple sclerosis after a first demyelinating event. *N Engl J Med*. 2003;349:139-145.

3. Brex P, Ciccarelli O, O'Riordan JI, Sailer M, Thompson AJ, Miller DH. A longitudinal study of abnormalities on MRI and disability from multiple sclerosis. *N Engl J Med*. 2002;346:158-164.

4. CHAMPS Study Group. MRI predictors of early conversion to clinically definite MS in the CHAMPS placebo group. *Neurology*. 2002;59:998-1006.

5. Confavreaux C, Hutchinson M, Hours MM, et al. Rate of pregnancy-related relapse in multiple sclerosis. *N Engl J Med*. 1998;339: 285-291.

6. Ebers G. Natural history of multiple sclerosis. *J Neurol Neurosurg Psychiatry*. 2001;71: 16-19.

7. Filippi M, Horsfield MA, Morrissey SP, et al. Quantitative brain MRI lesion load predicts the course of clinically isolated syndromes suggestive of multiple sclerosis. *Neurology*. 1994;44:635-641.

8. Fox EJ. Immunopathology of multiple sclerosis. *Neurology*. 2004;63(Suppl 6):S3-S7.

9. IFN-beta Study Group. Interferon beta-1b is effective in relapsing-remitting multiple sclerosis. I. Clinical results of a multicenter, randomized, placebo-controlled trial. *Neurology*. 1993;43:655-661

10. Jacobs L, Cookfair DL, Rudick RA, et al. Intramuscular interferon beta-1a for disease progression in relapsing multiple sclerosis. *Ann Neurol*. 1996;39:285-294.

11. Jacobs LD, Beck RW, Simon JH, et al. Intramuscular interferon beta-1a therapy initiated during a first demyelinating event in multiple sclerosis. *N Engl J Med.* 2000;343:898-904.

12. Johnson K, Brooks BR, Cohen JA, et al. Copolymer I reduces relapse rate and improved disability in relapsing-remitting multiple sclerosis: results of a phase III multicenter, double-blind, placebo-controlled trial. *Neurology.* 1995;45:1268-1276.

13. Kappos L, Clanet M, Sandberg-Wolheim M, et al. Neutralizing antibodies and efficacy of interferon beta-1a. *Neurology.* 2005;65:40-47.

14. Lennon VA, Wingerckuk DM, Kryzer TJ, et al. A serum autoantibody marker of neuromyelitis optica: distinction from multiple sclerosis. *Lancet.* 2004;364:2106-2112.

15. Lublin FD, Reingold SC, et al. Defining the clinical course of multiple sclerosis. *Neurology.* 1996;46:907-911.

16. Lucchinetti C, Bruck W, Parisi J, Scheithauer B, Rodriguez M, Lassman H. Heterogeneity of multiple sclerosis lesions: implications for the pathogenesis of demyelination. *Ann Neurol.* 2000;46:707-717.

17. Lucchinetti CF, Mandler RN, McGavern D, et al. A role for humoral mechanisms in the pathogenesis of Devic's neuromyelitis optica. *Brain.* 2002;125:1450-1461.

18. McDonald T, Compston A, Edan G, et al. Recommended diagnostic criteria for multiple sclerosis: guidelines from the International Panel on the Diagnosis of Multiple Sclerosis. *Ann Neurol.* 2001;50:121-127.

19. Noonan CW, Kathman SJ, White MC. Prevalence estimates for MS in the United States and evidence of an increasing trend in women. *Neurology.* 2002;58:136-138.

20. O'Connor KC, Bar-Or A, Hafler DA. The neuroimmunology of multiple sclerosis: possible roles of T and B lymphocytes in immunopathogenesis. *J Clin Immunol.* 2001;21:81-92.

21. Optic Neuritis Study Group. High- and low-risk profiles for the development of multiple sclerosis within 10 years after optic neuritis. *Arch Ophthalmol.* 2003;121:944-949.

22. Panitch H, Goodin DS, Francis G, et al. Randomized comparative study of interferon beta-1a treatment regimens in MS: the EVIDENCE trial. *Neurology.* 2002;59:1496-1506.

23. Pittock SJ, Mayr WT, McClelland RL, et al. Disability profile did not change over 10 years in a population-based prevalence cohort. *Neurology.* 2004;62:601-606.

24. Posonby A-L, van der Mei I, Dwyer T, et al. Exposure to infant siblings during early life and risk of multiple sclerosis. *JAMA.* 2005;293:463-469.

25. The PRISMS Study Group. Randomized, double-blind, placebo-controlled trial of interferon beta-1a in relapsing-remitting multiple sclerosis. *Lancet.* 1998;352:1498-1504

26. Rudick R, Fisher E, Lee JC, Simon J. Use of the brain parenchymal fraction to measure whole brain atrophy in relapsing-remitting multiple sclerosis. *Neurology.* 1999;53: 1698-1704.

27. Sadovnik AD. The genetics of multiple sclerosis. *Clin Neurol Neurosurg.* 2002;104: 199-202.

28. Schwarz S, Mohr A, Knauth M, Wildemann B, Storch-Hagenlocher B. Acute disseminated encephalomyelitis. *Neurology.* 2001;56: 1313-1318.

29. Trapp BD, Peterson J, Ransohoff RM, Rudick R, Mork S, Bo L. Axonal transaction in the lesions of multiple sclerosis. *N Engl J Med.* 1998;338:278-285.

30. van der Mei IAF, Ponsonby A-L, Dwyer T, et al. Past exposure to sun, skin phenotype, and risk of multiple sclerosis: case-control study. *Br Med J*. 2003:327:1-6.

31. Wallin MT, Page WF, Kurtzke JF. Multiple sclerosis in US veterans of the Vietnam era and later military service: race, sex and geography. *Ann Neurol*. 2004;55:65-71.

32. Wingerchuk DM, Weinshenker BG. Neuromyelitis optica: clinical predictors of a relapsing course and survival. *Neurology*. 2003;60:848-853.

33. Wray SH: Optic neuritis. In: Albert DM, Jakobiec FA, eds. *Principles and Practice of Ophthalmology*. WB Saunders Co; 1994: 2539-2568.

8. Questions

1. A 29-year-old woman with established relapsing-remitting multiple sclerosis presents to the Emergency Room complaining of bilateral leg weakness, stumbling and falling, bladder urgency and frequency, and profound fatigue. She has had these same symptoms with MS flares in the past.

Which of the following tests is NOT essential for assessment of this patient:

A. Neurological examination

B. MRI of the brain and spinal cord

C. Urinalysis and culture

D. Lumbar puncture

E. Physical examination

F. B. and D.

2. A 19-year-old woman presents with a two-year history of intermittent right-sided headaches, often associated with photophobia and phonophobia. On physical examination she has episcleritis in the left eye, and in the right eye has an afferent papillary defect, a central scotoma, red-green desaturation and loss of visual acuity (20/50). There is mild weakness of the right arm and leg.

Which of the following would not be typical findings associated with multiple sclerosis?

A. Red-green color desaturation

B. Loss of visual acuity

C. Central scotoma

D. Afferent pupillary defect

E. Episcleritis

3. A 58-year-old man with longstanding MS discontinues his interferon-beta injections, and over the subsequent six weeks develops severe aphasia, fatigue and right-sided weakness.

Which of the following would not be typical features of an MS flare?

A. Profound fatigue

B. Progression of symptoms over days or weeks

C. Severe aphasia

D. Deterioration after discontinuing prophylactic medication

4. A 32-year-old woman is referred for management of recently diagnosed multiple sclerosis. Review of her medical history is notable for two episodes of severe transverse myelitis and a history of possible optic neuritis. Brain MRI is reportedly normal. Laboratory studies include ESR 11, ANA + 1:512, CSF glucose 100 mg%, CSF total protein 330 mg%, CSF cell count 25 mononuclear cells.

Which of the following is most inconsistent with a diagnosis of multiple sclerosis?

A. A normal sedimentation rate

B. A normal brain MRI scan

C. Positive ANA

D. Cerebrospinal fluid protein = 330 mg%

5. A 46-year-old woman with longstanding systemic lupus erythematosis presents to the ER with lower extremity weakness and sensory loss, urinary urgency and frequency, and a T6 sensory level. Lumbar puncture reveals two oligoclonal bands unique to the CSF, normal glucose and protein, and no white blood cells. An NMO-Ig test is subsequently positive.

Which of the following are typical/common features of neuromyelitis optica?

A. Positive NMO-Ig

B. Persistent CSF oligoclonal bands

C. Systemic lupus erythematosis

D. All of the above

E. A. and C.

6. A 22-year-old woman is referred for evaluation of possible multiple sclerosis. Over the previous four years she has had frequent unilateral headaches, at times associated with tingling over the left half of her body. The headaches and tingling seem to occur more often in the week prior to menses. Heat or exercise also seems to be trigger factors. Brain MRI shows eight small (3-4 mm) white matter lesions, hyperintense on T2 weighted images and isointense on T1 weighted images.

Which clinical features occur in either MS or migraine?

A. T2 hyperintense white-matter foci on brain MRI

B. Exacerbation of symptoms in the premenstrual week

C. Eurologic symptoms may or may not coincide with headaches

D. Exercise or heat may exacerbate symptoms

E. All of the above

7. A previously healthy 18-year-old woman develops steadily progressive paraparesis, incontinence, and loss of sensation in the lower extremities over a five-year span, without any preceding flares. MRI of the brain is normal.

Which of the following is correct?

A. She likely has primary progressive multiple sclerosis

B. She has a "clinically-isolated syndrome" and has high risk of developing MS

C. Her evaluation should include tibial somatosensory evoked potentials

D. Multiple sclerosis is unlikely

E. MRI of the spine is unnecessary because she clearly has a myelopathy

8. A 23-year-old woman has typical features of MS on brain and spine MRI, and a history of two flares (optic neuritis, brainstem episode) consistent with MS. A thorough serologic evaluation is negative and there are no features of systemic illness.

Which of the following is correct?

A. "ABCR" prophylactic therapy can probably reduce the probability of future flares by about one-third

B. Prophylactic treatment is most effective after age forty

C. She should be advised not to become pregnant, because of the negative effects of pregnancy on her illness

D. It is highly likely that her children will develop the same illness

E. Her siblings have a 15% risk of getting MS

9. A previously healthy 25-year-old woman develops right monocular optic neuritis, and then makes a good recovery. Which of the following is correct?

A. If she has no additional flares within the next five years, she is not going to develop MS

B. If her baseline brain MRI is normal, she is not going to develop MS

C. If baseline cerebrospinal fluid is normal, she is not going to develop MS

D. Hot, humid weather might cause transient blurring of vision in the right eye

E. Persistence of a relative afferent papillary defect in the right eye after full recovery of visual acuity and color perception suggests a new injury

10. A 29-year-old woman develops bilateral optic neuritis, followed six months later by cervical myelitis. Two months after the myelitis she again develops optic neuritis. A cervical spinal cord lesion extends for four vertebral body lengths and NMO-Ig is positive. Which of the following is correct?

A. She has relapsing-remitting MS

B. She should receive chelation therapy

C. She is at risk of ultimately dying from respiratory complications of her illness

D. She is unlikely to have further flares

E. Potential for full recovery is excellent

Answers

1. F.
MRIs and lumbar puncture. MRIs are not essential for either MS flares or pseudoflares, unless another pathological process is suspected (eg, herniated disc), or in rare instances where contrast enhancement may be a useful clue; lumbar puncture is also unnecessary in a patient with an established diagnosis. CSF changes are not a reliable way of deciding if there is a flare. A U/A and culture should always be done as infection may accompany or provoke a flare.

2. E.
Episcleritis. Answers 1-4 are all typical features of optic neuritis, a common syndrome in patients with multiple sclerosis. Episcleritis is an inflammatory condition of the connective tissue between the conjunctiva and sclera that is associated with collagen vascular diseases but is not a typical feature of multiple sclerosis.

3. C.
Severe aphasia. Although significant neuropsychological deficits are not uncommon in patients with MS, aphasia would be very atypical. The history above is meant to suggest a mass lesion in the left hemisphere, rather than MS. Aphasia might be seen in patients with acute disseminated encephalomyelitis.

4. D.
CSF total protein =330 mg%. Although less than 10% of MS patients have a normal brain MRI, this is still much more common than a marked elevation of CSF total protein (>100 mg%). Positive ANA is common in MS, and the majority of MS patients have a normal ESR.

5. E.
Positive NMO-IG and systemic lupus erythematosis. Oligoclonal bands may occur transiently with NMO but are generally not persistent. About one-third of patients with NMO also have a collagen-vascular disorder.

6. E.
Brain MRI lesions in multiple sclerosis are generally larger than those seen in migraine, and have a somewhat different distribution (eg, MS lesions are periventricular, or involve the corpus callosum). MS patients may have headaches in association with flares.

7. D.
Primary progressive MS is extremely unlikely to begin at age eighteen. She does not have a clinically-isolated syndrome, because the time course (five years rather than weeks-months) and pattern (progression rather than flare) are incompatible. She does not need tibial somatosensory evoked potentials because the history and exam have already demonstrated that she has a myelopathy. MRI of the spine is necessary in order to rule out a compressive lesion or intrinsic cord tumor.

8. A.
She meets criteria for MS. The ABCR drugs (Avonex, Betaseron, Copaxone, Rebif) reduce flares by about one-third. Prophylactic treatment is most effective early in the illness, rather than after age forty. There is no net deleterious effect of pregnancy on MS. Her children have a low risk (about 4%-5%), as do her siblings.

9. D.
Elevated ambient temperature, fever, or fatigue may cause "pseudo-exacerbation" by causing conduction block in previously demyelinated tracts. Patients may develop their second flare years or even decades after their first episode. Patients with optic neuritis and normal baseline MRI have a 16% risk of MS by five years. Baseline cerebrospinal fluid is often normal in individuals who later develop MS. Persistence of the relative papillary defect is common, even when visual function seems otherwise restored to normal.

10. C.
She likely has the relapsing form of neuromyelitis optica, which has a one-third risk of death due to respiratory arrest from acute cervical myelitis. Chelation therapy has no proven benefit for NMO. She is likely to have further disabling flares with progressive, stepwise disability.

Chapter 26: Headache Evaluation and Treatment

Thomas Ward, MD

Contents

Introduction

"Headache" is not a diagnosis, it is a symptom with hundreds of possible causes. The fundamental approach to correct diagnosis, which then allows appropriate treatment, begins by deciding if the headache is secondary (ie, symptomatic, due to an underlying cause) or primary (a sui generis: not due to an underlying cause). In this chapter, we will discuss how to begin to make that distinction using the classical approach of careful history and examination followed by the judicious selection of tests to confirm or refute the initial diagnostic impression(s).

1. Approach to Diagnosis

In attempting to properly diagnose a patient with headache, the single most important thing to have is an accurate history. Occasionally, in the emergency room or with a delirious/demented patient, it may not be possible to obtain a reliable history. In that situation diagnosis is made much more difficult and possibly less certain. In those circumstances history should be obtained from previous records, family members, witnesses and anyone else who may have relevant information.

Key information to obtain includes whether this is a new headache or a recurrent headache, how long the headache(s) lasts, where it is located, what it feels like, how severe it is, whether there are associated symptoms (nausea/vomiting, photophobia/phonophobia), and how this headache began (gradual or sudden onset). One would like to know about any recent head/neck trauma. It is important to know what the patient was doing when the headache began (ie, was it during exertion?). What are the patient's other medical conditions? The presence of malignancy or AIDS suggests certain possibilities. If this is a recurrent headache, has there been a change in frequency, symptoms or severity? The behavior of a patient during the attack also provides important clues. A cluster headache patient may be agitated and pace about, while the migraineur prefers to lie quietly in a dark room.

"Red flags" or worrisome aspects of the history may increase the suspicion that a secondary headache is the problem. These include very sudden onset or onset during exertion, older patients/very young patients (>50 years old, <5 years old), worsening under observation, or increasing frequency/severity of pattern, any abnormality on neurologic examination (including the mental status), abnormal vitals signs, or seizures with headache. Mention should be made of the clinical clue "first/worst" headache. This is a little misleading, as for a given patient this description merely signals their worst-ever headache. However, a sudden onset headache, especially with vomiting and/or loss of consciousness, might suggest a subarachnoid hemorrhage (SAH) and bears careful consideration. Nonetheless, most cases of this sort will ultimately turn out to be severe migraine (crash migraine).

Once the history has been obtained, a careful examination should be done. This should include vital signs. Fever reliably measured (and not masked by antipyretics) may be a clue to the presence of infection or other serious conditions. Essential hypertension typically is not associated with headache, but paroxysmal elevations of blood pressure as seen with the tyramine reaction in patients on MAOIs, or with pheochromocytoma, or at the very high levels of malignant hypertension, certainly is associated with headache. A rising blood pressure with a falling pulse rate (Cushing reflex) suggests rising intracranial pressure, as with an expanding mass lesion or SAH. A rapid pulse might lead one to the diagnosis of hyperthyroidism or infection. As appropriate, examination of the head and neck usually follows, including observation for signs of trauma. A neurologic examination is next, including mental status, fundoscopic examination, inspection for signs of trauma (Battle's sign, raccoon eyes, etc.), cranial nerves, motor, sensory, cerebellar functions, station and gait, deep tendon reflexes, and plantar testing. General medical examination is also appropriate. A patient with a fever, tachycardia, new cardiac murmur, and petechiae with headache may have bacterial endocarditis, for example, with emboli to the brain and subsequent abscess formation.

Selection of testing depends upon the initial differential diagnosis generated by the history. In the absence of adequate history more testing may need to be done to cover the broad range of possible etiologies, especially those that might carry severe consequences if not promptly treated (eg, SAH, mass lesion, encephalitis/meningitis). Also, in settings such as the emergency room, where the patient may not be known to the physician, or who may be less likely to follow up, there is a lower threshold for obtaining tests.

The International Headache Society has published a classification to assist in headache diagnosis. This classification is now in its second edition, the *International Classification of Headache Disorders (ICHD-II)*. It is useful for both primary and secondary headaches and contains a collection of useful references as well (see References).

2. Pathophysiology

Much of what is known about headache pathophysiology comes from recent advances occurring with the advent of the triptans (Table 1). In the last 2 decades there has been an explosion of knowledge, mostly about migraine. Imaging has demonstrated an area near the periaqueductal gray that shows increased activity during and after a migraine. While it has been known for some time on clinical grounds that the hypothalamus must be involved in cluster headache due to its periodicity, PET scanning and MRI have demonstrated an area of abnormality in either the posterior hypothalamic gray

Table 1

The Triptans

Sumatriptan	Tablets: 100 mg, 50 mg, 25 mg Nasal spray: 5 mg, 20 mg s.c. injection: 6 mg
Zolmitriptan	Tablets and orally disintegrating tablets: 2.5 mg, 5 mg Nasal spray: 5 mg
Naratriptan	Tablets: 1 mg, 2.5 mg
Rizatriptan	Tablets and orally disintegrating tablets: 5 mg, 10 mg
Almotriptan	Tablets: 6.25 mg, 12.5 mg
Frovatriptan	Tablets: 2.5 mg
Eletriptan	Tablets: 20 mg, 40 mg

matter or in a nearby area (the subparafascicular nucleus of the thalamus).

The area of anatomic and physiologic convergence for headache is thought to be the trigeminal nucleus caudalis (TNC, spinal nucleus of V). There are indirect connections with the superior salivatory nucleus, which have parasympathetic outflow, thus explaining the ocular and nasal autonomic symptoms sometimes seen in migraine, cluster, and other headache syndromes. As the spinal nucleus of V runs down to the third cervical spinal level it becomes easier to comprehend how input from cervical structures might trigger headache. A patient with a unilateral severe headache such as migraine or cluster will often have a tender greater occipital nerve (C2, C3) on examination, and performance of a greater occipital nerve block will often alleviate these headaches. In such cases, the location of the underlying problem is undoubtedly elsewhere, but the peripheral site seems to be a way of "accessing" the circuit.

The phenomenon of cortical spreading depression (CSD) has been avidly studied since the time of Lashley and Leão. CSD moves across cortex at about 3 mm/min and is actually a wave of neuronal excitation followed by suppression of activity, accompanied with a transient increase, then sustained decrease in blood flow. Therefore, while there are vascular changes in migraine, they appear to be secondary to the neuronal changes. It is suspected that CSD is the pathophysiologic equivalent of migraine aura. Perhaps CSD also occurs in patients that do not have what is more commonly described as migraine aura, and may occur more frequently, even in those who only have, for example, blurry vision. CSD by orthodromic activation of the Vth cranial nerve causes activity in the TNC with the appearance of early response genes c-Fos and c-Jun. In turn, there is antidromic release from these unmyelinated trigeminal fibers of inflammatory neuropeptides from CGRP and substance P at numerous sites, including meningeal blood vessels. Sterile neurogenic inflammation occurs with these vessels dilating and becoming tender. Clinically, treating while only the first order trigeminal neuron is activated (typically when the headache is early and mild) tends to give better therapeutic outcomes. Left untreated, second order (trigeminotha-lamic) and third order (thalamocortical) neurons become activated. The clinical correlate of this central sensitization is cutaneous allodynia, where typically non-painful stimuli become quite painful and treatment outcomes at this stage are much less robust.

There are numerous other abnormalities which seem to be relevant to the genesis of migraine and other headaches. Subsequent to discovering that familial hemiplegic migraine appears to be due to an abnormality of calcium channels, it has been more broadly speculated that migraine is in part a channelopathy. There also seem to be abnormalities of glutaminergic transmission. It has also been reported that migraine patients have low brain magnesium. In that magnesium is an inhibitory ion, which tends to "plug" calcium channels, the concept of migraineurs having a hyperexcitable brain has been proposed. This may explain why migraine patients seem to be susceptible to certain triggers. The final common mediator for "vascular" headaches is thought to be nitric oxide (NO). The role of patent foramen ovale in migraine with aura remains uncertain.

One cannot discuss migraine pathophysiology without mentioning the role of serotonin (5-hydroxytrptamine, 5-HT). Years ago, Lance noted a fall in platelet levels of serotonin during a migraine attack with a commensurate rise in urine 5-hydoxyindoleacetic acid (5-HIAA, the metabolite of 5-HT) levels during an attack. In 1960, it was reported that 5 mg of serotonin administered during an attack would terminate a migraine but with impressive side effects. The triptan drugs such as sumatriptan are chemically similar to 5-HT but act primarily at 5-HT1D (on trigeminal neurons) and 5-HT1B (on blood vessel) receptors. These pharmacologic agents not only have been effective therapeutic agents but also have been used to study headache mechanisms. Response to treatment is not diagnostic, as there have been reports of patients with SAH transiently responding to agents such as dihydroergotamine and triptans. This suggests that in certain secondary headaches activation of the trigeminovascular system also occurs.

While much has been learned about the various mechanisms that generate head and facial pain, there is much that is not yet known. The most common headache, tension-type headache (TTH), is perhaps the least well understood. It is clinically defined as a headache without features of migraine. There may even be a difference between TTH in migraineurs (which responds to triptans) and TTH in nonmigraineurs (which is triptan-unresponsive). There is clearly much research yet to be done to elucidate the mechanisms of headache.

3. Testing

The most important parts of the evaluation of patients with headache and facial pain remain a careful and thorough history and examination. Tests are then ordered judiciously to confirm or refute the various choices in the differential diagnosis. The selection of specific tests will also be addressed below in the various diagnostic categories. In this section we will briefly review the more commonly chosen tests and list a few of their various advantages and limitations.

CT scan of the brain can be quite helpful in the emergency room. It is widely available and studies can be performed rapidly. Approximately 90%-95% of SAH will be visualized if performed within 24 hours of the hemorrhage. If SAH is being considered in the differential diagnosis, then a lumbar puncture must follow a negative CT scan. Due to limitations of the technology (photon dropout), CT scan does not visualize the posterior fossa nor the inferior middle cranial fossa well. Also, routine studies often do not include views of the sphenoid sinus. Therefore if clinical suspicion includes the region of the sphenoid sinus (eg, sphenoid sinusitis with consequent cavernous sinus thrombosis), it is important to request additional views.

MRI typically offers better visualization of the brain than CT scanning. Structures in the posterior fossa are better seen and sagittal views allow evaluation for abnormalities such as Chiari malformations. Magnetic resonance angiography (MRA) can help when aneurysm, vascular dissection and arteriovenous malformations (AVM) are possible, and magnetic resonance venography (MRV) may help if venous sinus thrombosis is being considered. MRI with gadolinium is felt to be more sensitive in the evaluation of multiple mass lesions such as metastatic disease.

Lumbar puncture (LP), properly performed, remains an important diagnostic tool in headache evaluation. The opening pressure may reveal intracranial hypertension or hypotension. Spectrophotometry adds sensitivity and accuracy in assessing the presence of xanthochromia. Routine studies including cell count/diff, protein, and glucose can help evaluate the presence of infection or inflammation. Further studies, including culture and PCR, may rule in/out specific infectious processes, and cytology for malignant cells is essential for the diagnosis of possible carcinomatous meningitis. LP may also be therapeutic in the case of idiopathic intracranial hypertension.

EEG has little role in the assessment of headaches in adults, and a small role in the assessment of headache in children. However, if seizure is thought to coexist with headache, then it is more useful. Postictal headaches are often migrainous and migraine has been known to trigger seizures. Conventional angiography occasionally still is useful in the diagnostic assessment of headache and the roles of CT angiography and CT venography are expanding.

Useful blood tests for headache diagnosis include CBC, ESR, electrolytes BUN/Cr, glucose, thyroid function studies, and Lyme testing. Other tests such as for HIV, carbon monoxide level, drug screen and arterial blood gases are appropriate in specific circumstances.

4. Secondary Headaches

Post-traumatic Headache

In the acute setting, post-traumatic headache and whiplash injuries are typically seen in the emergency room. A prompt and thorough history and examination are important. Diagnostic considerations to quickly consider include epidural/subdural hematoma (especially if there has been a concussion), intracerebral contusion or hematoma, arterial dissection (carotid or vertebral), SAH, basilar skull fracture, and cervical spine injury. C-spine fracture must be ruled out before moving the patient's neck. CT scan can rapidly exclude/include intracranial mass lesions.

Patients seen in the first minutes/hour after a concussion must be observed for a second loss of consciousness. This interval between a concussion and a second neurologic deterioration is called the "lucid interval" and suggests the presence of an epidural hematoma.

The evaluation of patients subsequent to a head or neck injury in the following days/weeks/months takes a somewhat different course. Post-concussion syndrome is common. Head and neck pain frequently coexist, as the same mechanisms that produce concussion also produce whiplash-type events. A history needs to be taken followed by an examination and a review of prior records. A concussion may be defined as a change in mental status due to trauma to the brain. Loss of consciousness is not required. Shear forces produced by acceleration/deceleration cause "diffuse axonal injury" and often particularly affect the upper brainstem. Injury to the dorsal raphe nucleus, periaqueductal gray, and reticular activation system may explain many of the subsequent symptoms including impaired sleep, impaired attention, and fatigue. Chronic input from injured cervical structures into the spinal nucleus of V may explain headache and neck pain, and with chronicity "central sensitization" may develop.

International Headache Society (IHS) classification guidelines from 2004 (ICHD-II) now require that the onset of post-traumatic headache begins within 7 days of the injury or of regaining consciousness therefrom. Some experts do recognize the occurrence of later-onset headaches. Headache is the most frequent symptom of post-concussive syndrome and neck pain frequently coexists. Secondary causes need to be ruled out, such as vascular dissection, chronic subdural hematoma, venous sinus thrombosis with intracranial hypertension, and hydrocephalus. MRI/MRA/MRV are most useful for these considerations. Lumbar puncture for opening pressure may also be indicated.

The headache of post-traumatic syndrome may mimic any of the primary headache syndromes. Most treatment, once underlying causes have been excluded, is symptomatic and given as one would for that primary headache type. Most cases resolve within a year and often before. Perhaps 20% remain chronic. In these cases, the possibility of the headaches being perpetuated by medication overuse/analgesic rebound needs to be entertained. Some of these patients will improve once the offending pain medications are stopped. Also, upper cervical nerve root entrapment (C2, C3) may cause delayed-onset, persisting, usually unilateral headache. These headaches may begin weeks or even a few months after the injury. Post-traumatic syndrome exhibits a multitude of symptoms including headache, neck pain, vertigo/tinnitus, altered cognition, neuralgia, personality change, anosmia, blurred vision, and sleep-wake cycle disturbances. A multidisciplinary approach is often best.

Mass Lesions

Intracerebral mass lesions such as meningiomas are often incidental findings. Intracranial mass lesions cause headache typically when they lead to obstruction of CSF pathways (eg, colloid cyst of the third ventricle), or cause increased intracranial pressure or traction on pain-sensitive structures. Primary and metastatic tumors, chronic subdural hematomas, and abscesses are the major considerations. The history will often reveal a story of a progressive headache, although headache as the sole presenting symptom of brain tumor only occurs in about half of such patients. Examination may reveal signs of raised intracranial pressure (papilledema, bilateral VIth nerve palsies, impaired upgaze) and there may be other abnormalities on the neurologic examination. Lesions in clinically silent areas of the brain such as the frontal lobes may initially present with few findings (abulia might be present), so if there is clinical suspicion even without abnormalities on examination, imaging should be obtained. MRI with contrast would be the preferred examination.

Treatment is directed against the underlying etiology with symptomatic treatment of the headache. Clinical experience suggests that features of such a headache in migraineurs are often reminiscent of their migraines.

Infections

Headache in the setting of infection may occur because of infection in or adjacent to CNS structures. It may also occur due to systemic infection (interleukin-1 causes headache). Peripheral infection is a frequent etiology of headache in pediatric emergency room patients. A careful history and examination will usually point to the source. Parameningeal sources such as otitis or sinusitis may cause meningitis, abscess or venous sinus thrombosis. Particular caution must be exercised in the evaluation of patients who may be immunosuppressed (on steroids, HIV). Chronic meningitis tends to cause a progressively worsening headache. The time course may be one of an acute or subacute problem. Examination may reveal fever (unless masked by antipyretics), and if meningitis is present, Brudzinski and/or Kernig signs (these signs of meningeal irritation are lost in deep coma). Mental status changes may prevent the patient from accurately describing the headache and the features of such headaches usually are severe and bilateral.

If meningitis or encephalitis in suspected, ideally a mass lesion should be excluded by CT or MRI scanning before proceeding to lumbar puncture. Treatment of headache in this setting is directed against the underlying cause, as well as symptomatic therapy for pain relief.

Stroke

Headache may occur in the setting of stroke and transient ischemic attack (TIA). A significant minority of patients with TIA and/or ischemic stroke may have headache, although the features may be nondescript. Headache, often severe and associated with nausea and/or vomiting, is a more consistent feature of intracerebral hematoma. Certainly, in a patient with risk factors for stroke who has a transient neurologic event, the possibility of TIA should be entertained, and a prompt workup/therapy initiated. TIA/stroke may also occur in the setting of vascular dissection. A history of neck trauma or of a predisposing condition such as fibromuscular dysplasia would increase the level of clinical suspicion. MRA or CTA are generally chosen as the imaging procedures. So-called "late-life migraine equivalents," as described by Fisher, are in the differential diagnosis, but I consider them a diagnosis of exclusion. Such events should be considered TIAs until proven otherwise.

The clinical presentation of SAH is one of the most dramatic in clinical medicine. "Thunderclap headache" may be the presentation of an expanding/thrombosing/leaking aneurysm or AVM. Aneurysmal leak may produce a sentinel (warning) bleed, which may be mistaken for migraine and the diagnosis missed. Alternatively, a catastrophe may occur as the initial presentation with the demise of the patient. Patients with SAH may lose consciousness, but if awake they may report severe headache with nausea/vomiting, stiff neck and back pain. The headache is usually bilateral and may pound.

The first-ever migraine may also present in this way, but is a diagnosis of exclusion. In patients with the possible presentation of SAH, a careful history is important, specifically wondering if there might have been a sentinel hemorrhage. Headache onset is usually sudden and sometimes occurs in the setting of exertion. CT scan is a useful screening test (unenhanced), and if negative should be followed by a carefully performed LP. The opening pressure should be recorded, xanthochromia evaluated, with cell counts and differential on the first and third tubes, and measurement of protein and glucose levels. It is important to remember that it may take up to 12 hours for blood to reach the lumbar region. Therefore, if the LP is performed before 12 hours from the ictus, it might be falsely negative. If clinical suspicion of a SAH is present, the LP either needs to be repeated at 12 hours or later, or an imaging procedure such as MRI/MRA or CTA should be accomplished.

Intracerebral hematoma also usually has a dramatic presentation. Headache is typically severe with nausea and/or vomiting. A history of hypertension may be present. Fever and hypertension as well as neurologic changes are often present on examination. CT scanning is quite useful, although MRI/MRA are often performed, looking for bleeding into an underlying lesion, such as a tumor or AVM. Repeat scanning to confirm resolution of the hematoma is appropriate. Typical sites for hypertensive hemorrhage include the putamen, pons, thalamus, cerebellum and centrum semiovale. Cerebellar hemorrhage deserves special mention. Close neurosurgical consultation is essential as the expanding mass may need to be evacuated if there is impending brainstem compression and/or increasing intracranial pressure.

Vasculitis

Headache may occur in the setting of intracranial vasculitis such as primary angiitis of the CNS or systemic lupus erythematosis (SLE). Appropriate blood testing and studies such as angiography, lumbar puncture, and even brain biopsy may be required. SLE seems to occasionally coexist with migraine and the exact relationship/mechanisms remain uncertain. CNS vasculitis may cause "beading" on angiography (the exact sensitivity of conventional angiography in this setting is unknown) and is expected to cause a CSF pleocytosis with elevated protein.

One entity that should always be considered in patients over the age of 50 with a new headache is giant cell arteritis (also known as temporal arteritis, cranial arteritis, Horton disease). It is the most common systemic arteritis in the elderly. Patients are usually older than 50 years and usually have an ESR over 50 mm/hr. Remember that steroids and NSAIDs can lower the ESR result. In GCA, headache is the most common symptom in about 90% of cases. The headache may take almost any form—be unilateral or bilateral, constant or intermittent—and mimic any of the primary headache patterns. It may coexist with polymyalgia rheumatica. Fever and weight loss may be present. Tender temporal arteries, jaw claudication, diplopia, and transient visual loss are just a few of the other possible symptoms. Undiagnosed/untreated cases of GCA have a significant risk of blindness and stroke.

Once the diagnosis is suspected on clinical grounds, steroids should be started immediately, often as prednisone at 60-80 mg per day. Biopsy of the superficial temporal artery is performed within 1-2 weeks. Selection of the side/site is based on clinical grounds but may be aided by ultrasound of the artery. A positive biopsy may reveal intimal proliferation with luminal stenosis, disruption of the internal elastic lamina, invasion and necrosis of the media by a mononuclear cell infiltrate, intraluminal stenosis, and sometimes granuloma formation with giant cells. Due to the patchy involvement of the vessels with "skip lesions," an adequate biopsy of several centimeters is best taken, and if negative the contralateral side should be biopsied.

Prednisone is gradually tapered once symptoms lessen, and symptoms and ESR are followed as the steroid dose is reduced. GCA is often self-limited, and therapy can be stopped after a number of months although late relapses have been reported. In cases where the steroid dosage cannot be adequately reduced ("steroid resistance"), other agents have been employed. Symptoms of PMR sometimes emerge as the steroid dose is tapered.

Toxic-Metabolic Causes of Headache

There are myriad toxic-metabolic causes of headache. Drugs are a notoriously common cause, especially vasodilators including hydralazine, agents used for erectile dysfunction, proton-pump inhibitors (PPIs), and nitroglycerin (a NO donor). Some NSAIDs may induce a chemical meningitis. While some headaches best respond to indomethacin (such as paroxysmal hemicrania), a major side effect of this drug in those that are not already so afflicted is to cause headache. Phenylpropanolamine and cocaine have been known to initiate headache by causing a secondary vasculitis. IVIG infusions have also been reported to cause headache, which often has migrainous features.

The role of interleukin-1 in the setting of infections causing headache has already been mentioned. Many other medical conditions are also associated with headache. Severe anemia, polycythemia, renal failure, hypoxemia and hypercarbia are well-known causes, as are hyper- and hypothyroidism. With an appropriate history of possible exposure, carbon monoxide poisoning should be considered. In females with a history of migraine, exposure to exogenous estrogen from oral contraceptives or hormone replacement therapy is a frequent culprit.

A thorough history supplemented by appropriate blood tests usually gives the correct diagnosis and correction of the underlying abnormality, or removal of the offending agent may benefit the patient. One scenario that merits special mention is so-called "analgesic-rebound" headache. This occurs only in migraineurs and seems to be related to use of any of a number of analgesics and other pain remedies including triptan drugs. Similar headaches occur in the setting of frequent ergotamine use. If a migraine patient uses these agents more than 2-3 days per week, the headache pattern may evolve from one of intermittent headache to chronic daily headache. The usual story is a worsening headache pattern and the use of more and more symptomatic medications. Preventive medications are often ineffective in this situation and the effective treatment entails cessation of consumption of the offending agent(s). Sometimes this requires hospitalization and the use of intravenous medications to control the withdrawal headache that may occur.

Neuralgias

Neuralgias are classically described as sudden "lancinating" electrical pains occurring along the distribution of a nerve or one or more of its branches. Sometimes the pain pattern is more complex, with a background of more persistent aching pain coexisting in the region of the neuralgic pain. There conditions are often caused by trauma to the nerve, surgery, infections, compression (by blood vessels or tumors), and demyelination. The pain may occur spontaneously or in association with triggers such as touching the area, chewing, swallowing, shaving, applying make-up, etc. Postherpetic neuralgia is a common affliction of the elderly and may involve the head. We shall focus on two other frequently seen entities, trigeminal neuralgia (tic douloureux) and occipital neuralgia.

The pain of trigeminal neuralgia may occur along any of the three branches of CNV, but most often in the first or second divisions. It may be classified as primary, which includes those cases felt to be due to "microvascular compression of the nerve" by blood vessels or perhaps viral infection; or secondary, which includes compression by mass lesions and demyelination (a more likely etiology in younger patients, especially if bilateral). Once the diagnosis is made, imaging—usually MRI/MRA—is performed to exclude a mass lesion and to look for evidence of demyelination. Treatment should be initiated promptly as the pain is excruciating. A clinical pearl is that rapid relief may be provided with intravenous phenytoin (or fosphenytoin). Patients often lose the benefits from this agent, so it is less often used for long-term management. Effective treatments include carbamazepine, baclofen, valproic acid, clonazepam, gabapentin, and in the setting of multiple sclerosis, misoprostol.

The occipital nerve (composed of fibers from C2) may mediate neuralgic pain. Occipital neuralgia is a unilateral posterior pain problem, with neuralgic pains and often a constant background discomfort. The nerve itself may be exquisitely tender. There may or may not be a history of antecedent trauma. This nerve is often also tender ipsilateral to a unilateral migraine or on the side of a cluster attack. An occipital nerve block may provide dramatic relief. One regimen is to use 1 cc of 1% lidocaine with 20 mg of depo-methylprednisolone. Surgical procedures directed towards this region are sometimes employed and the use of occipital nerve stimulators is being studied.

Miscellaneous Causes of Headache

Ocular, Dental, and Sinus Causes of Headache

Due to the pattern of innervation of the trigeminal system, much head pain is appreciated maximally in the region of the orbit. This does not mean that the origin of this sensation is in the eye, in fact the eye is usually not the source. Nonetheless, there are serious ocular sources of eye pain. While chronic glaucoma is usually painless, acute glaucoma can have a dramatic presentation. Eye pain is usually severe, the eye may appear reddened and the patient may see halos around objects. Nausea and vomiting may be associated. Tonometry will reveal elevated intraocular pressures. Urgent ophthalmologic consultation and treatment are necessary to preserve vision. Other ophthalmologic conditions which may cause eye pain include posterior scleritis and retrobulbar neuritis. Tolosa-Hunt syndrome also is well known to cause eye pain, but is uncommon. Eye pain and/or diplopia are commonly seen in GCA, presumably due to extraocular muscle ischemia.

Occasionally, dental disease may cause pain which has features of neuralgia; more often trigeminal neuralgia (and the controversial entity "pre-trigeminal neuralgia") may cause pain mistaken as emanating from a dental source. Often in dental disease there are clues to the problem such as local sensitivity to hot/cold, pain on chewing, etc. Careful examination and evaluation by a dental specialist may clarify the diagnosis and allow correct intervention. The temporomandibular joint is often a source of diagnostic confusion. Temporomandibular joint syndrome consists of clicking and popping of the joint, pain on use, and limitation of jaw opening (usually less than 30 mm in the midline). Treatment is most often symptomatic with rest, NSAIDs, and perhaps a bite splint. Surgery is rarely if ever needed. Dental consultation may be helpful.

Sinus symptoms cause frequent diagnostic confusion in headache patients. Chronic sinusitis rarely is a cause of headache. Acute sinusitis certain does cause headache. However, because of the reflex between the trigeminal nucleus caudalis and the superior salivatory nucleus, migraine patients and those with TACs such as cluster headache often experience sinus symptoms such as stuffiness and rhinorrhea, causing diagnostic confusion. Most "sinus headache" that headache specialists see is actually migraine. Acute purulent sinusitis should be confirmed by the presence of local pain, fever, drainage, perhaps elevated WBC and ESR, and abnormal imaging. MRI tends to overestimate the extent of sinus disease, thus CT scan is superior. Treatment includes analgesics, decongestants, antibiotics in refractory cases, and occasionally, surgery for refractory/recurrent cases.

Headache Due to High or Low Intracranial Pressure

Idiopathic intracranial hypertension (IIH) formerly was known as pseudotumor cerebi or benign intracranial hypertension. The former name was used because the patient looked clinically as though they had an intracranial mass with headache and papilledema yet they had no mass lesion. The latter name was inappropriate, as any entity that can cause visual loss is certainly not "benign." This entity may occur in the setting of head trauma, postpartum, dehydration, cancer, other hypercoaguable states, and with exposure to certain agents such as excess vitamin A, and perhaps others which are more controversial. It seems to be more common in obese females. Venous sinus thrombosis is being recognized with increasing frequency as a common etiology.

Patients with idiopathic IIH generally complain of bilateral constant headache, which may have migrainous features. Tinnitus is common, and they may have transient visual obscurations. Papilledema is frequently noted, although this condition may occur in the absence of papilledema, perhaps due to anatomic defects of the optic nerve sheath. Other findings on exam may include diminished visual acuity, loss of peripheral vision, bilateral VIth nerve palsies, and decreased upgaze. With this history and clinical presentation, an MRI/MRV should be obtained immediately. Once a mass lesion has been excluded, a lumbar puncture to measure an opening pressure should be performed. CSF pressures are typically higher than 240 mm H_2O (values from 180-240 are equivocal). Routine studies are normal in IIH. The LP is not only diagnostic but may be therapeutic (transient relief of headache). If venous sinus thrombosis is documented, further tests should include a thrombosis screen looking for the cause. Anticoagulation may be appropriate depending on the clinical circumstances. Intracranial pressure may be lowered with a number of agents, particularly acetazolamide (unless the patient has a history of nephrolithiasis or sulfa allergy). Weight loss is also advocated. Serial ophthalmologic examinations are necessary. Refractory cases where vision is at risk may require optic nerve sheath fenestration or ventricular shunting to preserve vision.

Intracranial hypotension in many ways is the converse of intracranial hypertension. The most common scenario is the "post-LP headache." After a lumbar puncture the patient develops a positional headache that is worse on sitting/standing and immediately improved with recumbency. It is felt to be due to diminished CSF volume with traction on pain-sensitive structures, as the intracranial contents "sag." Other causes include after surgery where the meninges are violated, and trauma (including CSF leak due to basilar skull fracture or fracture of the cribiform plate). Occasionally, intracranial hypotension may present as a postcoital headache, presumably due to a dural tear.

Early in the clinical course, the headache due to low CSF pressure maintains a close temporal relationship to sitting up/standing up and lying down, as noted above. With chronicity, this relationship becomes less closely temporally linked, and the headache more and more gradually appears as the patient is upright, and more slowly resolves with recumbency. MRI with gadolinium may show pachymeningeal enhancement and repeat LP will document low or unmeasureable pressures (even negative!). If the site of the leak is unknown, MRI, myelography or even radionuclide isotope scanning (Indium-111) may be necessary to reveal the location of the defect.

In the case of post-LP headache, the problem often responds to 1-2 days of strict bedrest. Failing that, an epidural blood patch is usually effective. Intravenous caffeine sodium benzoate has also been utilized. For other causes, the site of the leak often must be identified, then repaired, as in a dural root sleeve tear.

Migraine

Migraine affects about 10% of the population. The International Headache Society has published new diagnostic criteria (*ICHD-II*) for migraine without aura and typical aura with migraine (Table 2, 3). If the patient fulfills all the criteria for a particular diagnosis then the diagnosis is "definite;" if they miss a definite diagnosis by one criterion then they are categorized as "probable."

From a practical point of view, certain features aid in the clinical recognition of migraine. The history is usually one of intermittent disabling attacks with associated symptoms of nausea and/or vomiting, and perhaps light and sound sensitivity. Sometimes triggers can be identified and there is usually a family history of others with migraine (although they may be called "sinus headaches" or "sick headaches"). If one meets criteria for intermittent/low frequency migraine and has a normal neurologic examination, neuroimaging is not required.

Table 2

***ICHD-II* Criteria for Migraine Without Aura**

Diagnostic Criteria
A. At least 5 attacks fulfilling criteria B - D
B. Headache attacks lasting 4-72 hours (untreated or unsuccessfully treated)
C. Headache has at least two of the following characteristics: 1. Unilateral location 2. Pulsating quality 3. Aggravation by or causing avoidance of routine physical activity (eg, walking or climbing stairs)
D. During headache at least one of the following: 1. Nausea and/or vomiting 2. Photophobia and phonophobia
E. Not attributed to another disorder

Table 3

***ICHD-II* Typical Aura with Migraine Headache**

Diagnostic Criteria
A. At least 2 attacks fulfilling criteria B - D
B. Aura consisting of at least one of the following, but no motor weakness: 1. Fully reversible visual symptoms including positive features (eg, flickering lights, spots or lines) and/or negative features (eg, loss of vision) 2. Fully reversible sensory symptoms including positive features (eg, pins and needles) and/or negative features (eg, numbness) 3. Fully reversible dysphasic speech disturbance
C. At least two of the following: 1. Homonymous visual symptoms and/or unilateral sensory symptoms 2. At least one aura symptom develops gradually ≥5 minutes and/or different aura symptoms occur in succession over ≥5 minutes 3. Each symptom lasts ≥5 and ≤60 minutes
D. Headache fulfilling criteria B - D for Table 2 Migraine Without Aura begins during the aura or follows the aura within 60 minutes
E. Not attributed to another disorder

Migraine aura is the (usually) reversible neurologic phenomenon that may occur before or during the migraine, or sometimes without a headache (typical migraine aura without headache). Aura is most often visual (scintillating scotoma, photopsias, teichopsias/fortification spectra, others), less often cheiro-oral, and less often still hemiplegic. If two or more symptoms (except motor weakness) referable to the posterior circulation or from both hemispheres simultaneously manifest, then the migraine is called basilar-type. Aura symptoms typically last ≥5 minutes and ≤60 minutes. Seizures and TIAs may be in the differential diagnosis. Migraine aura lasting >60 minutes and aura beginning in middle age bear further investigation (for anticardiolipin antibodies, AVM, tumor and other possible etiologies).

There are 3 options in treating migraine: nonpharmacologic measures, acute/abortive treatment, and preventive medications. A peculiar phenomenon that seems to only occur in migraineurs is analgesic rebound. There may be over 5 million such patients in the United States alone. When migraine patients consume certain acute medications >2-3 days per week, some of them appear to "transform" from episodic migraine to more of a chronic tension-type headache pattern with superimposed migraine-like attacks. They usually tell a story of taking more pills yet having more headaches. It has been shown that in the setting of analgesic rebound preventive medications are less effective. Some of the medications that can cause this problem include acetaminophen, ibuprofen (personal observation), combination medications including butalbital and caffeine, short-acting narcotics, and triptan drugs. Caffeine alone and ergotamine may also cause rebound and/or dependency.

Nonpharmacologic measures include avoidance of triggers, regular meals (delaying/missing a meal is a common trigger), and regular/adequate sleep. It is important to remember that headache patients want and need education to understand what type of headache they have, to be reassured, and to be able to effectively participate in their care. The goal is "self-efficacy," ie, the patient can manage the attack without requiring a trip to the doctor's office or emergency room. Psychologic treatment including cognitive behavioral therapy, thermal and EMG-guided biofeedback has good support in the literature and is complementary to preventive medications. These measures are particularly useful in patients that are pregnant or planning to become pregnant, patients with a history of medication overuse/rebound, and in patients who prefer to avoid/limit medications.

Acute treatment is chosen to try to terminate an attack, or failing that, to lessen the symptoms, or to "rescue" the patient (stop vomiting and allow the patient to achieve sleep). Migraineurs often have more than one type of attack and therefore may need multiple treatment options to manage their various attack types. Oral formulations may be fine if there is time for them to work, but once severe nausea/vomiting occur, non-oral routes take precedence and become more appropriate, such as nasal sprays, suppositories, subcutaneous/intramuscular injections and intravenous formulations. The ideal is to terminate the attack and restore the patient to normal. The ergot drugs formerly were used for this goal but have largely been supplanted by the triptans (Table 1). When used properly they may terminate an attack. Typical nuisance side effects include a sensation of chest/neck tightness, paresthesiae and flushing. These agents vary in their efficacy and tolerability from patient to patient. A particular patient may need to try several agents before finding the optimal one. The treatment goal is to try to rapidly terminate the attack and associated symptoms and hopefully avoid headache recurrence. Triptans work best when the migraine is early/mild (before central sensitization occurs) and have fewer side effects when utilized at this time. They may work later in the attack but have been reported to fail once cutaneous allodynia develops. These drugs should be avoided in patients with coronary artery disease, uncontrolled hypertension, Prinzmetal angina (vasospastic angina), and severe Raynaud phenomenon. They are also contraindicated in hemiplegic and basilar-type migraine. When used with these restrictions they are remarkably safe.

NSAIDs taken early during the attack with an agent to restore GI motility, such as metoclopramide, may be effective. Naproxen sodium 550 mg is preferred to naproxen, which achieves a maximum blood level in two hours (naproxen) rather than one. Indomethacin suppositories 50 mg can be compounded or obtained from Canada. NSAIDs can be used in conjunction with triptans.

Much of the misery of a migraine attack is due to the attendant nausea/vomiting. Hydroxyzine pamoate and hydrozyzine HCl may be used orally or as intramuscular injection. Some utilize prochlorperazine orally or as suppositories, but due to the rather frequent occurrence of acathisia and dystonic reactions, promethazine may be preferable. Chlorpromazine suppositories (100 mg as the adult dose) may be compounded and utilized along with 25-50 mg of oral diphenhydramine. This regimen effectively stops vomiting and allows the patient to rest or achieve sleep, but like all neuroleptics should be used judiciously to lessen the risk of tardive movement disorders.

"Rescue" strategies enable the patient to stop vomiting and achieve sleep, which often will terminate an attack. Avoiding a call to the doctor in the middle of the night or a trip to the emergency room is a laudable goal. One inexpensive and effective regimen is 25 mg of promethazine as the suppository and 5-10 mg of oral diazepam.

Preventive medications are generally taken daily to make the headaches shorter/milder/fewer. The patient must keep a daily headache diary to help assess progress. Drug selection is based on coexistent/comorbid conditions (Table 4). The ideal choice will treat 2 or more conditions/symptoms that the migraine sufferer has without aggravating anything. The goal is to try to reduce the use of acute migraine medications to ≤2-3 days per week, thus avoiding analgesic rebound. For example, if the patient has mitral valve prolapse, tremor, or hypertension, a beta-blocker such as propranolol might be a good choice. Similarly, if cold extremities (Raynaud) are present a calcium channel drug might be appropriate. Valproate or topiramate would be good possibilities if the patient also had epilepsy, and valproate has been used in bipolar disorder. Amitriptyline is often chosen when depression is present. Details of the initiation of these agents can be found in the references. For those unwilling to use prescription agents there is support in the literature for vitamin B_2 (riboflavin), magnesium, Petasides hybridus, and coenzyme Q10. Recent evidence suggests that feverfew is probably not as effective as once believed. The role of botulinum toxin in headache treatment remains controversial.

Table 4

Conditions Comorbid With Migraine

Mitral valve prolapse (?patent foramen ovale)
Psychiatric conditions (anxiety, depression, bipolar disorder, phobias
Raynaud's phenomenon
Stroke
Epilepsy

Some mention should be made of the role of narcotics in migraine treatment. They are best reserved for occasional use in the pregnant migraine patient when other agents may be contraindicated. Similarly, they have a place in the treatment of patients who cannot use the triptans or NSAIDs. Elderly patients may be candidates, but migraine tends to be less common in the elderly. Meperidine is a serotonin reuptake inhibitor and seems to be a poor choice for migraine patients that are often on other agents that affect serotonin. Narcotics are usually very poor choices for patients with psychiatric comorbidity.

If a headache has not responded to the measures available to the patient, especially if there has been vomiting or if the features are not typical of the patient's usual migraines, a visit to the emergency room becomes necessary. An evaluation should be made to clarify whether the diagnosis for this attack is actually migraine. Migraineurs are in no way immune to having other types of headache such as those due to SAH, meningitis, etc. If the patient turns out to have an intractable headache, intravenous hydration and medications are chosen. Intravenous dihydroergotamine preceded by metoclopramide and sometimes diphenhydramine is particularly useful. Other remedies may be chosen depending on what has worked in the past and on associated medical conditions. Sometimes the patient must be admitted to the hospital for several days to get medical control and manage the pain. In either case, arrangements for appropriate follow-up are important.

Tension-type Headache

The *ICHD-II* also has criteria for the various categories of tension-type headache (TTH) (Table 5). The name is of historical interest but misleading as there is more "tension" in the muscles of migraineurs than in TTH patients. While the most common of the headache types, experienced nearly universally, it is not well understood. In fact, the *ICHD* defines it by symptoms that are not seen in migraine. Fortunately for physicians, patients with TTH usually treat themselves and infrequently present for medical care. NSAIDs and muscle relaxants have been advocated, as have physical measures. If prevention is required, amitriptyline is often chosen. Coexistent medical conditions may represent a therapeutic opportunity. When TTH coexists with migraine it often responds to the same medications utilized to treat migraine. This fact suggests that while TTH in migraineurs and nonmigraineurs is phenotypically similar, pathophysiologically it may be different.

Table 5

***ICHD-II* (Frequent Episodic) Tension-Type Headache**

Diagnostic Criteria
A. At least 10 episodes occurring on ≥1 but ≤15 days per month for at least 3 months (≥12 and ≤180 days per year) and fulfilling criteria B - D
B. Headache lasting from 30 minutes to 7 days
C. Headache has at least two of the following characteristics: 1. Bilateral location 2. Pressing/tightening (nonpulsating quality) 3. Mild or moderate intensity 4. Not aggravated by routine physical activity such as walking or climbing stairs
D. Both of the following: 1. No nausea or vomiting (anorexia may occur) 2. No more than one of photophobia or phonophobia
E. Not attributed to another disorder

Table 6

***ICHD-II* Criteria for Cluster Headache**

Diagnostic Criteria
A. At least 5 attacks fulfilling criteria B - D
B. Severe or very severe unilateral orbital, supraorbital and/or temporal pain lasting 15-180 minutes if untreated
C. Headache is accompanied by at least one of the following characteristics: 1. Ipsilateral conjuctival injection and/or lacrimation 2. Ipsilateral nasal congestion and/or rhinorrhea 3. Ipsilateral eyelid edema 4. Ipsilateral forehead and facial swelling 5. Ipsilateral miosis and/or ptosis 6. A sense of restlessness or agitation
D. Attacks have a frequency from one every other day to 8 per day
E. Not attributed to another disorder

Cluster Headache and Other Trigeminal Autonomic Cephalalgias (TACs)

Cluster headache is uncommon but highly rewarding to treat. Again, the *ICHD-II* has specific diagnostic criteria for this entity (Table 6), as well as the related TACs. Unlike migraine, cluster is more common in men. Most patients have the episodic form, which is characterized by bouts (periods of daily or near-daily headache attacks which may be multiple), separated by remissions during which headache attacks do not occur. The chronic form has either no remissions or less than 1 month per year of freedom from attacks.

The headache pattern is notable for periodicity, with bouts tending to recur at certain times of the year and attacks tending to occur at certain times of the day.

This has always suggested a problem in the hypothalamus and recent imaging has shown an abnormality in or near the posterior hypothalamic gray matter. Some of the attacks may awaken the patient from sleep. They tend to be of maximal intensity within 15 minutes of onset and are excruciating (the worst pain known). The pain is usually most intense in and around the eye. Associated autonomic symptoms are ipsilateral to the pain and include conjunctival injection, lacrimation, partial Horner syndrome (ptosis, miosis), nasal stuffiness, and rhinorrhea. A sense of restlessness and agitation is common and the patient may pace about. Attacks tend to last about 45 minutes.

Diagnosis is made mostly on history. Between attacks there is little to find on examination save for the occasional persisting partial Horner syndrome and perhaps a tender ipsilateral carotid artery. It is important to remember that cluster headache can be symptomatic and neuroimaging (MRI) is appropriate. Attacks of shortening duration or loss of episodicity (conversion to chronic cluster pattern) are especially worrisome and abnormalities of the pituitary/parasellar region should be considered.

Treatment of cluster headache is usually very rewarding both for the patient and the physician. At the start of a bout, a prednisone taper is often advocated, but this author favors an ipsilateral occipital nerve block to lessen the frequency/severity of the attacks. Agents used for an acute attack must act rapidly as the pain is maximal at onset or shortly thereafter and the attacks are fairly brief (about 45 minutes). Oral agents therefore make little sense. Sumatriptan 4-6 mg s.c. in appropriate candidates is ideal and often provides relief in under 15 minutes. It is limited to twice daily. Zolmitriptan nasal spray is a somewhat slower option. Oxygen administered as 100% FIO_2 by mask at ≥7 liters per minute for 15 minutes up to several times per day also is usually effective (flow rates as high as 12 liters per minute may be necessary and patients need to stop smoking). Transnasal butorphanol 1 puff (= 1 mg) acts rapidly but may be highly sedating and has addiction potential. Its use needs to be tightly monitored but represents an option for patients who cannot use sumatriptan until the attacks stop or prophylactic agents become effective. Lidocaine 4% 1 mL dripped into the ipsilateral nostril may also be effective.

Preventive agents for cluster headache include methysergide, verapamil, valproate, lithium and melatonin. Methysergide is no longer available in the United States. Patients using sumatriptan should not also use methysergide. Verapamil may be initiated, depending on the blood pressure, and adjusted with a customary maximum dose of 480 mg per day (although higher doses are sometimes used in refractory cases). EKG monitoring is appropriate when using verapamil, especially at higher doses. Lithium or valproate may be used singly or in addition to verapamil. Bedtime doses of melatonin (about 10 mg) may be added. Patients with unresponsive cluster sometimes improve after hospitalization for repetitive intravenous dihydroergotamine.

Refractory cases of chronic cluster sometimes come to surgical intervention. This approach needs to be highly individualized based on the patient. Elderly patients with shorter life expectancies may benefit from less invasive choices. Some procedures such as radiofrequency lesioning are directed at the trigeminal ganglion. The nerve has also been subjected to microvascular decompression or sectioning, sometimes with the nervus intermedius as well. Newer procedures which may hold promise include ipsilateral occipital nerve stimulation, vagal nerve stimulation, and deep brain stimulation.

There are numerous other headaches which bear some similarity to cluster headache but tend to be briefer. These include paroxysmal hemicrania (which responds dramatically to indomethacin) and short-lasting unilateral headache with conjuctival injection and tearing (SUNCT). These are well described in the *ICHD-II*.

6. Intractable Headache

When a patient, especially one with a prior history of intermittent headache, presents with daily or near-daily headache, a careful reassessment is necessary. Is this a new headache or worsening of a prior headache? All the potential secondary headache causes such as new development of a brain tumor or vasculitis need to be considered. Among the most difficult cases to treat are those that have the primary headache type new daily-persistent headache (NDPH).

The history should be reviewed in detail and the examination repeated. Previous imaging and other testing should be reviewed. Often it is appropriate to repeat studies if significant time has passed. This author has had numerous patients who had normal CT/MRI years earlier, that then developed a brain tumor.

MRI may reveal other causes of daily headache, including Chiari malformations and AVMs. Lumbar puncture for measurement of opening pressure and to rule out chronic meningitis is often necessary. Thyroid abnormalities are frequently associated with a worsening headache pattern. Persistent unilateral headaches should prompt consideration of hemicrania continua, which is listed in *ICHD-II* (and a brief trial of indomethacin), occipital neuralgia (and possibly an occipital nerve block), and upper cervical root entrapment of C2 and/or C3 (a CT-guided deep block should alleviate symptoms in such cases).

The thoughtful clinician will wonder if the headache problem is difficult, is the patient difficult, or both? Noncompliance with therapy is common, as is medication overuse/analgesic rebound. Undiagnosed/uncontrolled psychiatric conditions such as PTSD and personality disorders complicate management. Cyproheptadine given entirely at bedtime suppresses nightmares, improves sleep, lessens headache, and is the antidote for many of the side effects of SSRIs. Other medical conditions need to be addressed and managed effectively. The possibility of illicit drugs and medications (especially oral contraceptives/hormone replacement therapy) as culprits needs to be considered. In selected cases, a trial of long-acting chronic daily opioids such as methadone may be undertaken, but the majority of headache patients fail to do well on such regimens.

If outpatient management strategies fail, admission to the hospital may be effective. Ideally, this should be accomplished in a unit with experience in managing difficult headache conditions. Medications that may be causing analgesic rebound can be stopped. Phenobarbital can be substituted for butalbital (100 mg butalbital = 30 mg phenobarbital) and then tapered. Neuroleptics such as intravenous chlorpromazine preceded by diphenhydramine suppress withdrawal symptoms from narcotics. The repetitive intravenous dihydroergotamine protocol of Raskin can be dramatically effective, especially in cases of analgesic rebound, post-traumatic headache and intractable chronic cluster. During hospitalization, consultations may be obtained from Psychiatry, Pain, Behavioral Medicine, and other services. New medications can be initiated under medical supervision. Many patients will benefit from skilled inpatient evaluation and treatment.

7. References

1. Ward TN, Levin M, Phillips JM. Evaluation and management of headache in the emergency department. *Med Clin N Am.* 2001;85(4):971-985.

   (Very practical review of the fundamentals.)

2. Ward TN, Levin M. Diagnosis and pathophysiology of migraine. *Expert Rev Neurotherapeutics.* 2004;4(3):383-390.

   (Review of migraine pathophysiology with useful reference list.)

3. Weiller C, May A, Limmroth V, et al. Brainstem activation in spontaneous human migraine attacks. *Nature Med.* 1995;1(7): 658-660.

4. May A, Bahra A, Buchel C, et al. Hypothalamic activation in cluster headache attacks. *Lancet.* 1998;351:275-278.

5. Lashley KS. Patterns of cerebral integration indicated by the scotomas of migraine. *Arch Neurol.* 1941;46:331-339.

6. Leão AAP. Spreading depression of activity in cerebral cortex. *J Neurophysiol.* 1944;7: 359-390.

7. Woods RP, Iacoboni M, Mazziotta JC. Bilateral spreading cerebral hypoperfusion during spontaneous migraine headaches. *NEJM.* 1994;331:1689-1692.

8. Bolay H, Reuter U, Dunn AK, et al. Intrinsic brain activity triggers trigeminal afferents in a migraine model. *Nature Med.* 2002;8(2): 136-142.

9. Hoskins KL, Kaube H. Goadsby PJ. Central activation of the trigeminovascular pathway in the cat is inhibited by dihydroergotamine: a c-fos and electrophysiologic study. *Brain.* 1996;119:249-256.

10. Burstein R, Cutrer FM, Yarnitsky D. The development of cutaneous allodynia during a migraine attack: clinical evidence for the sequential recruitment of spinal and supraspinal nociceptive neurons in migraine. *Brain.* 2000;123:1703-1709.

11. Burstein R, Collins B, Bajwa Z, Jukubowski M. Triptan therapy can abort migraine attacks if given before the establishment or in the absence of cutaneous allodynia and central sensitization: clinical and preclinical evidence. *Headache.* 2002;42(5):390-391.

12. May A, Ophoff RA, Terwindt GM, et al. Familial hemiplegic migraine locus on chromosome 19p13 is involved in the common forms of migraine with and without aura. *Hum Genet.* 1995;96:604-608.

13. Welch KM, D'Andrea G, Tepley N, et al. The concept of migraine as a state of central neuronal hyperexcitablility. *Neurologic Clinics.* 1990;8(4): 817-828.

    (Thoughtful application of basic science to explain clinical manifestations of migraine.)

14. Curran DA, Hinterberger H, Lance JW. Total plasma serotonin, 5-hydroxyindoleacetic acid and p-hydroxy-m-methoxymandelic acid excretion in normal and migrainous subjects. *Brain.* 1965;88:997-1010.

15. Kimball RW, Friedman AP, Vallejo E. Effect of serotonin in migraine patients. *Neurology.* 1960;10:107-111.

    (Pivotal article of historical interest.)

16. Cady RK, Lipton RB, O'Quinn S, et al. Treatment of "mild" pain with sumatriptan in the spectrum of headaches in patients with disabling IHS migraine (Abstr). *Neurology.* 1999;52(Suppl 2):A205-206.

17. Ward TN, Levin M. Post-traumatic headache. In: Silver J, McAllister TW, Yudofsky SC, eds. *Textbook of Traumatic Brain Injury*. 2nd ed. Washington, DC: American Psychiatric Publishing; 2005;21:385-391.

18. Headache Classification Subcommittee of the International Headache Society. The International Classification of Headache Disorders. 2nd ed. *Cephalalgia*. 2004:24(Suppl 1):1-160.

(A "must-have" for those studying headache.)

19. Ward TN. Headache in cerebrovascular disease. In: Samuels MA, Feske S, eds. *Office Practice of Neurology*. New York, NY: Churchill Livingstone, 1996;1141-1144.

20. Fisher CM. Late-life migraine accompaniments as a cause of unexplained transient ischemic attacks. *Can J Neurol Sci*. 1980;7:9-17.

21. Ward TN, Levin M, Wong RL. Headache caused by giant cell arteritis: current treatment options. *Neurology*. 2004;6(6):499-505.

22. Ward TN. Medication overuse headache. *Prim Care Clin Office Pract*. 2004;31:369-380.

23. Ward TN, Levin M. Facial pain. In: Warfield C, Bajwa Z, eds. *Principles and Practice of Pain Medicine*. 2nd ed. New York, NY: McGraw-Hill; 2003:25;246-251.

24. US Headache Consortium Guidelines. www.aan.com

(Useful evidence-based review of data through 1997.)

25. Ward TN. Management of an acute primary headache. *Clin Neurosci*. 1998;5:50-54.

26. Ward TN. Providing relief from headache pain. Current options for acute and prophylactic therapy. *Postgrad Med*. 2000;108(3): 121-128.

27. Raskin NH. Repetitive intravenous dihydroergotamine as therapy for intractable migraine. *Neurology*. 1986;36:995-997.

28. Rapoport AM, Mathew NT, Silbertsein SD, et al. Zolmitriptan Spray in the acute treatment of cluster headache: A double-blind study. *Neurology*. 2007; 69: 821-826.

8. Questions

Match the comorbid migraine condition with the probable best preventive treatment agent(s):

1. Raynaud's phenomenon	A. Propranolol
2. Epilepsy	B. Amitriptyline
3. Depression	C. Topiramate
4. Mitral valve prolapse	D. Verapamil

5. "Red flags" in headache diagnosis include:

A. Sudden onset of headache

B. Very old or very young patients with headache

C. Headache worsening over time

D. Abnormalities on the neurologic examination

E. All of the above

6. A 32-year-old man was mowing the lawn on a hot summer's day. He suddenly experienced a severe holocranial headache, throbbing, with nausea and photophobia. The headache was "the worst" of his life. After a few minutes it became less severe but was still moderate in intensity. He reported to the emergency room, where you have been called to see him. The differential diagnosis of "thunderclap headache" includes all of the following except:

A. Hemicrania continua

B. Subarachnoid hemorrhage

C. Migraine

D. Venous sinus thrombosis

7. A 47-year-old man presents to your clinic with a recurrence of severe headache attacks. He is known to have episodic cluster headache and these attacks are typical for his cluster episodes. His bouts only last about 2-3 weeks so you do not feel prevention is necessary, but he needs therapy for the attacks that are now occurring about twice a day. Effective acute treatment of cluster headache might include all except:

A. Oxygen

B. Nitric oxide

C. Occipital nerve block

D. Sumatriptan

8. Effective preventive treatment of migraine might include all except:

A. Propranolol

B. Valproic acid

C. Trazodone

D. Amitriptyline

E. Topiramate

9. A 20-year-old female is seen in the headache clinic. Six weeks earlier she had been in a serious motor vehicle accident. She struck her head on the windshield (she was not wearing her seat belt) and was unconscious for about 20 minutes. She awoke at the scene with a moderately severe holocranial headache and neck pain. She has been sent to you because, if anything, her parents feel she is worse now than she was a few days after the accident. Post-traumatic syndrome typically includes all of the following except:

A. Headache

B. Neuralgia

C. Synkinesis

D. Altered cognition

E. Neck pain

10. Which of the following may be absent in idiopathic intracranial hypertension due to defects in the optic nerve sheath?

A. Headache

B. Papilledema

C. Diplopia

D. Raised intracranial pressure

11. Which triptan has the most routes of administration?

A. Ubiquitriptan

B. Zolmitriptan

C. Alwaytriptan

D. Sumatriptan

E. Eletriptan

12. A 64-year-old man comes to your office with a complaint of a new-onset headache beginning 3 weeks ago. The headache is holocranial and moderate in severity. He has noted some discomfort in his jaw when chewing. Yesterday he had a 10-minute episode of loss of vision in his left eye. You feel he may have giant cell arteritis. Which statement about giant cell arteritis (CGA) is false?

A. Patients always have ESRs over 50 mm/hr and are always over 50 y/o

B. Headache is the most common symptom

C. Prednisone is the most accepted treatment

D. Nonsteroidal drugs cannot be used alone to treat GCA

E. Stroke and blindness may result

13. Which test has the LEAST usefulness in headache diagnosis?

A. Lumbar puncture

B. Electroencephalography

C. CT scan

D. MRI

14. Which statement about "analgesic rebound" headache is false?

A. It seems to occur in migraineurs exclusively

B. Triptan drugs do not cause it

C. Preventive drugs do not seem to be very effective in this condition

D. Similar headaches occur with ergotamine overuse

15. The "first/worst" headache could be:

A. A migraine

B. A subarachnoid hemorrhage

C. Simply the worst headache of any type the patient has had

D. All of the above

16. Options being studied for medically refractory cluster headache include (may choose more than one):

A. Trepanation

B. Vagal nerve stimulation

C. Trepidation

D. Electro-convulsive therapy

E. Deep brain stimulation

F. Occipital nerve stimulation

G. Nontraditional acupuncture with Holme's refined needles

17. Which type of hypertension is thought to not be associated with headache?

A. Malignant hypertension

B. Essential hypertension

C. Paroxysmal elevations of blood pressure, eg, due to pheochromocytoma

D. Hypertensive crisis due to tyramine reaction with MAOIs

18. In patients with migraine that develop cutaneous allodynia, which statement is true?

A. They should wait to treat their headaches until cutaneous allodynia develops, so they are sure the headache actually is a migraine

B. Having cutaneous allodynia is good because once it occurs only painful stimuli will hurt

C. Treatment outcomes may be worse once cutaneous allodynia develops

D. Cutaneous allodynia occurs before a migraine starts

19. A 47-year-old man is found unconscious in the back of a church. He is brought by the fast squad to your emergency room. He is in coma. His temperature is 38° C, his respiratory rate is 34, his pulse is 96, and his blood pressure is 180/100. Ten minutes later his pulse is 56 with a blood pressure of 224/120. You suspect an expanding intracranial lesion, such as an intracranial hematoma, and order a CT scan of the brain. A rising blood pressure with a falling pulse rate is known as:

A. Intracranial syndrome of Levin

B. Pulsus paradoxicus of Cohen

C. Holmes rebound syndrome

D. Cushing reflex

E. None of the above

20. A patient in the emergency room who sustained a concussion with loss of consciousness awoke, and shortly deteriorated, with a second loss of consciousness, and thus might have been seen during the "lucid interval." The underlying condition is most often a:

A. Subdural hematoma

B. Subarachnoid hemorrhage

C. Epidural hematoma

D. Subhyaloid hemorrhage

21. A 35-year-old man has a constant left-sided dull headache, with superimposed jabs and jolt on the same side. He will also get 45-minute bouts of pounding left-sided headache during which his left eye waters. You correctly suspect hemicrania continua and prescribe:

A. Sumatriptan

B. Indomethacin

C. Dihydroergotamine

D. High-flow oxygen by mask

E. Transnasal butorphanol

22. Your patient with cluster headache has responded to prophylaxis with verapamil. He now only gets 1-2 attacks per week. He does not respond to oxygen treatment and requests something which works rapidly. Which triptan drug can be administered that works the fastest?

A. Zolmitriptan

B. Eletriptan

C. Almotriptan

D. Sumatriptan

E. Rizatriptan

23. A 14-year-old girl fell off her bicycle, not wearing a helmet, about 20 minutes ago, and was briefly unconscious. In your emergency room she initially was complaining of headache and was normal on examination but then she became drowsy, then unarousable with unequal pupils. You order:

A. A stat CT scan of the brain, C-spine films, and neurosurgical consultation

B. Mannitol and admit for observation

C. An electroencephalogram looking for non-convulsive status

D. Close observation and dihydroergotamine

Answers

1. D.
Verapamil, a calcium channel blocker, would help ameliorate Raynaud phenomenon, while beta-blockers might exacerbate it.

2. C.
Topiramate would be expected to help epilepsy.

3. B.
Amitriptyline helps depression.

4. A.
Propranolol may help mitral valve prolapse.

5. E.
All of the listed factors have been considered "red flags" that increase the likelihood of finding a secondary rather than a primary headache disorder.

6. A.
Thunderclap headache implies headache of sudden onset. Hemicrania continua is a constant left-sided headache which may vary in intensity.

7. B.
Nitric oxide may be the final common mediator of some headaches, including cluster and migraine. The other three treatment options may all be effective in treating a cluster headache attack.

8. C.
Trazodone is not known to be a preventive treatment for migraine. Its metabolite, m-cpp (meta-chlorophenylpiperazine) has been infused experimentally to cause migraine-like headaches.

9. C.
All of the other choices occur commonly in post-traumatic syndrome. Synkinesis means mass motion, ie, involuntary movement of multiple muscles.

10. B.
Actually, theoretically, all the features could be absent if the nerve sheath defects were large enough. The entity "increased intracranial hypertension without papilledema," however, has been thought to occur due to anatomic defects in the optic nerve sheath.

11. D.
Sumatriptan has the most—being available as a pill, nasal spray, subcutaneous injection, and in some countries as a suppository. Alwaytriptan and ubiquitriptan are not real medications. Zolmitriptan comes as oral formulations and a nasal spray. Other triptans only have oral formulations.

12. A.
Patients with GCA usually have elevated sedimentation rates and usually are over 50 years old. Uncommonly, younger patients may have the condition, and the ESR can be suppressed in patients already on steroids for other conditions or taking NSAIDs.

13. B.
Electroencephalography has limited utility in headache diagnosis unless one suspects coexistent seizures. Neuroimaging and CSF analysis, along with determination of CSF pressure, is far more useful.

14. B.
Triptan drugs have been reported to cause analgesic rebound/medication-overuse headache. The duration of the actual rebound headaches may be shorter with triptan drugs when withdrawn than for some of the combination analgesics.

15. D.
The "first/worst" headache has classically been taught to suggest subarachnoid hemorrhage, and it may have been seen when that occurs. Alternatively, however, the patient may simply be experiencing what for them is their worst headache ever, such as a sudden-onset migraine with vomiting.

16. B, E, F.

There are limited case series documenting the use of deep brain stimulation, occipital nerve stimulation, and vagal nerve stimulation for medically-refractory cluster headache. Trepanation is of historical interest and has been done for centuries with no documentation of real efficacy for primary headaches.

17. B.

Paroxysmal elevations of blood pressure to very high levels (as seen with pheochromocytoma and the tryamine reaction in patients on MAOIs), and very high sustained levels of blood pressure such as occur in malignant hypertension (with diastolic readings above 120 mm Hg) are associated with headache. Headache associated with essential hypertension is controversial but generally not regarded as a true cause-and-effect situation.

18. C.

Allodynia means, typically, non-painful stimuli are perceived as painful. For headache patients this means central sensitization has occurred with second and third order neurons active. Treatment outcomes are often suboptimal once this has occurred, especially with triptan drugs.

19. D.

The Cushing reflex manifests as a rising blood pressure and falling pulse rate.

20. C.

The "lucid interval" occurs in patients that have had enough of a head trauma to lose consciousness (concussion) and subsequently awaken (lucid interval), only to lose consciousness again with neurologic deterioration as the epidural hematoma enlarges. This is a neurosurgical emergency. Patients with a subarachnoid hemorrhage may have a sentinel hemorrhage from which they recover only to rebleed later (clearly not a concussion). Subdural hematomas are generally more leisurely venous bleeding and sometimes are without a clear history of head injury (although acute subdural hematomas as may occur in boxers, for example, follow a much more rapid course than the more common chronic subdural hematoma).

21. B.

Indomethacin is the treatment of choice for hemicrania continua. In fact, response to indomethacin is part of the *ICHD-II* criteria.

22. D.

Sumatriptan Bu subcutaneous injections works most rapidly for an acute cluster attack. Recent information suggests intranasal zolmitriptan may also work, but is not as fast. The other triptans only have oral formulations, which are not fast enough.

23. A.

This is the classic story of an epidural hematoma. It is an emergency. A stat CT of the brain and neurosurgical consultation may save her life. She may be starting to have brain herniation. She probably presented to the emergency room during the "lucid interval."

Chapter 27: Childhood Neurology

Philip Brunquell, MD

Contents

Covering all of Pediatric Neurology in a few pages is akin to pouring an ocean into a thimble. To approach this task, we will concentrate on a series of key clinical problems while seeking to avoid repetition of those topics (for example, epilepsy, neuromuscular disease and neonatal neurology) that are covered elsewhere in this volume.

1. Abnormal Cranial Size and Shape

Macrocephaly

Macrocephaly means that a patient's head circumference is greater than 2 standard deviations above the mean. To remember the causes, think of the name BETH:
B = big brain (megalencephaly);
E = extra-axial collections;
T = thick skull;
H = hydrocephalus.

Big Brain
Megalencephaly is either anatomic or metabolic. Anatomic megalencephaly is due to an increase in cell size or number without an underlying metabolic defect. Causes include:

The 2% of the normal population whose head size is more than 2 standard deviations above the mean. In these children, neurological examination, psychomotor development and cranial CT findings are all normal. Some patients in this group may be identified as having benign familial macrocephaly (autosomal dominant/polygenic).

Sotos syndrome. In these patients there is accelerated growth during the first three years of life and dysmorphism (frontal bossing, high-arched palate and hypertelorism). Genetic and sporadic forms of this condition exist.

Neurocutaneous disorders. Check the skin for signs of neurofibromatosis, tuberous sclerosis, incontinentia pigmenti, hypomelanosis of Ito, and epidermal nevus syndrome.

Achondroplasia. These patients show rhizomelic dwarfism, frontal bossing, midface hypoplasia, lumbar lordosis and restriction of elbow extension. The ventricles may also be enlarged. Inheritance is autosomal dominant.

Metabolic megalencephaly includes some gray matter diseases (mucopolysaccharidoses, gangliosidoses); white matter diseases (Alexander, Canavan, and Krabbe diseases, metachromatic leukodystrophy, and leukoencephalopathy with swelling and cysts); aminoacidopathies (for example, maple syrup urine disease and gluteric aciduria type I); and abnormalities of carbohydrate metabolism (glactosemia may produce megalencephaly via the development of brain edema).

Extra-Axial Collections

In benign enlargement of the subarachnoid spaces (external hydrocephalus) patients commonly present like those with benign macrocephaly but their CT scans are abnormal. While the subarachnoid spaces are capacious,ventricles may be normal or minimally enlarged. Subdural hematomas may result from trauma (both accidental and non-accidental), bleeding disorders, and occasionally after minimal or no documented trauma in patients with benign enlargement of the subarachnoid spaces. Subdural effusions can arise from meningitis, leukemia, trauma and dehydration.

Thick Skull

This may be encountered not only in primary bone dysplasias (for example: osteopetrosis, cleidocranial dyostosis, osteogenesis imperfecta) but also in systemic conditions such as rickets or anemia.

Hydrocephalus

This may be either of the communicating or non-communicating type. In the former the ventricular system communicates with the subarachnoid spaces while in the latter condition it does not. Communicating hydrocephalus arises from processes that produce substances that block the absorption of cerebrospinal fluid at the arachnoid villi (for example, blood from subarachnoid hemorrhage, inflammatory exudate from meningitis and neoplastic cells from meningeal malignancy), as well as from congenital structural abnormalities that block CSF flow distal to the ventricles (basilar impression, achondroplasia). Noncommunicating hydrocephalus may be secondary to a mass lesion (such as tumor, abscess or hematoma) as well as from congenital structural abnormalities (such as aqueductal stenosis, the Arnold-Chiari malformation, and the Dandy-Walker malformation).

Microcephaly

Patients with this condition have head circumferences that are more than 2 standard deviations below the mean. Microcephaly can be primary (formation of an abnormally small brain) or secondary (a normally forming brain is subject to adverse insult). For causes, think of the 3 Ps: Prenatal, Perinatal and Postnatal. While perinatal and postnatal causes result in secondary microcephaly, prenatal causes may be either primary or secondary. Prenatal primary microcephaly includes chromosomal abnormalities and malformations of cerebral development such as micrencephaly vera, anencephaly and holoprosencephaly. Secondary prenatal causes include vascular insult, toxin exposure and TORCH infections. Perinatal causes include infections such as meningitis or encephalitis, intracranial hemorrhage and vascular events including severe hypoxic-ischemic encephalopathy. Postnatal causes frequently arise from systemic diseases such as malnutrition, renal disease and cardiopulmonary dysfunction.

Abnormal Head Shape

This may arise prenatally from cranial deformation secondary to a constricted intrauterine environment. Conversely, it may occur in the absence of such constriction if there is abnormal brain development. The Dandy-Walker malformation, for example, can produce occipital prominence, while hydrocephalus typically results in frontal bossing. Postnatal positioning may result in skull deformation such as the occipital flattening seen in infants who are consistently placed in the recommended supine position.

A major cause of abnormal head shape is craniosynostosis. A clue that this is present is sutural ridging. By remembering that skull growth occurs perpendicular to suture lines, the resultant head shape can be predicted as per Table 1.

Craniosynostosis may be: 1.) isolated (both autosomal dominant and autosomal recessive varieties exist); 2.) associated with systemic diseases (for example hypothyroidism, polycythemia vera, rickets, and sickle disease), or 3.) occur as a component of a dysmorphic genetic syndrome (for example, Apert, Carpenter, and Crouzon syndromes). Surgical repair for craniosynostosis is necessary if the bony confinement is causing increased intracranial pressure. It is also sometimes undertaken for cosmetic repair.

2. The Hypotonic Infant

This is one of the classic problems in pediatric neurology. When approaching this, it pays to remember Murphy's Law: whatever can go wrong, will go wrong.

By this, we mean that abnormalities anywhere from the cerebral cortex to the muscle can cause hypotonia in the infant. Cerebral causes include chromosomal abnormalities (especially Prader-Willi syndrome and the trisomies), other forms of cerebral dysgenesis, acquired insults (most importantly neonatal hypoxic ischemic-encephalopathy), and metabolic diseases (for example, peroxismal disorders, infantile GM1 gangliosidosis, and acid maltase deficiency). Spinal cord disease may arise from traction injuries during breech or cephalic presentations. Anterior horn cell diseases include the spinal muscular atrophies (look for tongue faciculations and absent deep tendon reflexes in a child who otherwise appears alert), and poliomyelitis (suggested by a viral prodrome, bulbar signs and respiratory insufficiency). Peripheral neuropathies include the hereditary motor sensory neuropathies, giant axonal neuropathy, and congenital hypomyelinating neuropathy. The neuromuscular junction is the locus in both the familial, infantile and transitory forms of myasthenia gravis, botulism (with this condition check for internal and external ophthalmoplegia, constipation, and a history of tainted honey ingestion), hypermagnesemia (in infants whose mothers were treated with magnesium for preeclampsia),

Table 1

Skull Growth and Head Shape

Head Appearance	Suture(s) Fused	Head Type
Long, narrow	Saggital	Scaphocephaly
Wide	Both coronal	Brachycephaly
One side flattened	One coronal or one lambdoid	Plagiocephaly
Triangular with midforehead ridge	Metopic	Trigonocephaly
Pointed	All	Oxycephaly

and neuromuscular blockade secondary to aminoglycoside antibiotics.

In sorting through these many possibilities, it is helpful to divide them into three major categories:

1. ***Central*** (proximal to the anterior horn cell). This group accounts for the largest proportion of hypotonic infants.

2. ***Peripheral*** (diseases involving the anterior horn cell and distal structures, ie, peripheral nerve, neuromuscular junction and muscle).

3. ***Central and peripheral loci combined.***

Central causes should be highly suspected when:

A.) Abnormalities on the physical examination are not confined to the nervous system (for example, the presence of dysmorphism or multi-organ involvement).

B.) Abnormalities on the neurological examination are not confined to the motor system. Seizures, marked irritability with a high-pitched cry, cortical thumbing and scissoring of the lower extremities should all suggest a central cause.

C.) The motor examination shows:

i.) relatively normal strength in the face of low tone;

ii.) improvement in tone when the infant is stimulated;

iii.) the patient's postural reflexes (such as the Moro and tonic neck) are elicitable, and

iv.) deep tendon reflexes are exaggerated.

Peripheral causes should be suspected when:

A.) Other organ system involvement is lacking (exceptions occur);

B.) The patient appears socially attentive and interactive;

C.) The motor examination shows:

i.) weakness that is commensurate with the degree of hypotonia;

ii.) tone that doesn't improve upon stimulation of the infant;

iii.) nonelicitable postural reflexes, since they ultimately depend upon the integrity of the peripheral components of the motor pathway for their expression, and

iv.) deep tendon reflexes that are normal (for example, neonatal myasthenia gravis, congenital myopathies), or depressed/lost (for example, congenital muscular dystrophies, spinal muscular atrophies).

Conditions that produce hypotonia due to simultaneous central and peripheral involvement can be grouped into four main categories:

1. Combined central and peripheral disease when the former initially overshadows the latter. The most notable example is the infant who upon recovering from hypoxic ischemic encephalopathy with improving mental status and subsidence of seizures is then found to have diminished movement secondary to previously unrecognized anoxic damage to the spinal cord.

2. Peripheral disease that leads to secondary central involvement. For example, acute infantile spinal muscular atrophy, congenital myotonic dystrophy and x-linked myotubular myopathy may present with respiratory failure that can lead to a secondary anoxic cerebral insult.

3. Some predominantly peripheral diseases that have less dominant central involvement (such as neonatal myotonic dystrophy and familial dysautonomia).

4. Metabolic diseases such as mitochondrial disorders, lipid storage diseases, acid maltase deficiency, metochromatic leukodystrophy and Krabbe disease can simultaneously equally target both peripheral as well as central nervous system tissue.

3. Ataxia

The causes of ataxia in childhood are usually organized according to their temporal mode of presentation: acute, recurrent or chronic. Although this provides a convenient way of thinking about ataxia, in clinical practice the distinctions are not always clear-cut. For example, if you evaluate an ataxic child for what will ultimately prove to be the initial bout of recurrent disease you do not know for certain whether future relapses are in the offing or even if the episode of ataxia that you are witnessing will resolve. Similarly, brain tumors commonly produce a chronic progressive ataxia but their insidious development may not produce symptoms that are initially recognizable to family or friends. Symptoms may then reach a critical threshold that causes the disease to be perceived as an acute event. Finally, some of the metabolic forms of recurrent ataxia may not be met with complete recovery between attacks and with time these cumulative disabilities may merge into a chronic progressive illness.

Acute Ataxia

Neuroimaging is helpful to look for evidence of tumors, trauma and vascular disease. Since most brain tumors in children of ages 2-12 years reside in the posterior fossa (for example, cerebellar astrocytoma, ependymona, medulloblastoma) the ataxia can be readily explained by damage to the cerebellum and its pathways and/or to the concomitant development of obstructive hydrocephalus. However, it is useful to remember that the cerebellum has significant reciprocal connections with the cerebral cortex and thus it is not unusual for supratentorial tumors to also present with ataxia.

In children, ataxia may occur after minor trauma as well as following more serious insults such as posterior fossa hematoma or contusion. Ataxia may be a component of post-concussive syndrome in which neuroimaging findings may be normal although axonal injury may occasionally be detected on some T2-weighted MRI scans. Ataxia evolving in a child who has sustained neck injury should raise the prospect of infarction within the vertebrobasilar system. Other vascular causes of acute ataxia include non-traumatic stroke, hemorrhage secondary to a ruptured arterial venous malformation, and Kawasaki disease. The last is a systemic vasculitis that causes multiple brain infarctions and may respond to the administration of intravenous immune globulin. Five of the following six signs are required for diagnosis: fever, lymphadenopathy, rash, limb edema, erythema of the lips and oropharynx, and conjunctival congestion.

Acute cerebellar ataxia of childhood is thought to be an autoimmune process often triggered by a preceding viral infection, such as varicella or one of the enteroviruses. Recovery can take from days to months.

If the acute ataxia is conjoined with areflexia, weakness and cranial neuropathy in the absence of a space occupying lesion on neuroimaging, the Miller Fisher variant of Güillain-Barré syndrome should be considered. The presence of cyto-albuminic dissociation of the spinal fluid is supportive. Brainstem encephalitis can also produce ataxia with cranial neuropathies and can sometimes evolve to more diffuse disease with alterations of consciousness and seizures. Of the drugs that can cause acute ataxia, psychotropic medication, anticonvulsants and antihistamines are major suspects. Among patients with epilepsy, ataxia may be an ictal manifestation (especially in children with Lennox-Gastaut syndrome) or a postictal phenomena. If a child's ataxia is maximum at presentation and then clears over minutes to hours, a postictal effect from an unwitnessed seizure should be considered within the differential diagnosis.

Hysterical conversion reaction may present as unsteady gait. In astasia-abasia, the child sways from the waist, gait does not improve with the assumption of a wide base, and the child may manifest lurching movements. As with other conversion reactions in childhood, some of these patients may be victims of sexual abuse.

If you need a way to pull all of this together, remember: ***A Good Boy Eats His Spinach*** and ***Tiny, Tender Turnips.***

A = acute cerebellar ataxia of childhood;
G = Guillain-Barré syndrome;
B = brainstem encephalitis;
E = epilepsy;
H = hysteria;
S = stroke and other vascular causes;
T = tumor;
T = trauma;
T = toxins.

Recurrent Ataxias

The major conditions here are childhood multiple sclerosis, basilar migraine, benign paroxysmal vertigo, and certain genetic metabolic diseases. MRI and CSF findings are pivotal in the diagnosis of childhood multiple sclerosis in a manner similar to adults with the disease. A family history of migraine may offer supportive evidence for the presence of basilar migraine in a child. Unlike migraine, attacks of benign paroxysmal vertigo last only minutes but such patients may go on to develop migraine later in life. Two autosomal dominant recurrent ataxias are identified. Episodic ataxia type I is due to a mutation of the potassium channel on chromosome 12p. Symptoms typically commence in the first decade of life, last minutes to hours and, by the time the child is in the beginning of the second decade of life, myokymia may be evident. Treatment is with carbamazepine, phenytoin or acetazolamide. Episodic ataxia type II results from a mutation in the calcium channel gene on chromosome 19p. Onset is in the first or second decade of life. Treatment is with either acetazolamide or flunarizine.

The presence of metabolic disease should be considered in a child with recurrent ataxia. Primary considerations are pyruvate dehydrogenase deficiency, the intermittent form of maple syrup urine disease, and Hartnup disease. Pyruvate dehydrogenase deficiency should be considered in a child with recurrent ataxia who has lactic acidosis, a low lactate to pyruvate ratio and, at times, hyperalanemia. The diagnosis is confirmed by measuring enzyme activity in tissue such as cultured fibroblasts or leukocytes. Treatment includes the ketogenic diet, thiamine and acetazolamide. The intermittent form of maple urine disease is associated with elevated amounts of branch chain amino acids and keto acids during attacks and, like pyruvate dehydrogenase deficiency, the diagnosis is confirmed by measuring enzyme activity in cultured fibroblasts. Treatment consists of restriction of dietary protein, thiamine for those who are thiamine responsive, withholding of protein during an acute attack and if necessary peritoneal dialysis. Hartnup disease, an abnormality of tryptophan metabolism, results in aminoacideria with excretion of neural monoaminocarboxylic amino acids. Photosensitivity and a pellagra like skin rash are important clues. Treatment is with nicotinamide as well as a high protein diet.

Chronic Ataxias

Neuroimaging is essential to exclude brain tumors as well as congenital malformations such as basilar impression, Arnold-Chiari malformation, Dandy Walker malformation and other cerebellar dysplasias. Two syndromes involving the triad of opsiclonus, polymyoclonia and truncal ataxia are identified. One is a paraneoplastic process secondary to neuroblastoma. The tumor is usually confirmed by a magnetic resonance image of the chest and abdomen and documentation of elevation of homovanillic acid and vanillylmandelic acid in the urine. Tumor removal does not necessarily affect neurologic prognosis, and ACTH or oral steroids may provide neurological benefit to the majority of patients. The second condition, Kinsborne syndrome, is not associated with neuroblastoma, may respond to ACTH or oral steroids, and may be ultimately associated with diminished cognitive abilities.

A variety of genetic-metabolic conditions need to be considered in the child with chronic progressive ataxia. Several of the autosomal dominant spinocerebellar atrophies are diagnosable by trinucleotide repeat analysis. The presence of fat malabsorption, failure to thrive and, ultimately, retinitis pigmentosa should suggest abetalipoproteinemia. There are low levels of cholesterol and triglyceride in the plasma with absence of apolipoprotein B. Treatment is with dietary fat restriction and large doses of vitamin E. Friedreich ataxia is due to trinucliotide repeat expansion of the frataxin gene (chromosome 9q13). In addition to the ataxia, plantar responses are extensor, tendon reflexes are diminished and there is a loss of posterior column sensation. The majority of patients develop a cardiomyopathy. The presence of recurrent sinopulmonary infection in a child with progressive ataxia raises the prospect of ataxia-telangiectasia, an autosomal recessive disease localized to chromosome 11q 22-23. At times the telangiectasias may not appear for years after the onset of the ataxia. Oculomotor apraxia is another important clinical tip-off. Laboratory studies include elevated alpha fetoprotein, diminished immunoglobulins A, E or G, acanthocytes on the blood smear, a low erythrocyte sedimentation rate, and a positive molecular genetic test for the condition. Other laboratory measures that can be directed towards the child with chronic progressive ataxia include very long chain fatty acids and phytanic acid for adrenoleukodystrophy and Refsum disease, blood lactate and glucose-lactate tolerance for mitrochondrial disorders; white cell or fibroblast determination of hexosaminidase for GM2 gangliosidosis; arylsulfatase A and saposin B for juvenile metachromatic leukodystrophy; and carnitine acetyltransferase for carnitine deficiency. There are conditions associated with progressive ataxia in childhood that are likely metabolic, although the precise defect has not yet been identified. One example is the Marinesco-Sjögren syndrome, in which the ataxia is conjoined with cataracts and mental retardation.

4. Attention Deficit Hyperactivity Disorder

ADHD is the most common behavior disorder referred to pediatric neurologists. Prevalence rates range from 2%-16%, and males are affected twice as often as females. The cause of ADHD is not entirely known, but a dysregulation of central monoaminergic mechanisms and/or genetic influences may play a role. Fully 33%-75% of children with ADHD have symptoms that persist into adulthood.

The cardinal components of ADHD are: 1.) inattention, and 2.) hyperactivity-impulsivity. The balance of these symptoms may vary among patients such that one, the other, or both, dominate the clinical picture. As normal children will, from time to time, exhibit these same symptoms, clinical judgment must be used to determine whether symptom intensity reaches a threshold for diagnosis. This determination is usually made from analysis of teacher's reports, parents' description of the child's behavior at home, behavioral observations during the office visit (which, except in the most severe cases, may offer limited information), and the results of behavior rating scales submitted by the physician to teachers and parents.

The diagnosis of ADHD may be complicated by its association with other conditions, such as learning disabilities, tic disorder, oppositional-defiant disorder, anxiety disorder and bipolar disease. In every child who presents for evaluation of suspected ADHD, the history should be directed to these areas as well, even if the parents do not spontaneously raise concern.

The physical examination should ascertain whether there are any neurological signs to suggest that the child's behavior might represent the early stages of a neurodegenerative disease. Conversely, many neurological disorders, such as head trauma and encephalitis, may result in ADHD symptoms.

Although there is no laboratory test for ADHD, physical findings suggestive of hyperthyroidism or anemia should prompt appropriate laboratory testing. A history of pica warrants a lead level. If the child's inattentiveness coalesces into discrete episodes of staring and unresponsiveness, an EEG should be considered to help exclude absence epilepsy.

Educational planning is a foundation for treatment. It must be ascertained whether the child's class placement is appropriate for his aptitude. Structuring the classroom routine and creating as much of a distraction-free environment as possible is necessary. Special services to promote the development of study and organizational skills and if needed, to address specific learning disabilities, should be arranged. Psychological counseling can help with issues of self-esteem and socialization. Associated severe anxiety disorders and bipolar disease would warrant psychiatric consultation.

Pharmacotherapy is often considered for patients in whom educational and environmental adjustments are not sufficiently effective. Stimulants enhance attention span and reduce hyperkinesis in up to 70% of patients. Agents include methylphenidate (Ritalin®, Concerta®), D-amphetamine (Dexedrine®) and mixed dextroamphetamine and amphetamine salts (Adderall®). Pemoline (Cylert®) is infrequently used because of the risk of heptatoxicity. Clonidine or guanfacine are often considered in place of these agents for those children who have tics exacerbated by stimulants. Another option to stimulants is atomoxetine (Strattera™), thought to act by selective inhibition of the presynaptic norepinephrine transporter. There has been recent concern regarding suicidal ideation among patients treated with Strattera. Although antidepressants such as fluoxetine (Prozac®) and Wellbutrin® (bupropion) have been considered second-line drugs for ADHD, their safety in children is also currently being re-examined.

5. Cerebral Palsy

The term cerebral palsy denotes a nonprogressive disorder of motor function due to a lesion of the developing brain. It occurs in 1.2 to 2.5 children per 1000. When initially evaluating a child with suspected cerebral palsy, determining that the condition is nonprogressive is not always straightforward. Some degenerative disorders progress very slowly and thus may mimic cerebral palsy. Examples include Niemann-Pick disease type C, ataxia-telangiectasia, and the hereditary motor and sensory neuropathies. Conversely, although the brain lesions of children with cerebral palsy are static, clinical manifestations may change with the passage of time, thus suggesting a neurodegenerative process. For example, many patients with spastic forms of cerebral palsy may have had an initial period of low tone. Then, as the spasticity continues over the years, progressive contracture, joint instability and orthopedic deformity may ensue. Some patients with spastic diplegia develop an ataxic component to their motor disability. As the behavioral repertoire of children with cerebral palsy expands with age, learning and behavioral problems may emerge, triggering concerns for progressive disease. Given these complexities, serial examinations are needed to determine the type and degree of any motor or cognitive decline. One must be particularly suspect of a positive family history of "cerebral palsy," as this might well be the clue to the presence of a degenerative disorder.

Cerebral palsy is usually classified by the type and pattern of motor involvement. Spastic cerebral palsy includes hemiplegic, quadriplegic, and diplegic varieties. Hypotonic cerebral palsy may either be ataxic or choreoathetoid/dystonic.

In spastic hemiplegic cerebral palsy, the motor deficit may not be recognized during the first few months of life. The development of premature handedness (ie, hand preference before a year of age) is an important clue. Because the lower face receives bilateral cortio-bulbar involvement until birth, facial involvement is unusual. Periventricular hemorrhagic infarction is the most common underlying lesion in premature infants, while in term infants cerebral malformations, cerebral infarctions, and intracranial hemorrhages predominate. Congenital brain tumors are rare causes of spastic hemiplegia in infancy but can be excluded by the same neuroimaging used to disclose the more typical lesions. Up to a quarter of patients with spastic hemiplegic CP will have a homonymous hemianopia, 28% have mental retardation, and seizures occur in a third to a half of patients.

Spastic quadriplegic cerebral palsy results most often from multicystic encephalomalacia and brain malformations. Seizures occur in half of the patients. Dysarthria and dysphagia due to supranuclear palsy is common. Compared to patients with other forms of cerebral palsy, those with spastic quadriplegia have a higher likelihood of associated deficits in vision, hearing and learning.

Spastic diplegia involves leg weakness that is more prominent than arm weakness. This is more frequent in premature compared to term infants, with hypoxic-ischemic insult leading to periventricular leukomalacia being the primary cause. Parasagittal lesions, hydrocephalus and spinal cord lesions can also cause preferential leg involvement and should be considered in the differential diagnosis. Twenty-seven percent of patients have seizures, 43% have strabismus, and 30% or more have mental retardation.

Choreoathetoid/dystonic cerebral palsy can result from anoxia or jaundice; gross inspection of the basal ganglia may reveal a marbeled appearance ("status marmoratus"). Some degree of cortical involvement, such as cortical laminar necrosis, may be associated and be reflected clinically by corticospinal findings. A history of significant hyperbilirubinemia conjoined with hearing loss, choreoathetosis and restriction of upgaze (and sometimes lateral gaze) should raise concern for kernicterus. Because the appearance of extrapyramidal findings are delayed in these patients (often following a period of hypotonia), progressive degenerative neurological conditions are often considered in the differential diagnosis.

The pathophysiology of ataxic cerebral palsy is poorly understood. Only 28% of patients show posterior fossa abnormalities on neuroimaging, while 55% show lesions in the cerebral hemispheres. This is the least common form of cerebral palsy, although ataxia may be conjoined with other more common forms (see spastic diplegia, above).

The treatment of cerebral palsy is multidisciplinary. Early intervention programs offer individualized combinations of physical, occupational and speech therapy. Ophthalmologic and audiological assessments and follow-up are essential. Oral spasmolytic therapy is of limited benefit; botulinium toxin injections and selective dorsal root rhizotomy may be helpful for selected patients. For severe cases, surgery to relieve contracture may be necessary. Special education services with development of individual education plans are offered to the school age child who may also continue to receive the rehabilitative therapies in the school setting.

6. Psychomotor Regression

The loss of intellectual and/or motor skills previously acquired raises the prospect of an inborn error of metabolism. Although individually such errors are rare, collectively they are common. Nonetheless they are not the only causes of regression, and they therefore must be considered alongside a variety of other conditions. Of the chronic infections, the major considerations are HIV, the TORCH complex (toxoplasmosis, other—especially syphilis, rubella, cytomeglovirus, and herpes), and subacute sclerosing panencephalitis (SSPE). The latter is a chronic rubeola encephalitis marked by periodic discharges occurring every five to seven seconds on the EEG in association with myoclonic jerks. IgG and measles antibody titre are elevated in the CSF. Trauma can cause progressive decline when it is recurrent (eg, the athlete who suffers serial concussions; the child who is the victim of repeated abuse) or complicated by secondary processes (hydrocephalus, chronic subdural hematoma). Neuroimaging is helpful in excluding infiltrative neoplasms, vascular events (eg, from systemic lupus erythematosis or moyamoya disease) and demyelinating disease. Hypothyroidism and hypoadrenocorticism are the two commonest endocrine curses of regression, and they are eminently treatable. Uncontrolled seizures may result in an epileptic encephalopathy. Global decline may be an integral component of certain epilepsy syndromes such as the Lennox-Gastaut syndrome and the progressive myoclonic encephalopathies. At times, the cognitive impairment may be relatively more selective, as in the acquired epileptic aphasia of the Landau-Kleffner syndrome. Toxins that cause loss of function may be endogenous (eg, from hepatic or renal disease) or exogenous (lead, drugs of abuse, certain chemotherapeutic agents). The presence of autism and other forms of pervasive developmental disorders should be considered in children who develop eye contact avoidance, tactile defensiveness, stereotypic mannerisms, a desire for preservation of sameness, and loss of reciprocal social interactions. As in adults, a pseudodementia caused by depression can be seen in children. The diagnosis is usually established by recognizing both the affective and vegetative components of this condition.

The wide variety of metabolic errors causing regression include aminoacidopathies, organic acidemias, abnormalities in ammonia, carbohydrate and oxidative metabolism, and the "organelle" disorders (lysosomal, mitochondrial and peroxisomal diseases). The differential diagnosis is usually developed from the age of the patient at symptom onset, the predominant neuroanatomic level affected (eg, grey matter vs. white matter involvement), associated clinical findings, and the results of screening laboratory studies. Grey matter diseases present with early dementia and seizures. White matter diseases often demonstrate optic atrophy, spasticity, hyperreflexia and cortical blindness or deafness. Seizures, if they occur, appear later in the course of the disease.

By comparing those diseases that commence before two years of age with those that occur after, and by contrasting those with predominantly grey versus white matter involvement, a 2 x 2 matrix can be constructed as shown in Table 2.

Embedded within the list of gray matter diseases are the corencephalopathies which preferentially affect deep structures (basal ganglia, thalamic, brainstem and cerebellum). This accounts for the extrapyramidal signs that are characteristic of this group.

Because of symptom overlap among conditions within each of the gray and white matter categories, associated physical findings may help to refine the diagnosis. Sparse, wiry hair (pili torti) is seen in Menkes disease; dry short hair suggests late onset argininosuccinic-aciduria. Cataracts occur in oculocerebrorenal (Lowe) syndrome, galactosemia and cerebro-tendinous xanthomatosis. The macular cherry red spot is seen in GM1 and GM2 gangliosidosis, metachromatic leukodystrophy, Niemann-Pick disease, Farber disease, sialidosis type III, and the cherry red spot myoclonus syndrome. Neuronal ceroid lipofuscinosis, Refsum disease, Cockayne syndrome, abetalipoproteinemia, Hallervorden-Spatz disease and Kearns-Sayre syndrome can all produce pigmentary retinopathy. Optic atrophy is expected in metachromatic leukodystrophy, Krabbe disease, and Pelizaeus-Merzbacher disease by virtue of their white matter involvement.

Gingival hypertrophy is not confined to patients on phenytoin. It can be a clue to the diagnosis of mannosidosis, mucolipidosis II (I cell disease) and mucopolysaccharidoses types I through III.

Table 2

Grey Matter and White Matter Diseases

Gray Matter Diseases

Onset: Before Two Years	Onset: After Two Years
Infantile ceroid lipofuscinosis	Late infantile/juvenile ceroid lipofuscinosis
GM2 gangliosidosis (Tay-Sachs)	Juvenile GM 2 gangliosidosis
Niemann-Pick Type A	Neimann-Pick Type C
Gaucher Type II	Gaucher Type III
Mucopolysaccharidoses Types I, III	Mucopolysaccharidoses Types II, VII
Glycoprotein degradation disorders: Mannosidosis, infantile form Fucosidosis, infantile form	Glycoprotein degredation disorders: Mannosidosis, juvenile form Fucosidosis, juvenile form
Alpers disease	
Menkes disease	
Rett syndrome	
Carbohydrate deficient glycoprotein syndrome	
Most amino and organic acidopathies	Hallervorden-Spatz disease*
Leigh disease*	Huntington disease*
Lesch-Nyhan disease*	Wilson disease*

*corencephalopathies

White Matter Diseases

Onset: Before Two Years	Onset: After Two Years
Krabbe disease	Late onset Krabbe disease
Metachromatic leukodystrophy	Late onset metachromatic leukodystrophy
Neonatal adrenoleukodystrophy	Adrenoleukodystrophy
Alexander disease	Alexander disease
Canavan disease	Cerebrotendinous xanthomatosis

Angiokeratomas are cutaneous findings in Fabry disease and fucosidosis. Xanthomas of the Achilles tendon are seen in cerebrotendinosis xanthoanatosis. Visceromegaly is palpable in Niemann-Pick and Gaucher disease, GM1 gangliosidosis, glycogenoses, and Hurler syndrome.

Routine laboratory studies can often guide the selection of more specific tests. The CBC may show evidence of bone marrow suppression in patients with propionic and methylmalonic acidemias. Examination of the blood smear may show vacuolated lymphocytes in mannosidosis, fucosidosis, mucolipidosis II, aspartylglucosaminuria, early infantile GM1 gangliosidosis and Niemann-Pick disease, and the late infantile and juvenile forms of neuronal ceroid lipofuscinosis.

Hypoglycemia is seen in organic acidemias, glycogen storage disorders and fructose intolerance. The presence of hypoglycemia without ketosis should suggest a fatty acid oxidation disorder. The presence of reducing substances in the urine (Benedict's [Clinitest®] positive, but glucose oxidase negative) is a hallmark of galactosemia.

Hyperammonenia occurs with urea cycle disorders (look for respiratory alkalosis without ketosis); organic acidemias (clues: metabolic acidosis, ketosis, hyperglycinemia, hypeglycinuria); fatty and oxidation disorders (again, hypoglycemia without ketosis); dibasic amino transport defects; transient hyperammonenmia of prematures; and congenital lactic academia. In the latter condition, check the lactate/pyruvate ratio. If it is normal (<25), consider pyruvate dehydrogenose deficiency or a defect in gluconeogenesis. If elevated—especially if it is >35—a respiratory chain defect, pyruvatre carboxylase type A deficiency, or a mitochondrial myopathy may be responsible.

Metabolic acidosis can signal the presence of an inborn error of metabolism. First, check the anion gap. If it is normal, the problem is bicarbonate loss, either through the gut or the kidneys (renal tubular acidosis). If it is elevated, and there is no exogeneous source of acid (such as salicylate poisoning), then endogenous acid is accumulating. This occurs in organic acidemias, mitrochondrial encephalomyopathies, fatty acid oxidation disorders, and some aminoacidopathies (eg, maple syrup urine disease).

It should be cautioned that these routine biochemical markers may not be consistently present in patients with metabolic disease. For some, it is only under situations of stress, such as fasting, infection or surgery, that the derangements will be detectable.

Ultimately, the diagnosis will rest on more definite testing. This may include plasma and urine amino acids, urine organic acids, carnitine profile, acylcarnitine level (especially helpful in fatty acid oxidation disorders); urine mucopolysaccharides, plasma phytanic acid and very long chain fatty acids (for Refsum disease and other peroxismal disorders); bone marrow aspirate (for cells containing storage material as in Gaucher and Niemann-Pick disease); muscle or liver biopsy (for many of the mitochondrial diseases and carbohydrate disorders respectively); enzyme assay in leukocytes, fibroblasts, and other tissues (for many of the lysosomal diseases); and, increasingly, specific genetic testing (eg, mutation testing in the mitochondrial encephalomyelopathies).

7. Movement Disorders

Movement disorders are typically classified according to the character of the displacement of the body part. Tics are complex, stereotyped movements that can be at least transiently voluntarily suppressed. Myoclonus refers to muscle jerks that are very rapid. The movements of chorea are random, arrhythmic, nonstereotypical, migrate from one body part to another, and are often incorporated into voluntary movements. Ballismus, an extreme form of chorea, consists of flinging movements originating from the hip or shoulder girdle. Chorea is sometimes cojoined with athetosis, a slow, writhing movement involving preferentially the distal appendicular musculature. Tremor is an involuntary oscillating movement of fixed frequency, amplitude and force that is perpendicular to the axis of the extremity. Dystonia is a fixed posture caused by simultaneous contraction of agonist and antagonist muscles. There may be associated twisting and turning movements along the long axis of the extremity.

Tourette syndrome consists of both motor and vocal tics that tend to wax and wane, often with one type of tic being replaced by another over time. Half of the patients have ADD, and a third suffer from OCD. The symptoms may occur following a streptococcal infection, a sequence referred to as PANDAS (pediatric autoimmune neuropsychiatric disorders associated with streptococcal infections), and may be potentrated by stimulant medication or certain anticonvulsants (lamotrigine, carbamazepine). Treatment should be considered for children who are bothered by the tics, or whose symptoms are sufficiently severe to interfere with classroom or social performance. Haldol®, pimozide, fluphenazine and clonidine are therapeutic alternatives.

The differential diagnosis of chorea is broad. A perinatal history may help identify antecedents of cerebral palsy. Neuroimaging is used to exclude cerebral tumor, vascular conditions and Fahr disease. The latter is an autosomal dominant disease localized to chromasome 14q; the chorea is conjoined with encephalopathy and calcifications of the basal ganglia. Both viral encephalitis and bacterial meningoencephalitis may leave chorea in their wake, and readily available serum chemistries can check for metabolic evidence of hypernatremia, hypocalcemia, hypoparathyroidism, vitamin B_{12} deficiency, hyperthyroidism, systemic lupus erythematosis and Addison disease. Drugs that can induce chorea include anticonvulsants, antiemetics, neuroleptics, stimulants and oral contraceptives. Chorea occurs in 10% of children who undergo cardiopulmonary bypass surgery for congenital cyanotic heart disease.

A number of genetic disorders are marked by prominent chorea. When seen with developmental regression, acanthocytosis and normal lipoprotein levels think of neuroacanthocytosis. The same findings with abnormal lipoprotein levels should suggest abetalipoproteinemia (see the section on ataxia, above). Liver dysfunction with low copper and ceruloplasmin levels indicates that the chorea is likely due to Wilson disease. Mental retardation, self-mutilation and hyperuricemia points to Lesch-Nyhan disease. Chorea may be a component of ataxia-telangiectasia (see above). Recurrent sinopulmonary infections and oculomotor apraxia may signal this diagnosis. Chorea occurring in the wake of an acute encephalopathy or following hypotonia with developmental delay in megalencephalic infants heralds glutaric acidemia type 1. Machado-Joseph disease, one of the spinocerebellar ataxias, may include chorea. Paroxysmal choreoathetosis, often including dystonia, may be movement-induced (kinesiogenic) or nonkinesiogenic. The former episodes are brief, lasting less than 2 minutes, while the latter episodes can last from minutes to hours. As in adults with Huntington disease, dementia and emotional lability can be seen in children with the condition, although seizures and parkinsonian features are more common than in adults. Benign familial chorea is autosomal dominant, associated with normal intelligence, and improves with age.

Chorea, hypotonia and emotional lability developing weeks to months after a strep infection is characteristic of Syndenham chorea. Rheumatic heart disease develops in one-third of these patients, so penicillin prophylaxis is required. Haldol, valproate or benzodiazepines may help alleviate the chorea.

Many of the previously cited conditions associated with chorea can also produce dystonia, ie, perinatal cerebral injury, toxins, collagen vascular diseases, infections, strokes, tumors, Wilson disease, Huntington disease, Machado-Joseph disease, glutaric acidemia type I, and familial paroxysmal choreoathetosis. Four other conditions are of particular note. Dystonia with dementia, corticospinal tract involvement, retinitis pigmentosa, optic atrophy, and an MRI showing the "eye of the tiger" sign—ie, lucency in the globus pallidus—is indicative of Hallervorden-Spatz syndrome. The disease is autosomal recessive. Pathologically there is iron deposition in the globus pallidus and pars reticulata of the substantia nigra. Segawa disease is an autosomal dominant (14q) dopa-responsive dystonia with parkinsonian symptoms. The dystonia is worse in the evening hours and is exquisitely responsive to small amounts of L-dopa. Progressive spongy degeneration of the corpus striatum with variable involvement of the globus pallidus is seen in infantile bilateral striatal necrosis. Some forms of this condition are biotin-responsive. Idiopathic tortion dystonia may be familial (autosomal dominant, dystonia musculorum deformans) or sporadic. There is no intellectual or corticospinal involvement. Drugs used have included trihexyphenidyl, baclofen, carbamazepine, and benzodiazepines. To exclude Segawa disease, a trial of L-dopa is frequently employed.

Benign myoclonus may occur in response to exercise, anxiety and in sleep (hypnic jerks). Impairment of consciousness and/or associated epileptiform discharges on the EEG support myoclonic seizures. Many of the causes of chorea and dystonia can also produce myoclonus: trauma, stroke, hypoxia, infections, drugs and basal ganglia degenerations. Hepatic and renal failure can produce myoclonus, as can some of the lysosomal storage disorders. The syndrome of opsiclonus-myoclonus has been previously discussed (see chronic ataxia, above). Segmental myoclonus may be due to demyelinating disease or tumors. Brainstem involvement (central tegmental tract or dentato-olivary tract) can result in palatal myoclonus. Spinal myoclonus may be due to a cystic astrocytoma of the cord.

Tremor may be physiological and may be accentuated by stress, fatigue, exercise, drugs and hyperthyroidism. Familial essential tremor is autosomal dominant (localized to 3q 13 or 2p 25-p22), has a frequency of 4-8 hertz, occurs during activity, and if it interferes with daily living can be treated with propranalol, topiramate or gabapentin.

Spasmus nutans consists of head nodding (titubation), head tilt and nystagmus, that begins in the latter half of the first year of life and resolves within 1-5 years. Leigh disease and tumors of the anterior visual pathways can produce similar findings.

8. References

Books

1. Cohen ME, Duffner PK. *Weiner and Levitt's Pediatric Neurology.* 4th ed. Philadelphia, Pa: Lippincott, Williams and Wilkins; 2003.

   (The basics in outline form.)

2. Fenichel GM. *Clinical Pediatric Neurology: A Signs and Symptoms Approach.* 5th ed. Philadelphia, Pa: Elsevier Saunders; 2005.

   (Information-dense, elegantly written, and quite simply the best problem-oriented pediatric neurology text available.)

3. Swaiman KF, Ashwal S, Ferriero DM, eds. *Pediatric Neurology: Principles and Practice.* 4th ed. Philadelphia, Pa: Mosby Elsevier; 2006.

   (Massive, multi-authored, beautifully illustrated work. The definitive reference work in the field.)

Papers

1. DeMeyer W. Megalencephaly: types, clinical syndromes and management. *Pediatric Neurol.* 1986;2:321-328.
2. Opitz JM, Holt MC. Microcephaly: General considerations and aids to nosology. *J Craniofac Genet Dev Biol.* 1990;10:175-204.
3. Watemberg N, Silver S, Harel S, Lerman-Sagie T. Significance of microcephaly among children with developmental disabilities. *J Child Neurol.* 2002;17 (2):117-122.
4. Aviv RI, Rodger E, Hall CM. Craniosynostosis. *Clin Radiol.* (England) 2002;57(2): 93-102.
5. Ryan MM, Engle EC. Acute ataxia in childhood. *J Child Neurol.* 2003;18(5)309-316.
6. Parker CC, Evans OB. Metabolic disorders causing childhood ataxia. *Semin Pediatr Neurol.* 2003; 10(3):193-199.
7. Johnson HM. The floppy weak infant revisited. *Brain Dev.* (Netherlands). 2003;25(3): 155-158.
8. Prasad AN, Prasad C. The floppy infant: contribution of genetic and metabolic disorders. *Brain Dev.* (Netherlands). 2003;25(7): 457-476.
9. Biederman J. Practical considerations in stimulant drug selection for the attention-deficit/hyperactivity disorder patient – efficacy, potency and titration. *Today's Therapeutic Trends.* 2002;20(4):311-328.
10. Nelson KB, Grether JK. Causes of cerebral palsy. *Curr Opin Pediatr.* 1999;11:487-491.
11. Nelson KB. Can we prevent cerebral palsy? *N Engl J Med.* 2003;349(18):1765-1769.
12. Barness LA. An approach to the diagnosis of metabolic diseases. *Fetal Pediat Pathol.* 2004; 23(1):3-10
13. Delgado MR, Albright AL. Movement disorders in children: definitions, classifications and grading systems. *J Child Neural.* 2003;18 Suppl 1:S1-S8.
14. Jankovic J. Tourette's syndrome. *N Engl J Med.* 2001;345:1184-1192.
15. Louis ED. Essential tremor. *N Engl J Med.* 2001;345:887-891.

9. Questions

1. What do neurofibromatosis, achondroplasia and Sotos syndrome all have in common?

A. They all cause microcephaly

B. They are all causes of metabolic megalencephaly

C. They are all causes of anatomic megalencephaly

2. Causes of metabolic megalencephaly include some:

A. Grey matter diseases

B. White matter diseases

C. Inborn errors of metabolism

D. All of the above

3. Match the pattern of premature sutural synostosis with the resultant head shape.

1. Both coronal sutures	A. Scaphocephaly
2. Metopic suture	B. Plagiocephaly
3. All sutures	C. Oxycephaly
4. Saggital suture	D. Trigonocephaly
5. One coronal or one lambdoid	E. Brachycephaly

4. Indicate whether lack of the following physical findings points to a central (= C) or peripheral (= P) cause of infantile hypotonia.

1. Relatively preserved strength in face of hypotonia

2. Inability to elicit postural reflexes

3. Dysmorphism and/or multi-organ involvement

4. Improvement in tone with stimulation

5. Absent deep tendon reflexes

5. True or False?

Peripheral causes of infantile hypotonia are, collectively, more common than central causes.

6. The acute onset of astasia-abasia in a child suggests:

A. Medulloblastonia

B. Drug intoxication

C. A paraneoplastic syndrome

D. Conversion hysteria

E. Part-infectious demylinating disease

7. True or False?

Most brain tumors among children ages 2-12 are supratentorial.

8. True or False?

The attacks of benign paroxysmal vertigo in children typically last hours to days.

9. Episodic ataxia type I (EA-1):

A. Results from a mutation of the potassium charged gene

B. Results from a mutation of the calcium channel gene

C. Is associated with myokymia

D. May respond to propranolol

E. May respond to diamox

10. True or False?

Causes of recurrent ataxia include: Hartnup disease, maple syrup urine disease, and pyruvate decarboxylan deficiency.

11. A child with progressive ataxia has recurrent sinopulmonary infections, decreased serum IgG2 subclass, and elevated serum alpha fetoprotein. The most likely diagnosis is:

A. Friedreich's ataxia

B. Ataxia-telangietasia

C. Juvenile sulfatide lipidosis

D. Abetalipoproteinemia

E. Marinesco-Sjögren syndrome

12. A child with progressive ataxia has malabsorption, failure to thrive, retinitis pigmentosa and low levels of plasma cholesterol and triglycerides. The most likely diagnosis is:

A. Friedreich's ataxia

B. Ataxia-telangiectasia

C. Juvenile sulfatide lipidosis

D. Abetalipoproteinemia

E. Marinesco-Sjögren syndrome

13. Conditions that may be comorbid with attention deficit-hyperactivity disorder include:

A. Tic disorder

B. Learning disabilities

C. Oppositional-defiant disorder

D. Anxiety disorder

E. All of the above

14. True or False?

Up to 70% of children with attention deficit-hyperactivity disorders will respond to stimulants.

15. Periodic discharges occurring every 5-7 seconds on the EEG in association with myoclonic jerks in a dementing child suggests infection with:

A. Toxoplasmosis

B. Rubella

C. Rubeola

D. Cytomegalovirus

16. Pili torti is a clinical hallmark of:

A. Menkes disease

B. Wilson disease

C. Tay-Sachs disease

D. Lowe syndrome

E. GM1 gangliosidosis

17. GM2 gangliosidosis, Niemann-Pick disease and sialidosis type III all:

A. Are white matter diseases

B. Can produce a macular cherry red spot

C. Are peroxismal disorders

D. Are mitochondrial diseases

18. Diseases that can produce extrapyramidal findings include:

A. Leigh disease

B. Wilson disease

C. Lesch-Nyhan disease

D. Hallervorden-Spatz disease

E. All of the above

19. A child with developmental regression has gingival hypertrophy but is not on phenytoin. Diagnoses to consider are:

A. Mannoisidosis

B. Neuronal ceroid lipofuscinosis

C. Mucolipidosis II

D. Gaucher disease

E. Rett syndrome

20. True or False?

Metabolic acidosis due to an inborn error of metabolism is typically associated with a normal anion gap.

21. Hypoglycemia without ketosis suggests:

A. Wilson disease

B. Lesch-Nyhan disease

C. Transient hyperammonemia of the newborn

D. Late infantile ceroid lipofuscinosis

E. Fatty acid oxidation disorder

22. Conditions that are often comorbid with Tourette syndrome are:

A. Spasmus nutans

B. Attention deficit disorder

C. Myoclonus

D. Obsessive compulsive disorder

E. Striatal necrosis

23. Encephalopathy, choreoathetosis and calcifications of the basal ganglia suggest:

A. Huntington disease

B. Machado-Joseph disease

C. Fahr disease

D. Segawa disease

24. Drugs that can elicit choreoathetosis include:

A. Anticonvulsants

B. Antiemetics

C. Neuroleptics

D. Oral contraceptives

E. All of the above

25. Intellectual impairment choreoathetosis, self-mutilation, choreoathetosis and hyperuricemia are combined hallmarks of:

A. Dystonia musculorum deformans

B. Kinsbourne syndrome

C. Machado Joseph disease

D. Lesch-Nyhan syndrome

26. True or False?

All patients with Syndenham's chorea should receive antibiotic prophylaxis.

27. "Eye of the tiger" sign on cranial MRI is characteristic of:

A. Hallervorden-Spatz syndrome

B. Leigh disease

C. Huntington disease

D. Segawa disease

E. Dystonia musculorum deformans

28. The drug treatment of choice for Segawa disease is:

A. Biotin

B. Trihexphenidyl

C. L-dopa

D. Propranalol

E. Haloperidol

29. True or False?

A major cause of segmental myoclonus in children is cystic astrocytoma of the spinal cord.

30. Spasmus nutans includes:

A. Titubation of the head

B. Head tilt

C. Nystagmus

D. Tics

E. Chorea

Answers

1. C.

2. D.

3. 1. E.
   2. D.
   3. C.
   4. A.
   5. B.

4. 1. C.
   2. P.
   3. C.
   4. C.
   5. P.

5. False

6. D.

7. False

8. False

9. A., C., E.

10. True

11. B.

12. D.

13. E.

14. True

15. C.

16. A.

17. B.

18. E.

19. A. and C.

20. False

21. E.

22. B., D.

23. C.

24. E.

25. D.

26. True

27. A.

28. C.

29. True

30. A., B., C.

Chapter 28: Neonatal Neurology

Douglas J. Hyder, MD

Contents

1. Introduction

Neonatal neurology is concerned with neurological diagnoses and treatment occurring within the first few months of life. This chapter will focus on conditions which cause symptoms or signs during the neonatal period. All inherited conditions are present during the neonatal period, but most take a number of months or years before symptoms develop; these are discussed in other chapters. The chapter is organized around several symptoms such as hypotonia, seizures, etc. However, since the infant has a limited repertoire of symptoms, many conditions could be placed in more than one category.

2. History

Several sources are useful in obtaining an accurate history for a neonate. Information from a caretaker is most helpful: usually this is a parent, but in the hospitalized infant it may be a healthcare provider. In addition to questions regarding the onset, duration, type, extent and resolution of symptoms, information should be gathered about the pregnancy, labor and delivery.

Pregnancy Questions

- Did the mother receive routine care?
- Were there any problems with blood pressure, gestational diabetes, infection, or early labor?
- Did the fetus grow well?
- Were there concerns about the location and health of the placenta?
- Did the mother use any medications, smoke, drink alcohol, or use illicit drugs?
- Was an ultrasound done and was it abnormal?
- Was there an amniocentesis or other prenatal genetic testing?
- Are the parents blood relatives?

Labor and Delivery

- Were there any problems with the fetal tracing during labor?
- Was a scalp pH done?
- Was there any evidence of fetal distress?
- Were there any concerns at the time of delivery— meconium, tight nucal cord?
- Did the newborn need any resuscitation?
- What were the Apgar scores?

Additional history should be sought regarding any siblings or half siblings and any family problems, especially family members who suffered an early childhood death, developmental or learning problems, or early onset of seizures.

3. Physical Exam

Expectations for a neonate's neurological exam vary depending on gestational age. Most infants spend many hours sleeping; if possible, they should be observed and examined while awake. Premature infants tend to have low muscle tone. Term infants tend to have increased tone that will gradually decrease during the first year of life: normal posture for a term infant is flexed at the hips, knees and elbows. Tendon reflexes can appear somewhat brisk; crossed adduction will sometimes accompany the knee jerk; an extensor plantar response (Babinski) is normal; and 5-10 beats of nonsustained, symmetrical beats of ankle clonus can be seen. Primitive reflexes such as a plantar and palmar grasp, rooting, suck, and Moro should be symmetrically present. The asymmetric tonic neck reflex usually develops in the one month old, but an infant should be able to break out of this posture. Normal term infant head circumference is 34 cm. Term infants will have pupils that react to light and full horizontal eye movements. Esotropia, exotropia, and intermittent opsoclonus can be transiently present in normal infants. The cornea and lens of the eye should be clear. The fundi should be carefully examined for evidence of hypoplasia, atrophy, hemorrhage, or chorioretinitis. Retinoblastoma is one of the few tumors that can present at birth: the pupil will appear white and a mass will be present within the globe. Normal term infants will fix and briefly follow only close objects: an infant's visual acuity is estimated to be about 20/150. Head shape should be examined, and cranial sutures palpated. Anterior and posterior fontanelles should be soft and flat. Facial muscles should be symmetrically strong. In hypotonic infants, look carefully at the tongue to see if fasiculations are present: this is seen in infants with spinal muscular atrophy type 1.

Infants Develop (GA=gestational age):
Rooting 24 weeks GA

Galant (spinal incurvation) 24 weeks GA

Horizontal eye movements 25 weeks GA

Startles to sound 28 weeks GA

Moro reflex 28-30 weeks GA

Papillary reactivity 30 weeks GA

Grasp (palmar and plantar) 32 weeks GA
Sucking 34 weeks

Stepping reflex 37 weeks

Asymmetric Tonic Neck Reflex (ATNR) 40 weeks

Crossed leg extensor 40 weeks

4. Maternal Drug Use

History should be sought from the mother regarding medication and drug use, although this is not always forthcoming. Studies looking at the effects of maternal exposure are difficult because the exact dose, timing during the pregnancy, duration of fetal exposure, and genetic and environmental factors complicate assessment.

The fetal alcohol syndrome is identified by the constellation of clinical findings. Neonates are born small and remain so. Most have microcephaly and developmental delay. Facial features include: short palpebral fissure, epicanthal folds, midface hypoplasia, hypoplastic or smooth philtrum, and thin vermillion border of the upper lip. Conductive hearing loss and optic nerve hypoplasia occurs relatively commonly. Many will have limb abnormalities such as joint abnormalities, camptodactyly, or clinodactyly. About half have cardiac atrial septal defects. Longer term, behavioral and learning problems are encountered; however, the degree to which this is attributable to the alcohol exposure is unclear.

Fetal exposure to cocaine is thought to be associated with premature delivery of small for gestational age infants. There is an increased likelihood of placental abruption and fetal death. Neonates may have several neurological effects, such as microcephaly, agenesis of the corpus callosum, or septo-optic dysplasia. Other abnormalities such as schizencephaly, lissencephaly, heterotopias and myelomeningoceles may be causally related. There appears to be an increased risk of neonatal stroke, both nonhemorrhagic and hemorrhagic. Long-term behavioral and learning problems are seen; again, the degree to which this is causally related to cocaine exposure versus other factors is unclear.

All narcotics when taken for duration by the mother can cause low birth weight and a neonatal withdrawal syndrome. The withdrawal syndrome is characterized by jitteriness. This can sometimes be confused with seizures, although jitters can be stopped temporarily by limb flexion, and are not accompanied by abnormal eye movements or by ictal activity on EEG. Often video EEG monitoring is necessary to sort out the cause of the movements even when the intrauterine exposure is clear. Other features of intrauterine narcotic exposure include irritability, high-pitched cry, minimal sleeping, excessive sucking, and diarrhea. Seizures are thought to occur in 1%-2%. Treatment with gradually tapering doses of a narcotic agent, such as methadone, is sometimes indicated.

5. Traumatic Injuries

There are three general types of extracranial hemorrhage in a newborn:
Caput succedaneum is hemorrhagic edema of the scalp, usually the vertex, localized outside the cranial aponeurosis. Since the blood is in the scalp, it crosses suture lines. It is common after vaginal delivery and resolves without medical intervention.

Subgaleal hemorrhage occurs when blood is between the aponeurosis and the periosteum. This blood can spread beneath the entire scalp and into the neck. The mass is firm and fluctuant in the subcutaneous tissue, also crossing sutures lines. Potential concerns include skull fracture, coagulopathy (such as vitamin K deficiency), and development of hyperbilirubinemia secondary to reabsorption and breakdown of the hemorrhage.

Cephalohematoma is blood under the periosteum. This blood does not cross suture lines. It is more common following low and mid forceps deliveries. Cephalohematomas tend to be firmer and tenser than other types of extracranial hemorrhage. There may be an associated skull fracture or subdural hematoma.

Skull fractures are generally managed by neurosurgeons. Depressed skull fractures can be associated with subdural or epidural hematoma and these can cause signs of increased pressure (such as a fixed, dilated pupil) or seizures. If this is the case, neurosurgical intervention to remove the intracranial blood is considered.

Brachial plexus injury occurs in about 1 in every 1000 births. The injury is to the nerve roots, which are usually stretched, although they can be severed. Prognosis depends mostly on the degree of damage to the nerve sheath, axons and roots; injury to just the nerve sheaths has a much better prognosis than when the roots are severed. The main risk factors are a large fetal head, weight over 4.5 kg, difficult delivery causing fetal depression, and abnormal presentation such as shoulder dystocia or breech delivery. The most vulnerable roots are C5-8. An Erb's palsy involves C5-7, causing the shoulder to be internally rotated and adducted, the elbow to be flexed and pronated, and the wrist and fingers to be flexed. Erb's palsy is sometimes associated with diaphragmatic paralysis when C4 is involved. If the entire plexus is involved, the wrist and fingers will be extended and a Horner's sign (miosis and ptosis) may be present. Prognosis depends on the extent of the injury: those who will improve generally show signs of recovery within the first month, and infants who recover completely generally do so within 6 months. Peripheral nerve surgery is considered for those infants with extensive injury or those who do not show signs of recovery within about a month. The results of surgical intervention are encouraging: about half of infants referred for surgery will have some improvement. Physical therapy is often recommended, however, it is unclear the extent to which improvement is related to therapy or to time.

6. Neural Tube Defects

Primary neurulation during the third and fourth weeks of gestation results in the formation of the brain and spinal cord cranial to the lumbar region. Secondary neurulation resulting in the formation of sacral and coccygeal spinal elements starts around four to seven weeks of gestation and differentiation continues until after birth.

Neural tube defects and spinal dysraphisms occur when these processes are disrupted. Obstetricians screen for these conditions by checking maternal alpha-fetoprotein levels around the beginning of the second trimester. Elevated alpha-fetoprotein levels can be caused by open neural tube defects, esophageal or duodenal atresia, omphalocele, congenital kidney problems, fetal death, and multiple gestation pregnancies. Ultrasound is also used to exam the fetus for open neural tube defects at the beginning of the second trimester. A folate supplement taken by women prior to and during early pregnancy reduces the risk of a neural tube defect by 60%-70%.

Occult dysraphisms are disorders of secondary neurulation where the skin is intact over the lesion. Vertebral defects occur in 85%-90% of occult dysraphisms. Dermal lesions such as a dimple, tract, hair patch, hemangioma, or subcutaneous mass occurs in about 80% of occult dysraphisms. MRI is the preferred method of diagnosis.

Anencephaly is a failure of anterior neural tube closure resulting in a large defect in the skull and little structure to the neural elements cranial to the brainstem. About 75% of infants are stillborn. Of those born alive, at least 40% will be dead after 24 hours. Endotracheal intubation can extend survival to several days or a few weeks. Brainstem functions such as papillary response, eye movements, auditory response and gag reflexes may be present. Management is supportive. Some infants are considered for organ donation.

Encephalocele is a partial failure of anterior neural tube closure resulting in a skull defect and neural elements extending through the defect. Most encephaloceles are occipital; other sites are seen but less commonly. A Chiari III malformation is an occipital encephalocele (containing cerebellum) with a myelomeningocele. Encephaloceles are frequently associated with other cerebral malformations such as heterotopias. Management is neurosurgical.

Myelomeningocele is a partial failure of posterior neural tube closure resulting in defects of the vertebrae and neural elements partially or entirely protruding through the skin. The majority of myelomeningoceles are lumbar (including thoracolumbar, lumbar or lumbosacral). Depending on the spinal level, motor, sensory and sphincter function may be affected. Some will have brainstem symptoms such as apnea, swallowing difficulty, or a poor gag reflex. Those with sacral lesions have a better chance of becoming ambulatory and not developing scoliosis than those with lumbar lesions. Hydrocephalus occurs in about 90% of infants with lumbar myelomeningoceles: this is best assessed by palpation of the fontanelle, serial measurement of head circumference, and imaging such as cranial ultrasound or CT. Early surgical closure of the defect, antibiotics to prevent infection, and shunting hydrocephalus (if indicated) are generally considered to result in the best outcomes, although these interventions are certainly dependent upon the exact clinical situation. Overall survival is around 85%. About 75% of survivors are ambulatory. About 75% of survivors have an IQ >80. About 75% will develop a latex allergy. Many children with myelomeningocele will develop precocious puberty.

7. Large Head, Increased Intracranial Pressure

Two genetic conditions, Canavan and Alexander, cause macrocephaly in infants, although the macrocephaly usually takes 6 months to develop. Canavan disease is caused by a deficiency of N-acetylaspartoacylase. Neonates will have poor visual fixation, irritability and poor suck. Hypotonia, weakness, nystagmus, and failure to attain milestones then become apparent, unfortunately culminating in spasticity, blindness, psychomotor regression and death. Developmental retardation and macrocephaly associated with hypotonia usually leads to MRI which demonstrates diffuse white matter abnormality. An increased level of N-acetylaspartic acid is present in the urine. Treatment is supportive and genetic counseling is indicated since prenatal diagnosis is possible.

Alexander disease is caused by a mutation on 17q leading to deficiency in NADH-ubiquinone oxidoreductase flavoprotein-1. This results in macrocephaly, spasticity, psychomotor retardation and seizures. Optic atrophy does not occur. MRI shows white matter, basal ganglia and thalamic abnormalities. Molecular testing is available. Treatment is supportive.

Increased intracranial pressure in a neonate presents with irritability, lethargy, poor feeding and failure to thrive. On exam the fontanelles are full and sometimes one or both pupils are fixed and dilated, and an external ophthalmoplegia (usually abduction deficit), low pulse and high blood pressure is present. Head circumference should be checked and compared with previous measurements of that child and age-related norms. A large head circumference argues against an acute etiology since it takes time for the skull bones to grow large. Papilledema is uncommon in neonates because the fontanelles are open, thus providing some relief for the elevated pressure.

Evaluation of a large head usually consists of an imaging study. If the imaging study is negative or fever is present, or other signs of infection, lumbar puncture is indicated.

A positive imaging study could reveal hydrocephalus, a brain tumor, or a vein of Galen aneurysm. None of these is generally managed by a neurologist in isolation.

Hydrocephalus in a neonate is usually caused by aqueductal stenosis (narrow aqueduct of Sylvius), although in premature infants it is most commonly secondary to intraventricular hemorrhage. Management is by a neurosurgeon and usually involves CSF diversion, generally with a ventriculo-peritoneal shunt. Common complications of shunt placement are infection and blockage.

Neonates may develop nearly any type of brain tumor, although teratomas are more common in this age group than tumors such as medulloblastoma, astrocytoma, ependymoma and choroid plexus tumors. Outcome for tumors that affect neonates is generally poor, with the exception of choroids plexus papilloma. Choroid plexus papilloma is a tumor of the choroid plexus that is apparent on imaging as an intraventricular mass; if complete removal is possible, outcome is very good. The most common brain tumor of neonates is teratoma. Even with optimal surgical and adjuvant treatment, mortality is high.

Vein of Galen aneurysm presents in the neonatal period with the combination of macrocephaly and congestive heart failure. A cranial bruit is often present occiptally. Hydrocephalus may be present secondary to CSF outflow obstruction. Management usually involves a combination of intravascular embolization and surgery.

If brain imaging is negative, a neonate with increased intracranial pressure should be evaluated for infection. Two types of meningitis are recognized in the neonate: early onset (<5 days of life) and late onset (>5 days of life). Early onset meningitis is most commonly caused by *Escherichia coli* and group B beta hemolytic *Streptococcus*. Late onset meningitis is most commonly caused by E *coli, Streptococcus, Listeria monocytogenes*, or Gram-negative enteric bacilli such as *Pseudomonas* or *Klebsiella*. As in other age groups, meningitis is diagnosed with demonstration of the organism. Newborns with meningitis will usually have dramatically abnormal CSF; usually there are thousands of leukocytes and either very high (>1000 mg/dL) or very low (<30 mg/dL) white blood cell levels. Newborn CSF is different than adults: there are normally a few white cells (0-20 leukocytes/mm_3). CSF protein concentration is higher than in adults, ranging from 40-130 mg/dL; this is especially apparent in premature infants. Similarly, CSF glucose measurements in neonates are higher, usually between 35-55 mg/dL; again, this is especially apparent in premature infants. When the organism is demonstrated, treatment is focused on that organism. Empiric treatment varies, but ampicillin and gentamicin is a common combination for infants with suspected sepsis and meningitis. Depending on the organism, mortality can be quite high, especially with Gram-negative infections. Neurological sequelae occur in 30%-50% of survivors; these include hydrocephalus, cerebral palsy, mental retardation, epilepsy and deafness.

Abnormal CSF in an infant with seizures, lethargy, feeding difficulty, hepatomegaly, hyperbilirubinemia and bleeding raises the question of herpes simplex infection. This is usually acquired during delivery from an infected mother. While the majority occurs as a reactivation of maternal genital herpes, about one-third may be the first episode of genital herpes. Empiric treatment with acyclovir is indicated until a herpes infection is excluded, usually by PCR testing.

In a similar fashion, neonates with congenital syphilis can present with meningitis, although this is usually after the first two weeks of life. Hepatosplenomegaly, hyperbilirubinemia, lymphadenopathy and anemia are important clues. Neurological signs include seizures, cranial nerve palsies, hydrocephalus and stroke. Bone changes on x-ray are periostitis (periosteal elevation of the bone) and osteochondritis (ragged appearing metaphyses). Treatment is usually with penicillin.

8. Germinal Matrix – Intraventricular Hemorrhage

Premature infants, usually those with birth weight less than 1500 g, may develop a hemorrhage into the periventricular region (germinal matrix) and blood products may extend into the ventricular system. The pathogenesis is multifactorial, but immaturity of cerebral blood flow autoregulation may lead to bleeding as a consequence of cerebral blood flow increases, decreases, or fluctuates. Other factors include an increase in cerebral venous pressure and disturbances in platelet and coagulation. As respiratory care of premature infants has improved, the incidence of periventricular-intraventricular hemorrhage (PIVH) has decreased. Generally, PIVH occurs in the first several days of life.

The grading system used for PIVH is:

Grade I: subependymal hemorrhage

Grade II: intraventricular hemorrhage without ventricular dilation

Grade III: intraventricular hemorrhage with ventricular dilation

Grade IV: same as grade III with a coexistent hemorrhagic infarction of the brain parenchyma

Grade I PIVH may be asymptomatic and discovered only with routine cranial ultrasound. More severe grades can present with lethargy, hypotonia and signs of increased intracranial pressure. Seizures can develop, especially in grade IV lesions.

Hydrocephalus can develop and is thought due to outflow obstruction at the level of the arachnoid villi. Serial lumbar punctures or an external ventricular drain are sometimes sufficient to allow recovery of normal CSF reabsorption mechanisms; however, sometimes a ventricul-peritoneal shunt is necessary.

Short-term implications of PIVH depend on grade. Mild PIVH is associated with a mortality rate of about 5% and a risk of progressive ventricular enlargement of 5%. Severe IVH has a mortality rate of 50% and about 80% will develop progressive ventricular enlargement. Long-term outcome of PIVH also depends on grade.

The incidence of neurological sequelae is 5% for those with Grade I, 15% for Grade II, 35% for Grade III and 90% for Grade IV. For those with severe PIVH, almost all have motor deficits (cerebral palsy) and about 85% have cognitive abnormalities.

9. Hypoxic-Ischemic Encephalopathy (HIE)

HIE is a major cause of acute and chronic neurological injury. Although considered together, hypoxemia and ischemia are separate events. Hypoxemia in a neonate is caused by intrauterine asphyxia, postnatal respiratory insufficiency, or a left to right shunt either related to a cardiac defect or persistent fetal circulation. Therefore, HIE can be caused by antepartum, intrapartum or postpartum events. The brain is not the only organ affected: other sensitive systems such as the kidneys and liver are dysfunctional in severe cases.

Three major types of neuronal ischemia and necrosis are recognized: diffuse, cerebral cortical and deep nuclear (basal ganglia), and deep nuclear and brainstem. The distribution of the injury is apparent on ultrasound, CT scan or MRI. In its most common chronic form, HIE leads to periventricular leukomalacia (PVL), a severe disruption of the white matter with associated atrophy and hydrocephalus. PVL is usually apparent on MRI imaging after the neonatal period, usually when an infant or toddler is being assessed for developmental delay.

In the neonatal period, HIE is characterized by mild and severe forms. Stupor, coma, seizures, hypotonia or hypertonia with dystonia, ocular motor disturbances, and difficulties with sucking and swallowing are described. Long-term sequelae in survivors include mental retardation, spastic quadriparesis, and seizure disorders. If the basal ganglia are affected, choreoathetosis or dystonia may be prominent symptoms.

While a distinction needs to be made between mental retardation and spastic diplegia or quadriparesis, there is high comorbidity. In one study, a normal IQ was seen in 68% of those with spastic diplegia but only 14% of those with spastic quadriparesis. Severe mental retardation was seen with 17% of those with spastic diplegia but with 54% of those with spastic quadriparesis.

Measures to prevent HIE include prevention of intrauterine asphyxia by obstetricians, maintenance of good respiratory status, maintenance of adequate perfusion, serum glucose, body temperature and controlling seizures.

10. Hypotonia

Hypotonia in infants may be caused by dysfunction of the brain, spinal cord, neuro-muscular junction, or muscle. Peripheral neuropathies are uncommon in neonates, except in the setting of trauma. Regardless of cause, infants with hypotonia appear similar: legs are abducted, arms either extended lying next to the torso or flexed beside the head. Moving the joints is met with little or no resistance. The head lags when the infant is pulled to sit, and when sitting the head limply falls forward. When infants are hypotonic *in utero* they may develop arthrogryposis; these infants have a variety of joint contractures and hip dislocation is frequent. Careful attention should be paid to information about the pregnancy labor and delivery. Other diagnostic clues are tendon reflexes, pupillary light reflex, pectus excavatum (from weak chest wall muscles) and liver enlargement.

Central Causes of Hypotonia

Neonatal hypotonia from brain dysfunction is usually apparent on history or physical. Infants with asphyxia, infection or other serious systemic problems are frequently hypotonic. If the infant's mother was treated with magnesium for preeclampsia, the infant will be hypotonic until their serum magnesium returns to normal. Clues to central causes of hypotonia are fisting (thumbs are enclosed by the other fingers in a tight fist), scissoring (legs adduct and cross when vertically suspended), and brisk tendon reflexes. Chromosome studies are indicated if the infant is dysmorphic and hypotonic.

Oculocerebrorenal (Lowe) syndrome is characterized by hypotonia, hyporeflexia, vision problems secondary to cataracts or glaucoma, and renal tubule dysfunction leading to metabolic acidosis. Cataract formation may be delayed until after the neonatal period. Diagnosis is based on demonstration of metabolic acidosis, proteinuria, aminoaciduria, and MRI findings of demyelination. Treatment is supportive, with the most severely affected dying. Milder forms will cause slow growth, mental retardation, kidney problems and late-onset cataract formation. Some benefit from alkalinization, carnitine and mineral supplements.

Cerebrohepatorenal (Zellweger) and neonatal adrenoleukodystrophy are peroxisomal disorders characterized by dysmorphic facies (high forehead, hypertelorism, full cheeks, micrognathia, high arched palate, and flat nasal bridge), hypotonia, seizures, cataracts, pigmented retinopathy, hepatomegaly, and renal impairment. Brain MRI will show white matter abnormalities and migrational defects. Diagnosis is based on demonstrating a high serum level of very-long chain fatty acids. Treatment is supportive.

Leigh syndrome is a mitochondrial disorder characterized in infants by hypotonia, weakness, central hypoventilation, external ophthalmoplegia (pupil spared), facial weakness, and poor feeding. Blood levels of lactate, pryruvate and alpha-ketoglutarate are present. MRI demonstrates decreased signal in the midbrain, basal ganglia and periventricular white matter. Treatment attempts include vitamin (thiamine, vitamin E), coenzyme Q10, and carnitine supplements.

Familial dysautonomia (Riley-Day) syndrome, a defect in chromosome 9q, is characterized by hypotonia, hypoactive reflexes and absent corneal reflexes, absence of tears, feeding difficulty, temperature and blood pressure instability, absence of fungiform papillae of the tongue, and abdominal distention. Diagnosis is based on recognition of the constellation of symptoms and chromosome analysis. Treatment with synthetic parasympathomimetics such as bethanechol helps with some symptoms in some patients.

Prader-Willi syndrome is an abnormality of chromosome 15q causing hypotonia, hypogonadism, mental retardation, short stature and obesity. Neonates will have a poor suck, feeding problems and failure to thrive. Tendon reflexes are absent or depressed. Both chromosomes 15 are from the father in Prader-Willi syndrome. If the abnormal chromosomes are maternally inherited, the child will develop Angelman syndrome.

Spinal Cord Causes of Hypotonia

Neonatal spinal cord injuries are most likely related to delivery; however, automobile accidents can cause cord injuries as well. The main risk factor for spinal cord injury at delivery is breech presentation. Presentation and evaluation is not significantly different from cord injuries in older people. Spine MRI is the preferred diagnostic modality.

Spinal muscular atrophy type 1 (SMA) is a genetic disorder localized to 5q causing loss of motor neurons in the spinal cord and brainstem. Pupillary light reflex is preserved. The infantile form causes hypotonia, weakness, areflexia, tongue fasciculations and eventual respiratory failure. Serum creatinine kinase is usually normal. Diagnosis is based on clinical findings and chromosome analysis. Most infants die within the first 6 months of life. Treatment is supportive.

Neuromuscular Junction

Infantile botulism is caused when the spore *Clostridium botulinum* (or a related *Clostridium* species) is not killed in an infant's stomach. An infant's stomach pH is higher than that of children or adults. The toxin prevents release of acetylcholine. Living near active construction or honey ingestion are the most common sources of the spore. Infants present with constipation, hypotonia, weakness, difficulty eating, ptosis, and eventually respiratory failure. Pupils are dilated and react poorly to light. External ophthalmoplegia is seen in a minority of cases. Muscle stretch reflexes are preserved. Diagnosis is confirmed EMG findings and isolation of the organism and toxin in the stool. Use of botulism immune globulin (BIG) is very expensive, but shortens hospital stay.

Two main types of myasthenia are seen: genetic syndromes and a transitory syndrome occurring in about 15% of infants born to mothers with myasthenia caused by passive antibody transfer. Genetic myasthenic syndromes present with hypotonia, weakness, respiratory and feeding difficulties, and sometimes with ocular findings. Acetylcholine receptor antibodies are not present in genetic syndromes, in contrast to the transitory syndrome. Diagnosis is based on EMG findings and in some cases response to edrophonium. Depending on the underlying defect, some genetic myasthenic syndromes respond to neostigmine or pyridostigmine. Myasthenia related to passive transfer of maternal antibodies is treated with plasma exchange (if severe) or neostigmine.

Congenital Myopathies

There are a large number of congenital myopathies that may present in neonates who are weak and hypotonic. In many cases serum creatine kinase is normal and diagnosis is suspected from EMG findings. Diagnosis of the exact myopathy rests on muscle biopsy. None of the congenital myopathies are treatable except with physical therapy and other supportive measures.

Metabolic Myopathies

Acid maltase deficiency (Pompe disease) is caused by a defect on chromosome 17q resulting in skeletal and cardiac muscle weakness and brain dysfunction. Acid maltase dysfunction causes accumulation of glycogen in the central nervous system and muscle. Infants present with hypotonia, congestive heart failure, hepatomegaly, decreased awareness and absent tendon reflexes. Skeletal muscles have a doughy or rubbery consistency. Diagnosis is based on recognizing cardiomegaly, hepatomegaly and congestive failure associated with weakness and muscle biopsy. Research protocols are sometimes available to attempt to circumvent the biochemical abnormality.

11. Metabolic Disorders

Of the many described metabolic disorders, only a few present in the neonatal period. Some have already been described as presenting with hypotonia. The remainder is a diverse group of disorders that can be divided into deficiencies of carbohydrate, amino acid, organic acid and urea cycle metabolism. Disorders of fatty acid metabolism, such as carnitine opalmitoyltransferase 2 deficiency and very-long chain acyl-coenzyme A dehydrogenase deficiency, usually present in older children who have painful exercise intolerance.

There is no set definition of hypoglycemia in a neonate since normal serum glucose is dependent on gestational age and the age of the infant. Generally, serum glucose levels less than 40 mg/dL should at least raise the possibility of hypoglycemia. Premature and neonates less than 24 hours old can normally have even lower levels. Early onset hypoglycemia can be associated with neonatal asphyxia, intracranial hemorrhage or maternal diabetes, whereas late onset is caused by hypothyroidism, and inborn errors of metabolism present in the first days. Symptoms of neonatal hypoglycemia include apnea, bradycardia, jitteriness, poor feeding, vomiting, hypotonia, seizures and coma.

Neonates with disorders of amino acid metabolism will appear healthy at birth, but feeding difficulties, lethargy, hypotonia and seizures will develop after they begin eating. Maple syrup urine disease (MSUD), so named because of their characteristic maple syrup odor, is caused by deficiency of the metabolism of the branched chain amino acids leucine, isoleucine and valine. Diagnosis is based on checking serum amino acid concentrations and demonstrating increased concentrations of the branched amino acids. A variant form of MSUD responds to thiamine supplementation. Other cases are managed with a special diet low in branched chain amino acids, with some success at controlling long-term neurological sequelae.

Organic acid disorders elevate serum ketones and lactate-causing acidosis. Of the many types of organic acidurias, three presenting in the neonatal period will be discussed: isovaleric, methylmalonic, and propionic acidemia. These are all detected by demonstrating metabolic acidosis, and finding abnormalities in the urine organic acids.

Isovaleric acidemia presents in a similar way to MSUD, except the infant's odor is described as "sweaty feet." Diagnosis is suspected with demonstration of isovaleric acid in the urine. Dietary restriction, in particular restriction of leucine intake and levocarnitine supplements, has benefited some children.

Methylmalonic acidemia presents in neonates as lethargy, feeding intolerance, vomiting, hypotonia, dehydration and respiratory distress. Many will be pancytopenic and many will have intracranial hemorrhage. Infants will have a metabolic acidosis, ketosis, hyperammonemia, and high urine and serum methylmalonic acid. Some infants respond to cobalamin. Other treatments include dietary restrictions and levocarnitine supplements.

Propionic acidemia may present with seizures and hepatomegaly in addition to symptoms much like methylmalonic acidemia. Diagnosis is based on demonstrating increased serum levels of glycine and propionic acid and urine levels of glycine, methylcitrate and beta-hydroxyprionic acid. Treatment is with diet and levocarnitine. Antibiotics can also be administered to decrease colonic bacterial production of propionic acid.

Urea cycle disorders present with lethargy, vomiting, and hypotonia even before being fed. Coma and seizures will then occur in untreated infants. Diagnosis is based on demonstrating hyperammonemia without organic acidemia. Of the urea cycle disorders, ornithine transcarbamoylase deficiency is an X-linked trait. Arginase deficiency does not present in infancy. The others are autosomal recessive: carbamyl phosphate synthetase deficiency, citrullinemia, argininosuccinic acidemia, and arginiemia. Strategies to reduce serum ammonia include an intake of essential amino acids, encouraging alternate nitrogen excretion with sodium benzoate and phenylacetic acid. Arginine supplements are necessary in urea cycle disorders other than arginase deficiency.

12. Neonatal Seizures

Cortical and subcortical immaturity makes infants unable to sustain organized generalized epileptiform discharges, so generalized tonic-clonic and absence seizures do not occur. Neonates can develop clonic, tonic, or myoclonic seizures, and these are generally considered ominous neurological symptoms in a newborn. Clonic seizures appear as rhythmic jerking of focal or multifocal muscle groups. Focal seizures in neonates can be caused by focal lesions (such as an infarct), or more widespread insults (such as asphyxia, infection, hemorrhage, hypoglycemia). Tonic seizures consist of asymmetric posturing of the trunk or eye deviation. Myoclonic seizures appear as rapid jerks of muscles.

Video EEG is the diagnostic modality of choice. The expectation for the EEG tracing is dependent upon gestation age: the normal background activity of a premature is very different than a full-term infant. Ictal epileptiform activity in a neonate is either:

1. Focal spike or sharp wave discharges;

2. Focal rhythmic discharges;

3. Focal low frequency discharges;

4. Multifocal discharges.

An important distinction from adult EEG tracings is that a neonatal focal EEG abnormality need not be associated with focal pathology. Electrographic seizures often occur without any clear convulsive movements; this generally carries a poorer prognosis than electric seizures with behavioral changes.

Diagnosis of neonatal seizures leads to an investigation of etiology. Common etiologies include:

1. Asphyxia related to hypoxic-ischemic encephalopathy;

2. Hypocalcemia (may be accompanied by hypomagnesemia);

3. Hypoglycemia, usually defined as serum glucose less than 30 mg/dL, depending on gestational age. Maternal diabetes is a risk factor.

4. Hyponatremia or hypernatremia;

5. Intracranial hemorrhage;

6. Congenital infection such as toxoplasmosis, rubella, cytomegalovirus, coxsackievirus B, herpes simplex, HIV;

7. Postnatal infection;

8. Congenital malformation of the brain;

9. Metabolic disorders;

10. Withdrawal from maternal drugs;

11. Inadvertent injection with a local anesthetic during delivery (intended for episiotomy anesthesia).

Work-up for neonatal seizures will usually include an EEG, CBC, serum electrolytes, ammonia, bilirubin, liver function tests and blood culture. If a metabolic disease is suspected (peculiar odor, food or protein intolerance, acidosis, alkalosis, lethargy, stupor), an arterial blood gas, serum amino acids, and urine organic acids are indicated. Spinal fluid examination is usually a good idea if the etiology is unclear or if infection is suspected (fever, apnea, lethargy).

Congenital infections are usually associated with other systemic signs, such as microcephaly, jaundice, rash, hepatomegaly and chorioretinitis.

Congenital malformations of the brain are usually diagnosed with MRI, although more malformations can be diagnosed with ultrasound. The most common neuronal migration and neuronal organization abnormalities are:

1. Polymicrogyria (excessive sulci);

2. Neuronal heterotopias (abnormal collections of gray matter in the white matter);

3. Schizencephaly (cleft usually running radially from the ventricle to the brain surface);

4. Lissencephaly/pachygyria (underdeveloped cortical layers leading to absent sulci or very large gyri);

5. Holoprosencephaly (cerebrum is a single large cavity with an undivided prosencephalic vesicle with undivided thalami);

6. Hydranencephaly (cerebral hemispheres are almost absent, leaving a sac-like structure filled with fluid).

Although rare, infants with seizures related to inadvertent injection with local anesthetic will present with bradycardia, apnea, hypotonia and seizures. They will generally have mydriasis, absent lateral eye movements, and papillary light reflexes.

Treatment of neonatal seizures involves addressing the underlying cause. If no treatable cause is readily apparent, phenobarbital is the usual drug of first choice. A serum level of 20 mg/mL is achieved with two 10 mg/kg boluses. Maintenance dosage is usually 5-6 mg/kg/day. Phenytoin can be added if an additional anticonvulsant is necessary. Neonates will usually require a higher dose (on a mg/kg/day basis) because of their rapid metabolism of phenytoin. The usual loading dose of phenytoin is 15 mg/kg.

The prognosis for neonates with seizures depends on the underlying condition. In general, infants with transient conditions (electrolyte disturbance) or treatable conditions (sepsis) will have a better prognosis than those with brain malformation, congenital infections, and untreatable inherited metabolic disorders.

Other EEG Abnormalities

Sick infants can have intra-ictal abnormalities, including EEGs demonstrating isoelectric, low voltage, burst suppression or excessive discontinuity: these usually imply a poor prognosis. Both term and preterm infants will normally have sporadic spikes and sharp waves. Abnormal spikes and sharp waves include those that are focal, persist through all sleep states, or are rolandic positive sharp waves. Rolandic positive spikes and sharp waves are often associated with white matter disease such as periventricular leukomalacia or intraventricular hemorrhage; these are not usually associated with seizures.

Sick neonates will often have repetitive stereotyped movements that may be thought to represent seizures. Described movements include sucking, lip and tongue movements, odd postures, pedaling movements, blinking, nystagmus and apnea. A video EEG usually sorts this out. Myoclonus not associated with epileptiform discharges can occur in sick neonates.

13. References

1. Arzimanoglou A, Guerrini R, Aicardi J. *Aicardi's Epilepsy in Children*. 3rd ed. Philadelphia, Pa: Lippincott Williams & Wilkins; 2004.
2. Browne TR, Holmes GL. *Handbook of Epilepsy*. 3rd ed. Philadelphia, Pa: Lippincott Williams & Wilkins; 2004.
3. Fenichel GM. *Clinical Pediatric Neurology*. 5th ed. Oxford: Elsevier; 2005.
4. Menkes JH. *Textbook of Child Neurology*. 4th ed. Media, Pa: Lea & Febiger; 1990.
5. Thompson JA, Filloux FM, Van Orman CB, Swoboda K, Peterson P, Firth SD, Bale JF Jr. Infant botulism in the age of botulism immune globulin. *Neurology*. 2005;Jun 28;64(12): 2029-2032.
6. Volpe JJ. *Neurology of the Newborn*. 4th ed. Philadelphia, Pa: Saunders; 2001.

14. Questions

1. All of the following reflexes are normal in a newborn except:

   A. Moro reflex

   B. Parachute reflex

   C. Rooting

   D. Grasp

2. Opsoclonus in a newborn is a sign of:

   A. Blindness

   B. Retinoblastoma

   C. Normal finding

   D. Hydrocephalus

3. Infants with fetal alcohol syndrome will be unlikely to have:

   A. Abnormal facial features

   B. Heart defects

   C. Normal hearing

   D. Joint abnormalities

4. Cephalohematoma is differentiated from subgaleal hemorrhage based on:

   A. Presence of skull fracture

   B. Blood respects suture lines

   C. Coagulation work-up

   D. History of difficult delivery

5. Brachial plexus injury can be associated with all the following except:

   A. Involvement of cervical roots 5 through 8

   B. Signs of spontaneous improvement

   C. Require surgical correction

   D. Be associated with Horner syndrome

6. Which answer is incorrect?

Treatment of myelomeningocele involves:

   A. Assessment of current functional status

   B. Serial lumbar punctures to control hydrocephalus

   C. Use of antibiotics to control infection

   D. Caution with latex products

7. Increased intracranial pressure in neonates:

   A. Presents with visual difficulty from papilledema

   B. Always causes an increased head circumference

   C. Is treated with a ventriculo-peritoneal shunt

   D. Is a complication of newborns with intraventricular hemorrhage

8. Brain tumors in infants:

A. Need not be diagnosed because there is no treatment

B. Choroid plexus papilloma is amenable to surgical resection

C. Teratoma is the most common and carries the best prognosis

D. Are usually secondary to neurofibromatosis type 1

9. The most common type of meningitis in a neonate is:

A. Hemophilus influenza

B. Toxoplasmosis

C. Neisseria meningitidis

D. *E coli*

10. You are asked to see a neonate with a grade IV intraventricular hemorrhage. When discussing with the family, all of the following are false except:

A. Caused by an extension of intraventricular blood into the brain

B. Associated with long-term motor deficits

C. Improved by early shunting

D. Treated with adjusting ventilator FiO_2 to as close to 21% as possible

11. A one-week-old infant presents with hypotonia, cataracts, metabolic acidosis and proteinuria. Diagnosis is most likely:

A. Oculocerebrorenal (Lowe) syndrome

B. Cerebrohepatorenal (Zellweger) syndrome

C. MELAS syndrome

D. Prader-Willi syndrome

12. An infant presents with hypotonia, difficulty feeding, labored breathing and crossed eyes. Other symptoms and signs of botulism would not be:

A. Constipation

B. Nonreactive pupils

C. Demonstrating botulinum toxin in the stool

D. Tongue fasciculations

13. An infant presents with hypotonia, large liver, and congestive heart failure. Diagnosis is most likely:

A. Cerebrohepatocardiac syndrome

B. Acid maltase deficiency

C. Spinal muscular atrophy type II

D. Infantile myasthenia

14. A four-day-old infant presents to the emergency department with a seizure at home. The infant now appears ill, but is not seizing. Correct advice is:

A. Load with phenobarbital 10 mg/kg

B. Obtain an EEG

C. Obtain metabolic studies

D. Recommend use of rectal diazepam if another seizure occurs

15. EEG studies in neonates are:

A. Similar to adult tracings

B. Characterized by a burst-suppression pattern

C. Indicated for repetitive movements such as lip smacking

D. Unlikely to have spike and sharp waves

16. The obstetrician reports a new mother received methadone during the pregnancy. Her infant appears jittery and the NICU observed movements suggestive of seizures. All are true except:

A. 1%-2% of infants exposed to narcotics *in utero* will have seizures as a neonate

B. Video EEG is useful to exclude the diagnosis of seizures

C. Physical exam will likely show irritability, high-pitched cry and minimal sleeping

D. The infant may benefit from low-dose benzodiazepines to help them sleep

17. You are called to the NICU to evaluate an infant with a large head and congestive heart failure. You immediately suspect the cranial ultrasound will show:

A. Aqueductal stenosis

B. Vein of Galen aneurysm

C. Meningoencephalitis

D. Pheochromocytoma

18. As part of routine pre-natal care, an ultrasound reveals hydranencephaly. Symptoms likely to be present at birth are:

A. Poor APGAR scores resulting in a need for resuscitation

B. Severe hypertonia, especially in the lower extremities

C. Diffuse hypotonia

D. Normal findings

19. An emergency room physician contacts you regarding a three-week-old infant with a seizure and a fever. They do not wish to do a lumbar puncture because the infant is irritable and there is a strong family history of febrile seizures. You suggest:

A. They keep trying to do the lumbar puncture before using any antibiotics

B. They discharge the infant home with round-the-clock Tylenol® to prevent additional febrile seizures

C. They obtain a blood culture, give antibiotics and then obtain CSF

D. Check the urine for unusual concentrations of amino acids since this is a typical history of propionic acidemia

20. An infant male presents and develops lethargy and vomiting. On exam he is hypotonic. He has not yet been fed, but serum ammonia is elevated. You are very concerned because:

A. He has the signs and symptoms of ornithine transcarbamoylase deficiency

B. He will likely have too many branched chain amino acids in his urine sample

C. He will soon be diagnosed with arginase deficiency

D. He is likely to have schizencephaly

Answers

1. B.

The parachute reflex does not develop until 6-9 months of age. The other reflexes should be present and symmetrical: if not, the concern for a neurological problem increases. Keep in mind, however, the cerebral hemispheres of an infant are immature, so extensive damage can be present but these reflexes can be intact. This is especially apparent in infants with hydranencephaly – they often appear perfectly normal in the neonatal period!

2. C.

Opsoclonus, due to immaturity, usually disappears within the first month of age, however, it can sometimes linger until 6 months of age. Opsoclonus, myoclonus and ataxia can be a manifestation of neuroblastoma, however, this is rare; when it is present it is seen in toddlers and school-aged children.

3. C.

In utero alcohol exposure causes a broad range of clinical features depending on the amount, duration and timing of the exposure. The most common effects, (occurring at a rate of about 90%) are: growth deficiency, microcephaly, developmental delay, short palpebral fissures, hypoplastic philtrum, thin vermilion upper lip. Other common manifestations (about 75%) are short, upturned nose, midface hypoplastia, conductive hearing loss, and optic nerve hypoplasia. About half will have epicanthal folds, abnormal palmar creases, or joint abnormalities.

4. B.

A cephalohematoma is blood under the periosteum, thus it will respect sutures, in contrast to a subgaleal hemorrhage where the blood is between the aponeurosis and the periosteum and can therefore cross suture lines. The concern with both a cephalohematoma and subgaleal hemorrhage is that there may be an associated skull fracture. With subgaleals, also worry about coagulopathies and the development of hyperbilirubinemia secondary to reabsorption and breakdown of the extensive hemorrhage.

5. B.

The common brachial plexus injury involves C5-8. If the injury is not severe, improvement is usually seen within the first month following delivery. With more severe injuries, miosis and ptosis (Horner sign) can be present because there is concomitant injury to the paravertebral ganglionic chain housing sympathetic fibers. Surgery is sometimes considered when a complete avulsion occurs.

6. B.

The lumbar spine is anatomically abnormal in people with myelomeningocele, so it would be quite difficult to safely do a lumbar puncture. While usually managed by a neurosurgeon, it's important to know that survival in people with myelomeningocele is dramatically improved if there is careful attention to controlling infection and managing hydrocephalus. Latex allergies are also relatively common in those with myelomingocele; the reason is not entirely known but may be related to increased mucosal exposure.

7. D.

Blood in the ventricles interferes with CSF reabsorption, so hydrocephalus is a complication of intraventricular hemorrhage. Infants do not have papilledema because the pressure is modulated by the skull's ability to expand – in contrast to the adult skull. Increased pressure doesn't always cause a large head because it takes time for the bones to grow larger. A ventriculo-peritoneal shunt is reserved for only the most serious cases.

8. B.

Choroid plexus papilloma presents with a large intraventricular mass and is curable by surgical resection. While ominous in many cases, there are treatments for brain tumors in infants and children. Teratoma, unfortunately, carries a bad prognosis. While the incidence of brain tumors is higher in children and adults with neurofibromatosis type 1, these are very rarely diagnosed in neonates.

9. D.

Gram-negative organisms such as *E coli* are relatively more common than the other organisms listed. It is important to have a working knowledge of which organisms most commonly cause meningitis in various age groups – this will guide the choice of empiric antibiotics until a definitive cause is identified, ideally with a CSF culture. Remember herpes infections can be seen in neonates too.

10. B.

Grade IV hemorrhage is the combination of an intraventricular hemorrhage and a hemorrhagic infarct of the brain. It is most commonly a complication of extreme prematurity and almost always results in the motor deficits of cerebral palsy. Early shunting and using 21% oxygen are not believed to be helpful.

11. A.

The key here is recognizing that cataracts are only seen in oculocerebrorenal (Lowe) syndrome. One of the challenges of neonatal neurology is that many conditions will present in similar ways. In contrast to day-to-day medical practice, a test question will need to include the diagnostic clues that will help differentiate one condition from another.

12. D.

Tongue fasiculations are seen with spinal muscular atrophy type 1 (SMA-1). The other clue to botulism is non-reactive pupils secondary to the botulinum toxin. Infants with SMA-1 have normal pupil reactivity and ocular motility.

13. B.

Acid maltase deficiency or Pompe disease presents with these symptoms. The gene involved is dysfunctional, causing an enzyme deficiency in alpha-glucosidase (GAA), which is necessary to metabolize glycogen. Fortunately, alglucosidase alfa has been recently developed for the treatment of Pompe disease. There is no condition called cerebrohelpatocardiac syndrome. SMA type 2 usually presents in children aged 6-12 months, not in neonates. Infantile myasthenia does not cause a large liver or congestive heart failure.

14. C.

In the initial management of neonatal seizures, look for common etiologies such as metabolic conditions. If the serum sodium or glucose, etc., is abnormal, then the treatment is aimed at addressing the underlying cause. Certainly, if metabolic abnormalities are not identified, then obtaining an EEG or using medications would enter into the discussion.

15. C.

Seemingly harmless repetitive movements *in neonates*, such as lip smacking, can be secondary to seizures. A video EEG is often the most straightforward way of sorting this out: the movement in question can be observed with the EEG tracing. Neonatal EEGs are decidedly different than adult tracings.

Very premature infants can have a burst-suppression pattern, however, with increasing maturity, the record will normally become continuous.

16. D.

Using a gradually tapering dose of a narcotic such as methadone will likely be more useful than a benzodiazepine. Infants exposed to narcotics will often present with jitteriness, irritability, high-pitched cry, minimal sleeping and diarrhea. About 1%-2% will have seizures and a video EEG will help sort out if the movements are jitters or seizures.

17. B.

Vein of Galen aneurysm presents with macrocephaly (the aneurysm is a space occupying lesion increasing ICP and thus head circumference) and congestive heart failure. With congestive heart failure present, aqueductal stenosis is less likely. A cranial ultrasound is not the diagnostic test of choice for meningoencephalitis. Pheochromocytomas are not intracranial tumors.

18. D.

Infants with hydranencephaly often appear quite normal at birth. The normal neonate isn't using much more than spinal and brainstem reflexes, so it usually takes a few months for infants with hydranencephaly to start appearing clinically different from those with infant cerebral hemispheres.

19. C.

Generally speaking, infants with meningitis will be bacteremic. While it's useful to have CSF and the results of a CSF culture, it is clinically more important to get antibiotics into an infant with suspected meningitis without delay.

20. A.

OTC deficiency presents with lethargy, vomiting and hypotonia. The serum ammonia is elevated even if the infant has not had a protein feeding. Arginase deficiency does not present in neonates. The serum ammonia is not elevated in either maple syrup urine disease or schizencephaly.

Chapter 29: Neuro-ophthalmology

Susan M. Pepin, MD

Contents

1. Afferent System

History and Examination of the Patient with Afferent Complaints

Unexplained visual loss or subnormal visual acuity commonly brings a patient to the ophthalmologist or neurologist. The history and examination can help identify the cause as optical, neural or psychogenic. Optical disturbances are the result of refractive errors or irregularities of the media including the cornea, lens and vitreous. Common media opacities include cornea scarring or edema from past injuries, infections or dystrophies. Surface irregularities from dry eyes or blepharitis are common findings in patients. Cataracts are lens opacities that can be noted as a sudden onset if the patient covers one eye for some reason. Neural etiologies involve the visual pathway from the retina to the visual cortex. The timing and progression of visual loss, whether or not it is unilateral or bilateral, as well as the association or lack of association with pain are important clues that can point the clinician to different approaches in solving the diagnostic problem.

Examination of the Afferent System

Visual Acuity Testing

Simple tests in the office can be used to adequately assess the patient's visual acuity. A Snellen card can be used to determine near acuity. One eye should be examined at a time by placing an occluder over the other eye or using an eye patch to ensure proper closure. Refractive needs can be met by having the patients wear their spectacles. This becomes particularly important after forty years of age when patients can began to have symptoms of presbyopia, a decline in the ability to change the eyes' focal point to near targets. The pinhole test is an imperfect but helpful added test to determine if visual problems are caused by aberrations of the ocular media. Most ocular occluders have an arm with multiple pinholes. By concentrating on one hole, the patient is allowing a narrow light path that produces a limited blur circle on the retina. An improvement in the measured acuity through a pinhole indicates that uncorrected refractive error or ocular media irregularities such as certain cataracts are the cause of previously measured acuity. The finding can then be confirmed by full refractive attempts with an eye care specialist.

Color Testing

Color plates can be used to test color vision one eye at a time and bring out differences in the eyes indicative of optic nerve disease. Bilateral color deficits can be due to bilateral optic neuropathies, congenital color blindness, or retinal disease such as cone dystrophies. In the absence of commercial test materials, brightly colored red, yellow and blue objects can prove useful in the examination. In the color saturation test, a red stimulus is presented to each eye separately. The patient reports whether the red looks "brighter" or "richer" to one eye versus the other eye.

Amsler Grid Testing

A patient's complaint of distorted vision or warped figures (metamorphopsia) can be tested easily in the office with an Amsler grid. A grid of black lines on a white background is presented to the patient, one eye at a time, at reading distance (14 inches). When held at one-third of a meter from the patient, each square of the grid subtends 1 degree of visual field. The patient's report of bent, distorted lines or squares being larger or smaller indicates a retina disturbance in the macula which anatomically corresponds to central vision. Significant disturbance on the viewing of an Amsler grid warrants evaluation with detailed ophthalmoscopy and possible fluorescein angiography to diagnose retinal disease.

Pupil Testing

The swinging-light pupil test is an accurate and objective method to detect asymmetric optic nerve disease (Table 1). If the pupil in one eye dilates consistently or shows a reduced constriction to the light, a relative afferent pupillary defect (RAPD) or Marcus Gunn pupil is noted. Although extremely dense unilateral cataracts, total retinal detachments in one eye, or severe amblyopia in one eye may confuse the test, a relative defect should be taken as an indication of asymmetric or unilateral optic nerve disease.

Visual Fields

The pattern of visual field loss is an important clinical finding in attempts at localizing the pathology of afferent vision loss. The anatomy of the visual pathways makes visual field testing a powerful and simple clinical tool. Hemianopic field loss which

Table 1

Performing the Swinging-Light Pupil Test

Dim the room illumination
Have the patient fixate in the distance at a target and warn them not to look at the near light stimulus
Use a bright light stimulus (flashlight is often too dim)
Direct the light from below the eyes
First assess the response of each pupil to light
Move the light briskly and evenly from eye to eye several times

respects the vertical meridian indicates disease from the chiasm and posteriorly. Nonhemianopic field defects are caused by optic neuropathies or retinopathies. Clinical testing of the visual field can involve the central 30-degree radius or the peripheral field beyond 30 degrees. The central field can be tested with the Amsler grid, confrontation techniques (Table 2), tangent screen or bowl perimetry. Testing the peripheral visual field requires a bowl perimetry machine, either a kinetic, manual Goldmann machine or an automated machine.

Interpretation of Visual Field Defects

The visual field has a reversed and inverted relationship to the retina in each eye. The superior visual field stimuli fall on the inferior retina, the inferior visual field on the superior retina, the nasal visual field on the temporal retina, and the temporal visual field on the nasal retina. The ganglion cells from the ten-layered retina form the retinal nerve fiber layer which converge and become the optic nerve. The fibers from the macula (corresponding to central vision) form the papillomacular bundle and enter the temporal aspect of the optic disc (Figure 1). Optic neuropathies can affect these fibers and result in central, cecocentral (central depression connected to the blind spot) or paracentral scotomas. The fibers from the retina more temporal to the fovea (the center of the macula) enter the superior and inferior poles of the disc. Damage to these fibers can result in arcuate scotomas that respect the horizontal meridian or nasal steps (field cuts on the nasal side of the visual field), typical of glaucomatous disease. The nerve fibers that enter the nasal aspect of the optic disc travel straight to the optic nerve and result in a wedge-shaped temporal scotoma that do not necessarily respect the horizontal meridian.

The nasal retinal fibers of each eye cross in the optic chiasm and join the temporal fibers in the contralateral optic tract. Temporal fibers remain uncrossed. Most often a chiasmal lesion (typically a pituitary lesion) will cause a bitemporal hemianopia due to the location of the decussating nasal fibers (Figure 2). The lower retinal fibers project through the optic nerve and chiasm to lie laterally in the optic tracts, while the upper fibers lie medially. Lesions behind the chiasm (retrochiasmal) result in homonymous hemianopias. Posterior lesions that are closer to the occipital visual cortex tend to show more identical features in shape and size, described as congruity. Optic tract lesions tend to have incongruous homonymous hemianopias.

Figure 1

Nerve fiber anatomy of the retina

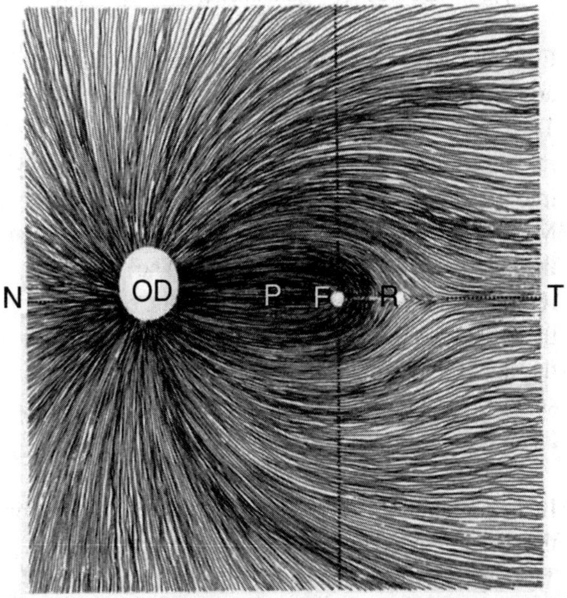

Figure 2

Anatomy of the visual pathway

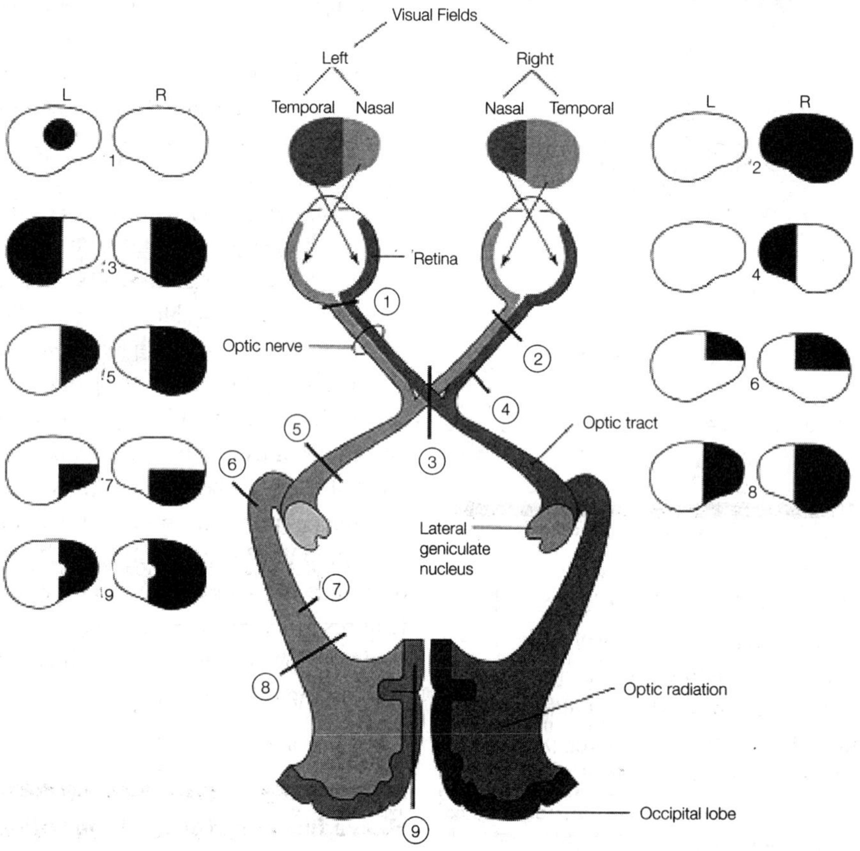

www.homestead.com/emguidemaps/files/vision.htm

From the lateral geniculate body, there is a superior and inferior separation of fibers in the temporal lobe. The inferior fibers from the ipsilateral inferotemporal and contralateral inferonasal retina run anteriorly into the temporal lobe, forming what is known as Meyer's loop, which lies approximately 2.5 cm from the anterior tip of the temporal lobe. The superior retinal fibers run posteriorly in the optic radiations of the parietal lobe. This separation can allow a "pie in the sky" midperipheral contralateral homonymous superior quandrantanopia field defect when there is an anterior temporal lobe lesion.

In the parietal lobe there is a 90-degree correction for the rotation that occurred through the optic chiasm. The superior retinal fibers lie superiorly in the optic radiation, while the inferior retinal fibers lie inferiorly in the optic radiation. Parietal lobe lesions often affect the superior fibers initially and result in contralateral inferior homonymous quandrantanopia, in convenient contrast to temporal lobe lesions.

Finally, in the visual cortex of the occipital lobe, the macula of the retina is represented at the posterior tip of the lobes. This area is also a watershed zone in the distribution between the middle and posterior cerebral arteries. The mesial surface of the occipital lobes contains the representation of the midperipheral and peripheral, which is supplied only by the posterior cerebral artery.

The visual information used by both eyes together is contained in the central 60-degree radius. Each eye has a temporal crescent that is only represented by the far nasal retina, which travels to the most anterior mesial surface of the occipital lobe. For

Table 2

Performing Confrontational Visual Field Test

Occlude one eye of the patient
Allow approximately one meter between the patient and the examiner
Ask the patient to look at the examiner's nose and hold steady fixation
Present between one and four fingers sequentially in all four quadrants, varying the number, in a static manner at approximately 20 and 30 degrees from fixation
A double simultaneous stimulation on both sides of the vertical meridian can identify visual field inattention
Repeat the test with the patient's other eye occluded

these anatomical reasons, if a patient is found to have a spared temporal crescent with an homonymous hemianopia, an occipital lobe lesion should be present.

Finally, the questions that may be answered with a thorough assessment of the patient's visual field findings include the following:

1. Is the field defect unilateral or bilateral?

2. Does the visual field reveal a pattern that allows an anatomical location of a lesion of the visual pathway?

Anterior and Posterior Examination of the Globe
A flashlight or pen light examination can reveal pathologies that indicate the need for a slit lamp or in-depth ophthalmic evaluation. Difficulty viewing the posterior pole (retina and optic nerve) may be due to corneal opacification, anterior chamber inflammation (uveitis), lens opacity (cataracts), or blood or inflammation in the vitreous cavity. A dulled or asymmetric red light reflex can detect unilateral or bilateral media opacities. A view of the posterior pole can reveal optic nerve abnormalities such as nerve pallor or hyperemia, as well as disc cupping or edema with blurring of the nerve margins at the normal boundary of the optic nerve and the surrounding retina. Direct ophthalmoscopy can also allow the detection of retinal hemorrhages, exudates from leaking vasculature, drusen from macular degeneration, and cherry red spots from arteriolar occlusion.

Optic Neuropathies

The diagnosis of the optic nerve as the site of pathology when a patient complains of vision loss can often be made on the history and clinical findings. The clinical features of optic neuropathies include decreased measured visual acuity not attributable to refractive error, abnormal color vision, visual field deficit with pattern of optic nerve disease, afferent papillary defect in asymmetric or unilateral disease, and often an abnormality of the appearance of the optic nerve. This final finding includes both ends of the spectrum, from pallor to marked edema or hyperemia. The spectrum of this clinical finding is great, and viewing a large number of the normal and abnormal spectrum of nerve appearances will greatly assist the clinician in correlating the nerve appearance with pathologic diagnoses.

The differential diagnosis of optic neuropathies includes the following:

1. Ischemic

2. Traumatic

3. Hereditary (Table 3)

4. Compressive (Table 4)

5. Infiltrative/inflammatory (Table 5)

6. Demyelinating

7. Toxic (Table 6)

8. Nutritional (Table 7)

Table 3

Hereditary Optic Neuropathies

Leber's hereditary optic neuropathy
Dominant optic atrophy (with progressive hearing loss and ataxia or congenital deafness)
Recessive optic atrophy (DIDMOAD or Wolfram syndrome)
Optic atrophy with hereditary ataxias (Friedreich ataxia, Marie ataxia)
Optic atrophy with hereditary sensorimotor neuropathy (Charcot-Marie-Tooth disease)

The evaluation of a painless, progressive, bilateral optic neuropathy should include neuro-imaging with magnetic resonance imaging with Gadolinium enhancement to better visualize the optic nerves and anterior visual pathway. In addition, a complete blood count, a serum vitamin B_{12} level and folate level should be considered. Finally, if the patient's history is appropriate or there is any doubt, a urine heavy metal screen, syphilis serologies and Leber's hereditary optic neuropathy mitochrondrial DNA mutation analysis can be ordered. Although there is no proven medical therapy for hereditary optic neuropathies, appropriate intervention can be given for deficiencies, exposures or infectious causes.

Ischemic Optic Neuropathy

Anterior ischemic optic neuropathy (AION) is believed to be caused by ischemic infarction of the anterior portion of the optic nerve. Clinically, there is sudden, painless vision loss in the middle-aged to older patient. Acutely, optic nerve edema is present and often described as pallid edema to distinguish the edema from the hyperemic nerve of inflammatory conditions. In addition, peripapillary flame hemorrhages and attenuated arterioles can be present. Optic atrophy/pallor then develops over weeks that can be diffuse or in a sectoral pattern. Classically, a small cup to disc ratio or the so-called "disc at risk" appearance of the optic nerve anatomy has been noted to be prevalent in patients with AION. The association with underlying vascular risk factors such as hypertension, diabetes and smoking is controversial and need not be found to make a comfortable diagnosis of AION. The visual field defects classically have an altitudinal pattern respecting the horizontal meridian, but central, cecocentral or arcuate defects can be found as well.

Table 4

Causes of Compression Optic Neuropathies

Tumors Meningioma Glioma Pituitary tumor Craniopharyngioma Lymphoma Metastasis
Infectious sinus disease (mucocele)
Inflammatory or sinus disease
Bone disease (fibrous dysplasia, osteopetrosis)
Thyroid eye disease
Vascular disease Carotid artery aneurysm Cavernous sinus fistula Arteriovascular malformations

Table 5

Causes of Inflammatory or Infiltrative Optic Neuropathies

Inflammatory Sarcoidosis Churg-Strauss Systemic lupus erythematosis Sjögren syndrome Inflammatory bowel disease Relapsing polychondritis Polyartertis nodosa
Infectious Syphilis Tuberculosis Aspergillus Lyme disease Cryptococcal meningitis
Neoplastic Lymphoma Leukemia Carcinomatous meningitis Plasmacytoma
Paraneoplastic Disease

Table 7

Nutritional Deficiencies Associated with Optic Neuropathies

B_1 deficiency (thiamine)
B_6 deficiency
B_{12} deficiency
Folate deficiency

Table 6

Common Causes of Toxic Optic Neuropathies

Ethambutol
Isoniazid
Streptomycin
Chloroquine
Digitalis
Chloramphenicol
Ethanol
Amiodarone
Glue sniffing
Thallium
Heavy metals (lead, mercury, arsenic, etc.)
Vincristine

An ischemic optic neuropathy in a patient under the age of 40 is less typical and warrants consideration of further workup. Assessment of blood glucose and neuroimaging are frequently indicated.

It is extremely important for the clinician to be aware of the differences between a nonarteritic optic neuropathy and an arteritic anterior ischemic optic neuropathy. An arteritic anterior ischemic optic neuropathy associated with giant cell or temporal arteritis is an emergency that requires prompt diagnosis and treatment. Because giant cell arteritis can present with an anterior ischemic optic neuropathy, any patient over 50 years of age should be questioned about the clinical features symptoms of giant cell (Table 8). In situations where the clinician is suspicious of the possibility of temporal arteritis, an erythrocyte sedimentation rate (ESR) and possible C-reactive protein tests should be ordered. Results of the ESR are usually greater than 50 mm/hr by Westergren method in untreated patients with temporal arteritis. The patient should be referred for temporal artery biopsy, which allows confirmation of the diagnosis. Treatment is initiated

Table 8

Clinical Features of Giant Cell Arteritis

Age above 50 years (median age 75)
Headache (4%-100%)
Fatigue (12%-97%)
Anorexia (14%-69%)
Jaw claudication (4%-67%)
Scalp or temporal artery tenderness (28%-91%)
Weight loss (16%-76%)
Fever
Muscle aches or weakness
Polymyalgia rheumatica

with IV or po steroids, lasting up to 6 months with steroid tapering adjustments made in conjunction with ESR reduction.

An ischemic optic neuropathy without acute disc edema is referred to as a posterior ischemic optic neuropathy. Such a presentation is atypical, and other causes of optic neuropathies must be considered and adequately evaluated. Conditions that have been associated with posterior ischemic optic neuropathy include severe blood loss or prolonged hypotension, giant cell arteritis, radiation therapy and surgical complications.

Traumatic Optic Neuropathy

Traumatic optic neuropathy (TON) occurs after direct or indirect impact injury to the head, face or orbit. The mechanism is not known but proposed mechanisms include compression or direct mechanical injury, hemorrhage or vascular injury. TON can manifest with unilateral or bilateral vision loss in the range of 20/20 to no light perception. A swollen optic nerve can be seen, but commonly the fundus appears normal at initial evaluation. With unilateral vision loss, a relative afferent papillary defect is present. If a traumatic optic neuropathy is suspected, CT neuroimaging should be done to allow detailed examination for bone fragments and hemorrhage. Other causes of vision loss must be considered, such as rupture of the integrity of the globe (open globe), traumatic cataract, anterior chamber hyphema, vitreous hemorrhage retinal commotion, or retinal detachment. Such injuries can require significant medical treatment or surgery.

Because the natural history of traumatic optic neuropathy has not been adequately studied, the natural history is not known. There has been no large, randomized, prospective trial to assess treatment for TON. Three treatment approaches can be considered: steroids alone, steroids with orbital decompression surgery, and surgery alone. A meta-analysis of treatment results found that recovery of vision was better in patients who underwent treatment compared with observation. No difference in improvement was found between the various treatment modalities (Cook, 1996).

Medical treatment for TON consists of corticosteroids but there have been no well-controlled, prospective studies to define the details of therapy. Many authors have advocated the use of high-dose IV corticosteroids due to the data available on the use of high-dose methylprednisolone after central nervous system injury. Table 9 outlines a treatment approach for suspected traumatic optic neuropathy.

Optic Neuritis

Optic neuritis is the term used to describe an optic neuropathy that has a demyelinating, inflammatory or infectious etiology. The most common etiology in a young adult (less than 40 years of age) is idiopathic or demyelinating disease. These patients experience an acute, usually unilateral decline in visual acuity or loss of visual field. Pain with eye movement is reported in approximately 90% of cases. The optic nerve can appear swollen (35% with "anterior optic neuritis") or normal (65% with "retrobulbar optic neuritis"). A relative afferent papillary defect and diminished color vision (dyschromatopsia) are usually present. These patients often experience improvement over 6 weeks to near normal acuity, although defects in contrast sensitivity can usually be detected. With patients that have these findings and therefore appear to have "typical" optic neuritis, neuroimaging with enhanced MRI studies can be a valuable predictor of multiple sclerosis. Imaging should be considered to assess the risk of future neurologic events and to aid in the treatment decision process.

When a patient is suspected to have an optic neuritis with "atypical" features (Table 10), further workup including lumbar puncture as well as CXR, syphilis serology, and tests for collagen vascular diseases should be done to consider other causes of optic neuropathies and disorders that are associated with optic neuritis (Table 11).

The Optic Neuritis Treatment Trial (ONTT) was the first well-controlled, prospective clinical trial to consider the efficacy of steroid treatment for optic neuritis (Beck, 1992). Table 12 summarizes the treatment results.

Neuroretinitis

Neuroretinitis refers to the clinical findings of decreased vision with swelling of the optic nerve, hard exudates from vascular leakage in a star pattern in the macular due to the anatomy of the nerve fiber layer, and often vitreous cell. Some authors prefer the use of the terminology optic disc edema with a macular star (ODEMS) for idiopathic disease. Authors have speculated that ODEMS is the result of a viral illness or an immune mediated process as it is usually benign and self-limited. When an infectious etiology is suspected or documented, the term neuroretinitis is applied (Lee, 1998). Neuroretinitis often occurs in young adults (20-40 years). It is often painless but it can be associated with headache, retrobulbar pain or pain with eye movement, allowing the confusion with a diagnosis of optic neuritis. Infectious agents associated with neuroretinitis include viruses (herpes simplex and zoster, hepatitis B, mumps and Epstein-Barr), bacteria (*Bartonella henselae,* tuberculosis, Lyme, syphilis), fungi (histoplasmosis), and parasites and protozoa (toxoplasmosis and toxocara). When considering a diagnosis of neuroretinitis, it is important to ensure other causes of macular star formation are not present, such as artery occlusions, papilledema, severe hypertension or infiltrative disease.

Table 9

Treatment of Traumatic Optic Neuropathy

Consider other globe and orbit etiologies of post-traumatic vision impairment
Perform a cantholysis of the lateral canthus if the contents of the orbit are tense from high pressure
Consider drainage of subperiosteal hematoma if present on CT scan
Begin IV methylprednisolone with a 30 mg/kg bolus followed by 5.4 kg/kg/hr for 48 hours
If vision improves, start oral taper of steroids with po prednisone
If vision declines, consider surgical decompression of the optic canal

Table 10

Clinical Features of Atypical Optic Neuritis

Greater than 50 years of age
No pain or discomfort with eye movement
Bilateral disease with close temporal onset in an adult patient
Lack of visual acuity improvement or worsening of vision
History or clinical findings suggestive of other systemic illness

Papilledema and Idiopathic Intracranial Hypertension

The term papilledema should be reserved for disc swelling that is caused by increased intracranial pressure. Optic disc swelling can describe any type of problem until the etiology is understood from the history and neuro-ophthalmic exam. It is important to note that disc swelling may not be apparent with increased intracranial pressure if optic nerve atrophy is present. Some patients may have unilateral swelling or asymmetric swelling, so the clinician cannot rely on the presence of bilateral optic nerve swelling before the diagnosis of a process causing increased intracranial pressure is considered. Up to 10% of patients with elevated intracranial pressure will not develop optic nerve swelling due to the variant of anatomy without the meninges extending to the back of the globe.

Disc swelling must be distinguished from normal variants of optic nerve anatomy or elevated discs due to optic nerve head drusen (pseudopapilledema). Ophthalmoscopic findings that can assist in distinguishing papilledema from pseudopapilledema include the following (Glaser, 1990):

1. Small to absent central cup
2. Vessels arising from the central apex of the disc
3. Anomalous branching pattern of the vessels
4. Discernable venous pulsations
5. Irregular disc margins
6. Absence of superficial capillary telangiectasia
7. Absence of peripapillary hemorrhages
8. Absence of exudates or cotton wool spots

Buried drusen often can be confirmed with photography due to the property of autofluorescence or by CT imaging or ultrasound due to the presence of calcification. Drusen are not apparent on MR imaging. The presence of myelinated nerve fibers or a crowded disc in a patient with hyperopia can also cause the appearance of pseudopapilledema.

Certain symptoms in the presence of bilateral optic nerve swelling should raise the suspicion of increased intracranial pressure. The patient may complain of brief episodes only lasting seconds when the vision in one or both eyes dims or blackens, particularly when there is a postural change (transient visual obscurations).

The causes of increased intracranial pressure include the following:

1. Idiopathic intracranial hypertension (IIH or pseudotumor cerebri)
2. Intracranial hypertension associated with drugs, pregnancy or systemic disease
3. Intracranial tumors
4. Intracranial hemorrhage/subarachnoid hemorrhage
5. Intracranial infection with abscess

Table 11

Systemic Diseases Associated with Optic Neuritis

Sarcoid
Inflammatory bowel disease
Systemic lupus erythematous
Infections (Lyme, Bartonella henselae, Whipple disease, syphilis, tuberculosis, viruses, fungi, toxoplasmosis)
Sinus infection or inflammation
Postvaccination

Table 12

Optic Neuritis Treatment Trial Results

High-dose IV methylprednisolone (250 mg q 6 hours for 3 days) followed by oral steroids (accelerated visual recovery compared to oral steroids alone or placebo but provided no long-term benefit to the patient's vision)
Oral prednisone alone was associated with an increased rate of new attacks of optic neuritis
Treatment was well tolerated
IV steroids followed by oral steroids (reduced the rate of development of clinically definite multiple sclerosis during the first 2 years but by 3 years the treatment effect had subsided) (Beck, 1995)

6. Meningitis/encephalitis

7. Venous obstruction/thrombosis

Thorough neuro-ophthalmologic history and examination allows the directed work-up in patients with suspected papilledema. The following tests should be considered:

1. Blood pressure measurement to assess for malignant hypertension causing bilateral optic nerve swelling and hemorrhages

2. Neuroimaging

3. MR angiography or venography if arteriovenous malformations or venous thrombosis is suspected

4. If neuroimaging reveals no structural lesions or hydrocephalus, lumbar puncture should be performed with:

   • Accurate evaluation of opening pressure;

   • Cell count and differential, chemistries (glucose and protein);

   • Cytology if suspicious for malignancy;

   • VDRL if appropriate.

Intracranial Hypertension (Pseudotumor Cerebri)

The criteria for intracranial hypertension include the following:

1. No evidence of intracranial abnormality such as mass or hydrocephalus on neuroimaging except an empty sella or smaller than normal ventricles;

2. Increased intracranial pressure as measured by lumbar puncture;

3. Normal CSF composition.

Patients with intracranial hypertension often present with symptoms of headache, nausea, transient visual obscurations, diplopia, pulsatile tinnitus and dizziness. The incidence of the disorder peaks in the third decade with a strong preponderance of obese females. The problem occurs less frequently in children and lean adults. There have been reported associations of systemic diseases, vitamin deficiencies and excesses, pregnancy and exogenous agents that should be considered in all patients with intracranial hypertension as attention to the associated factor can aid in the treatment of the disorder. Table 13 lists many of the reported etiologies of intracranial hypertension.

In patients that are found to have cerebral venous obstruction, the underlying, associated condition must be addressed. Such obstruction is typically related to trauma, childbirth, hypercoaguable states or middle ear infections.

The pathophysiology of intracranial hypertension remains under investigation. Absorption of cerebral spinal fluid (CSF) across the arachnoid granulations into the dural venous sinuses may be impaired. The large number of obese patients has led to the theory that abdominal pressure is a factor in these patients. Hormonal abnormalities have been considered and specific endocrine dysfunction may be involved. The role of cerebrospinal fluid pulsatility and hydrocephalus is being explored (Madsen, 2006). For some patients, the disease may be self-limited,

Table 13

Associated Etiologies of Intracranial Hypertension

Pregnancy
Endocrine dysfunction
Systemic lupus erythematosis
Vitamin A (>100,000 U/day)
Tetracycline
Nalidixic acid
Cyclosporine
Oral contraceptives
Cyclosporine
Use of or withdrawal from systemic corticosteroids

Table 14

Management of Idiopathic Intracranial Hypertension

After diagnosis and initial stereo optic disc photos, monthly to q 3 month serial exams for visual acuity, papillary exam, color testing, visual field testing and fundoscopic examination
Acetazolamide (Diamox sequels 500 mg) tapered up to 2-4 grams per day
Weight loss
Consideration of other analgesics for headache management
Surgical treatment Optic nerve sheath fenestration or neurosurgical shunting procedure if vision loss progresses, with full medical management, or if patient cannot tolerate medical therapy (Corbett, 1989).

particularly with strong efforts at weight loss and the use of minor analgesics. However, the natural history can be one of severe vision loss.

The treatment for idiopathic intracranial hypertension should be tailored to the patient's symptoms if vision loss progresses, with full medical management, or if patient cannot tolerate medical therapy (3 plus grams of Diamox®), may require surgical intervention (Corbett, 1989). Surgical options currently include lumboperitoneal or ventriculoperitoneal shunting procedures or optic nerve sheath decompression (Spoor, 1993). Gastric bypass surgery in patients with severe obesity is also being performed (Sugerman, 1999). Table 14 outlines a rational treatment plan.

2. Efferent System

History and Examination of the Patient with Efferent Complaints

Diplopia is another common complaint of patients who present the neurologist or neuro-ophthalmologist. The following questions about the patient's history can help direct further investigations:

1. Is the diplopia monocular or binocular? In other words, does the double image go away if either eye is occluded? It is important to ask whether each eye was tested alone, as covering the eye with a cause for monocular diplopia will also allow the resolution of symptoms.

2. Does the double vision vary depending on which field of gaze the patient is looking? (comitant versus incomitant diplopia)

3. Are the images placed side by side (horizontal), up and down (vertical), or obliquely?

4. Is the double vision present all of the time or is it intermittent?

5. Does fatigue or other factors bring the double vision to the attention of the patient?

Patients may be unaware as to the timing of the onset of the problem and frequently mistake double vision for blurred vision. Other associated symptoms should also be considered such as pain, numbness, coordination problems, eyelid and orbital appearance changes, weakness and other signs or symptoms of other cranial nerve or brainstem dysfunction. Figure 3 shows the relationships of the cranial nerves involved in eye movements.

Examination of the Efferent System

Pupils

While the swinging light pupil test is a measure of the afferent system, it is important to remember that an asymmetry in pupil size (anisocoria) can be pathologic and reflect an efferent dysfunction. The amount of anisocoria should be compared in ambient light and dark. The inequality of papillary size in common, physiologic anisocoria remains the same in light and dark. Old photographs of the patient or past license pictures can be useful to confirm that an anisocoria is long standing. An anisocoria that is greater in light suggests that the larger pupil has a parasympathetic abnormality. Anisocoria that is more prominent in the dark implicates the smaller pupil as having sympathetic dysfunction consistent with a Horner syndrome.

Figure 3

Cranial nerve anatomy

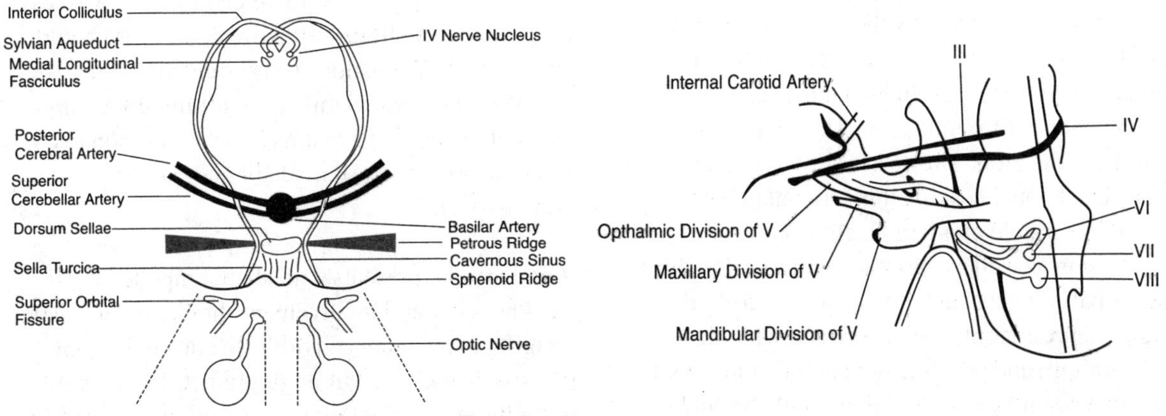

http://umed.med.utah.edu/neuronet/lectures/2002/neuro_opthpics/Basics10.jpg

Eyelids

Examination of the eyelids should include assessment of their appearance, their functioning in both opening (levator muscle) and closing (orbicularis oculi), as well as their position compared to the other eyelid and to the globe.

Ocular Motility and Alignment

The ocular motility exam requires observation of the eyes in primary gaze as well as ductions (one eye at a time) and vergences (two eyes together). Subtle abnormalities in versions can be seen as a relative delay in the movement of one eye. The delay can be brought out with the repetitive movements induced by the optokinetic nystagmus drum. In addition, misalignment of the two eyes in primary and eccentric gaze should be noted (strabismus). If monocular double vision resolves with the use of a pinhole, refractive error or media opacity should be evaluated as the cause of the problem. In order to accurately use eye movements as useful information for the accurate topographical diagnosis of brain disease, both slow and fast eye movements must be examined systematically including ocular alignment, range of movement, ability to hold eccentric gaze, saccades, smooth pursuit, vestibulo-ocular responses, optokinetic responses and vergence (Kaminski, 2002).

Third Nerve Palsies

The third cranial nerve (oculomotor nerve) supplies the medial, superior and inferior recti, the inferior oblique muscle, as well as the levator muscle that opens the eyelid. The nerve also contains parasympathetic fibers that supply the sphincter of the iris and the ciliary body (Figure 4). The clinical features of a complete, peripheral third nerve palsy include ptosis (drooping eyelid), a dilated, fixed pupil and the globe sitting in a "down and out" position at rest. Palsies of the third cranial nerve can result in variable ptosis, adduction, elevation and depression as well as variable pupil size. If a third nerve palsy is associated with other neurologic signs, neuroimaging (MRI with and without gadolinium) and possible lumbar puncture should be done. On imaging, attention should be paid to areas suggested by the associated neurologic signs and symptoms. Table 15 lists the localization of third or oculomotor nerve lesions.

Figure 4

Third nerve nucleus (III)

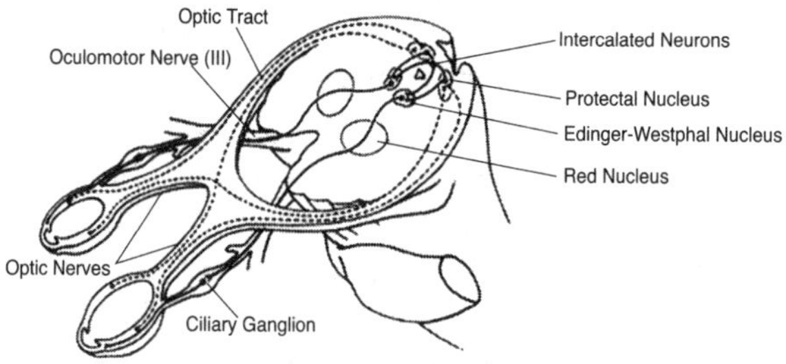

A patient who presents with normal pupil function and complete palsies of the muscles controlled by the third nerve is most commonly caused by ischemia, often thought to be related to diabetic disease. There is a lack of damage to the periphery of the nerve where the majority of the pupillomotor fibers run. Adults with diabetes who develop a pupil-sparing third nerve palsy do not need angiography due to a threat of aneurysm. Patients who do not have diabetes or those who do not show improvement in the palsy after three months should have neuroimaging to consider a compressive etiology. A work-up for diabetes should also be done. The patient should be followed closely initially, as patients with an aneurysm may have delayed papillary involvement. In older patients (greater than 55 years of age) with other systemic symptoms suggestive of temporal arteritis (headache, weight loss, fatigue, polymyalgia rheumatica), an ESR should be obtained. A Tensilon® test should also be considered if fatigue or variability are prominent components of the patient's history, or examination to consider the possibility of myasthenia gravis (see section on MG).

A patient who presents with an incomplete CN III weakness or pupil involvement should undergo MR imaging of the brain and orbits to consider a compressive lesion. An MR angiogram, CT angiogram or traditional angiogram is necessary if neuro-imaging alone does not reveal a lesion, in order to evaluate for the possibility of an aneurysm or dural-cavernous sinus fistula. If neuroimaging reveals

Table 15

Third Nerve Lesions and Their Clinical Findings

Oculomotor nucleus: ipsilateral complete CN III palsy, contralateral ptosis and superior rectus weakness
Oculomotor subnucleus: isolated muscle weakness
Isolated levator subnucleus: bilateral ptosis
Paramedian mesencephalon: ipsilateral ptosis and contralateral eyelid retraction
Isolated oculomotor fascicle: partial or complete CN III weakness with or without pupil involvement
Oculomotor fascicle, red nucleus, superior cerebellar peduncle: ipsilateral CN III weakness with contralateral ataxia and tremor (Claude syndrome)
Oculomotor fascicle and cerebral peduncle: ipsilateral CN III weakness and contralateral hemiparesis (Weber syndrome)
Oculomotor fascicle and red nucleus, substantia nigra: ipsilateral CN III weakness with contralateral choreiform or involuntary limb movements or tremor (Benedikt syndrome)
Cavernous sinus lesion: painful or painless CN III weakness with or without other cranial neuropathies of CN IV, VI and V1, CN III weakness with small pupil (Horner's syndrome), primary aberrant CN III regeneration
Superior orbital fissure lesion: CN III weakness with or with out other cranial neuropathies of CN IV, VI, V1, proptosis
Orbital lesions: complete, superior or inferior CN III branch weakness, often accompanied by visual loss, proptosis, lid swelling, conjunctival chemosis (Brazis, 1996)

meningeal enhancement, a lumbar puncture should be performed to assess for meningeal processes. Table 16 lists the more common causes of oculomotor nerve palsies.

Fourth Nerve Palsies

The fourth cranial nerve (CN IV) (trochlear nerve) innervates the superior oblique muscle whose function is to depress, intort and abduct the eye. The CN IV nucleus lies in the dorsal aspect of the caudal midbrain beneath the inferior colliculus. It is directly next to the more rostral portion of the third nerve nucleus. The fascicle is short and runs dorsally around the periaqueductal gray to cross within the anterior medullary velum below the pineal gland. It is the only cranial nerve that exits on the dorsal surface (Figure 5). It has the longest intracranial course and passes between the superior cerebellar artery and the posterior cerebellar artery. It then runs in the subarachnoid space paralleling the tentorium. It travels within the lateral wall of the cavernous sinus and enters the superior orbital fissure

Table 16

Causes of Oculomotor (CN III) Palsies

Nerve infarction (from diabetes or giant cell arteritis)
Congenital
Trauma
Neoplasm (meningiomas, chordomas, metastases, primary tumor of the third nerve)
Infarction
Hemorrhage
Aneurysm (posterior communicating artery, internal carotid)
Inflammation (orbital or cavernous sinus)
Migraine

above the annulus of Zinn to enter the superior oblique muscle in the superior medial orbit.

Fourth nerve palsies cause a vertical misalignment of the globes that manifests as a vertical or oblique, binocular diplopia. Due to the actions of the superior oblique, the hyperdeviation is ipsilateral to the palsy in primary position and is worsened by contralateral gaze and ipsilateral head tilt. Patients often take a compensatory head tilt to the opposite side.

The differential diagnosis of fourth nerve palsies includes myasthenia gravis, thyroid eye disease or other restrictive strabismus syndromes causing vertical misalignment of the eyes, such as muscle fibrosis following retrobulbar anesthetic injection for eye surgery, scleral buckling surgery for retinal detachment repair, or orbital trauma causing bone fractures and subsequent muscle entrapment. When a fourth nerve weakness is suspected due to the pattern of deviation in different positions of gaze, a distinction must be made between a newly acquired fourth nerve palsy and a congenital fourth nerve weakness that may be manifesting with symptoms of diplopia later in life (decompensating congenital fourth nerve palsy). Table 17 lists common features of congenital fourth nerve palsies.

Table 17

Features of Congenital/ Decompensating Fourth Nerve Palsies

Head tilt (often best viewed in old photos such as a license the patient may possess on exam)
Cyclotropia of the eye without symptoms of image tilting
Vertical fusional amplitudes that are greater than 6-8 prism diopters
Facial asymmetry in the area of the superior orbital rims (hypoplasia on side of head turn)

Figure 5

Fourth nerve nucleus (IV)

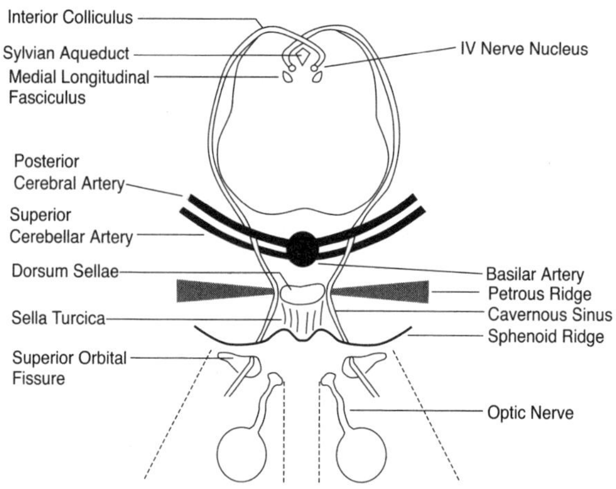

If a patient has a fourth nerve weakness and other signs of neurologic disease, further evaluation is needed, including testing for myasthenia gravis if fatigue is a component, and neuroimaging. Neoplasms and infection can affect the fourth nerve from the nucleus to the orbit. Fourth nerve palsies can also occur with multiple sclerosis or inflammatory disease (Tolosa-Hunt), aneurysms, or arteriovenous malformations. Isolated fourth nerve palsies that are not keeping company with other neurologic disease are often caused by trauma. Patients greater than 50 years of age with vasculopathic risk factors such as diabetes may have ischemic fourth nerve palsies which do not require neuroimaging as long as there is improvement over the following 6-8 weeks. If a patient does not have risk factors or has worsening or unresolved symptoms after 6-8 weeks, neuroimaging should be performed. A Tensilon test for myasthenia gravis should be considered if change in symptoms occurs (Burde, 2002).

Sixth Nerve Palsies

The sixth cranial nerve controls horizontal conjugate gaze. The sixth nerve nucleus contains both motor neurons for the lateral rectus and interneurons that travel by the medial longitudinal fasciculus (MLF) to the contralateral medial rectus subnucleus of the third nerve. (The nucleus is located in the

Figure 6

Abducens nucleus (VI)

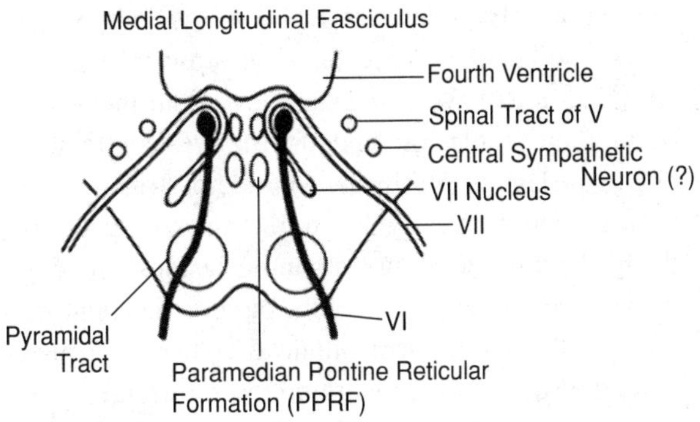

sixth). The nerve fascicle leaves the brainstem and enters the prepontine cistern of the subarachnoid space, coursing vertically along the clivus over the petrous apex of the temporal bone. It is tethered at the petroclinoid ligament in Dorello's canal. It then enters the cavernous sinus medial to the ophthalmic division of the fifth (trigeminal) cranial nerve and lateral to the internal carotid artery. It enters the orbit to the lateral rectus through the superior orbital fissure.

A sixth nerve palsy causes an ipsilateral abduction deficit (globe turning away for the nose) with an esodeviation that is worse in the direction of the weakness. Because the eyes diverge to look in the distance and require symmetric use of the lateral recti, sixth nerve palsies are worse in the distance and sometimes not symptomatic at near.

Due to the intracranial anatomy of the course of the VIth nerve, sixth nerve palsies can be the result of significant head trauma. The palsy may be considered congenital if the patient was born with the abduction deficit or it is noted in the first three months of life (Mobius syndrome). Duane retraction syndrome can mimic sixth nerve palsies and should be distinguished. Orbital disease or myasthenia gravis can also mimic sixth nerve palsies and should be considered. Patients older than 55 years of age with vasculopathic risk factors can be considered to have ischemic sixth nerve palsies unless the ocular deviation does not resolve significantly by 12 weeks.

It is again useful to distinguish sixth nerve palsies that have no other neurologic symptoms or signs (isolated) from those that have other cranial neuropathies, brainstem signs, headache, or pertinent systemic disease (nonisolated). Nonisolated sixth nerve palsies or patients without vasculopathic risk factors require neuroimaging with MRI, with close attention to the area suggested by associated signs or symptoms. The more common etiologies of nonvasculopathic sixth nerve palsies are listed in Table 18. Patients should also be considered for more extensive evaluation, including complete blood count, fasting blood glucose, blood pressure evaluation and lumbar puncture, depending on their history and other findings.

Supranuclear Palsies

The common disorders of gaze are caused by disease of the brainstem, cerebellum and cerebral hemispheres. Horizontal eye movements are generated in the pons and vertical eye movements are generated in the midbrain (Leigh, 1999).

Horizontal Gaze Abnormalities

The sixth nerve nucleus in the pons is adjacent to the horizontal gaze center, containing both motoneurons, which run in the sixth nerve to the lateral rectus muscle, and internuclear neurons which cross the midline and ascend in the medial longitudinal fasciculus (MLF) to medial rectus motoneurons in the third nerve nucleus. Premotor commands for saccades, pursuit, vestibular and optokinetic movements must project to the sixth nerve nucleus. Vergence commands project directly to the third nerve nucleus. Initiation of horizontal saccades occurs in burst neurons from the paramedian pontine reticular formation (PPRF). Input from the lateral semicircular canals of the vestibular system synapse in the medial vestibular nucleus, which project to the sixth nerve nucleus. Pursuit and optokinetic input project from the cerebellum to the sixth nerve nucleus.

Table 18

Common Etiologies of Sixth Nerve Palsies

Nuclear (horizontal gaze palsy)
- Demyelinating disease
- Infarction or ischemia
- Neoplasm
- Trauma
- Mobius syndrome

Fascicular
- Demyelinating disease
- Trauma
- Infarction
- Neoplasm

Subarachnoid Space
- Trauma
- Vascular abnormality
- Complication from lumbar puncture, shunting procedure, cervical traction or spinal or epidural anesthesia
- Carcinomatous meningitis
- Infection
- Inflammatory disease
- Neoplasm
- Increased intracranial pressure (IIH)
- Subarachnoid hemorrhage

Cavernous Sinus
- Neoplasm
- Inflammatory (Tolosa-Hunt syndrome)
- Infectious
- Internal carotid aneurysm
- Cavernous sinus fistula
- Cavernous sinus thrombosis

Orbit
- Neoplasm
- Infectious
- Inflammatory
- Trauma (Lee 1998)

Horizontal gaze abnormalities occur when there is a lesion in the pathway that controls horizontal eye movements. Unilateral restriction of voluntary horizontal conjugate gaze to one side is usually due to contralateral frontal lobe disease or ipsilateral pontine damage. Eyes deviate toward the side of the lesion. Doll's eye (oculocephalic) testing and caloric stimulation will overcome gaze deviations induced by supranuclear lesions and turn the eyes contralateral to the lesion. Pontine lesions do not overcome the tonic deviation. A conjugate horizontal gaze palsy to the ipsilateral side occurs in pontine lesions affecting the abducens nucleus and/or the paramedian pontine reticular formation. Horizontal gaze palsies are often caused by demyelination, trauma, hemorrhage, infarction, tumors or infection. Patients with horizontal gaze palsies require neuroimaging, and an EEG if a seizure disorder is suspected.

Lesions in the MLF block transmission from the contralateral VI nerve to the ipsilateral third nerve nucleus and result in internuclear ophthalmoplegia (INO). Clinically, there is adduction weakness on the side of the MLF lesion and monocular nystagmus of the abducting eye. Usually medial rectus function is intact when convergence is stimulated. The MLF also carries vertical vestibular and pursuit commands so that asymmetries of the vestibuleocular reflex may become apparent with rapid head movements. Combined lesions of one abducens nucleus or PPRF and the ipsilateral MLF cause impairment of all horizontal conjugate movements except for abduction of the contralateral eye ("one-and-a-half" syndrome).

INO is caused by pathology affecting the medial pontine or midbrain parenchyma. There can be associated brainstem signs and symptoms. Unilateral or bilateral INO in a younger adult is often due to demyelinating disease. Unilateral INO in an adult over 50 is most likely due to brainstem vascular disease. The pattern of extraocular muscle weakness of myasthenia gravis can mimic a true INO (pseudo INO), as can Güillain-Barré syndrome and Fisher syndrome.

INO is caused by pathology affecting the medial pontine or midbrain parenchyma. There can be associated brainstem signs and symptoms. Unilateral or bilateral INO in a younger adult is often due to demyelinating disease. Unilateral INO in an adult over 50 is most likely due to brainstem vascular disease. The pattern of extraocular muscle weakness of myasthenia gravis can mimic a true INO (pseudo-INO), as can Güillain-Barré syndrome and Fisher syndrome.

Clinical tests on a patient with an INO can be tailored to the circumstances of the presentation. Neuroimaging is warranted if the patient does not have known multiple sclerosis and has an isolated INO or has associated brainstem signs. A Tensilon test can be performed if there is variability or other ocular signs of myasthenia gravis, such as fatigue or ptosis. In older patients without vasculopathic risk factors, temporal arteritis should be considered when systemic symptoms are present (fatigue, headache, temporal tenderness, jaw claudication, joint ache). If an ESR is elevated, a temporal artery biopsy should be obtained. In rare cases with negative neuroimaging, syphilis serology, B_{12} level, drug levels and lumbar puncture may be indicated.

Vertical Gaze Abnormalities

Motoneurons in the third nerve nucleus and the trochlear nucleus innervate muscles that move the eyes vertically. Both nuclei receive afferent input from vestibular, smooth pursuit, optokinetic and saccadic systems (Leigh, 1999). The vertical saccade command starts in burst neurons in the rostral interstitial nucleus of the medial longitudinal fasciculus (riMLF), which lies dorsomedial to the red nucleus at the junction of the midbrain and the thalamus. There is bilateral innervation for upward movement but downward motoneurons have unilateral innervation. The interstitial nucleus of Cajal is required to hold eccentric vertical gaze. These axons are projected through the posterior commissure to the contralateral motoneurons. Vestibular input, optokinetic and vertical pursuit signals arise from the medulla to the midbrain.

Patients with tumors or strokes in the midbrain involving the riMLF just rostral to the third nerve nucleus and dorsomedially to the red nucleus can have palsies of down gaze. Lesions that are more dorsal and contiguous with the posterior commissure cause an up gaze palsy. The group of findings in patients with pretectal lesions is called the dorsal midbrain syndrome, the Sylvian aqueduct syndrome, or Parinaud syndrome, and include primary position vertical nystagmus and vertical gaze abnormalities (see Table 19 for list).

Table 19

Clinical Findings of the Dorsal Midbrain Syndrome

Up gaze limitation
Down gaze limitation (variable)
Tonic downward deviation of the eyes ("setting sun sign")
Primary position up and downbeat nystagmus
Impairment of convergence and divergence
Convergence-retraction nystagmus
Skew deviation (hypertropia often on the side of the lesion)
Bilateral upper eyelid retraction
Large pupils with light-near dissociation

The causes of vertical gaze problems include tumors of the pineal area, thalamus, midbrain, third ventricle or Sylvian aqueduct. Midbrain or thalamic infarction or hemorrhage is also common. Multiple sclerosis and neurodegenerative diseases can affect this area, as can any infectious or inflammatory cause. Finally, metabolic diseases, drugs such as barbiturates and neuroleptics, as well as trauma from neurosurgical procedures can result in the syndrome. The studies indicated in patients with vertical gaze abnormalities should be tailored to the history and other findings. If there is no evidence of myasthenia gravis, degenerative or metabolic disease, neuroimaging with attention to the mesencephalon, thalamus and ventricular system is necessary to consider structural lesions. If a dorsal midbrain syndrome develops in a patient after a shunting procedure for hydrocephalus, shunt revision may be necessary even if neuroimaging reveals no ventricular dilatation. If no other etiologies are found and neuroimaging is normal, Whipple disease evaluation (biopsy of intestine for evidence of *Tropheryma whippelii*), syphilis serologies, and B_{12} level should be considered.

Skew Deviation

When a vertical misalignment does not follow a pattern of a cranial neuropathy, myasthenia gravis, or restrictive or inflammatory disease, a supranuclear dysfunction should be considered. An acquired vertical ocular misalignment due to imbalance of the vestibular input to ocular motoneurons and the interstitial nucleus of Cajal is called a skew deviation. Skew deviations can be caused by peripheral or central problems. Central pathology occurs more frequently anywhere in the posterior fossa (brain stem and cerebellum). Because skew deviations can be comitant or incomitant, and torsional complaints are common, it can be difficult to distinguish skew deviation from a fourth nerve palsy. Skew deviations are sometimes seen with internuclear ophthalmoplegia. Common causes include multiple sclerosis, trauma, tumor or infarction.

Ocular Myasthenia Gravis

Myasthenia gravis (MG) is an autoimmune disorder in which the acetylcholine receptor sites for neuromuscular transmission are blocked by immune complexes. For this reason it is characterized by worsening symptoms, with fatigue and weakness. Symptoms generally improve with rest. Fifteen percent of myasthenic patients have clinical involvement that is restricted to the ocular muscles. Most patients with MG develop neuro-ophthalmic problems during the course of the disease. While spontaneous remissions can occur in up to 10% of patients in the first year after diagnosis, within six months of presentation more than half of patients develop generalized disease (Kupersmith, 2003).

The most common sign of MG is ptosis, which may be unilateral or bilateral. Lid height tends to vary and lower after exertion, in the evening or after prolonged up gaze. Cogan's lid twitch has been described, which is a brief over-elevation of the upper eyelid with an upward saccade during down gaze. The patient may have varying diplopia, which can appear to be in any pattern of a cranial neuropathy, isolated muscle weakness, total ophthalmoplegia, or supranuclear disturbance. Orbicularis oculi weakness has also been noted in most patients with ocular myasthenia. Common systemic symptoms include dysphagia, dysarthria and dyspnea, as well as weakness of the jaw, neck, trunk and limb muscles, warranting emergent treatment. Graves disease is estimated to occur in 5% of MG patients.

Diagnosis based on clinical suspicion can often be confirmed by pharmacological, serological, or electrophysiologic testing. A rest test (consisting of a set amount of time resting prior to examination with eyes closed) and an ice test (application of cold pack or ice to the closed lids for a set amount of time) have been described to be useful in some patients. The administration of intravenous edrophonium chloride (Tensilon®) in the office—an acetylcholinergic agent that briefly overcomes the receptor block—can alleviate some or all of the symptoms for approximately 60 seconds. Major side effects are rare, but the patient should be warned that edrophonium can cause abdominal pain, nausea, vomiting and salivation. Atropine sulfate (0.4 mg) should be available at the time of the test should bradycardia or respiratory arrest occur. Consultation with the patient's primary doctor should be considered prior to the test if the patient has significant cardiac disease. Several variations of administration of Tensilon are used by different clinicians. One approach is to give increments of 2 mg, then 4 mg, then another 4 mg, stopping if a response is found. Another approach is to give the dose in two 5 mg boluses (1.0 cc). If the eyelid elevates or the motility improves, the test is considered positive. The more dramatic clinical findings allow a discernable endpoint, and the test should not be undertaken if the patient is asymptomatic on examination. A negative test does not exclude the diagnosis. Strong clinical suspicion warrants repeating the test at a later date.

Three types of acetylcholine receptor antibody (AChR Ab) tests are available: binding, blocking and modulating. Binding antibodies are present in 80%-90% of generalized patients but only 50% of patients with ocular myasthenia. In generalized patients with negative AChRAb serologies, 30% have been found to be positive for antibodies directed against a muscle specific kinase (MuSK). Ocular myasthenic patients do not seem to have antibodies to MuSK. Antistriational muscle antibodies can be found and are thought to be a possible marker for thymomas, which rarely occur, in isolated ocular disease.

Treatment of myasthenia gravis includes systemic cholinesterase inhibitors, corticosteroids and other immunomodulators. Only 20%-40% of patients have a significant improvement in their ocular symptoms on daily Mestinon®. Alternatively, prednisone is used, with varying regimens. Doses can be raised gradually from 10-20 mg to 50-60 mg until symptoms are under control. Patients can require continued use of steroids years after the initiation of treatment. Several retrospective studies have suggested that steroid treatment reduces the risk of generalized disease (Sommer, 1997). The response to corticosteroid treatment varies in patients with generalized myasthenia gravis, but 80% have significant improvement of weakness in the first month of treatment. Thymectomy can sometimes be helpful in the treatment of generalized disease but is only done in a limited number of patients with ocular MG. Azathioprine has also been found to be beneficial for patients with generalized and ocular MG (Sommer, 1997).

Thyroid Eye Disease

Thyroid eye disease (TED), or orbitopathy (Graves disease), is typically found with hyperthyroidism but can be seen with hypothyroidism or in patients without findings of thyroid abnormalities. Importantly, the course of the eye problems does not necessarily reflect the activity of the thyroid disease or the effectiveness of the thyroid treatment. It is an autoimmune inflammatory problem without a known cause.

The clinical signs and symptoms of TED may be extremely asymmetric between the two orbits. Symptoms include a red eye, although pain is limited to symptoms of severe dryness and exposure keratopathy. The signs may include proptosis of the globe, eyelid retraction, lid lag, restrictive myopathy, optic neuropathy and elevated intraocular pressure. If the extraocular muscles are involved symmetrically, the patient may not experience diplopia. The majority of patients have asymmetric disease that leads to the symptoms of diplopia. The inferior rectus is most commonly involved, followed by the medial and then the superior rectus. If the muscles are severely inflamed at the apex of the orbit, the optic nerve may be compressed, leading to compressive neuropathy. The patient may experience blurred acuity and decreased color vision. Visual field testing may reveal central or arcuate defects. Optic disc appearance can range from edema to pallor (indicating long-standing compression on the nerve). The clinical external appearance of the orbit may appear normal in rare cases even when there is compression of the nerve at the apex.

The eye signs are critical in the diagnosis of TED because thyroid function tests can be normal. The extraocular muscles are visualized by CT scan or MRI coronal views. Classically, the tendons of the extraocular muscles are spared and only the muscle body shows enlargement. This finding is in contrast to inflammatory orbital myositis, which does involve the muscle insertion. The differential diagnosis of proptosis and a red eye in addition to TED includes orbital pseudotumor/inflammatory disease, carotid cavernous fistula and orbital masses.

In addition to adequate control of thyroid hormone abnormalities, treatment of TED must be tailored to the problems the patient is experiencing. Clinical evidence of optic nerve dysfunction must be addressed promptly. Orbital disease can be treated with corticosteroids in the range of 1.0 to 1.5 mg/kg of prednisone. Radiation therapy in the range of 20 Gy in 2 Gy fractions can also be used when the compression at the orbital apex is critical. Finally, orbital decompression surgery may be needed when there is progressive visual loss from compressive optic neuropathy. Adequate lubrication for dry eyes and exposure due to lid abnormalities is needed, and ranges from frequent natural tears and ointments at night to tarsorrhaphy (surgical partial closure of the lids) when the corneal disease is severe enough to warrant greater intervention. Double vision can be managed with patching one eye or prisms in spectacles until the muscle fibrosis is complete and the misalignment of the eyes is stable. Strabismus surgery can be performed to reposition the globe for realignment. Lid surgery to address lid retraction should occur only after orbital or strabismus surgery (Kazim,1991).

Nystagmus and Ocular Oscillations

The ability to maintain the eyes with stability on a target can be interrupted by problems with the cerebellum or vestibular pathways. Stability should be observed in primary position of the eyes as well as directions of eccentric gaze. If the eyes drift from fixation, a saccade is generated to place fixation back on an object. Nystagmus is a repetitive movement of the eye that can be to-and-fro with smooth sinusoidal oscillations (pendular nystagmus) or a slow component with a quick corrective jerk phase (jerk nystagmus). The more common early onset nystagmus and acquired nystagmus forms will be described (Leigh, 1999).

Congenital Nystagmus

Congenital nystagmus is usually noticed early in life. Clinically it appears as an involuntary, conjugate, horizontal oscillation of the eyes. The intensity increases on lateral gaze and becomes right-beating in right gaze and left-beating in left gaze. Unlike adult onset nystagmus, patients do not complain of oscillopsia. A null point is often found and the patient may take a head position to place primary gaze in this position. The clinician must determine in initial evaluation if there is evidence of a problem with the visual tracking or evidence of optic nerve pallor. Such abnormalities require neuroimaging. Most commonly, congenital nystagmus occurs alone but can be associated with sensory visual loss in patients with albinism, Leber congenital amaurosis, aniridia, achromatopsia or optic nerve hypoplasia (Brodsky, 1996).

Latent Nystagmus

Latent nystagmus can appear early in life and occurs when one eye is occluded and binocular fixation is interrupted. The fast beat of the horizontal nystagmus is toward the viewing eye. Latent nystagmus occurs in cases of strabismus, most often esotropia. Manifest latent nystagmus describes the movement characteristic of latent nystagmus, which is present when both eyes are open and is the most common form of nystagmus in early life.

Spasmus Nutans

The nystagmus of spasmus nutans can be monocular or binocular. The clinical appearance is horizontal and rapid nystagmus of low amplitude. The patient sometimes displays head nodding or abnormal head positioning. Spasmus nutans resolves usually by the sixth year of life. It can be impossible to distinguish from other more problematic conditions of childhood, and patients usually require neuroimaging to rule out other disease. Although rare, small amplitude nystagmus of one eye in childhood can be a sign of a chiasmal glioma. The eye with the nystagmus may have an afferent pupillary defect or poor vision.

Gaze-Evoked Nystagmus

In patients with gaze-evoked nystagmus, eccentric gaze cannot be maintained and the eyes drift back to the center. A saccadic corrective movement with the fast phase in the direction of gaze repositions the eye. The nystagmus is usually symmetric to the left and the right. Gaze-evoked nystagmus is the most common type of acquired nystagmus and can be benign in elderly patients or on extreme eccentric gaze. The finding is also common in patients on anti-seizure medications or due to ethanol use. Lesions must be considered in the brainstem or cerebellum if the gaze-evoked nystagmus is asymmetric.

Downbeat Nystagmus

Patients with acquired downbeat nystagmus have lost the ability to hold vertical gaze. Loss of the symmetric, tonic input from the anterior semicircular canals results in an upward drift of the eyes. Corrective downward saccades are generated. It is most often found in primary position but increases in amplitude in down gaze. Patients usually have significant oscillopsia symptoms. Fifty percent of patients with downbeat nystagmus are found to have structural lesions at the cervicomedullary junction. MR imaging with sagittal images through the foramen magnum should be done. The more common causes of downbeat nystagmus include:

1. Arnold-Chiari malformation
2. Demyelination/multiple sclerosis
3. Tumor at the foramen magnum
4. Trauma

5. Cerebral vascular accident

6. Spinocerebellar degenerations

7. Brain stem encephalitis

8. Drugs such as lithium, antiseizure meds

9. Nutritional deficiency (Mg, parenteral feeding, Wernicke encephalopathy)

10. Syrinx

The approach to downbeat nystagmus relies on complete neurologic examination and neuroimaging to diagnose the etiology when possible. Convergence can dampen the nystagmus and base-out prisms may be tried to abate oscillopsia symptoms. Other medicines, such as clonazepam and baclofen, can be administered, although there has been limited reported success (Leigh, 1994).

Upbeat Nystagmus

With upbeat nystagmus, the fast component of the movement is upward in primary gaze as well as lateral gaze. The nystagmus may be large or small amplitude and often increases in upgaze. Similar to downbeat nystagmus, a pathologic lesion is not always identified. Most patients have intrinsic brainstem disease, often from demyelination or cerebral vascular disease. Abnormalities in the anterior cerebellar vermis or any posterior fossa lesion may be recognized, making upbeat nystagmus a less useful sign for localization of brain pathology.

Periodic Alternating Nystagmus

Periodic alternating nystagmus (PAN) describes a jerk nystagmus present in primary gaze that demonstrates a cycle of movement with the fast component to one side for 1-2 minutes and then slowly reverses to the other side. Due to the periodicity, the change can be overlooked in a rapid exam. PAN can be congenital or acquired. Cerebellar or posterior fossa disease may be present with a proposed vestibulocerebellum pathology, allowing a shifting null point for the nystagmus. PAN can be seen with temporary poor vision (eg, vitreous blood from diabetic disease). Baclofen may be useful in the treatment of PAN that is acquired.

See-Saw Nystagmus

See-saw nystagmus describes a rare pendular eye movement with a conjugate rotary movement but a disconjugate vertical movement. One eye moves upward and intorts while the other eye moves downward and extorts. See-saw nystagmus can be seen with suprasellar lesions such as craniopharyngiomas and bitemporal field deficits. Congenital absence of the chiasm or chiasmal gliomas may also produce see-saw nystagmus (Druckman, 1966).

Ptosis

Ptosis is a drooping of the upper eyelid often defined as a height of less than 2 mm from the center of the pupil (Small,1989). Downward displacement of the lid can be caused without true ptosis (pseudoptosis) for a variety of reasons listed in Table 20. Ptosis can be stable and long-standing (likely congenital) or acquired. Congenital ptosis can be unilateral or bilateral and associated with other abnormalities. The most common form results from dystrophic development of the levator muscle. Table 21 lists forms of congenital ptosis. Marcus Gunn jaw-winking is a synkinetic movement of the eyelid that occurs with jaw movement. The clinician must be aware of the potential for sensory amblyopia due to occlusion if the lid height blocks the pupil or induces significant astigmatism to the corneal surface. If a ptosis is new, the patient requires evaluation for specific etiology. Table 22 lists the causes of acquired ptosis.

Pupil Abnormalities

Two muscles of the iris control the size of the pupil. The sphincter muscle is innervated by parasympathetic nerves that originate in the Edinger-Westphal nucleus (EW) in the midbrain, which is part of the oculomotor nucleus. The light reflex excites the EW nucleus by afferent neurons from retinal ganglion cells which travel to the pretectal area. Information from one eye is carried by the optic nerve to the chiasm, where half of the fibers cross to the contralateral tract. Approximately two-thirds of the way along each optic tract, some of the fibers leave the tract to enter the brachium of the superior colliculus and synapse in the pretectal region. Intercalated neurons from the pretectal area then travel bilaterally to the EW nucleus. The stimulated parasympathetic fibers from the EW nucleus travel with the oculomotor nerve (III) with the inferior division through the superior orbital fissure to synapse in the ciliary ganglion in the orbit, and finally to the iris sphincter muscle, which on contraction brings the iris tissue closer to the center of the pupil.

The dilator muscles of the iris which open the pupil to a larger size are innervated by sympathetic nerves in a three-neuron pathway. The first-order neurons originate in the posterior hypothalamus and travel through the brainstem to the C8-T8 level of the spinal cord. The second-order neuron fibers then exit the cord and enter the paravertebral sympathetic chain. These preganglionic neurons terminate in the superior cervical ganglion at the base of the skull. The third-order neuron fibers enter the skull on the internal carotid artery. In the cavernous sinus, the fibers join the ophthalmic nerve, traveling to the orbit through the superior orbital fissure to the pupil dilator muscles and to Muller's muscle of the upper eyelid and the lower lid retractors.

The strongest influence on the size of the pupil is the amount of ambient light. Pupils become smaller as people age. Very small pupils can be the result of

Table 20

Causes of Pseudoptosis

Lid retraction of the contralateral eye
Hemifacial spasm or blepharospasm
Volitional splinting
Microphthalmia
Hypoglobus (downward displacement of the globe)
Hypertropia
Apraxia of lid opening
Aberrant regeneration of the facial nerve

Table 21

Congenital Ptosis

Isolated
Ocular defects Strabismus/amblyopia Epicanthus Congenital cataracts Anisometropia Nasolacrimal duct/punctual defects
Neurogenic (third nerve palsy)
Synkinesis (Marcus Gunn jaw winking)
Myogenic (congenital fibrosis syndrome)
Myasthenia gravis

Table 22

Causes of Acquired Ptosis

Mechanical (tumors, cicatricial scarring, infiltration, inflammation, levator aponeurotic disinsertion, contact lenses, giant papillary conjunctivitis)
Myogenic (external ophthalmoplegia, myotonic dystrophy, long-term steroid eye drops)
Neurogenic (third nerve palsy, Horner syndrome, migraine, apraxia of lid opening, Miller-Fisher syndrome)
Neuromuscular (Botulism, myasthenia gravis
Traumatic

narcotic use, topical drops such as pilocarpine, or pontine hemorrhage. Very large pupils can be caused by parasympathetic block by topical or systemic medicine, often inadvertently applied to the eye with a finger. It is important to remember that pupils can become an irregular shape due to trauma, past eye inflammation (anterior uveitis), or eye surgery. Rarely, migraine sufferers can present with segmental dilation of a pupil that resolves over minutes, and has been called a tadpole pupil due to its shape. Young people with a history of headaches can also experience episodes of an enlarged pupil (mydriasis) that is accompanied by blurry vision and discomfort but resolves spontaneously, referred to as benign episodic papillary mydriasis.

Anisocoria

Anisocoria is a difference in the size of the two pupils in an individual, sometimes caused by efferent pathology (Thompson, 1976). Approximately 20% of people have a difference in pupillary size that is noticeable to the eye (0.4 mm) (physiologic anisocoria). Anisocoria is more common as we age, making its presence in children more concerning. Physiologic anisocoria is equal in light and dim illumination.

Horner Syndrome

A disruption along the sympathetic pathway to dilate the pupil produces a Horner syndrome, which includes a ptosis and a miosis (small pupil) on the ipsilateral side. The upper eyelid is lower (ptotic) but not closed, and the lower eyelid may be slightly higher (reverse ptosis) due to the paresis of Muller's muscle and lid retractors with disruption of the sympathetic input. The anisocoria is more prominent in dim illumination. The affected side shows a lag in dilation of the pupil, compared to the other side with more anisocoria found after the lights are dimmed than 20 seconds later. Anhidrosis affects the entire ipsilateral side of the face with a central first-order neuron disruption. With postganglionic lesions from the superior cervical ganglion to the eye, anhidrosis is absent or limited to the forehead. Congenital Horner syndrome has iris heterochromia (difference in color/pigmentation) with the involved side having a lighter iris.

A careful history and neurologic exam can help localize a Horner syndrome. Accompanying central neurologic symptoms such as ataxia, weakness, numbness or nystagmus can point to a first-order neuron lesion. Cough, neck mass or hemoptysis can raise the suspicion for a second-order neuron disruption. Third-order neuron disruption can be accompanied by numbness in the distribution of the fifth cranial nerve (V1) or diplopia from sixth cranial nerve disease.

Dysfunction of the sympathetics to the eye can be confirmed and localized pharmacologically with topical eye drops. Cocaine is used because it blocks the reuptake of norepinephrine released at the neuromuscular junction of the iris dilator muscle and increases the amount of norepinephrine available at the terminal to stimulate the muscle. Cocaine will cause dilation in a normal eye but fail to cause dilation if the patient has a Horner syndrome. Hydroxy amphetamine, which causes release of norepinephrine from the presynaptic terminal, can be used on a separate office visit to further localize the lesion. The pupil will dilate after hydroxyamphetamine drops, a normal pupil or a preganglionic

Table 23

Pharmacologic Testing for Horner Syndrome (Oculosympathetic Paralysis)

Defect	Drug	Abnormal Pupil	Normal Pupil
Horner syndrome	Cocaine 10%	Fails to dilate	Dilates
Preganglionic	Hydroxyamphetamine 1%	Dilates	Dilates
Postganglionic	Hydroxyamphetamine 1%	Fails to dilate	Dilates

Horner syndrome. In a postganglionic Horner syndrome, the nerve terminal degenerates and the pupil will dilate poorly. Table 23 lists the results of the pharmacologic testing.

Localization of a Horner syndrome has important implications for the etiology of the disorder. First-order neuron disruption can be caused by central nervous system disease such as tumors, upper cervical spinal disease, neurosurgical procedures and vascular occlusion in the lateral medulla. Second-order neuron lesions can be caused by apical lung tumors, past chest surgery, metastases, trauma to the brachial plexus or thoracic aneurysms. Third order neuron lesions can be caused by internal carotid artery dissection, past neck surgery, extension of tumors into the cavernous sinus or degenerative changes in the wall of the carotid artery.

A new Horner syndrome that is accompanied by pain requires attention because spontaneous dissection of the internal carotid artery can present in this way and can result in stroke. MRI of the neck may reveal intramural hemorrhage. MR angiography or traditional cerebral angiography may be needed to provide more definitive evidence of a dissection. These patients need urgent evaluation and anticoagulation. Other workup can be guided by the results of pharmacologic testing and imaging of the head, neck and lung apices can be directed appropriately. Cluster headaches can be associated with ipsilateral Horner syndrome, which may resolve but also may become permanent with repeated episodes (Digre, 1992).

Adie's Tonic Pupil

Tonic pupils can occur acutely in young people, approximately 70% female. The clinical findings include sluggish, segmental pupillary response to light but better response to near effort, followed by a slow redilatation. Tonic pupils are caused by damage to the postganglionic parasympathetic fibers. The problem occurs unilaterally 80% of the time, but approximately 4% of patients per year have involvement of the other eye. Histologically, the ciliary ganglion has a reduction in ciliary ganglion cells in patients with tonic pupils. The Holmes-Adie syndrome describes tonic pupils with diminished deep tendon reflexes and orthostatic hypotension. Rarely, systemic conditions may be associated with tonic pupils, including herpes zoster, varicella, syphilis and temporal arteritis.

A tonic pupil becomes supersensitive to parasympathetic solutions, allowing diluted pilocarpine (0.1%) to be used to diagnose the problem. A normal pupil will constrict only slightly or not at all to dilute pilocarpine, while an Adie's pupil will constrict more than a normal pupil. Patients may have symptoms from difficulty with accommodation or photosensitivity. Dilute pilocarpine may be helpful in managing the latter symptom (Flach, 1984).

Third Nerve Palsy

With a third nerve palsy with pupil involvement, the anisocoria is maximized in bright light. Without function of the pupillary sphincter muscle, pupil size depends on the level of sympathetic stimulation. The pupil involvement aids in the diagnosis of acute third nerve palsies and is usually accompanied by varying degrees of ptosis and limitation of ocular motility. If the pupil is involved, an aneurysm at the junction of the internal carotid and posterior communicating arteries must be considered with thorough imaging. An aneurysm is unlikely if the pupil is not involved and all of the other third nerve functions are completely involved.

Pupillary Light-Near Dissociation

Light-near dissociation describes the situation when the near response of pupil constriction exceeds the reaction to light. The etiologies include bilateral afferent disease, midbrain disease causing loss of pretectal light input to the EW nucleus, diabetes, Adie's pupil and aberrant third nerve regeneration.

Conclusion

Performing a thorough neuro-ophthalmic examination can allow accurate localization of a lesion or limit the diagnostic possibilities that the clinician must consider. The information obtained from such an examination when a patient has visual complaints can be crucial in focusing additional testing such as neuro-imaging, intervention or treatment.

3. References

1. Beck R. The optic neuritis treatment trial: three year follow-up results. *Arch Ophthalmol.* 1995;113:136-137.

2. Beck R, Cleary PA, Anderson MA, et al. A randomized, controlled trial of corticosteroids in the treatment of acute optic neuritis. *N Engl J Med.* 1992;326:581-588.

3. Brazis P, Masdeu JC, Biller J. *Localization in Clinical Neurology.* Boston, Mass: Little Brown; 1996.

4. Brodsky M, Baker RS, Hamed LM. *Pediatric Neuro-Ophthalmology.* New York, NY: Springer; 1996.

5. Burde R, Savino PJ, Trobe JD. *Clinical Decisions in Neuro-Ophthalmology.* St Louis, Mo: Mosby; 2002.

6. Cook M, Levin LA, Joseph MP, Pinczower EF. Traumatic optic neuropathy: a meta-analysis. *Arch Otolaryngol Head Neck Surg.* 1996;122: 389-392.

7. Corbett J, Thompson HS. The rational management of idiopathic intracranial hypertension. *Arch Neurol.* 1989;46:1049-1051.

8. Digre K, Smoker WRK, Johnston P, et al. Selective MR imaging approach for evaluation of patients with Horner's syndrome. *AJNR.* 1992;13:223-227.

9. Druckman R, Ellis P, Kleinfeld J, et al. Seesaw nystagmus. *Arch Ophthalmol.* 1966;76:668-675.

10. Flach A, Dolan BJ. Adie's syndrome: A medical treatment for symptomatic patients. *Ann Ophthalmol.* 1984;16:1151-1154.

11. Glaser J. *Neuro-ophthalmology.* Philadelphia, Pa: JP Lippincott; 1990.

12. Johnson L, Krohel GB, Madsen RW, et al. The role of weight loss and acetazolamide in the treatment of idiopathic intracranial hypertension. *Ophthalmology.* 1998;105:2313-2317.

13. Kaminski H, Leigh RJ. Neurobiology of eye movements: from molecules to behavior. *Ann NY Acad Sci.* 2002 ;956:1-619.

14. Kazim M, Trokel S, Moore S. Treatment of acute Graves orbitopathy. *Ophthalmology.* 1991;98:1443-1448.

15. Kupersmith M, Latkany R, Homel P. Development of generalized disease at 2 years in patients with ocular myasthenia gravis. *Arch Neurol.* 2003;60:243-248.

16. Lee A, Brazis PW. *Clinical Pathways in Neuro-Ophthalmology: An Evidence-Based Approach.* New York, NY: Thieme; 1998.

17. Leigh R, Averbuch-Heller L, Tomsak RL, et al. Treatment of abnormal eye movements that impair vision: strategies based on current concepts of physiology and pharmacology. *Ann Neurol.* 1994;36:129-141.

18. Leigh R, Zee DS. *The Neurology of Eye Movements.* New York, NY: Oxford University Press; 1999.

19. Madsen JR, Egnor M, Zou R. Cerebrospinal fluid pulsatility and hydrocephalus: the fourth circulation. *Clin Neurosurg.* 2006;53:48-52.

20. Sommer N, Sigg B, Melms A, et al. Ocular myasthenia gravis: response to long term immunosuppressive treatment. *J Neurol Neurosurg Psychiatry.* 1997;62:156-162.

21. Spoor T, McHenry JH. Long-term effectiveness of optic nerve sheath decompression for pseudotumor cerebri. *Arch Ophthalmol.* 1993;111: 632-635.

22. Sugerman H, Felton WI, Sismanis A, et al. Gastric surgery for pseudotumor cerebri associated with severe obesity. *Ann Surg.* 1999;229: 634-640.

23. Thompson H, Pilley SJ. Unequal pupils: A flow chart for sorting out the anisocorias. *Surv Ophthalmol.* 1976;21:45-48.

4. Questions

1. Sixth nerve palsies can be the result of all of the following EXCEPT:

   A. Decompensating

   B. Cavernous sinus thrombosis

   C. Trauma

   D. Vascular disease/idiopathic

2. A tumor in the left temporal lobe would most likely affect which quadrant of the patient's left eye visual field?

   A. Inferionasal

   B. Superonasal

   C. Inferotemporal

   D. Superotemporal

3. The characteristics of spasmus nutans in childhood may include all of the following except:

   A. Head nodding

   B. Torticollis

   C. Low amplitude horizontal nystagmus

   D. Poor vision in one eye

4. Vision loss in one eye associated with a normal initial appearance of the optic nerve could be found in the all the following diagnoses except:

   A. Optic neuritis

   B. Traumatic optic neuropathy

   C. Leber's hereditary optic neuropathy

   D. Anterior ischemic optic neuropathy

5. All of the following are causes of pseudoptosis EXCEPT:

   A. Aberrant regeneration of the facial nerve

   B. Neurofibroma of the lid

   C. Lid retraction of the contralateral eye

   D. Microphthalmia

6. A 25-year-old obese woman presents with headache and dizziness. Examination reveals bilateral optic nerve swelling. The next appropriate step would be which of the following?

   A. Obtain the opening pressure on lumbar puncture

   B. Refer to a nutritionist for concentrated weight loss efforts

   C. Obtain ENT consultation

   D. Start Diamox sequels qPM

   E. Order MRI of the brain

7. A 79-year-old woman complains of headache and fatigue and is found to have an adduction weakness when looking to the right, and nystagmus of the left globe in abduction. An appropriate next step in her care would be:

   A. Perform a Tensilon test

   B. Lumbar puncture

   C. Obtain ESR

   D. Perform a temporal artery biopsy

   E. Obtain syphilis serologies

8. Which of the following cannot be concluded from the Optic Neuritis Treatment Trial?

A. Treatment with corticosteroids is well-tolerated in patients with few major side effects.

B. Oral prednisone alone did not improve the visual outcome after optic neuritis.

C. Long-term benefit is found from the use of corticosteroids in the setting of optic neuritis associated with demyelinating disease.

D. IV followed by oral corticosteroids reduced the rate of development of clinically definite multiple sclerosis during the first two years but this effect subsided by three years.

9. Which of the following is not true about the edrophonium (Tensilon) administration test?

A. The test can be performed in the office if precautions are taken.

B. False positive responses occur rarely.

C. A negative test excludes the diagnosis of myasthenia gravis.

D. Frequent side effects of the test include salivation and abdominal cramping.

10. A patient who measures 20/20 visual acuity in both eyes but has poor color vision in the right eye (dyschromatopsia), and a right relative afferent pupillary defect, has a problem with which anatomic structure?

A. Left retina

B. Right retina

C. Left optic nerve

D. Right optic nerve

E. Right optic tract

11. A patient with a new pupil size difference, neck pain and ptosis needs which diagnostic test urgently?

A. Administration of dilute pilocarpine topically

B. Carotid Doppler study

C. MRA of the neck and brain

D. Visual field testing

12. All the following statements are true about Adie's tonic pupils except:

A. The abnormal pupil becomes supersensitive to dilute pilocarpine

B. Patients are asymptomatic

C. Patients may have diminished deep tendon reflexes

D. Systemic conditions may be associated with the disorder

13. The most common visual field defect following a nonarteritic anterior ischemic optic neuropathy is:

A. Nasal step

B. Arcuate

C. Cecocentral

D. Altitudinal

14. The following statements are true about internuclear ophthalmoplegia EXCEPT:

A. Lesion involves the medial pontine or midbrain parenchyma

B. Common ocular motility disturbance in patients with demyelinating disease

C. Can occur bilaterally

D. Treatment involves neuroleptics

15. In order to hold eccentric vertical gaze, which structure must be intact?

A. Rostral medial longitudinal fasiculus

B. Interstitial nucleus of Cajal

C. Sylvian aqueduct

D. Corpus collosum

16. A 67-year-old hypertensive man presents with a painless, nonprogressive loss of vision in his right eye and is found to have pallid swelling of the right optic nerve with flame hemorrhage, and an inferior altitudinal visual field defect of the right eye. A diagnostic test that should be performed urgently is:

A. MRI of the brain

B. Neuro-imaging of the orbits

C. ESR

D. CBC

E. None of the above

17. True or False: Thyroid function studies can be normal even when a patient has thyroid eye disease.

18. Clinical signs and symptoms of thyroid eye disease include all of the following except:

A. Proptosis

B. Diplopia

C. Visual field loss

D. Nystagmus

E. Dry eyes

19. True or False: Cocaine topically fails to dilate a normal pupil which is not involved in a Horner syndrome.

20. Clinical findings in a dorsal midbrain syndrome include all of the following except:

A. Convergence-retraction nystagmus

B. Up-gaze limitation

C. Inability to adduct the eyes

D. Bilateral upper eyelid retraction

Answers

1. A.

2. B.

3. D.

4. D.

5. B.

6. E.

7. C.

8. C.

9. C.

10. D.

11. C.

12. B.

13. D.

14. D.

15. B.

16. E.

17. True

18. D.

19. False

20. C.

Chapter 30: Neuro-otology: Dizziness and Hearing Loss

Morris Levin, MD

Contents

1. Dizziness & Vertigo

Introduction — Terms and Definitions

The complaint of "dizziness" is notoriously nonspecific. Patients may use the term to mean a lightheaded presyncopal perception, a sensation of movement, a sensation of imbalance, or a generalized feeling of anxiety, to name several possibilities. Knowing and distinguishing among the possible connotations of the word dizziness can help sort out what can often be a daunting problem.

These are some constellations of dizziness descriptions we hear from patients:

1. "spinning, tilting, listing, rolling, falling"
2. "unsteadiness, imbalance, swimming feeling"
3. "floating, near-fainting, lightheadedness"
4. "blurry vision, hazy"
5. "disoriented, confused, spacey, dreamlike"
6. "anxious, tense"

The first group of symptoms, relating to a sense of movement, are descriptions of vertigo, defined as a sensation of movement of oneself or objects around oneself, generally accompanied by nausea, malaise, and dysphoria.

"Unsteadiness" or "imbalance" may result from vertigo, but more commonly these terms relate to an ataxic state (due to dysfunction in cerebellum, frontal lobes, dorsal columns or connections).

"Lightheadedness" and similar terms generally imply a presyncopal state. Here the implication is that there is a decrease in blood flow or oxygen to the brain as may occur in hypotension, cardiac arrhythmia, etc. Other descriptions elaborating on a complaint of dizziness may indicate any of a myriad of problems including neuropathy, poor visual acuity, diplopia, panic disorder, dementia, confusional state, excessive somnolence, dissociative feelings, and somatization (see Table 1). Hence, the first step in evaluating patients with dizziness is to determine whether it is due to true vertigo or another etiology.

Table 1

Diagnostic Implications of Patients' Descriptions of Dizziness

Described Symptoms	Diagnostic Implication
Spinning, tilting, listing, rolling, falling	Vertigo — vestibular dysfunction
Unsteadiness, imbalance, swimming	Ataxia
Floating, near-fainting, lightheadedness	Presyncope
Blurred vision	Visual dysfunction
Disorientation	Possible dementia
Anxiety	Possible panic disorder, phobia

Figure 1

Inner ear

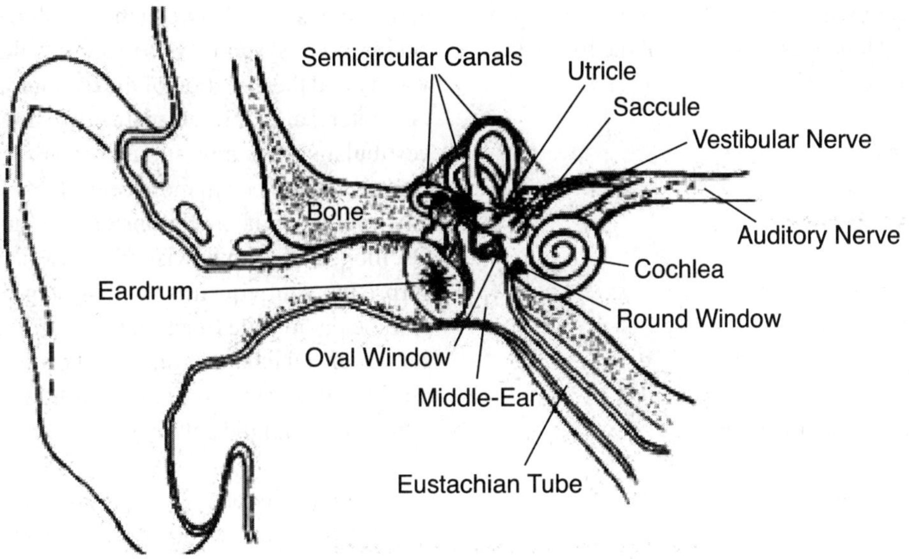

http://www.mossfoundation.org/images/inner-ear.jpg

Anatomy of the Vestibular System and Localization of Lesions

Vertigo is essentially a symptom of vestibular system malfunction, the anatomy of which is complex, with many sites of modulation and interconnections. Below is a summary of the anatomical physiology of the vestibular system from labyrinth to the cortex (see Figure 1).

The sensory organ for angular and linear acceleration is the membranous labyrinth. It is an organ composed of canals filled with the high potassium fluid, endolymph. The membranous labyrinth is housed, along with the cochlea, in the petrous portion of the temporal bone. Perilymph is the high sodium content fluid filling the space between the bony labyrinth and the membranous canals (see Figure 2).

The body of the primary bipolar neuron in the vestibular system lies within the vestibular ganglion (Scarpa ganglion). Peripheral processes synapse with hair cells in the labyrinth (saccule, utricle or semicircular canals). Hair cells in the ampullae of the 3 perpendicular semicircular canals sense movement of endolymph and thus sense angular motion. Hair cells in the utricle and saccule attach to an otolith and sense linear movement. The central processes of the bipolar cells constitute the vestibular nerve which runs with the auditory nerve, forming the acoustic nerve.

The acoustic nerve enters the skull at the internal auditory meatus, traverses the cerebellopontine angle (CPA), and then enters the brainstem at the pontomedullary junction. Vestibular fibers then terminate in 4 vestibular pontine nuclei (lateral, medial, inferior and superior). These nuclei interconnect with cerebellar and spinal systems, cranial nerves III, IV, and VI, and with cortical areas. The lateral (Deiter's) vestibular nucleus sends axons down the ipsilateral lateral vestibulospinal tract to innervate antigravity (extensor) muscles of the lower extremities. The inferior vestibular nucleus sends fibers to the flocculonodular lobe of the cerebellum via the inferior cerebellar peduncle. The medial and superior vestibular nuclei are connected via the median longitudinal fasciculus to ocular motor nuclei (III, IV, VI) and are responsible for, among other things, the oculocephalic ("doll's-eyes") reflex (tendency for eyes to remain conjugately fixed in one direction of gaze).

Dysfunction anywhere in vestibular system can produce vertigo. Hence lesions in any of the following locations may lead to it:

- Labyrinths
- VIII nerve
- Cerebellopontine angle
- Cerebellum
- Vestibular nuclei in brainstem
- Cortical centers

Several symptoms typically occur with vertigo—nausea, malaise, diaphoresis, anxiety and visual changes. Nausea is said to occur because of "sensory conflict"— the vestibular system providing information different from that coming from visual input and somatosensory systems. However, there are a number of connections between the vestibular system and autonomic centers which must play a role. Nystagmus is a common sign, presumably due to the connections between the vestibular nuclei and ocular motor systems. It is usually of the "jerk" variety and the direction of the nystagmus is usually only lateral and/or rotational with lesions in the vestibular system or vestibular nerve. Vertical nystagmus can be seen in more central lesions (generally implying bilateral brainstem dysfunction). Oscillopsia ("jumping vision") may occur (though surprisingly infrequently) with nystagmus. When extraocular muscle function is impaired, diplopia can occur. Diaphoresis and lightheadedness are also ascribed to sensory conflict, as well as direct stimulation of autonomic pathways.

Labyrinthine disease generally presents without hearing loss and there are usually no neurological findings. The patient often feels propelled to the side of the lesion. Lesions of the vestibular nerve often present with hearing loss as well. Cerebellopontine angle lesions may present with dysfunction of other cranial nerves in the vicinity – VII, VII, IX,

Figure 2

Inner ear schematic

A. Vestibular system summary; B. Arterial supply of the inner ear

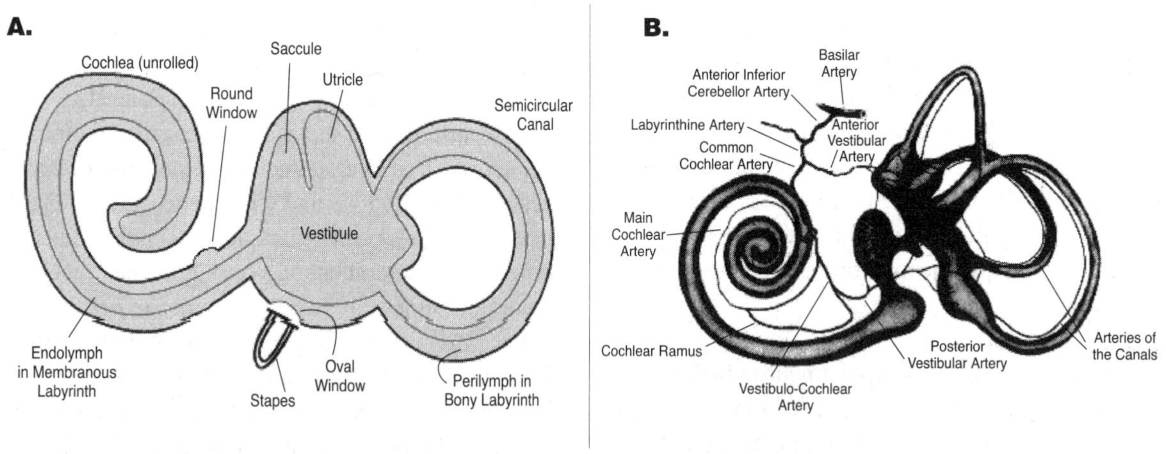

A: http://thalamus.wustl.edu/course/audvest.html B: http://www.bme.jhu.edu/labs/chb/disorders/aica.html

and X – as well as ataxia if there is cerebellar involvement. Hearing loss is common. Brainstem lesions typically produce multiple cranial nerve signs, long tract signs (body sensory and motor changes), and ataxia. Cerebellar lesions generally produce ataxia but in some patients distinguishing gait difficulty due to vertigo from an ataxic gait can be challenging. Cortical lesions may be accompanied by aphasia and other cognitive deficits, visual field deficits, hemisensory and hemimotor abnormalities, and seizures.

History Taking in the Dizzy Patient

Lightheadedness due to decreased cerebral perfusion is generally easy to exclude historically, but symptoms can be unclear. Chest pain, dyspnea, palpitations, history of syncope and use of medications which lower blood pressure and/or pulse (or produce orthostasis) are important clues. The sensation of imbalance (indicating cerebellar or positional sense dysfunction) should be tested apart from a sense of motion. Worsening by position change suggests vestibular dysfunction. Changes in hearing, vision and other cranial nerve mediated function, along with a history of weakness or incoordination suggest more diffuse cranial nerve, brainstem or cerebellar involvement. A history of migraine or even a family history of migraine may suggest a migrainous etiology. A history of psychiatric illness or psychiatric symptoms is important to elicit. Time course, drug exposure, infections, trauma, history of stroke or risk factors for stroke are all important details to investigate.

Examination of the Patient with Vertigo

General examination including supine and standing blood pressure and pulse measurement are essential. A thorough head and neck exam should be done. Especially important is the otoscopic exam, looking for otitis, varicella vesicles, and other signs of infection or inflammation. Mastoids should be checked for tenderness. Carotid arteries should be palpated and auscultated. A thorough neurological exam must be done, with careful attention to cranial nerve and cerebellar/gait function.

Nystagmus is a very helpful finding on exam. As noted above, vertical nystagmus usually indicates central vestibular dysfunction, and purely horizontal or rotatory nystagmus suggests peripheral vestibular dysfunction. Pendular nystagmus is usually congenital (and more likely to cause oscillopsia). Upbeat nystagmus can occur with lesions at the pontomedullary junction. Downbeat nystagmus can occur with lesions at the craniocervical junction.

Provocative maneuvers like rapid head turning or Dix-Hallpike testing can be extremely helpful. The aim is to induce fluid movement in the semicircular canals to produce symptoms and signs on exam. The rapid head-turning maneuver is performed by asking the patient to quickly rotate the head to the side while maintaining fixation on the examiner's nose. In normal subjects, there will be instantaneous compensation and the eyes will appear not to move at all from their fixed gaze. With vestibular dysfunction, there will be a delay and a quick saccade (or several) to "catch up." Patients may report the induction or worsening of vertigo.

The Dix-Hallpike maneuver is done by asking the patient to quickly transition from sitting to lying supine with the head turned to one side and hanging 30 degrees below the plane of the examination table. If the patient experiences vertigo and any of his/her typical accompanying symptoms, it is good evidence that the patient has vestibular dysfunction. (A rule of thumb is that the dysfunctional vestibular system is the one pointed downward during the symptomatic provocative test.) Then, a number of other symptoms and signs point the examiner toward localizing vestibular problems in peripheral versus more central areas (see Table 2). For example, peripheral causes of vertigo such as labyrinthine inflammation will generally cause horizontal or rotatory nystagmus which is moderately severe, often accompanied by nausea, and diminishes over time. More central causes can produce multidirectional nystagmus, without fatigability.

Diagnostic Testing in Vertigo

An audiogram is helpful to assess for hearing loss. MRI with gadolinium (with attention to CPA, internal auditory canal, cerebellum and brainstem) is often helpful for the evaluation of possible central causes of vertigo. Brainstem auditory evoked potentials may be useful for early detection of audiovestibular pathway dysfunction.

Electronystagmography is a way to quantify vestibular response (nystagmus) to cool and warm ear irrigation. The procedure consists of recording from eye electrodes, which detect nystagmus while cold water is injected into the external auditory canal. (Cold water induces currents in endolymph which suppress the ipsilateral horizontal semicircular canal, and eyes deviate toward that side, with a correcting nystagmus in the opposite direction.)

Rotational testing and posturography are also sometimes used in advanced labs and can provide additional information about vestibular dysfunction.

Symptomatic Treatment of Vertigo

Pharmacological treatments fall into 4 major categories: anticholinergics, antihistamines, benzodiazepines, and neuroleptics (see Table 3). The antihistamines meclizine and dimenhydramine are effective but may not be potent enough in some cases. Their use can also be limited by sedation. The anticholinergic scopolamine is significantly more potent, and is available in transdermal patch as well as oral formulation. A number of patients experience dysphoria and even hallucinosis, so caution must be exercised. Benzodiazepines are limited in that the therapeutic dose is very close to the sedating dose. However, diazepam can be useful in the dose range of 5-10 mg q 4-6h prn (as tolerated). Neuroleptics, such as promethazine (dose – 25 mg q6h prn) are also useful and presumably act by their dopamine blocking actions. The serotonin acting antiemetic ondansetron is helpful in some patients.

Physical treatments lack serious adverse effects and can be helpful for selected patients. The simplest approach is to ask patients to direct the eyes toward the position that induces vertigo and hold that gaze as long as possible. When this becomes tolerable (after a few days), the next steps involve head turning while attempting to keep focus in one direction, and eventually standing and walking during the exercises (using caution!).

To address the possibility that vertigo is related to the pathological accumulation of granules in the endolymph of the labyrinthine canals, a number of maneuvers have been designed to "reposition" these granules, including the Epley canalith repositioning

Table 2

Provocative Testing for Vertigo (Hallpike, Barany, et al)

Peripheral Pattern	Central Pattern
Vertigo intense	Vertigo mild
Short duration of nystagmus	Nystagmus may persist
Nystagmus may fatigue	No fatiguing of nystagmus with multiple trials
N&V intense	Nausea less common
Nystagmus: fixed direction	Nystagmus may change direction
Nystagmus: usually horizontal or diagonal	Nystagmus direction can include vertical
Latency of several seconds	No latency

Table 3

Pharmacologic Treatment of Vertigo

Class of Drug	Drug	Typical dose	Adverse effects
Anticholinergic	Scopalamine	.2 mg po q6h Transdermal 1q3d	Mental status changes
Antihistamine	Meclizine	2.5-25 mg po tid	Sedation
	Dimenhydramine	2.5-25 mg po tid	Sedation
Neuroleptic	Promethazine	2.5-25 mg po tid	Sedation, dyskinesia
Benzodiazepine	Diazepam	2-5 mg po tid prn	Sedation, addiction

maneuver (see Figure 3). The goal is to move these canaliths into the utricle where acceleration will not induce an endolymph current. These maneuvers often need to be repeated many times, and during initiation of these programs patients can become uncomfortable.

Diseases Presenting with Vertigo

There are many potential causes of vertigo, as listed in Table 4. The most common cause is motion sickness, which is transient and rarely comes to the attention of the neurologist. Below are descriptions of some of the more common or important entities presenting with vertigo.

Benign Positional Vertigo (BPV)

This very common condition consists of recurrent (usually brief) episodes of positional vertigo, in some cases following trauma, prolonged unusual head positions, or prolonged bed rest. The etiology is unclear but a long proposed mechanism suggests that otoconia (minute calcific granules) settled in the cupula of the posterior canal (cupulolithiasis) are dislodged when the head turns quickly; this sets endolymph into motion, leading to perception of motion; as otoconia are dispersed, repeated head-turning produces less dramatic responses. Granules probably coalesce in other parts of the semicircular canals (canaliths) and can induce vertigo after position change in certain planes depending upon the individual canal.

In BPV, vertigo occurs with head turning or body position change, and patents often report worsening of symptoms when lying down. Hearing is usually spared and neurological examination is typically normal. In some patients the stimulus for vertigo need only be mild movement and thus the condition can become very disabling.

Figure 3

Epley canalith repositioning maneuver

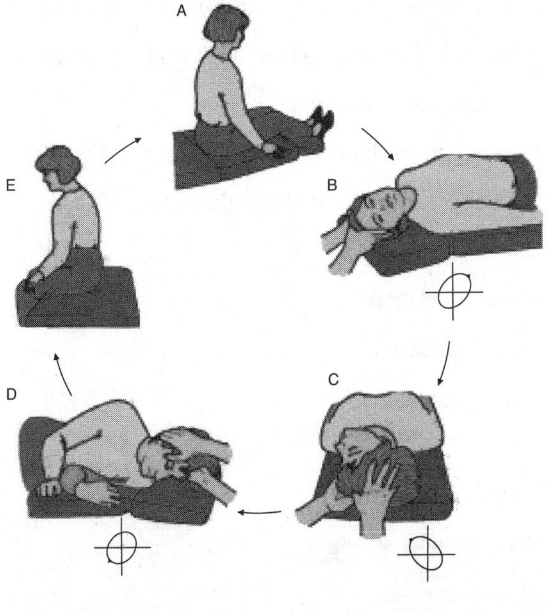

Table 4

Causes of Vertigo

Benign positional vertigo
Medication effect
Inner ear infection/inflammation
Vestibular neuronitis /viral labyrinthitis
Bacterial otitis
Meniere disease
Post-traumatic vertigo
Psychogenic/phobic vertigo
Perilymphatic fistula
Brainstem or vestibular ischemia or CVA
Autoimmune disease of inner ear
Lymphocytic infiltration of inner ear
Cogan syndrome
Herpes zoster oticus – Ramsay Hunt syndrome
Acoustic neuroma and other CPA tumors
Complex partial
Migraine
MS - brainstem plaque
Brainstem neoplasm, hemorrhage or AVM
Meningitis (carcinomatous, TB, fungal, bacterial
Arnold-Chiari syndrome
Neurosyphilis – labyrinth infection, meningitis, arteritis
Intralabyrinthine hemorrhage (leukemia, trauma)
Sarcoidosis
Hyperventilation
Hypothyroidism
Hypoglycemia
Carcinoid syndrome
Cardiac arrhythmia
Pheochromocytoma
Motion sickness

Treatment is often successful, particularly when physical techniques, like the canalith repositioning maneuvers, are combined with symptomatic pharmacological treatment. Fluctuations in symptoms will occur, necessitating adjustments in therapy. Patients need to be advised to use caution with respect to activities like driving. Prognosis is usually good even without treatment, although persistent symptoms are reported in some cases.

Vertigo as a Medication Effect

Historically, patients with this cause of vertigo will relate the initiation of new medication or a dosage change at the time of the onset vertigo and related symptoms. A number of medications are reported to cause dizziness (see Table 5), but those with a pronounced tendency to produce true vertigo include: aspirin, phenytoin, aminoglycosides, and cisplatin. Many medications that cause vertigo can lead to hearing loss as well. For example, aminoglycosides damage the cochlear hair cells as well as labyrinthine structures, so hearing loss generally accompanies vestibular symptoms.

Inner Ear Infections and Inflammation

Vestibular neuronitis presents with a single episode of severe vertigo and nausea, which abates in 48-72 hours. The etiology is unknown, but it is thought to be due to inflammation of the vestibular nerve. Patients complain of relatively acute awareness of severe vertigo exacerbated by virtually any movement. Unlike BPV, symptoms are also present at rest (without head position change). There are usually no accompanying neurological symptoms and hearing is spared.

Viral labyrinthitis is a proposed condition presenting identically to vestibular neuronitis, but an infectious etiology is suggested by the general observation in many patients of a recent viral syndrome. Because of the similarities, many feel that viral labyrinthitis and vestibular neuronitis describe the same entity.

Diagnosis is made in these conditions based on the acute onset of vertigo and nausea, with differential diagnostic possibilities of brainstem or labyrinthine ischemia, perilymphatic fistula, bacterial infection,

Table 5

Medications and Toxins Which Can Cause Hearing Loss, Tinnitus or Vertigo

Antibiotics	
	Aminoglycosides – streptomycin, etc.
	Chloramphenicol
	Erythromycin
	Tetracycline
	Vancomycin
Anti-inflammatory Analgesics	
	Aspirin
	Nonsteroidal anti-inflammatory medications
Chemotherapeutic Agents	
	Actinomycin
	Bleomycin
	Cisplatin
	Mechlorethamine
	Methotrexate
	Vincristine
Diuretics	
	Furosemide
	Bumetanide
	Ethacrynic acid
Quinine Derivatives	
	Quinine sulfate
	Quinidine
	Plaquenil
	Mefloquine
	Chloroquine
	Atabrine
Others	
	Aminophylline
	Heavy metals – mercury, lead
	Heterocyclic antidepressants
	Calcium channel blockers
	Carbamazepine
	Propranolol
	Levodopa
	Caffeine

migrainous vertigo (first occurrence), Ménière disease, Ramsey Hunt syndrome of zoster involvement of VIII nerve, and labyrinthine hemorrhage. BPV and Ménière diseases are generally ruled out by the lack of recurrence, but some cases of vestibular neuronitis do recur in mild form.

Treatment is usually not necessary as symptoms are self-limited. Symptomatic treatment may help patients remain comfortable. Corticosteroids may be helpful if symptoms do not abate.

Bacterial otitis is characteristic for ear pain, hearing loss, vertigo, fever, and malaise, with signs of systemic illness. So, when it causes vertigo it is usually distinguishable from vestibular neuronitis. Examination generally reveals an erythematous tympanic membrane (TM). Thus, an important diagnosis to exclude is zoster infection of the ear (the Ramsey Hunt syndrome), which may produce erythema of the TM without the pathognomonic vesicular eruption. Treatment is systemic antibiotics, but residual vertigo can persist in some patients.

Ménière Disease

This illness is characterized by attacks of vertigo, nausea and vomiting, fluctuating hearing loss and tinnitus. The etiology of this syndrome is apparently an increase in the volume of endolymph which distends the semicircular canals and other portions of the labyrinthine system. The paroxysmal nature of the attacks may be related to occasional ruptures of the labyrinthine membranes with fluid and electrolyte shifts.

The spells of vertigo are often sudden and can last for up to an hour or so. Hearing loss and tinnitus can occur early in the disease, but may develop later, making the diagnosis challenging since symptoms otherwise mimic other causes of labyrinthine vertigo. Other symptoms include sudden falls of unknown etiology, a sensation of fullness in the ear, and even mild to moderate headaches. Ménière disease most often begins in the forties, but may occur at younger or older ages.

On exam, patients are often very uncomfortable, preferring to stay in their one best position. Lateral nystagmus is present, and the hearing loss is of the sensorineural pattern with reduction in both air and bone conduction of sound. Audiograms show low frequency hearing loss early in the course of the disease and high frequency hearing loss later. Neuroimaging is generally noncontributory.

Treatment with antihistamines, anticholinergics, or benzodiazepines is usually effective. Antiemetics are often necessary. The long-promoted salt-restricted diets and use of diuretics have never been shown conclusively to work in Ménière disease, but some patients do seem to respond.

For refractory cases with significant hearing loss, invasive procedures are considered if the pathology is clearly limited to one side. These include labyrinthectomy, and injection of streptomycin or corticosteroids transtympanically. Sectioning of the vestibular portion of the VIII nerve is sometimes attempted. Some have recommended creation of a shunt between the endolymph and the subarachnoid space with various techniques, with the aim of reducing the increased endolymph pressure. Others have postulated that a vascular compression of the vestibular nerve is causal in Ménière disease, and have suggested surgery aimed at decompression of the nerve, akin to trigeminal nerve decompression in procedures advocated for trigeminal neuralgia.

Interestingly, the majority of patients with Ménière disease tend to spontaneously stabilize after several years, although lasting hearing loss often remains.

Perilymphatic Fistula

This entity is due to a generally post-traumatic formation of a connection between the bony labyrinth and the middle ear (or mastoid), usually at the oval or round windows. Head trauma, whiplash, barotrauma and noise trauma have all been reported as causes. Even exercise, straining, coughing or sneezing have been postulated as causes. The incidence of this condition is not clear and there is still considerable controversy over the existence of spontaneous cases.

Pathophysiology is supposed to involve the alteration in balance between the endolymph and the perilymph as a result of the fistula, which then causes disturbances in fluid dynamics of the labyrinthine canals leading to vertigo and the other symptoms.

Diagnosis is difficult, particularly distinguishing PF from Ménière disease, which can also be considered to be related to an imbalance between endolymph and perilymph. In PF there is usually a sudden onset, often following a Valsalva maneuver or other sudden pressure change, of any or all of the following: vertigo, disequilibrium, a sense of fullness in the ear, hearing loss, tinnitus, nausea and vomiting. Hyperventilation or valsalva induce or worsen vertigo in some patients. The tinnitus can be reported as "roaring" or "whooshing" noise.

Sensorineural hearing loss can be found. Neuroimaging testing is generally normal, but in post-traumatic cases it is necessary to rule out bony fractures (temporal bone). Micro-endoscopic procedures and radioisotope labeling of perilymph are new procedures being investigated for diagnosis.

Bed rest and avoidance of Valsalva maneuvers is typically advised. Spontaneous healing of the fistula can occur after the acute injury. Meclizine and scopolamine can sometimes help. Surgical closure can help some patients, although hearing loss may not improve. A complication of PF is meningitis, since there is a patent connection (the cochlear duct) between the perilymph and the CSF in many people.

Post-traumatic Vertigo

This can follow head injury or whiplash injury and can lag for several days following trauma. When trauma is severe, fracture of the temporal bone may be suspected. When no major bony trauma occurs, the etiology of the vertigo is considered to be secondary to non-penetrating labyrinthine trauma, perhaps related to dislodgement of otoconia.

Post-traumatic vertigo generally improves within a few days. However, it can persist as a part of the post-concussion syndrome and mimic BPV.

Brainstem or Vestibular Ischemia

The labyrinth is supplied by branches of the internal auditory artery (IAA), which is usually a branch of the anterior inferior cerebellar artery (AICA). Sometimes the IAA is a direct branch of the basilar artery, and rarely, it is a branch of the posterior inferior cerebellar artery (PICA). IAA has three terminal branches, the anterior vestibular artery which supplies the anterior and lateral SCC; the cochlear-vestibular artery, which has two branches, the posterior vestibular artery which supplies the posterior SCC and the saccule, and a cochlear branch which supplies the base of the cochlea (high-frequency tones); and a pure cochlear artery which supplies the apex of the cochlea (low-frequency tones). As a result, occlusion of the basilar artery, AICA, IAA, or vestibular branches (particularly the anterior vestibular artery) can cause vertigo due to labyrinthine ischemia (see Figure 4). The presence or absence of hearing loss depends on where the occlusion is. Possible contributing factors include atherosclerosis, hypercoagulable states (such as sickle cell anemia, polycythemia, and macroglobulinemia), and embolic conditions.

Vestibular nerve infarction is another possible cause of vertigo. In the internal auditory canal, the vestibular nerve is supplied by arteries which supply the dura and petrous bone. In the CPA, it receives blood supply from an anastomosis of branches of AICA, PICA and vertebral arteries.

Labyrinthine ischemia presents acutely and may mimic vestibular neuronitis. Hearing loss may suggest Ménière. History of TIA or stroke, or presence of risk factors for cerebrovascular disease, can be suggestive, but with small infarctions, diagnosis may be elusive. After the initial symptoms abate, a condition similar to BPV may ensue, presumably due to necrosis related formation of canaliths in the semicircular canals.

Brainstem strokes can cause vertigo on the basis of damage to vestibular nuclei, which are supplied by the vertebrobasilar system, particularly the PICA. Brainstem TIAs and strokes which cause vertigo are diagnosed by syndromic accompaniments due to other cranial nerve nuclei ischemia (facial numbness, diplopia, dysarthria, Horner syndrome, etc.), and long tract signs like hemiparesis and hemibody sensation loss.

Autoimmune Disease of Inner Ear – Cogan Syndrome

Lymphocytic infiltration of inner ear can occur in Cogan syndrome, which consists of interstitial keratitis of the eye, and audio-vestibular symptoms including vertigo, ataxia, nystagmus, and hearing loss. Cardiovascular, musculoskeletal, and gastrointestinal symptoms can also occur.

An autoimmune mechanism is presumed in this condition. Interestingly, the presence of antineutrophil cytoplasmic antibody (ANCA) has been reported.

Presentation usually begins with inflammatory eye disease. Symptoms progress within days, however, to include vertigo and hearing loss. Diagnostic testing can reveal abnormal ESR, WBC, and C-reactive protein, and there may be thrombocytosis or anemia. A slit-lamp examination is essential. Cortico steroids (systemic and ophthalmic) as well as immunosuppressants have been used, but efficacy is not proven. Visual and hearing loss can be permanent.

Herpes Zoster Oticus — Ramsay Hunt Syndrome

Vertigo, disequilibrium, hearing loss, ear pain and facial paralysis are the presenting features of zoster infection of the ear. Vesicles are seen in the pinna, external auditory canal, or tympanic membrane. The infection can track to the brainstem and cause encephalitis.

Diagnosis is generally straightforward, but the vesicular eruption may be absent or difficult to appreciate. In some instances only erythema of the auditory canal or TM may be seen, suggestive of bacterial otitis.

Treatment consists of oral or IV acyclovir. Corticosteroids have not been proven effective but are often given in the hope of hastening recovery and preventing permanent facial weakness and hearing loss. Analgesics are often necessary for ear pain.

Acoustic Neuroma and Other CPA Tumors

Acoustic neuroma, meningioma, epidermoid, cholesteatoma, and metastatic tumors can all occur in the CPA and cause vertigo, hearing loss, and tinnitus. Acoustic neuromas are by far the most common tumor in this area (>90%). They arise from Schwann cells and almost always originate in the vestibular portion of the VIII nerve, in or near the internal auditory canal. They can occur as part of von Recklinghausen disease (neurofibromatosis type II). Some acoustic neuromas can undergo malignant transformation, although this is rare. Other mass lesions in this region include epidermoid tumors, meningiomas, cholesteatomas, and metastatic tumors.

Compression of other cranial nerves can occur, including V, VII, IX and X. As a result, hearing loss, facial pain, facial weakness and ataxia are common presentations.

Complex Partial Seizure – "Tornado Seizure"

Epileptic vertigo has been postulated to result from a seizure focus in or near the primary vestibular cortical zones – the superior lip of the intraparietal sulcus, the temporal-parietal border regions, and particularly the posterior superior temporal lobe ("temporal neocortex"). Auditory hallucinations or distortions can also occur in these patients.

EEG and MRI scan of the head are useful tests. Treatment with anticonvulsants like carbamazepine is usually effective. When EEG is normal, a trial of an anticonvulsant medication is reasonable in suspected cases.

Migraine

Vertigo is a very common accompaniment of migraine and it can occur even without head pain, lasting generally up to several minutes. Nausea may or may not be present. Diagnosis should be entertained in anyone with recurrent bouts of vertigo, particularly if there is a history of recurrent headaches or a strong family history of migraine. In some patients, other features of brainstem dysfunction such as ataxia, dysarthria, and diplopia and visual changes consistent with occipital lobe dysfunction can co-occur. Many of these cases are considered to have "basilar migraine," which is a still poorly understood variant of migraine perhaps related to oligemia in the posterior circulation.

Treatment with anti-migraine medications, including cyclic antidepressants, beta-blockers, calcium channel blockers, valproate, and topiramate can be gratifying.

Psychogenic/Phobic Vertigo

This is usually situational (eg, being in a mall, on a bridge, in certain social situations), and is often not clearly true vertigo. However, some patients do report definite sensations of movement. Accompanying symptoms are helpful but not pathognomonic: a sense of doom, paresthesias, diaphoresis, hyperventilation, and palpitations. History of anxiety disorder, especially panic disorder, is suggestive.

Treatment should include psychotherapy, but medications can help, including benzodiazepines, SSRI medications, and other anxiolytics. Behavioral medicine therapy, including relaxation techniques, can be very useful as well.

Other Causes of Vertigo

A number of other causes of vertigo may be encountered, including the following:

- MS – brainstem plaque in the region of vestibular connections
- Brainstem neoplasm, hemorrhage or AVM
- Meningitis—carcinomatous, TB, fungal, bacterial
- Arnold-Chiari Syndrome
- Neurosyphilis —labyrinth infection, meningitis, arteritis
- Intralabyrinthine hemorrhage (leukemia, trauma)

- Sarcoidosis
- Hyperventilation
- Hypothyroidism
- Hypoglycemia
- Carcinoid syndrome
- Cardiac arrhythmia
- Pheochromocytoma

Clues to the Accurate Diagnosis of Patients with Vertigo

1. Vestibular neuronitis is usually not just positional (may occur at rest), and is usually self-limited.
2. Ménière disease usually involves hearing loss and/or tinnitus eventually.
3. With perilymphatic fistula there is almost always a hearing loss, and there is almost always an antecedent incident like weight-lifting, barotrauma, scuba diving, forceful nose-blowing, etc.
4. With meningeal infection and/or inflammation there is usually meningismus, headache, and other cranial neuropathies.
5. CPA region masses generally also cause hearing loss and onset is usually slow (although sudden symptoms may result from hemorrhage into the mass).
6. Vertebrobasilar ischemia usually involves other signs of brainstem dysfunction, such as facial numbness, diplopia, dysarthria, Horner syndrome, visual field loss, hemibody sensory or motor loss, etc. This is true also for brainstem tumors.
7. Patients with migrainous vertigo usually have a history (or strong family history) of migraine.

2. Hearing Loss and Tinnitus

Anatomy of Hearing

The neuroanatomy of auditory processing shares some features with that of the vestibular system. The primary bipolar neuron of the hearing pathway has its body in the spiral ganglion. Peripheral processes terminate in hair cells in the organ of Corti in the cochlear duct inside the cochlea. The cochlear duct, like the semicircular canals, is also filled with endolymph.

Hair cells sense sound at specific frequencies (highest frequencies are transduced at the base, lowest at the apex). Central processes of the bipolar cells constitute the cochlear nerve, which runs with the vestibular nerve forming the acoustic nerve.

The acoustic nerve enters the skull at the internal auditory meatus, traverses the cerebellopontine angle (CPA), and then enters the brainstem at the pontomedullary junction. Cochlear fibers terminate in the cochlear nucleus, which is composed of two parts. The dorsal cochlear nucleus is responsible for high frequency sounds, and the ventral cochlear nucleus is responsible for low-frequency sounds. Axons are then sent via the lateral lemniscus to both ipsilateral and contralateral inferior colliculi. Fibers then project to medial geniculate body. The medial geniculate then projects to the primary auditory cortex in the temporal lobe (aka, Heschl gyrus; transverse temporal gyrus; Brodman area 41) (see Figure 5).

There are several places where bilateral connections occur, including: 1) Probst commissure, which interconnects the lateral lemnisci; and 2) the trapezoid body with fibers connecting the right and left cochlear nuclei. Therefore, unilateral lesions central to the cochlear nucleus will not cause deafness.

The stapedius muscle, which retracts the stapes from the round window and dampens loud sounds, is innervated by a branch of VII. The tensor tympani muscle, innervated by V, is attached to the malleus and TM and it too dampens loud sounds. Dysfunction of this dampening reflex causes hyperacusis, which is usually unpleasant. Sensation in the external auditory canal is carried by a number of cranial nerves: V(3), VII, IX, and X.

Lesions anywhere in the auditory system can produce hearing loss (or tinnitus) including:

- Cochlea
- VIII nerve
- Colliculus
- Medial geniculate body
- Auditory cortex

Unilateral cortical lesions do not affect hearing, although they can result in difficulty with sound localization or identification of sounds. Bilateral temporal lobe lesions can result in hearing loss, but this is unusual. However, in patients with previous temporal lobe injury that subsequently experience a contralateral auditory cortex insult, deafness can indeed occur.

Figure 4

Hearing pathway

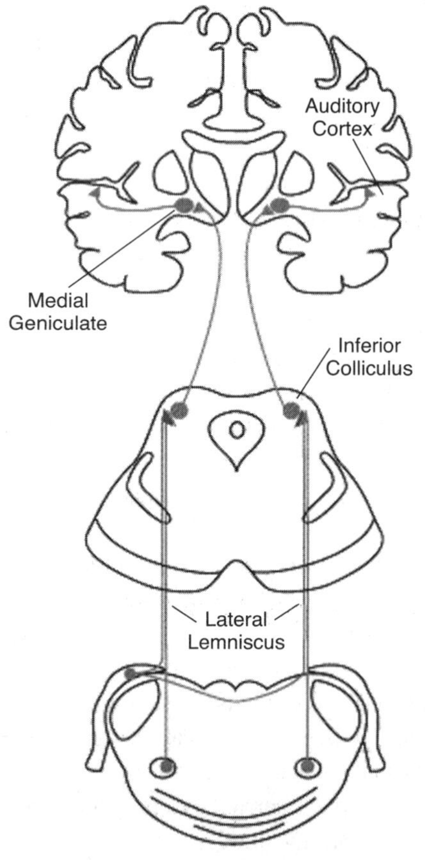

Examination of the Patient with Hearing Impairment

Speech discrimination is a good place to start and can also be quantitatively measured in the lab. Testing for hyperacusis (abnormally increased recruitment or poor stapedius function) can be helpful.

Bedside tests of hearing include Weber test, Rinne test, and Schwabach test:

- Weber – 512 Hz tuning fork placed midfrontally; patient is asked where sound is loudest (perceived louder on the side of a sound conduction problem, because ambient noise is blocked).
- Rinne – 512 Hz tuning fork placed on the mastoid, then the ear (normally air conduction is better: if conductive loss, bone>air, if sensorineural problem, air>bone, although both decreased).
- Schwabach – also with tuning fork, compare patient's bone conduction with that of the examiner.

A good way to use these tests is to consider typical findings in the two major types of hearing loss:

1. hearing loss occurring as a result of a sound conduction problem: Rinne test will reveal bone>air conduction in the affected ear and Weber test will reveal that the tone is louder in the affected ear because ambient noise is reduced due to sound conduction problems;

2. hearing loss occurring because of a cochlear nerve problem: Rinne test will reveal air>bone conduction and Weber test will reveal that the tone is louder in the normal ear. Schwabach test is then used to confirm the conclusion (see Table 6).

Hysterical or factitious deafness can sometimes be detected by watching for a blink to loud sound, or some other change in behavior when loud sounds are delivered.

Testing in the Patient with Hearing Impairment

Audiometry

Pure tone audiometry is done as an initial test in most people with suspected hearing loss. An audiogram is created displaying the patient's threshold for sound at different frequencies, showing the difference between left and right ear stimulation. High-frequency loss suggests sensorineural deafness; low-frequency loss suggests a conductive or cochlear problem. A number of other audiological tests can be done including tests of abnormal recruitment and tone decay. Stapedius muscle function can be assessed by measuring the air pressure in the auditory canal after a loud sound.

Brainstem auditory evoked responses (BAERs) are helpful in evaluating hearing problems (see Figure 6). Only the first 5 waveforms are used clinically, and can help to assess different portions of the auditory pathway. A mnemonic for NCOLIMA may help in recalling the presumed origin of the 7 waves commonly denoted on BAER:

N – cochlear Nerve

C – Cochlear nucleus

O – Superior olive/trapezoid body

L – Lateral lemniscus

I – Inferior colliculus

Figure 5

Brainstem auditory evoked potentials

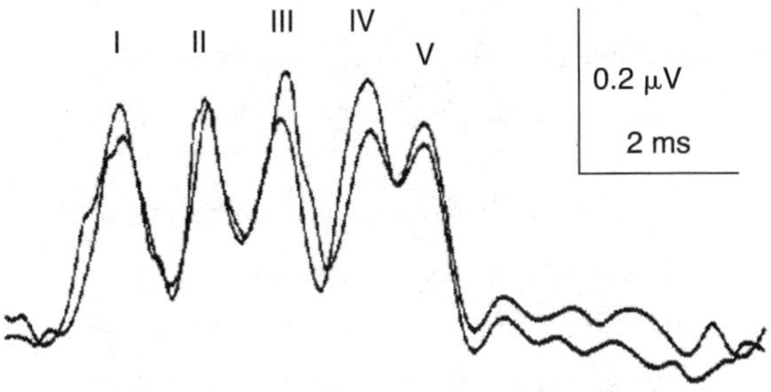

M – Medial geniculate body

A – Auditory cortex

MRI and CT scanning are essential if there is any suspicion of a mass lesion, infection or inflammation, which may be causing hearing loss. CT may be best in suspected bony disease, but MRI with and without gadolinium is superior in most cases.

Differential Diagnosis of Hearing Impairment

It is useful to subdivide causes of hearing loss into three categories based on localization: 1.) Sound conductive problems in the region of the outer and middle ear; 2.) Cochlear and cochlear nerve dysfunction; and, 3.) Nuclear (brainstem) dysfunction, as well as more rostral sites of dysfunction (see Table 7).

Table 6

Bedside Exam in Hearing Loss

Condition	Weber	Rinne	Schwabach
Normal	Nonlocalized	Air>bone	Similar to examiner
Cochlear nerve lesion	Louder in normal ear	Air>bone	Reduced in affected ear
Conduction	Louder in affected ear	Bone>air	Reduced in affected ear

Table 7

Causes of Hearing Loss

Conductive (Problem with transforming and conducting sound to the cochlea)

1. Obstruction of the external auditory canal by cerumen, foreign body, or atresia
2. Thickening or perforation of the tympanic membrane (TM) due to infection or trauma
3. Chronic otitis media
4. Obstruction of eustachian tube leading to serous otitis media
5. Otosclerosis
6. Cholesteatoma
7. Glomus tumor—arising from the jugular bulb and eroding into the nearby middle ear
8. Temporal bone tumor, fracture, or Paget disease
9. Trauma to the TM or middle ear

Sensorineural (Disease of the cochlea, cochlear nerve, or acoustic nerve)

1. Ischemia to the cochlea
2. Tumors—acoustic neuroma, cholesteatoma, meningioma, epidermoid, metastatic tumors
3. Infection/inflammation—meningitis, syphilis, sarcoidosis
4. Noise or physical trauma to the inner ear
5. Medication toxicity
6. Meniere disease
7. Perilymphatic fistula

Central (Due to lesions of the cochlear nuclei or their cortical connections)

1. Brainstem tumor (eg, pontine glioma)
2. Brainstem stroke
3. Demyelinating disease
4. Congenital malformations – Chiari malformation, Klippel-Feil

Selected Diseases Presenting with Hearing Loss

Otosclerosis

This is the most common form of hearing loss in adults. It is felt to be an autosomal dominant trait with incomplete penetrance. Pathophysiology involves overgrowth of bony material around the oval window, eventually encasing the stapes. Microsurgery aimed at reversing this has proven effective in some cases.

Noise-induced Hearing Loss

This is the result of hair cell loss as a result of single occasion or long-standing exposure to loud noise. Prevention is the key to treatment in these cases, as permanent or progressive hearing loss tends to result from repeated exposure.

Congenital and Other Hereditary Deafness

The majority of these are autosomal recessive traits. In a number, the connexin-26 gene on chromosome 13 is involved. Most involve peripheral organs of hearing but VIII nerve aplasia or degeneration can also occur. Refsum disease and several mitochondrial diseases (Kearns Sayre, MELAS) are characterized by deafness.

Susac Syndrome

This is a rare but fascinating syndrome seen in young women which presents with encephalopathy, visual loss, and hearing loss. Pathologically it is a microvasculopathy affecting the brain, retina and cochlea and while the pathophysiology is not yet clear, it seems to be an immune related vasculitis. MRI reveals areas of signal change in grey and white matter. Brain biopsy can demonstrate perivascular inflammatory changes and infarctions. Treatment choices include corticosteroids, anticoagulation, immunomodulators, plasmapheresis, and intravenous immunoglobulins, but evidence is lacking regarding efficacy.

Cerebrovascular Causes of Hearing Loss

The cochlea is supplied by branches of the internal auditory artery (IAA), which is usually a branch of the anterior inferior cerebellar artery (AICA). Sometimes the IAA is a direct branch of the basilar artery and rarely, it is a branch of the posterior inferior cerebellar artery (PICA). IAA has three terminal branches: the anterior vestibular artery which supplies the anterior and lateral SCC; the cochlear-vestibular artery, which has two branches, the posterior vestibular artery which supplies the posterior SCC and the saccule, and a cochlear branch which supplies the base of the cochlea (high-frequency tones); and a pure cochlear artery which supplies the apex of the cochlea (low-frequency tones). As a result, occlusion of the basilar artery, AICA, IAA, or cochlear branches can cause deafness in one ear (see Figure 4). Possible contributing factors include atherosclerosis, hypercoagulable states such as sickle cell anemia, polycythemia, macroglobulinemia, and embolic conditions.

Diagnosis is reasonable when there is a history of TIA or stroke and if infarction is seen in the brainstem on MRI. When the occlusion is distal there may only be hearing loss with or without vertigo, and confirming the diagnosis is difficult. Treatment is aimed at preventing future ischemic injury to the CNS.

Treatment of Hearing Loss

Treatment of reversible hearing loss of course depends on identifying the cause and treating it. The treatment of irreversible hearing loss, such as age related and noise induced hearing loss, relies on sound amplifying technology. Hearing aids, which are available in numerous varieties including in-ear and outside ear placement, are the most convenient options, but other amplifying tools (speakers, telephone and computer attachments, etc.) are available. When this approach fails in cases of severe hearing impairment, cochlear implants are an option. Here electrodes designed to stimulate the cochlear nerve are implanted near the organ of Corti, which are connected to an implanted external sound transducing system.

Tinnitus

Tinnitus is defined as an unwanted noise not due to a source in the environment. Descriptions include: "roaring," "ringing," "buzzing," "high pitched tone," and "whooshing." Some patients describe the sound as "like listening to the ocean in a shell." Lesions can be in the temporal bone, outer ear, middle ear, cochlea, or auditory nerve.

The differential diagnosis list includes: noise-induced hearing loss, Ménière disease, ototoxic medications, acoustic neuroma and other CPA masses (see Table 8). Palatal myoclonus and stapedius muscle spasm are rare causes, and induce a clicking sound rather than a single pitch or hum. Pulsating tinnitus necessitates a search for a cause of turbulent blood flow such as a carotid or vertebral bruit, dural AVM or fistula, and vascular tumors (eg, glomus tumor). Pseudotumor cerebri is known to cause pulsatile tinnitus as well. Most medications that cause hearing loss can also cause tinnitus, including salicylates, quinidine, and aminoglycosides. Other medications and substances known to cause tinnitus include aminophylline, indomethacin, and caffeine.

Treatment of Tinnitus

Medication is generally ineffective but anxiolytics and anticonvulsants have been tried. Masking devices ("white noise" producing machines) can help. When tinnitus persists it can lead to quite a bit of frustration and depression as well as significant sleep deprivation. In these cases, soporific medication and perhaps antidepressant medications may be useful.

Table 8

Causes of Tinnitus

Nonpulsatile
Hearing loss
Otosclerosis
Foreign body or cerumen in auditory canal
Meniere disease
Acoustic neuroma or other CPA mass lesion
Ototoxic medications
Substances – eg, caffeine, alcohol
Head injury
CPA region mass

Pulsatile
Hypertension
Carotid or other arterial bruit
Persistence of stapedial artery
Dural arteriovenous malformation or fistula
Intracerebral arteriovenous malformation
Vascular tumors (eg, glomus tumor)
Pseudotumor cerebri
(Idiopathic intracranial hypertension)
Palatal myoclonus
Stapedial muscle spasm
Temporomandibular dysfunction
Psychogenic – depression, anxiety, fibromyalgia

3. Conclusion

Vertigo and hearing loss often appear together due to the proximity of anatomical structures subserving vestibular and auditory functions. Differential diagnosis in both conditions can be challenging and requires careful history and exam skills as well as judicious use of laboratory tools. Treatment of vertigo is often successful with a combination or physical and pharmacological techniques. Hearing loss is best treated by prevention or early intervention, but new technology is leading to improved results.

4. References

1. Baloh R. Vestibular neuritis. *New England Journal of Medicine*. 2003, 348:1027-1032.

2. Baloh RW. Episodic vertigo: central nervous system causes. *Current Opinion in Neurology*. 2002, 15(1):17-21.

3. Brandt T, Stedden S, Daroff RB. Therapy for benign positional vertigo revisited. *Neurology*. 1994, 44:796-800.

4. Bronstein AM. Vision and vertigo: some visual aspects of vestibular disorders. *Journal of Neurology*.2004, 251(4):381-387.

5. Cogan DG. Syndrome of nonsyphilitic interstitial keratitis and vestibulo-auditory symptoms. *Archives of Ophthalmology*. 33:144-149, 1945

6. Do TH, Fisch C, and Evoy F. Susac Syndrome: Report of four cases and review of the literature. *Am J Neuroradiol*. 25:382–388 2004

7. Epley J. The canalith repositioning procedure for treatment of benign positional vertigo. *Otolaryngol Head Neck Surg*. 1992, 7:399-404.

8. Furman J, Cass, SP. Benign Positional Vertigo. *New Eng Jourl Med*. 1999, 341:1590-1596.

9. Johnson G. Medical Management of Migraine-Related Dizziness and Vertigo. *Laryngoscope*. 1998, 108(1) Supplement 85):1-28.

10. Levin M. Dizziness. In: *Neurology Clinical Case Studies*. Edited by Levin M. Columbus, OH: Anadem; 2003:29-38.

11. Nadol J. Hearing Loss. *New Eng Jour Med*. 1993, 329(15):1092-1102.

12. Neuhauser H, Leopold M, vonBrevern M. The interrelations of migraine, vertigo and migrainous vertigo. *Neurology*. 2001, 56:436-441.

13. Pappas DG, Jr. Autonomic related vertigo. *Laryngoscope*. 1658, 113(10):1658-1671.

14. Saeed S. Diagnosis and treatment of Ménière's disease. *Brit Med Jour*. 1998, 316:368-372.

15. Traccis S, Zoroddu GF, Zecca MT, Cau T, Solinas MA, Masuri R. Evaluating patients with vertigo: bedside examination. *Neuro Sci*. 2004, 25(1).

16. Troost BT. Vestibular migraine. *Current Pain & Headache Reports*. 2004, 8(4):310-314.

17. von Brevern M, Radtke A, Clarke AH, Lempert T. Migrainous vertigo presenting as episodic positional vertigo. *Neurology*. 2004, 62(3):469-472.

18. Weider DJ. Treatment and management of perilymphatic fistula: a New Hampshire experience. *Am J Otol*. 13(2):158-66, 1992

19. Yueh B, Shapiro N, MacLean CH, Shekelle PG. Screening and management of adult hearing loss in primary care: scientific review. *JAMA*. 289(15):1976-85, 2003 Apr 16, 289(15):1976-1985.

5. Questions

1. Scarpa ganglion contains:

A. Unipolar primary auditory neurons

B. Bipolar primary auditory neurons

C. Unipolar primary vestibular neurons

D. Bipolar primary vestibular neurons

E. Both vestibular and auditory neurons

2. Each of the following is connected functionally to the brainstem vestibular nuclei EXCEPT:

A. Flocculonodular lobe of the cerebellum

B. Cerebellar hemispheres

C. Median longitudinal fasciculus

D. Oculomotor nucleus

E. Abducens nucleus

3. A patient with a mass compressing the labyrinthine apparatus might exhibit:

A. Fixed direction horizontal pendular nystagmus

B. Fixed direction vertical nystagmus

C. Horizontal and occasional vertical nystagmus

D. Alternating left and right lateral nystagmus

E. Fixed direction horizontal and rotatory nystagmus

This case refers to the next 3 questions:

A 28-year-old man awakens with acute severe positional vertigo with nausea. On exam, he has horizontal nystagmus, worse on Hallpike maneuver with head turned to the right. Vertigo and nausea gradually subside over the next 48 hours.

4. Which of the following is the most likely diagnosis?

A. Vestibular neuronitis / labyrinthitis

B. Ménière disease

C. Perilymphatic fistula

D. Benign positional vertigo

E. Brainstem stroke

5. Where is the probable site of the lesion?

A. L labyrinthine system

B. R labyrinthine system

C. L Pons

D. R Pons

E. R Oval window

6. Which of the following medications would be LEAST useful?

A. Diazepam

B. Dimenhydramine

C. Carbamazepine

D. Scopolamine

E. Meclizine

7. What is the proposed mechanism of benign positional vertigo (BPV)?

A. Dislodgement of labyrinthine membrane

B. Endolymph leak

C. Perilymph leak

D. Labyrinthine ischemia

E. Calcific granulation in the cupula

8. All of the following medications are known to induce vertigo EXCEPT:

A. Chloroquine

B. Furosemide

C. Acetaminophen

D. Phenytoin

E. Gentamycin

9. All of the following may induce pulsatile tinnitus, EXCEPT:

A. Dural arteriovenous malformation

B. Glomus tumor

C. Pseudotumor cerebri

D. Ménière disease

E. Palatal myoclonus

10. A 44-year-old man describes bouts of severe positional vertigo, which is often abrupt and disabling. Exam reveals only some moderate hearing loss on the right. The pathophysiology of the most likely diagnosis in this case is thought to be:

A. Endolymph leak

B. Perilymph leak

C. Overabundance of endolymph

D. Inflammation of the vestibular nerve

E. Brainstem encephalitis

11. A 52-year-old woman had a prolonged bout of sneezing, following which she developed vertigo, but no other symptoms. A likely diagnosis is:

A. Vertebral dissection

B. SDH

C. Perilymph fistula

D. Venous thrombosis of the labyrinth

E. Inner ear hematoma

12. Where is the most likely site of the lesion in the case above?

A. Oval or round window

B. Cochlear aqueduct

C. Petrous bone

D. Saccule

E. Utricle

13. A young woman complains of spells of vertigo and tinnitus over the past 4 years, with more recent progressive hearing loss. She has been diagnosed with Ménière disease but has not responded to treatment. She also complains of recurrent eye infections, anemia, and an abnormal ECG. A possible missed diagnosis is:

A. Cogan syndrome

B. Susac syndrome

C. Familial Ménière disease

D. Acoustic neuroma

E. Migraine

14. The condition above is due to:

A. Syphilis

B. Interstitial keratitis

C. Vasculitis

D. Bacterial infection

E. Nutritional neuropathy

The following case applies to the next 2 questions:

A 28-year-old woman complains of earache, vertigo and malaise for 2 days. Examination of the ear reveals marked erythema of the right tympanic membrane, and facial weakness on the R.

15. The most likely diagnosis is:

A. Bacterial otitis media

B. Basal meningitis

C. Otitis externa

D. Idiopathic Bell palsy

E. Ramsey Hunt syndrome

16. The cause of this illness is:

A. Staph or strep bacteria

B. Herpes zoster virus

C. Lymphoma

D. Herpes simplex virus

E. Epstein Barr virus

17. A 59-year-old man has noted progressive hearing loss on the right. MRI of the head following gadolinium infusion reveals a mass lesion in the right cerebellopontine angle. Possibilities include the following EXCEPT:

A. Meningioma

B. Metastatic tumor

C. Dermoid

D. Schwannoma

E. Cholesteatoma

18. A patient with a history of epileptic seizures begins to have spells of vertigo and altered mental state. If these spells represent partial seizures, where is a likely focus?

A. Prefrontal cortex

B. Mesial temporal lobe

C. Posterior superior temporal lobe

D. Anterior occipital lobe

E. Cingulate gyrus

19. A 54-year-old man has the following results on his bedside testing:

Weber test reveals that the tone is louder on the right. Rinne test reveals bone>air conduction on the right side. What is the most likely cause of his hearing dysfunction?

A. Conduction deficit on the R

B. Conduction deficit on the L

C. Sensorineural deficit on the R

D. Sensorineural deficit on the L

E. Central hearing dysfunction

20. An army veteran has had bilateral hearing loss since his tour of combat duty as a tank officer. The mechanism is probably based on damage to the:

A. Bony labyrinth

B. Tympanic membrane

C. Hair cells of the cochlea

D. Stapes bone

E. Stapedius muscle

Answers

1. B.
Scarpa ganglion is the ganglion containing primary afferent neurons of the vestibular system. The spiral ganglion contains primary afferent neurons of the auditory system. Both auditory and vestibular primary afferents are bipolar neurons.

2. B.
The eight vestibular nuclei of the brainstem have extensive connections to cerebellar, spinal, and ocular motor centers and nuclei. Cerebellar connections are mainly vermian, not hemispheric.

3. E.
Labyrinthine lesions tend to produce jerk horizontal and rotatory nystagmus, whereas more central (brainstem) lesions tend to produce vertical as well as horizontal/rotatory nystagmus. Alternating horizontal nystagmus would implicate bilateral vestibular dysfunction such as seen in toxic metabolic states. Pendular nystagmus is generally seen in congenital visual/ocular deficits and other central lesions.

4. A.
With acute onset of vertigo, significant nausea, horizontal nystagmus, and gradual resolution, this case is a typical presentation of vestibular neuronitis or labyrinthitis. Certainly Ménière disease could conceivably present in a similar fashion initially, but eventually hearing loss is present. Brainstem stroke generally produces other deficits. BPV is brief and positional. Perilymphatic fistula presents acutely, but it generally follows some sort of trauma (sneezing, barotrauma, etc.) and does not abate.

5. B.
Labyrinthitis/vestibular neuronitis is thought to involve the labyrinth and perhaps primary afferents. Generally, in labyrinthine causes of vertigo, symptoms are exacerbated with the affected side pointed downward during Hallpike maneuver.

6. C.
Benzodiazepines (eg, diazepam), antihistamines (eg, meclizine), and anticholinergics (eg, scopolamine) are all useful agents in vertigo. Although not one of the choices in this question, neuroleptics

like promethazine can improve the nausea and vomiting that often accompanies vertigo (as well as the vertigo itself). However, antiepileptic medications, such as carbamazepine, have not been useful.

7. E.
The etiology of BPV is still unclear but it is believed that minute calcific granules coalesce and settle in the cupula of the posterior canal. They are dislodged when the head turns quickly; this sets endolymph into motion, leading to perception of motion.

8. C.
There are a number of medications known to induce vertigo and/or hearing loss, including quinine derivatives, salicylates, NSAIDs, antibiotics, diuretics, and chemotherapeutic agents, but acetaminophen has not been implicated as a cause of vertigo.

9. D.
The vascular glomus tumor and dural AVMs can cause audible pulsations by virtue of the high flow lesions lying near the hearing apparatus. Palatal myoclonus causes an audible rhythmic clicking sound. Pseudotumor cerebri causes pulsatile tinnitus for unclear reasons, but it is a very common symptom in this disease. Ménière is not known for an association with pulsatile tinnitus.

10. C.
This case is likely Ménière disease, thought to be caused by an excess of fluid in the labyrinthine system, hence the synonym "endolymph hydrops." Perilymph is the fluid surrounding the semicircular canals.

11. C.
The history of severe vertigo preceded by pressure trauma is very suggestive of perilymph fistula, which is believed to occur in most cases at the oval or round window.

12. A.
Perilymph fistula is believed to occur in most cases at the oval or round window.

13. A.
Cogan syndrome is a lymphocytic infiltration of the inner ear accompanied by interstitial keratitis of the eye. Hearing and vestibular symptoms including vertigo, ataxia, nystagmus, and hearing loss all occur. Cardiovascular, musculoskeletal, and gastrointestinal symptoms can also occur. Susac syndrome is a microvasculopathy which causes encephalopathy, visual loss and hearing loss.

14. B.
An autoimmune mediated interstitial keratitis is presumed as the primary cause of Cogan syndrome.

15. E.
While this case sounds convincing for otitis media (erythema of the TM, earache, malaise), the vertigo and facial weakness are classic for Ramsey Hunt syndrome. Basal meningitis may cause several cranial nerve palsies, but ipsilateral VII and VIII dysfunction with the ipsilateral TM inflammation suggests something more focal.

16. B.
Ramsey Hunt syndrome is felt to be due to involvement of VII +/- VIII by the Herpes zoster virus.

17. C.
Epidermoid tumors are slow-growing benign tumors, and are found in the CPA or parasellar region. Schwannomas, cholesteatomas, and meningiomas can all be found in the CPA as well as metastases. Dermoids are teratomas which are not generally found in the CPA region.

18. C.
Vertigo as a manifestation of partial seizure activity is quite rare, but when it happens the focus is generally in the temporal neocortex, particularly in the posterior superior portion of the temporal lobe, as opposed to the more well known temporal seizure foci in medial temporal areas.

19. A.

This patient localized the tuning fork tone to the right on Weber testing. That could mean that there is a conduction problem on the right masking ambient noise and leading to greater perception on the right of the bone-conducted sound from the tuning fork. If that is true, then bone conduction should be better than air on that side, which turns out to be true as tested by Rinne procedure.

20. C.

Noise induced hearing loss is due to sound pressure damage to the hair cells in the organ of Corti of the cochlea. This is an unfortunately irreversible process and the only good treatment is prevention (ear protection).

Chapter 31: Behavioral Neurology/ Neuropsychiatry

Deborah N. Black, MD, FRCP(C)

Contents

1. Introduction

The problem of neurology is to understand man himself.
— Dr. Wilder Penfield

Behavioral neurology/neuropsychiatry cuts across the disciplines of neurology and psychiatry to consider all aspects of cognition, behavior and affect in relation to brain function. The conditions of interest in behavioral neurology/neuropsychiatry may be deficit syndromes such as aphasia, apraxia, and agnosia, or "productive syndromes," such as panic or aggression caused by disinhibition of regulatory circuits.

Just as in other branches of neurology, neuroanatomy provides the scaffolding for cognitive operations, and cognitive operations provide the scaffolding for behavior. In contrast to other branches of neurology, however, the complex brain functions underlying cognition, behavior and affect cannot be precisely mapped onto brain anatomy. Cognition, behavior and affect reflect the activity of multiple neural networks distributed across wide brain regions engaging in iterative interactions ("parallel distributed processing"). Disruption of a functionally interconnected network at any point can cause a similar clinical picture. For example, amnesia can result from a lesion in the hippocampus or its affiliated structures. The "dysexecutive" frontal lobe syndrome can follow a lesion of the frontal cortex or its subcortical connections (Table 6).

The anatomical and neurochemical circuits that mediate normal brain function also mediate abnormal brain function. Normal memory and its pathological variant, amnesia, point to the hippocampus and its connections. Motivated behavior and its pathological variant, apathy, point to a disorder of the anterior cingulate and its connections. The frontal and temporal lobes are particularly relevant to psychosis, whether idiopathic or following traumatic brain injury. Knowing the circuits and their normal functions enables understanding of their pathological variants.

In recognition of the neuroanatomical foundation of normal and abnormal brain function, this chapter uses a functional anatomical approach to organize the major symptoms and signs of normal and abnormal higher brain function. The behavioral neurology of the cerebellum and corpus callosum is not considered here; pertinent references are included below.

On a historical note, the United Council for Neurologic Subspecialties approved Behavioral Neurology and Neuropsychiatry as a single subspecialty in June, 2004.

2. The Frontal Lobes

Overview

The prefrontal area of the brain – so named to distinguish it from the motor and speech areas of frontal cortex – governs attention, the monitoring of the external and internal milieu; intention, the shaping of behavior in accordance with internal motivation and external context; and execution, the orchestration of complex sensorimotor sequences in a seamless path toward a goal. The Russian neuropsychologist Alexsandr Luria related prefrontal activity to programming motor behavior, inhibiting immediate responses, abstracting, problem solving ability, verbal regulation of behavior, reorienting behavior according to consequences, temporal integration of behavior, personality integrity, and consciousness.

Three major areas of prefrontal cortex are relevant to behavioral neurology/neuropsychiatry:

Dorsolateral Prefrontal Cortex

The dorsolateral frontal cortex is closely associated with "executive" functions: synthesizing information, planning and implementing strategies, problem-solving, reasoning, "top-down" control of attention, and working memory.

Working memory (synonyms: short-term memory; "scratchpad" memory) is an attentional function that enables retaining and manipulating limited amounts of information (5 to 7 items) for a short period of time, usually seconds to a few minutes. Working memory is involved in remembering a telephone number or the number of a page in an index. This remarkable cognitive capacity allows us to perform cognitive operations such as goals, plans, and intentions independent of immediate environmental contingencies.

Orbitofrontal Cortex

The orbitofrontal cortex is involved in emotional regulation and inhibition of impulsive and aggressive behavior in accordance with internalized rules. The orbitofrontal and anterior cingulate cortex are major cortical hubs where inputs from the limbic system, basal ganglia, and cortical association regions converge.

Anterior Cingulate Cortex

Through its connections with limbic structures, midline thalamic nuclei, and other areas of prefrontal cortex, the anterior cingulate cortex plays a major role in motivation.

Major Afferents and Efferents (Figure 1)

Three distinct parallel circuits link prefrontal cortex with the basal ganglia, substantia nigra and thalamus before returning to their cortical sites of origin. The major cortical excitatory neurotransmitter is glutamate. Dopamine, acetylcholine, serotonin, GABA, and numerous neuropeptides serve as neurotransmitters and neuromodulators in the basal ganglia and thalamus. Glutamate is the major excitatory neurotransmitter closing the circuit from the thalamus back to layer IV of the prefrontal cortex. Thalamocortical fibers travel in the anterior limb of the internal capsule.

All areas of prefrontal cortex have extensive reciprocal connections with parietal, temporal and occipital association cortex. These extensive intracortical connections enable the frontal cortex to exert "top down" control over activity in other cortical areas, consistent with the role of the frontal lobes in the integration of sensory information, in planning, directing attention, regulating affect, and organizing movement.

The orbitofrontal and anterior cingulate cortex are reciprocally connected with limbic structures including amygdala, nucleus accumbens and hippocampus. The anterior cingulate is the cortical termination of Papez circuit originating in the hippocampus. Dense interconnections between the anterior cingulate and supplementary motor cortex allow communication between cognitive and motor systems.

The entire frontal cortex receives a dense dopaminergic innervation from the ventral tegmental nucleus, which lies dorsomedial to the substantia nigra in the midbrain. This ventral tegmental-frontal dopamine pathway is the mesocortical dopamine circuit, in contrast to the mesolimbic and striatal dopamine circuits discussed below. Dopamine in the frontal cortex is believed to mediate working memory attention and self-monitoring

Figure 1

Fronto-subcortical circuits

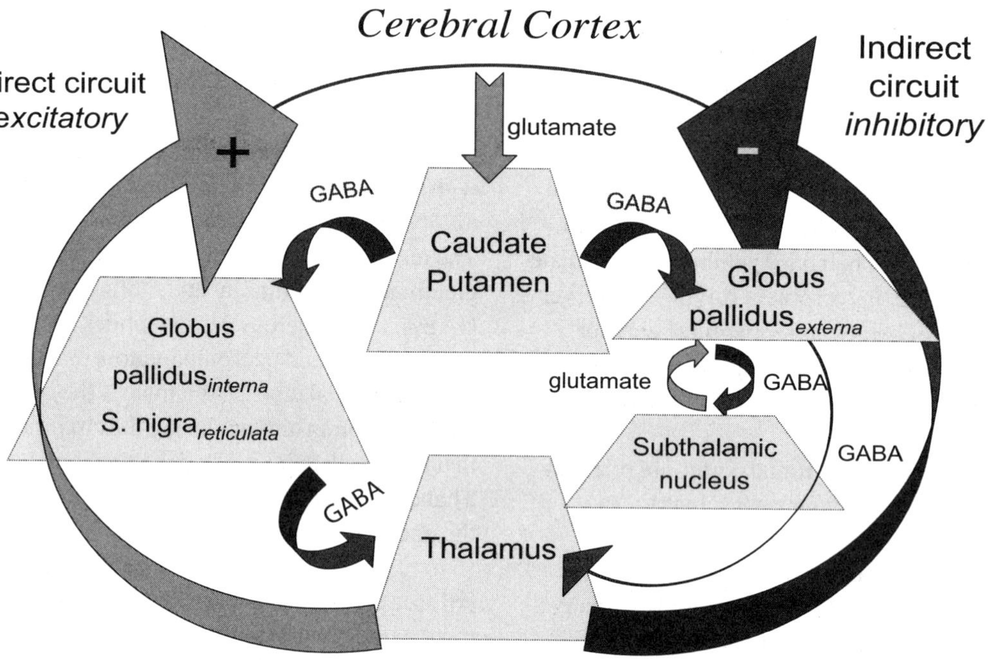

and error correction in cognitive operations. Dopaminergic activity in the anterior cingulate cortex is critical to the initiation of goal-directed behavior.

Clinical Signs of Frontal Lobe Disorders (Table 1 and Appendix 4)

Although frontal lobe syndromes are divided into dorsolateral ("executive"), anterior cingulate ("motivational"), and orbitofrontal ("social") disorders, frontal disorders rarely occur in isolation. For example, it is not uncommon for an apathetic patient to swear or strike out if frustrated. This symptomatic overlap reflects the interconnectivity of prefrontal regions and the lack of anatomical specificity of lesions.

Environmental Dependency

All frontal disorders share loss of internal guidance of behavior. The "environmental dependency" of the frontal patient may take the form of impulsiveness without regard to consequences, imitation behavior, or inability to call up memories, or to initiate or suppress responses voluntarily.

Dysexecutive Syndrome

The dysexecutive syndrome implies dysfunction of the dorsolateral frontal cortex. Planning is impaired; thinking is concrete and bound by immediate contingencies. Difficulty adapting to changing contingencies is reflected in perseveration: the purposeless iteration of behavior. Reasoning is erroneous and self-monitoring is deficient. Working memory dysfunction is seen as losing train of thought and distractibility (eg, forgetting a task in midstream, or the subject of a sentence). Common signs of dorsolateral prefrontal cortex dysfunction are failure to self-administer medication, follow recipes, keep appointments, handle finances, and other activities of daily living. One of my elderly patients stopped meticulously recording her husband's epileptic seizures as she developed Alzheimer disease.

Table 1

Behavioral Disorders Associated With Prefrontal Cortex

Dorsolateral
Perseveration
Impaired ability to generate problem-solving strategies
Impaired ability to use symbols (eg, concreteness)
Reduced mental control; behavior guided by automatic and overlearned reponses
Depression
Memory retrieval deficit
Orbitofrontal
Disinhibition
Impulsiveness
Lack of social tact
Impairment of insight
Impairment of empathy
Mood lability, depression, hypomania
Personal neglect
Anterior Cingulate
Apathy
Lack of spontaneity
Motor inactivity
Impaired task maintenance
Poor self-monitoring and correction
Perseveration
Memory retrieval deficit

Disinhibition

Orbitofrontal cortex dysfunction is associated with impulsive, aggressive behavior and violations of social rules ("acquired sociopathy"), as in the famous case of Phineas Gage. Gage was a responsible 25-year-old foreman overseeing the construction of a railroad line in Cavendish Vermont. On September 13, 1848, while using a tamping iron to pack explosives into a rock, an uncontrolled explosion propelled the tool through his left cheek and behind his left eye, shattering his upper jaw before passing through the top of his head. Gage was knocked over, but within minutes he was able to be transported back to his boarding house while seated in a horse cart. One day later *The Boston Post* reported that Gage was "alive... in full possession of his reason, and free from pain." Gage was attended by Dr. Martyn Harlow, a young country surgeon. Dr. Harlow provided the first report of the profound personality change that ensued:

"He is fitful, irreverent, indulging at times in the grossest profanity, manifesting but little deference for his fellows, impatient of restraint or advice when it conflicts with his desires, at times pertinaciously obstinate, yet capricious and vacillating, devising many plans of operation, which are no sooner arranged than they are abandoned in turn for others appearing more feasible. A child in his intellectual capacity and manifestations, he has the animal passions of a strong man..."

Gage was unable to return to his former job as foreman. He worked at odd jobs and appeared at Barnum's museum. In 1860, he developed epileptic seizures and died, destitute, in San Francisco. In 1867, Gage's body was exhumed and sent to Dr. Harlow, who donated his skull to the Harvard Medical School. Subsequent neuroimaging reconstructions by Hannah and Antonio Damasio and colleagues in 1994 and by Ratiu and Talos in 2004 have suggested that the left anterior frontal lobe, and possibly the right as well, were extensively damaged.

Behavior change following orbitofrontal damage may take the form of irritability, aggressive outbursts, inappropriate sexual behavior, tactless remarks, violations of social rules (eg, theft, public urination or masturbation), or facetious jocularity (Witzelsucht) that may be confused with mania. Imitation and utilization behavior are signs of environmental dependency. Utilization behavior is the tendency to pick up or use objects in sight. Lhermitte described a patient who, seeing his stethoscope, picked it up and began examining him. Insight and empathy are shallow; mood is labile. Although patients may be able to recognize and articulate behavioral guidelines, they are not able to use these rules to guide their behavior. Disordered and disorderly behavior may be the only signs of orbitofrontal injury, since this brain region is not associated with elementary sensory, motor, or language functions. IQ, language, memory, and other cognitive functions may be intact, leading to a striking discrepancy between intellect and behavior.

Apathy

Deficient activation of the anterior cingulate and its subcortical connections results in apathy, broadly defined as lack of motivation (Table 6). The apathy syndrome is defined by its three major dimensions: cognitive (lack of interest); motor (lack of action, or inertia); and affective (lack of concern, pleasure, and empathy). Apathy lies on a spectrum of severity, with abulia and akinetic mutism at its extreme end. The apathetic patient typically shows psychomotor slowness and lack of spontaneity. The facial expression is bland, affect blunted, and speech monotonous, sparse and unelaborated. The patient requires prompting to initiate and to sustain activity. They may sit alone, apparently indifferent to social interactions, pleasure and pain. Mental imagery, thought and fantasy are impoverished (vide psychique). The ability to retrieve previously-memorized information is impaired ("frontal amnesia"), and events of the past are telescoped.

Lesions and Differential Diagnosis of Frontal Lobe Disorders

The frontal lobes may be damaged by direct trauma, by primary or secondary brain tumors, or by stroke involving anterior branches of the middle cerebral artery. Rupture of an anterior communicating artery aneurysm may cause frontal damage by hemorrhage, by secondary vasospasm, or by hydrocephalus. Other causes of frontal impairment include chronic alcohol abuse, degenerative dementias (Alzheimer disease and fronto-temporal dementia), a variety of infectious causes including neurosyphilis, acquired immune deficiency syndrome, Jacob-Creutzfeldt disease, and toxic-metabolic encephalopathies.

Frontal dysfunction is a principal component of multiple other conditions: normal aging, attention deficit disorder, autism, obsessive compulsive disorder, Tourette syndrome, schizophrenia, and subcortical disorders affecting frontal-subcortical circuits.

In clinical practice, anxiety, depression, disturbed sleep, chronic pain, and medication side effects are the "Big 5" associated with reversible attentional impairment.

Intermittent explosive disorder and antisocial personality disorder need to be distinguished from the "acquired sociopathy" of orbitofrontal lesions.

Clinical Assessment of Frontal Functions (Appendices 2 and 3)

Although formal neuropsychological testing is valuable, careful clinical assessment can reveal signs of frontal dysfunction in most cases where it is suspected. Since the Folstein Mini-Mental Status Examination is not sensitive to frontal dysfunction, a normal Mini-Mental Status score does not rule out frontal lobe impairment. A comprehensive approach to clinical diagnosis includes the following:

- Obtain a careful longitudinal description of behavior (Table 1). Inquire about family history, head trauma, substance abuse, medical conditions, sleep, medications, anxiety and depression.

- Observe behavior as the patient enters the exam room. Keep in mind that the structured setting of the office or hospital and the presence of a white coat may contain behavior that would be inappropriate in a less structured setting.

Assess level of arousal by observing behavior, facial expression, responsiveness to the environment, and degree of stimulation required to elicit a verbal or behavioral response. An optimal level of arousal is necessary for accurate cognitive assessment; conversely, any degree of attentional impairment will affect all other cognitive functions. Apathetic patients may require repeated cueing to respond, or their response may trail off in mid-task.

Observe for imitation behavior. Imitation behavior is tested by asking the patient to follow a command (eg, holding out their hands while the examiner performs another gesture, such as, tapping hands on head). Imitation behavior, or echopraxia, is present when the patient echoes the examiner's behavior.

Imitation behavior is sometimes seen during visual field testing where, after being told to look straight ahead and point to your moving finger, the patient stretches out their arms to imitate your gesture.

To look for utilization behavior, lay out an assortment of objects on the desk and observe the patient's response. I use paper and pencil, small change, a stapler, my reflex hammer, and candy. Any tendency to pick up or use the objects without asking permission or out of context should be noted.

Assess the capacity to sustain attention by having the patient perform a continuous task such as reciting the alphabet or counting out loud. A variant is to ask the patient to tap every time they hear the letter "A" in a string of letters presented one a second.

Working memory is assessed with digit span, months in reverse, days of the week in reverse, subtractions of serial 7s, or the letters of the word "world" in alphabetical order. Normal forward digit span is 7 ± 2. I like to ask the patient to reverse their personal telephone number. More difficult tasks rely on the capacity to maintain attention on two tasks simultaneously; for example: mental alternation of letters and numbers from 1A to 5E, or mental rehearsal of 3 words while counting backward by 3s for 15 to 30 seconds. These tasks also evaluate capacity to inhibit rote, overlearned, and automatic responses. Typical "frontal" errors are: December, November, October ... November, December; or: 1A, 2A, 3A... Many people make minor errors on serial 7s; if the task is too difficult, try an easier one.

Self-monitoring, judgment and complex reasoning are assessed by inquiring about awareness of behavior, the reason for medical evaluation, and future plans. Mathematical problems such as, "How many quarters in $1.75?," assess complex reasoning.

Verbal fluency is a language task which is also sensitive to active retrieval from memory, a frontal function. Category fluency (eg, asking the patient to name as many animals, or foods, as possible in 1 minute), is easier than semantic fluency (eg, words beginning with the letter F or P). Obviously, performance on semantic fluency requires intact language functions. Normal verbal fluency is 15 ± 5 words in 60 seconds.

Recall of a list of 3 to 5 words also measures ability to retrieve previously-learned information from memory. Most patients can remember a list of words equal to their forward digit span minus one. Poor spontaneous recall, and improved performance with cueing, suggest impaired cognitive activation rather than hippocampal-based amnesia (0).

Alternating manual and written tasks assess set shifting, ie, the ability to alternate strategies. The bimanual Ozeretski task requires the patient to simultaneously fist one hand and open the other, then reverse. One-hand alternating tasks include the fist-ring and the Luria palm-fist-cut sequence. Have the patient rehearse the movements with you five times, then ask the patient to execute the movements alone. It is important not to provide verbal cues while demonstrating these tasks, since the point is to see whether the patient is capable of generating an internal program independently. Patients with frontal dysfunction have a verbal-manual dissociation, ie, they are unable to use language to guide their behavior. Perseveration, intrusions from previous tasks, alteration of sequence or inability to activate both hands simultaneously are seen with frontal dysfunction. If the patient has difficulty, providing a verbal cue (eg, "fist, ring," "one, two, three," or "palm, fist, cut") may improve performance in patients with less severe frontal impairment.

Written alternating tasks include alternating M-N, triple loops, circle-square-triangle, or the more difficult ramparts task. Draw the alternating square-triangle sequence once, then ask the patient to continue drawing the same sequence to the end of the page. If the patient has difficulty, make the task rule explicit ("first the square, then the triangle"). Note perseveration, intrusion, simplification (eg, drawing a series of 3s rather than 3 loops), distractibility, drawing on top of the model ("closing in"), poor effort, and alteration of sequence.

Abstraction is assessed with proverbs and analogies. Frontally impaired patients tend to give concrete responses (eg, train and bicycle: wheels; plums and cherries: seeds); or they may insist that a train and a bicycle are not the same, suggesting difficulty with set shifting and a stimulus-bound response.

The clock-drawing task reflects visual-spatial organization, a non-dominant parietal function, as well as the dorsolateral prefrontal functions of planning and organization. Several useful clock scoring systems exist. Patients with dorsolateral frontal dysfunction may show perseveration (drawing many circles or multiple hands), poor planning of number placement, or attraction to the salient stimulus: When asked to indicate 11:10, the minute hand is placed on the 10 instead of the 2 (Figure 2).

The go-no go task is sensitive to orbitofrontal dysfunction. One version of this task is to ask the patient to tap twice every time the examiner taps once, and to tap once when the examiner taps twice. A more difficult version is to have the patient tap twice when the examiner taps once, but to withhold tapping when the examiner taps twice. Impulsive errors such as tapping every time, or imitating the examiner, are characteristic of orbitofrontal dysfunction.

Signs of frontal lobe impairment on neurological examination include: motor impersistence (opening the eyes when told to keep them closed, failure to maintain hands outstretched or tongue protruded), peeking at the stimulus in the peripheral visual field instead of maintaining visual fixation, grasp, suck and snout reflexes, imitation or utilization behavior. One of my patients stood with their coat half off, one arm in the sleeve, until prompted to remove their coat. These deficits reflect impaired task initiation and maintenance. Paratonia, or Gegenhalten, is a fluctuating, quasi-voluntary increase in muscle tone, a form of motor negativism, related to inability to suppress the automatic tendency to resist. Patients may appear indifferent or unconcerned when confronted with these lapses, or may not be able to suppress them.

Examine olfaction because of the proximity of the orbitofrontal cortex to the olfactory bulbs and tracts.

Careful fundoscopic and visual field examination may show an asymmetrical field cut or optic disc pallor suggesting a lesion of the optic nerves or chiasm.

Figure 2

Clock drawing in frontal lobe disease

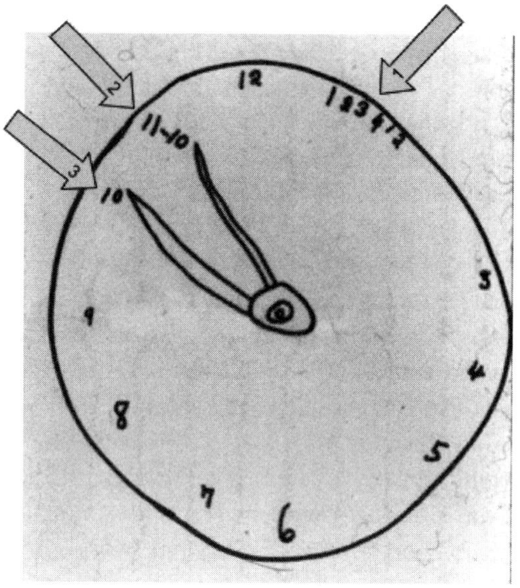

This clock was drawn by a 66-year-old woman with fronto-temporal dementia. Asked to "draw a clock, show all the numbers, and set the time to 10 after 11," this clock shows difficulty with planning of number placement (arrow 1), automatic behavior, ie, a tendency to write "11-10" rather than illustrating the time with hands (arrow 2), and "attraction to the salient stimulus," ie, inability to disengage from the 10 in order to place the minute hand next to the 2 (arrow 3).

Neuroimaging should always be obtained for suspicion of orbitofrontal injury. SPECT scanning may be more helpful than CT or MRI in showing orbitofrontal hypometabolism.

Treatment of Frontal Lobe Disorders

Patients with frontal lobe disorders have profound impairment of self-regulation, and may require a structured, supervised setting to oversee basic hygiene and self-care. The "Big 5" are potentially reversible with appropriate treatment. Stroke, head trauma, subcortical disorders, intoxications, schizophrenia, and subcortical disorders have specific therapies.

Treatment of aggressive, impulsive behavior relies on containing the behavior by appropriate environmental constraints and enhancing central serotonergic activity. Pharmacological options include selective serotonin reuptake inhibitors (SSRIs), lithium, buspirone, anticonvulsant mood stabilizers (carbamazepine, sodium valproate), high-dose beta blockers (propranolol, pindolol, atenolol), atypical neuroleptics such as aripiprazole, clozapine, olanzapine, quetiapine, risperidone and ziprasidone, or alpha-adrenergic agonists (clonidine or guanfacine).

Cholinesterase inhibitors may improve agitation and apathy in Alzheimer disease. Recent studies suggest that these agents may also improve cognition in traumatic brain injury, subcortical stroke and multiple sclerosis.

Antidepressant medication is the first choice where apathy accompanies depression. SSRI medications and the typical neuroleptics may promote apathy because of their antidopaminergic properties. Buproprion, fluoxetine, sertraline, and duloxetine are relatively stimulating antidepressants.

Other pharmacological options for treating apathy include bromocriptine 5-90 mg/day; pergolide 5-90 mg/day; amantadine 100 mg bid to tid; and levodopa-carbidopa 100/25 mg 2-10 times a day. Start with the lowest dose and titrate gradually to clinical effect. High doses may be required. Complications include psychosis, hallucinations and delirium. The best outcomes occur when cortical function is relatively intact.

Psychostimulants, alone or in with dopaminergic agonists, include methylphenidate 10 to 90 mg/day, and d-amphetamine 10-60 mg/day. Adrenergic side effects (tachycardia, weight loss, insomnia) may occur. Modafinil, 200-400 mg/day, is an alternative medication which simulates physiological wakefulness.

3. Disorders of the Basal Ganglia and Their Projections

Overview

Although the basal ganglia are known for their motor functions, they also play a key role in nonmotor integrative functions, including reward prediction, attention, and switching of response strategies. Because of the extensive cortical, thalamic, and limbic affiliations of the basal ganglia, cognitive, mood and behavioral changes accompany all basal ganglia disorders.

Major Afferents and Efferents

The caudate, putamen and nucleus accumbens comprise the striatum. The striatum, globus pallidus and subthalamic nucleus comprise the basal ganglia.

The dorsal striatum receives glutamatergic input from the frontal cortex and a dense dopaminergic projection from the substantia nigra pars compacta. Striatal axons containing GABA, enkephalin and substance P project to the globus pallidus. The globus pallidus sends GABAergic fibers to the mediodorsal thalamus. The circuit is closed with a glutamateric projection from thalamus back to frontal cortex.

In addition to frontal afferents from the anterior cingulate and orbitofrontal cortex, the ventral striatum receives limbic afferents from the insula, amygdala, and hippocampus as well as a dense dopaminergic projection from the ventral tegmentum. Fibers from the ventral striatum project to the mediodorsal thalamus which projects back to the anterior cingulate and orbitofrontal cortex. The mediodorsal thalamus also participates in reciprocal connections with limbic structures. The ventral striatum is thus a critical link between motivational processes linked to the limbic system (0) and motor output systems of premotor and motor cortex.

Clinical Signs of Dysfunction of the Basal Ganglia and Their Projections

In addition to their motor signatures, disorders of the basal ganglia and their subcortical pathways share disturbance of cognition, mood and behavior.

Subcortical Dementia

Psychomotor slowing, impairment of executive functions, insight and judgment, apathy, and pseudobulbar affect accompany most disorders of the basal ganglia and their subcortical connections. Subcortical lesions which disrupt frontal-subcortical circuits cause functional deactivation of prefrontal cortex (diaschisis) and produce a "dysexecutive syndrome" which is qualitatively similar to a disturbance of cortical function. This constellation of motor and cognitive signs is sometimes termed subcortical dementia (Table 6).

Depression

Depression is the most common neuropsychiatric disturbance associated with disorders of the basal ganglia and their subcortical pathways. Anxiety, euphoria, irritability and disinhibition, and less frequently mania, are also seen.

Lesions of the Basal Ganglia and Their Projections

Ischemia

Ischemia of small penetrating branches of the middle and posterior cerebral arteries may cause transient ischemic attacks or focal neurological deficits. Hypertension is usually present. Examination may show variable combinations of pseudobulbar palsy, pyramidal tract signs, lower extremity paratonia, a plantar grasp reflex, and gait apraxia. Frequently confused with primary Parkinson disease, "lower half parkinsonism" does not respond to levodopa.

The term, "vascular depression," refers to the association of depression with extensive white matter ischemic changes in elderly patients. Cognitive impairment with prominent psychomotor slowing is universal.

Parkinson disease

The triad of rest tremor, rigidity, and bradykinesia suggests Parkinson disease. Thirty to 40% of Parkinson patients will develop dementia, and 40% are depressed. Cognitive deficits, present in the majority of patients without overt dementia, are related to dopaminergic dysfunction in frontal-subcortical pathways. These consist of bradyphrenia (slowing and effortful initiation of mental processes) and difficulty shifting motor and perceptual set, characteristic of frontal executive systems impairment.

Dementia associated with Parkinson disease is associated with Alzheimer type plaques and tangles in the cerebral cortex, cortical Lewy bodies, and cortical cholinergic deficiency related to degeneration of the nucleus basalis of Meynert. Patients with predominantly akinetic-rigid Parkinson disease are more prone to dementia than those with predominant rest tremor.

Sleep disturbance, nightmares, well-formed visual hallucinations, confusion and delusions comprise the psychosis of Parkinson disease, which occurs in approximately 30% of patients. Psychosis is associated with dopaminergic treatment and is also correlated with age, cognitive impairment, sleep disturbance, severity of motor symptoms, and the apolipoprotein ε-4 allele.

Other non-motor features of Parkinson disease include anxiety, mood swings in concert with on-off fluctuations, apathy, disturbed sleep, obsessionalism, hypersexuality, and pathological gambling; the latter is related to high-dose dopaminergic medication.

Lewy Body Disease

Parkinsonism with prominent visual hallucinations, delusional psychosis, and episodic pronounced fluctuations in attention and vigilance suggest Lewy body disease. Typically, dementia precedes the extrapyramidal disorder; less frequently, dementia is followed by the appearance of extrapyramidal signs within 12 months of diagnosis. Marked exacerbation of extrapyramidal signs after conventional neuroleptics is typical of Lewy body disease and should raise diagnostic suspicion.

The clinical features of Lewy body disease reflect the distribution of the pathological changes: dementia correlates with neuritic plaques and Lewy bodies in the cerebral cortex; psychosis correlates with Lewy bodies in limbic structures (with relative sparing of hippocampus); parkinsonism correlates with Lewy bodies in the substantia nigra. There is also a pronounced cortical cholinergic deficit.

Cognitive testing shows memory impairment, prominent visuospatial disturbance, and frontal dysfunction. Diagnosis can be difficult in early stages. One of my patients presented with the complaint of palinopsia and driving errors; rigidity and poor balance appeared over the next months.

Depression is present in 50%-70% of patients with Lewy body disease. REM sleep behavior disorder, Capgras syndrome (delusional misidentification), and myoclonus are more frequent than in Parkinson disease, while rest tremor is unusual.

Progressive Supranuclear Palsy (PSNP)

PSNP is characterized by vertical gaze apraxia, axial rigidity, dystonic dysarthria and a subcortical pattern of dementia. Apathy and depression are prominent; less often, obsessive behavior or disinhibition with bulimia, sexually inappropriate behavior, or aggressiveness occur. The cognitive inertia of PSNP is generally more severe than in Parkinson disease. These clinical signs reflect the accumulation of neurofibrillary tangles containing tau protein in basal ganglia, substantia nigra, midbrain oculomotor nuclei, upper pons, and dentate nucleus of the cerebellum. Despite evidence of dopaminergic hypoactivity in the basal ganglia and a diffuse cholinergic deficit throughout the brain, response to neurotransmitter replacement or augmentation therapy is minimal or absent due to degeneration of the post-synaptic receptors in PSNP.

Corticobasal Degeneration

Corticobasal degeneration presents with striking asymmetrical ideomotor apraxia (0), rigidity, dystonia, myoclonus and parietal cortical sensory loss. These signs eventually become bilateral. Uni- or bilateral pyramidal tract signs, oculomotor paralysis and pseudobulbar palsy occur in advanced stages. The alien limb phenomenon may also be seen.

A disproportionately severe dysexecutive syndrome is combined with signs of visuospatial disorientation, hemispatial neglect, or dysphasia. Apathy and depression are present in 75% of patients; irritability and agitation are common, while hallucinations and delusions are uncommon. Ballooned neurons containing tau-positive inclusions are found in the anterior cingulate and insular cortex, basal ganglia, substantia nigra, midbrain and upper brainstem monoaminergic nuclei, with relative sparing of hippocampus and thalamus.

Huntington's Chorea

Huntington's chorea results from an autosomal dominant expansion of the CAG trinucleotide sequence on the short arm of chromosome 4. Thirty-nine to 86 repeats (normal 6-34) confer a "gain of function" mutation associated with cytoplasmic accumulation of mutated huntingtin protein. Mutated huntingtin disrupts transcriptional regulation of several neurotrophic proteins, neurotransmitter receptors and intracellular signaling systems in the frontal cortex and basal ganglia. Clinically, Huntington's chorea presents with the triad of dementia, personality change, and chorea. Mood disorders, personality change and cognitive decline may precede chorea by a decade or longer. Personality change takes the form of irritability, anger, intermittent explosive disorder, antisocial behavior, mood lability, disinhibition, and apathy. Forty percent of patients are depressed; suicide occurs in 5%-10% of patients at a frequency 2 to 4 times the general population. A schizophreniform psychosis with delusions, auditory hallucinations and thought disorder occurs in 25% of patients. Cognitive deterioration occurs in all patients. A retrieval-type memory deficit appears early. Apathy with psychomotor slowing, executive system dysfunction and visuospatial impairment are prominent.

Tourette Syndrome and Obsessive Compulsive Disorder

The simple and complex motor and vocal tics of Gilles de Tourette syndrome overlap extensively with obsessive-compulsive disorder. Approximately 30% of individuals with Tourette syndrome have comorbid obsessive-compulsive disorder. Other comorbid conditions associated with Tourette syndrome include attention deficit disorder, conduct disorder, self-injurious behavior, explosive rage, substance abuse, anxiety and mood disorders. Subtle difficulties with visuomotor integration, impaired fine movements, and executive dysfunction are present in some individuals. Genetic studies of families show extensive genetic and phenotypic overlap between Tourette syndrome and obsessive compulsive disorder, both of which are believed to reflect imbalance between excitatory and inhibitory frontal-subcortical circuits and inefficient frontal modulation of motor activity and cognition.

Other Disorders

Other disorders of the basal ganglia and their subcortical connections characterized by motor, cognitive, and psychiatric symptoms include *Wilson disease; Fahr disease; olivopontocerebellar atrophy, striatonigral degeneration, Shy-Drager syndrome); dementia pugilistica ("punch-drunk syndrome"); catatonia; encephalitis lethargica; neuroacanthocytosis; carbon monoxide, manganese and cyanide poisoning*. Dyskinesia, choreiform movements, tremor and rigidity in neuroleptic-naïve schizophrenics attest to the involvement of the basal ganglia in the pathophysiology of *schizophrenia*.

Differential Diagnosis of Cognitive and Behavioral Changes Associated With Basal Ganglia Disorders

There is extensive clinical overlap among the motor signs and cognitive impairment shared by the disorders of the basal ganglia and their subcortical projections. The pattern, distribution, time course, and associated features (eg, extreme neuroleptic sensitivity and fluctuations in Lewy body dementia; limb apraxia in corticobasal degeneration) help with clinical diagnosis.

The mood and cognitive deficits of vascular depression overlap with endogenous depression. Apathy, irritability, disturbed sleep and appetite occur in both endogenous and secondary depression. However, disorientation, incontinence, and gait impairment are not present in endogenous depression, and should raise suspicion of secondary depression.

Development of extrapyramidal signs months to years after the diagnosis of depression suggests Parkinson or Lewy body disease.

Depression may precede clinical signs of Alzheimer disease by months to years. Up to 30% of Alzheimer patients also have extrapyramidal signs, most commonly rigidity and gait impairment.

Clinical Assessment of Disorders of the Basal Ganglia and Their Projections

Four features distinguish the cognitive impairment of subcortical disorders from the disturbance of "instrumental" functions (language, praxis, gnosis) in cortical disorders:

- the invariable presence of motor signs in subcortical disorders;
- prominent cognitive slowing, shown as increased latency to verbal response, generalized psychomotor inertia, poverty of affect and verbal output;
- deficient memory retrieval with preserved recognition;
- absence of signs of cortical dysfunction.

The presence of motor signs in a patient with cognitive impairment is a marker of subcortical neurological disease and an indication for neuroimaging.

Verbal fluency, combined with a mental concentration task (days of the week or months in reverse, mental alternation of letters and numbers) and the clock drawing task is a particularly helpful screen for the cognitive slowing and executive deficits of frontal-subcortical disorders.

Dubois et al described the "clapping sign" in PSNP. The patient is asked to clap their hands 3 times as quickly as possible. Patients with PSNP are unable to inhibit the tendency to clap 4 or 5 times, suggesting difficulty terminating an overlearned motor program.

Treatment of Disorders of the Basal Ganglia and Their Projections

Response of cognitive and behavioral features of Parkinson disease to dopamine supplementation and to cholinesterase inhibitors is variable. Optimization of the extrapyramidal disorder with levodopa or dopamine agonists may produce psychosis and confusion in patients with underlying cognitive impairment. Psychosis responds to reduction of the dopaminergic load combined with quetiapine in the range of 25 to 200 mg/day or clozapine 25 to 100 mg/day.

Lewy body disease responds poorly to levodopa. Amantadine combined with a cholinesterase inhibitor may produce dramatic functional improvement.

Antidepressant medication is the first-line treatment for primary or secondary depression. A stimulating antidepressant such as buproprion, fluoxetine or sertraline should be used if apathy and psychomotor slowing are present; if agitation, restlessness and sleep disturbance are present a sedating antidepressant such as fluvoxamine or mirtazepine is appropriate. Some Parkinson disease patients have a positive psychotropic response to selegeline.

Where the etiology of depression is in doubt, an empirical course of antidepressants or electroconvulsive therapy (ECT) may improve mood and expose the underlying cognitive impairment. Response to antidepressant medication is less robust in vascular than in endogenous depression, and prolonged post-ECT confusion is frequent.

A psychostimulant such as methylphenidate, low-dose amphetamine, or modafinil can be added to antidepressant medication to target apathy and cognitive inertia.

Psychostimulant medication may be combined with low-dose typical or atypical neuroleptics to treat comorbid attention deficit disorder and tics in Tourette syndrome. Recent research has established that methylphenidate and amphetamine do not exacerbate tics.

Tricyclic antidepressants should generally be avoided in the elderly patient because of potential anticholinergic worsening of cognition. However, judicious use of low-dose amitriptyline or nortriptyline may improve sleep and reduce hypersalivation in the parkinsonian patient.

D2 blocking agents such as haloperidol may decrease the chorea of Huntington disease, but may worsen cognitive impairment. Risperidone may be helpful. Agitation, aggression and anxiety respond to benzodiazepines, buspirone and lithium. Depression responds to antidepressant medications or ECT.

Dopamine blocking agents suppress tics in Tourette syndrome, while serotonin reuptake inhibitors are helpful for obsessions and compulsions in OCD.

4. The Temporal Lobes, Amnesia and Epilepsy

Overview

The temporal lobes contain a group of tightly interconnected structures which constitute the limbic system. Although its anatomical and functional boundaries are imprecise, the limbic system is generally considered to include the following structures:

- Core limbic structures: amygdala and hippocampus, situated in the mesial temporal lobes;
- Cortical limbic structures: insula, temporal poles, piriform cortex (the primary olfactory projection area) and entorhinal cortex;
- Subcortical limbic structures: hypothalamus; basal forebrain including ventral striatum, septal nuclei and nucleus accumbens; limbic nuclei of the thalamus (anterior nuclear group, dorsomedian, pulvinar, and midline nuclei).

The basic roles of the limbic system include: binding of new and previous experience into memories; integration of memory with basic drives (eg, hunger, sex) and autonomic responses; the orchestration of social and affiliative behavior; perception of smell, taste and pain.

The plasticity and interconnectivity of limbic structures, which are necessary for learning and memory, also confer vulnerability to kindling and to rapid spread of epileptic activity. Kindling refers to a gradual reduction in seizure threshold as a result of repeated subthreshold stimulation. The majority of focal epilepsies in the adult originate from limbic structures, principally hippocampus and amygdala.

Hippocampus, Memory and Amnesia

Memory refers to the capacity to store and retrieve information. Memory is classified into declarative and procedural types. *Declarative* (*synonym: explicit*) memory includes *semantic* (*synonym: verbal*) memory (recall of facts and events), and *episodic* (*synonym: autobiographical*) memory. *Procedural* (*synonym: implicit*) memory refers to the acquisition of motor skills and habits outside conscious awareness, eg, learning to play the piano, to ski, or to drive.

The process of memory acquisition involves encoding, ie, the laying down of a memory trace; and *consolidation*, ie, the process whereby the newly-acquired memory trace is committed to long-term storage within distributed neural networks ("engrams") in association cortices.

The hippocampus (*Gr: seahorse*) is crucial for both the encoding and consolidation of declarative memory. Subcellular events underlying memory consolidation include release of glutamate, protein synthesis, and the formation of new synapses. In contrast to the role of the hippocampus in declarative memory, acquisition of procedural memory involves basal ganglia and cerebellum.

The frontal lobes and amygdala also participate in the acquisition of declarative memory. Working memory holds the memory trace "on line" to enable further processing within the hippocampus. Reciprocal connections between hippocampus and amygdala enable the amygdala to modulate hippocampal activity during the encoding of emotional events. Noradrenaline seems to be a crucial neurotransmitter in the enhancement of affect-laden memories. We have all had the experience of vividly remembering emotional events, such as weddings or car accidents. Preferential recall of salient events with potential impact on survival allows prediction and mental modeling of future similar events.

Retrieval of consolidated memories requires the integrity of hippocampus and prefrontal cortex. The prefrontal contribution is the activation and selection of information. The hippocampi coordinate retrieval of engrams. Retrieval of semantic memories activates the left lateral temporal cortex. The right prefrontal cortex and temporal pole are specialized for the retrieval of episodic and spatial memories.

Unilateral removal or destruction of the hippocampus is without major clinical repercussions provided the other side is intact. Bilateral hippocampal destruction causes severe and permanent anterograde amnesia with sparing of procedural memory, as in the famous case of H.M. described by Scoville and Milner in 1957 following temporal lobectomy for intractable epilepsy (see References).

Major Afferents and Efferents of the Hippocampus

Afferents to hippocampus from all areas of association cortex converge on the entorhinal cortex; perforant fibers from the entorhinal cortex form synapses with the dentate gyrus and pyramidal neurons of the hippocampus.

Papez circuit is the major hippocampal outflow, which forms the fornix. The fornix bundle arches over the thalamus to synapse in the mammillary bodies of the hypothalamus. The mammillothalamic tract is a further projection from the mammillary bodies to the anterior thalamic nuclei. Other collaterals of the fornix terminate in the anterior cingulate gyrus and septal nuclei in the basal forebrain. Reciprocal connections from the cingulate re-enter the hippocampus via the entorhinal cortex. A lesion anywhere in Papez circuit can produce an amnestic deficit.

Clinical Signs of Memory Dysfunction

Anterograde Amnesia (Table 2)

Anterograde amnesia is a disruption of semantic memory resulting in the inability to form new memories. Procedural memory is typically intact.

Confabulation is common in amnestic disorders, presumably to compensate for mnemonic lacunae. More fantastic and implausible stories are associated with signs of frontal impairment.

Retrograde Amnesia

Retrograde amnesia is a permanent loss of previously-acquired semantic or autobiographical information (eg, the date of Christmas or one's anniversary) or inability to access such information. The latter is seen frontal lobe impairment, and can be improved with cueing.

Lesions Associated With Amnesia

Alzheimer Disease

Amnesia is the most common early sign of Alzheimer disease, related to accumulation of plaques and tangles in mesial temporal lobe structures. Minimal cognitive impairment (MCI) is diagnosed if cognitive testing shows only isolated memory impairment. Patients with MCI convert to Alzheimer disease at a rate of 15% per year. Serial mental status examinations may show stable memory impairment for several years, followed by progressive deterioration of other higher cortical functions compatible with Alzheimer disease. Recent studies suggest that early use of anticholinesterase inhibitors may retard the conversion of MCI to Alzheimer disease

Post-traumatic Amnesia

PTA is nearly universal following concussion and other major head injury. PTA is the most common cause of amnesia in clinical practice. Mesial temporal structures are vulnerable to contusion and

Table 2

Psychogenic Amnesia versus Transient Global Amnesia

Psychogenic Amnesia	Transient Global Amnesia
Loss of personal identity	Personal identity retained
Anterograde memory intact	Anterograde memory impaired
Memory loss selective (eg, personal identity, relatives, specific events or period of time)	Memory loss not selective
No temporal gradient	Temporal gradient (anterograde > retrograde)
Associated depression and anxiety	Emotional factors not prominent
Lack of emotional concern with amnesia	Distress and repeated queries common
Incidence highest 20s to 40s	Incidence highest 50s to 70s

compression against the tentorium of the dura. Retrograde amnesia includes the moment of impact and several minutes to several years previously. Anterograde amnesia disrupts learning and memory consolidation. As the amnesia recedes, the patient is left with a mnemonic lacune for the impact and surrounding events. The duration of anterograde and retrograde amnesia is inversely correlated with cognitive outcome following head injury.

Epilepsy Involving Memory

Seizure discharges arising from the hippocampus can cause illusions of familiarity (*déjà vu*), illusions of unfamiliarity (*jamais vu*) and sudden vivid memories often accompanied by an associated affect which reflects amygdala activation.

Transient Global Amnesia (TGA)

TGA is characterized by dense anterograde amnesia and variable retrograde amnesia lasting 1 to 24 hours. Personal identity is retained, in contrast to psychogenic amnesia. Unlike psychogenic amnesia patients, TGA patients are distressed by their memory loss; repeated queries are characteristic. Onset is usually between 50 and 70 years. Triggers reported in some cases include exposure to cold water, sexual intercourse, physical exertion, emotional stress, pain, and Valsalva maneuver. A history of migraine or risk factors for cerebrovascular disease may be present. Bilateral ischemia of mesial temporal structures has been demonstrated in a few cases. The neurobehavioral history (Table 2) may reveal preceding head injury or a history of metabolic disturbance, substance abuse or withdrawal to suggest a toxic-metabolic confusional state. EEG and neuroimaging should always be obtained to rule out partial complex seizures, herpes encephalitis or tumor.

Wernicke-Korsakoff Syndrome

A history of alcohol abuse and malnutrition is present in most cases. The acute illness is characterized by delirium, nystagmus, oculomotor paresis and ataxia; peripheral neuropathy is frequent. Supplementation with thiamine may salvage cerebral function in some cases. After 3-6 months 2/3 of patients show signs of Korsakoff syndrome, characterized by a severe anterograde amnesia, confabulation and an apathetic frontal syndrome which contrasts with the bizarre and fantastic content of the confabulations. Retrograde amnesia frequently extends over several years to several decades.

Anoxia and Hypoglycemia

The hippocampi are vulnerable to cerebral anoxia and hypoglycemia because of their high metabolic requirements. Post-anoxic amnesia is supported by history of cardiopulmonary arrest, and may be accompanied by other signs of cortical impairment.

Herpes Simplex Encephalitis

The herpes simplex virus type I has an affinity for limbic structures, including the hippocampus, amygdala, and orbitofrontal cortex. The diagnosis is supported by a history of fever, headache, seizures, obtundation and nuchal rigidity with a lymphocytic CSF pleocytosis. Although amnesia is the most common sequela of herpes simplex encephalitis, other signs of temporal lobe dysfunction may also be present, such as epilepsy, Klüver-Bucy syndrome , aphasia or visuospatial impairment.

Psychogenic Amnesia

Psychogenic amnesia (PA) is classified as a dissociative disorder. Onset may be sudden, triggered by an emotionally charged situation. The distinguishing feature is amnesia for personal identity (e.g., name, address, family members, or a specific period of time). Memory loss may also be selective for emotionally charged information such as the whereabouts of one's spouse. Depression and anxiety are frequent, but their presence should not obviate a thorough investigation for other causes of amnesia. Malingering should also be suspected. Psychogenic amnesia usually lasts 24 to 48 hours, although dissociative fugue states may last several weeks. Differences between PA and transient global amnesia are shown in Table 5. Although the pathophysiology of PA is not fully known, PA is no less a brain-based disorder than transient global amnesia, and the diagnosis of PA should not lead to the spurious distinction between organic and psychiatric disorders.

Other Disorders

Other causes of amnesia include: infarction of the anterior choroidal or posterior temporal artery; temporal lobectomy; primary or secondary neoplasm involving the hippocampi or fornix; paraneoplastic encephalitis; electroconvulsive therapy.

Differential Diagnosis of Amnesia

Patients with hippocampal damage have impaired recall of words and figures and sometimes also of the task, reflecting impairment in encoding and consolidation. Performance does not improve with cueing. In contrast, the performance of patients with amnesia related to dysfunction of frontal and frontal-subcortical circuits improves when the patient is presented with a category cue or a multiple choice enabling recognition of the previously learned item.

Clinical Assessment of Memory

It is important to ascertain attention before testing memory to make sure that the patient has sufficient attentional resources to encode the stimulus, since encoding is necessary for memory acquisition. Aphasia and motivational state also influence verbal memory ability.

To test verbal memory present a list of words slowly, around 1 word a second. Most patients can remember a list of words equal to their forward digit span minus one. If forward digit span is 6, the patient should be able to remember a list of 5 words. Instruct the patient to repeat the list when you have finished. Record the number of trials until all the words are repeated. Normally, retention improves with repetition; a flat learning curve suggests deficient attention. Inform the patient that you will ask them to recall the list in 5 to 10 minutes. If recall is deficient, give a category cue (eg, "the name of a color"). If a category cue is insufficient, ask the patient to select the correct word from a multiple choice ("red, blue, or green").

Test visual memory by having the patient copy a series of shapes or the abridged Rey figure (Appendix 2). Patients with defective visual memory may copy the figure adequately but be unable to reproduce it accurately after 5 minutes. Patients with dysfunction of the non-dominant parietal lobe may show distortions or omissions on the copying task but preserved memory on delayed recall.

Treatment of Amnesia

Therapy of memory dysfunction depends on accurate diagnosis and correction of the underlying cause. Cognitive strategies for the treatment of amnesia should be tailored to the individual patient's needs and combined with environmental adaptation. Helpful strategies include writing down appointments, daily events, and messages, use of an agenda, written reminders, and association of new information with old memories. Repetition is helpful when memory loss is not severe (eg, "Today is Thursday, December 2"). The indications for acetylcholinesterase inhibitors (donepezil, rivastigmine and galantamine) beyond Alzheimer disease are presently being explored.

Amygdala, Mood and Affect

The amygdala is a collection of mesial temporal nuclei, which play a critical role in the channeling of drive and affect. The amygdala responds within 100 to 200 milliseconds to emotionally salient stimuli, even before conscious recognition occurs. Through its multiple connections with other limbic structures, orbitofrontal and cingulate cortex, sensory association cortex and hypothalamus, the amygdala engages the neural circuitry for the emotional coloring of perception, memory and experience and associated autonomic reactions.

The amygdala projects reciprocally to the ventral striatum and thalamic dorsomedian nucleus This limbic—ventral striatal circuit parallels the frontal—striatal—thalamic—frontal loops.

The major dopaminergic input in the limbic—ventral striatal ("mesolimbic") circuit arises from the ventral tegmental nucleus adjacent to the substantia nigra in the midbrain. Dopaminergic activity in the mesolimbic circuit is linked to the expectation and experience of reward and to the initiation of goal-directed behavior. Cocaine, amphetamine and other substances of abuse induce marked release of dopamine in the nucleus accumbens. Abnormal dopaminergic activity in the mesolimbic circuit is associated with psychosis, and this pathway is a major target of neuroleptic medication.

Noradrenergic inputs to the amygdala arising from the locus ceruleus in the rostral pons facilitate the acquisition and retention of emotionally relevant experience.

Clinical Signs of Amygdala Dysfunction

Epilepsy

Epileptic discharges originating in the temporal lobes may be associated with paroxysmal dread, panic or sudden rage. Directed aggression is, however, rare during temporal lobe seizures. Experiential ictal phenomena include memory flashbacks, visual and auditory hallucinations, vertigo, or the sense of an unseen presence. Epilepsy arising at the temporal, parietal, and occipital junction has been linked to out-of-body experiences and to "autoscopy," the hallucinated vision of one's own body seen from without. Autonomic ictal phenomena include gustatory and olfactory hallucinations, often of an unpleasant nature; nausea; epigastric sensations; abdominal pain; flushing; salivation; heaviness in the chest; tachycardia or palpitations; sexual and urinary sensations. Complex psychiatric phenomena include episodic psychosis, a beclouded confusional state resembling delirium, and (rarely) paroxysmal aggression.

Epileptic phenomena are usually abrupt in onset and offset, brief (seconds to minutes), spontaneous, and stereotyped. The surface EEG may be normal when the seizure originates in mesial temporal lobes and basal forebrain. Telemetry monitoring and depth electrode recordings should be considered in all cases where epilepsy is suspected but not confirmed by conventional surface EEG. Response to an empirical trial of anticonvulsant medication may corroborate the clinical suspicion of epilepsy.

Interictal Personality Disorder of Geschwind

The major symptoms of this controversial entity include: deepened emotionality, philosophical, religious and occult preoccupations, sense of personal destiny, humorlessness, irritability, hypergraphia, hyposexuality, circumstantiality, and social viscosity (a tendency to prolong social encounters beyond reasonable limits). The author Fyodor Dostoyevsky, and the painter Vincent van Gogh, both epileptic, are often cited as examples. In practice, it is unusual to find all elements present in the same patient. The incidence among the epileptic population is unknown, since studies and case reports tend to come from academic centers not necessarily representative of the community-dwelling epileptic population. Although elements of the interictal personality disorder may also be present in persons with other neurological and psychiatric disorders, the presence of these features, particularly hypergraphia, should prompt a search for temporal lobe pathology. The pathophysiology may reflect enhancement of affective-cognitive associations related to altered limbic activity.

Postictal Psychosis

Following a flurry of seizures, a "lucid interval" lasting several days gives way to disorientation, insomnia, anxiety, dysphoria, delusions, and hallucinations. The sensorium may be clear or altered, leading to suspicion of non-convulsive status epilepticus or a toxic delirium, but no metabolic cause or anticonvulsant toxicity can be identified. The EEG is normal in 50% of patients; in the remainder, EEG is epileptiform or diffusely slow. Post-ictal psychosis typically lasts days to several months, may resolve spontaneously, and may recur in one-third of patients. There is often a history of refractory epilepsy. Pathophysiology is felt to reflect post-ictal inhibitory mechanisms involved in seizure suppression, possibly involving sensitization of limbic dopamine receptors. Treatment is with low-dose neuroleptics and benzodiazepines in addition to the usual anticonvulsant regimen.

Interictal Psychosis of Epilepsy

A chronic or episodic schizophreniform psychosis occurs in 10%-15% of patients with temporal lobe epilepsy, usually after an average interval of 14 years. Distinction from primary schizophrenia relies on the following factors: low frequency of formal thought disorder and negative symptoms; a more variable course with periods of remission, and encapsulation of the psychotic symptoms.

Risk factors for chronic interictal psychosis include earlier age at onset of epilepsy, borderline intellectual functioning, and family history of psychosis.

Lateralization of the seizure focus has not been consistently associated with risk of interictal psychosis.

Conventional treatment of interictal psychosis is with neuroleptics. Chlorpromazine, loxapine and clozapine are the most likely to lower seizure threshold. Blumer has emphasized the dysphoric aspect of interictal psychosis of epilepsy, which may respond to combined tricyclic and selective serotonin reuptake inhibitors.

Klüver-Bucy Syndrome

Klüver-Bucy syndrome was originally produced in monkeys following bilateral surgical ablation of the amygdalae. Features: indiscriminate sexual activity; oral exploration of inedible objects; placidity; "hypermetamorphosis" (excessive attention to visual stimuli); and visual agnosia ("psychic blindness"). These elements are all related to inability to distinguish between motivationally relevant and irrelevant stimuli. In the human, emotional indifference and hyperphagia are common. Aphasia, amnesia, or dementia are associated in most cases. Etiologies include herpes simplex encephalitis, frontotemporal dementia, tumor, head trauma, and cerebral anoxia.

Post-traumatic Stress Disorder

Features: Persistent re-experiencing of a traumatic event in the form of flashbacks, hypervigilance, disturbed sleep, avoidance of trauma-associated stimuli, and generalized emotional numbing. Intense activation of the amygdala during the traumatic event causes pathological enhancement ("overconsolidation") of the traumatic memory, which is subsequently re-experienced, both spontaneously and in response to minor environmental stimuli. Functional imaging shows persistent hypermetabolism of the amygdala in the resting state as well as hypometabolism of orbitofrontal and cingulate cortex involved in the regulation of conditioned fear. The recognition of the role of noradrenergic activity in the basolateral amygdala in the consolidation of emotional memory has led to promising research on the use of propranolol in the aftermath of the traumatic event.

Intermittent Explosive Disorder

Features: Sudden attacks of explosive, destructive rage occurring after minimal or no obvious provocation occur in intermittent explosive disorder and with a variety of brain lesions interfering with behavioral control: mental retardation, intoxication, injury to the orbitofrontal cortex. Directed aggression is uncommon in temporal lobe epilepsy. It is more likely to occur in the post-ictal period if the confused patient is forcibly restrained. The neurobiology of IED is probably related to release of amygdalo-hypothalamic pathways from inhibitory modulation with consequent display of an innate rage response. IED symptoms may respond to sodium valproate or selective serotonin reuptake inhibitors.

Panic

The intense fear, dizziness, chest tightness, trembling, paresthesias and derealization associated with a panic attack can resemble a partial complex seizure. Activation of hippocampus and amygdala is common to both disorders. Where diagnosis is in doubt, video telemetry monitoring of an attack or an empirical trial of anticonvulsant medication may be helpful.

Organic Delusional Syndromes

Capgras syndrome is the delusion that close others have been replaced with identical-appearing imposters. In reduplicative paramnesia the patient believes they are simultaneously present in two different places. They may claim that their present location has two different names or that they are next to one another. Capgras syndrome and reduplicative paramnesia are most common after traumatic brain injury. Dementing disorders, tumors, stroke and toxic confusional states are other causes. These delusional syndromes reflect a mismatch between perception and affect, in which the perception of a familiar person or a place is not associated with a feeling of familiarity, leading to a profound sense of estrangement.

5. The Left Hemisphere, Aphasia and Apraxia

Overview

Aphasia is a disturbance of linguistic processing resulting from an inability to translate speech sounds, printed words and thoughts into words and sentences. Aphasia is distinct from word deafness, from dysarthria, and from the disordered thinking of schizophrenia. In addition to verbal communication, aphasia also disrupts other cognitive processes which depend on language, such as the ability to calculate and to reason. Here the term aphasia is used to include less severe or partial disorders of language (dysphasia).

Apraxia is a disruption of the production of complex learned skills or gestures not caused by weakness, loss of sensation, or inability to understand the request. Apraxia is more common after left than after right hemisphere injury, reflecting the role of the left hemisphere in the programming and control of complex sequential movements involving both sides of the body.

Major Afferents and Efferents

In 99% of right-handed individuals, and approximately two-thirds of left-handed individuals, the brain speech centers are in the left hemisphere; in the remainder of left-handed individuals language functions are bilateral.

Cortical speech centers: Broca's area in the left inferior frontal gyrus; and Wernicke's area in the posterior third of the superior temporal gyrus. Broca's and Wernicke's areas are connected by a band of white matter, the arcuate fasciculus (Figure 3).

The superior temporal gyrus contains primary auditory cortex lying in Heschl's gyrus. This region is contiguous with Wernicke's area, where meaning is extracted from speech sounds and visual symbols.

Apraxia results from disruption of a left hemispheric network involving the inferior parietal lobule and the motor and supplementary motor cortex. The parietal area integrates visual, auditory and somesthetic information to encode a sensory representation of the intended movement; the frontal cortex encodes a motor plan of the intended movement. The motor plan is transferred to the right hemisphere via the corpus callosum. Disconnection of the sensory and conceptual representation of a movement from anterior motor pathways results in apraxia.

Figure 3

Speech cortex

Patients with transcortical sensory aphasia are capable of repeating words they hear but cannot understand. This may be mediated by the direct connection between Wernicke's and Broca's areas. This aphasia is caused by damage to the posterior language area. Wernicke's aphasia, the loss of comprehension of spoken language, loss of ability to read (silently) and write, and distortion of articulate speech, is caused by damage to both Broca's and Wernicke's areas.

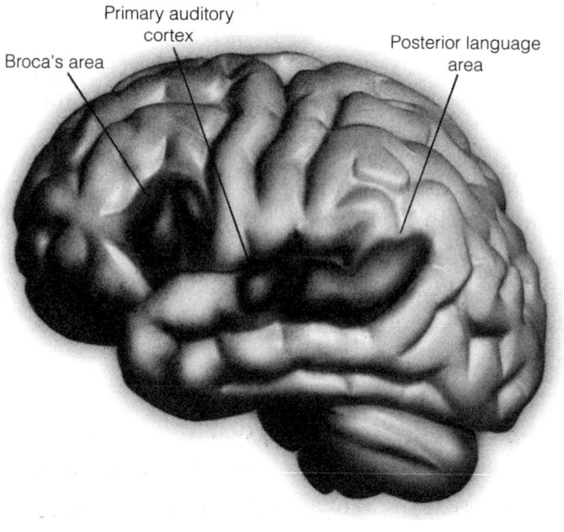

Clinical Signs: Aphasia (Figure 4 and Appendix 4)

Broca's Aphasia (Synonyms: Expressive Aphasia; Motor Aphasia)

Speech is slow, effortful, telegraphic, non-fluent, dysarthric and agrammatical with numerous word-finding pauses. Naming of nouns is better preserved than verbs and conjunctions (and, or, if, but). Comprehension is intact, although sophisticated testing shows subtle difficulties understanding passive voice and complex syntax. Repetition, naming, and writing are impaired.

Associated abnormalities: Right face and arm paresis and apraxia of voluntary facial movements.

Wernicke's Aphasia (Synonyms: Receptive Aphasia; Sensory Aphasia; Jargonophasia)

Damage to Wernicke's area disrupts the decoding and translation of auditory and visual symbols into language. Speech is fluent or accelerated and well articulated, but numerous paraphasic errors and neologisms, of which the patient is unaware, may render speech unintelligible. Paraphasias may be *semantic* (substitution of one word for another (eg, "ring" for "comb"), or *phonemic* (substitution of an unintended sound into a word, eg, "trable" for "table"). Naming, comprehension and repetition are impaired.

Associated abnormalities: If the lesion is confined to Wernicke's area there may be no associated facial or limb paresis, but a right superior quadrantanopia and disruption of cortical sensation such as graphesthesia, two-point discrimination, and stereognosis are common.

Conduction Aphasia

The responsible lesion involves the left parieto-temporal cortex and subadjacent arcuate fasciculus, disconnecting Broca's area anteriorly from Wernicke's area posteriorly. Comprehension is intact, but naming and repetition are impaired, with multiple phonemic paraphasias.

Associated abnormalities: Right facial weakness is usually present.

Global Aphasia

Global aphasia is the result of an extensive lesion in the left hemisphere. All aspects of language production are impaired, including naming, comprehension, repetition, reading, and writing. A few stereotyped words or phrases may be used propositionally, eg, "yes-yes-yes." Overlearned, automatic sequences such as the alphabet, nursery rhymes, prayers, and the ability to sing and to swear may be preserved. The ability to respond to whole-body commands such as "Sit up!" is said to be intact, although I have never observed this phenomenon.

Global aphasia may be present at the outset of a large left middle cerebral artery stroke, later evolving into a Broca's, Wernicke's, or conduction aphasia, depending on the major site of infarction.

Associated abnormalities: Right hemiparesis, hemianopia, and a sensory deficit are invariably present.

Transcortical Aphasia

Transcortical aphasia is distinguished from Broca's, Wernicke's, conduction and global aphasia by preservation of the capacity to repeat.

The lesion causing *transcortical motor aphasia* involves the supplementary motor area and frontal cortex adjacent to Broca's area. Speech is non-fluent and naming is impaired; repetition is intact.

The lesion causing *transcortical sensory aphasia* involves the temporal or parietal cortex adjacent to Wernicke's area. Speech is fluent and comprehension is impaired; repetition is intact.

Alexia Without Aphasia (Synonym: Word Blindness) (Table 6)

A lesion in the left occipital cortex and splenium of the corpus callosum disconnects the decoding of visual word forms from Wernicke's area and associated components of the language network. Patients are able to write and can understand words spelled out loud or written on their palm but are unable to read their own written words. Associated abnormalities: right homonymous hemianopia; achromatopsia (rare).

Word Deafness

Word deafness is caused by a lesion of Heschl's gyrus, which disconnects primary auditory cortex from the language network. The ability to recognize spoken language is lost in the absence of any other language deficit. In contrast, auditory agnosia is the inability to recognize environmental non-verbal sounds. Cortical deafness includes both word deafness and auditory agnosia. These patients are unable to recognize any sounds despite normal hearing.

Figure 4

Classification of the aphasias

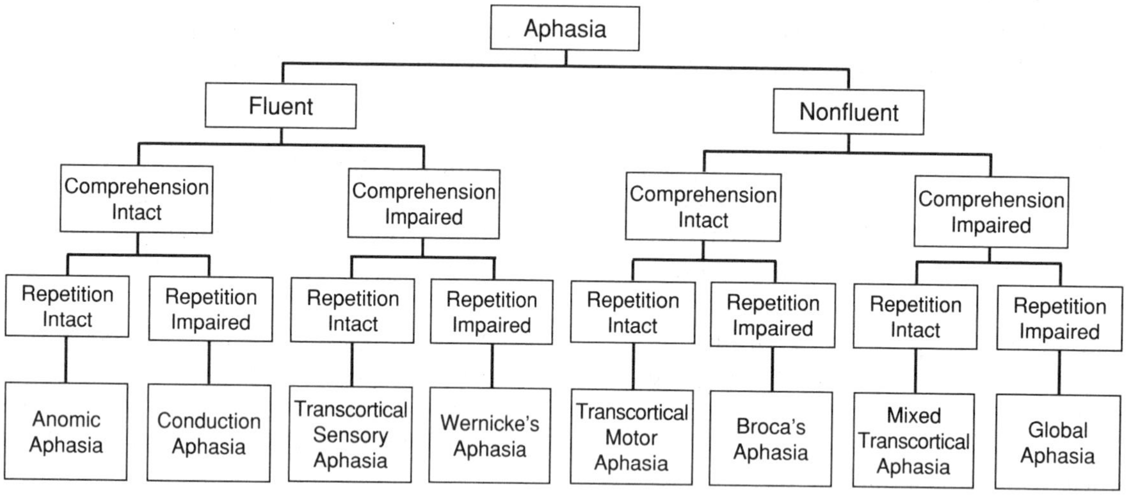

Gerstmann Syndrome

Features: Agraphia; acalculia; finger agnosia (inability to recognize and name individual fingers); right-left confusion. The responsible lesion involves the left angular gyrus adjacent to Wernicke's area (Appendix 4). Some degree of aphasia is usually present.

Subcortical Aphasia

Aphasia with lesions of the thalamus and basal ganglia closely resembles transcortical sensory aphasia. Dysarthria, impaired speech initiation, right hemiparesis and right motor neglect are frequent. Motor neglect refers to underuse of one side in the absence of paresis or sensory impairment; clinically seen as a disinclination to use the affected limbs (Appendix 4).

Clinical Signs: Apraxia (Appendix 4)

Following the conception of Leipmann in the early 1900s, apraxia is divided into three major types: ideational, ideomotor, and limb kinetic apraxias. In practice, the distinction between these types may be problematic.

Ideational Apraxia (Synonym: Conceptual Apraxia)

Loss of the conceptual linkage between tools and their uses and disruption of functional sequences. For example, patients may try to eat soup with a fork or brush their teeth without putting toothpaste on the brush. When asked to show how to use a hammer, patients may make the movements for writing. Alzheimer disease is the most common cause of ideational apraxia.

Ideomotor Apraxia

The inability to execute voluntary movements which can be performed spontaneously, eg, waving good-bye, whistling, lighting a match. Spatial, temporal and sequencing errors cause distortion and disruption of transitive (involving tools) and intransitive (without tools) actions on both sides of the body.

Apraxia of facial movements is a variant of ideomotor apraxia. The responsible lesion involves the face area of the left motor cortex. Broca's aphasia is usually present.

Limb Kinetic Apraxia

Loss of the "kinetic melody" of learned movement patterns. Skilled voluntary movements, particularly those involving the hands and individual fingers, appear clumsy, effortful, faltering and unpracticed.

Other Types of Apraxia

Callosal apraxia. A lesion of the corpus callosum, Broca's area or left motor cortex and deep underlying white matter disrupts transfer of the movement plan elaborated in the left hemisphere to the right motor cortex. Pantomime to command, imitation, and object use are intact on the right but apraxic in the left extremities. Broca's aphasia and right hemiparesis are usually present.

Constructional apraxia. Disruption of spatial orientation reflected in distortion of drawing or block assembly and difficulty navigating in three-dimensional space. Sometimes associated with dressing apraxia, constructional and dressing apraxias are not apraxias in the strict sense, but reflect disturbance of spatial and body representation as a result of a lesion in the right (non-dominant) parietal lobe (Appendix 4).

Gait apraxia. Apraxia of walking is the characteristic motor signature of normal pressure hydrocephalus and multi-infarct dementia. Agility and coordination are intact when the patient is tested in the supine position. While standing, the patient's feet appear to be stuck to the floor (thus the term "magnetic gait"); steps are short and faltering and balance impaired. Movement sequences such as foot tapping, stepping up on a stool and turning are particularly difficult. In distinction to Parkinson disease, the upper body is typically spared in gait apraxia.

Lesions Causing Aphasia and Apraxia

Responsible lesions include:

Head injury; stroke or a transient ischemic attack involving branches of the middle cerebral artery. The left posterior cerebral artery is involved in alexia without aphasia. Epilepsy originating from left hemisphere language areas is associated with speech arrest, forced thinking, palilalia, stuttering, verbal automatisms such as moaning or repeating a word or phrase, and aphasia. Primary or secondary brain tumors, migraine aura, and degenerative dementias are also associated with aphasia and apraxia. Primary progressive aphasia is a variant of Pick disease in which there is an insidious and progressive aphasia sparing other cognitive functions. Alzheimer pathology or focal spongiform degeneration are less common causes of primary progressive aphasia. Unilateral ideomotor and limb kinetic apraxia is a common presenting feature of corticobasal degeneration.

Differential Diagnosis of Aphasia

Careful bedside examination of language is essential to distinguish aphasia from dysarthria, especially since both may be simultaneously present.

Aphasia may be mistaken for confusion, especially if semantic paraphasia causes the patient to respond "February" instead of "April," or if phonemic paraphasia causes garbed, unintelligible speech. Examination may show paraphasias, word-finding difficulties and focal neurological deficits in the aphasic patient, and attentional impairment and disorientation in the confused patient.

In the absence of "positive" epileptic signs such as facial or limb clonus, epileptic speech disruption may resemble a transient ischemic attack. Epileptic activity on EEG and a positive response to intravenous lorazepam or diazepam help establish the diagnosis of epilepsy.

Differential Diagnosis of Apraxia

Aphasia and elementary disorders of movement and sensation must be ruled out before apraxia is diagnosed. Visual agnosia may resemble apraxia if it causes the patient to select the wrong tool for the task. If the patient can name the tool after visual inspection, visual agnosia is unlikely.

Limb kinetic apraxia, which is most clearly seen in the distal extremities, should not be confused with the gross, oscillatory tremor of the trunk and proximal extremities in cerebellar disorders.

Clinical Assessment of Aphasia

The presence of aphasia in a right-handed person invariably implies a lesion involving the left cerebral hemisphere. Lesion localization is less precise when aphasia occurs in a left-handed person.

Aphasia limits conclusions about cognitive impairment based on clinical cognitive assessment because of the linguistic demands of most tasks. Language should therefore be assessed early in the clinical cognitive examination.

Examination of language includes the following components:

Observe spontaneous speech for fluency, latency to initiate speech, word-finding pauses, paraphasias, syntax, prosody (speech melody and rhythm), paraphasias, articulation, and content. Automatic speech may be preserved, even when propositional speech is severely affected.

Test naming of common objects (eg, spoon) and less common objects (eg, paper clip). Include different categories such as colors, actions, and body parts. Anomia is common to all aphasias, but can also occur in toxic-confusional states and frontal-subcortical disorders where access to the verbal lexicon is slowed. Observe for semantic and phonemic paraphasias and circumlocutions. If the patient is unable to provide the correct name, check for comprehension by asking them to mime its function. In visual agnosia, the patient may not be able to name an object presented in the visual modality but is able to provide the correct name after being allowed to touch the object.

Comprehension is closely dependent on attention. Use simple one-step verbal commands, followed by 2- and then 3-step commands and complex sentences. Also test comprehension of written commands.

To test repetition, begin with short and simple phrases and proceed to longer, complex sentences. Repetition span (the number of words correctly repeated) is usually one word longer than digit span. Conduction aphasia, impaired attention, and hearing all decrease the ability to repeat.

Reading is evaluated for individual letters, words, and whole sentences. I ask the patient to read a large-print paragraph from a magazine, then summarize it. Reading ability varies with educational level. Make sure that the patient is wearing eyeglasses and that illumination is adequate.

Test spontaneous sentence writing and writing to dictation. Like reading, writing depends on educational level. Writing is impaired in aphasia and in motor disorders interfering with coordination. Writing on the far right of the page may provide an important cue to the presence of left hemispatial neglect.

Verbal fluency is discussed in Section 1, Clinical Assessment of Frontal Disorders.

Assess calculation, right-left orientation, and finger recognition. Ask the patient to identify individual fingers of their own and the examiner's hands. Gerstmann syndrome is present if agraphia is also present, although elements of Gerstmann syndrome may occur separately. Assess addition, subtraction, multiplication and division with paper and pencil problems commensurate with educational level. I assess right-left orientation by crossing my arms, asking the patient to identify my right or left hand. A simpler variant is without crossing, or asking the patient to identify their own right or left hands.

Clinical Assessment of Ideational, Ideomotor and Limb Kinetic Apraxia

An approach to the diagnosis of apraxia includes the following:

Observe spontaneous behavior during common tasks (eg, washing, shaving, writing, eating).

Ask the patient to produce movements to command. Movements should include simple tasks (eg, picking up a utensil) and complex sequences (eg, squeeze toothpaste onto toothbrush and brush teeth; open a bottle and pour liquid into a glass; take a pipe out of the pocket, light it and smoke it).

Include movements of the face (whistle, wink, pucker lips; puff out cheeks; drink through a straw), as well as sequences that do not involve use of tools (blow a kiss; salute; sign of the cross; wave goodbye).

The movements should be carried out with actual tools and to pantomime. Pantomime is more difficult since it requires a mental formulation of the task. "Substitution of body part for object" refers to the inability to separate pantomime from actual tool use, so that the patient, asked to imitate combing their hair, touches their head with their hand, implying defective activation of motor programs.

If there are errors in tool use and pantomime, the patient is asked to imitate the examiner performing the task.

Make sure the patient understands the task by asking them to choose thc correct task among several performed by the examiner.

Note organization, orientation of hand to tool, fluency and sequencing. Test each side separately.

Treatment of Aphasia and Apraxia

Speech and language therapy for aphasia and occupational therapy for apraxia are cornerstones of treatment. Early initiation of therapy is correlated with better outcome.

Left anterior lesions are highly correlated with depression, which should be routinely suspected and treated.

Dopaminergic and cholinergic augmentation combined with speech and language therapy have been reported to be helpful in small series of patients with motor aphasia.

Prognosis for recovery is related to the nature of underlying lesion, age, and severity of impairment.

6. The Right Hemisphere, Attention, and Spatial Orientation

Overview

The right hemisphere in right-handed individuals is specialized for spatial attention to both sides of intra- and extrapersonal space. In contrast, the spatial attentional functions of the left hemisphere direct attention primarily to contralateral (right) hemispace. Although the right hemisphere is dominant for spatial attention in most right-handed individuals, in left-handed individuals crossed or mixed dominance is more likely.

The right hemisphere is also specialized for the interpretation and expression of non-verbal communication. The non-verbal, "paralinguistic" aspects of language include speech prosody and associated facial expression and gestures. Prosody refers to variations in the pitch, emphasis, timing and volume of speech. Consider the differences between a disk jockey broadcasting on a rock station, a parent reading a bedtime story to their 3-year-old, and the robotic tones of a voice synthesizer. The paralinguistic elements of language convey crucial meaning beyond vocabulary, grammar and syntax. Expressive prosody is an anterior right hemisphere function, while receptive prosody, the ability to comprehend meaning through speech melody, resides in the posterior right hemisphere. The organization of the non-verbal aspects of language in the right hemisphere thus parallels Broca's and Wernicke's speech centers in the left hemisphere. People with Asperger syndrome and acquired right hemisphere disorders resulting in loss of proficiency in the non-verbal aspects of communication are at a major social disadvantage. The clinician examining a patient with right hemisphere damage should not infer the affective state of the patient without considering the possibility that dysprosody may disrupt the patient's ability to communicate their emotional state effectively. (For further reading on aprosodia and non-verbal aspects of communication, see the chapter by Ross in References.)

Major Afferents and Efferents

The neural network for spatial attention consists of multiple densely connected nodes.

The *brainstem reticular activating system* mediates

arousal via connections with intralaminar and midline thalamic nuclei and the thalamocortical relay system. The midline thalamus projects to the anterior cingulate, a frontal area critically involved in motivation. Direct brainstem-neocortical pathways bypassing the thalamus include a dopaminergic projection from substantia nigra/ventral tegmentum, a serotonergic projection from the raphe nuclei, and a noradrenergic projection from the locus coeruleus. The neocortex also receives a dense cholinergic projection from the nucleus basalis of Meynert in the basal forebrain. Descending inhibitory signals from all areas of neocortex modulate the strength of the arousal response; in this way, repeated exposure to a novel stimulus produces habituation.

The *right prefrontal and posterior parietal cortex* exert "top down" control of attention to select and manipulate specific aspects of the environment while ignoring irrelevant stimuli. The right parietal cortex contains neurons which integrate the sensory and kinetic aspects of a stimulus, such as gazing and reaching toward a specific food object. The right frontal eye fields and inferior frontal lobe coordinate orienting and exploratory movements of the eyes, head and limbs.

The *amygdala and anterior cingulate cortex* bias the value of the stimulus in accordance with motivational state: food is more important when you're hungry. Damage to the anterior cingulate is associated with apathy, in which stimuli, even motivationally relevant ones, fail to evoke the appropriate response.

Modality-specific neurons in primary and association neocortex respond selectively to stimuli in their respective sensory fields, for example, face-recognition neurons in inferotemporal cortex, language-sensitive neurons in auditory association cortex.

Clinical Signs of Right Hemisphere Dysfunction

Neglect

Neglect is seen almost exclusively after right hemisphere lesions involving any component of the posterior parietal, prefrontal and limbic attentional network and their subcortical thalamic and striatal connections.

The patient behaves as if the left side of space or their own limbs don't exist and aren't important. They may eat only food on the right side of the plate, fail to read words on the left side of the page, shave only the right half of their face or dress only the right half of their body. There may be a gaze preference toward the right, and they may fail to orient to people or other stimuli on their left side. Spontaneous drawing and writing may be shifted toward the extreme right of the page.

Neglect tends to resolve spontaneously after a median duration of 2 to 7 months.

"Right Parietal Lobe Syndrome"

Although neglect can occur alone, left hemianopia, hemihypesthesia or hemiparesis, and extinction to simultaneous visual or tactile stimulation are frequently associated. The constellation of constructional and dressing apraxia , neglect, and anosognosia (denial or unawareness of illness) is sometimes referred to as the "right parietal lobe syndrome" (Appendix 4).

Lesions of the Right Hemisphere Attentional Network

Stroke, primary or secondary brain tumors, and degenerative dementias are the most common etiologies of right hemisphere dysfunction. Focal seizure discharge or post-ictal neuronal exhaustion causes reversible functional disruption of cortical activity. The white matter lesions of multiple sclerosis may disrupt intracortical or cortical-subcortical connections. Hemilateral neglect is a rare consequence of toxic-metabolic encephalopathies, subdural hematoma and head injury.

Differential Diagnosis

Unilateral neglect needs to be distinguished from visual agnosia which can cause spatial disorientation. Visual agnosia is not associated with extinction or with behavioral signs of neglect.

Clinical Assessment of Neglect

Observe the patient's spontaneous dressing, eating, gaze, motor orientation to environmental stimuli, and limb preference.

Inquire about getting lost at home, in the neighborhood, while driving or shopping.

The patient's description of the inside of their house or a familiar public place may reveal poverty or absence of detail on the left.

Extinction exists if there is an accurate response to unilateral stimulation but consistent lack of perception of the left-sided stimulus during bilateral simultaneous stimulation. Extinction can be modality specific, so it is important to test different modalities, ie, visual, auditory, and tactile.

Asked to bisect the middle of a horizontal line, the patient with unilateral neglect shows a consistent bias toward the right. Pointing to the midline of the body is displaced toward the right. A tactile stimulus on the left limbs may be reported as coming from the right (allesthesia); reading, writing and drawing may be displaced toward the right side of the page or the patient may fail to read words on the left side of a paragraph.

Motor ("intentional") neglect is suspected if the patient's failure to use their left limbs spontaneously can be overcome with vigorous encouragement; similarly, they may fail to explore objects placed in the left hand.

Suspect constructional apraxia if the patient is unable to draw the interlocking pentagons on the Folstein Mental State Examination, a house, a bicycle, a flower, or copy a 3-dimensional cube. In general, patients with left hemisphere lesions retain the overall proportions of a drawn figure but omit details, while patients with right hemisphere disorders retain details but distort the overall configuration. If neglect is present, the left side of objects such as the abridged Rey figure may be omitted, or the left-half of the clock drawing may be devoid of numbers.

Check for dressing apraxia by observing the patient's approach to putting their arms in sleeves and aligning the garment correctly with their body. A more difficult task is to hand the patient their coat inside out and observe their approach to putting it on.

Treatment of Neglect

The presence of neglect is a poor prognostic factor for recovery after stroke. Verbal cueing and sensory stimulation on the left provide only short-lived improvement. Patching the right eye or immobilizing the right limbs are also not consistently helpful.

7. Cortical Disturbances of Visual Perception

Overview

Visual agnosia is defined as visual perception stripped of meaning. In the absence of aphasia, blindness, dementia or impaired vigilance, the patient is unable to recognize visual stimuli. Visual agnosia is modality-specific, so that recognition is intact in other sensory channels.

Although we will only consider the visual agnosias here, keep in mind that agnosia can occur in the tactile and in the auditory domains as well.

Astereognosia and *agraphesthesia* refer respectively to inability to identify shapes or written symbols by touch in the absence of a deficit of elementary sensation. *Asomatognosia* refers to inability to recognize one's own body. Asomatognosia is sometimes associated with delusional misidentification of body parts as not belonging to oneself or as belonging to someone else; anosognosia and other features of the right parietal syndrome are commonly present. *Auditory agnosia* is discussed in Section 5, The Left Hemisphere, Aphasia and Apraxia.

All agnosias are disconnection syndromes in the sense that primary sensory percepts are disconnected from the association areas necessary to link percepts to meaning.

Major Afferents and Efferents

The perceptual encoding of faces and objects is a function of the visual association cortices.

The fusiform face region of the inferotemporal cortex is specialized for recognition of facial features and for other classes of objects. This area is linked to superior and lateral temporal cortex, amygdala, and hippocampus, which figure in contextual memory and affect.

There are two neurally and functionally distinct visual systems. A ventral stream of projections from primary visual cortex to inferotemporal cortex is involved in object identification ("what it is"). A dorsal stream of projections from primary visual cortex to posterior parietal cortex provides online control of the movements required to execute motor plans in three-dimensional space ("where it is").

Clinical Signs of Cortical Disturbances of Visual Perception (Appendix 4)

Visual Object Agnosia

Apperceptive agnosia. The patient is able to see color, movement, dimension and intensity but cannot distinguish one form from another (eg, a circle and a square) or copy or match objects in the visual modality. Identification through other sensory modalities is intact. Vision is subjectively blurred. Alexia is usually present. The lesion involves extensive bilateral areas of occipitotemporal visual cortex.

Associative agnosia. In contrast to apperceptive visual agnosia, perception for elementary forms is intact and patients can copy and match similar visual stimuli, but object recognition is impaired. The impairment may affect specific classes of objects such as tools. Recognition is intact in other sensory modalities (eg, voice, touch). Prosopagnosia, achromatopsia, and alexia are frequently associated. Bilateral lesions involve the medial occipoto-temporal cortex and inferior longitudinal fasciculus connecting the occipital and temporal lobes (Appendix 4).

Prosopagnosia

A type of associative visual agnosia distinguished by inability to recognize familiar faces, including one's own face, despite normal vision. Oliver Sacks' *The Man Who Mistook His Wife For A Hat* is an example of prosopagnosia. Unlike associative agnosia, recognition of objects belonging to a generic class ("that's a cow") is intact, but identification of individuals (cows, persons, cars) is impaired. Prosopagnosia is believed to be a disturbance of visual face memory. Because connections between the ventral visual pathway and the amygdala are intact, patients with prosopagnosia can identify facial emotion and they generate a galvanic skin response to a familiar face, implying intact non-verbal processing of facial identity. Identification by other specific features (eg, hair color, voice) is intact. The lesion site in prosopagnosia is controversial. Most patients have bilaterally symmetric lesions of occipital association cortex which interrupt the sensory processing of facial features upstream of the fusiform face area 0, although cases have been reported after unilateral lesions, more often on the right.

Associated features include: Superior quadrantic visual field defect, achromatopsia, alexia, and Bálint syndrome.

The 3 major components of Bálint syndrome are:

- ***Simultagnosia***, the inability to perceive more than one visual stimulus at a time;

- ***Optic ataxia*** ("misreaching"), the inability to reach for an objects under visual guidance; and

- ***Optic apraxia***, the inability to volitionally shift gaze from one target to another.

Simultagnosia, the core symptom of Bálint syndrome, is an impairment of visual attention rather than a true agnosia. The object of vision shifts unpredictably from quadrant to quadrant and may vanish suddenly as fixation shifts. Inferior quadrantanopia may be present. The lesion responsible for Bálint syndrome involves parieto-occipital cortex bilaterally, affecting the dorsal ("where it is") visual stream (Table 6).

Anton syndrome

Anton syndrome is denial of blindness. The cortically blind patient with bilateral lesions of the occipital cortex or optic radiations confabulates answers to questions concerning visual information. Dementia or delirium are usually associated.

"Blindsight"

Patients with a lesion of the occipital cortex or optic radiations may retain the ability to localize flashes of light and coarse objects in the blind visual field without conscious awareness. Blindsight is believed to reflect sparing of alternative visual pathways including parietal association cortex, superior colliculi and pulvinar.

Alexia without aphasia ("word blindness") is discussed in Section 5, The Left Hemisphere, Aphasia and Apraxia.

Lesions of the Cortical Visual System Associated with Visual Agnosia

Etiologies include: Embolic stroke involving the posterior cerebral artery; glioma of the splenium of the corpus callosum invading the occipital lobes; and bilateral occipital epileptic foci. Bálint syndrome is most commonly caused by watershed infarctions or metastases in the middle and posterior cerebral artery territories.

Differential Diagnosis of Cortical Disturbances of Vision

Aphasia is the major differential diagnosis for visual agnosia. The aphasic patient knows what an object is and how to use it, is able to manipulate it or choose logically connected items (eg, a match and a candle; key and lock; hammer and nail). The agnosic patient, in contrast, is unable to name a visual stimulus, but can name stimuli presented in the auditory or tactile mode.

Bálint syndrome may be mistaken for visual agnosia, but patients with Bálint syndrome can recognize and name objects – one at a time.

Individuals with Bálint syndrome have difficulty dressing because they are unable to coordinate the orientation of their clothes in relation to their body or correct their error under visual guidance. Unlike dressing apraxia caused by right parietal lesions, Bálint syndrome is not associated with unilateral neglect.

Hysterical blindness may simulate blindsight. However, optokinetic nystagmus provoked by moving a measuring tape horizontally in front of the patient is preserved in hysterical blindness, indicating intact cortical vision.

Clinical Assessment of Cortical Visual Disturbances

Examine elementary visual functions (pupils, visual fundi, acuity, and visual fields).

Establish that the patient possesses a sufficient degree of alertness to collaborate with the clinical examination and that they are not aphasic.

Ask the patient to describe an object and demonstrate its use. Suspect visual agnosia if object identification is impaired to sight but intact to touch or hearing (eg, keys jangling; familiar voice).

Ask the patient to copy and match similar visual stimuli. These capacities are impaired in apperceptive agnosia but intact in associative agnosia.

Check for simultagnosia by asking the patient to describe a complex visual scene. I use magazine pictures which contain objects of different visual classes (eg, faces, animals, and cars) as well as different colors to check for achromatopsia.

A. The finger-nose test may reveal optic ataxia.

B. Voluntary saccades may reveal optic apraxia.

Use of optokinetic nystagmus in the examination of the hysterically blind patient is described above 0.

Treatment of Cortical Visual Disturbances

Compensatory rehabilitation strategies for visual agnosia include providing the patient with additional cues in other sensory domains such as manipulating objects or providing a verbal description to circumvent the recognition disorder.

8. Appendices

Appendix 1

The Neurobehavioral Questionnaire

Hand, Foot, and Ocular Dominance

Write, throw ball, kick ball, bat, strike a match, cut with scissors, shovel, fork, hammer, brush teeth, unscrew lid of jar, look through camera

Perinatal History

Pregnancy complications
Prematurity or term
Perinatal period

Developmental History

Psychomotor milestones
Coordination (sports, running, jumping, accident prone)

Educational History

Years education
Grades repeated
Problem subjects
Learning difficulty
Attention disorder in childhood

Neurological History

Epilepsy
Traumatic brain injury
Migraine
Meningitis, encephalitis

Social History

Behavioral disorder in childhood
Relationships with peers
Substance abuse

Family History

Neurological illness
Psychiatric illness
Hereditary diseases

Appendix 2

Clinical Cognitive Assessment

Orientation

Date (month, day, year)
Time of day
Season
Kind of hospital
Name of hospital
Duration of hospitalization
Floor or unit
Name of doctor

Attention and Concentration

Serial 7s from 100
1-A, 2-B, 3-? ... (pt. starts again to 5-E)
w-o-r-l-d in reverse
Variant: w-o-r-l-d in alphabetical order (Leopold, NA et al. *Neurol.* 1997;49:1521)
Days of week in reverse
Months in reverse
Patient's telephone number in reverse
Digit span (normal 7 ± 2 forward; 5 ± 2 reverse). Start low, increase until patient consistently makes errors. Digit span is the number of digits repeated without error.
- 37990
- 35923
- 4-9-6-1
- 5-3-9-1
- 3-8-6-7-2
- 7-6-2-3-8
- 4-2-6-7-3-8
- 9-3-1-6-8-7
- 3-5-4-8-9-6-2
- 1-5-8-7-2-3-9
- 7-1-6-8-2-4-3-5

Language

Spontaneous speech. Observe fluency, latency to initiate speech, word-finding pauses, paraphasias, syntax, prosody, paraphasias, articulation, and content
Naming (objects, colors, actions, body parts, including fingers)
Comprehension
Show me the door... the window... the chair
Show me your left thumb ... your right hand
Touch your left thumb with your right hand
Put the pen on the watch
Touch the watch with the pen
Touch the keys and then the pen
Touch the pen before touching the keys
Touch the pen but not the keys
Put the pen between the watch and the keys
Take the watch and pass me the pen
Take the pen with your right hand and with your left hand put the keys on the watch
Is this said by a disciplined or an undisciplined person?: I am unaccustomed to disobeying rules
Take the paper in your right hand, fold it in half, and put it on the floor
Is your name Green?
When you get dressed do you put on your socks before your shoes?
If a lion and a tiger have a fight and the lion is killed by the tiger, which animal is dead?
Is the brother of my wife a man or a woman?
If I had lunch after cleaning the house, which did I do first?
Finger naming
Repetition
- "He is there"
- "The ship sailed into the port to escape the storm"
- "First field T-shirt"
- "First British Field Artillery"
- "No ifs, ands, or buts"
- "Massachusetts Constitution"
- "The cat always hid under the couch when dogs were in the room"

I only know that John is the one to help today
Reading (letters, words, sentences)
Writing (spontaneous and to dictation)
Automatic speech (prayers, alphabet, days of the week, counting, singing)

(continued)

Appendix 2 *(continued)*

Clinical Cognitive Assessment

Memory

Verbal memory
- Long-term
  - Orientation
  - Word list recall at 5 minutes
  - What did you have for lunch?
  - Recent news items
  - Sentence recall at 5 minutes:
  - The sun rises in the east; In May the apple trees blossom.
- Retrograde
  - How long have you been hospitalized?
  - Past medical history
  - What did you do yesterday?
  - Date of birth
  - Children's names
  - Name and address

Visual memory
- Abridged Rey figure (copy; immediate; delayed recall at 5 minutes)

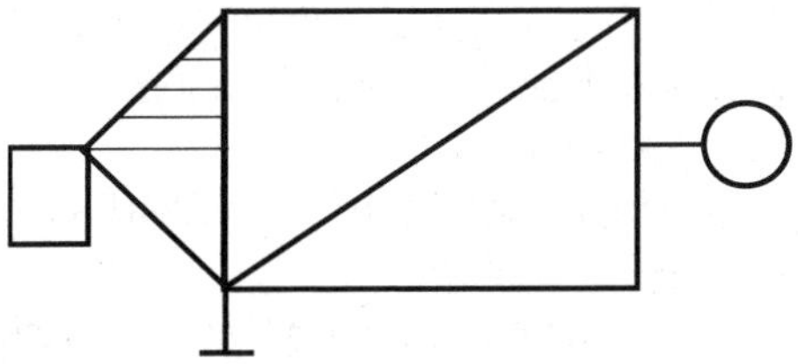

Constructions

Clock drawing (Instructions: Draw a clock and put in all the numbers. Set the time to 10 past 11)
Three-dimensional cube
Bicycle
House
Pentagons from the Folstein Mini-Mental status Examination
Six-point star

Calculation

Addition
Multiplication (8 x 7)
Division (434/7 ... 150/25 ... 550/25)

Praxis

Spontaneous use
- Observe patient using fork and knife, pen, hammer, key, toothbrush
- Evaluate the right and left hands separately

Use to verbal command and pantomime
- Transitive (tool-based): scissors; fork and knife; comb; toothbrush; drinking straw; hammer
- Intransitive (non-tool based): scratch head; knock on door; screw in light bulb; tie shoelaces; hitchhike; military salute; applaud; sign of the cross
- Facial intransitive gestures (blow out match; drink through straw; close eyes; cough; stick out tongue; blow a kiss; whistle)
- Complex sequences (fold letter, stamp it, put it in envelope, seal it; light a candle with a match; open bottle and pour liquid into a glass; take pipe out of pocket, light it and smoke it)

Imitation
- Meaningful gestures (screw in light bulb; hammer a nail)
- Nonmeaningful gestures (touch fingers to thumb in succession; double rings with thumb and index; "devil's horns"; inverted "devil's horns" (one hand facing up-one hand facing down)

Matching (hammer and nail; toothbrush and toothpaste; paper and pen)

Identification. Ask the patient to identify the gesture that you pantomime (eg, hammering, using a screwdriver)

(continued)

Clinical Cognitive Assessment

Frontal Functions

Note inertia, apathy, irritability, lability, impulsivity, rigidity, perseveration, disinhibition, imitation and utilization behavior
Insight (awareness of illness, eg, reason hospitalized); long-range plans; personal and family needs; life goals
Attention and concentration (above)
Utilization behavior
  Set out pitcher and glass; crayons and paper; staple and paper; syringe; sunglasses; small change; packet of Life Savers®; reflex hammer; stethoscope
Imitation behavior
  Examiner removes lab coat
  Touch my finger (while examiner puts hand on head)
  Touch your ear (while examiner touches nose)
  Make a fist (while examiner claps once)
  What's this called? (while flexing wrist)
Planning
  Clock drawing (See Constructions, above)
Abstractions
  Analogies (apple-pear; dog-lion; North-West; piano-violin; air-water; reward-punishment; fly-tree; dress-coat; table-chair; truth-beauty; boat-car; watch-ruler; bee-wasp; poem-statue)
  Proverbs
    The early bird gets the worm
    Don't cry over spilt milk
    If the shoe fits wear it
    A stitch in time saves nine
    The grass is greener on the other side
    Still water runs deep
    People who live in glass houses shouldn't throw stones
    When the cat's away the mice will play
    When in Rome do as the Romans
    A rolling stone gathers no moss
    The appetite comes in eating
    A smooth sea never made a skilled mariner
    Birds of a feather flock together
    A watched pot never boils
    Too many cooks spoil the broth

Complex reasoning
  How many quarters in $1.75?
  The father is 27-years-old, the mother is 2 years younger and their son is 20 years younger than the mother. How old is grandpa if his age is the sum of the father, mother and son combined? (57)
  The price of canned peas is two cans for 31 cents. What is the price of one dozen cans? Ask if failure: 6 x 31 = ($1.86)
Judgment
  Joe Blow, president of a railroad company, receives the annual report which says that train accidents cause injuries to people in the last car. So Joe Blow decides to remove the last car in every train. What do you think of his decision?
  Joe Blow's feet are so big he can't get his pants on over them. So he decides to put his pants on by putting them over his head. What do you think of his decision?
Verbal fluency
  Semantic fluency [Words beginning with F or P in 1 minute; no proper nouns (normal 15 ± 5)]
  Categorical fluency [Animals; items in supermarket (normal 15 ± 5)]
Alternating sequences. Test right and left hands separately
  Bimanual alternation palm-fist (Ozeretski task)
  Fist-ring
  Touch shoulder-extend arm with ring
  3-step Luria sequence (palm-fist-cut)

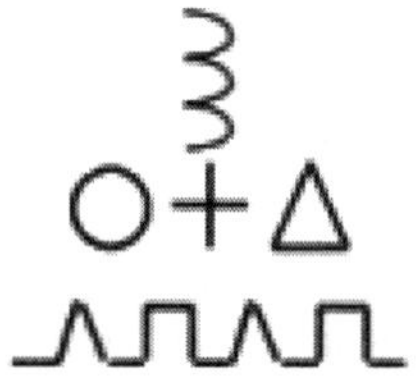

  Alternate tapping twice, then three times
  Tap twice with right hand, once with left, then reverse
  Alternating drawing figures
  MNMNMN

(continued)

Appendix 2 *(continued)*

Clinical Cognitive Assessment

Impulsiveness
- Standard Go/No-go: When I tap once, you tap twice; When I tap twice, you tap once. Have patient repeat instructions to demonstrate understanding.
- Alternative go/no-go: When I tap once, you tap twice; When I tap twice, you do nothing. Have patient repeat instructions to demonstrate understanding.
- Alternative go/no-go: When I say "Stop," you tap; When I say "Tap," you do nothing. Have patient repeat instructions to demonstrate understanding.

Appendix 3

The Neurobehavioral Examination

Head Circumference

Use standard head circumference chart to estimate percentile

Olfaction

Cloves, coffee, lemon, soap
Avoid noxious substances
Frontal signs
Motor impersistence
(maintain visual fixation, eye closure, tongue protrusion, arm elevation >5 seconds)
Paratonia (synonym: Gegenhalten)

Palmomental

Snout
Sucking
- To visual stimulus: mouth opens as patient sees stimulus approaching
- To tactile stimulus: in response to touch at corner of mouth

Rooting
Glabellar tap (normal <5 blinks)
Palmar and plantar grasp
Note whether patient able to "let go" (inhibit the grasp) while examiner exerts traction

"Soft Signs" of Neurodevelopmental Origin

Erratic ocular pursuits
Synkinesis of eye and head movements
Subtle choreiform movements of outstretched upper limbs
Clumsiness on fine motor tasks
Overflow movements (eg, elbows moving during forearm pronation-supination)
Mirror movements
Dystonic posturing of upper extremities while walking on tiptoe or on heels, jumping, or hopping
Right-left confusion
Paratonia
Sensory abnormalities (below)

Sensory Tests of Frontal-Parietal Dysfunction (Test right and left hands separately)

Extinction to simultaneous stimulation
(With patient's eyes closed, apply a light touch to ipsilateral cheek and dorsum of hand. Alternate cheek, hand, or both. Abnormal if patient perceives only "face" after 5 simultaneous touches to face and hand)
Visual, tactile, auditory
Face-hand test
Graphesthesia (Numbers between 1 and 9 drawn on palm)
Coin estimation (penny, nickel, dime, quarter)

Appendix 4

Behavioral and Cognitive Syndromes and Associated Brain Regions

Sign or Syndrome	Brain Region
Alexia without aphasia	Left occipital cortex and splenium of corpus callosum
Anosognosia	Right posterior parietal
Anterograde amnesia	Hippocampus, fornix or medial forebrain septal nuclei
Apathy	Anterior cingulate gyrus, nucleus accumbens, globus pallidus, thalamus
Bálint syndrome	Bilateral occipitoparietal cortex
Broca's aphasia	Left inferior premotor and prefrontal cortex
Conduction aphasia	Arcuate fasciculus
Constructional apraxia	Right parietal
Depression	Left anterior frontal cortex, caudate, and fronto-subcortical projections
Disinhibition	Orbitofrontal cortex and subcortical projections
Dressing apraxia	Right parietal
Dysprosody	Right premotor and prefrontal area
Frontal dysexecutive syndrome	Dorsolateral prefrontal cortex
Gerstmann syndrome	Left angular gyrus adjacent to Wernicke's area
Ideational apraxia	Left hemisphere (localization uncertain)
Ideomotor apraxia	Left fronto-parietal
Impulsiveness	Orbitofrontal cortex
Limb-kinetic apraxia	Left hemisphere (localization uncertain)
Mania	Right frontal cortex, caudate, thalamus
Memory retrieval deficit	Dorsolateral prefrontal cortex
Motor neglect	Dorsolateral prefrontal cortex, anterior cingulate, thalamus
Obsessions	Orbitofrontal cortex and subcortical projections
Perseveration	Multiple frontal areas
Prosopagnosia	Bilateral occipital association cortex and subadjacent white matter
Sensory neglect	Right posterior parietal, thalamus
Spatial disorientation	Right parietal
Transcortical motor aphasia	Supplementary motor area and frontal cortex adjacent to Broca's area
Transcortical sensory aphasia	Parieto-temporal cortex adjacent to Wernicke's area
Visual agnosia (all types)	Bilateral occipitotemporal cortex
Wernicke's aphasia	Posterior third of the superior temporal gyrus

8. References

Frontal Lobe Disorders

1. Fogel BS. The significance of frontal system disorders for medical practice and health policy. *Journal of Neuropsychiatry and Clinical Neurosciences*. 1994;6:343-347.

   (Helpful in understanding practical implications of frontal disorders not adequately captured by the Folstein Mini-Mental Status Examination.)

2. Mega MS, Cummings JL. Frontal-subcortical circuits and neuropsychiatric disorders. *Journal of Neuropsychiatry and Clinical Neurosciences*. 1994;6:358-370.

   (Review of the functional neuroanatomy of frontal-subcortical circuits.)

3. Cummings JL, Benson DF. Psychological dysfunction accompanying subcortical dementias. *Annual Review of Medicine*. 1988;39:53-61.

   (Profile and pathophysiology of subcortical dementias.)

Limbic System Functional Neuroanatomy

4. Trimble MR, Mendez MF, Cummings JL. Neuropsychiatric symptoms from the temporolimbic lobes. *Journal of Neuropsychiatry and Clinical Neurosciences*. 1997;9:429-438.

   (Review and clinical approach to interictal psychosis.)

5. Blumer D, Wakhlu S, Montouris G, Wyler AR. Treatment of the interictal psychoses. *Journal of Clinical Psychiatry*. 2000;61: 110-122.

Nonverbal Aspects of Communication

6. Ross ED. Affective prosody and the aprosodias. In: Mesulam M-M, ed. *Principles of Behavioral and Cognitive Neurology*. 2nd ed. New York: Oxford University Press; 2000:316-331.

Cognitive Functions of the Cerebellum

7. Schmahmann JD. Disorders of the cerebellum: ataxia, dysmetria of thought, and the cerebellar cognitive affective syndrome. *Journal of Neuropsychiatry and Clinical Neurosciences*. 2004;16:367-378.

Clinical Cognitive Screening Instruments

8. Nasreddine ZS, Phillips NA, Bédirian V, et al. The Montreal Cognitive Assessment (MoCA): A Brief Screening Tool For Mild Cognitive Impairment. *Journal of the American Geriatric Society*. 2005;53:695-699.

   (New cognitive screening instrument validated against standardized neuropsychological tests. Highly sensitive to mild cognitive impairment. Takes approximately 10 minutes to administer. Includes frontal functions.)

9. Leopold NA, Borson AJ. An alphabetical 'WORLD': a new version of an old test. *Neurology*. 1997;49:1521-1524.

10. Dubois B, Slachevsky A, Litvan I, Pillon B. The FAB: A frontal assessment battery at bedside. *Neurology*. 2000;55:1621-1626.

    (A 10-minute standardized screen for frontal lobe disorders including conceptualization, mental flexibility, motor programming, sensitivity to interference, inhibitory control, and environmental autonomy. French neurology in the tradition of Lhermitte.)

Landmark Papers in Behavioral Neurology/Neuropsychiatry

11. Harlow JM. Passage of an iron rod through the head. *Boston Medical and Surgical Journal*. 1848;39:389-393.

12. Lhermitte F, Pillon B, Serdane M. Human autonomy and the frontal lobes. Part I. Imitation and utilization behavior: a neuropsychological study of 75 patients. *Annals of Neurology*. 1986;19:326-334.

13. Lhermitte F. Human autonomy and the frontal lobes. Part II. Patient behavior in complex and social situations: the "environmental dependency syndrome." *Annals of Neurology*. 1986;19:334-350.

14. Scoville WB, Milner B. Loss of recent memory after bilateral hippocampal lesions. *Journal of Neurology, Neurosurgery and Psychiatry*. 1957;20: 11–21.

Textbooks

15. Mesulam M-M. *Principles of Behavioral and Cognitive Neurology*. 2nd ed. New York, NY: Oxford University Press; 2000.

(Dense; contributions from multiple authors. The best overall summary of behavioral neurology.)

16. Cummings JL, Mega MS. *Neuropsychiatry and Behavioral Neuroscience*. New York, NY: Oxford University Press; 2003.

(Emphasis on psychiatric concomitants of neurological disease. Excellent illustrations, summary tables and differential diagnoses.)

9. Questions

1. A 33-year-old long-distance truck driver in good health sustained a mechanical neck injury as she was attaching a heavy load. Over the following months, during which she was receiving physical therapy for ongoing neck pain, she complained of difficulty remembering route plans and recent events, irritability, and insomnia. She fears she is developing Alzheimer disease. Neurological examination is normal. Which of the following bedside cognitive tests is most likely to be abnormal?

A. Alternating hand sequences

B. Verbal fluency

C. Digit span

D. Clock drawing

2. Neuroimaging in a 74-year-old man with a 6-month history of gait disturbance and occasional falls shows enlarged lateral ventricles and attenuation of periventricular white matter. Which of the following clinical signs is not likely to be present in this patient?

A. Visual extinction to simultaneous stimulation

B. Psychomotor slowing

C. Perseveration

D. Apathy

3. A 67-year-old patient with a history of poorly-controlled hypertension complains of poor memory. She is able to recall 2 of 5 words after 5 minutes, but 5 of 5 with cueing. You inform her:

A. There's nothing wrong with her memory

B. She has Alzheimer disease

C. She needs to see a psychiatrist

D. She needs better control of her blood pressure

4. A 54-year-old man with an extensive legal history is brought to the emergency room for "confusion." Your cognitive assessment shows that he is alert. There are no signs of aphasia. He is disoriented to date, place, and personal identity. You suspect:

A. Acute alcohol intoxication

B. Subdural hematoma

C. Psychogenic amnesia

D. Temporal lobe epilepsy

5. An 81-year-old woman has been getting lost in her home. She is oriented to date and time. Verbal memory and verbal fluency are intact. She is unable to copy the abridged Rey figure. Brain imaging is most likely to show:

A. Diffuse atherosclerosis

B. A right posterior parietal lesion

C. Marked cerebral atrophy

D. A large pineal cyst

6. A 60-year-old patient has a 2-year history of depression, insomnia and occasional falls. Examination shows bilateral plantar grasp reflexes. The most appropriate next clinical step is:

A. Obtain neuroimaging

B. Return for re-examination in 9 months

C. Prescribe sleeping pills

D. Prescribe a helmet and knee guards to prevent injury

7. After a flurry of seizures, a 25-year-old retarded man on anticonvulsant polypharmacy presents with insomnia, disorientation, visual hallucinations and extreme anxiety. The most likely diagnosis is:

A. Post-ictal psychosis

B. Non-convulsive status epilepticus

C. Anticonvulsant toxicity

D. Adjustment disorder

8. A 26-year-old motorcyclist sustained a severe closed head injury. One year later she is apathetic. Outbursts of verbal abuse limit attempts to return to work. Brain CT shows bifrontal atrophy. You should:

A. Encourage her to get a job

B. Refer her for insight-oriented psychotherapy

C. Obtain more brain imaging studies

D. Consider a trial of psychostimulant medication

9. Two weeks following a left middle cerebral artery embolic stroke, neurological examination shows sparse, halting speech with word-finding pauses and marked dysnomia, but your patient can repeat the phrase, "No ifs ands or buts." You diagnose:

A. Broca's aphasia

B. Wernicke's aphasia

C. Transcortical motor aphasia

D. Malingering

10. A 76-year-old homeless man is brought to the emergency room by the police. He is babbling continuously and incoherently. You can make out only an occasional word. He is not able to provide any history. He does not repeat short phrases. He does follow most simple verbal commands. The best clinical diagnosis is:

A. Conduction aphasia

B. Jargonophasia

C. Schizophasia

D. Transcortical sensory aphasia

11. A right-handed patient complains of clumsiness of their right hand. Examination shows awkward use of utensils and disruption of handwriting with intact language, motor and sensory examination. You suspect:

A. Early Parkinson disease

B. Ideomotor apraxia

C. Alien hand syndrome

D. Subcortical stroke

12. A 45-year-old woman with metastatic breast cancer complains of blurred vision. She appears blind, although corrected visual acuity is 20/30. She is unable to locate buttons on her clothes or eating utensils. When attempting to reach out and touch objects she misses them. When shown pictures in a magazine she only identifies one item at a time. The diagnosis is:

A. Prosopagnosia

B. Apperceptive visual agnosia

C. Hysterical blindness

D. Bálint syndrome

Answers

1. C.

2. A.

3. D.

4. C.

5. B.

6. A.

7. A.

8. D.

9. C.

10. A.

11. B.

12. D.

Chapter 32: Neurologic Complications of Medical Disorders

Barbara Koppel, MD
Gokhan Akfirat, MD

Contents

1. Cardiac Disease Complications

There is constant interplay between the body, which supports the functions of the brain, and the consequences of the body's disorders on the nervous system. Conversely, as the brain controls many bodily functions some of the disorders of the brain will produce problems of systemic activity. In this chapter we will review conditions of various organ systems that affect the nervous system, including pathophysiology, clinical findings and differential diagnosis, diagnostic testing and treatment.

The brain requires a continuous energy supply (glucose and oxygen) that is provided by the heart's action. Therefore, the neurologic complications of cardiac disease are caused by interruption of this energy supply. These complications can be focal (stroke and transient ischemic attack), or global (syncope, seizure, hypoxic-ischemic encephalopathy, dementia), and also can occur after cardiac surgery. Brain abscess can complicate cyanotic congenital heart disease.

Cerebrovascular Complications

Pathophysiology

A cardiac origin for emboli is found in 20% of ischemic strokes. Another mechanism is indirect, when decreased cardiac output due to failure or arrhythmia combines with incomplete occlusion or stenosis in neck or cerebral vessels to produce a low flow state that will cause strokes in a particular vessel territory, or hypoperfusion in watershed infarcts.

Structural problems in the heart that can lead to emboli include atrial fibrillation with atrial thrombus formation, cardiomyopathy (especially the dilated type), and acute myocardial infarction with mural thrombus in the left ventricle, left atrial tumor (myxoma), valvular heart disease (after streptococcal or during active infection (endocarditis)), malignancy (marantic endocarditis), lupus (Libman-Sacks endocarditis), atrial septal aneurysm, and patent foramen ovale, with thrombus formation surrounding the hole or clots from the legs passing through the hole. Mitral valve prolapse, another common abnormality in young adults, is questionable as a cause of stroke.

Paroxysmal arrhythmias occur in young patients with abnormal electrical (His bundle) systems, thyroid disease, and toxic states such as fever or caffeine overuse. The incidence of abnormal rhythms, such as non-valvular atrial fibrillation, goes up exponentially after age 50, probably due to ischemic heart disease.

Clinical Findings and Differential Diagnosis

Embolic stroke presents with the sudden onset of a major focal deficit, while the patient is awake. Headache and seizures are not unusual. The deficit may clear in the ensuing hours, if the embolism breaks up, or improve if more distal vessels become affected. A history of recent chest pain, palpitations or intermittent tachycardia is sometimes present.

Diagnostic Tests

The diagnosis of embolic stroke can be made by imaging, with the CT showing an area of hypodensity in the territory of a blood vessel. The anterior circulation is more often involved, although cerebellar infarcts (without brainstem involvement) are due to cardiac emboli about half the time. Hemorrhagic conversion, with petechial blood seen in part or all of the same distribution as the initial stroke, occurs in 20% of patients by the first day. MR with diffusion-weighted imaging is more sensitive for both initial detection of stroke and for detecting hemorrhagic conversion, which is eventually seen on MR in up to 705 of patients, especially those who are elderly or who have a large infarct.

The nature of the cardiac abnormality is established by imaging the heart, using echocardiography performed through the anterior chest wall (TTE) to image the left ventricle and through the esophagus by swallowing the device (TEE) to image the left atrium and its appendage, or to look for a patent foramen ovale. The addition of saline bubble injection will also facilitate imaging of a patent foramin. EKG should be done in the initial assessment of all stroke patients, to search for coexisting myocardial infarction and arrhythmia. Twenty-four hour Holter monitoring can uncover intermittent dysfunctions in heart rhythm. Telemetry is useful in unstable patients or when arrhytmias are suspected but not present on initial EKG. Angiogram of the aorta or heart vessels may be required in special instances, but this procedure carries the risk of recurrent stroke.

Treatment
In rare circumstances, an embolic clot can qualify for attempted dissolution with intravenous or intraarterial tissue plasminogen activator (tPA), or retrieval through an angiographically placed catheter (Merci device). Most treatment of stroke due to cardiac pathology is directed at preventing future stroke, and involves anticoagulation with warfarin, with or without initial use of heparin. INR should be maintained near 2.5 unless there is structural valve pathology, in which case 3-3.5 is the preferred range. Conditions that make the long-term use of anticoagulation dangerous include dementia, unsteady gait, uncorrectable bleeding source, extreme old age, and unreliability of compliance with laboratory testing to maintain the correct dose.

Bleeding is the major concern with anticoagulant therapy. Age over 75 years increased the risk of major hemorrhage to 4.2% per year (RR = 2.6), compared to 1.7% per year in the younger population.

Nonvalvular atrial fibrillation has recently been studied, and antiplatelet therapy with aspirin, which reduced stroke risk by 22%, was found to be as effective as anticoagulation (WARRS trial). In patients with other cardiac causes of stroke under the age of 65, aspirin or other antiplatelet therapy is preferred.

Encephalopathy

Pathophysiology
When the entire brain is deprived of blood supply, diffuse cognitive dysfunction ensures.

Clinical Findings
Depressed consciousness can range from lethargy to deep coma or "brain death." If severe and prolonged ischemia has occurred, seizures and myoclonus are present, along with alteration of consciousness. If mild and transient, short-term cognitive dysfunction, sometimes requiring formal testing to uncover, is present. Some patients with prolonged cardiac failure have permanent dementia.

Diagnostic Testing
Diagnostic tests for encephalopathy due to cardiac disease are functional rather than structural and include electroencephalography or prolonged EEG monitoring. In comatose patients, patterns ranging from normal to most severely abnormal, include normal background, diffuse low amplitude slowing, burst suppression, alpha-coma (where alpha is seen in atypical, non-occipital, areas), and isoelectric. These patterns are usually non-reactive, ie, painful stimulation is given by the technician, and no change in frequency or amplitude of background is seen. Intermittent or continuous generalized epileptiform discharges are common and do not necessarily produce seizures.

In extreme cases, cerebral blood flow studies such as nuclear scans or angiography will document the lack of flow above the intracranial portion of the carotid and vertebral circulations.

Treatment

Restoration of effective circulation, if done sufficiently early, may reverse encephalopathy. Hypothermia with external cooling devices is benefi-

Figure 1

Brain CT of anoxic encephalopathy

Noncontrast scan reveals diffuse cerebral and cerebellar edema with hypodensities in cerebellar hemispheres and lentiform nuclei bilaterally, and effacement of the mesencephalic cistern, cisterna magna, aqueduct and fourth ventricle, consistent with herniation.

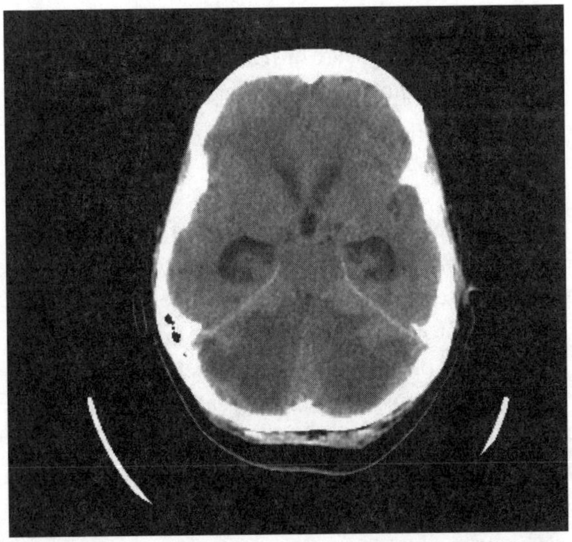

Figure 2

Electroencephalogram of anoxia (brain death)

18-channel electroencephalogram in the same patient, 48 hours after respiratory failure due to drug and alcohol overdose, showing no cerebral activity, rhythmic EKG, and respirator and muscle artifact.

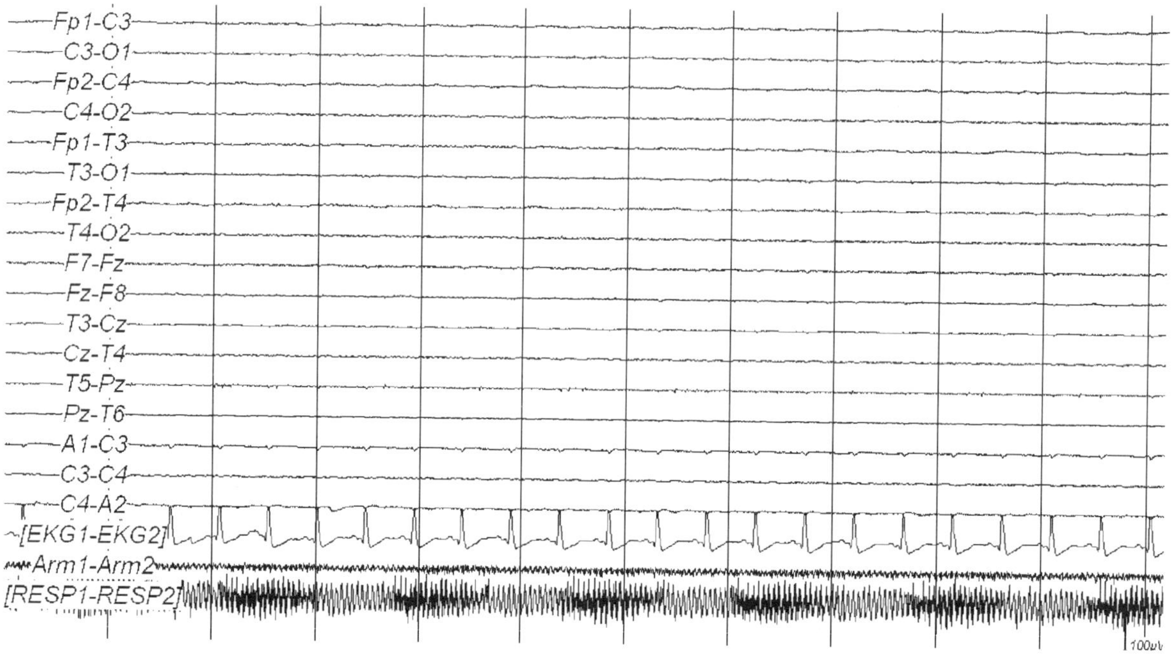

cial in reducing the incidence of vegetative state. Similarly, metabolic derangement after shock (liver or kidney failure) can be treated with dialysis or hematologic exchange with the potential to improve mentation. Epileptiform patterns on EEG monitoring should be treated but are difficult to stop, and their treatment does not always correlate with recovery.

Syncope

Transient, self-limited interruptions of cardiac output result in generalized cerebral ischemia, leading to brief (<30 seconds) loss of consciousness without following prolonged confusion. The circumstances and position of the patient immediately before the event yield important clues to its cause. Cardiac syncope is usually caused by a dysrhythmia such as sick sinus syndrome, Ward-Romano syndrome, or Jervell-Lange-Nelson syndrome, but obstruction of cardiac outflow can be responsible. Indirect involvement of the heart is seen in neurocardiac syncope, such as vasovagal, reflex or situational syncope, which are much more common.

Pathophysiology

The pathophysiology of neurally mediated syncope is due to sudden drop in cardiac output, usually due to bradycardia or even arrest, peripheral decrease in vascular tone, such as in prolonged standing, or combinations of both. Vasovagal syncope, where an upsetting event such as the sight of blood, trauma, elevator enclosure, or other shock provokes the event, is most common in the young or those with prolonged standing or overheating. Specific reflex syncopes can also be provoked by coughing, swallowing, micturition, or defecation. Pressure on the carotid sinus from a tie or tight collar, or neck rotation, causes syncope in other patients who are usually older than the first group. Orthostatic hypotension, a feature of some neurodegenerative diseases such as

Shy-Drager syndrome, Parkinson disease, and autonomic neuropathy, is common but does not usually lead to syncope. Seizure-induced cardiac arrest is present in Panayiotopoulos syndrome. Cardiac syncope in some cases is the result of obstruction of blood flow at the outlet of the heart, such as aortic stenosis, or extreme heart failure, such as is seen in severe cardiomyopathy, or after large or repeated infarctions. In most cases, syncope is the result of an abnormal heart rhythm. Arrthythmias can be slow or fast and are generated in the atrium, sinoatrial node, or ventricle. Ventricular tachycardia or fibrillation usually occurs in the context of serious heart failure, although a rare syndrome of nocturnal death is reported in young men from Southeast Asia, and other young patients have been described with the Brugada syndrome. The cause is suspected to be dysplasia in the right ventricle, or an underlying sodium channel defect in familial cases. Another ventricular dysrhythmia that is a rare cause of sudden death or syncope in young people, the long QT interval syndrome, is sometimes due to deletion of chromosome 22q11.2 in the velocardiofacial syndrome, or may be triggered by emotional or physical distress, or some medications.

Clinical Findings and Differential Diagnosis

Syncope begins with a brief premonitory phase of light-headedness, dizziness, or impending doom, during which the patient shows outward signs of autonomic dysfunction such as sweating or pale, gray skin. Vision begins to lose color and blur or fade, and nausea or the urge to urinate or defecate is felt. If the patient is unable to lie down or otherwise abort the event, a loss of muscle tone leads to slumping and falling. Usually the eyes roll up, and brief tonic posturing, a few beats of clonic arm movements, or mouth twitching can be seen. Consciousness is regained within a minute, with no "post-ictal" headache, injury or prolonged disorientation. A review of the immediately preceding circumstances provides important clues to the diagnosis, and specific questions should be asked related to palpitations, rapid heart beat, prolonged standing or straining (Valsalva maneuver). When there are no specific triggers, prior nausea or malaise, and the patient faints without being upright, the heart should be suspected as the cause. Physical findings are usually obtained after the event, and can include cardiac murmurs, an abnormal pulse, and drop in blood pressure on standing. If witnesses are present during a syncopal event, other brainstem signs should be sought.

The differential diagnosis of cardiac syncope mainly includes generalized seizure, which is more prolonged, has a different type of prodrome or aura that is stereotyped for each patient, has more prolonged abnormal movements, salivation and automatisms, a higher propensity for injury, and after the event a prolonged period of confusion, headache or muscle pain. Incontinence occurs with both. Atonic seizures, as seen in Lenox-Gastaut or other childhood epileptic syndromes, may initially be confused with syncope, especially as the history is difficult to obtain. This diagnosis is not difficult to make, as these events are frequently recurrent and appear in the setting of static encephalopathy.

Vertebrobasilar insufficiency, a form of TIA that can interrupt the reticular activating system in the brainstem, is distinguished from pure syncope by the presence of other signs of brainstem dysfunction. When triggered by arm exercise, subclavian steal, where flow in the vertebral artery is reversed, can rarely lead to loss of consciousness. Basilar migraine may cause LOC but the slow evolution of symptoms and other brainstem signs, such as dizziness or vertigo, set it apart from syncope.

Diagnostic Testing

Diagnostic testing includes tilt table analysis to distinguish neurocardiogenic syncope from pure cardiac syncope. Patients are tilted up to 70 degrees for at least 20 minutes, during which time isoprotenerol may be given. Loss of consciousness if accompanied by the patient's usual symptoms is diagnostic, and monitoring of the heart during the test distinguishes cardioinhibitory causes as opposed to vasodepression. In patients where cardiac syncope is more likely, the testing must start with electrocardiography. Since most abnormal rhythms are brief, prolonged testing with exercise, either with 24-hour Holter monitor or implantable loop recorders for more prolonged analysis, can provide clues, but only if the detected abnormal rhythm is accompanied by symptoms. Abnormal rhythms include bradycardic patterns (Stokes-Adams attacks), and tachy patterns such as fibrillation; neither necessarily cause syncope. Invasive electrophysiologic testing carries some risk and is only used in preparation for ablation of abnormal conduction tissues. Outflow problems such as aortic stenosis are observed on echocardiography. The electroencephalogram (EEG) is not generally required for diagnosis of syncope. An interruption in heartbeat is followed by background flattening and slowing or emergence of large slow waves. ECG should always be recorded simultaneously with EEG in order to determine if a seizure has triggered an arrythmia. Ninety percent of seizures are accompanied by sinus tachycardia, with less than 1% of seizures accompanied by bradycardia or asystole.

Treatment
Syncope is self-limited; supportive measures such as lying down with leg elevation are often the only management needed. In cases of serious arrhythmia, especially slowing or uncontrolled rapid rates, pacemaker insertion may be needed. Even more rarely, a cardiac defibrillator is required.

Neurologic Complications of Cardiac Surgery

Stroke, encephalopathy and compression neuropathies can all follow heart surgery.

Pathophysiology (Stroke)
Stroke can result from thrombotic material breaking off from the heart and interrupting large vessels of the brain. In addition, patients with high-grade carotid stenosis who will have low cardiac output during surgery presumably could suffer perioperative stroke without emboli. Therefore, preoperative screening with carotid duplex led to performance of simultaneous CABG and carotid endarterectomy. A recent metanalysis of Canadian patients showed a risk of stroke of 6.8% in those undergoing combined surgery, compared to 1.8% with the same carotid stenosis having CABG alone, suggesting the combined procedure is counterproductive.

Clinical Findings and Differential Diagnosis
Focal neurologic deficit with occasional obtundation if herniation ensues (usually these strokes are large) is seen immediately or in the post-operative week.

Diagnostic Testing
CT or MRI will show a stroke, especially if diffusion-weighted images are used, and it is necessary to exclude hemorrhagic transformation. Echocardiography after valvular surgery may be helpful. Electrocardiograms can look for abnormal rhythms or ischemic changes, as troponins may be elevated by surgery itself.

Treatment
Thrombolytic therapy cannot be used, but interventional techniques to remove a clot may prove useful. Massive swelling may require craniectomy. Heparin is useful in preventing future embolic events.

Pathophysiology (Encephalopathy)
Despite technical improvements—such as reduced time on the bypass pump and better filters, neuroprotective techniques such as lowering of body temperature to cool the brain, and careful management of blood pressure during the operation—cardiac surgery is followed by a relatively high rate of transient cognitive dysfunction (up to 30%). In rare patients, this difficulty in episodic (short-term) memory and learning persists. In others a delayed progressive dementia develops in the ensuing years, especially in patients with preexisting stroke or risk factors for cerebrovascular disease, which may or may not be attributed to the operation.

Clinical Findings and Differential Diagnosis
Acute confusional state or inability to regain consciousness after anesthesia is withdrawn are the presenting signs of postoperative encephalopathy.

Differential diagnosis includes sepsis or other infection and seizure activity. Metabolic encephalopathy from renal or hepatic failure can also appear the same as ischemic encephalopathy from heart failure secondary to surgery.

Diagnostic Testing
Electroencephalography is useful to rule out nonconvulsive status epilepticus, which may be reversible with treatment. Analysis of electrolytes and renal function is also helpful. Imaging can exclude bilateral cortical events.

Pathophysiology (Neuropathy)
Ulnar neuropathy can follow prolonged procedures if the arm (elbow) is not properly cushioned or stretched too far laterally. Lower brachial plexus stretching when the arms are placed above the head,

beyond 90 degrees, leads to weakness of the distal arms and hands.

Clinical Findings and Differential Diagnosis

New numbness or weakness in the distribution of a peripheral nerve, or branch of the plexus, especially if excess fluids were infused, or care was not taken during limb positioning.

Diagnostic Testing

Nerve conduction velocities around the elbow and at Erb's point, or at other pressure points, can establish the diagnosis.

2. Respiratory Disease

Control of respiration is overseen by the nervous system, with normal regulation controlled by the medulla. Neurogenic pulmonary edema can occur after a generalized seizure, subarachnoid hemorrhage, or any sudden increase in intracranial pressure. This is due to increase in sympathetic outflow, which can decrease cardiac output, increase pulmonary vascular pressure and capillary permeability, or produce slowed respiration, hypoventilation, or even apnea. Other abnormal patterns of respiration seen in central nervous system pathology include Cheyne-Stokes respiration, with periods of increasing amplitude alternating with decreasing amplitude and apnea for several seconds; ataxic respiration with irregular amplitude and frequency of respiration, seen with pontine dysfunction; and apnea, seen in medullary lesions. Central apnea is probably responsible for sudden infant death syndrome (SIDS) and sudden unexplained death in epilepsy (SUDEP). Parkinson disease, olivoponto-cerebellar dysfunction, and other extrapyramidal syndromes also disrupt respiration, especially causing poor respiratory excursion. Respiratory dyskinesias can also cause diaphragmatic flutter or segmental myoclonus and can present as seizures. Ventilatory failure is also found in lesions of the spinal cord above C3-4 and of the peripheral nervous system, including Güillain-Barré syndrome, botulism and ciguatera toxin poisoning.

Hypoxic/Anoxic Encephalopathy

Pathophysiology

The brain cannot be deprived of oxygen for more than 1 minute without initiating a cascade of calcium influx leading to neuronal death.

Clinical Findings and Differential Diagnosis

Signs of anoxia include obtundation and coma, with myoclonus and seizures. Chronic hypoxia such as seen in chronic pulmonary disease or altitude sickness can present with frontal lobe dysfunction such as poor judgment and apathy, memory dysfunction, headache, or hallucinations. After anoxic injury, action-provoked myoclonus and ataxia can persist, requiring elevation of serotonin levels, along with dementia, gait dysfunction and seizures (Lance-Adams syndrome).

Diagnostic Testing
Electroencephalography can provide clues to prognosis and detect seizure activity. CT scans show diffuse hypodensity, especially in the brainstem and cerebellum, with cerebral edema in severe cases.

Treatment
Supportive therapy is given while waiting for recovery. Amphetamines have been tried, but response is not yet proven. After many years of a minimally conscious state, placement of stimulators in the thalamus has improved the level of function in isolated patients.

Hypercapnia

Pathophysiology
Pickwickian syndrome and obstructive sleep apnea lead to excess levels of pCO_2.

Clinical Findings
Symptoms include headache that is migrainous or similar to that seen in benign intracranial hypertension, visual loss due to papilledema, and in extreme, acute cases, depressed level of consciousness.

Treatment
Treatment includes reduction in ambient carbon dioxide levels by improving ventilation or avoiding sleeping under excessive blankets. If associated with sleep apnea, ventilatory support in the form of C-PAP or bi-PAP respirators can solve the hypercapnia. Sedatives must be avoided as the adverse effect of respiratory depression exacerbates the underlying problem.

Hypocapnia
Acute hypocapnia is one of the most common causes of dizziness. The light-headedness, fingertip and perioral parasthesias, and in extreme cases syncope, can all be reproduced after less than 30 seconds of hyperventilation in people who have low pCO_2 levels due to chronic hyperventilation.

Pathophysiology
Although constriction of major blood vessels supplying the brain is the traditional explanation of cerebral symptoms, cellular effects such as calcium shifts and changes in oxygen delivery also play a role. Breathing oxygen to relieve pain in acute cluster or migraine is thought to work through the induction of hypocapnia.

Treatment
Rebreathing air to elevate carbon dioxide levels by using a paper bag, or holding one's breath, is sufficient to relieve symptoms, but the underlying anxiety should be addressed to prevent future attacks.

3. Hepatic Disease

Liver failure causes a neuropsychiatric syndrome that ranges from mild clumsiness and inadequate performance of psychometric tests to acute coma and herniation from cerebral edema. The latter is due to fulminant hepatitis or necrosis. Chronic liver failure or portosystemic shunt formation (bypassing the hepatic circulation) cause the more common metabolic encephalopathy.

Pathophysiology

When the liver malfunctions, ammonia cannot be converted to urea and instead accumulates in the serum, from which it can cross into the brain. In patients with normal liver parenchyma but portal hypertension, the presence of portal-systemic shunting allows substances to avoid detoxification in the otherwise normal liver. Ammonia has long been suspected of being the primary toxin that causes the encephalopathy in liver failure, but other toxins have been proposed to explain those cases where ammonia levels were not elevated in the serum or CSF. NH3 acts directly on the membrane of neurons, as well as affecting the production of glutamine, which competes with the excitatory transmitter glutamate. Mercaptan, another toxin produced by bacteria in the intestine, interferes with the sodium-potassium-ATPase activity in the brain, as well as being metabolized to the inhibitory transmitter taurine. Gluconeogenesis may be impaired in patients with poor liver function. Finally, increased inhibitory tone due to upregulation of $GABA_A$ receptors, excess presence of gamma-aminobutyric acid (GABA), or abnormal synthesis of the naturally occurring benzodiazepine-like substances (DBI, diazepam binding inhibitor) leads to depression of function. Problems with decreased availability of branched chain amino acids due to excess tryptophan saturating the transporters across the blood-brain barriers leads to depletion of glutamate and build-up of serotonin and catecholamines. As the blood-brain barrier becomes more permeable, and neuronal and glial membranes lose their integrity, the brain swells, cerebral perfusion falls, and severe intracranial hypertension causes herniation and death. Cerebral edema is present in 75% of patients with grade IV encephalopathy.

Clinical Findings

Hepatic encephalopathy is more common in chronic than acute liver failure, with ascites and jaundice. Early signs of encephalopathy include inability to concentrate, yawning and drowsiness, lack of judgment, irritability or other mood changes, often with delusions, hallucinations or agitation. The pathognomonic sign of motor dysfunction is asterixis, a failure to maintain extensor tone with hands stretched upward, known as "liver flap," but other findings frequently encountered include tremor, ataxia and dysarthria. Hyperreflexia is common, but Babinski sign and myoclonus are less frequent. Grade I encephalopathy is the inability to perform higher cortical functions as fluently as usual, grade II is mild obtundation, III is stupor and IV is deep coma, occasionally with decerebrate posturing. Long-standing liver failure can lead to non-Wilsonian hepatolenticular degeneration, a dopamine deficiency state that resembles Parkinson disease.

Diagnostic Tests

NH_3 is generally elevated in the serum and CSF, but does not show an exact correlation with degree of encephalopathy. Serum tests for biliary obstruction, such as elevated AST and GGTP, may be normal in patients with cirrhosis, while tests of liver function such as prothrombin time (INR) are elevated. The EEG is slow, with paroxysmal bursts of high voltage 1.5-3hz slowing seen bifrontally. Triphasic sharp and slow waves are also maximal in the frontal regions, but epileptiform activity is otherwise absent. CT shows atrophy (after recovery from), or edema acutely in cases of Grade IV encephalopathy, and MRI shows increased globus pallidus signal on T1-weighted images, as well as cerebral edema. Brain biopsy or pathology shows giant astrocytes (Alzheimer type II astrocytes) in the cortex.

Treatment

Ammonia production can be decreased by reducing the substrate of its formation (low protein diet, correction of gastrointestinal bleeding), eliminating bacteria from the large and small intestine through the use of nonabsorbable antibiotics (neomycin or metronidazole), or by increasing transit time through the gut and changing its acidity to convert more ammonia to ammonium (lactulose). Although controversial, the use of branched chain amino acids such as leucine, valine and isovaline is occasionally effective. Flumazenil, a benzodiazepine antagonist, can be used to temporarily awaken patients. Chronic hepatolenticular degeneration is treated with dopa agonists such as bromocriptine. In fulminant cases of liver failure, standard efforts to reduce elevated intracranial pressure such as mannitol, hyperventilation, and maintenance of the head above 30 degrees are worth trying, but liver transplant may be the only option.

4. Renal Disease and Electrolyte Disorders

The failure of the kidneys to clear the body's toxins, including but not limited to ammonia, causes an encephalopathy similar to that described by liver failure when acute. When long-standing, uremia leads to peripheral neuropathy, the movement disorder of restless leg syndrome (which may be related to the neuropathy or to the encephalopathy), and dementia. Causes and complications of renal failure, including diabetes, hypertension, heroin use, and poor platelet function raise the incidence of cerebrovascular events, both hemorrhagic and ischemic. Finally, the treatment of renal failure by dialysis or transplant also has neurologic consequences.

Encephalopathy

Pathophysiology

Despite the evidence provided by dialysis, in which the clearing from the body of water-soluble molecules leads to improvement in cognitive function, the exact toxin responsible for uremic encephalopathy is still not clear. A normal transmitter such as glutamine, or organic acids, that accumulate due to failure of its breakdown in the kidneys, may be responsible. Fluid shifts can cause cerebral edema or dehydration. Blocked transport systems in the brain interfere with acquisition of necessary amino acids and other products that normally cross through the choroid plexus. Anemia, responsive to erythropoietin, contributes to the overall lack of initiative. The rapidity of rise rather than the absolute number of BUN and creatinine correlates with the degree of encephalopathy.

Clinical Findings

Symptoms of uremia include slowing of cognitive processes with apathy, and inability to concentrate or initiate mental tasks. These fluctuate in degree from mild fatigue and confusion to coma, often without relationship to degree of azotemia or treatment. Delusions and hallucinations are seen in patients with delirium. Focal complaints are not unusual and do not necessarily imply hemorrhage, stroke or subdural hematoma. Seizures, partial or generalized are much more common in uremic than other forms of metabolic encephalopathy. Cortical irritability also causes multifocal myoclonus, an arrhythmic, asymmetric twitching. Meningeal signs are present in up to a third of patients (although generalized increase in tone must be excluded from specific nuchal rigidity on flexion). Other motor abnormalities are common, including asterixis, limb ataxia, and poor fine motor function, hemiparesis, and ataxic gait. Speech is often soft and dysarthric.

Neuropathy, Restless Leg Syndrome and Muscle Cramps

Pathophysiology

Uremic neuropathy is axonal, with secondary segmental demyelination, presumably due to failure to maintain the perikaryon of the nerve axon. The putative toxin is not simply excess urea, as dialysis does not always lead to improvement in neuropathy. Malnutrition, with vitamin deficiencies such as pyridoxine (B_6) and biotin, has also been proposed. Accumulation of amyloid, especially distal to the AV fistula used for dialysis, produces pressure neuropathy; the fistula may also cause neuropathy by ischemia. Calcium derangement may cause muscle cramps or tetany.

Clinical Findings

Seventy percent of chronic renal failure patients experience neuropathy, but it may be asymptomatic. Burning feet and dysesthesia to light touch, numbness in stocking-glove distribution, and distal weakness are signs of neuropathy. Restless legs are characterized by the urge to kick or stretch the leg in order to relieve a creeping, crawling sensation, usually

Figure 3

Electroencephalogram of hepatic encephalopathy

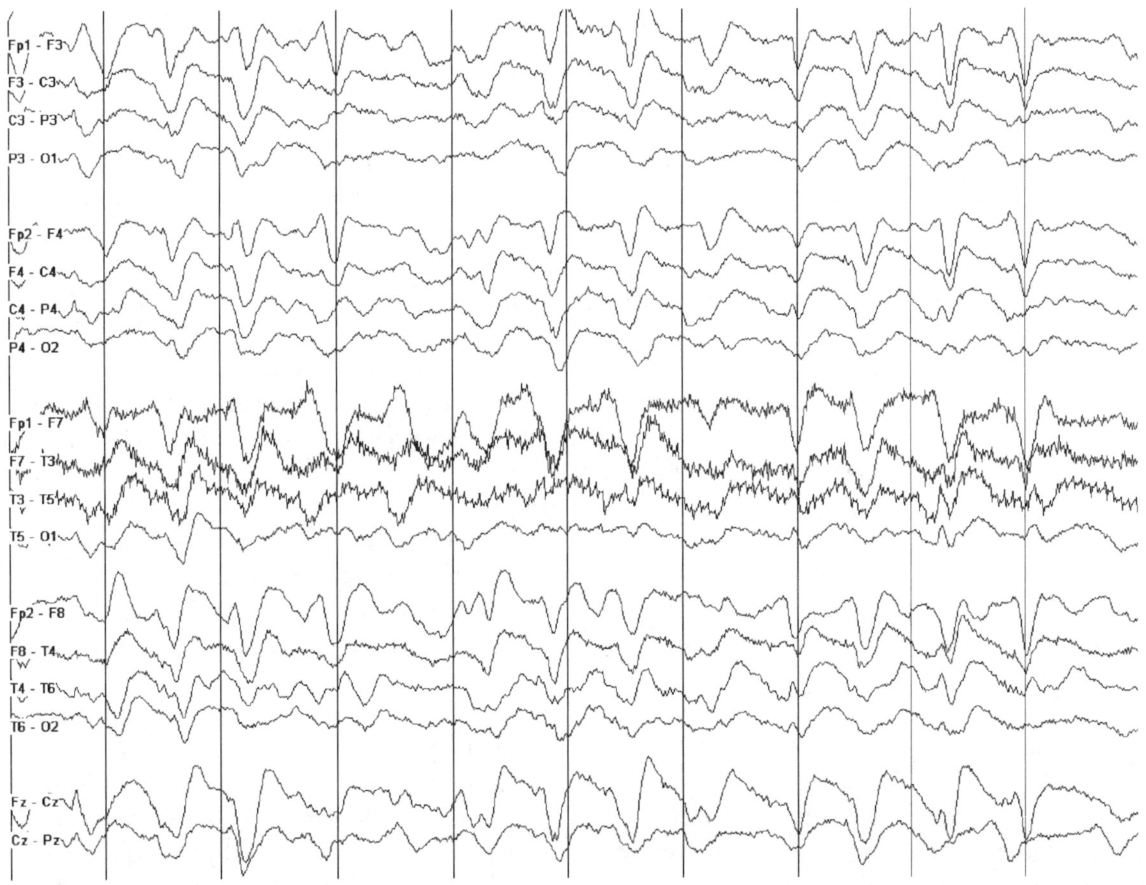

while trying to sleep. Muscle cramps are painful spasmodic contractions, often in the calf. Rarely, flaccid quadriplegia is seen.

Diagnostic Tests
Nerve conduction velocities are slow and compressive palsies related to amyloid deposition or fluid overload produce focal slowing (eg, carpal tunnel syndrome).

Treatment
Dialysis eventually helps, although true symptom resolution is best seen with renal transplant. Vitamin supplements or liberalization of protein intake in the diet alleviate some of the pain of neuropathy. Cramps don't respond well to potassium or calcium supplementation. Symptomatic treatment with anticonvulsants such as gabapentin must be done carefully, as this is metabolized in the kidneys and requires dose adjustment. Restless legs syndrome responds to dopamine agonists and benzodiazepines.

Electrolyte Disturbances: Sodium
Hypernatremia is defined as a serum sodium above 145 mEq/L, but neurologic symptoms are not usually seen below 160 mEq/L. The elderly and children below age 3 are most likely to suffer from this, either due to fluid loss from external perturbations (heat, gastroenteritis, poor sweating), or internal dysregulation due to lack of thirst or access to water. The amount of sodium is determined by hormones that are secreted in the hypothalamic pituitary axis and act on receptors in the kidneys.

Hyponatremia is defined as a serum sodium below 130mEq/L, (mild) to <115 (severe), with symptoms correlating with the rapidity of decline from normal.

Pathophysiology
Hypernatremia develops when vasopressin and antidiuretic hormones fail to regulate the loss of sodium from the kidneys to compensate for restricted intake of water or loss of water from other causes. The elderly are especially susceptible, and those hospitalized patients who suffer from fever or diarrhea, or who are kept "NPO" for testing or procedures, or who continue to use diuretics without adequate access to water, are subject to a multiplication of these insults. In patients without an obvious explanation, CNS lesions in the hypothalamus or pituitary may be responsible. Diabetes insipidus from head trauma can also cause hypernatremia.

The brain actually shrinks during hypernatremia, when osmotic shifts of water leave the glia and neurons to return to the circulation. This can cause hemorrhage in the parenchyma, subarachnoid or subdural space. This was responsible for permanent neurologic sequalae or death in 20% of children in one series. Fluid shifts during extreme hypernatremia or corrective rehydration cause generalized seizures, myoclonus, and movement disorders. Muscle breakdown is very rare.

Hyponatremia occurs when salt is wasted due to inappropriate ADH secretion, which can be due to brain or lung masses, adrenal insufficiency or heart failure, or increased tubular sensitivity to normal amounts of ADH, medication side effects, excessive water drinking, or iatrogenic errors in fluid replacement, including bladder lavage with water instead of physiologic fluids. Fluid shifts due to osmotic gradients in the brain cause cerebral edema and seizures, especially in patients who also have hypomagnesemia, or generalized hypotonia in patients with hypokalemia as well.

Clinical Findings
Loss of skin turgor and dryness are clues to the presence of dehydration. Confusion and lethargy are the earliest signs of dehydration and hypernatremia, with progression to stupor and coma if untreated. Abnormal movements such as tremor and asterixis are not unusual, and rigidity is similar to that of neuroleptic malignant syndrome. Seizures are common, and intermittent generalized muscle weakness is rare.

Hyponatremia causes confusion, drowsiness or stupor, generalized seizures or myoclonic twitching, with eventual hypothermia and respiratory failure, with herniation and coma due to increased brain edema. The latter is associated with drops within 24 hours.

Diagnostic Tests
Analysis of serum sodium is key, with frequently repeated checks during correction. BUN and creatinine will also be elevated in dehydrated patients. Urine sodium levels will determine the cause of hypernatremia, with high levels in attempts to con-

serve salt and water (small amounts of highly concentrated urine), and low levels in the dilute urine of diabetes insipidus, and low levels in dehydration. Generalized atrophy is seen on CT or MR, which may also reveal underlying hypothalamic or pituitary pathology responsible. Transient increases in signal are rarely seen in the thalamus of severely hypernatremic patients.

Treatment

Careful rehydration with intravenous fluids is required for hypernatremia. Seizures and myoclonus do not require anticonvulsants.

For hyponatremia, careful fluid replacement with normal saline is required, as overly rapid replacement can cause central pontine myelinolysis, while edema and herniation can occur while waiting to correct sodium levels.

Electrolyte Disturbances: Potassium

Unlike the central effects of sodium perturbation, potassium's effects are mainly on the muscle. Paralysis is found in both hyperkalemia and hypokalemia.

Pathophysiology

Episodic weakness of variable degree of the arms and legs that lasts several minutes is caused by genetic disorders on chromosome 17q13 (hyperkalemic periodic paralysis), 1q32, or rarely, same as above (hypokalemic periodic paralysis), and 17q23 (Andersen syndrome, HyPP with cardiac arrthymia). The involved genes form portions of the ion channel, including the α subunit of the sodium channel, the dihydropyridine-sensitive L-type calcium channel, and the inwardly rectifying potassium channel, all found on muscle tissue. In addition to these genetic diseases with symptoms provoked by stressors such as carbohydrate-rich foods or glucose and cold (hypo-) or rest after exercise, fasting and ingestion of foods rich in potassium (hyper-), any condition that changes the serum potassium below 3.0mEq/L or above 5.5mEq/L can cause muscle weakness. Urinary and intestinal losses, often medication related, and hyperthyroidism (especially in Asian patients) lead to hypokalemia and uremia; potassium-sparing diuretics and extreme intake of potassium lead to the former. Channels that use ions to cause muscle contraction and relaxation will be affected adversely by extreme changes in the ion content of the serum; either provoking repetitive firing leading to myotonia, or inactivation leading to weakness.

Clinical Findings

Weakness that ranges from mild to extreme occurs without sensory symptoms or mental status changes. Cramps do not accompany the weakness but can be present at other times. Measurement of serum potassium during the attack makes the diagnosis. Careful history taking for activities and food ingested the day before (as hypokalemic PP usually comes on in sleep), or immediately before for hyperkalemic PP, helps teach how to avoid future attacks as well as making the diagnosis.

Diagnostic Tests

Measurement of serum potassium is essential. If DNA testing is available, the responsible gene can be established, once it has been established that there is abnormal potassium during attacks of weakness. Otherwise, the old-fashioned provocative test giving glucose and insulin intravenously to cause an attack can induce low potassium and high sodium in the serum; this is not without risk. In patients with hypokalemic PP without the gene present, hyperthyroidism should be measured, especially if the patient is of Asian origin. Creatine kinase becomes elevated relative to the duration and severity of symptoms. Rhabdomyolysis can occur. In hyperkalemic periodic paralysis, myotonia can be detected using EMG even when not seen clinically.

Treatment

This is simpler in the hypokalemic forms, where either food or supplements containing potassium, starting with 20mEq and repeating as needed, abort attacks. Attacks may be prevented by chronic use of acetazolamide, a carbonic anhydrase inhibitor, or potassium-sparing diuretics such as spironolactone. If hypokalemia is due to thyrotoxicosis, this must be treated, and similarly renal or intestinal disease addressed.

Electrolyte Disturbance: Calcium

Like sodium and potassium, calcium is involved in membrane stabilization and normal neuronal and muscle cell function. Therefore, changes of plasma levels outside a narrow range lead to dysfunction in the peripheral and central nervous system. The most frequent, hypercalcemia, produces lethargy, while hypocalcemia produces muscle irritability with cramps and spasms.

Hypercalcemia

Pathophysiology

Serum levels of calcium are determined by its absorption in the intestine, excretion or resorption in the kidney, and ongoing deposit and resorption from bone, under regulation by parathyroid hormone. Normal range is 8-10mg/dL, and neurologic symptoms begin above 11-12 mg/dL (2.9-3mmol/L). The regulators include parathyroid hormone, cholecalciferol, and calcitonin. Most cases (75%) of hypercalcemia are due to malignancies, especially breast and lung cancer and multiple myeloma, which directly destroy bone in metastases or increase parathyroid hormone levels. Adenomas of the parathyroid gland itself cause primary hyperparathyroidism.

Clinical Findings

Coma is found in very high levels (>15mg/dL), while more common signs include depression, confusion or lethargy and constitutional "slowing" leading to constipation, nausea, or anorexia and increased urination. There may be cardiac arrhythmias or short QT interval on EKG. Hyperparathyroidism, even with only mild hypercalcemia, has been associated with brainstem dysfunction. Apnea is occasionally the only sign of hypercalcemia in children.

Peripheral symptoms include a proximal myopathy with weakness and easy fatiguability, cramps and parasthesias. Carpal tunnel syndrome, especially in uremic patients with hypercalcemia, is increased.

Diagnostic Tests

EMG shows fibrillations, indicative of myopathic or neuropathic changes. Muscle biopsy shows atrophy. Once hypercalcemia is discovered, with repeated testing to rule out laboratory error, the underlying cause is sought by measuring parathyroid hormone, especially in chronic cases, and then seeking adenomas. Malignancies with bone metastases or lung or kidney tumors which secrete hormones inducing hypercalcemia, together with parathyroid disease, account for 90% of cases of hypercalcemia. Vitamin D intoxication, granulomatous disease, thiazide use, and renal failure with aluminum intoxication account for hypercalcemia in rare cases.

Treatment

Lowering the serum calcium level by use of saline and diuretics temporarily helps; surgery for underlying malignancy or adenoma provides permanent resolution.

Hypocalcemia

Chronic hypocalcemia in adults is seen in renal failure and acute pancreatitis. Acute hypocalcemia can complicate thyroid or parathyroid surgery, and is rarely found in neonates. Hypocalcemia is also a common complication of acute pancreatitis.

Pathophysiology

Membrane instability due to inadequate calcium accounts for most symptoms of hypocalcemia, both chronic and acute. Intracranial calcifications found in the basal ganglia (Fahr disease) in the hypoparathyroidism that is usually responsible for hypocalcemia presumably interrupt basal ganglia connections, leading to chorea and parkinsonism. Low magnesium contributes to exaggerated reflexes and twitching in hypocalcemia.

Clinical Findings

Tetany is an involuntary muscle spasm that may be painful or painless; since the most common locations are wrist or foot, it is often referred to as carpopedal spasm. It may be elicited by tapping the facial nerve just in front of the ear, causing facial spasm (Chvostek's sign), or by occluding the brachial artery for three minutes with a sphygmomanometer and watching for wrist spasm (Trousseau's sign). Hyperventilation also elicits tetany, usually after perioral and fingertip parasthesias. Myopathy can occur, as well as deafness.

Abrupt drops in serum calcium cause seizures (generalized or focal) and irritability or agitation, with extreme cases appearing delirious. Chronic hypocalcemia can present with dementia, choreoathetoid movements, or rarely, parkinsonism. Benign intracranial hypertension has been reported; the mechanism is unknown.

Diagnostic Tests

Measurement of serum calcium gives the diagnosis and extent of the problem. Albumin, phosphorus and magnesium should also be measured. EEG may be slow, with rare epileptiform activity. Creatine kinase elevation and myopathic changes on EMG are rarely seen. A lowered threshold of excitability of the nerve to stimulation (Erb sign) is also found in some cases. CT (in cases of hypoparathyroidism-induced hypocalcemia) shows intracranial calcifications, especially in the basal ganglia. ECG abnormalities include prolonged QT interval and nonspecific ST-wave changes.

Parathyroid hormone levels must be measured, as hypoparathyroidism accounts for most cases of hypocalcemia. In pseudohypoparathyroidism, with normal or elevated levels of PTH, the hormone is antagonized at the cellular level, which is one cause of short stature and mental retardation. Some cases have been associated with the Kearns–Sayre syndrome and muscle phosphorylase deficiency (presumably due to failure of calcium to activate phosphorylase kinase).

Treatment

Increasing serum calcium is accomplished by vitamin D and calcium supplements given orally. (Neonates require intravenous treatment.)

Electrolyte Disturbance: Magnesium

Magnesium is an important ion in the nervous system, as it is needed for the function of intracellular enzymes and modulates synaptic transmission both centrally and peripherally.

Hypomagnesemia

This resembles hypocalcemia, and is often found with it. Clinical findings include recurrent seizures, delerium, myoclonus and tetany, especially when serum magnesium concentrations fall below 0.8 mEq/L.

Pathophysiology

Low magnesium levels in the body are a result of decreased intake (starvation), absorption (sprue), or increased output (diuretics, alcoholism, renal tubular acidosis). Low serum levels are found in up to 10% of hospitalized patients, but the intracellular content may be normal, and neurological effects tend to occur only in those with levels below 1.2 mEq/L. Hypomagnesemia may contribute to parathyroid hormone dysfunction responsible for hypocalcemia, or the lack of response of patients with low calcium levels to calcium replacement. Hypomagnesemia is a complication of cisplatin.

Clinical Findings

Low levels of magnesium in the serum (<1.8, but generally symptoms require <1.2meq/L) cause the same symptoms described in hypocalcemia. These reflect irritability, with peripheral involvement causing tetany with carpopedal spasm, and central involvement causing seizures or confusion. Muscle weakness can be chronic or acute, but may be due to co-existing hypokalemia or hypophosphatemia, or mitochondrial myopathy. Focal deficits are occasionally present.

Diagnostic Tests

Serum levels make the diagnosis, and other neurologic tests are not indicated as this is a transient. To determine the cause in patients with no obvious risk factors, further analysis of kidney function is mandated.

Treatment

In convulsing patients, parenteral administration of magnesium salts (magnesium sulfate) is required, with calcium gluconate on hand to counteract transient hypermagnesemia, which causes respiratory muscle paralysis. Oral supplementation with magnesium gluconate is sufficient for milder and chronic cases.

Hypermagnesemia

Although much rarer than hypomagnesemia, elevated levels have been described with chronic renal dysfunction, magnesium overuse (as in antacids) or as an iatrogenic complication of treatment of eclampsia. Levels >5 mEq/L cause nervous system depression.

Clinical Findings

These involve the muscles, causing paralysis, and in extreme cases leads to respiratory insufficiency. On examination, the earliest sign is depressed deep tendon reflexes. Lethargy can occur with very high serum magnesium levels (> 8 mEq/L), but patients can be asymptomatic with much higher levels, reflecting the difference between intracellular and serum concentrations.

Pathophysiology

Blockade of neuromuscular transmission is responsible for the paralysis of hypermagnesemia. Similar interference with synaptic transmission centrally can cause CNS depression, but much higher levels of magnesium are required.

Treatment

Interruption of the supply of magnesium in patients with renal failure, or those given magnesium for eclampsia, will correct most cases. Hydration and diuretics speed the process.

5. Hematologic Disorders and Complicatons of Cancer

Erythrocyte Disorders

Sickle Cell Disease

Stroke in children who have sickle cell disease occurs in 7%-15% of homozygous patients.

Pathophysiology

In patients who are homozygous for the both hemoglobin S gene, an abnormal β-globin chain in which the glutamic acid substitutes for valine at the sixth amino acid position is produced, and when the red cell is deoxygenated, polarization of hemoglobin occurs. This distorts the shape of the erythrocyte, rendering it too stiff to travel through arterioles and capillaries, leading to ischemia throughout the body and brain. The incidence of stroke in SS disease is 0.6 per 100 patient years for SS, and the cumulative risk of stroke by age 45 is 24% for SS patients and 10% for SC patients. Sickle-β-thalassemia causes stroke one-tenth of the incidence of SS disease. Strokes are ischemic in children, whose mean age of first occurrence is 8 years, while hemorrhage is more common in patients over age 20. In addition to older age, elevated WBC count (not necessarily infection) and decreased hemoglobin concentration are risk factors for hemorrhagic stroke.

Arteries of all sizes become thickened due to intimal proliferation, resembling vasculitis to some extent. In addition to this intracranial stenosis that leads to stroke during periods of hypoperfusion, the deformed sickle cells have trouble passing through smaller caliberdistal arterioles, leading to sludging.

Hemorrhage can occur into an infarct, or due to subarachnoid hemorrhage due to aneurysm formation, especially in more distal vessels.

Clinical Findings

Typical strokes occur in an unusually young population of African or African-American descent. Hemorrhage occurs in up to 40% of cases. Cognitive impairment even in the absence of stroke is common, manifesting as learning disability or psychologic difficulty. Infarctions of individual nerves or the spinal cord present with appropriate findings. Seizures occur in up to 12% of SS cases, and may present with or follow stroke or infection, especially meningitis. Meperidine, a common analgesic used in painful crisis, lowers the seizure threshold. SC disease causes a retinopathy in 58% of patients, and hearing loss is more common than with SS disease. Rarely, myelopathy is caused by cord compression from extramedullary hematopoiesis.

Diagnostic Testing

Stroke is diagnosed by neuroimaging. CT scan shows cortical hypodensity or hemorrhage, either in the subarachnoid space or into the infarcted territory. Atrophy develops in time. Magnetic resonance imaging (MRI) shows infarcts, in large vessel territory in 72%, and the remainder in small vessel. Asymptomatic older infarcts are seen frequently. Angiography (even intravenous injections for CT-angiography) should be avoided due to the high complication rate of stroke or sickle cell crisis, but in prior studies has shown large vessel pathology and segmental narrowing. MR angiography has been positive for stenosis in children even below 4 years of age. Carotid and transcranial Doppler studies demonstrate reduced flow. EEG shows focal or diffuse slowing and occasional epileptiform activity.

Treatment

Symptomatic stroke prevention has been partially accomplished by maintaining HbS<30% of total hemoglobin using frequent blood transfusions. Although the rate of recurrent stroke is lowered to 10% by regular transfusion compared to 46%-90% within 3 years of the first event without it, alloimmunization and iron overload can be serious problems. In SS patients screened by transcranial Doppler ultrasonography, prophylactic transfusion can be started even before a first stroke in patients with abnormal transcranial Doppler ultrasonography. Butyric acid and hydroxyurea have also been used to lower fetal hemoglobin concentration. Bone marrow transplantation can be curative.

Thalassemia

Another genetic disease due to defective production of the α-globin chain is α-Thalassemia, which produces a hemolytic in individuals of Mediterranean or Asian descent. Most neurologic symptoms, including dizziness and graying of vision, are due to anemia and respond to transfusion. This nonspecific dizziness occurs in 20% of patients, polyneuropathy (mainly affecting motor nerves) also is reported in 20%, headaches or seizures in 13%, and paroxysmal myopathy is rarely described. Extramedullary hematopoiesis can lead to cord or cauda equina compression, which responds to transfusion and radiation therapy. Blood analysis provides the diagnosis.

Pathophysiology

Excess red blood cells (hematocrit >45mg/mL) can be due to the myeloproliferative disorder *P vera*, to pulmonary hypoventilation, cyanotic heart disease or high altitude, or lesions that secrete erythropoietin such as cerebellar hemangioblastoma or hypernephroma. Neurologic symptoms include stroke, headache, tinnitus, dizziness, blurred vision, cognitive impairment, paresthesias, and a predominantly sensory axonal neuropathy.

Repeated phlebotomy or chemotherapy reduces the blood viscosity by lowering the hematocrit.

Clinical Findings

Most neurologic symptoms, including dizziness and graying of vision, are due to anemia and respond to transfusion. In addition to this nonspecific dizziness which occurs in 20% of patients, polyneuropathy (mainly affecting motor nerves) is reported in 20%, headaches or seizures in 13%, and paroxysmal myopathy in rare sufferers. Extramedullary hematopoiesis can lead to cord or cauda equina compression, which responds to transfusion and radiation therapy.

Diagnostic Testing

Blood analysis for hemoglobin type provides the diagnosis in anemic patients.

Treatment

Transfusion and in cases of extramedullary hematopoeisis, radiation, are helpful in symptom control. Bone marrow transplant is also performed.

Treatment

Repeated phlebotomy or chemotherapy reduces the blood viscosity by lowering the hematocrit.

Platelet Disorders

Thrombocythemia (Essential)

An elevated platelet count (> 600,000/mm^3) causes dysfunction, with a predisposition to both hemorrhage and thrombosis in arterial and venous circulations. This most often causes headache, paresthesias, visual blurring, TIA or stroke, and seizures. CNS bleeding is very rare.

Antiplatelet agents, including aspirin, clopidogrel or dipyridamole, or medications that lower platelet numbers, including hydroxyurea and anagralide, generally work, but in major thromboembolic events, platelet pheresis should be performed.

Thrombotic Thrombocytopenic Purpura

Although there is a paucity of platelets, in TTP there is intravascular clumping of platelets leading to transient neurologic deficits or global confusion, renal failure and fever, which is often fatal. Patients tend to be younger (mean age of 40) and this may accompany other autoimmune states: hemolytic uremia syndrome, especially following *E coli* infection, or can occur in HIV infection. As antibodies against or congenital deficiency of von Willebrand factor-cleaving protease are responsible, treatment with plasma exchange or IVIg therapy is highly successful, especially if there are no strokes or hemorrhages found on CT. CSF protein may be elevated. Chemotherapy or corticosteroids may be required to maintain remission after plasma exchange or IVIg.

Heparin-induced Thrombocytopenia (HIT)

This immune-mediated disorder starts 5 or more days after initiation of heparin in a patient not previously exposed. Platelet counts fall <100,000/μL, followed by arterial or venous thrombosis (including stroke) in up to 3% of cases. IgG binds to heparin/platelet factor 4 complex, which activates platelets. Treament consists of stopping heparin and substituting danaparoid or argatroban.

Antiphospholipid Syndrome

Two antibodies (aPLs) most associated with stroke are the anticardiolipin antibody and the lupus anticoagulant, which can be inherited, drug-induced or otherwise acquired. Stroke and thrombosis elsewhere in the body are found in patients under age 50.

Pathophysiology

The cause of stroke when aPL or LA are present is multifactorial, including platelet binding, endothelial binding, altered thrombomodulin, inhibition of natural anticoagulants such as protein C and S, vasculopathy of intracranial vessels, or in the case of lupus anticoagulants, inhibition of coagulation pathways. In addition, cardiac emboli are associated with antiphospholipids. The important antibodies belong to the IgG class, as IgM can be "innocent" bystanders of infection or inflammatory states.

Clinical Findings

Recurrent thrombotic events, beginning usually before the age of 45, can occur throughout the body or brain, with cerebral venous thrombosis producing headache and seizures along with hemorrhagic strokes outside of arterial territories. Arterial ischemic events also occur, especially in the eye, digits and lungs, as well as the brain. Murmurs due to Libman-Sacks endocarditis or other valvular lesions may be present. Skin mottling due to cyanosis, ie, livedo reticularis, may be seen on the legs or arms. Migraines or, in some patients, headaches secondary to benign intracranial hypertension occur. Myelopathy and chorea may occur. Recurrent miscarriages happen to mothers with anticardiolipin antibody syndrome.

Diagnostic Testing

A prolonged activated partial thromboplastin time (aPTT), which does not correct with mixing of plasma from which platelets have been extracted, is a marker of lupus anticoagulant. IgG anticardiolipin antibodies of >40 phospholipid units must be measured more than once by ELISA. Low platelets, hemolytic anemia, false positive VDRL, a low titer of positive antinuclear antibodies and C4 (complement) deficiency are other indicators. Cardiac echo can reveal verrucous vegetations on the valves or mural thrombi.

Treatment

Anticoagulation is often used, although aspirin has worked as well in older, unselected patients. Immunosuppression with azathioprine, cyclophosphamide or cyclosporin, modulation with IVIg, plasmapheresis and anti-idiotype antibodies or corticosteroids have all been tried. Rarely, anticoagulation must be combined with immunosuppression.

Blood Cell Dyscrasias

Leukemia

Acute lymphoblastic leukemia with WBCs >150,000/mm^3 can lead to stroke by leukostasis occluding cerebral blood vessels. Rarely, hemorrhage is caused by blasts infiltrating endothelial walls. Indirectly, treatment of leukemia can predispose to CNS infection by decreasing white blood cell count.

Clinical Findings
Leukematous meningitis can cause cranial nerve V or VII palsies or focal numbness or weakness due to clumping of leukemic cells compressing the nerve roots; intracerebral metastases (chloromas) are rare, but when they involve the skull or facial bones they can cause facial palsy. If they are in the epidural space of the spinal cord there will be symptoms of cord compression at that level. Infiltration of the hypothalamus by leukemic cells presents with diabetes insipidus, or obesity due to hyperphagia.

Treatment
Treatment is directed against the primary leukemia, using radiation or intrathecal chemotherapy with methotrexate or cytosine arabinoside. Emergency leukopheresis to lower the blast count may be necessary in thrombotic states.

Plasma Cell Dyscrasias

Multiple myeloma, Waldenström macroglobulinemia (with IgM paraprotein), and amyloidosis all produce B cells, to variable degrees, which may be asymptomatic or change to chronic lymphocytic leukemia.

Pathophysiology
Monoclonal gammopathy of unknown significance (MGUS) is associated with a demyelinating peripheral polyneuropathy (sensory or motor) due to IgM antibody activity against myelin-associated glycoprotein, axonal sulfatides or chondroitin sulfate.

Clinical Findings
When myeloma involves bones of the vertebral column, the most frequent neurologic complication is radiculopathy or cord compression. Sometimes the bones are not involved but instead masses appear within the spinal canal to produce cord compression. Plasmacytoma can produce polyneuropathy, or amyloid deposition can cause individual neuropathies such as carpal tunnel syndrome. POEMS (polyneuropathy, organomegaly, endocrinopathy, M protein, and skin changes) is a rare complication of myeloma or plasmacytoma.

Hyperviscosity is also found with Waldenström macroglobulinemia, causing symptoms similar to those of polycythemia vera or thrombocytosis. In the Bing-Neel syndrome, plasma cell invasion of perivascular spaces leads to leukoencephalopathy.

Either sensory or motor polyneuropathy is indirectly produced by these dyscrasias. Cauda equine syndromes cause flaccid neurogenic bladder, sexual dysfunction, radicular pain and weakness in the legs, and higher locations of compression cause spastic paraparesis that evolves slowly.

Treatment
Treatment involves plasmapheresis, IVIg or removal of an isolated plasmacytoma for neuropathies, and radiation for root or cord compression, that also helps control bone pain. Immunosuppression or chemotherapy can prevent recurrence.

Myelofibrosis

Spinal cord or cerebral compression may be caused by masses related to the extramedullary hematopoiesis that accompanies myelofibrosis. If located in the orbit, exophthalmous will be seen.

Coagulation Disorders

Hematologic disorders such as the inherited "thrombophilias" (Protein C, Protein S, Antithrombin III deficiencies and Factor V Leiden and prothrombin 20210A mutations) account for 1% of ischemic strokes and up to 15% of strokes in patients under age 45. The latter has only been known to cause venous thrombosis, but arterial thrombosis, mainly of the carotid artery, is found with Protein C, S, and antithrombin III deficiencies. Stroke itself and anticoagulation can produce alterations in the levels of the above factors, so caution is advised in making the diagnosis too quickly, although newer genetic testing such as THROMBX® Evaluation II, performed by Athena Diagnostics, can look for antigens to Protein C, S, Factor VII and V and antibodies to anticardiolipin antibodies in the presence of anticoagulation.

Pathophysiology

Antithrombin III deficiency (AT III), found in 1:2-5,000 people, is either acquired (GI losses, nephrotic syndrome, DIC, extreme blood loss) or inherited through an autosomal dominant pattern. This glycoprotein binds to heparin and inactivates coagulation proteases such as thrombin. Protein C is a natural anticoagulant that is activated when thrombin is produced with the endothelial cofactor thrombomodulin to form activated protein C. Protein S, a vitamin K-dependent protein, helps this activation, which in turn inactivates factor V to turn off the coagulation process. A mutation in factor V Leiden can similarly interfere with protein C's function. DIC, liver or kidney disease (nephrotic syndrome), birth control pills, warfarin use and leukemia can cause these deficiencies or dysfunctions.

Clinical Findings

Venous infarcts in the brain, causing variable deficits, seizures, headache and, in the case of major sinuses, obtundation, are the hallmark of the "hypercoagulable" states. Infarcts elsewhere in the body occur in unusual sites such as the mesenteric circulation or arms, instead of the deep veins of the legs and lungs. A patent foramen ovale raises the risk of stroke in these circumstances by a factor of 10. Events known to trigger thrombosis in predisposed individuals include pregnancy, dehydration, immobilization, infection and surgery. A family history is found in the inherited forms.

Diagnostic Testing

CT and MR scans show hemorrhagic venous infarcts with loss of sulci. MR venogram, angiography or contrast-enhanced CT show clots in the sinuses, including the delta sign in the posterior sagittal sinus. All the above factors can be measured in the blood, but reliable values are not obtained for several months after an event, especially once anticoagulation with warfarin is present.

Treatment

Anticoagulation with heparin or warfarin is used only after a clinical thrombotic event, except in rare instances of patients with known factor deficiencies (by a positive family history) who are at risk of stroke due to pregnancy, major surgery or trauma, or prolonged bed rest. Warfarin loading should be avoided, as distal thromboemboli can lead to necrosis of fingers and adipose tissue. Duration of therapy is usually at least 3 months after an event unless contraindicated, and may be required for the patient's entire life if the event was severe enough. Stressors such as cigarette smoking and oral contraceptive use should be avoided. Heparin does not work in antithrombin III deficiency. These patients will need AT III concentrate during times of crisis. Supplements of folic acid may help the homocysteinemia that accompanies protein C deficiency in some patients.

Pregnancy

Venous thrombosis is part of eclampsia, occurring immediately before or in the first four weeks after delivery. On MRI, eclampsia is accompanied by T2 hyperintensities in the back of the brain but with no definite posterior circulation stroke. It is otherwise determined by hypertension, proteinuria and seizures. Hemorrhage is possible due to backed up elevation in the brain. Treatment is aspirin or heparin, as warfarin is contraindicated during pregnancy.

Hemophilia

Lack of clotting factors leads to hemorrhage anywhere in the body, both spontaneous or after minimal trauma. Neurologic symptoms correspond to the site of bleeding in the brain, spinal cord, peripheral nerve or muscle.

Cerebrovascular Complications of Cancer

Ischemic Complications

The hypercoagulable state that accompanies some malignancies, such as pancreatic cancer, leads to venous and arterial thrombotic infarcts. This also occurs if metastases interfere with the liver's ability to make coagulant factors.

Emboli can break from atrial myxomas or from nonbacterial thrombotic endocarditis, especially in the presence of adenocarcinoma or lymphoma. Tumor emboli can evolve into cerebral metastases.

Lymphoma located within small blood vessels causes multiple small strokes and dementia (neoplastic angioendotheliomatosis).

After radiation therapy to the neck for malignancy, severe atherosclerosis can cause stenosis of the carotid artery, leading to TIA or infarction. Endarterectomy is technically difficult, with poor healing, so intravascular stent placement is the optimal treatment.

Hemorrhagic Complications

Leukemia is associated with DIC, and the coagulopathy causes either hemorrhage or multiple strokes, leading to encephalopathy. This is diagnosed by measuring an increase in fibrin split products.

Depression of platelet function from chemotherapy (there is no growth factor available for platelets, as there is for neutrophils and red blood cells) makes the brain vulnerable to bleeding when levels fall below 20,000/mm^3. Subdural hematoma occurs with metastatic deposits to this space. Certain metastases (lung, hypernephroma, thyroid, melanoma, choriocarcinoma) that are very vascular with hyperdense appearance on CT are more likely to bleed even under normal hematologic conditions.

Even with normal coagulation and platelet function, some high-grade gliomas or metastatic tumors (melanomas, lung carcinomas, choriocarcinomas and hypernephromas) are likely to bleed.

Lastly, invasion of the wall of an artery may produce a subarachnoid or intracerebral hemorrhage. Hemorrhage should be treated with recombinant factor VII, as surgery is extremely difficult due to bleeding complications.

6. Vasculitides and Collagen Vascular Diseases

As a group of conditions characterized by inflammatory changes in the circulatory system, ischemic and hemorrhagic strokes are the predominant cause of nervous system disability in the vasculitides, but other manifestations will be discussed as well. Some are primary to the CNS, and secondary vasculitides refer to nervous system involvement in systemic collagen vascular disease, such as lupus, sarcoid, Behçet's and others.

Primary CNS Vasculitis

These are limited to the nervous system, the most common being giant cell (temporal) arteritis. Smaller vessels are involved by granulomatous angiitis, known as PACNS, which causes stroke or obtundation in younger people.

Pathophysiology

The size of the blood vessel that is involved determines where the pathology in the nervous system will occur, inclusive of the brain, peripheral nerve and muscle. Table 1 gives the condition, blood vessel size, and laboratory tests useful in diagnosis. The differential diagnosis of primary vasculitides includes multiple sclerosis, primary CNS lymphoma, encephalitis or migraine, amyloid angiopathy, vasospasm after subarachnoid hemorrhage or sympathomimetic use, and other vasculopathies such as malignant hypertensive encephalopathy, post-radiation, and cyclosporine use.

These conditions are immune-mediated but not always "auto-immune"; extrinsic causes include infection, cocaine or amphetamine use and other toxins. Granuloma formation, a hallmark of sarcoidosis, can occur within blood vessels or act as a mass. Blood vessels are damaged by the deposition of immune complexes, endothelial attacks by anticardiolipin or antineutrophil cytoplasmic antibodies, cytotoxic T cell, or cytokine directed activity and strokes can also be produced by platelet clumping brought on by the action of anticardiolipin antibodies. In the CNS, these produce infarcts of variable size, seizures, psychosis (rarely) and dementia, which rarely involves the spinal cord. In the PNS, these produce individual nerve infarcts when the vaso nervosum artery is occluded, leading to mononeuritis multiplex.

Table 1

Features of Syndromes with Primary or Secondary Vasculitis

Disease	Vessel Size	Laboratory and Radiographic Findings	
PACNS	S,M,L Granulomata stenosis, beads	CSF:10WBC, Pro>100 Culture Ag,Ab+Olig oclonal bands	MR: subcortical ↑signal T2, meningeal enhancement, mass lesion+/- MRA, SPECT changes
SLE	S art, vein, cap Rare stenoses in Lg arteries (Vasculitis rare)	Pancytopenia, +ANA, +/- antiCardiolipin +n-ds DNA homogeneous), +Sm or RNP (speckled) +RNA (nucleolar), anti ribosomal P ↓Complement during flare CSF: ↑protein, few lymphs, IgG, oligoclonal bands	Hemmorrhage w/vasculitis CT, MRI: nonspecific ↑signals w.m., resembles hypertensive Rare abnormal angio, MRA. Atrophy (dissuse involvement) PET ↓metabolism
APA	Rare vasculities, M, L thrombosis	+Antiocardiolipin Ab (IgG, IgM), +LA or ↑pTT, ↓plt	Multiple cortical and subcortical strokes SPECT diffuse & focal↓
WG	Arterioles, venules, rare, M,L	AnticANCA>>pANCA Kidney, lung, sinus involvement	Sinusitis
RA	Any size, near involved meninges	+RF	Enhancement meninges, pachymeningeal, plaque, hemorrhage
SS	S, outside CNS	Anemia, ↑ESR, +RF, +ANA, antiRo(SSA), La(SSB) hyper-globulinemia	MS life lesionis
Behcet	Cap, veins, often brainstem	CSF: few L or N, s1↑ Pro, oligoclonal bands	Meningeal thickening, Sm irregular lesions brainstem, spinal cord, deep wm
Cogan	Aorta, Any	Eye findings, CSF lymphs	Rare cavernous sinus thrombosis

(continued)

Table 1 *(continued)*

Features of Syndromes with Primary or Secondary Vasculitis

Disease	Vessel Size	Laboratory and Radiographic Findings	
PAN	S,M, branch pt. Aneurysms	↑ESR, ↑WBC, anemia anemia +HepB, B, HIV pANCA	Single or multiple strokes, often normal, irreg vessels with aneurysms on angiogram
TA	M, L carotid (external) rare intracranial	↑ESR, ↑CRP	Rare infarct, angiogram beading

ANA=antinuclear antibody, APA=antiPhospholipid antibody, c-ANCA=cytoplasmic-staining antineutrophil cytoplasmic autoantibody, pANCA=perineuclear staining ANCA, GA=granulomatous angiitis, LA=lupus anticoagulant, PACNS=primary angiitis central nervous system, PAN=polyarteritis nodosa, pTT=prothrombin time, RA=rheumatoid arthritis, SS=Sjogren syndrome, TA=temporal arteritis, WG= Wegener's granulomatosis

Giant Cell Arteritis

Clinical Findings

Giant cell arteritis (GCA) affects 42-270/million adults over 50 years of age, and is the most common vasculitis. It presents with headache or visual symptoms caused by retinal vein ischemia, or diplopia caused by ischemia of cranial nerves to the extraocular muscles, accompanied by muscle pain in half the cases (polymyalgia rheumatica). Other symptoms are jaw claudication, alopecia due to scalp involvement, fever, anorexia, sweats and anemia, with elevated ESR or C-reactive protein in almost all patients.

Diagnosis

Diagnosis is made by temporal artery biopsy (guided by Doppler or angiogram) or response to high-dose prednisone. After 3 months, this can be tapered, with continued treatment of NSAIDs symptomatically.

Primary angiitis of the central nervous system, or granulomatous angiitis, affects small- and medium-sized vessels of the brain and sometimes meninges, with the multiplicity of involvement leading to headache, confusion or obtundation rather than specific stroke syndromes. Seizures occur rarely. Diagnosis can take up to 6 months, especially if biopsy proof is required. Benign, self-limited disease is seen in some patients, relapsing disease in others, and severe patients progress to death despite immunosuppression.

Serologies will be negative in primary vasculitides, other than antibodies to viruses that trigger them, such as hepatitis B and C, borrelia, syphilis, tuberculosis, HIV, CMV and herpes varicella. CSF shows elevated protein (median 177mg%) and lymphocytic white blood cells (mean 77/mm^3) with IgG synthesis and oligoclonal bands. Angiography shows segmental narrowing and dilatations or vascular occlusions with collateral formation, but is normal in up to 44 percent. MRI with MRA are normal or show multiple areas of damage, with enhancing areas. Diagnosis depends on biopsy of involved parenchyma or meninges. Immunosuppression is the treatment, including high- dose corticosteroids, but success is variable.

Takayasu's arteritis shares histopathology (granulomatous inflammation) with GA, but the vessel involved is the aorta and its branches, and aneurysms are seen in addition to endothelial changes, leading to subclavian steal, global hypoperfusion, or stroke, especially in the carotid territory in 1/3 cases (others have infarcts in other arterial territories such as the brachial artery). It usually occurs in Asian women, under age 50, including children.

Systemic Vasculitides Involving the Nervous System

Nervous system dysfunction, often stroke, is a feature of several diseases, with location varying according to the disease and vessel size. Other symptoms are present based on other areas of the body's involvement—often circulatory dysfunction, such as kidney damage in PAN, lung involvement in sarcoid, or joint involvement in SLE.

Examples of various systemic vasculitides are discussed as follows:

Polyarteritis nodosa involves medium-sized vessels, usually in the nerves, and causes mononeuritis multiplex or sensory and motor neuropathy, with less than one-quarter of patients also having CNS disease such as stroke, seizures, encephalopathy, or cranial nerve palsies. Hepatitis B infection is found in up to 50 percent. Vessel damage produces intimal obliteration by fibrin deposits or proliferation and aneurysms.

Kawasaki disease, associated with viral infection in children, also involves medium-sized vessels and produces seizures and facial palsy in addition to stroke. Other features include conjunctivitis, reddening of the tongue, and oropharynx, adenopathy and coronary artery disease. Treatment is aspirin and intravenous immunoglobulins.

Wegener's granulomatosis involves small vessels and causes changes similar to hypertensive leukoencephalopathy, or dural thickening near sinuses and orbits, meningitis, or other granulomata. In addition, there must be at least two other symtoms: oral ulcers or nasal discharge, abnormal chest x-ray, hematuris, or arterial wall involvement by biopsy. C-ANCA is usually present in the serum. In addition to the usual immunosuppression or steroid use, the antibiotic co-sulfamethoxazole is used.

Churg-Strauss syndrome also is characterized by small vessel involvement of either the peripheral (polyneuropathy) or central nervous system, sometimes hemorrhage, and ischemic optic neuropathy. It is accompanied by asthma, allergy, and eosinophilia with sinusitis and pulmonary infiltrates. C-ANCA is present.

Cryoglobulinemia is characterized by immune complex deposition that leads to polyneuropathy.

Behçet disease involves small vessels, including arterioles and venules, or large vessels in the form of venous sinus thrombosis. After headache, generalized weakness and signs of cerebellar or brainstem ischemia, dementia and seizures are seen rarely. Aseptic meningitis may be present. Other features include uveitis and mucus membrane ulcerations (genital and mouth most often). Heparin and anticoagulation are indicated in venous thrombosis; treatment otherwise consists of steroids and immunosuppression, or modulation with thalidomide and interferon-α. Cogan syndrome can mimic Behçet, but also has prominent eye and vestibular features, caused by keratitis and uveitis, and involves vessels of any size. Untreated diseases have up to 90% mortality rates.

Pathophysiology

These are autoimmune diseases whose symptoms depend on vessel size involved and accompanying areas of the body that are affected.

Diagnosis

Serologic tests give clues to the disease, along with angiography when indicated, or biopsy.

Treatment

As in all immune-mediated disease, treatment includes corticosteroids, and standard immunosuppression with methotrexate, cyclophosphamide and chemotherapeutic agents. Options after failure of conventional treatment include the monoclonal antibody rituximab, the anti-tumor necrosis factors infliximab, etanercept, mycophenolate mofetil, and anticoagulation as indicated.

Secondary Vasculitides Associated with Collagen-Vascular Diseases

Systemic lupus erythematosis causes nervous system disease in prevalence rates that vary from 15%-85%, reflecting subtle problems such as cognitive and psychiatric dysfunction. Seizures and psychosis are the only problems included in classification criteria, these being the most specific. The American College of Rheumatology listed 19 possible neuropsychiatric syndromes of lupus, with one series finding headache occurring most frequently (24%), stroke (14.5%), mood disorders (16%), cognitive disorders (11%), seizures (8%), psychosis (8%), anxiety (4%), and acute confusion (4%), with lesser incidences of neuropathy, mononeuritis multiplex, myelopathy, chorea, central and peripheral demyelination, myasthenia and cranial neuropathies. Anticardiolipin and antiphospholipid antibodes lead to vessel damage not always accompanied by inflammatory changes, and platelet clumping, causing thrombosis. Therefore, ischemia must be prevented by using antithrombotics or anticoagulation instead of simply using immunosuppression.

Rheumatoid arthritis rarely directly involves the nervous system, and when it does it is due to chronic meningitis from inflammation, leading to complications. Indirect pressure from bony pathology such as atlantoaxial subluxation, vertebral collapse or nerve compressions from pannus formation can occur.

Progressive systemic sclerosis can involve the fifth or other cranial nerves, in addition to neuropathy from microvascular ischemia.

Sjögren syndrome can frequently involve the nervous system (up to 20%), leading to myelopathy from spinal cord involvement and motor neuron disease, optic neuropathy, polyneuropathy, or cranial neuropathy and diffuse CNS involvement similar to that of SLE. Non-neurologic symptoms include salivary and lacrimal gland dysfunction.

Sarcoidosis may present with neurologic features, such as facial nerve palsy, and eventually 5%-15% of patients will show symptoms of CNS or PNS involvement. Hypothalamic involvement can lead to diabetes insipidus, and other signs reflect the location of meningeal thickening or granuloma formation.

Vasculitis Secondary to Conditions Other than Collagen-Vascular Disease

Infection, especially viruses such as hepatitis and HIV, and herpes viruses such as varicella, indirectly cause vasculitis. Cancer, especially lymphoma and some leukemias, likewise can cause it, and indirect paraneoplastic syndromes have also been described with small cell lung, renal, gastric and endometrial cancers, leading to peripheral neuropathy. Vasculitis has been set off by exposure to amphetamines, cocaine, heroin, ergotamines and LSD, and by sympathomimetic drugs found in diet and decongestant aids. Angiography or biopsy are often required to make the diagnosis. Antiviral treatment is indicated in vasculitis accompanying encephalitis, such as herpes.

7. Bone Disease

Paget Disease (Osteitis deformans)

Skeletal abnormalities cause compression of cranial nerves or parts of the brain or spinal cord, in addition to pelvic and tibial involvement.

Pathophysiology
Weakened but enlarged bones occur in this condition of excessive bone formation and resorption. These compress nearby areas.

Clinical Findings and Differential Diagnosis
Nonspecific head pain is often present. The cranial nerve most frequently affected is the eighth, leading to deafness; facial palsy follows in frequency, and other cranial nerves exiting at the base of the skull can be impaired or compressed. Similarly, paraparesis can emerge after spinal column involvement. Brainstem symptoms due to severe basilar impression occurs with Arnold-Chiari I syndrome.

Seizures can occur even with normal calcium. Accelerated atherosclerosis is also symptomatic in some patients.

Diagnostic Testing
Routine x-rays are diagnostic, with the skull showing increased and decreased bone densities, leading to overgrowth of bone with a fluffy appearance. CT can show basilar invagination and skull expansion. MRI shows mottling in the diploic space of the skull and impingement on the nerves or dens.

Treatment
Intranasal calcitonin inhibits the osteolytic process, strengthening bone. Disodium etidronate is also used.

Achondroplasia

Dysplasia of the entire skeleton leads to short stature with skull enlargement. The cause is a mutation in the fibroblast growth factor receptor 3 gene (FGFR3). In addition to cord compression from disc disease or spinal stenosis, hydrocephalus can occur with obstruction of CSF outflow. Ataxia and medullary dysfunction are caused by compression of the posterior fossa. Mentation is usually normal.

8. Nutritional Disorders and Toxins

The nervous system is vulnerable to deficiencies during development, such as folate deficiency causing neural tube deficits, and later in life, especially affecting the peripheral nerves, spinal cord and vermis of the cerebellum. Thiamine deficiency causes short-term memory deficits (Korsakoff syndrome) after an illness characterized by confusion, nystagmus and ataxias (Wernicke syndrome). In addition to the vitamin deficiencies listed in Table 1, special circumstances affect the nervous system, such as myopathy in anorexia nervosa, myopathy or paralysis from hypokalemia related to diarrhea, and ataxia and peripheral neuropathy from gluten enteropathy (celiac sprue) (although the ataxia may be autoimmune rather than nutritional, as anti-Glu antibodies are diagnostic). Inflammatory bowel diseases cause demyelinating neuropathy, myopathy, and at times thrombembolic events involving the central nervous system. B_{12} deficiency in patients with overgrowth of the small intestine or lack of gastric receptors (pernicious anemia) leads to the combined systems disease of the posterior columns (sensory symptoms and sensory ataxia), corticospinal tract (myelopathy), peripheral neuropathy, and dementia.

Bariatric surgery, especially the bypass operation using the Roux-en-Y procedure (not the band placement done laproscopically), is associated with up to 15% of neurologic complications, including minor ones such as carpal tunnel and meralgia parasthetica. Shortly after surgery, an encephalopathy with myalgias, incontinence, and acute polyradiculoneuropathy has been described with normal thiamine levels and no ophthalmic features of Wernicke encephalopathy. Patients who fail to continue injections of vitamin B_{12} have developed optic neuropathy after 1 year, and myelopathy involving the posterolateral cord, a mean of 10 years post-operatively. This presents with gait ataxia, spasticity with positive Babinski signs, urinary urgency, and leg weakness, with additional sensory loss to pin and temperature in a stocking glove pattern in about 50 percent. Peripheral neuropathy, which can develop in the absence of myelopathy, is also slowly progressive occurring about 10 years post-operation. Although some patients are found to be deficient in B_{12} or copper, these syndromes can occur in patients receiving proper vitamin supplementation, and do not always respond to supplementation started late.

Pathophysiology

Co-factors necessary for myelin formation or upkeep are found in vitamins and minerals, and their absence leads to central, spinal cord, or peripheral nerve degeneration.

Clinical Findings

These reflect the part of the nervous system involved, and vary with the nutrient that is implicated; reviewed in Table 2.

DiagnosisSerologic analysis can detect many deficiencies, while some, such as celiac disease, require antibody (anti-Glu Ab) testing.

Table 2

Vitamin Deficiencies

Vitamin	Neurologic Signs and Symptoms	Systemic Signs Lab Abnormalities	Treatment
B_{12} (cobalamin) combined system disease	Demyelination of posterior and lateral columns leads to ataxia, myelopathy and + Romberg sign. Peripheral neuropathy leads to burning feet and hands. Dementia, optic neuropathy, anosmia or dysgeusia, orthostatic hypotension. Congenital: mental retardation, seizures, microcephaly. Acquired: nitrous oxide or metformin exposure, vegan diet, bacterial overgrowth in intestine. Pernicious anemia: achlorhydria or antibodies against intrinsic factor.	Anemia, hair loss, vitiligo, weight loss, sore tongue B_{12} <200 pg/mL ↑methylmalonic acid, homocysteine Axonal pattern on NCV, +/-abnormal evoked potential MRI ↑T2 in thoracic cord, enhancement Schilling test	1000 mcg IM daily x 1 wk, then weekly for one month, then monthly. Oral absorption not reliable with PA. Nasal spray may work.
B_1 (thiamine) Dry beriberi/ Wernicke/ Korsakoff	Neuropathy-numbness or weakness, hands involved more than feet Wernicke encephalopathy (confusion, delerium, nystagmus and EOM palsies, ataxia) Korsakoff syndrome (chronic short term memory failure)	H/o alcoholism, nausea, anorexia or bariatric surgery. Low thiamine or RBC transketolase MRI: symmetric hyperintense signal in midbrain and thalamus, 3rd & 4th ventricles, PAG	IV or IM thiamine 1000 mg daily, then 100 mg po daily
Folate	Congenital-neural tube defects	Myelomeningocele, spina bifida, anencephaly	Prenatal supplementation, especially in women using aniepilepetic medication

continued

Table 2 *(continued)*

Vitamin Deficiencies

Vitamin	**Neurologic Signs and Symptoms**	**Systemic Signs Lab Abnormalities**	**Treatment**
Multiple vitamins	Polyneuropathy Optic neuropathy (predisposed by mitochondrial DNA mutations)	Axonal neuropathy ↑vulnerability to pressure palsies	Multiple vitamins (oral) Abstinence from alcohol, nicotine
Nicotinic acid (Niacin)	Pellagra: delirium, amnesia Peripheral neuropathy	Alcoholics	Nicotinic acid therapy
Vitamin D	Developmental delay, tetany	Osteomalacia	Vitamin D supplement ↑sunlight exposure
Vitamin E	Spinocerebellar symptoms, abnormal EOMs (reverse INO, nystagmus Neuropathy, ↓reflexes	Vitamin E <0.5 mcg/dL NCV: ↓SNAP; delay SSEP	100 mg/kg α-tocopherol daily
B_6 (Pyridoxine)	Sensory neuropathy, axonal loss associated with use of Isoniazid for treatment for tuberculosis Infantile seizures	↓amplitude sensory>motor EEG: Hypsarrthymia	Supplement with 50 mg daily. Avoid pyridoxine
Copper	Myelopathy/neuropathy (rare)	Zinc toxicity Bariatric surgery	Copper supplement

Table 3

Toxin's Effects on the Nervous System

Toxin	Brain D/E/H/MR/ A/Sz*	Basal Ganglia P/Dy/C My/T	Spinal Cord	Muscle	N-M Jx	Nerve a-autonomic s-sensory m-motor
Alcohol	All	Rare PC		√		√
Aluminum	Dialysis D/E	My				
Arsenic	E,H, Coma					√(s,>m)
Bismuth	Coma, Sz	My				
Botulism						
Carbon Monoxide	E	P,C, Tic				
Cyads	D	P	ALS			
Cyanide	Sz, coma	P,Dy,C				
Lead	E/MR	My,T	?ALS			√(motor)
Manganese	D	P/D/T				
Marine-	Sz (domoic) acid	Temor				(sciguatera) (m,a, puffer) (m,shellfish)
Mercury	D,E	My,T	?ALS			
Mushrooms	E,H	My			√	√
Organophas-phates	E			√		
Solvents	E,H,A,Coma	P,D, My		√		√(m+s)
Tetanus		My			√	
Thallium						√(s>m)
Venoms	E (scorpion)			√	√	√(all)

**D=dementia, E=encephalopathy, MR=mental retardation, A=ataxia, Sz=seizures*
***P=parkinsonism, Dy=dystonia,C=chorea, My=myoclonus,T=tremor*
+ Solvents include methanol, carbonsdisulfide, n-hexane, toluene

9. References

1. Bronster DJ. Neurologic complications of cardiac surgery: current concepts and recent advances. *Curr Cardiol Rep*. 2006;8(1):9-16.

2. Brust JCM. *Neurologic Complicationsn of Substance Abuse*. Philadelphia: Lippincott, Williams & Wilkins; 2006.

3. DiComite G, Sabbadini MG. Neurological involvement in rheumatological diseases. *Neurol Sci*. 2005;26:S9-S14.

4. Dobbs MR, Wicklund MP. Toxic and environmental neurology. *Neuro Clinics*. 2005;23: 321-521.

5. Engel J, Jr, Pedley TA, eds. *Epilepsy: A Comprehensive Textbook*. Philadelphia: Lippincott, Williams & Wilkins; 2008

6. Foster B, Rosenthal E, Marques S, et al. Primary systemic vasculitis: treatment of difficult cases. *Lupus*. 2006;15:143-7.

7. Juhasz-Pocsine K, Rudnicki SA, Archer RL, Harik SI. Neurologic complications of gastric bypass surgery for morbid obesity. *Neurology*. 2007;68(21):1843-50.

8. Rowland LP, ed. *Merrit's Neurology*. 11th ed. Philadelphia, Pa: Lippincott Williams & Wilkins; 2005.

9. Riordan SM, Williams R. Treatment of hepatic encephalopathy. *N Engl J Med*. 1997;337: 473-479.

10. Selnes OA, McKhann GM. Neurocognitive complications after coronary bypass surgery. *Ann Neurol*. 2005;57:615-621.

11. Wijdicks EFM, Cranford RE. Clinical diagnosis of prolonged states of impaired consciousness in adults. *Mayo Clin Proc*. 2005;80(8): 1037-1046.

12. Williams O, Brust JC. Hypertensive Encephalopathy. *Curr Treat Options Cardiovasc Med*. 2004 Jun;6(3):209-216.

10. Questions

1. 46-year-old man with history of cardiomyopathy with decreased ejection fraction, alcohol abuse and crack cocaine use is admitted after he had a prolonged seizure. On exam he has normal mental status and cranial nerves but appears blind with good pupillary reflexes, normal muscle strength in all extremities, symmetric 2/2, DTRs, decreased stereognosis, and graphesthesia with normal primary sensation and bilateral Babinski signs. Which of the following is the likely CT scan finding?

A. Border zone infarctions between the territories of the middle and posterior cerebral arteries

B. Left MCA infarction

C. Bilateral ACA infarctions

D. Dorsal pontine infarction

E. None of the above

2. What is the etiology?

A. Hypoperfusion of the brain

B. Cardiogenic emboli

C. Left ICA stenosis >90%

D. Small vessel ischemic disease

E. None of the above

3. What could have contributed to the patient's clinical picture?

   A. Bilateral carotid stenosis

   B. Decreased ejection fraction

   C. Prolonged seizure

   D. None of the above

   E. All of the above

4. After cardiac bypass surgery, a 69-year-old man became confused and lethargic with paraparesis. On second post-op day, Neurology is consulted for altered mental status. EEG shows 6Hz generalized slowing without epileptiform activity. On exam, he has paraplegia with sensory level up to T8 in pinprick and touch sensations, and intact vibration sense. Babinski sign is present bilaterally. This shows:

   A. Hepatic encephalopathy

   B. Left MCA infarction

   C. Post-surgery encephalopathy

   D. Peripheral neuropathy

   E. None of the above

5. What is the most likely cause for his weakness?

   A. Anterior spinal artery infarction

   B. Left ACA infarction

   C. Lumbar disc herniation

   D. Peripheral neuropathy

   E. Popliteal artery occlusions

6. A 55-year-old woman starts her car in her attached garage, and then goes to the adjacent kitchen. The next day she is found by the neighbors, and is confused, complaining of headache, and the EMS notices red skin. This shows:

   A. Carbon monoxide poisoning

   B. Dysautonomia

   C. Heat stroke

   D. Psoriasis

   E. Complicated migraine

7. A 48-year-old obese, hypertensive man presents to clinic with excessive daytime sleepiness, waking up feeling like he had never slept at all, with mild headache. He says he wakes himself up with loud snoring, which started after he gained 40 lbs. during the past 2 years. On exam, he has BP of 145/95, decreased visual acuity, and mild papilledema. He was involved in an accident when he fell asleep driving.

   Which of the following would be the most helpful test in diagnosing this patient?

   A. Multiple sleep latency test

   B. Polysomnogram

   C. CT head

   D. MRI brain

   E. EEG

8. Which of the following is not an appropriate treatment for this patient?

A. CPAP

B. Weight loss

C. Amphetamines

D. Benzodiazepines

E. Uvulopalatopharyngoplasty

9. Where is the respiratory center?

A. Left parietal lobe

B. Red nucleus

C. Substantia nigra

D. Nucleus ambiguous and solitary tract nucleus (medulla)

E. Globus pallidus and putamen

10. A 28-year-old man who works at an automobile body shop comes with wrist drop. On exam, he has weakness of the extensor hand muscles in the radial nerve distribution. What is the most likely cause for his wrist drop?

A. Manganese intoxication

B. Methyl alcohol intoxication

C. Lead intoxication

D. Carbon monoxide poisoning

E. Mercury intoxication

11. Which of the following would be an appropriate treatment?

A. Chelation with IV dimercaptopropanesulfonic acid

B. Chelation with calcium EDTA

C. Physical and occupational therapy

D. All of the above

E. Vitamin C

12. A 36-year-old man with history of VP shunt placement as a child for obstructive hydrocephalus was reported to collapse, and now has altered mental status with respiratory insufficiency. Chest x-ray shows pulmonary edema. Which of the following is likely to cause the chest x-ray findings?

A. Seizure

B. Subarachnoid hemorrhage

C. Acute increased ICP

D. Heart failure

E. All of the above

13. A 72-year-old man presents to clinic with forgetfulness and imbalance for the past 6 months. On exam, MMSE is 24/30, there is gait ataxia, decreased visual acuity, and decreased sensation in the lower extremities. What is the most likely cause for the patient's clinical presentation?

A. Alzheimer disease

B. Hyperthyroidism

C. Dementia with Lewy bodies

D. Spinocerebellar ataxia

E. None of the above

14. What are the lab findings?

A. Low TSH, high free T4

B. High MCV, methylmalonic acid and anemia

C. Low potassium, high sodium

D. Triphasic waves on EEG

E. Cryoglobulinemia

15-19. Match the nutritional deficiency:

15. B_1 deficiency	A. Wernicke's encepahalopathy
16. B_6 deficiency	B. Dementia
17. B_{12} deficiency	C. Sensory neuropathy
18. Magnesium deficiency	D. Nystagmus, cerebellar ataxia
19. Vitamin E deficiency	E. Seizure

20. A 14-year-old African-American female with history of sickle cell disease is admitted for right hemiparesis and aphasia. MRI with DWI confirms left MCA infarction. Which of the following is correct?

A. Cumulative risk of stroke by age 45 is 24% for SS patients and 10% for SC patients.

B. Hemorrhagic stroke is more common in patients over age 20 than younger patients.

C. Elevated WBC count and decreased hemoglobin concentration are risk factors for hemorrhagic stroke.

D. Ischemic strokes are more common in children with mean age of first occurrence 8 years.

E. All of the above.

21. A 50-year-old woman with a history of bariatric surgery (Roux-en-Y procedure) in 1995 presents with difficulty walking, stiff legs, dizziness and parasthesias in the feet. She had a 100-pound weight loss, with BMI now 27, and she denied hypertension and diabetes. There was social alcohol use (1-2 glasses wine on weekends) and no smoking. She had been taking a multivitamin daily since the surgery, and had no other medications. Physical exam included no back or neck tenderness with FROM, -Lhermitte sign, normal mental status and cranial nerves, strength normal in arms and 4/5 proximally in legs with increased tone, reflexes 2/2 arms, 3/3 knees, and 4/4 ankles with upgoing toes. Gait was wide-based, spastic with difficulty turning. Vibratory and position sense and pinprick sensation were decreased in the feet, and Romberg was positive.

The patient's deficits involve which parts of the nervous system:

A. Cerebellum

B. Parietal lobes

C. Spinal cord

D. Muscle

E. Nerve roots

22. The most likely deficiency is:

A. Vitamin D

B. B_{12}

C. Estrogen

D. Zinc

E. Calcium

23. If she had received injections of B_{12} and copper supplementation without improvement, what would be required to reverse these symptoms?

A. Rebanding of the stomach

B. Lengthening the loop and correcting a blind loop

C. Parenteral nutrition

D. Providing higher doses of vitamins

E. Physical therapy

Answers

1. A.
Border zone infarct. Because both arms hemispheres are affected, one arterial territory could not be responsible for the findings. The low ejection fraction due to cardiomyopathy, combined with prolonged seizure, would lead to a watershed infarct from hypoperfusion of vulnerable areas.

2. A.
Hypoperfusion of the brain would cause vulnerable areas to infarct. This often includes the area between the parietal and occipital lobes, producing cortical blindness.

3. E.
All of the above, in combination, could contribute to the hypoperfusion in this territory.

4. C.
Post-surgery encephalopathy, which is associated with cardiac surgery, would cause confusion and lethargy with generalized slowing on the EEG, but not the weakness.

5. F.
Anterior spinal artery infarct, which can occur with aortic artery ischemia or emboli from the cross clamping of the aorta during bypass surgery, is known to cause paraplegia with Babinski signs, and possible preservation of function in the dorsal columns.

6. A.
CO poisoning produces hypoxic encephalopathy with transformation of oxygenated hemoglobin to methemoglobinemia, leading to red skin.

7. B.
Polysomnography would demonstrate the apneic events that are causing sleep disruptions with insufficient time spent in REM and Stage 3 and 4, and excessive daytime sleepiness. Multiple sleep latency testing is for narcolepsy, with rapid entry into REM sleep (< 2 minutes). CT and MRI show structural lesions which are not part of sleep apnea. Routine EEG without measurement of respiratory muscle activity would not demonstrate the cause of the drowsiness.

8. A.
CPAP, or continuous positive airway pressure, produces an air column that supports the soft tissues of the nasopharynx, allowing free entry of oxygen and preventing apneas. BiPAP would work as well, and weight loss may allow the airway to remain open without support. HCTZ is a safe antihypertensive. Benzodiazepines, whether taken for anxiety or sleep, could be dangerous without airway support.

9. D.
The medulla, including the nucleus ambiguous and solitary tract nucleus, is where the respiratory center is located.

10. B.
Lead poisoning in the adult produces motor neuropathy, most often involving the radial nerve. In the developing nervous system, brain damage is more likely, producing seizures and developmental disability.

11. D.
Chelation and physical therapy are appropriate treatments for lead poisoning.

12. E.
A sudden increase in ICP can cause increased vagal nerve outflow, which leads to left heart failure and pulmonary edema. This is usually found with repeated seizures, but can occur with one, or SAH, or any rapidly developing increased ICP.

13. E.
None of the listed diagnoses cause all the clinical findings.

14. B.
B_{12} deficiency causes increased MCV and anemia, and increased methylmalonic, which is a co-factor in myelin formation, therefore involving many systems (brain, cord, peripheral nerves). Hypothyroidism would cause forgetfulness and ataxia but not the decreased sensation.

15. A.
B_1 or thiamine deficiency causes Wernicke encephalopathy (and neuropathy).

16. C.
Pyridoxine deficiency (and extreme excess use) causes peripheral neuropathy, especially in patients taking INH for treatment of tuberculosis.

17. B.
B_{12} deficiency causes dementia in addition to other effects on the nervous system.

18. E.
Magnesium deficiency, with its effect through calcium, can produce seizures.

19. D.
Vitamin E deficiency produces nystagmus (or reverse INO with failure to abduct and nystagmus in the adducting eye) and ataxia.

20. E.
All of the statements concerning sickle cell stroke are true.

21. C.
Although peripheral neuropathy is the most common problem after bariatric surgery, especially newer procedures that do not involve intestinal bypass, the symptoms this patient describes are consistent with myelopathy.

22. B.
B_{12} deficiency is the most common nutrient that is deficient after bariatric surgery, although copper can also be involved.

23. B.
Encephalopathy and myelopathy (and peripheral neuropathy) have been described in patients who have used vitamin supplements regularly, and reversal of the intestinal bypass may be the only way to correct the neurologic symptoms.

Chapter 33: Surgical Neurology

Tarek A. H. Radwan, BMedSci, MBBChir
Jeffrey A. Cohen, MD

Contents

1. Neurosurgical Trauma

Coma of Anatomical Cause

Of all patients who present with coma of unknown origin in a general hospital emergency room, the causes are as follows:

- 30% drug overdoses
- 35% mass lesion
- 35% diffuse metabolic causes

Securing the ABCs (airway, breathing and circulation), followed by expeditious imaging of the head by CT scanning, is therefore mandatory to exclude those that require any surgical intervention as a matter of emergency. Additionally, toxicology screening, treatment on severe electrolyte abnormalities, especially hyponatremia and breaking seizures in status epilepticus, form the cornerstones of managing the comatose patient.

The neurologic assessment of the comatose patient, although necessarily thorough once completed, should initially focus on those aspects that will give the maximum amount on information in the first two minutes, and therefore are highly reproducible in a repeated fashion for serial exam purposes.

The scheme for a basic quick coma neurologic exam includes the three elements found in Table 1.

In the documentation of the consciousness level, it is imperative to document the: a.) time of the examination; b.) exact stimulus applied to patient; and c.) the exact response obtained when the stimulus was applied. The Glasgow Coma Scale (GCS) (Table 2) is a recognized scale for this purpose.

Table 1

Neurological Assessment of Coma

Function	Response
Glasgow Coma Scale	Eye opening Motor response Verbal response
Brain Stem Function	Pupillary reactions Corneal responses Spontaneous eye movements Oculocephalic responses Oculovestibular responses Respitory pattern
Motor Function	Motor response Muscle tone Tendon reflxes Seizures

Table 2

Glasgow Coma Scale

Eye Opening	4 = Spontaneous 3 = To speech 2 = To pain 1 = none
Best Verbal	5 = Oriented 4 = Confused 3 = Inappropriate words 2 = Incomprehensible sounds 1 = None
Best Motor	6 = Obeys commands 5 = Localizes to pain 4 = Withdrawal/flexion; does not localize 3 = Flexion (abnormal) 2 = Extension 1 = None

Head Injuries

The importance of head injuries does not need underscoring, neither from the devastating effects it has on the individual and the family, nor the cost to society in terms of long-term care cost and productive life years lost in what are mostly young, productive patients.

Of all trauma deaths in the US, one-half are due to closed head injuries, a total of 75,000 deaths per year. For severe head injury (GCS 3-8 after resuscitation), here is overall outcome based on the trauma coma data bank: ~ 45% good outcome (good recovery or moderate disability, GOS 1-2); ~ 20% poor outcome (severely disabled or vegetative, GOS 3-4); ~ 35% dead

Up until relatively recently, the admission GCS was the criteria for head injury. Mild, moderate and severe head injuries over the last 30 years have been defined as GCS of 13-15, 9-13, and equal or less than 8, respectively. The increased use of early sedation, intubation, and ventilation, especially in the field, has decreased the value of the full GCS for the purposes of early classification. The computed tomographic scan (CT) has come to be the standard radiologic investigation of the acutely polytraumatized patient, both for neurologic as well as other injuries.

The Head Injury CT

The computed tomographic scan (CT) has come to be the standard radiologic investigation of the acute traumatized patient. It is extremely sensitive to picking up acute lesions of surgical significance, namely skull fractures, hemorrhage/hematoma, as well as contusional injury. There are also a significant number of radiologic signs on the CT scan that can be used to infer either mass effect locally, eg, tentorial edge herniation, as well as intracranial pressure generally. Some of these signs are more discriminatory than others.

Discriminatory Findings on Head Injury CT

- Presence or absence of mass lesions (SDH, EDH, ICH)
- Presence and size of midline shift (no shift, shift 6-10mm, shift >10mm)
- Status of basal cisterns (interpeduncular, ambient, prepontine, quadrigeminal; present, compressed, or absent)
- Presence of intraventricular blood/hemorrhage (IVH)
- Presence of traumatic subarachnoid hemorrhage (tSAH)

Focal Head Injuries

Skull Fractures (Figure 1.1, 1.2, 1.3)
A simple classification scheme of fracture is as follows:

Linear
Linear skull fractures are usually sustained as a result of direct impact, typically falls; and, in general, with intact skin or a clean wound do not require any intervention. These can present only occasional problems of fracture growth over time in infants with open sutures. Healing is uniformly satisfactory.

Depressed
Depressed skull fractures are those that involve more than one linear fracture and result in bony depression below the level of the inner table of the calvarium. These are highly variable in appearance and implications. These also heal satisfactorily, if there are not complications (see below).

Complicated
Usually these are depressed fractures (on occasion linear) that have adverse modifying factors. These include skin laceration with contamination (technically an *open* fracture with risk of osteomyelitis); depression beyond the inner calvarial table of at least full bone thickness; dural laceration (with or without cerebral penetration); and penetration of air sinuses with potential for CSF leakage and meningitis. Internal fractures of air sinuses into the cranial

cavity also have to be considered open fractures in the same vein. The most dangerous areas for fractures are those that directly cause injury to the dural venous sinuses, eg, occipital fractures over the torcula, which can lead to venous sinus thrombosis and cerebral infarction. Fractures of the petrous temporal bone, especially those close to or involving the condylar fossa (also usually the mandible), can cause internal carotid artery injury in its petrosal genu segment.

Fracture Hematoma

All fractures bleed from the diploic space of the fractured bone (as with any other bone), and therefore can form a *fracture hematoma* in "orthopaedic" terminology. These are often referred to as *venous epidurals*. On the whole, these usually lack any significant pressure to cause symptoms, but must be differentiated from an arterial epidural (see below).

Hematoma

EDH–Epidural Hematoma

The commonest cause is rupture of the middle meningeal artery at its course within its groove in the squamosal portion of the lateral temporal bone. It is usually associated with a fracture, whether linear or depressed. As an arterial hemorrhage, there may be a period of time of temporary hematoma stabilization after the initial injury, followed by rehemorrhage and expansion of this to cause a significant mass. This is seen clinically as the so-called lucid interval.

Generally speaking, this process occurs between 4 and 6 hours from the moment of injury. This is the rationale for neurologic observation for 12-24 hours, and nowadays to repeat CT scans (if the initial scan was hyper-early, ie, less than 4 hours).

Location is all important with epidurals: a low temporal epidural can quickly cause uncal herniation and third nerve palsy with somnolence, whereas a high frontal epidural may be totally asymptomatic.

SDH–Subdural Hematoma

As with EDH, location is all important (see above). Typically, SDH occurs due to brain translation or rotation, with tearing of the cortical bridging veins, or in some severe cases the actual cortical surface veins. These are venous in nature and so not high in pressure effect, but will insidiously accumulate volume.

IVH and TSAH–Intraventricular Hemorrhage and Traumatic Subarachnoid Hemorrhage

These typically occur as kinetic energy is transmitted to vascular structures, in particular those transitioning from a CSF location to fixed structures with consequent rupture. Traumatic SAH is therefore seen usually on the convexity where small arteries are torn, and IVH is seen most sensitively in the dependent part of the ventricle in the inferior-most tip of the occipital horns.

Contusional Injury

Contusional brain injury occurs as a consequence of blunt traumatic injury to the cortex and subcortical white matter from impact with part of the containing calvarial wall. Commonly, this is seen in the basal frontal lobes from laceration of the brain on the irregular grooves on the floor of the anterior fossa floor, in the anterior temporal lobe and pole from the direct deceleration impact onto the anterior middle fossa, and the uncus from the medial tentorial edge. Classically, contusion occur on the opposite side of the calvarium from a fracture, due to the rapid deceleration of the moving brain; but they can also be seen directly under fractures, especially depressed fracture.

Diffuse Head Injury

Diffuse Axonal Injury (DAI) is technically a post-mortem neuropathological diagnosis, but has been in popular clinical use to denote the likely cause of a patient's coma. This describes a classic high velocity acceleration-deceleration injury pattern. There is rupture of axonal processes that traverse the neuropil in an up-and-down direction from cortex to brain stem. Often no imaging abnormality is seen on CT, or tiny petechial "salt & pepper" hemorrhages can be seen due to rupture of the very small vessels accompanying those axons.

This most commonly is seen in the subcortical white matter. More severe velocities and rotational momentum also in the deep white matter, midbrain and brain stem can, however, leave minimal evidence on CT, but devastating clinical effects with a patient in deep coma without any obvious radiologic abnormalities. MRI, especially with blood-sensitive sequences such as gradient recall echo (GRE) and susceptibility weighted imaging (SWI) has a much higher sensitivity for such injuries, but its use is essentially for prognostic purposes.

The treatment of severe head injuries in the ICU setting is covered in the section on Neurosurgical Critical Care.

Post-traumatic Seizures Risk Factors

- GCS < 10
- Cortical contusion
- SDH
- EDH
- ICH
- Depressed skull fracture
- Penetrating head wound
- Seizure in 1st 24 hrs

The use of prophylactic anti-convulsants decreases the rate of early seizures (in the first week post injury), but *does not affect the rate of late developing seizures*.

Figure 1.1

Skull fractures

a.) EDH showing the classic "lens" shape underlying a fracture of the temporal bone; b.) different patient with a depressed skull fracture with underlying SDH and midline shift; c.) the same patient as in (b.) demonstrating extension of SDH into middle fossa with pressure on temporal lobe and tentorial herniation (patient had third nerve palsy on left). The abundance of pneumocephalus is seen associated with a basal skull fracture.

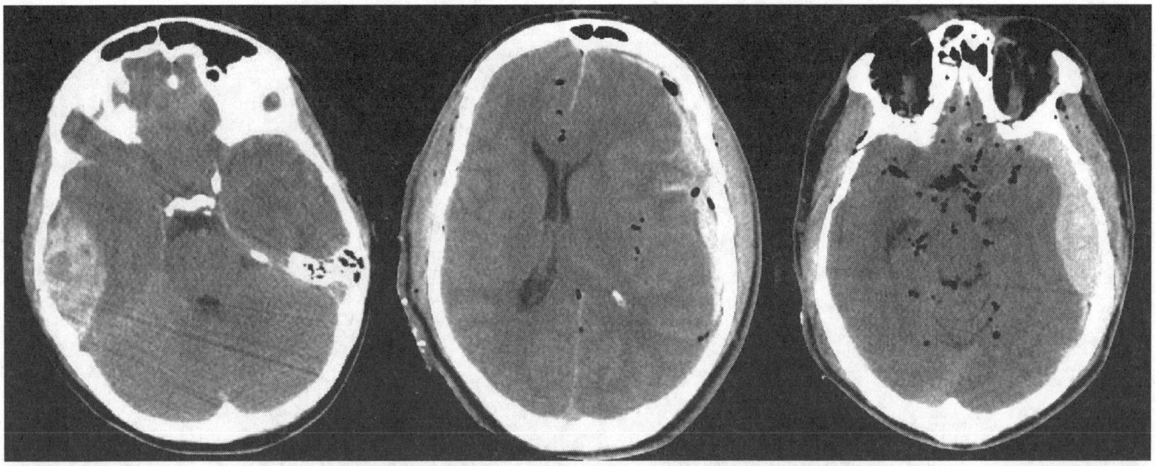

Figure 1.2

Occipital skull fracture

A seemingly benign linear occipital skull fracture, but associated with this was contre-coup contusions in the frontal lobes. These made a massive hemorrhagic transformation over only two hours (middle and right hand picture).

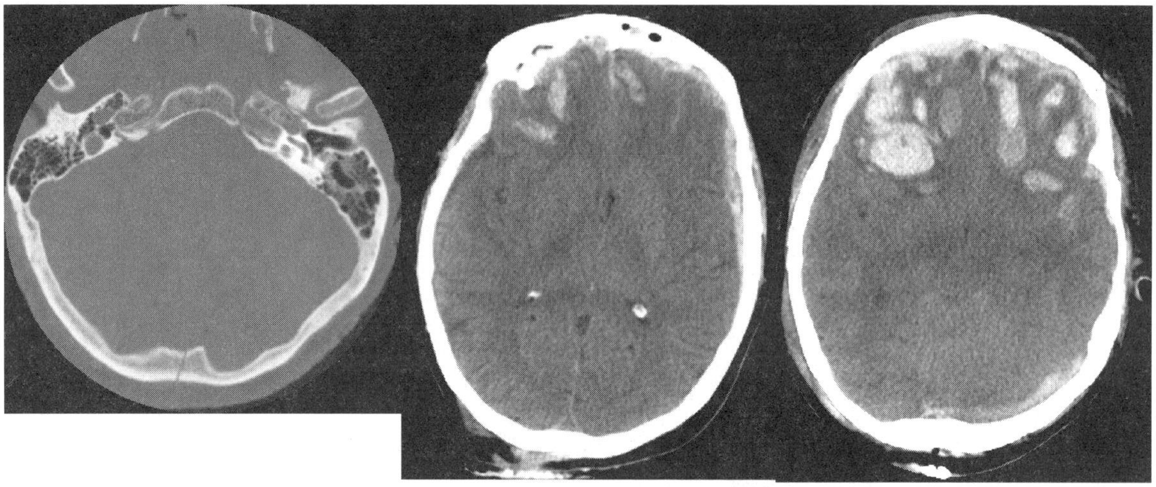

Figure 1.3

Diffuse axonal injury

Diffuse axonal injury, with multiple petechial contusions on CT, more easily demonstrated on gradient recall echo (GRE) MRI. The same patient six weeks later with encephalomalacia of the injured brain.

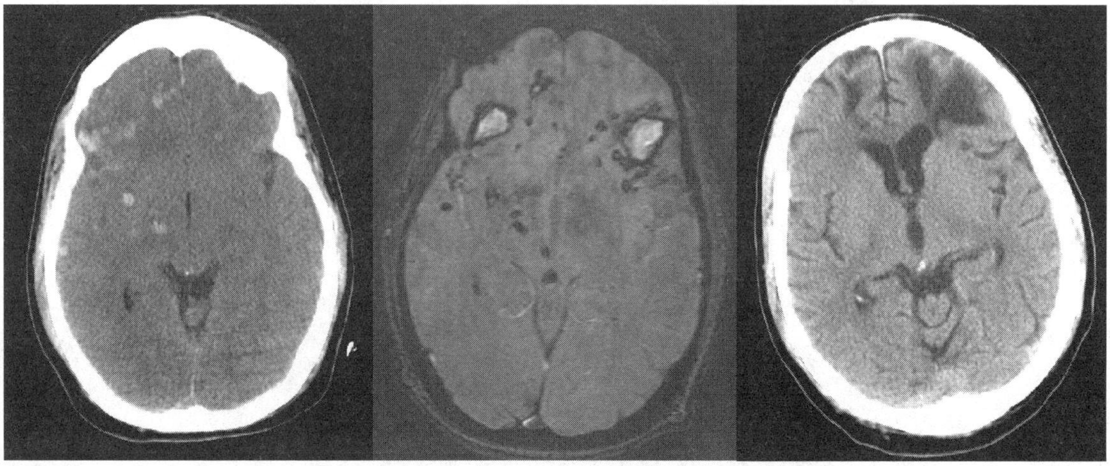

Spinal Injuries (Figures 1.4, 1.5)

Instability

Spinal instability can be considered in terms of either neurologic or mechanical terms. The latter may occur through:

- fractures
- congenital anomalies (failures of formation or segmentation)
- spondylolisthesis
- iatrogenic damage to the spine
- degenerative changes in the spine

The unstable spine is not able to resist physiological loads without resulting in abnormal movements (the mechanical), pain (subjective), or neurological deficit.

Stability is usually defined on the basis of pattern of fracture, its probable mechanism, how many columns are involved, and alignment, and neurological compromise—if any—sustained.

Simple osteoporotic compression fractures in the midthoracic spine can be considered "stable," while bilateral facet dislocation is a highly "unstable" injury. A full catalogue of fracture classification is beyond the scope of this chapter.

Cord Injury (Syndromes)

Spinal injury can result in any combination of (as well as lack of) neurological dysfunction of the nerve roots or the spinal cord. It is imperative that the spinally injured patient undergoes a thorough neurological examination that documents the full function of the examinable tracts of the spinal cord.

A good example of a system that assists with the documentation of this examination is the ASIA classification system (Table 3), as it has prognostic implications for the patient (see section on neurosurgical scales). It is vital to establish whether the patient has a complete or incomplete lesion.

Table 3

ASIA Impairment Scale

Grade	Classification	Neurologic Function
A	Complete	No motor or sensory function is preserved in the sacral segments S4-S5.
B	Incomplete	Sensory but not motor function is preserved below the neurological level and includes the-sacral segments S4-S5.
C	Incomplete	Motor function is preserved below the neurological level, and more than half of key muscles below the neurological level have a muscle grade less than 3.
D	Incomplete	Motor function is preserved below the neurological level, and at least half of key muscles below the neurological level have a muscle grade of 3 or more.
E	Normal	Motor & sensory function normal.

The neurological examination in spinal cord injury has been classified into some distinct syndromes (Table 4). These in general are incomplete lesions.

Treatment of Spinal Cord Injury

Primary treatment is essentially the same as head injury with maintenance of ABC's and ensuring adequate perfusion to prevent secondary injury. This is especially true when there is neurogenic shock, and the need for resuscitation and inotropic support as appropriate for bradycardia and hypotension due to sympathetic output loss. The mainstay of medical treatment is good supportive care with attention to detail, especially in the realm of nursing such as non-pressure bedding, bladder care, skin care, deep venous thrombosis prophylaxis, pulmonary management to ensure adequate weaning for high cervical quadraparetic patients, as well as early physiotherapy and physiatry to ensure early rehabilitation potential and the prevention of contracture development.

Use of Steroids

The use of steroids remains controversial even among experts. The results of the National Acute Spinal Cord Injury Studies (NASCIS I) suggested a benefit of administering methylprednisolone within 8 hours of injury. NASCIS II and III investigators found that in patients treated earlier than 3 hours after injury, the administration of methylprednisolone for 24 hours was best. In patients treated 3-8 hours after injury, the use of methylprednisolone for 48 hours was best. Tirilazad was equivalent to methylprednisolone for 24 hours. The administra-

Table 4

SCI Clinical Syndromes

Syndrome	**Definition and Presentation**
Cord Concussion	Transient neurologic deficit localized to the spinal cord that fully recovers without any structural injury. Usually characterized by congenital narrowing of the canal in an otherwise well young person.
Central Cord	Disproportionately greater motor deficit in the upper limbs than lower. Usually results from hyperextension in spondylosis.
Brown-Séquard	Spinal cord hemisection. Usually penetrating trauma or spondylosis. Ipsilateral motor paralysis and loss of posterior column function. Contralateral dissociated sensory loss (loss of pain and temperature and preserved light touch).
Anterior Cord	*aka Anterior spinal artery syndrome.* Paraplegia (or quadriplegia below C7) with dissociated sensory loss (loss of pain and temperature with preserved two-point discrimination).
Conus Medullaris	Bilateral symmetric saddle sensory deficit; sensory dissociation. Symmetric motor loss, fasciculations can be present. Prominent early autonomic symptoms (bladder areflexia). Mix of upper and lower motor neuron signs.
Cauda Equina	Unilateral/bilateral sensory loss. Radicular type pain may be most prominent symptom. Typically motor and sensory asymmetric. Can involve autonomic nerve.

Figure 1.4

Vertebral body burst fracture

Vertebral body burst fracture with bifacetal dislocation, a highly unstable injury with a high rate of neurologic injury (incredibly, this patient was intact). The arrows demonstrate the burst fracture with retropulsed bone in the canal, interspinous process widened gap, and the dislocated "jumped" facets.

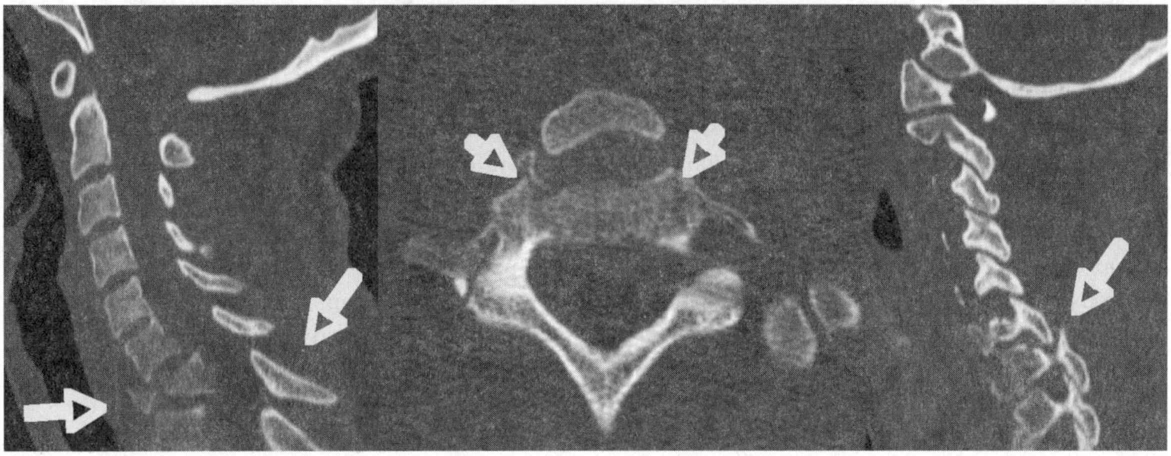

tion of steroids remains an institutional and physician preference in spinal cord injury. Meta-analyses of the literature could not identify any study that replicated the original studies.

Surgery

Surgical reduction and decompression of nerve roots may improve the neurologic recovery rate if traction reduction is unsuccessful in facet dislocation. In spinal cord injury, surgery remains controversial in terms of any improvement in neurologic prognosis. This is especially true in central cord syndrome resulting from trauma superimposed on a background of spondylosis.

In pure traumatic injury in young patients, however, anecdotal evidence abounds with improvements after surgical decompression, although no controlled studies have looked into this.

On the other hand, surgical treatment of the instability of the mechanical/vertebral elements ensures early mobilization when possible of the patient, and potentially mitigates further continuing mechanical injury. The timing of surgical decompression of complete lesions is not uniformly established.

Figure 1.5

Spinal cord injury due to hyperflexion

Spinal cord injury due to hyperflexion injury with high cord signal. This patient was a 16-year- old footballer, who became quadriplegic with a C5 sensory level.

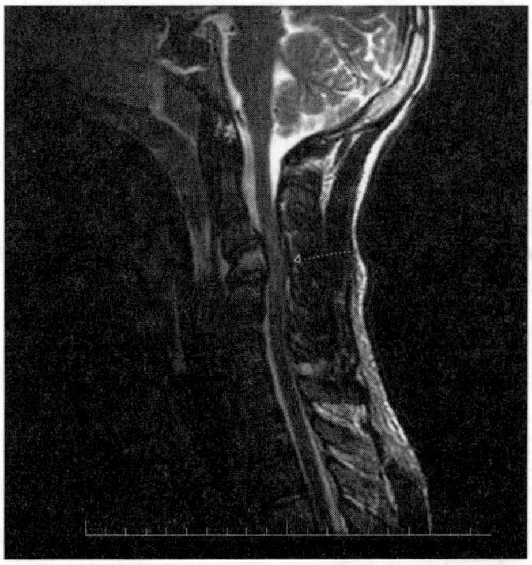

2. Neurosurgical Emergencies (Non-traumatic)

Intracerebral Hemorrhage

Intracerebral hemorrhage (ICH), also "hemorrhagic stroke," is a term used to imply intra-axial blood, denoting the hemorrhage is either parenchymal or ventricular, or both. It is a common reason for referral to a neurosurgeon.

Demographics

This is the second commonest form of stroke but the most lethal, presenting with headache and typically progressing over minutes to hours with signs of raised intracranial pressure (vomiting and altered conscious level). The expansion of the clot volume occurs in about one-third of cases within the first 3-6 hours of onset. Its incidence is about 15/100,000, or twice the incidence of subarachnoid hemorrhage.

Risk Factors

The major risk factor is age, with incidence doubling every decade of life till age >80. Others include hypertension, male gender, previous history of stroke of any sort, alcohol consumption, and sympathomimetic drug use.

Etiology

Consider "structural" (abnormalities of macrovasculature such as aneurysm, AVM, cavernoma, or tumor and traumatic vascular injury) vs. "non-structural" (such as hypertensive, amyloid angiopathy, hemorrhagic conversion of ischemic stroke, and coagulopathy). The second group is commoner overall.

Location

Location is highly significant both for the implied etiology as well as whether the lesion is "surgical" vs. "non-surgical." Supratentorially, ICH can be located centrally (eg, corpus striatum, putamen, thalamus) versus peripherally (lobar or limited cortical/subcortical white matter). Infratentorially, ICH can also be located centrally (vermian), in the cerebellar hemispheres or the brain stem. The third localization of ICH is ventricular, which typically is extension of blood complicating either of the "central" hemorrhage of supra- or infratentorial origin.

Imaging

The initial test of choice is a non-contrast CT head. Imaging needs then to further direct whether there is a surgical lesion: ie, mass effect from a lobar hemorrhage or an angiographically visible aneurysm or arteriovenous malformation. Catheter angiography or CT angiography (CTA) is necessary if the ICH satisfies certain criteria, namely lobar or surface hemorrhage, young patient (<55) without a clear cause, no hypertension (history or presentation), and a clear surgical candidate.

Surgery

The primary reason for referral to a neurosurgeon remains the consideration for surgical treatment of mass effect. The diagnostic process immediately focuses on eliminating a potential structural (vascular) cause that requires surgical treatment urgently. To this end, cerebral angiography is performed. CT angiography has superseded catheter angiography as first-line due to its advantages of speed and non-invasiveness, together with comparable accuracy of diagnosis in the acutely unstable patient. In the patient without a clear cause even on angiography, continued search should take place for a low-flow lesion or an underlying tumor, such as a cavernoma, by MRI scan. If there is very early edema out of keeping with the clot volume, with extension into the white matter, suspicion for an underlying neoplasm must prompt an MRI scan pre- and post-contrast administration. In some cases, where there is still suspicion for a neoplasm (usually lymphoma) with an equivocal MRI due to blood products, a delayed contrast MRI would be useful at 4-6 weeks.

Indications for Angiography (or CTA)

- Lobar or surface hemorrhage
- Young patient (<55) without clear cause
- No hypertension (previous or on presentation)
- Potential surgical candidate

Factors Favoring Surgery

- Those with structural lesion – such as an aneurysm or AVM that requires surgery.
- Young patients (<55) with major mass effect from a lobar hemorrhage

- Cerebellar hemorrhage
- Intraventricular extension – place an external ventriculostomy

Factors Against Surgery

- Very elderly (>75)
- Centrally located clot
- Large hematoma volume (>60mls)
- No ventricular extension
- Coma (GCS <8)

Good quality evidence for the aggressive management of non-structural ICH is lacking.

In most studies, surgical management of non-structural ICH was associated with a worse outcome, both functional and mortality (Figure 2.1).

The mainstay of medical treatment is aggressive blood pressure control to preset limits, keeping in mind the hypertensive patient's need for a higher baseline blood pressure for cerebral perfusion maintenance, while controlling BP extremes. Intravenous continuous infusions (such as nicardipine or nitrates) are often needed in the acute phase of hypertension in an effort to limit the potential for hematoma expansion.

Other medical therapy is warranted as for any stroke patient, including physiotherapy to prevent contractures, aspiration and skin pressure precautions, and bladder care.

Prognostic Pointers

Various authors have focused on important predictors of survival and morbidity:

The most important prognostic factors were:

- Level of consciousness at presentation (GCS <8 or GCS ≥9)
- Hematoma volume – powerful predictor (<30ml do well, >60ml do poorly)
  GCS <8 AND volume >60ml = 91% mortality
  GCS ≥9 AND volume <30ml = 19% mortality
- Hydrocephalus, posterior fossa ICH, first day MAP (>145 mm Hg)—worse prognosis

Hematoma *enlargement* likely with:

- admission shortly after onset
- heavy drinkers
- irregularly-shaped hematoma
- decreased level of consciousness
- low serum level of fibrinogen

High risk for deterioration in:

- Hydrocephalus
- Vermian hematoma

Hydrocephalus predictive of mortality in two studies:

- With hydrocephalus – 51% hospital mortality, 21% went home
- Without hydrocephalus – 2% hospital mortality, 35% went home
- Another study: Hydro and GCS<8: survival = 11%
  No hydro and GCS>8: survival = 100%

Figure 2.1

Large volume ICH

A large volume deep ICH with ventricular extension in the dominant hemisphere of a 72-year-old patient who presented with a GCS of 5 and bilateral extensor posturing. The patient had been on aspirin and clopidogril for multiple cardiac stents. An example of a non-surgically salvageable presentation. Ultimately, the family elected to institute comfort measures only.

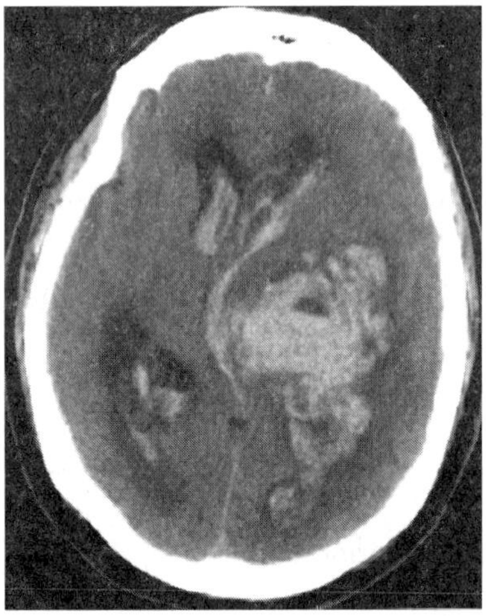

Acute Hydrocephalus (Figure 2.2)

Acute hydrocephalus describes a condition where ventricular dilatation (with the possible exception of slit ventricle patients), together with raised intracranial pressure, both occur in an acute setting with rapid neurological decompensation.

The patient shows signs of raised intracranial pressure, usually in the following order:

Headache, nausea, confusion and apathy to examiner; vomiting, somnolence, difficulty rousing; difficulty with upgaze or 4th or 6th nerve palsy; coma with pupillary changes, and other herniation signs.

The acute onset of hydrocephalus can be from many primary pathologies:

- Intraventricular hemorrhage (IVH)
- Ventricular shunt obstruction
- Meningitis
- Tumor
- Post-traumatic
- Post-operative (acoustic, cerebellar tumor)

Treatment
The treatment is strictly urgent and surgical, namely, placement of an external ventricular drain (or shunt if desirable), typically in the right frontal horn of the lateral ventricle to relieve the pressure, followed by addressing the primary pathology. In an emergent scenario with a patient who has a shunt obstruction, aspiration from the shunt reservoir or even cannulating the ventricle with a spinal needle may be life saving. If the hydrocephalus is caused by a cerebellar mass lesion in a relatively stable patient, the placement of the ventriculostomy may be delayed to be done in the operating room for fear of causing upward herniation.

Acute Myelopathy and Cauda Equina

Acute Myelopathy
Acute myelopathy is defined as sudden onset spinal cord dysfunction, and is usually referred to as cord compression, signifying a surgically remediable compressive lesion.

The commonest cause of non-traumatic acute cord compression in practice tends to be that associated with blood (spinal epidural hematoma) or tumor or both, followed by infective causes, such as spinal epidural abscess.

Documentation of the exact sequence of clinical deterioration and the detailed neurologic exam (including sacral nerve and autonomic function) is vital.

Figure 2.2

Acute hydrocephalus

Note ballooning of the third ventricle and dilatation of the temporal horns (not typically seen on such a low cut). Treatment with urgent ventriculostomy has been carried out (right-hand image).

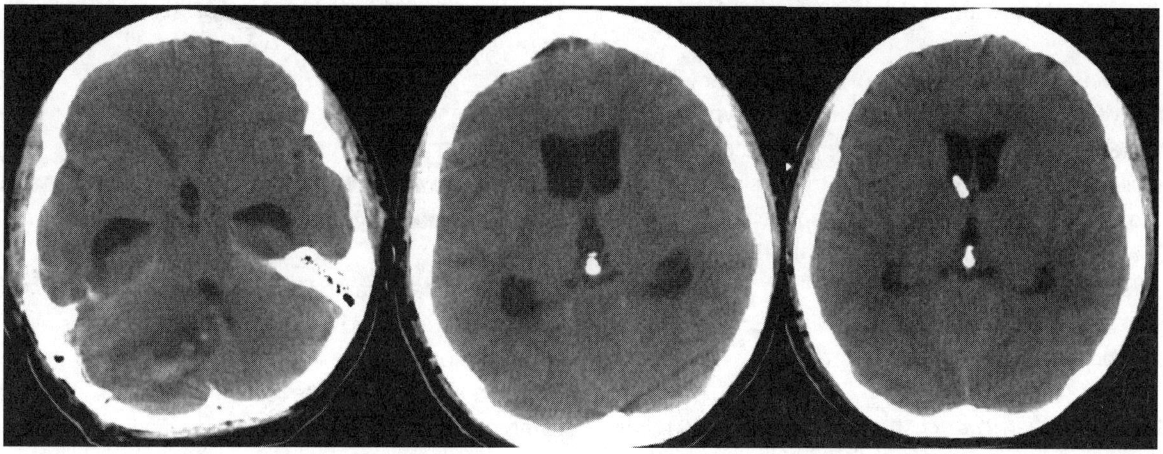

Tumorous cord compression tends to be due to epidural lesions, with the commonest being metastases from multiple myeloma, lymphoma, prostate and breast cancer. These are often chemotherapy and radiotherapy-sensitive tumors, and therefore before embarking on surgical decompression, one has to consider the speed of neurological deterioration. If this is subacute, it can be reversed with urgent radiation therapy alone. Administration of very high-dose steroids (dexamethasone 50-100mg) reduces pain in 85%, and may produce transient neurologic improvement.

The neurologic deficit and time with the deficit are prognostically important for any surgical decompression. Total paralysis (with a complete clinical cord lesion) present greater than 24 hours duration is essentially not surgically recoverable.

Additionally, the location and stability of the metastases in the spinal canal is also an important surgical consideration. Dorsally located lesions are easily accessible; vertebral body lesions with purely ventral compression are more involved. The latter necessitate a more difficult anterior procedure with vertebral body resection and reconstruction (higher morbidity for the elderly). This may become necessary if there is severe spinal instability in the face of recurrence after maximal radiation therapy.

Spinal epidural hematoma (SEH) occurs rarely as a spontaneous entity, and sometimes in association with anti-coagulation or antiplatelet agent use, trauma or an epidural hemorrhagic tumor (such as renal cell carcinoma). Again, documentation of speed of neurologic deterioration and the very rapid surgical decompression of the spinal cord is warranted. Most SEH's can be evacuated by a straightforward dorsal laminectomy approach, although a significant number will be "long segment" hematomas necessitating multiple "skip laminectomies." The single prognostic factor for neurological recovery in SEH is the time to surgical decompression with delayed presentation (beyond 8 hours) carrying a grim prognosis for recovery of function.

Cauda Equina Syndrome (Figure 2.3)

A syndrome that develops due to compression of the cauda equina nerve roots.

It is important to differentiate this from a conus medullaris spinal cord lesion. (See spinal cord syndromes in Neurosurgical Trauma section.)

The most acutely emergent of etiologies for CES is that of a herniated midline lumbar disk, typically on a background of previous, more moderate disk prolapse or canal stenosis (aka Central Disk syndrome).This is, however, rare—on the order of 1%-2% of all herniated lumbar disks that come to surgery.

The possible findings are:

Sphincter disturbance: urinary hesitance and retention is most consistent, although incontinence can be seen, either urinary or fecal. Anal tone is diminished in 60 percent.

Saddle anesthesia: the most common sensory deficit. Once complete perineal anesthesia develops, patient tends to be at risk of irreversible bladder paralysis.

Motor weakness: usually significant and asymmetric involving more than one nerve root.

Sciatica +/- low back pain: the commonest context is a patient with bilateral sciatica; prognosis may be worse if the history is of sciatica pain resolving, then saddle numbness developing.

Investigation
Urgent non-contrast MRI of the lumbar spine is the test of choice.

Surgical Treatment

- Emergent surgical decompression of the cauda equina.
- Bilateral laminectomy is performed for wide exposure (of the usually tense midline disk) and complete diskectomy.
- Emergent surgery is associated with a higher rate of inadvertent durotomy and nerve injury.

Timing of surgery is much debated with evidence in both directions, but in practice most surgeons would aim for either emergent decompression (including in middle of the night), or on the next available morning list within 6-8 hours of presentation of a true classic cauda equina syndrome.

Figure 2.3

Cauda equina syndrome

This patient had bilateral lower limb radiculopathy and difficulty voiding, and could not feel himself passing urine. The patient underwent laminectomy and diskectomy with complete resolution of all his symptoms.

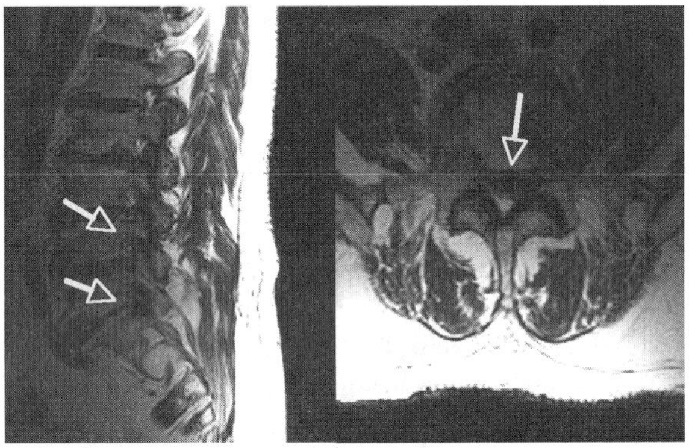

Infection

Cerebral Abscess (Figure 2.4)
A cerebral abscess is a walled-off infection within the brain that forms in distinct stages. Infection can occur by contiguous spread (otitis media, mastoiditis, paranasal sinusitis or dental infection) or via hematogenous routes (infective endocarditis, pneumonia). Any of these can result in localized abscess formation, meningitis, empyema, or any combination thereof. Most abscesses are caused by pyogenic organisms. One-third of patients have polymicrobial

abscesses. Most frequently isolated are *streptococci* and *staphylococci*, although Gram-negatives are on the rise.

Four stages have been described in abscess evolution: early cerebritis, late cerebritis, early capsule formation, and late capsule formation:

1. *Early cerebritis (3-5 days):* unencapsulated congested brain tissue, some necrotic foci.

2. *Late cerebritis (>3-5 days):* focal reaction, central necrosis, inflammatory ring, lasts 5-14 days.

3. *Early capsule stage:* well-delineated capsule, central necrosis, mass effect subsiding, early gliosis.

4. *Late capsule stage:* inner inflammatory layer, middle collagen layer, outer gliotic layer, lasts months.

Initially, CT scan of the head may show ill-defined edematous white matter, and with contrast a ring-enhancing lesion is seen. MRI has a higher sensitivity, as it can show better detail of the capsule and cerebral inflammatory reaction, better delineating whether there is complete encapsulation (stage 3). Diffusion sequences are typically diagnostic with restricted diffusion.

Treatment consists of ideally organism-directed antibiotic therapy involving:

- Systemic cultures

- Urgent stereotactic aspiration of only fully encapsulated abscesses (for culture)

- Induction of broad spectrum intravenous antibiotic therapy

- Maintenance of intravenous antibiotic therapy for minimum of 6 weeks with regular imaging

- Treatment of the primary source of infection

Figure 2.4

Brain abscess

This patient had an odontogenic source for his brain abscess. Note the ring-enhancement and the restricted diffusion on the DWI. The last image shows complete resolution with no further contrast enhancement after stereotactic aspiration, dental extractions, and antibiotic treatment for 12 weeks.

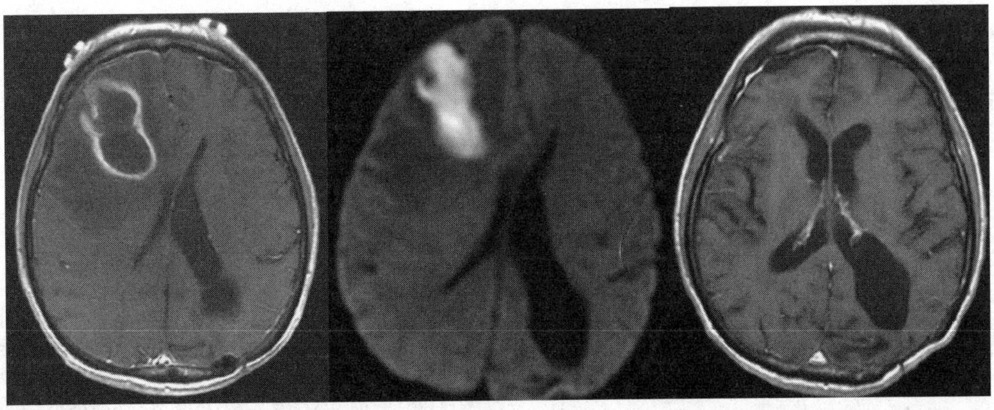

Cerebral Blood Flow, Cerebral Blood Volume and ICP

Basics

- The adult brain comprises ~2% of body mass, but utilizes ~20% of basal oxygen consumption (50 ml/min).
- Mean resting cerebral blood flow (CBF) in adults is about 50 ml/100 g/min.
- Synaptic transmission is abolished when CBF is below 15 ml/100 g/min.
- Neuronal maintenance of membrane potential is lost below 10 ml/100 g/min.
- If CBF remains reduced at above levels, permanent neurological damage may ensue within minutes.
- Whole brain oxygen consumption ~ 3.5 ml of oxygen/100 g of brain tissue/min.

Cerebral Blood Flow and Cerebral Blood Volume (CBF, CBV) (Figures 3.1, 3.2, 3.3)

- Cerebral blood flow is maintained to meet the brain's significant demands for oxygen and glucose.
- CBF is related to cerebral perfusion pressure (CPP) and cerebrovascular resistance (CVR) as follows:

  CBF = CPP / CVR where CPP = Mean arterial pressure (MAP) – Intracranial pressure (ICP) – venous pressure (VP).

- Manipulation of CBV can rapidly reduce ICP if intracranial hypertension exists.
- CBV does not change in parallel with CBF.
- Concept of flow-metabolism coupling: increased metabolic demand (CMR O2) increases CBF, CBV and ICP.

Figure 3.1

Factors affecting CBF

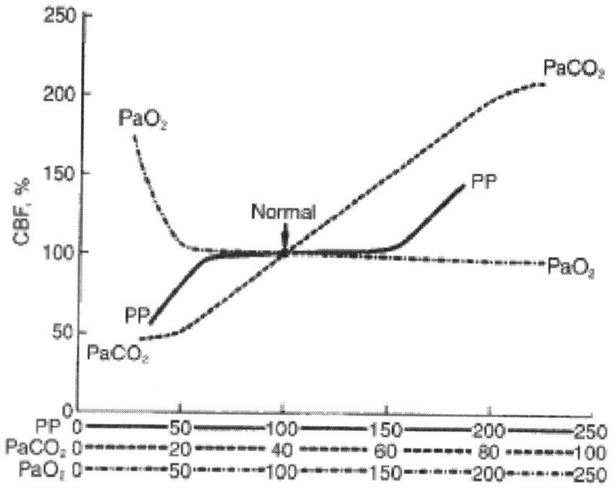

Figure 3.1: Gupta AK, Summors AC. Notes in Neuroanaesthesia and Critical Care. 2001. Cambridge University Press. Reprinted by permission.

Figure 3.2

ICP volume buffering

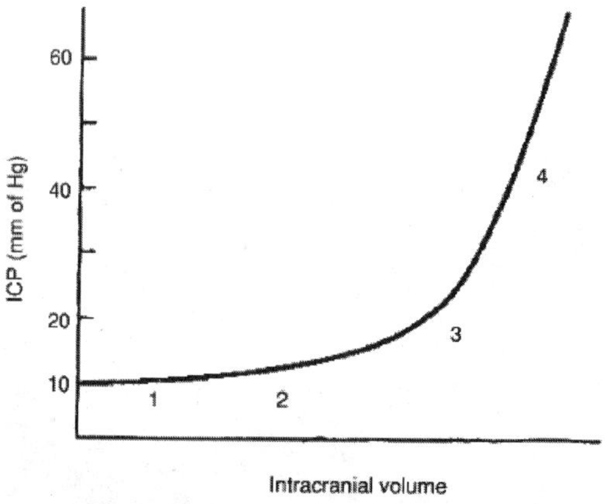

Figure 3.2: Gupta AK, Summors AC. Notes in Neuroanaesthesia and Critical Care. 2001. Cambridge University Press. Reprinted by permission.

Figure 3.3

The effect of CO_2 on CBF maintenance

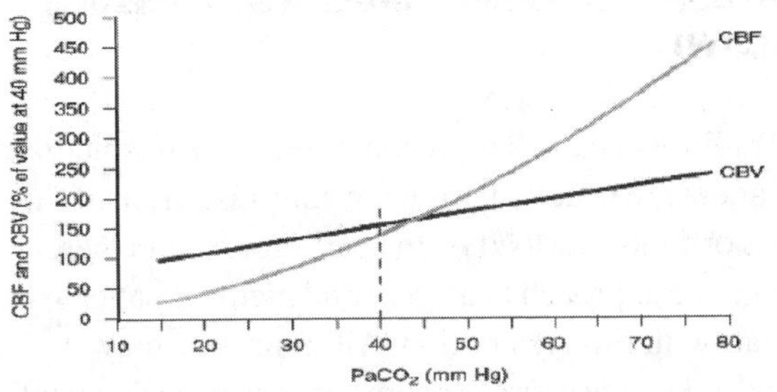

Figure 3.3: Gupta AK, Summors AC. Notes in Neuroanaesthesia and Critical Care. *2001. Cambridge University Press. Reprinted by permission.*

ICP

- The Monro-Kellie doctrine dictates that the intracranial contents are enclosed in a rigid cranial vault, and that these contents are essentially 3 compartments: brain (tissue), blood (in vessels), and cerebrospinal fluid (ventricles and cisterns).
- Raised ICP causes secondary brain injury through a variety of mechanisms (mechanical, vascular, metabolic).
- Volume buffering is important in maintaining normal ICP.
- In raised ICP:
  — changes to the CSF space is a major compensatory factor.
  —manipulation of CBV can rapidly reduce ICP.
- CBV does not change in parallel with CBF.
- pCO_2 is a powerful influence on CBV.
- Maintenance of CPP is just as important (arguably more important) than lowering ICP.

Neuroanesthesia: Agents and Effects (Table 5)

The principle of general anesthesia is to induce the "triad" of analgesia (to abolish nociceptive appreciation and sympathetic reflexes); hypnosis (to induce unconsciousness); and muscle relaxation (to eliminate movement). The induction of anesthesia is usually achieved in exactly that order. Usually an intravenous opiate is given, followed by the intravenous hypnotic (the "anesthetic" agent), and finally the paralytic/muscle relaxant, which is rapidly followed by endotracheal intubation and mechanical ventilation.

A classical approach for an elective ICU-type intubation is fentanyl, propofol, and rocuronium.

Alternatively, a "rapid sequence" approach may involve fentanyl, thiopentone, and suxamethonium.

All anesthetic agents (hypnotics, analgesics or paralytics) have hemodynamic, respiratory and metabolic effects that have to be tailored to achieve the optimal neuroanesthetic environment, be it in the neurosurgical operating room or the neurocritical care unit.

The overall aims are to maintain CBF (and hence tissue perfusion and oxygenation), control ICP (preventing spikes), and lower cerebral metabolism, as well as achieve paralysis. In an acute trauma situation, the basic focus of advanced life support must initially start with the ABC's (airway, breathing and circulation).

The ideal intravenous agent for neuroanesthesia should have the following properties:

- Allows for early neurological assessment by rapid recovery of consciousness.
- Easy and rapid titratability.
- Minimal effects on other systems, eg, cardiovascular, respiratory, renal, hepatic.
- Analgesic.
- A favorable effect on cerebral haemodynamics.

—Reduction in CMR coupled with CBF.

—No increase in CBV (and hence ICP).

—Maintain vasoreactivity to CO_2.

—Maintain cerebrovascular autoregulation.

—Not lowering seizure threshold.

Specific Electrolytes Derangements

Electrolyte derangements occur in neurosurgical patients as they do in all critically-ill patients. I concentrate here, however, on those who are seen with increased frequency and are therefore typical (and practical) issues in management. By far the commonest of electrolyte derangements seen in neurosurgery are those in sodium hemostasis.

Hyponatremia and Cerebral Salt Wasting (CSW)

Traditional causes of hyponatremia in a hospitalized patient are usually iatrogenic administration of fluids or fluid overload from heart failure, and therefore the approach to a "general" medical patient is to start with fluid restriction. Although this may indeed by the cause for some neurosurgical patients, the vast majority will actually be fluid depleted. This traditional approach could therefore be potentially dangerous.

Table 5

Effects of Anesthetic Agents on Blood Flow and Metabolism

Anesthetic agent	Primary action	CBF	CMRO2	Other effects
Propofol	$GABA_A$ +, NMDA -	↓ CBF	↓ $CMRO_2$	
Etomidate	$GABA_A$ +	↓ CBF	↓ $CMRO_2$	Adrenal suppression
Barbiturates (Thio)	$GABA_A$ +	↓ CBF	↓ $CMRO_2$	Cardiodepression
Benzodiazepines	$GABA_A$ +	↓ CBF	↓ $CMRO_2$	
Halothane volatile	In, Vh, Mu	↑ CBF 5	↓ $CMRO_2$	Most "neuro-friendly"
Ketamine	NMDA -	↑ CBF 4	↑ $CMRO_2$	ICP, dissociative anesthesia
Enflurane	In, Vh, Mu	↑ CBF 3	↓ $CMRO_2$	Lowers seizure threshold
Isoflurane	In, Vh, Mu	↑ CBF 2	↓ $CMRO_2$	
Nitrous oxide	In, Mu	↑ CBF 1	↑ $CMRO_2$	Risk of neumocephalus

Numbers 1-5 indicate degree to which each agent increases cerebral blood flow (5 highest, 1 least).
The only agents to increase both CBF & CMRO2 are Ketamine and NO.

The most important first step is to assess the patient's volume status, and to recognize that cerebral salt wasting (CSW) is exceedingly common in all neurosurgical patients (especially where there is intracranial blood, eg, in subarachnoid hemorrhage). This describes a condition where there is excessive loss of sodium in the renal tubules in association with diuresis and volume depletion, the so-called diuresis-natriuresis syndrome.

The hyponatremia (with concomitant volume depletion) in CSW has been associated with both increased rates of vascular vasospasm after subarachnoid hemorrhage, as well increased size of infarcts from vasospasm. Additionally, in trauma patients the treatment of CSW-hyponatremia (with hypertonic saline) has been associated with reduction in post-traumatic cerebral edema, ICP values and herniation syndromes.

Indeed, more recent literature suggests that the use of hypertonic saline (typically 3% NaCl) in addition to maintenance of normovolemia can reduce total numbers of ICP spikes in traumatic closed head injury patients.

Thus it is imperative that neurosurgical patients with hyponatremia are not treated with fluid restriction blindly.

The treatment for cerebral salt wasting is volume repletion by administration of initially normal (0.9%) saline, and serial sodium determinations. Should the sodium fail to come up over a reasonable period of time or there be concern about neurological sequelae of a low sodium, then hypertonic (typically 3% saline) can be given intravenously by continuous infusion until a normal upper range sodium is reached. The usual fastest dose of 3% saline administered is 50-60 ml/hour. The fastest safe rise allowable for Na is typically 0.5 mmol/L/hour.

Hypernatremia

This is a less common scenario in neurosurgical patients, and is usually seen in either hypotonic volume depletion in the context of diabetes insipidus, or in iso- or hypervolemic states after the administration of normal or hypertonic saline, or in elderly patients with drug-induced hyponatremia (diuretics, carbamazepine). In traumatic closed head injury, this can be iatrogenically induced in the course of hypernatremic hyperosmolar therapy. The latter is now increasingly established as one of the strategies to prevent/attentuate cerebral edema or progression of contusion volume increases over the first few days after head injury in the neurocritical care unit. The targets of hypernatremia hyperosmolar therapy typically see a sodium rise to 150-155 with serum osmolality of ~310-320, although specific protocols vary between neurocritical care units.

Continuous intravenous infusions are typically used, but the use of boluses of 3% saline is also gaining in popularity for periodic ICP rises, and also to save the overuse of mannitol, since overzealous use of the latter has been reported to be associated with paradoxical brain swelling where the blood-brain barrier has been broken down. Mannitol, in addition, induces a rapidly diuretic effect that may also cause transient volume depletion and hypotension in patients with borderline hemodynamic instability, especially if inotrope-dependent or septic.

The "Triple" Response

This is a triphasic response of central diabetes insipidus (DI) that is occasionally encountered after surgical resection of pituitary tumors or craniopharyngioma.

Phase 1: injury to pituitary reduced ADH with classic DI with polyuria, polydipsia and a rise in serum Na and osmolality.

Phase 2: cell death liberates ADH over the next 4-5 days, with transient normalisation of or even SIADH-like water retention.

Phase 3: reduced or absent ADH with return to transient or longer-term classic DI.

The importance of recognition of this triphasic response is that, if iatrogenic fluid replacement is being administered, to keep up with high urinary outputs (sometimes in excess of 1L/hour), especially during the first phase, or when administering vasopressin therapy. As the patient crosses over into the second phase and the urine output drops, the extra fluid administration and vasopressin effect would cause a precipitous hemodilution, with the danger of a rapid fall in Na concentration, potentially causing seizures and other negative sequelae, such as central pontine myelinolysis.

Mechanical Ventilation

Delivery of oxygen (DO_2) can be calculated from this formula:

DO_2 (in mL O_2/min) = CO x O_2 content
(CO = cardiac output)

The purpose of mechanical ventilation is to achieve movement of gases in and out of the airways and to adequately cause gas exchange, primarily oxygenating the blood and removing carbon dioxide, with the minimum of collateral complication.

Mechanical ventilation starts, however, from a non-physiologic basis. This basis is the initial paralysis, sedation and intubation of a patient, followed by the application of positive pressure to inflate the airways. This is in contradistinction from physiologic spontaneous ventilation that is achieved by diaphragmatic and intercostal muscle contraction and production of a vacuum effect with negative intrathoracic pressure causing air movement into the airways. All mechanical ventilation is, therefore, based on pressure in order to achieve flow, and subsequently gas exchange.

The following points are a basic *aide memoire* to understanding ventilation:

1. All mechanical ventilation is by definition positive pressure.

2. In an intubated patient, their natural upper airway resistance and respiratory muscles are essentially eliminated (ie, no natural PEEP or resistance to airway collapse).

3. In order to achieve flow, there has to be a potential difference, ie, an inspiratory pressure and an expiratory pressure.

4. The simplest bellow system is the model of a ventilator. Peak inspiratory pressure (PIP) is applied on a background of positive end expiratory pressure (PEEP), air moves during this inspiratory pressure application, then is allowed to recoil back, but only to the lower end expiratory pressure.

5. Basic ventilator settings (pressure control) are: Rate (with ratio of inspiration), PIP, PEEP, and fraction of inspired oxygen (FiO_2). Oxygen is an actively transported gas of haemoglobin with poor solubility, therefore more "gas" pressure has to be applied to get oxygen into the blood stream. It is the mean airway pressure (MAP) and FiO_2 (effective partial pressure of oxygen) that determine how much oxygenation occurs.

6. Carbon dioxide is a passively transported highly soluble gas, so the minute-volume of gas moved easily determines the amount of CO_2 cleared (so combinations used to vary CO_2 in the blood include changes in respiratory rate or tidal volume).

In the mechanically ventilated patient, non-physiologic pressures are iatrogenically induced in the alveoli, which almost always lead to some element of increased pulmonary vascular resistance, leading to a minor pulmonary hypertension (and hence, paradoxically, less flow in the pulmonary vessels). This means that all ventilated patients have a ventilation-perfusion mismatch by definition. The pulmonary hypertension and mismatch can be significant in ARDS patients.

Pressure/Volume Settings

PC = pressure control; VC = volume control; PRVC = pressure regulated volume control.

The simple bellow system is a description of a pressure-control ventilator, very commonly used in ventilating neonates. More sophisticated variations on these principles include other settings:

Volume control, where tidal volume is the primary parameter set and the pressures allowed to "ride," is typically used to achieve a predetermined minimal minute volume for that individual based on weight (usually 10ml/kg for children and ~ 5-7.5ml/kg for adults). This can lead to high ventilation pressures if there is increased stiffness in the system, eg, ARDS.

A further format of ventilation uses a computer calculation based on the fact that the volume-pressure curve is not linear, and will essentially try to deliver the volumes set, but by stepwise increments in volume.

Rate-control Settings

IMV (intermittent mandatory ventilation): Basically mechanical ventilation in a totally paralyzed fully-ventilated patient (patient does no work).

SIMV (synchronized intermittent mandatory ventilation): A backup rate (and minute volume) is reserved that is the minimum that the patient has to achieve, when the ventilator "kicks in," otherwise the patient determines the rate of his respiration (if above SIMV rate). Used usually when patient is not paralyzed. Also used as a "wean-mode."

CPAP-PS: a spontaneous mode where no rate is set for the patient to achieve (although most modern ventilators have backup rates anyway). Every breath the patient takes though has a pressure-support applied to it during respiration to aid inflation of the lungs. PEEP remains as preset. Also used as a "wean-mode" next down from SIMV.

CPAP = spontaneous mode, no pressure support is given, but PEEP is maintained. Two types of CPAP are differentiated, "active" provided by the ventilator, and "passive" provided by a simple valve at the end of tubing with gas flow without a ventilator. Again, a "wean-mode."

Invasive and Multimodality Monitoring: ABP, CVP & PAC, ICP, SjO_2

ABP Monitoring

Monitoring of arterial blood pressure is necessary for all patients in the neurocritical care unit. This allows estimate of the cerebral perfusion pressure (CPP) from the equation: MAP-ICP = CPP.

A key technical point on invasive ABP monitoring is the importance of measuring MAP that is relevant to the cerebral circulation. This is best accomplished by rezeroing the transducer at the level of the distal carotid artery entering the cranium—typically approximated by the level of the ear lobe.

Measurements at the level of manubro-sternal angle, as is standard in general critical care, misses the point of measuring cerebral blood pressure (and hence inferring) perfusion pressure, as this could potentially give a falsely elevated "normal" number.

ABP catheter placement also has the added benefit of allowing frequent arterial blood gas determinations to drive mechanical ventilation therapeutic changes to optimize pCO_2 and pO_2 to achieve the desirable lowering of CBV and improved tissue perfusion and oxygenation.

CVP and PA Catheter Monitoring

"The Foley catheter is the poor man's CVP catheter, and the CVP catheter is the poor man's PA catheter."

—English medical school saying.

The measurement of filling pressure is absolutely mandatory in any critically ill patient, where manipulations are made to ensure adequate blood pressure and cerebral blood flow. Knowledge of the volume status allows adjustment of further resuscitation fluid administration or treatment with pressor/inotropic agents. This is no more true than in unstable neurosurgical trauma or in septic patients. The critical minute-by-minute adjustments can be profoundly influential on ICP and CPP. Additionally, in those on high PEEP ventilation pressures, it allows an estimate of how much more fluid needs to be given for perfusion maintenance.

As the above saying indicates, the ideal measurement device would indicate left ventricular preload directly. A CVP pressure measurement is that of the right atrium, and as such is only a very rough approximation of filling pressure in the left atrium, provided a set of conditions are met (eg, a healthy young patient with concordant ventricular function). Since the vast majority of trauma patients fall in this category, many critical care units suffice with a CVP line. This falls apart for a sick patient with pulmonary hypertension from ARDS, or an older patient with poor left ventricular function or valvular disease. In those cases, the closest measure of filling pressure is a pulmonary capillary wedge pressure obtained by a pulmonary artery catheter (aka, Swann-Ganz catheter). In some neurocritical units, this is the standard method of volume monitoring. This, of course, gives more superior data, as well as other useful information, such as the ability to calculate cardiac output and estimate of systemic resistance, both helpful in the systemically vasodilated septic patient on inotropic agents.

ICP Monitoring

Intracranial pressure monitoring is a standard way of monitoring post-head injury patients with a poor neurologic exam, especially when they are sedated for airway protection. Intracranial hypertension has been associated with raised mortality and morbidity in post-head injury patients. Furthermore, ICP rises are used as triggers for further investigative imaging and therapeutic surgical interventions to relieve either compartmental pressure (eg, a focal hematoma) or generalized global intracranial hypertension from swelling. Monitoring is performed via either solid-state transducer or fluid column system, after drilling the skull table and entering (typically) at least the subdural space. Extra-dural pressure monitoring is inaccurate and is prone to artefact.

ICP "bolts" are fibre-optic transducers that employ the piezo-electric effect to measure pressure. Commonly used systems include Camino® and Codman® fibre-optic catheters. These are secured to the skull table with a concentric threaded hollow screw, the "bolt" part, with the fine-tipped fibre optic catheter threaded through into the subdural space or brain parenchyma.

Cannulation of the ventricular spaces is the other method employed for ICP measurement by placement of an external ventricular drain, alternatively known as "ventriculostom."

Key Points on ICP Monitoring

All solid state systems have a time-dependent "drift" tendency, and become increasingly inaccurate with time.

In general, a "fluid system" is essentially the gold standard when transduced correctly. In addition, a ventriculostomy allows both diagnostic pressure monitoring as well as therapeutic CSF drainage for reduction of ICP.

**(For an excellent and more detailed explanation of all the above, and measurement methodology, refer to Gupta & Summors, 2001.)*

$CMRO_2$

While CPP maintenance is important, this is only one parameter affecting cerebral oxygen delivery. CBF and blood oxygen contents are the prime parameters.

CPP is the potential difference determining CBF, but flow is also determined by cerebral vascular resistance. Cerebral oxygen demand is governed by metabolic rate, and neurons with high activity levels require greater amounts of oxygen than those which are quiescent. $CMRO_2$ describes this global value and this is related to cerebral blood flow and oxygen extraction fraction by the following formula:

$$CMRO_2 = CBF \times OEF \times SaO_2$$

The Fick principle can be used to measure the amount of oxygen extraction based on measurements of the arterial and venous oxygen content.

ICP and CPP values hence give little idea about the overall state of the injured brain and provide no information on oxygen delivery and utilization.

Multimodality monitoring combines other methods, including combination of jugular venous bulb oximetry and transcranial Doppler ultrasound, to understand the state of the cerebral circulation and oxygen consumption. These are methods that are increasing in popularity in academic neurocritical care units, as they can be employed with relative ease at the bedside in the ICU. Other more research-oriented approaches include PET and Xenon-based CT investigating global and focal cerebral blood flow—but these have thus far proven too cumbersome for routine clinical use.

SjO_2 Monitoring

The monitoring of venous oxygen saturation is performed at the clinically dominant jugular bulb by placement of a catheter in a retrograde fashion up the internal jugular vein, up to the jugular bulb at the skull base. The mixed venous oxygen saturation (SjO_2) of blood leaving the brain is measured, which is normally in the range 50%-75%. Solving the Fick equation for SjO_2 gives:

$SjO_2 = SaO_2$ - (Oxygen Consumption / Cardiac Output x Hb x 1.39)

When there is an imbalance between oxygen consumption and delivery, SjO_2 falls. If the SjO_2 falls below 50% (without a fall in arterial oxygen saturation—SaO_2), this implies either a fall in CBF or a rise in oxygen utilization (higher $CMRO_2$).

In the presence of maintained CPP, reduced CBF implies increased cerebrovascular resistance (CVR). The latter can be caused by vascular spasm, a common occurrence after brain injury. This can be significantly aggravated by hyperventilation.

Thus, an indication for SjO_2 is whenever there is prolonged hyperventilation, or where extreme hyperventilation (generally below pCO_2 of 35 torr) is deliberately utilized as part of ICP control measures.

Additionally, SjO_2 is useful as part of multi-modality monitoring when burst suppression with barbiturates is used to reduce $CMRO_2$ in patients who have refractory intracranial hypertension not responsive to standard therapy. SjO_2 increases to 85% or beyond are associated with either a hyperemia with a rise in cerebral blood flow, shunting of blood away from neurons, or a severe decrease in $CMRO_2$ (impending cell death/brain death).

Treatment of Raised ICP (Table 6)

- Moderate hyperventilation reduces CBF and brain volume.
- Excess hyperventilation may cause vasoconstriction with critical reduction in CBF to already compromised areas and focal ischemia.
- Intravenous anesthetics generally decrease cerebral metabolism, CBF and ICP.
- Inhalational agents are all cerebral vasodilators.
- The overall effect on CBF depends on a balance between the concentration of the inhalational agent and the degree of hyperventilation.

"HHH" Therapy

This is the therapeutic modulation utilized in the treatment of symptomatic cerebral vasospasm, typically in the wake of aneurysmal subarachnoid hemorrhage (SAH). It consists of: hypervolemia, hemodilution and induced hypertension. The hypervolemia (typically to CVP of at least 10-14 in a non-ventilated patient) is induced to replace volume and

Table 6

Treatment of Elevated IVP

First-Line Measures
- Elevate head to 30 degrees
- Relief of potential venous obstruction, minimize PEEP
- $paCO_2$ 30-35 mmHg, ICP <20; CPP >65-70
- Initial mannitol 0.5-1.0 g/kg single dose (and Q 6 prn)
- Maintain euvolemia, monitor CVP
- Ventriculostomy (for ICP monitoring & drain CSF as appropriate)
- Analgesia (small doses of opiates)
- Sedation (propofol preferable to benzodiazepines)
- Temperature maintenance 35-37°C

Second-Line Measures
- Induced hypothermia
- Hyperventilation $paCO_2$ 20-25 (must monitor SjO_2)
- Hyperosmolar therapy, 3% saline (target osmolality 310-320, Na ~150)
- EEG burst suppression with barbiturates

Aggressive Measures
- Decompressive craniectomy
- Resection of infarcted brain (+/- lobectomy)

Modified from Neurosurgery—Principles and Practice. *Moore AJ, Newell DW, eds.*

maintain filling pressures adequate for cerebral perfusion (20% of CO) in the wake of a condition of unusual diuresis and natriuresis that occurs after SAH. Hemodilution is performed (typically to hematocrit of ~30-33) to improve the rheologic properties of blood for enhanced flow, and induced hypertension aims to effectively push more blood through a heightened cerebral vascular resistance to maintain the same flow. In many cases, the target SBP in a patient with a protected aneurysm is around 180, although up to 200 is induced in some cases, if the patient is not already "auto-hypertensing." Inotropic agents such as phenylephrine, noradrenaline or dopamine are typically used in the setting of invasive CVP or PAC and arterial BP monitoring.

Brain Stem Death

Brain stem death may only be diagnosed in patients with apneic coma resulting from known irreversible intracranial pathology. This is most frequently seen in:

- Severe head injury.
- Intracranial hemorrhage.
- Cerebral edema with brain stem herniation.
- Hypoxic-ischemic encephalopathy.

Before the diagnosis of brain stem death may be made, the following must be excluded:

- Hypothermia (< 35°C).
- Abnormal $PaCO_2$.
- Depressant drugs with a potential to cause unconsciousness.
- Severe hypotension.
- Major derangements of endocrine, biochemical and metabolic values.

Brain Stem Death Criteria*

Absence of:

- pupillary light reflex—the corneal reflex
- the vestibulo-ocular reflex
- the gag reflex
- motor reflexes with brain stem arcs
- reflex response to bronchial stimulation
- any respiratory effort or spontaneous respiration for minimum of 2 minutes in the presence of:
- preoxygenation
- normo- or hypercarbia
- exclusion of the above factors

* *Commonly accepted amongst clinicians, but always check the exact statement of the law in the state where you practice.*

4. Vascular Neurosurgery

Cerebral Aneurysms

Incidence: Cerebral aneurysms are found in ~1.5% in autopsy series. They are the most common cause of non-traumatic subarachnoid hemorrhage (SAH). They cause death and disability in 18,000 patients/year in North America. There is an increasing cache of incidentally diagnosed aneurysms with increased use of imaging for common symptoms.

Age: Aneurysms rarely rupture in the 1st decade. The rupture incidence increases with age (20% between 15-45), and peaks at 55-60 years.

Gender: There is a clear female predominance ~1.6:1

Presentation: The classic symptom of SAH is sudden onset headache (in good grade patient).

Other symptoms include: meningismus, nausea, vomiting, confusion, focal deficit, coma. Mortality in the first week approaches ~27% in untreated cases.

Genetics: Aneurysms are mostly sporadic, with multiple aneurysms occurring in 15% of patients with a known aneurysm. An autosomal dominant variety is present in some families. Patients with polycystic kidneys have a 7%-16% chance of harboring cerebral aneurysms. An increased incidence in: Ehlers-Danlos, coarctation of the aorta, Marfan syndrome.

Investigation: CT head scan – good quality, high resolution (sensitivity > 95% at 48 hours).

– sensitivity highest closest to time of ictus, drops after 48 hours.

Lumbar puncture (for classic history with negative CT, especially if delayed).

CT angiography (sensitivity > 95% in detecting aneurysms as small as 2.2mm).

Conventional catheter angiography (the "gold standard").

Location: Anterior circulation (85% overall): 35% anterior communicating artery; 30% ICA bifurcation/ PCoMA; 20% MCA.

Posterior circulation (15% overall): 10% basilar artery apex, 5% others.

Mycotic aneurysms: rare, usually MCA territory-Traumatic aneurysms: rare, usually ACA territory.

Treatment of Subarachnoid Hemorrhage

The treatment of subarachnoid hemorrhage focuses on initially securing the aneurysm by surgery or endovascular techniques to prevent rebleeding with its high mortality risk. Prior to securing the aneurysm, treatment to lower blood pressure extremes is mandatory. Vigilant monitoring is warranted in an intensive care or level 3 care environment, aiming at rapid recognition and therapy of the many complications of subarachnoid hemorrhage. After rebleeding, the top two complications are hydrocephalus (typically from 12-24 hours after the ictus) and cerebral vasospasm (from day 3 to 14).

Hydrocephalus is treated with placement of a ventriculostomy to divert CSF. Vasospasm is monitored with transcranial arterial Doppler ultrasound and is treated initially with HHH therapy (see section on neurocritical care), then, if neurologically symptomatic, with endovascular balloon angioplasty and intra-arterial vasodilators (such as nicardipine, or papaverine). Nimodipine, a cerebrovascularly-selective dihydropyridine calcium channel blocker, is routinely administered to SAH patients (60 mg every 4 hours) for prevention/attentuation of vasospasm after studies had shown it to be associated with improved outcome.

Medical complications of SAH include diuresis, cerebral salt wasting, diabetes insipidus (especially after rupture of AComA aneurysms), arrythmias and ECG changes, myocardial stunning with troponin leak, and neurogenic pulmonary edema; all of which require vigilance and rapid recognition and treatment.

Surgery

Craniotomy and microsurgical clipping across the neck is the oldest and most definitive "gold standard" method of treating cerebral aneurysms. For the vast majority of anterior circulation aneurysms, a pterional craniotomy is performed, allowing access to the basal circle of Willis to allow clipping. For AComA aneurysms, additional exposure may be necessary with removal of the orbitozygomatic bar, especially if the aneurysm is superiorly projecting.

Endovascular Coiling

Endovascular coiling of intracranial aneurysms is now routinely employed for certain subgroups of aneurysms, whether ruptured or incidental. A number of factors favor the endovascular approach. Anatomical factors include the aneurysm's configuration with dome-to-neck ratio (>2 recommended), posterior circulation aneurysms in surgically morbid locations such as basilar apex aneurysm. Host factors include poor clinical grade SAH, and elderly (>75) with multiple comorbidities. Factors unfavorable for coiling include large hematoma with mass effect where surgical decompression is warranted, giant aneurysm, and complex aneurysm anatomy with wide neck or vessels off the aneurysm requiring reconstruction of the parent vessel. For incidental aneurysms, especially posterior circulation, or elderly patients, endovascular coiling in good hands makes intuitive sense.

Incidental Aneurysms

A few large series with long-term follow-up attempted to determine the natural history of incidental (unruptured) aneurysms. The international study of unruptured intracranial aneurysms (USUIA), amongst others, tried to stratify this risk (Table 7).

Table 7

ISUIA Reported 5-Year Cumulative Rupture Rates According to Size and Location of Unruptured Aneurysm

Aneurysm diameter	**<7mm**		**7-12mm**	**13-24mm**	**25mm**
	SAH -	**SAH +**			
Cavernous ICA (n=210)	0	0	0	3%-0%	6%-4%
Anterior circulation (n=1037)	0	1%-5%	2%-6%	14%-5%	40%
Posterior circulation (n=445)	2%-5%	3%-4%	14%-5%	18%-4%	50%

Anterior circulation = ACA, AComA, ICA (not cavernous), or MCA.

Posterior circulation = posterior communicating artery or vertebrobasilar 5-year cumulative haemorrhage rates by aneurysm site (parent artery), size, and group (for aneurysms <7 mm). About 90% of all unruptured aneurysms were in the anterior circulation for the combined cohort (ie, groups 1 and 2).

Modified from Wiebers DO & ISUIA investigators, 2003.

Significant risk factors also cited by Juvela apart from aneurysm size, location, and SAH-status were patient age and cigarette smoking.

All available data taken together suggests the following:

Highest risk category:
Posterior circulation aneurysms, Aneurysm >25mm

Lowest risk category:
Anterior circulation aneurysms, Size <5mm

Currently accepted recommendations are:

- All symptomatic unruptured aneurysms should be treated
- Incidental aneurysms need to be considered on a case-by-case basis (size, age, health/comorbidity, location).
- Microsurgical clipping and endovascular coiling should be considered as complementary.
- A low-risk elective clipping procedure (in a high volume center of excellence) is preferable for an unruptured aneurysm.

The following would be a reasonable statement of an accepted recommendation for 1st choice treatment for each category of patient (setting the limits):

- Microsurgical Clipping: Young patient, with a small anterior circulation aneurysm (Figure 4.1).
- Endovascular Coiling: High risk / elderly patient, with a posteriorly projecting basilar apex aneurysm (Figure 4.2).

(Source: Solomon R., personal communication)

Figure 4.1

Microsurgical clipping

SAH in a 50-year-old woman secondary to ruptured left vertebral artery aneurysm, with 2 other incidental middle cerebral artery aneurysms; the former was coiled, and she was shunted for hydrocephalus. She then returned for clipping of the left (simple) MCA and then the right (complex) MCA aneurysm in two further surgeries. The complex right aneurysm is seen with multiple vessels coming directly from it, and required parent vessel reconstruction.

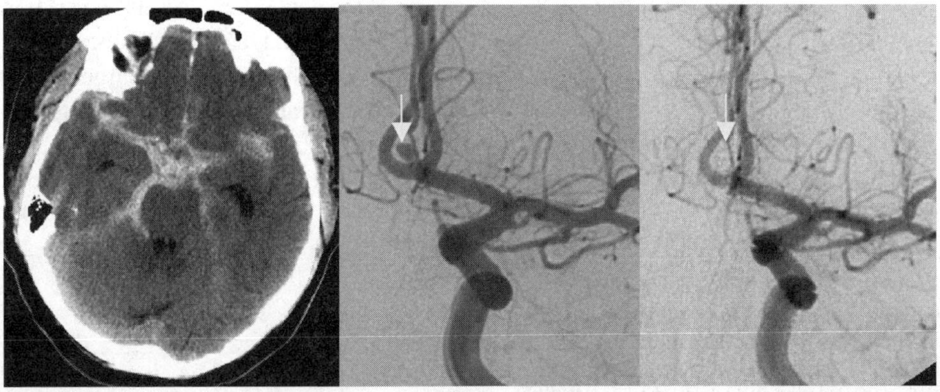

Courtesy of Dr. Clifford Eskey, Department of Neuroradiology, DHMC.

Figure 4.2

Endovascular coiling

SAH in a 50-year-old man secondary to ruptured anterior communicating artery aneurysm successfully coiled (arrows). Note the mild temporal horn dilatation signifying early hydrocephalus.

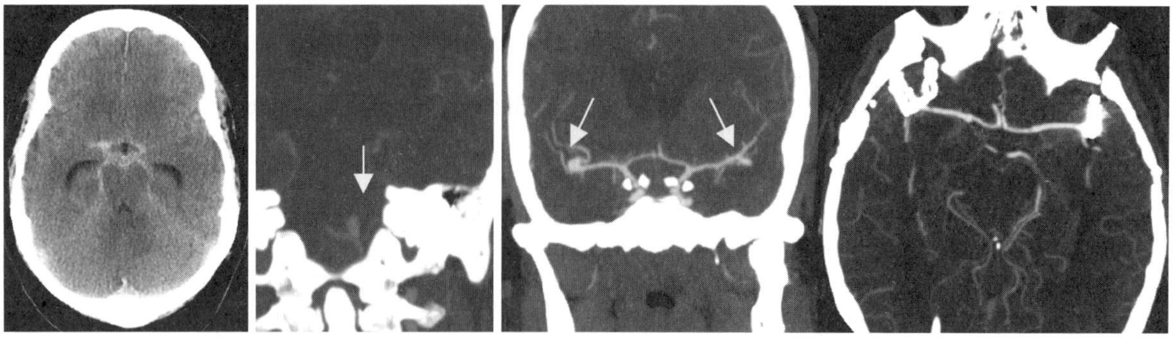

Courtesy of Dr. Clifford Eskey, Department of Neuroradiology, DHMC.

Arteriovenous Malformations (Figure 4.3)

Incidence: ~1%

Age: typically 20-40.

Presentation: Seizures, headache (occasionally migraine-like), stroke-like symptoms, hemorrhage, incidental.

Genetics: mostly sporadic, except Hereditary Hemorrhagic Telangectasia syndrome.

Risk of Rupture

The accepted risk of spontaneous rupture of AVM's may be low, in the order of 1% per year.

In natural history follow-up, predictors for hemorrhage appear to be hemorrhagic presentation, increasing age, deep brain location, and exclusive deep venous drainage.

The most influential factor for AVM rupture is a hemorrhagic presentation.

Annual haemorrhage rates vary from 0.9% for an unruptured superficial lesion with superficial venous drainage to as high as 34% for a lesion with all 3 risk factors. Lifetime risk of rupture can be significant in a young patient, but expectant management can also be justified in low grade, low risk lesions.

Endovascular Treatment

Endovascular embolization is the injection of a liquid embolic material (Onyx® is an example), which moulds itself to the shape of the AVM and excludes this from the circulation. As primary treatment, this has proved disappointing in long-term studies, but further development of embolic materials is improving this continuously. Endovascular embolization is primarily employed to obliterate some of the network of vessels in an AVM, in preparation for surgical resection, reducing the hemorrhagic risks and morbidity of surgery. Coiling of associated intranidal aneurysms is also possible now with Guglielmi detachable (GDC)-type of coils, again improving the conditions for surgical resection.

Surgical Excision

Surgical resection, when possible, is the oldest and most definitive method of treating AVM's. Risks of surgery are considered to be high for AVM's located in deep eloquent brain with deep venous drainage. Sometimes one is left with "no option" but total surgical resection, eg, in a superficial frontal lobe lesion with hematoma and mass effect. On occasion, surgery is not an option, eg, an unruptured deep brain stem lesion. Preoperative accurate embolization of the AVM can significantly reduce the intraoperative hemorrhagic risks and hence the morbidity of surgery. *It is mandatory to obtain angiography (CTA or catheter) on any intracerebral hemorrhage with the hallmarks of a potential AVM.*

Surgical resection carries a 1%-2% mortality with a 5%-10% morbidity, both of which are highly dependent on the grade of the lesion and preoperative neurologic status.

Stereotactic Radiosurgery

Stereotactic radiosurgery (SRS) of AVM's is increasing in frequency of use with more general application of SRS to non-tumor pathologics in thc central nervous system. Data is mixed for the efficacy of SRS for AVM's due to lack of long-term follow-up in a disease with a low natural history, especially unruptured AVM's. The non-invasive nature of the modality, however, lends itself to easy application in an asymptomatic condition (incidentals) and for highly morbid locations (deep white matter, basal ganglia). This is typically used for lesions <3cm in diameter, with 2-year occlusion approximately 85%, but at the cost of a hemorrhage rate of 10.5% in the 2 years until the AVM is obliterated.

Cervical Carotid Stenosis

Carotid stenosis is the narrowing of the internal carotid artery, typically seen right at the common carotid-internal carotid bifurcation segment due to eddy current and non-laminar flow. The narrowing is typically caused by an atheroma that can be fibrofatty or calcific plaque-like, causing atherosclerosis of the vessel. There is lipid deposition by low-density lipoprotein, typically oxidized, together with vessel intimal injury allowing fibroblast migration and smooth muscle hypertrophy. This results both in mechanical bulk taking up luminal space, as well as loss of the natural thromboresistance of the vascular wall and potential for platelet aggregation and thrombus formation and propagation.

Figure 4.3

Arteriovenous malformation

Superficial ICH in a 40-year-old male is seen on CT head. CTA shows a suspicious cortical draining vein appearing to fill directly from the distal ACA branches. Catheter angiography confirms that this vein fills in late arterial phase, ie, an AVM.

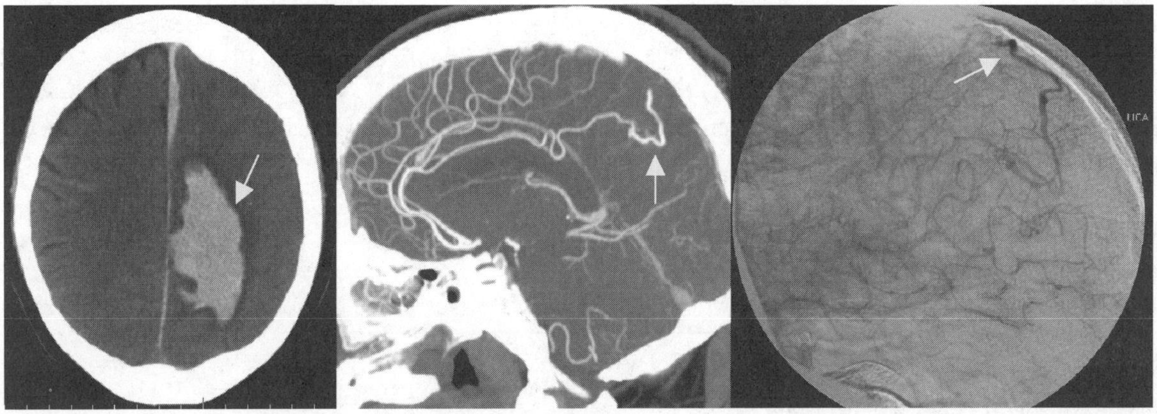

Clinically, this can be asymptomatic or present as either stroke, or transient ischemic attacks (TIA) of various types. These result in intermittent or permanent deficits. More readily nowadays, MRI imaging is demonstrating diffusion abnormalities in acute strokes at much earlier than CT used to (the earliest around 5-8 hours).

Risk Factors
Risk factors include hypertension, smoking, diabetes, previous strokes or cardiac disease.

- In asymptomatic patients with carotid stenosis (ie, carotid bruit), the risk of ipsilateral stroke with medical management is 2.1%/year (ACAS study).
- In symptomatic patients with carotid stenosis (TIA, stroke), the risk of ipsilateral stroke with medical management is 13%/year (NASCET study).
- The risk of a subsequent stroke is clearly higher in patients who present with stroke (versus a TIA) and less in those patients who present amaurosis fugax as their TIA symptom rather than another form of TIA.

Therapy
- Surgical carotid endarterectomy
- Endovascular stenting
- Medical management with cholesterol-modulating agents and antiplatelet agents (aspirin, clopidogrel).

The literature studying therapies for carotid stenosis is summarized as follows:

Stenosis was diagnosed by carotid Doppler and stratified into 3 grades:

Mild (aka low grade)	<30%
Moderate	30%-69%
Severe (aka high grade)	70%-99%

Symptomatic ICA Stenosis
The North American Symptomatic Carotid Endarterectomy Trial found the following:

The mean risks outlined in the study were:

- 13% per year risk of ipsilateral stroke with medical management
  (quoted 26% on a 2-year basis)
- 4.5% per year risk of ipsilateral stroke with surgical management
  (quoted 9% on a 2-year basis)
- 17% absolute risk reduction over 2 years.

- Risk of major or fatal stroke: 13% per 2 years in medical arm vs. 4.5% per 2 years in surgical arm.
- In centers who have a perioperative stroke and death rate of <6%; the cross-over time in which the benefits of surgery will be realized is 3 months.
- Risk reduction is greatest with the higher degrees of stenosis (90%-99%).

Asymptomatic ICA High-grade Stenosis
Our most up-to-date evidence comes from the asymptomatic carotid atherosclerosis study (ACAS).

The mean risks outlined in the study were:

- 1.2% for arteriographic complication in high-grade stenosis
- 2.3% for periop risk of stroke/death from CEA (95% confidence interval 1-3)
- 3.5% cumulative mean risk of surgery. (95% CI 2-5.3)

The stroke risk reduction was significant at 5 years, reducing the risk from 11% to 5%. It takes 5 years to accumulate the benefit from CEA, with the risk being taken upfront with surgery. No one over 80 was included in this study. This would tend to favor offering surgery to a patient only if the surgical risk for that particular patient is squarely below the 3% mark.

5. Degenerative Spine Disease

Lumbar Disc Disease

Prolonged axial back (and neck for that matter) pain is a common reason for referral to the spinal surgeon. Lumbar degenerative disk disease is usually associated with symptoms prolonged for more than 12 weeks. It is thought to occur as a product of a series of events from disk dehydration, and incompetence of the disk dorsally, with resulting loss of height and abnormal stresses on the adjacent endplates. The latter degenerative process continues with endplate sclerosis (aka MODIC changes) and osteophyte formation, as well as hypertrophy/arthropathy of the facet joints. There can be progressive loss of lordosis, which continues to further exacerbate the process. The axial pain generator remains unknown in lumbar (or cervical) degenerative disease due to the extensive changes that occur in multiple structures. Some authors advocate the incompetent disk itself as the predominant pain generator. This may partly explain the explosion in diskectomy and fusion surgeries that have occurred over the last 15 years for low back pain, despite no change in the incidence of the disease.

Presentation

Typically prolonged history of low back pain is followed by development of leg pain in a "sciatica" distribution. The radiculopathy commonly involves L5 or S1 (Figure 5.1). Dehydrated (low signal on T2) disks may be noted, with or without disk bulges or frank herniation seen on imaging.

Non-operative Treatment

Analgesics in the form of NSAIDs and opioids are used in the acute flare-up of symptoms. Other modalities include short courses of corticosteroids, as well as percutaneous epidural steroid injections that assist with dampening the inflammatory irritation of the nerve root. Active physical therapy has an important role in the treatment of these patients (after the acute flare has resolved). The latter forms the basis of various functional restoration programs that aim to strengthen paraspinal muscles and educate patients on spine care and maintenance of function, and eliminating the spiral into disability.

Indications for Surgical Diskectomy

Pure axial pain, whether in the lumbar or cervical spines, is rarely in isolation an indication for surgery. In fact, the teaching had been that even radiculopathy is uncommonly an indication for surgical diskectomy. This is because of the rather benign natural history of spontaneous improvement in at least 75% of cases of radiculopathy within an 8-12 week period.

The case for surgery had been to decompress compressed nerves where the patient had failed (or was unwilling to undergo) non-operative treatment (physiotherapy, epidural injections, oral steroids), or felt that they needed the rapid improvement that surgery can offer for lifestyle or employment purposes. On the other hand, surgery has a real complication rate, including CSF leak, repeat disk herniation, nerve root injury, and epidural scarring with permanent dysesthetic pain syndrome.

The most recent of clinical trials addressing the non-operative vs. operative treatment of lumbar disk radiculopathy has been the Spine Patient Outcomes Research Trial (SPORT). Its conclusions were as follows: "Patients in both the surgery and the non-operative treatment groups improved substantially over a 2-year period. Between-group differences in improvements were consistently in favor of surgery for all outcomes and at all time periods but were small and not statistically significant except for the secondary measures of sciatica severity and self-rated improvement. Because of the high numbers of patients who crossed over in both directions, conclusions about the superiority or equivalence of the treatments are not warranted based on the intent-to-treat analysis."

Cervical Spondylosis

Cervical spondylosis is the degenerative change seen in the cervical spine producing narrowing of the overall central spinal canal or nerve root foramina (Table 8). This can include various degenerative changes, including one or more of disc degeneration, loss of height, posterior vertebral osteophytic lipping, uncovertebral, and facet joint disease (Moore & Blumhardt, 1997). It commonly presents with radiculopathy and/or myelopathy. Cervical spondylotic myelopathy (CSM) is a very common source of disability in the elderly, on the order of 24% of all patients over 50 presenting with nontraumatic myelopathic symptoms.

The myelopathy can be associated with a classic "cord syndrome" or a combination of these.

Significantly, several other conditions may present in a fashion similar to CSM. It is important to exclude these because they may explain lack of neurological improvement after surgery.

Table 8

Syndromes Typical of Cervical Spondylosis Presentation

Cord Syndrome	Symptoms
Transverse	Spasticity, numbness, sensory ataxia, potential sphincter involvement
Motor	Spasticity & weaknes — minimal or no sensory change
Central	Severe motor and sensory change arms worse than legs; Lhermitte phenomenon on neck motion
Brown-Sequard	Ipsilateral spastic weakness or paralysis contralateral numbness or analgesia
Brachalgia and Cord	Predominant upper limb pain long tract/spastic symptoms in legs

Modified from Baron & Young, 2007.

Figure 5.1

Diagrammatic axial sections of the spinal cord demonstrating the somatotropic orientation of the spinal tracts. The white matter tracts anteriorly show a medial to lateral positioning of cranial to caudal segmental levels (C = cervical, T = thoracic, L = lumbar, S = sacral), while the opposite is true of the dorsal columns with cranial segments laterally placed to the more medial caudal segments.

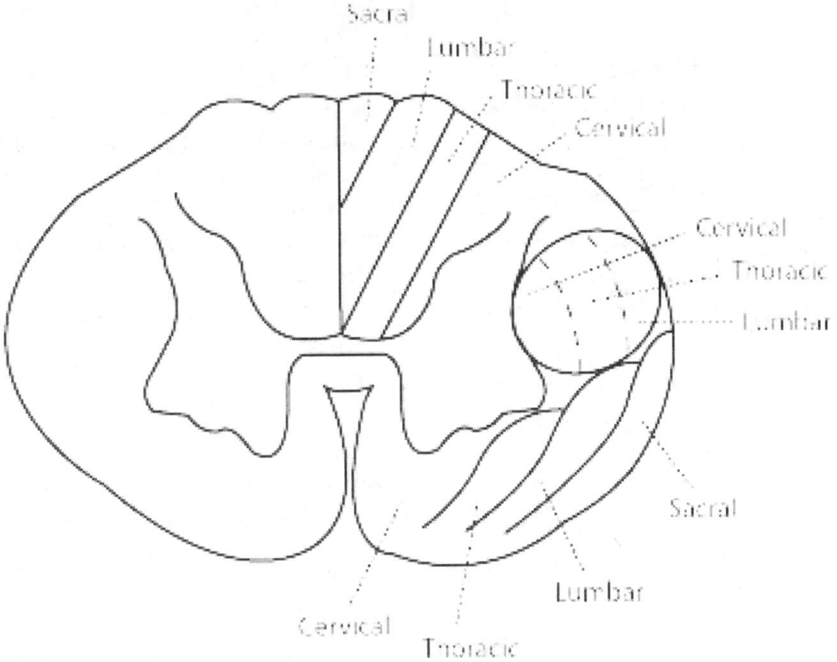

Reproduced by permission. Shedid & Benzel, 2007.

Differentials

ALS, MS, Syringomyelia, NPH, Vitamin B_{12} deficiency, tumor.

Radiculopathy

Spondylosis can present with radicular symptoms, both sensory or motor, with the former being commoner. This is not infrequently polyradicular, as the degenerative lateral recess and foraminal stenotic disease is often multilevel and bilateral. This can create diagnostic uncertainty regarding the etiology, often being confused with brachial plexus syndromes and peripheral compressive neuropathies (especially carpal tunnel syndrome). Electromyography and nerve conduction studies can be invaluable in evaluating a polyradicular syndrome of presentation.

Myelopathy (CSM)

The natural history of CSM is variable. A classical review by Nurick in 1972 reviewed the natural history as "the course of disease may be very prolonged. Long periods of non-progressive disability are the rule, and a few progressively deteriorating courses exceptional." He saw the disability from CSM due to canal stenosis as established early with little deterioration over time. Epstein reviewed cervical myelopathy patients in groups, and found in the non-operated group 36% with improvement and 64% without improvement. In the latter he found 26% with clinical deterioration over time. An older series by Clark in 1959 had clearer definition, especially of speed of symptomatic deterioration. Essentially the majority 75% had a series of episodes of symptoms (2/3rd deteriorated, 1/3rd unchanged), 20% had slow, steady progression of symptoms, and

5% had rapid onset of symptoms. There remains no definitive agreement on the issue of CSM natural history to date.

Treatment Options

- Observation – especially if patient has been stable for a prolonged period of time without evidence of progressive myelopathy.

- Surgery – for progressive myelopathy, especially urgent once gait or sphincter function is affected.

Surgical Options

Surgery is considered for patients who have evidence of spinal instability or neurologic deficit from spondylosis, especially evidence of progressive myelopathy. The latter, especially gait dysfunction (and even more for autonomic dysfunction) once started cannot be fully reversed with surgery. The target of surgery is to halt progression of myelopathy (although patients do make improvement in their functional ability). Surgery is also considered in those patients who present with sensory or motor radiculopathy and have failed non-operative treatment.

Surgery consists of decompressive procedure to free the spinal cord or nerve roots. This may or may not be coupled together with a stabilization procedure of some sort, whether instrumented or not. Put simply, there are anterior (anterior cervical diskectomy (usually with fusion) and foraminotomy) or posterior (laminectomy/laminoplasty) approaches to decompression.

Various factors are considered, especially where the primary compressive element is, the patient's constitutional condition, and biomechanics of the particular spine degenerative process, eg, the absence/presence of lordosis, and the presence of fixed stenosis versus a mechanical dynamic irritation.

Absolute indications for surgery do not exist in the very slowly worsening or even clinically static patient, with no high quality evidence indicating long-term benefit. In the United States, however, the trend has been to operate for any progressive symptoms.

6. Functional Neurosurgery

Stereotaxy

Stereotaxy is a Latin derivation of the meaning of placement within physical space, while stereotactic means literally "to touch in space." The two terms are used interchangeably and describe the method used in neurosurgery for locating points within the brain using an external, three-dimensional frame of reference, usually based on the Cartesian coordinate system. Essentially the brain is placed within a "box" of three-dimensional space and each discrete point can then be given an x, y and z coordinate. When the patient's head is placed within a stereotactic frame (the Leksell Model G frame is currently the most popular), and scanned in an MRI or CT, each point on the scan can be located in real space through a registration process that defines the transformation from scan space to real space and vice versa.

Frame-based stereotaxy allows the targeting of very small (2-5mm) structures with great accuracy by varying the trajectory and angles to avoid eloquent or vital structures but maintaining the tip of the probe at the target. This tool has been used for a variety of applications, such as aspiration of cysts or abscess, biopsy of deep brain tumors, and the making of highly selective iatrogenic lesions, or the placement of electrodes to stimulate deep functionally significant structures.

Frameless stereotaxy (aka neuronavigation, image-guided neurosurgery) registers the patient's head with fiducial markers scanned in the preoperative MRI or with natural skull landmarks for localization. This has allowed similar uses as frame-based systems, but with the addition of usability in the open surgical environment, enabling accurate localization of lesions to make craniotomy openings ever smaller and less morbid; and allowing more complex volumetric resection of tissue both for tumors and cortical tissue in epilepsy surgery.

Deep Brain Stimulation

Lesioning has been historically used to try to control the symptoms of a variety of movement disorders, before and after the advent of stereotaxy. The latter revolutionized the field leading to accuracy, and further accidental discoveries were made of which structures to target. Irving Cooper accidentally discovered ligation of the anterior choroidal artery, leading to improvement of symptoms of a Parkinson disease (PD) patient by producing a pallidal vascular lesion. From then on, pallidotomy was used for Parkinson, followed shortly by thalamotomy for both PD and tremor. Our understanding of some of the circuitry has led to the use of other targets in the motor system to control patients' symptoms.

Deep-brain stimulation with implanted electrodes simulates the effects of lesioning without destroying brain tissue, and has now almost supplanted lesioning as a method of effecting neuromodulation. Its mechanism is uncertain, but suggested mechanisms include activation of inhibitory neurons, depolarization blockade, suppression of abnormal neuronal firing patterns, and local inhibitory neurotransmitter release (eg, GABA).

Parkinson Disease

Parkinson disease motor dysfunction is thought to be related to increased neuronal activity in the subthalamic nucleus and the globus pallidus pars internus. Lesions made (and now DBS) in these structures have been found to improve motor function in monkeys with induced parkinsonism and patients with Parkinson disease, although they have been associated with neurologic deficits, especially when they are created bilaterally.

DBS has also become established for the treatment of other motor disorders such as essential tremor and dystonia; while it remains under clinical investigation for other disorders, such as obsessive-compulsive disorder, epilepsy and depression. The field is ever-expanding with more understanding of the circuitry of these disorders (Table 9).

Table 9

A Number of Deep Brain Stimulation Targets Utilized with Good Clinical Effects

Disease	Target for DBS
Parkinson Disease	GPi, STN
Dystonia	GPi
Essential Tremor	Vim Thalamus
Epilepsy	Anterior thalamus, STN
Obsessive-compulsive Disorder	Target for DBS
Depression	Area 25, Cingulate Gyrus (subgenual)

STN = subthalamic nucleus, Gpi = globus pallidus internus, Vim = ventralis intermedius nucleus of thalamus.

Surgical Treatment of Pain

Trigeminal neuralgia is a classic example of a condition where neurosurgical treatment of pain has revolutionized the care of the patient. Various procedures had been performed for this, but in summary, the following are the procedures currently done for the relief of trigeminal pain.

Ablative Procedures – Rhizolysis and Rhizotomy for Trigeminal Neuralgia

Percutaneous transfacial retrogasserian glycerol rhizolysis has been performed since the accidental discovery by Hakanson that glycerol injected into the trigeminal cistern had an ablative effect on the pain fibers, leading to improvement of trigeminal neuralgia. Similarly, radiofrequency trigeminal rhizotomy depends on a differential vulnerability of pain and touch fibers to thermocoagulation.

The approach to the two procedures is essentially the same, except for the material used to achieve rhizolysis. A needle is introduced percutaneously through the cheek of the patient under light sedation following a trajectory aimed at entering foramen ovale. On the lateral radiograph, the needle is seen to be directed toward the radiographic intersection of clivus and petrous bone.

As soon as foramen ovale is penetrated, often CSF is obtained and a small amount of radio-opaque contrast is injected confirming cisternal position. Glycerol is then injected into the trigeminal cistern (typically 0.3 mls). Radiofrequency ablation is done in the same way, except a radiofrequency probe is inserted through the needle once in position and this is used to heat the nerve by a standard protocol; eg, 60°C for 60 seconds twice to ablate its function.

Balloon compression is also performed for trigeminal neuralgia in a similar way, and is especially helpful in first-division pain (although is also helpful for multidivisional pain) because the unmyelinated fibers that mediate the blink reflex are preserved by the mechanical injury generated by the balloon.

Other ablative procedures done for superior division pain have also included superior orbital nerve avulsion. All ablative procedures are generally relatively low-risk and low-cost, and can be performed repeatedly with periodic success for most patients, especially the elderly, highly comorbid patient and multiple sclerosis patient. Complications can, however, include meningitis, recurrence of neuralgia, dysesthesiae, neuroparalytic keratitis, and anesthesia dolorosa (a severe constant, burning, aching pain that is refractory to all treatment).

Modulative/decompressive Procedures

Microvascular decompression (MVD) of the trigeminal nerve, since being pioneered by Jannetta, has become the commonest decompressive procedure performed for cranial neuralgia. The procedure is also performed to treat a host of other neurocompressive syndromes, including hemifacial spasm, vertigo, tinnitus, glossopharyngeal neuralgia, and spasmodic torticollis.

MVD of the trigeminal nerve involves a posterior fossa retromastoid craniectomy and the operative removal of the impingement of a vascular loop from its pressure on the trigeminal nerve in the prepontine cistern. The commonest vessel encountered is the anterior inferior cerebellar artery (AICA), followed by the superior cerebellar artery (SCA).

Such a posterior fossa procedure is reserved for severe neuralgia refractory to most other measures (prolonged medical therapy and other ablative procedures) and anticipated survival is >5 years. The morbidity associated with craniotomy is higher for the elderly and frail. Results are good with often long-lived relief (70%) at 10 years in some long-term follow-ups.

"Last Resort" Procedures

The so-called last resort procedure for seemingly refractory neuralgia to all measures, including previous MVD (and perhaps redo MVD), is the irreversible intradural trigeminal nerve section.

Epilepsy

Twenty percent of epilepsy patients continue to have seizures despite optimum treatment with antiepileptic medications (AEDs). Our understanding of the semiology, electrophysiology and more specifically the anatomical substrate of a great number of seizure syndromes has undergone major expansion in the last 20 to 30 years. The accuracy of imaging, especially MRI, in elucidating the anatomical substrate of lesional causes of seizures, has recategorized some syndromes away from the "idiopathic" or "cryptogenic" category to potential surgical lesions. Examples of this are low-grade gliomas and cavernomas.

Additionally, more accurate diagnosis of mesial temporal sclerosis (MTS) has led to ever more surgeries to resect these as foci, making this not only the most common procedure performed for epilepsy worldwide, but also the most successful, with long-term seizure freedom rates of 66 percent.

Multimodality Work-up

This is generally employed for the patient being considered for potential epilepsy surgery in an established program. The rationale for this is to further characterize the semiology, electrical signature, and anatomical localization of the seizure, as well as investigate potential adverse effects of proceeding with the next investigative or therapeutic surgical step (eg, speech-sided dominance).

Non-invasive tests

- *CT scan*

- *MRI scan:* imaging modality of choice, especially good at detecting MTS.

- *Video-EEG:* long term monitoring allows correlation of clinical seizure with electrical signature and potential localization

- *PET (positron emission tomography):* interictally obtained this can show hypometabolism on the side of the seizure focus.

- *SPECT (single photon emission tomography):* this is utilized to demonstrate hyperemia during the ictal event, helping to localize the site of onset.

- *WADA Test (aka intracarotid amytal test):* utilized to lateralize the language dominant hemisphere and assess ability of the other hemisphere to maintain memory when isolated.

Invasive tests

Video EEG from intracranial electrodes: These can be placed in various either brain surface (usually subdural) or depth electrodes. The former are placed through burrholes with small durotomy or large craniotomy; while the latter are placed stereotactically, classically into the hippocampus and mesial temporal lobe. Combinations of these can be placed in arrays to obtain coverage of all potential seizure foci previously suggested by the non-invasive data (imaging, scalp EEG, clinical semiology).

The three basic types of procedure performed for epilepsy are:

Resections

Resection of epileptic focus: higher chance of complete seizure control.

- Anterior temporal lobectomy

- Amygdalo-hippocampectomy

- Neocortical resections

- Resection of lesion in secondary epilepsy (eg, AVM, cavernoma, tumor).

Disconnections

Used for eloquent brain or to separate the electrical activity of the two hemispheres.

- *Corpus callosum section (callosotomy)*: Performed for drop attacks (most disabling) or for multiple bilateral foci.

- *Hemispherectomy:* Performed for unilateral seizures (multiple hemispheric lesions and profound contralateral hemispheric deficit) – eg, congenital hemiplegia syndrome, Rasmussen's.

- *Multiple subpial transections:* Performed for partial seizure foci from eloquent cortex.

- *Short interval (~5mm) transections* to interrupt horizontal seizure spread and spare vertical fibers.

Neuromodulative Procedures for Epilepsy

These are currently considered "fall-back" procedures, which are employed when resective or disconnection surgery is not possible due to poor localization on EEG data, or when the patient is not willing to accept the risks of intracranial surgery.

- *Vagus nerve stimulation:* Used for eloquent brain or to separate the electrical activity of the two hemispheres. The exact mechanism is unknown, but takes advantage of the protean relay projections and monosynaptic connections of the vagal nuclei and fibers. The locus coeruleus and raphe nucleus are thought to be key intermediaries, as bilateral lesions of these centers abolish the seizure-suppressing effects of VNS therapy in animal models.

7. Neurosurgical Oncology

The basic tenet of neurosurgical oncology, as for the rest of medicine, is first to do no harm. The aim is not to leave the patient with any new neurological deficits as a direct result of surgery. The standards are being raised ever higher by improving technologies, from microsurgical techniques and the use of the operating microscope to neuronavigation for accuracy and frameless stereotaxy. Furthermore, increased use of multimodality treatment with improved functional outcome for the individual patient has now become the standard in many neuro-oncology centres.

The aims of surgical therapy for tumors in the nervous system are much more circumscribed than in other systemic surgeries. These aims can be thought of in terms of a therapeutic ladder with steps in the following order: 1.) to establish a histologic diagnosis; 2.) to perform cytoreductive surgery (aka "debulking") of the tumor mass either to relieve mass effect, or lower tumor burden, or both (achieving surgical "tumor control"), and 3.) to complete macroscopic and microsurgical resection to improve neurologic function. How far one is able to climb up this surgical ladder will vary from lesion to lesion, patient to patient, and more importantly in intracranial surgery from location to location, depending on the achievement of securing tumor control or complete resection paid for by the price in morbidity (or mortality) for the patient.

Neurosurgical Multimodality Therapy

Neurosurgery is perhaps unique in the surgical specialities in that the development of many modalities that do not involve the surgical act of cutting tissue have come directly as a result of developments by neurosurgeons of the technology to achieve control of lesion, often in deep and hard-to-reach targets in the human brain or skull. Those modalities heavily applied in neuro-oncologic disease include:

Standard open surgical approaches
Craniotomy and resection of simple convexity meningioma remains a standard procedure.

Expanded surgical approaches
Improvements in skull base techniques now allow resection or at least partial resection and reconstruction in previously unresectable lesions.

Frame-based stereotactic techniques
Frame-based stereotactic systems have been in common neurosurgical use since 1951. These allow the accurate (+/- 1mm) targeting of deep lesions to obtain biopsies with great accuracy.

Neuronavigation, frameless and robotic stereotaxy
These have enabled achievement of highly accurate localization of even small tumors and margins of tumors involving or abutting eloquent brain structures. Examples of commonly used neuronavigation systems include Stealth Station® and Brainlab®. Further enhancement via robotic microscopy has allowed accurate volumetric resections of subtle low-grade lesions. An example of such a system is the Surgiscope®.

Ventricular access devices
These devices, sometimes known by their eponyms such as Ommaya or Rickam reservoir, are relatively frequently placed for intrathecal chemotherapeutic therapy of tumors spreading along the cerebrospinal fluid pathways. This is typically performed for primary (PCNSL) or secondary central nervous system lymphoma. The catheter is usually located in the non-dominant (usually right) frontal horn or the lateral ventricle.

Intra-tumoral chemotherapy
The placement of chemotherapy wafers within tumor cavities are currently used for some high-grade gliomas. An example is Gliadel® (BCNU wafers) for glioblastoma. Some concerns about the heightened wound complication rate have tempered early enthusiasm for its use.

Stereotactic radiosurgery

Focused beam gamma knife or linear particle accelerator particles are being used with frame systems to target small lesions, or those deep-seated with an unacceptable open surgical morbidity. Examples include acoustic neuromas and small metastases.

Stereotactic biopsy vs. resection

The biopsy of lesions, especially intrinsic brain tumors, for a histological diagnosis, prior to making a decision to resect, has a place in cases when there is diagnostic uncertainty. This is especially true of deep lesions in eloquent brain (eg, thalamic glioma), in areas where primary surgery has highly morbid risks (eg, pineal region), or where an alternative non-surgical approach is best used (eg, lymphoma).

Brain Tumors

Extra-axial Tumors

Generally, tumors that occur without the substance of the brain parenchyma involve the dural meninges, the cranial nerve sheaths (so-called neurolimmomas) or the bony calvarial structure. By far the commonest of all these lesions are meningiomas, followed closely by schwannomas of the eighth and fifth cranial nerves. Extra-axial tumors generally cause symptoms by causing mechanical pressure on the brain or cranial nerves, and when aggressive in biology can cause frank brain invasion.

Meningiomas

The vast majority of meningiomas are benign in biology, with a slow-growth course, and rarely invade the substance of the brain, thus presenting the potential for a surgical cure.

These arise from arachnoid cap cells. Common locations are anywhere where there is double-folding of dural edges, such as associated with the falx cerebri, tentorium cerebelli, and the corresponding dural venous sinuses. Other common locations include the cerebello-pontine angle, cranial nerve foramina, cribriform plate, medial middle fossa/sphenoid wing, and very occasionally in an intraventricular location. As with any intracranial benign tumor, the prime limiting factor for resection and morbidity from meningioma is location. Cushing and Eisenhardt's 1938 classification used location as the main factor, since 85%-90% are located supratentorially, of which 25% are parasagittal/falcine, 19% convexity, and 17% sphenoid ridge.

Microsurgical resection remains the gold standard primary modality for treatment of meningioma. Various factors influence the extent of resection of meningioma, the most important three being location (especially in the posterior fossa), vascularity (where preoperative embolization can be employed), and involvement of the dural venous sinuses. The latter can lead to post-operative venous congestion or frank thrombosis leading to venous infarction and neurological deficit, particularly in the parasagittal/falcine location. Adjuvant treatments are usually reserved only for meningiomas showing atypia on histology, or those in surgically unresectable locations (eg, in cavernous sinus). Stereotactic radiosurgery is now increasingly utilized as the primary treatment modality for small lesions (typically <2cm) in high medical-risk patients and lesions in surgically morbid locations, eg, in complex skull base lesions.

Incidental Meningiomas

Incidental meningiomas are found in increasing frequency due to higher frequency of neuroimaging utilization. In the elderly, asymptomatic population, serial imaging without intervention is an accepted modality of treatment.

Schwannoma

The commonest are vestibular and trigeminal schwannomas, followed by other cranial nerves.

The former are traditionally the commonest cerebellopontine angle tumor. Cranial nerve schwannomas are usually isolated lesions, but have a high incidence in the autosomal dominant condition neurofibromatosis type 2 (NF2), where they can be bilateral and associated with meningiomas and ependymomas. Hence, NF2 is also named the multiple inherited schwannomas, meningiomas, and ependymomas (MISME) syndrome. These tumors arise from the nerve sheath or neurilemma and consist of Schwann cells in a collagenous matrix, with histologically elongated spindle cells that can either be in a loosely-packed (Antoni A) or tightly-packed (Antoni B) configuration. The commonest symptom of a vestibular schwannoma is sensory neural hearing loss, with others including facial weakness being less common at presentation.

The resection of schwannoma, which is technically separate from the nerve axons/fascicles, is unfortunately fraught with potential risk of nerve injury, as these fascicles are oftentimes highly stretched over the tumor or intertwined within the tumor mass. The most often used surgical approaches to resection of a vestibular schwannoma are the suboccipital retrosigmoid (the commonest with a good chance of hearing preservation), and the translabyrinthine (this drills out the entire bony labyrinth for access and therefore usually only employed where there is no serviceable hearing). Surgical morbidity is primarily from potential for facial nerve injury, with other risks including brain stem injury, hydrocephalus and CSF leak. Stereotactic radiosurgery is now increasingly used as primary therapy, with literature suggesting satisfactory tumor control (defined variably) for small lesion (typically <2cm), with the limitation often being the radiation dose at the tumor margin next to the brain stem. For large lesions where surgery achieves subtotal resection (significant proportion), SRS is used as adjuvant therapy to the residual.

Sellar/Parasellar

Mostly extra-axial to brain, but usually considered in a category of their own. Sellar tumors are overwhelmingly of pituitary origin, primarily adenomas. Parasellar tumors are typically either suprasellar (eg, craniopharyngiomas involving the pituitary stalk or hypothalamus), or of the various structures surrounding the sella. The latter can be as diverse as developmental cysts (Rathke's pouch remnant) and notochordal bone tumors (chordoma), benign dorsum sella meningiomas to more aggressive nasopharyngeal carcinomas invading through the sphenoid sinus.

Treatment of benign pituitary tumors is primarily dependent on the endocrine syndrome. For example, prolactinomas are primarily treated by medication, eg, bromocriptine, or analogues such as cabergolide, with surgery saved for non-responders or those with medication intolerance. Growth hormone and corticotroph adenomas are primarily treated by trans-sphenoidal surgical resection. Non-functioning tumors typically present with visual changes of bitemporal field loss that necessitates surgical decompression.

Surgery with serial imaging is the commonest treatment for benign well-differentiated tumors, with chemotherapy, radiotherapy and even stereotactic radiosurgery saved for more histologically aggressive tumors, or those showing faster imaging growth than expected (especially in surgical morbid locations such as the cavernous sinus).

Intra-axial Tumors—Supratentorial/Infratentorial

Intra-axial lesions are located intrinsically within the brain parenchyma. The commonest of these lesions are metastatic lesions from systemic cancers with primary neuroglial tumors coming a close second in adults. Conversely, in children brain tumors are the second most common form of childhood cancer and the leading cause of morbidity and mortality from cancer in children.

Metastases

This is the commonest intraxial tumor in adults. Many primary tumors are the classic sources of brain secondaries: bronchogenic carcinoma, malignant melanoma, renal carcinoma, breast carciconma, and colonic carcinoma.

Metastatic lesions tend to be associated with a disproportionately large amount of white matter edema to their size. In metastases with mass effect, the primary aim is to decompress the brain and achieve a total macroscopic resection. In very small tumors or multiple lesions with a known or plausible primary on non-CNS imaging, biopsy of the primary is warranted, followed by chemoradiotherapy for the primary. Whole brain radiation therapy is then given per the institutional protocol. In cases of diagnostic uncertainty or without a clear primary, surgical biopsy, or resection where possible is performed.

Generally, resection can be performed for one, two, or even up to three easily accessible lesions where there is probable achievement of systemic disease freedom.

In lymphoma, the primary role of surgery is essentially diagnostic, as the tumor is highly chemosensitive. Steroids should be withheld in the neurologically-stable patient, even with edema on imaging if there is likelihood of lymphoma as the diagnosis, as this would cause lysis of cells and render the histological appearance of the tumor undiagnostic. This is especially true in small stereotactically-obtained biopsy samples.

High-Grade Glioma

The commonest primary cerebral neoplasm in adults. Presentation is typically with progressive neurologic deficit (usually motor), headache, or seizure (in that order). The term high-grade glioma describes a group of histopathologically defined aggressive glial tumors. These comprise: glioblastoma multiforme (GBM), anaplastic astrocytoma (AA), anaplastic oligodendroglioma (AO), anaplastic oligoastrocytoma or "mixed" glioma, gliosarcoma, and possibly gemistocytic astrocytoma (GA). These tumors show heterogeneity of glial cell differentiation but share a characteristic of diffuse invasiveness into surrounding brain and an extremely poor prognosis for survival beyond 2-3 years. As for metastatic lesions, the primary aim is to decompress mass effect and obtain accurate histologic diagnosis without increasing the patient's neurological deficit burden.

The secondary aim is to achieve complete macroscopic resection. Surgical technique for high-grade lesions is usually through internal debulking, followed by subtotal resection (or near total in non-eloquent brain). In deep-seated diencephalic lesions (eg, thalamic), often biopsy is all that can be achieved surgically. The issue of whether to resect versus biopsy only high-grade lesions in frail patients with multiple comorbidities is still a debated topic. The standard of care nowadays is for high-grade lesions to almost uniformly receive adjuvant chemoradiation (including the oral agent Temozolamide) treatment, depending on the patient's functional status, with the cutoff usually being around a Karnofsky of 75 (see the Karnofsky scale in the section on scales). The loss of the 1p19q allele is tested for in predominantly oligodendroglial tumors, as it predicts improved responses to chemotherapy.

Low-Grade Glioma

The term low-grade glioma (LGG) describes a group of intrinsic glial tumors arising from astrocytes, oligodendrocytes, or ependymal cells. They are characterized by well differentiation, a slow growth pattern, and particular radiologic appearances as compared to HGGs. The use of the clinical term LGG is sometimes reserved for low-grade (eg, pilocytic) astrocytomas, but within the World Health Organization criteria, oligodendrogliomas, ependymomas, gangliogliomas and pleomorphic xanthoastrocytomas are also included. LGGs tend to present in relatively younger patients (less than 40), and usually with epilepsy. The aim with these is to obtain resection of enhancing areas or FLAIR lesions (as many do not enhance). Radiation is withheld for lesion without histologic atypia. Often these are followed for years, and will recur or even progress to a higher grade on subsequent biopsies (the concept of tumor progression).

Spinal Tumors

Spinal tumors can be classified anatomically as either extradural (ED), intradural extra-medullary (IDEM), or intra-medullary (IM) lesions.

Extradural

Metastases

The spine is the commonest location for skeletal metastases, with metastatic lesions being the commonest tumors in the spine (98%). By far the commonest primaries are breast, prostate, lung and lymphoma (the first two being osteoblastic).The treatment for many is primary radiotherapy in addition to hormonal treatment. Radiation is effective even in cases of subacute cord compression, where most patient's symptoms are usually axial pain with limited numbers with myelopathy. In cases where there has been acute neurologic deterioration, surgical decompression may be warranted.

Bone tumors
Multiple myeloma, plasmacytoma, and other rare benign tumors, such as osteoid osteoma and osteoblastoma.

Intradural-Extramedullary

Meningioma
Meningioma is the commonest intradural extramedullary lesion in adults, followed closely by ependymoma and neurofibroma. Mostly located in the thoracic spine, and these present with insidious myelopathy. Their resection follows the same principles as for intracranial meningioma, namely that of defining the location and excluding the blood supply early in the surgery. The vast majority can be resected clean off the spinal cord via dorsal laminectomy, with additional transpedicular exposures for more laterally located lesions. Intraoperative bleeding can be a major issue for some, however, but preoperative endovascular embolization is not commonly used. Recurrences are seen but typically take 6 years in follow up studies.

Intramedullary

Spinal cord glioma (astrocytoma and glioblastoma)
These lesions are uncommon, but their resection involves usually a midline myelotomy along the dorsal funiculus and intratumoral debulking. The strategy involves usually obtaining an accurate frozen-section tissue diagnosis intraoperatively as soon as the tumor is identified, to set the limits and targets of resection. In high-grade lesions, no resection is warranted due to the risk of producing further neurological deficit. In cases where the patient already has a complete cord syndrome below the lesion, especially with ascending neurological signs, some surgeons have advocated complete resection and even cord transection.

In low-grade astrocytoma (30%), however, cytoreductive debulking is performed, but complete resection is often not possible due to difficulty of discerning normal from abnormal tissue, and radiation is used as adjuvant treatment. Ependymoma (30%) is a special case where there is often a plane allowing resection of tumor from normal cord.

Ependymoma
Myxopapillary ependymoma is the commonest lesion found at the conus medullaris, typically in young patients (third and sixth decade peaks). A complete surgical resection in often possible by coagulating and dividing the filum terminal above, then below, the lesion.

8. Pediatric Neurosurgery

Hydrocephalus

The most common cause of hydrocephalus in childhood is post-hemorrhagic hydrocephalus secondary to prematurity. Others include aqueductal stenosis, meningomyelocele, post-meningitis or post-traumatic.

The introduction of ventriculo-peritoneal shunting has completely changed the natural history of survival and morbidity of hydrocephalus. Shunted, otherwise normally developed children can lead next to normal lives. Literature suggests, however, that on the whole, shunted children still have a decreased life expectancy than average, and this may be due to the subgroups with other associated congenital anomalies.

Premature birth (especially before 30 weeks of gestation) predisposes to hemorrhage within the germinal matrix area of the diencephalon, the area located medially between the cauda nucleus and the thalamus in the subventricular area. Hemorrhage here dissects into the ventricle resulting in intraventricular hemorrhage (IVH). Although there is likelihood of spontaneous resorption of the blood, nevertheless some children end up with progressive ventricular dilatation and macrocephaly. Shunting is usually performed after there is documentation of symptoms (which can be non-specific in the neonate, from poor feeding all the way to seizures and obtundation), or for progressive macrocephaly over time, the latter witnessed by increases in head circumference on an age-appropriate centile chart over time.

The preferred method of shunting is ventriculo-peritoneal, although the terminus can be placed into the pleural cavity, or even the atrium. Nowadays, these other options tend to be second-line, or in complicated cases with proven problems with peritoneal shunting, for example, multiple complex abdominal operations.

Brain Tumors

Brain tumors are the most common cause of solid cancers, and the most common cause of cancer morbidity in children. Except for craniophayngioma, the vast majority of childhood brain tumors have a strong predeliction for the posterior fossa.

The commonest brain tumors are as follows in the supratentorial and infratentorial spaces:

Craniopharyngioma

This is more correctly termed a "tumor-like" malformation of the hypothalamic region, but tends to grow like a biologically benign tumor. The cells arise from rests of Rathke's pouch of the embryological primitive buccal origin from the pharynx, to sella turcica and the suprasellar area at the floor of the third ventricle.

It constitutes 3% of all intracranial tumors; 5%-10% of all childhood tumors; and has a bimodal age distribution peak at ages 5 to 14 (with smaller peak in adults at 50-74). Incidence is 0.13 cases per 100,000 per year in the US, with approximately 350 new cases diagnosed annually countrywide. Its location is purely intrasellar in 5%, intra and suprasellar in 20%, and suprasellar (with third ventricular extension) in 75% of cases.

Typically it is seen with a mixed solid-cystic appearance (latter predominates) and calcification. Presentation in children is seen with growth failure, hypopituitarism (including diabetes insipidus), and hydrocephalus signs and symptoms if obstructing the third ventricle.

Treatment of craniopharyngioma has changed philosophy in the past 30 years. Previously aggressive surgical resections achieved "good results," but at the cost of leaving children with hypothalamic hyperphagia, severe behavioral disturbances, and often poor conscious level, with operative mortalities approaching 20% and relapses still up to 60%. Nowadays, less aggressive surgery is performed and adjuvant radiation is the mainstay of therapy. Aggressive radiation in the older child with tumor doses of 5000-5500 cGy are given in 20-25 fractions, but the younger child (under 3) remains a management problem. The primary role for surgery is CSF diversion to relieve hydrocephalus, and drain the cystic component, often leaving catheters for repeated aspiration, or instillation of various agents used for tumor control (such as mitomycin). Endocrine follow-up and long-term pituitary replacement is necessary. Long-term control of approximately 80%-95% at 5-20 years, and a low risk of long-term morbidity is reported following the above principles.

Medulloblastoma (PNET)

Also known as primitive neuroectodermal tumors, these comprise 40% of all posterior fossa tumors in children, and are almost universally karyotypically abnormal lesions. They are commonest at ages 3-5 years, with a second peak at 7-8. They present with irritability, lethargy, and decreased social interaction (60%), intermittent vomiting (40%), and headache (40%) (usually worse in the morning). Physical findings commonly reveal papilledema and midline ataxia in up to 50%-60%. Imaging shows hyperdense homogeneously enhancing mass on CT scan and a heterogeneous mass with ill-defined margins arising from the vermis, filling the fourth ventricle, with hydrocephalus in up to 80%. The entire neuraxis is imaged to detect spinal metastases, which may occur via subarachnoid dissemination (33% at diagnosis). Corticosteroids are given. Surgical resection is through a midline suboccipital approach, with ventriculostomy rarely necessary preoperatively due to risk of upward herniation. Goals of surgery are to achieve radical tumor resection, when possible, and to restore normal CSF outflow. Five-year survival is around 75%+ with adjuvant posterior fossa and neuraxis radiation therapy. Temporary posterior fossa mutism is seen postoperatively in up to 20% of children.

Cerebellar Astrocytoma

These low grade tumors (mostly pilocytic WHO grade I lesion) comprise 40% of all posterior fossa tumors in children, commonest at ages 5-10. The commonest presenting symptoms in order are ataxia (lateral cerebellar findings); headaches; nausea; with vomiting developing later. These tumors are usually discrete, indolent lesions associated with cyst formation and a mural nodule, although 20% are midline/solid. 75% are associated with hydrocephalus. Therapy is based on administering steroids, and surgical resection with CSF diversion as necessary. Pilocytic astrocytomas carry a >95% cure rate.

Brain Stem Glioma

Gliomas in the brain stem comprise 10%-20% of all pediatric posterior fossa tumors. They can present at any age, but more commonly >5. Their presentation can be vague, with constitutional symptoms such as lethargy before neurological symptoms are recognized, typically multiple cranial nerve palsies (commonly 5th, 6th and 7th cranial nerves); and motor and cerebellar impairment. The lesion is typically a diffuse nonenhancing pontine lesion with contiguous spread; 30% or less with hydrocephalus. CSF diversion is done for the latter. Focal dorsally exophytic lesions, or those protruding into the 4th ventricle, can be tackled surgically for resection or biopsy and have a better prognosis. Focal radiotherapy is the cornerstone of treatment, with doses in the range 50-60 Gy with hyperfractionation. Surgery is not possible for totally intrinsic diffusely infiltrating tumors, which carry a mortality of 90% within 18 months.

Ependymoma

These are the commonest 4th ventricular tumor and are 10%-20% of all posterior fossa lesions in children (third after medulloblastoma and astrocytoma), with peaks in those <3 years old. Like medulloblastoma, often sixth, seventh, and eight cranial nerve palsies can be present, as well as other signs, such as torticollis and ataxia. Usually enhancing inhomogeneously, and may be laterally placed; approximately 50% have associated hydrocephalus. Treatment of pediatric ependymomas may include surgery, radiation therapy, and chemotherapy. Preoperative placement of a CSF shunt is often required, as well as screening of the neuraxis for CSF seeding. Surgery is the mainstay of therapy, and total resection is recommended if possible. Survival is variable: 40%-80%; there are often postoperative cranial nerve palsies. Ependymomas are considered to be relatively radiosensitive, and radiation therapy to the neuraxis seems to increase the survival period and delay recurrence for several years. Given the caveat about irradiating the under 5's (see above): some protocols have given younger children chemotherapy to allow saving of radiation until they are older.

Chiari Malformation (aka Hind Brain Hernia)

Chiari malformation is the name given to a variety of anomalies associated with tonsillar descent from the posterior fossa through the foramen magnum. These can be simply considered as a spectrum of developmental anomalies leading to a hind-brain hernia.

The exact cut-off for the amount of tonsillar descent diagnosis of a Chiari malformation is controversial, especially when this is asymptomatic. Generally, 5mm beyond the foramen magnum (ie, the line drawn from basion to opisthion) is the minimum considered necessary for considering a diagnosis, although most <5mm are asymptomatic. 6-12mm descents of the tonsils can be on average 30%-50% symptomatic. Four types of this anomaly are described, generally from the simplest Type I with minimal associated anomalies up to Type IV.

Type I: Caudal displacement of cerebellar tonsils below foramen magnum.

Type II: Caudal displacement of the cerebellar vermis, IVth ventricle, and lower brain stem below foramen magnum, associated with myelodysplasia/ myelomeningocele and supratentorial anomalies (callosal dysgenesis, and neuronal migration abnormalities).

Type III: Caudal displacement of the cerebellum and brain stem into a high cervical meningocele or occipital encephalocele, with some of the Type 2 anomalies.

Type IV: Cerebellar hypoplasia—of questionable relation to the others.

Their clinical manifestation can be protean, and potentially dependent on other associated anomalies of the cranium, craniovertebral junction and dysraphic spine, as well as the spinal cord conditions.

Examples of bony anomalies include:

- Klippel-Feil anomaly, Atlanto-occipital Assimilation (incomplete ossification of the atlas), and basilar invagination.

- Neuraxial abnormalities can involve the cerebrum (hydrocephalus, polymicrogyria, cortical heterotopia, colpocephaly), midbrain (aqueductal stenosis, tectal beaking), or brain stem (caudal displacement of pons, medulla and basilar artery, stretching of lower cranial nerves, and cervicomedullary kinking).

Surgical treatment involves one or more of the following:

- Posterior fossa bony decompression (for the mildest forms, as this has the lowest morbidity/complication rate)
- C1-C2 laminectomy (possibly more levels)
- Durotomy, sectioning of tight dural band, duroplasty
- Diathermy shrinking of redundant cerebellar tonsils
- Plugging of 4th ventricular obex
- Syringo-cavitary shunts
- Ventriculoperitoneal shunts

9. References

Neurosurgical Trauma

Denis F. The three column spine and its significance in the classification of acute thoracolumbar spinal injuries. *Spine*. Vol 8 (8). 1983.

White A, Panjabi M. *Clinical Biomechanics of the Spine*. 2nd ed. Philadelphia: Lippincott; 1990.

Larson SJ, Maiman S. Surgery of the Lumbar Spine. High dose methylprednisolone in the management of acute spinal cord injury—a systematic review from a clinical perspective. *Spinal Cord*. Vol. 38 (5); 273-286, May 2000.

Greenberg M. *Handbook of Neurosurgery*. Thieme; 2003.

Neurosurgical Emergencies (Non-traumatic)

Broderick JP, Brott TG, Duldner JE, Tomsick T, Huster G, Kothari R. Volume of Intracerebral Hemorrhage. A powerful and easy-to-use predictor of 30-day mortality. American Heart Association. *Stroke*. Vol. 24, 987-993.

Diringer M, et al. Hydrocephalus associated with ICH. *Stroke*. 1998: 29(7); 1352-1357.

Greenberg M. *Handbook of Neurosurgery*. 6th ed. Thieme; 2006.

Fogelholm R. Prognostic Value and Determinants of First Day Mean Arterial Pressure in Spontaneous Supratentorial Intracerebral Hemorrhage. *Stroke*. 1997: 28(7); 1396-1400.

Fujii Y. et al. Deterioration after ICH. *Stroke*. 1998: 29(6); 1160-1166.

Phan T. Hydrocephalus and ICH, et al. *Stroke*. 2000: 31(9); 2157-2162.

Mendelow AD, Gregson BA, Fernandes HM, Murray GD, Teasdale GM, Hope DT, Karimi A, Donald M, Shaw M, Barer DH, for the STICH investigators. Early surgery versus initial conservative treatment in patients with spontaneous supratentorial intracerebral haematomas in the International Surgical Trial in Intracerebral Haemorrhage (STICH): a randomised trial. Lancet. Vol. 365, Issue 9457, 29 January 2005, Pages 287-297.

Youmans Neurological Surgery. Winn HR, ed. 5th ed. Elsevier Inc. 2004.

Neurosurgical Critical Care

Moore AJ, Newell DW, eds. *Neurosurgery—Principles and Practice*. Springer; 2004.

Gupta AK, Summors AC. Notes in *Neuroanaesthesia and Critical Care*. 2001. Greenwich Medical Media Ltd., 137 Euston Road, London NW1 2AA.

Greenberg M. *Handbook of Neurosurgery*. 6th edition. New York: Thieme; 2003.

Citow, et al. *Comprehensive Neurosurgery Board Review*. Thieme; 2000.

Youmans Neurological Surgery. Winn, HR, ed. 4th Edition. Elsevier Inc. 2003.

Vascular Neurosurgery

Juvela S. Treatment Options of Unruptured Intracranial Aneurysms. *Stroke*. 2004;35:372-374.

Stapf C, Mast H, Sciacca RR, Choi JH, Khaw AV, Connolly ES, Pile-Spellman J, Mohr JP. Predictors of hemorrhage in patients with untreated brain arteriovenous malformation. *Neurology*. 2006;66:1350.

Spetzler, Martin. A proposed grading system for arteriovenous malformations. *Journal of Neurosurgery*. 65, Oct. 1986, pp. 476-483.

Wiebers DO & ISUIA investigators. Unruptured Intracranial Aneurysms: Natural History, Clinical Outcome, and Risks of Surgical and Endovascular Treatment. *Lancet*. Volume 362, Issue 9378, 12 July 2003: 103-110.

Endarterectomy for Asymptomatic Carotid Artery Stenosis. *JAMA*. 273(18), 10 May 1995:1421-1428.

North American Symptomatic Carotid Endarterectomy Trial. *NEJM*. 325(7), 15 August 1991:445-453.

Degenerative Spine Disease

Ahn NU, Ahn UM, Ipsen B, An HS. Mechanical Neck Pain and Cervicogenic Headache [Diagnosis and Treatment of Cervical Spondylosis: Overview]. *Neurosurgery*. 60(1) Supplement. January 2007, pp S1-21-S1-27.

Clark ER, P. Cervical myelopathy: A complication of cervical spondylosis. *Brain*. 1956(79): p. 483.

Epstein, JE. The surgical management of cervical spinal stenosis, spondylosis, and myeloradiculopathy by means of the posterior approach. In: *Cervical Spine Research Society: The Cervical Spine*. 2nd ed. 1989, J.B. Lippincott Co.: Philadelphia.

Moore AP, Blumhardt LD. A prospective survey of the causes of nontraumatic spastic paraparesis and tetraparesis in 585 patients. *Spinal Cord*. 35:361-367, 1997.

Nurick S. The pathogenesis of the spinal cord disorder associated with cervical spondylosis. *Brain*. 1972(95): pp. 87-100.

Nurick S. The natural history and the results of surgical treatment of the spinal cord disorder associated with cervical spondylosis. *Brain*. 1972(95): 101-108.

Shedid D, Benzel EC. Cervical Spondylosis Anatomy: Pathophysiology & Biomechanics. [Diagnosis and Treatment of Cervical Spondylosis: Overview]. *Neurosurgery*. 60(1) Suppl., January 2007: S1-7-S1-13.

Baron EM, Young WF. Cervical Spondylotic Myelopathy: A Brief Review if Its Pathophysiology, Clinical Course, and Diagnosis. *Neurosurgery*. Volume 60(1) Suppl., January 2007: S1-35-S1-41.

Weinstein JN, Tosteson TD, Lurie JD, Tosteson ANA, Hanscom B, Skinner JS, Abdu WA, Hilibrand AS, Boden SD, Deyo RA. Surgical vs. Nonoperative Treatment for Lumbar Disk Herniation. The Spine Patient Outcomes Research Trial (SPORT): A Trial. *JAMA*. Vol. 296 No. 20, November 22/29, 2006.

Functional Neurosurgery

Hakanson S. Trigeminal neuralgia treated by the injection of glycerol into the trigeminal cistern. *Neurosurgery*. 1981;9:638-646.

Greenberg M. *Handbook of Neurosurgery*. 6th edition. New York: Thieme; 2003.

Schulder M, Gandhi CD. *Handbook of Stereotactic and Functional Neurosurgery*. Marcel Dekker, Inc. New York, 2003.

Téllez-Zenteno JF, Dhar R, Wiebe S. Long-term seizure outcomes following epilepsy surgery: a systematic review and meta-analysis. *Brain*. 2005: 128; 1188–1198.

Neurosurgical Oncology

Greenberg M. *Handbook of Neurosurgery*. 6th edition. New York: Thieme; 2003.

DeMonte F, Al-Mefty O. Meningiomas. In: Kaye AH, Laws, Jr. ER. Brain Tumors. Churchill Livingstone. 1995.

10. Questions

Neurosurgical Trauma

1. The following are accurate descriptions of the injury given except:

   A. Depressed skull result in bony depression above the level of the calvarium.

   B. An open skull fracture can only be sustained from a fracture with overlying laceration.

   C. Cerebral contusions usually occur contrecoup to the side of the fracture.

   D. Diffuse axonal injury is technically a postmortem neuropathological diagnosis.

   E. Gaping scalp lacerations usually involve the galea aponeurotica.

2. On trauma CT head imaging, all of the following are discriminatory findings except:

   A. Subdural hematoma.

   B. Patent basal cisterns.

   C. Blood in the third ventricle.

   D. Periventricular white matter hypoattenuation areas.

   E. Blood in the sulci along the convexity.

3. Regarding the development of extra-axial and contusional injury, which of the following is accurate?

   A. Lucid interval refers to the time after 12 hours from injury when an EDH is more likely to develop.

   B. Translation and rotational shear of bridging veins is thought to be the mechanism for SDH formation.

   C. Kinetic energey is typically transmitted only to fixed intracranial structures.

   D. Intraventricular hemorrhage is most sensitively detected in the frontal horns on CT.

   E. Skull fracture and middle meningeal artery rupture typically cause SDH.

4. All of the following can contribute to spinal instability except :

   A. Spondylolisthesis

   B. Fractures

   C. Ligamentous injury

   D. Para-spinal muscle spasms

   E. Congenital pars defect

5. In the treatment of spinal cord injury, the following modalities are known to influence outcome:

   A. Surgical decompression has to led improved outcome from central cord syndrome.

   B. Steroids have been proven to benefit cord injury in Class I studies.

   C. Cauda equina syndrome can be treated with steroids and lumbar orthosis.

   D. Urgent traction and reduction may improve the neurologic outcome of jumped facets with radiculopathy.

   E. Surgical decompression and fixation in the complete cord injured patient is done primarily as it allows the cord to recover.

Neurosurgical Emergencies

1. A 22-year-old patient presents signs and symptoms of meningitis and is empirically started on ceftriaxone, vancomycin and metronidazole. He makes initial improvement, but then at 48 hours deteriorates with decreased conscious level, is following commands but is confused, and falls asleep whenever he is not addressed in a strong voice and stimulated. You note that he has a right-sided 6th nerve palsy. You obtain a CT scan which shows minimal increase in the size of the lateral ventricles, but a third ventricle with 7mm diameter and prominent temporal horns. On checking the initial gram stain, this was negative, but an addendum is now reading scant "AAFBs seen." Which is the most appropriate next step in management?

   A. Repeat the LP immediately and send more CSF to confirm the result.

   B. Start isoniazid intravenously as monotherapy.

   C. Consult neurosurgery emergently for placement of a ventriculostomy.

   D. Start rifampicin followed by isoniazid.

2. An 88-year-old hypertensive man is admitted with a 7 cm intracerebral hemorrhage centered in his left putamen, and insula. There is major mass effect and midline shift of 20mm. The hemorrhage has already filled all ventricles—including the 4th—with some brain stem compression. The patient is GCS 4 with extension only to painful stimuli, and sluggish pupils bilaterally, but no oculocephalics or corneals. Based on the evidence from the literature, what would you advise the family, who want only good quality of life for their father? (You are a neurologist in a small hospital 2.5 hours from Dartmouth.)

   A. Immediate helicopter transfer to Dartmouth neurosurgery, as you give them hope that "they can fix him."

   B. Intubate the patient immediately without talking to the family, who are physically present.

   C. Tell the family he has no realistic chance of survival or good quality of life and comfort measures are appropriate.

   D. You ask the ER physician to place a ventriculostomy to relieve the hydrocephalus and ventricular blood (he left a neurosurgery residency a year ago and is accomplished with the procedure).

   E. You start phenytoin for seizure prophylaxis.

3. A 70-year-old woman presents with a dense right hemiplegia in upper and lower limbs and face. She had been on warfarin but it turns out she had not taken it for over a week. CT head demonstrates a 3cm ICH centred within the internal capsule and corpus striatum on the left. Her BP is 200/100. Her INR is 1.4. The most important aspect of this patient's management is:

   A. Obtain a CTA to rule out the chance of a deep-seated AVM.

   B. Neurosurgical consultation for a stereotactic aspiration of the hematoma.

   C. Urgent BP control with intravenous nicardipine or nitrates.

   D. Administer FFP to correct her coagulopathy.

4. A 78-year-old man with known prostate carcinoma complains of severe back pain and numbness in his legs, which came on over 48 hours. To your exam, he is without objective motor deficit, but has very brisk reflexes with upgoing plantars and patchy pinprick numbness in a non-dermatomal distribution in both legs. You obtain an MRI of his whole spine, which shows 2 extradural and 1 vertebral body metastases, with the largest at T11 causing cord pressure and obliteration of the thecal sac. There is little doubt about the diagnosis of prostatic metastases. What do you suspect the first-line treatment is for this patient with impending cord compression?

   A. Urgent surgical decompression of his extradural lesion.

   B. Ordering a thoracolumbar spine orthosis.

   C. Steroid administration at large doses and urgent radiation therapy.

   D. DVT prophylaxis.

5. A 42-year-old patient presents with mild headache and fever of 38.7. He says he has had multiple teeth extracted for odontogenic abscesses in the last week, and cultures were obtained by the dental surgeon. He was on oral penicillin V at standard doses. On exam he has no focal findings. Brain MRI suggests infection with an area of enhancement and restricted diffusion. The neuroradiologist says there is some cerebritis, which appears very early without an encapsulated abscess. What the most appropriate next management step in this case?

   A. Urgent stereotactic aspiration of the diffuse brain lesion with culture.

   B. Blood cultures x2, start meningitic doses of triple antibiotics, and call the dentist for previous culture results.

   C. Look for a cardiac source with an echocardiogram.

   D. Continue the oral penicillin.

   F. Start phenytoin for seizure prophylaxis.

6. A 39-year-old woman presents to the ER with a complaint that her left leg is numb. She had previously had troublesome back pain and sciatica in the same leg, but yesterday she noted that both back and leg pain was gone and her leg became numb instead. When you enquire about bowel and bladder function, she says passing urine has been a little slow but she had had a gynecologic procedure which she attributes this to. She also states that she noted numbness in her vagina while placing a tampon. She has no other difficulties with gait and her exam demonstrates patchy sensory loss around her perineum. The most appropriate next step in management.

   A. Book her a clinic appointment the next day for nerve conduction studies.

   B. Refer her to a gynecologist for workup of her bladder neck problems.

   C. Book her an appointment in the spine center in the next couple of days.

   D. Obtain an urgent MRI of her lumbar spine in the ED.

Neurosurgical Critical Care

1. Synaptic transmission in the adult brain at 37 C is abolished when CBF falls below:

   A. 5 ml/100 g/min.

   B. 15 ml/100 g/min.

   C. 20 ml/100 g/min.

   D. 30 ml/100 g/min.

2. pCO_2 causes changes in CBF through which mechanism:

   A. Its effect of displacing O_2 from the cerebral blood vessels

   B. Its effect on the $CMRO_2$

   C. Its potent influence on CSF production & absorption

   D. Its powerful influence on CBV

3. A 35-year-old patient comes through the ED with a severe headache and CT head showing massive cisternal subarachnoid hemorrhage. Her lab work shows a sodium of 129. The most appropriate therapy would be:

   A. Start fluid restriction at a maximal daily intake of 1.5 L PO.

   B. Give her salt tablets immediately.

   C. Start intravenous hypertonic (3%) saline at 10 ml / hr.

   D. Start intravenous normal (0.9%) saline at 40 ml / hr.

   E. Start intravenous normal (0.9%) saline at 125 ml / hr.

4. Which of the following anesthetic agents is contraindicated for a trauma patient with potential for raised intracranial pressure?

   A. Sevoflurane

   B. Isoflurane

   C. Ketamine

   D. Thiopentone

   E. Propofol

5. The ideal anesthetic agent used in neuroanesthesia should have all the following ideal properties except:

   A. Lower vasoreactivity to CO_2.

   B. Maintain cerebrovascular autoregulation.

   C. Not lower seizure threshold.

   D. Cause no increase in CBV.

   E. Reduce $CMRO_2$ coupled with CBF.

Vascular Neurosurgery

1. A 35-year-old presents with sudden onset worst headache of her life, then precipitously deteriorates into a coma with GCS 6. What is the most appropriate next step in her management?

   A. Obtain an MRI scan of her brain immediately with stroke protocol.

   B. Intubate the patient to secure her airway.

   C. Send her factor V Leiden screen stat.

   D. Call her family to inform them of what has happened.

   E. Transport the patient to CT yourself for a stat CT head.

2. An 88-year-old man comes to your neurology clinic. He underwent an MRI brain scan because "his CP thought he could have water on the brain, causing his incontinence." The MRI shows no evidence of hydrocephalus or strokes, but demonstrates a 20mm basilar apex aneurysm. The patient's neurological exam is entirely normal in your office, and he asks what your advice would be to treat this aneurysm. He seems very risk averse and he says "I just wanna go when my time is up, doc." Your advice would be :

   A. To monitor the aneurysm with MRI / MRA in 2 years time.

   B. Strongly recommend he has microsurgical clipping as neurosurgery is so good nowadays.

   C. Treat his blood presure and discharge him from your clinic back to his PCP's care.

   D. Consult neurosurgery stat.

   E. Advise endovascular coiling and offer him regular monitoring with MRI/MRA in 6 months.

3. A 55-year-old man comes to your clinic because of an abnormal carotid ultrasound result. This was a study his PCP ordered to follow on a previous one that showed 30% stenosis of his ICA at the time he had his quadruple cardiac bypass procedure. He is now very well and is neurologically asymptomatic. The report of the Doppler study reads severe stenosis 80%-99% of the right internal carotid artery. What is your advice for this gentleman?

   A. Keep taking your aspirin and plavix, and raise your atorvastatin to 80mg a day.

   B. I will refer you to a neurosurgeon for consideration of endarterectomy.

   C. We need to obtain an MRI scan of your brain.

   D. We need to check your labs, especially a thrombosis screen.

4. Place the following incidental aneurysms in descending order of their risk of rupture and subarachnoid hemorrhage using the ISUIA data:

   A. 22mm AcomA aneurysm

   B. 8mm MCA aneurysm

   C. 5mm cavernous ICA aneurysm

   D. 15mm basilar artery tip aneuryms

5. A 45-year-old male has a headache while at work. He has a CT head that shows a 3.5 x 3.5 cm intraparenchymal hemorrhage. CTA shows a 4cm AVM in the right frontal lobe, with drainage into the thalamostriate vein. Quantify the Spetzler-Martin grade for this lesion to assist with evaluating his surgical risk of resection of this AVM.

   A. Grade 1

   B. Grade 2

   C. Grade 3

   D. Grade 4

Degenerative Spine

1. The definite pain generator in low back pain is:

   A. The disk

   B. The facet joints

   C. The ligamentum flavum

   D. As yet unidentified

2. Regarding the treatment for lumbar radiculopathy:

   A. Surgery is advised before 6 weeks of pain has passed for best results.

   B. Trials have shown surgery to have significant long term superiority to non-operative treatment.

   C. Surgery allows more rapid improvement of radiculopathy.

   D. Microsurgical diskectomy eliminates patient's back pain.

3. In clinical assessment of cervical spondylosis:

   A. Neck pain indicates worse disease process.

   B. Ipsilateral spastic weakness and contralateral numbness is classic for anterior cord syndrome.

   C. Multilevel radiculopathy can be confused with brachial plexopathy.

   D. Myelopathic signs such as a Hoffman's are pathognomonic for CSM.

4. In considering the natural history of cervical spondylotic myelopathy:

   A. Almost all patients will eventually need a decompressive procedure.

   B. Laminectomy has been effective at reversing the myelopathy.

   C. Multiple sclerosis can coexist with CSM.

   D. Motor neuron disease can be clinically differentiated from CSM in the short term.

5. In considering surgical decompression for cervical spondylotic myelopathy:

   A. Loss of lordosis is unfavorable for dorsal laminectomy.

   B. Anterior cervical diskectomy and fusion is preferred for 1 level radiculopathy with preserved lordosis in a 19-year-old female.

   C. Elderly patients always require a combined posterior and anterior fusion.

   D. A congenitally narrow canal is usually associated with loss of lordosis.

Functional Neurosurgery

1. Stereotaxy allows precise localization of small neuroanatomical targets in the brain through mapping every scan point to a point in real anatomical space; this process is called:

   A. Transformation

   B. Translocation

   C. Registration

   D. Stereoencephalotomy

   E. Neuronavigation

2. Which of the following are potential complications of percutanous trigeminal rhizolysis procedures?

   A. Carotid artery injury

   B. Dysesthesiae

   C. Neuroparalytic keratitis

   D. Meningitis

   E. Anesthesia dolorosa

3. What is the preferred target for DBS for a patient with PD who has more trouble with "off" periods as his predominant symptom?

   A. Cingulate gyrus

   B. GPi

   C. STN

   D. Anterior thalamus

   E. Vim thalamus

4. What vessel is the most common to be found compressing the trigeminal nerve at MVD for trigeminal neuralgia ?

   A. MCA

   B. Basilar

   C. SCA

   D. AICA

   E. PICA

5. What is the most successful procedure in achieving seizure freedom for medically refractory epilepsy?

   A. Frontal heterotopia resection

   B. Vagal nerve stimulation

   C. Temporal lobectomy for MTS

   D. Neuropace cortical stimulation

   E. Corpus callosotomy

6. Corpus callosum section is effective in:

   A. Infantile hemiplegia syndrome.

   B. Completely abolishing seizure transmission.

   C. Reducing the disability from drop attacks.

   D. Gelastic seizures.

   E. Cingulate gyrus seizures.

Neurosurgical Oncology

1. The following are all characteristics of meningiomas except:

   A. They arise from arachnoid cap cells.

   B. They are benign slow-growing tumors.

   C. Parasagittal/falcine location is the commonest.

   D. They are increasingly found as incidental lesions on scans for other reasons.

   E. The gold standard treatment is stereotactic radiosurgery.

2. The following primary tumors are all classic sources of brain secondaries except :

   A. Malignant melanoma

   B. Breast carcinoma

   C. Multiple myeloma

   D. Bronchogenic carcinoma

   E. Colonic carcinoma

3. Low-grade gliomas commonly present in young patients less than 40 years old with:

   A. Isolated cranial neuropathies.

   B. Headache and raised intracranial pressure.

   C. Hemorrhagic stroke.

   D. Seizures.

   E. Multiple sclerosis like optic neuritis.

4. Which is the best modality of treatment for an 88-year-old man with a 2cm Meckel's cave meningioma presenting with trigeminal neuralgia?

   A. Whole brain radiotherapy.

   B. Microsurgical resection with skull base approaches.

   C. Stereotactic radiosurgery.

   D. Microvascular decompression of the trigeminal dorsal root entry zone.

   E. Stereotactic biopsy.

5. Match the most appropriate neurosurgical diagnostic/treatment modality to the pathology:

A. Frame based stereotactic biopsy
B. Open craniotomy with neuronavigation
C. Awake craniotomy-language mapping.
D. Ommaya ventricular access device

1. Glioma abutting Heschel's gyrus
2. Primary CNS lymphoma with CSF seeding
3. 1cm deep thalamic lesion
4. 3cm convexity meningioma

Pediatric Neurosurgery

1. A 6-year-old child presents to your pediatric neurology practice with intractable vomiting over the last 4 weeks. He has had multiple general gastrointestinal work-ups, including upper GI endoscopy that yielded no abnormalities. His mother says he has been clumsier lately, having been previously an expert tree climber. You do a full neurologic exam and find only signs of mild truncal ataxia. The most appropriate next step in management is:

   A. Refer him to physiotherapy for his clumsiness.

   B. Perform a lumbar puncture looking for cells and protein.

   C. Send him home with a potential diagnosis of benign positional vertigo.

   D. Administer intravenous ondansetron in an age-appropriate dose.

   E. Obtain an MRI of his brain emergently.

2. A 5-month-old infant is seen by you while on a general pediatric rotation for routine check-up. It turns out he was born prematurely, and his corrected gestational age is 2 ¾ months. His mother says he had brain hemorrhage when on the neonatal unit in France, where he was born before the family located to the U.S. The mother says he has done well, but she has noticed his head is larger that her first child, who was born normally. You perform a neurological exam, which is normal. The child's head circumference is 2cm above the 99th percentile for his corrected age. The most appropriate next step in management is:

   A. Emergent referral to a neurosurgeon a 5pm on Friday afternoon.

   B. Perform a lumbar puncture for opening pressure.

C. See the child again in clinic in 2 weeks with a repeat head circumference.

D. Arrange an urgent MRI brain of the child within 24 hours.

E. Reassure the mother that his exam is normal and she is worrying unnecessarily.

3. A 10-year-old child presents to your pediatric neurology practice, having been seen at multiple pediatric clinics with unexplained weight loss, and lethargy. She absolutely denies that she is anorexic or is vomiting. Furthermore, she says that he throat is more "scratchy" than usual, which she found strange, as this appears worse with water; and that she has seen her right eye drooping on occasion. As part of her previous work-ups she had a normal CT head by report. Upon neurological exam, you note a very subtle ptosis and anisocoria, and are unsure about whether she has asymmetric shoulder shrug. She has bilateral pathologically brisk reflexes. Your suspicion is now higher for:

A. A diagnosis of Lyme disease.

B. Remitting relapsing multiple sclerosis.

C. Child abuse with conversion disorder.

D. A brain stem glioma not seen on the non-contrast head CT.

4. A 15-year-old child is noted on well-child check to have not gone into puberty, with Tanner 1 genitals and short stature for his age, well below the 2nd centile. His parents are tall. They are worried about him. You take a history from the child himself, and he tells you he has been drinking a lot of coke lately, and having to leave class at school to urinate every 2 hours. The rest of the child's examination is normal except for slightly blurred optic disk margins on fundoscopy. You order a CT head scan, which shows:

A. Normal calibre ventricles.

B. Calcified cystic lesion above the sella with moderate hydrocephalus.

C. A 1.5cm lateral cerebellar hemisphere tumor.

D. Abnormal thickening of his calvarial vault.

5. A 14-year-old girl presents with symptoms of difficulty swallowing, voice changes, and tongue and facial numbness. Your exam elicits nystagmus, pharyngeal, and palatal weakness, and asymmetry of tongue movements, with patchy sensory loss in trigeminal distribution. MRI brain and C spine shows Chiari malformation with tonsillar descent at 11mm below the foramen magnum, and a high cervical syrinx that extends into the lower medulla. The first-line surgical treatment for this girl's condition is:

A. Syringoperitoneal shunt.

B. Syringopleural shunt.

C. Suboccipital posterior fossa bony craniectomy only.

D. Suboccipital posterior fossa craniectomy and duraplasty.

E. Fourth ventricular peritoneal shunt.

Answers

Neurosurgical Trauma

1. B.
An open skull fracture can also be sustained from fracture of the sinuses (communicated with paranasal spaces = "open").

2. D.
Periventricular white matter changes are not discriminatory or predictive on a trauma head CT.

3. B.
All the other options are inaccurate. Specifically, "lucid interval" refers to the time, usually before 6 hours, when a patient is likely to deteriorate from expansion of an EDH. Kinetic energy can be transferred to any of the structures in the skull; it is the differential velocities that cause injury at points of fixation. IVH is most sensitively detected in the occipital horns. Skull fracture and middle meningeal rupture typically cause EDH, not SDH.

4. D.
Paraspinal muscle spasm or even tenderness is not an independent predictor of spinal instability.

5. D.
Urgent traction and reduction in jumped facets should be carried out urgently, as this can influence nerve root recovery. The influence (and even whether, and timing of) surgical decompression in central cord syndrome is highly controversial. Steroids have not been proven to influence outcome in class I studies. The NASCIS studies remain disputed even amongst experts. Cauda equina syndrome is a neurosurgical emergency. Surgical decompression and fixation in the complete cord injury is done primarily to aid the nursing of these patients, not for their neurologic outcome.

Neurosurgical Emergencies

1. C.
This patient has acute hydrocephalus, with already a 6th nerve palsy marking increased intracranial pressure. He requires an emergent placement of an external ventriculostomy by a neurosurgeon. An LP would be dangerous and could precipitate foramen magnum herniation (so-called "coning"). The other options of starting anti-tuberculous treatment are appropriate, (as he appears to have TB meningitis with hydrocephalus) after treating the life-threatening emergency.

2. C.
It is appropriate to advise the family of the extremely grim prognosis for this patient's survival or functional outcome according to the literature. It is inappropriate to emergently intubate the patient or make an emergent transfer without talking to the family (where they are physically present), or to give unrealistic expectation about surgical outcomes in such a patient.

3. B.
This patient has a hypertensive "central" hemorrhage, and her warfarin is not an issue (she has not taken it, and her INR is normal). She is not coagulopathic, and therefore not in need of FFP. Angiography is not indicated for this clearly hypertensive lesion. Urgent BP control is the most important aspect of the management here. There is no evidence for surgery in such a lesion.

4. C.
This patient has no motor neurologic deficit and an extradural mass with some sensory changes in an acute/subacute setting. The treatment is steroids and urgent radiation therapy. Surgery is not necessarily indicated; B. and C. may also be done as part of the treatment but are not the first-line.

5. B.
Early cerebritis (the precursor of a cerebral abscess) is a neurological emergency. The treatment should be urgent blood cultures, and commencing meningitic CNS doses of appropriate antibiotics, as well as looking up all other available culture data to drive therapy. Surgery is not indicated for cerebritis and may actually be detrimental, with potential for hemorrhage from friable brain; C. and E. are also appropriate next steps after cultures.

6. D.
This young lady has symptoms suggestive of cauda equina syndrome (CES). An urgent MRI of the lumbar spine is absolutely indicated to rule out a central disk with thecal compression. All the other options are inappropriate responses to an emergency such as this.

Neurosurgical Critical Care

1. B.
Synaptic transmission in the adult brain at 37 C is abolished when CBF falls below 15ml/100g/min. 50ml/100g/min is the normal resting value for adult brain.

2. D.
pCO_2 causes changes in CBF through its cerebral vasodilatation mechanism that causes powerful influence on CBV.

3. E.
This patient has cerebral salt wasting with mild hyponatremia. The initial treatment is to hydrate with maintenance NS (125ml/hr is appropriate), then consider the use of 3% saline if the Na is not improving or further falling. The treatment in A. with fluid restriction is potentially dangerous, as the patient has both CSW and diuresis from the SAH.

4. C.
Ketamine has the effect of increasing CBF and $CMRO_2$, and therefore can actually raise ICP, and therefore is contraindicated.

5. A.
The ideal "neuro" anesthetic agent should not lower vasoreactivity to CO_2. It should maintain it.

Vascular Neurosurgery

1. B.
A patient in coma with GCS 6 should undergo the basics of advanced life support, with securing the ABC's (airway, breathing, circulation) before proceeding with any other treatment or investigative tests.

2. E.
Incidental aneurysms are commonly discovered on work-ups for other conditions, in this case for possible NPH. A 20mm basilar apex aneurysm is a high-risk lesion according to the ISUIA study. Given the patient's age and location of the aneurysm, it is appropriate to at least offer endovascular treatment and regular MRI/MRA monitoring, with the next scan as early as 6 months. It is also acceptable to accept the patient's wish, at 88, not wanting any treatment or follow-up, but the best option here is to make the offer of treatment. The other options are inappropriate.

3. B.
Asymptomatic severe stenosis (80%-99%) of the ICA has been shown to benefit from endarterectomy in the ACAS study.

4. The incidental aneurysms in descending order of their risk of rupture and subarachnoid hemorrhage using the ISUIA data are:

D. 15mm basilar artery tip aneuryms
1. – (18.4%)

A. 22mm AcomA aneurysm
2. – (14.5%)

B. 8mm MCA aneurysm
3. – (2.6%)

C. 5mm cavernous ICA aneurysm
4. – (0%; no risk, cavernous ICA do not cause SAH)

5. C.
This is a S-M Grade 3 lesion. Total of (Size (3-6cm)=1, Deep=2, Non-eloquent = 0).

Degenerative Spine

1.D.
The definite pain generator in low back pain is as yet unidentified

2.C.
Surgical diskectomy only allows rapid improvement of symptoms in the short term, it does not

influence the long-term outcome significantly (results of SPORT trial).

3. C.
Multilevel radiculopathy can be confused with brachial plexopathy, and is often a reason for EMG / NCS testing. Neck pain has no relationship to disease severity. Ipsilateral spastic weakness and contralateral numbness is classic for Brown-Sequard. Myelopathic signs such as a Hoffman's are seen in myelopathy of any cause.

4. C.
Any neurodegenerative condition can exist with CSM, especially notable are MS and MND, which can confuse the clinical picture and lead to surgery without improvement. Laminectomy (or any decompressive procedure) is not known or proven to reverse myelopathy. It is only hoped to halt its progression.

5. A.
Loss of lordosis puts the spine at risk of progressive kyphotic deformity and potential instability if a laminectomy (a potentially destabilizing procedure) is performed. In a young patient (19 y/o) with single level disease, it is preferable to preserve the disk and only remove the limited herniated segment through a posterior procedure. A combined posterior and anterior fusion is a highly morbid procedure, and great thought should be given to this before subjecting an elderly patient to this. A congenitally narrow canal is usually associated with normal lordosis and early stenotic symptoms.

Functional Neurosurgery

1. C. Registration is the correct term.

2. F. All are potential complications of percutanous trigeminal rhizolysis procedures.

3. C. STN is the preferred target for PD patients with prolonged trouble with "off" periods.

GPi is used for dyskinesia predominant symptoms. Vim thalamus is used for tremor and cingulated gyrus for depression.

4. D. The anterior inferior cerebellar artery (AICA) is the commonest compressive vessel seen in trigeminal neuralgia at MVD. The second is the superior cerebellar (SCA).

5. C.
Temporal lobectomy is by far the most successful procedure in achieving seizure freedom for medically refractory epilepsy of temporal lobe origin. Corpus callosotomy does not eliminate seizures, but does diminish drop attacks. Multiple heterotopia resection has a poor control rate for seizures. Vagal nerve stimulation is considered "rescue therapy" to lower seizure frequency only. Neuropace neuromodulation is still experimental, undergoing clinical trials.

6. C.
Corpus callosum section is effective in reducing disability drop attacks. It is not effective in completely abolishing seizure transmission, or in infantile hemiplegia syndrome, due to the presence of other commissural fibres in the latter, typically treated by hemispherectomy. Gelastic seizures are mostly associated with hypothalamic hamartomas, and the surgery involves excision only for easily accessible exophytic lesions. Callosal section plays no role.

Neurosurgical Oncology

1. E.
The gold standard treatment for meningiomas remains microsurgical resection.

2. C.
Myeloma does not metastasise to brain, but is commonly seen in the axial skeleton/spine.

3. D.
Low-grade gliomas are relatively more common in the under 40-year-olds, and tend to present with seizure disorder/epilepsy. It is rare for them to present with raised ICP symptoms.

4. C.
Stereotactic radiosurgery is the most non-invasive and appropriate modality for this small lesion. Skull base surgery is highly morbid for this age group and this small sized lesion.

5. A. – 3; B. – 4; C. – 1; D. – 2.

Pediatric Neurosurgery

1. E.

This is the classic presentation of a medulloblastoma or other midline cerebellar (vermis) tumor in a child. Intermittent vomiting and midline ataxia are the keys in the history given. Often the former is investigated through a GI service first, because of concern re GERD, but this child is too old for infantile GERD. Referral to physiotherapy is inappropriate. A lumbar puncture is contraindicated and potentially dangerous; BPV is not an appropriate diagnosis in this age group. The most appropriate response is to obtain an urgent MRI brain scan with and without contrast.

2. C.

Periventriculatr hemorrhage of prematurity is a risk factor for development of hydrocephalus, but this is uncommon to present late (as is the history). Usually a high-grade hemorrhage would have developed hydrocephalus much earlier. The concern about the macrocephaly is valid, but this needs documenting over more points in time than a single clinic visit. In the presence of normal neurologic findings and normal fontanelle, it is appropriate to see the child with HC measurements every 2 weeks for 8-12 weeks to see if there is any progressive increase, or if this is static. The macrocephaly could be familial or entirely benign. Emergent referral and emergent MRI brain is not appropriate, and lumbar puncture is unnecessary and invasive. Reassuring without stipulating the child has to be followed is also an inappropriate strategy.

3. D.

Non-specific symptoms are disproportionately seen in brain stem gliomas in children. The "scratchy" throat with liquid dysphagia points to a bulbar dysfunction, and the ptosis, anisocoria and long tract signs are serious additional signs. Before a diagnosis of Lyme's can be made in a child with no history of tick bite or rash (this can have disparate neurological signs), one first needs to rule out a structural bulbar/brain stem etiology in a child. MS is not typically seen in this age group. Conversion disorder is an inappropriate diagnosis in the presence of incontrovertible neurological signs (anisocoria).

4. B.

The story of growth failure and hypogonadism for a child expected to have entered puberty is classic for a craniopharyngioma. The blurred optic disk margins in this is a serious pointer to potential for intracranial hypertension due to hydrocephalus (a common complication at presentation of craniopharyngioma). The imaging finds on CT are classically a suprasellar calcified mixed cystic solid lesion with hydrocephalus. Cerebellar tumors do not present like this.

5. D.

The standard approach in this classic combination of Chiari I and symptomatic syrinx is to perform a posterior fossa craniectomy decompression and duraplasty. Bony decompression alone would be considered insufficient for high grade tonsillar descent and syrinx.

Chapter 34: Psychiatry for Neurologists

Ronald L. Green, MD

Contents

1. Psychiatric Examination of the Neurology Patient

In many ways, several aspects of the psychiatric examination of the neurology patient are similar to psychiatric examination of all patients, in the sense that the domains covered are similar. In addressing any psychiatric issues the patient may have, the domains to investigate include history of any current psychiatric problems, including any current or ongoing stressors, past psychiatric history and a psychiatric "review of systems." By the latter, I refer to screening for psychiatric problems not mentioned in the course of the patient describing current and past psychiatric illness episodes—in other words "rule outs."

A caveat at the outset of an examination is to be certain whether the patient is capable of understanding the examiner's questions, which can be rapidly assessed—say in the case of a hospitalized patient—by asking why the patient is in the hospital. If the patient cannot answer this question reasonably well, then the subsequent questions need to be adjusted accordingly.

Assume, for the sake of discussion, that history yielded current and past depressive episodes. One would then ask if there is also any history of:

1. Hypomanic or manic episodes. The best way to elicit this is first to ask if the patient knows what hypomania or mania is, and if the patient answers in the affirmative, ask for a description of the patient's definition of these conditions, then ask if the patient has had any such episodes. If the patient does not know what these disorders are, then provide the patient examples of the clusters of symptoms of these disorders, then ask if any such episodes have occurred. The symptom cluster seen in mania is listed below under *DSM-IV-R* criteria for a manic episode in the section on bipolar affective disorder. This strategy of asking the patient whether she or he knows what the disorder in question is, and proceeding as above, is applicable to all of the "rule out" inquiries below.

The point is that one should not assume the patient cannot answer the question about whether she or he knows what a given disorder is, and or that the patient will not be able to describe whether she or he has had such a disorder. The possible exception would be an angry paranoid patient who would not take well to being asked directly if they are deluded. In this case, one might ask such a patient if they feel they are in any danger.

2. The other disorders about which to inquire, using the above strategy, are fear-related disorders such as panic, generalized anxiety, social phobia and post-traumatic stress disorder, attention deficit disorder, obsessive-compulsive disorder, eating disorder, and drug or alcohol abuse disorders.

The remaining questions in the history taking are similar to any medical examination. (See chapter 2 on the examination of the neurology patient.)

I would add these caveats:

1. Inquiries regarding family history should include the question, "Has anyone in your family had psychiatric illness, including drug and alcohol abuse and, if so, which family members, and what are/were the diagnoses, if known?" Also ask if there have been any suicides in the family.

2. Social history should start with asking patients how they regard their upbringing, then specific questions about any abuse. If abuse has occurred, one should inquire about any emotional legacy of the abuse (ie, eliciting post-traumatic disorder symptoms). Inquiries should also be made about school grade completed, work history, legal problems, military service, and relationships history. I often also ask, "What are the worst and best things that ever happened to you?" This frequently yields important information which all other examiner questions may not reveal.

Assessment of patient safety is of course of paramount importance. This issue is covered below in the section entitled "Diagnosis of Major Depressive Disorder." This is not to imply that safety assessment is solely important to depressive disorders. The approach to patient safety described in the depressive disorder section is applicable to assessment of patients with all medical and psychiatric disorders.

Finally, in addition to a physical examination, a mental status examination should be done. This should include assessment of general appearance, alertness and attention, psychomotor activity (retardation or agitation), mood, affect, speech characteristics (any latency to onset, rate, rhythm and volume), thought process and content, perceptual experiences, and violent ideation of any kind. See the discussion below in the section on major depressive disorder for in-depth consideration of assessment of danger to self or others. Finally, there's a Mini-Mental Status Examination (MMSE), the components of which can be found in the texts referenced at the end of this chapter. Keep in mind that responses to MMSE questions need to be judged against educational level achieved, and degree of cooperativeness and intelligence, best gauged by a patient's vocabulary. Also keep in mind that the MMSE is only a subset of the mental status examination.

Table 1 defines some of the key terms relevant to mental status examinations.

Table 1

Definitions of Some Key Terms Used in the Mini-Mental Status Examination

1. *Mood*: How a patient feels in response to a question such as "How would you describe your mood or spirit?" Relevant to assessment for mood disorders.

2. *Affect*: What you infer a patient's mood is based on their appearance and behavior. Relevant to assessment for mood disorders.

3. *Thought process*: As the patient speaks, are the ideas expressed goal-directed and coherent? Are thoughts expressed in a tangential nature (patient takes off on tangents unrelated to the subject at hand)? Or is there circumstantiality (patient veers off topic but ultimately returns to the subject at hand)? Or is there looseness of associations, meaning that thoughts expressed by the patient do not logically follow one another? Relevant to assessment of psychotic disorders, delirium and other disorders.

4. *Thought content*: The themes on which the patient focuses including presence of any paranoid thinking and delusions (false beliefs). Relevant to assessment of psychotic disorders, delirium and other disorders.

5. *Perceptual abnormalities*: Either hallucinations (percepts of voices, sounds, objects or scenes that are not present) or illusions (distortions of objects or scenes that are present). Relevant to assessment of psychotic disorders, delirium and other disorders.

6. The word psychosis is a very general term which refers to mental states in which the patient has hallucinations, delusions or bizarre behavior. Psychotic symptoms can be manifestations of several psychiatric disorders, such as schizophrenia and mania, and medical disorders such as delirium and dementia.

2. The Psychiatric Disorders

An exhaustive review of the many psychiatric syndromes is beyond the scope of this chapter. Far and away, depressive disorder will be the most common psychiatric disorder encountered by neurologists. Therefore, depressive disorder will be given the most thorough attention. Only highlights of the several other major psychiatric disorders will be reviewed and some such as eating and sleep disorders and others will be omitted entirely. Covering the field of psychiatry in a single chapter is not possible. Admittedly, the decisions about what to and what not to include were arbitrary to a degree. My hope was to include the most common disorders likely to be encountered by neurologists.

Disorders of Mood

There are several mood-related psychiatric disorders. See Table 2 for a list of these disorders, in decreasing order of frequency.

Table 2

The Most Common Disorders of Mood

1. Major depressive disorder.
2. Dysthymia.
3. Adjustment disorder with depressed mood.
4. Substance abuse induced mood disorder.
5. Bipolar disorder, types 1 & 2.
6. Schizoaffective disorder.
7. There are other disorders of mood such as cyclothymia. These are too infrequent to be considered in this chapter.

General Considerations

The reader is referred to *DSM-IV-R* for specific criteria for each mood disorder listed. Due to its high prevalence (see below), we will focus primarily on major depressive disorder.

A given patient may have several of the conditions listed in Table 1, although it should be noted that if a patient has a major depressive episode and no history of hypomania or mania (both described below), the patient is said to have unipolar affective disorder. If the depressed patient does have a history of hypomania or mania, the patient has bipolar affective disorder. Of course, if a relatively young person has a major depressive episode, the person may develop hypomania or mania. A patient in her or his twenties has about a 5% likelihood of having a hypomanic or manic episode at some point later in life. Thus, such a patient will prove to have bipolar affective disorder. This possibility is heightened if the young depressed patient has a family history of bipolar affective disorder. This possibility has important implications for the treatment of a depressive episode as discussed below.

These scenarios bring up the issue of cross-sectional diagnosis vs. longitudinal diagnosis. As just cited, a depressive episode may be imbedded in unipolar or bipolar disorder. Analogously, any given psychotic episode may be imbedded in one of several disorders. Several other psychiatric disorders are subject to this type of complexity.

The confound of comorbid alcohol or substance induced mood disorder is discussed in Table 3.

Table 3

***DSM-IV-R* Criteria for Major Depressive Episode**

A. Five (or more) of the following symptoms have been present during the same two- week period and represent a change from previous functioning; at least one of the symptoms is either: (1.) depressed mood, or (2.) loss of interest or pleasure (ie, anhedonia).

1. Depressed mood most of the day, nearly every day, as indicated by either subjective report (eg, feels sad or empty) or observation made by others (eg, appears tearful). (In children and adolescents, this may be characterized as an irritable mood.)
2. Markedly diminished interest or pleasure in all, or almost all, activities most of the day, nearly every day.
3. Significant weight loss when not dieting or weight gain (eg, a change of more than 5 lbs. of body weight in a month), or a decrease or increase in appetite nearly every day.
4. Insomnia or hypersomnia nearly every day.
5. Psychomotor agitation or retardation nearly every day.
6. Fatigue or loss of energy nearly every day.
7. Feelings of worthlessness or excessive or inappropriate guilt nearly every day.
8. Diminished ability to think or concentrate, or indecisiveness, nearly every day.
9. Recurrent thoughts of death (not just fear of dying), recurrent suicidal ideation without a specific plan, or a suicide attempt or a specific plan for committing suicide.

B. The symptoms do not meet criteria for a Mixed Episode.

C. The symptoms cause clinically significant distress or impairment in social, occupational, or other important areas of functioning.

D. The symptoms are not due to the direct physiological effects of a substance (eg, a drug of abuse, a medication) or a general medical condition (eg, hypothyroidism).

E. The symptoms are not better accounted for by bereavement, ie, characterized by marked functional impairment, morbid preoccupation with worthlessness, suicidal ideation, psychotic symptoms, or psychomotor retardation.

DSM-IV-R Criteria for Major Depressive Episode

Epidemiology

The lifetime prevalence of a major depressive episode is about 15% in the United States, being significantly more common in women. Dysthymia is likely even more common but the prevalence is unknown since a vast number of people with dysthymia do not seek treatment. There is less certainty about the prevalence of the other disorders listed in Table 2.

Clinical Presentation

The majority of patients with major depression will complain of depressed mood as the principal symptom. Not infrequently, however, irritability, fatigue and other such symptoms may be dominant in a depressive episode and depressed mood may be minimal or absent. Anhedonia, in contradistinction, is invariably present to one degree or another. This is defined as a diminished ability to enjoy activities one usually has to make no effort to enjoy. Anhedonia is of course not specific to depression as many factors can cause it—stress, disease, and the like. Depression is also invariably accompanied by a lowering of self-esteem. In mild depression this may be manifest by a lowering of self-confidence, while in severe depression that has shaded into psychosis, there may be delusional expressions of self-loathing. The many other possible symptoms and duration criteria can be found in the *DSM-IV-R* criteria enumerated above.

Major depression also frequently causes cognitive dysfunction. This can be severe, mimicking dementia. This condition is called pseudodementia. Cognition will clear when the depression is treated effectively.

One symptom not mentioned amongst the criteria for major depressive disorder in the *DSM-IV-R*, but well worth pointing out, is diurnal mood variation. This refers to feeling worse (mood-wise) upon awakening and the rest of the morning, with some mood lightening as the day unfolds. This is often expressed as "trouble getting going" in the morning. To signify depression, this pattern must be a departure from the patient's customary function. That is, some people normally have trouble getting going in the morning, often expressed as "I'm not a morning person." Which is not to say that such a person cannot get depressed. The point is that if a "non-morning person" develops diurnal mood variation (DMV) as part of a depressive episode, her or his morning will be more bleak than usual.

About 50% of patients with major depression have DMV. The diagnostic utility of being aware of DMV is that the question of the presence or absence of major depression often comes up in treating people with medical illnesses including neurological illnesses. All of the symptoms of depression can be caused by these illnesses, but none of them can cause DMV. Therefore, if present, DMV is a strong indication that a patient has major depressive disorder and should be treated accordingly. DMV is likely to be caused by an abnormal pattern of daily fluctuations in serum cortisol that occur in many patients with major depressive disorder.

The most severe form of major affective disorder is depressive stupor, also known as catatonic stupor. It was thought formerly that this state occurred in schizophrenia. Depressive stupor often has its onset in a depressive episode in which a prominent feature is psychomotor slowing, often associated with increased speech onset latency. One will sometimes watch this state gradually deepen into catatonic stupor, in which there is no speech or movement, although the patient is fully conscious and aware of what is occurring in his or her environment. One classic feature of depressive stupor is "waxy flexibility." The finding is that if the examiner raises a hand of a catatonic patient, then lets go of the hand raised in space, the hand will remain in the elevated state. The fact that electroconvulsive therapy (ECT) is virtually always curative of depressive stupor supports the idea that this state is a disorder of mood. ECT is effective in mood disorders but much less so in schizophrenia.

Another presentation of mood disorder is seasonal affective disorder (SAD). In unipolar depression, the most common pattern is increased depressed mood as the day shortens in the fall. Carbohydrate craving and hypersomnia also occur frequently as part of this syndrome. In patients with bipolar disorder, a common pattern is for the patient to have depression in the fall and hypomania or mania in the spring. The depression phase can often be prevented or attenuated by light therapy used early in the fall. The most effective approach is 2 hours of therapeutic light exposure each morning. A commercially available visor fitted with battery-powered lights is probably the most convenient light treatment, since one can go about one's morning routines and all the while experience the light exposure. This is far more acceptable to most people than sitting in front of a bank of lights for two hours each morning.

A final consideration regarding mood disorders is the well-known fact that many medical and neurological illnesses can present with solely depressive symptoms. Two such examples, among many, are hypothyroidism and frontal lobe tumors.

Diagnosis of Major Depressive Disorder

A common screening instrument which patients can fill out while awaiting their appointment is the Patient Health Questionnaire 9 (PHQ-9). This questionnaire targets major depressive disorder (*http://www.nyc.gov/html/doh/downloads/pdf/csi/depressionkit-clin-questionairre.pdf*). A commonly used clinician performed rating scale is the Hamilton Rating Scale for Depression (*http://apps.cignabehavioral.com/web/basicsite/provider/treatingBehavioralConditions/HamiltonRatingScaleforDepression.pdf*). Both of these scales have been shown to be valid and reliable.

Armed with the information and caveats provided above and with a *DSM-IV-R*, making a diagnosis of major depressive episode (MDE) is not difficult.

The steps are:

1. Review medical records for past episodes of psychiatric problems.

2. Perform a full psychiatric examination. Elicit the presence or absence of the *DSM-IV-R* criteria for a MDE.

3. Perform a mental status examination, which if MDE is present, should reveal at the least an anxious or depressed appearing person. This is not always the case, as many people are able to mask their internal emotional state. There may or may not be psychomotor symptoms such as agitation or psychomotor slowing. There may or may not be cognitive impairment as revealed in a Mini-Mental Status Examination (*http://www.chcr.brown.edu/MMSE.pdf*). Psychotic symptoms such as hallucinations and delusions should be sought out. Finally, assessment of suicide/homicide risk needs to be made (see below).

4. Perform a physical examination and obtain the laboratory studies necessary to exclude non-psychiatric diseases which can present with depressed mood. Urine screening for substance use is usually necessary.

5. If the patient will permit, obtain corroborating information (such as about substance abuse which the patient may have kept from you) from the patient's significant others.

The diagnosis does not depend upon the absence of precipitating stressors because at least half the episodes of major depression are occasioned by stressor(s).

Assessment of danger to self or others:

Whole texts are devoted to this subject. I will highlight some key principles:

1. Nobody in my opinion wants to die, the only exception being those with political or religious motivations. Even the terminal cancer patient in great pain wishes, rather than dying, that the pain would subside and the cancer remit. It is rather the prospect of interminable pain, whether physical or the intense emotional pain that can occur in depressive states, which causes the sufferer to wish to die.

2. Most patients recognize that their suicidal thoughts are caused by depressive illness and will let an examiner know about these thoughts. They may not volunteer them but will almost always reveal them if asked. There are—rarely, fortunately—depressed patients that have decided to commit suicide and will veil their intentions. Most of these people do not seek help in the hours before they commit suicide, although they may have in the recent past.

3. The factors which predict a heightened risk of suicide in patients with major depression are enumerated in all standard psychiatric texts: single, adolescent or elderly, comorbid substance or alcohol abuse, past history of suicide attempts, psychotic stigmata, family history of suicide and access to lethal means. Suicide plans that are likely lethal and suicide intent are among the most important elements that predict risk of suicide.

4. Depressed patients do not commonly wish to harm others but there are enough cases in the news of depressed patients who kill others to warrant inquiries to the patient about this.

Treatment

The first consideration is whether hospitalization is necessitated by suicide risk, psychosis, inanition due to nutritional neglect, or other grievous reasons.

1. Somatic methods include antidepressant medications, electroconvulsive therapy (ECT), and in recent years transcranial magnetic stimulation; implant of a vagus nerve stimulator and deep brain stimulation have become available. Antidepressant medication is the most common approach.

2. Cognitive-Behavioral Therapy (CBT) has been shown to be effective in treatment of mild-to-moderately severe depression.

3. CBT can be combined with somatic treatment and the two work better together than medication alone.

If the clinician decides to recommend antidepressant medication, there are several matters to consider:

1. If the patient has been treated for depression in the past with a medicine that was effective, then this medicine should be used again. If this is not the case, but if a first degree relative (parents, siblings, and children) with depression has been treated successfully with medication, then the patient should be treated with the same medication. The patient may not have this family information but should be asked to look into this, although at times patients may be averse to talking with certain relatives about their problems.

2. Careful inquiry should be made as to whether the patient has ever had hypomanic or manic episodes (see below regarding tips for inquiry into these often elusive symptoms). Additional needed information is whether or not there is family history of hypomania or mania. Should either the patient or a first degree relative have a history of hypomania or mania, one needs to proceed especially cautiously in the use of antidepressants. These patients are at risk for developing so-called pharmacologic-induced hypomania or mania.

3. The agents used to treat depression are thought to produce their therapeutic effects by their actions on the brain's serotonin, noradrenergic and dopamine systems. Some, such as fluoxetine (a selective serotonin reuptake inhibitor [SSRI]), acts on only one of these systems (serotonin), while others act on all three (eg, duloxetine).

4. Aside from prior treatment or family history clues as described above, there is no way to predict which antidepressant will be effective in a given patient. About 60% of patients with major depressive disorder respond to SSRIs, so they are used most often in initial treatment. Dosing strategies are available from multiple sources. There is a growing evidence base such as that produced by the STAR-D trials (see *http:/www.psych.org//news_room/ press_releases/0666stardresults110120 06.pdf*) on how to approach the patient who does not respond to the first tried antidepressant. The recommendations of STAR-D are available on the referenced website so will not be reviewed here, except to note that these measures include a variety of augmentation strategies (ie, various augmenting agents used with any given antidepressant). Augmentation agents include triiodothyronine (T3), lithium, buspirone, pindalol, tricyclic antidepressants, combining antidepressants, and others. Monotherapy with tricyclic antidepressants and monoamine oxidase inhibitors are also used in refractory depression, as is ECT. The relatively recent development of ECT that delivers a brief (.5 msec) and ultrabrief (.3 msec) pulse width, which result in significantly less memory impairment than the standard 1 msec pulse width, may increase the use of ECT in refractory depression. As indicated above, vagal nerve stimulator, transcranial magnetic stimulation and deep brain stimulation are being studied as approaches to refractory depression.

Etiology
Some dyregulation of monamine neurotransmitter systems has long been thought to underlie depressive disorder. This idea is based primarily on the fact that antidepressant medications pertubate these systems. Recent neuroimaging evidence has emerged that dysregulation of neural circuits involving dorsolateral prefrontal cortex and subgenual prefrontal cortex (both targets of monoamine projections from the brainstem) may represent the fundamental "lesions" that cause symptoms of depressive illness. The hippocampus has also been shown to be involved. This may explain some of the cognitive deficits often seen in depression.

Another exciting line of research has revealed that certain polymorphisms of the gene that codes for the manufacture of the serotonin transporter protein confer a heightened risk of depression under conditions of stress.

Dysthymia
See *DSM-IV-R* for the criteria for this diagnosis. In essence, this disorder represents a chronic smolder-

ing condition, which does not disable, as can major depression, but rather can rob life of its full enjoyment. There may be neuro-vegetative symptoms (eg, changes in sleep and appetite, etc., but if present are fewer in number and often of less severity than those seen in major depression). The prevalence is likely much higher than can be ascertained, because people with this condition often do not seek help unless they develop a major depressive episode. The diagnosis is, in these cases, made in retrospect by the patient and the treating clinician. Not infrequently, patients were not aware of being dysthymic, thinking their chronic pessimistic mood is how life is experienced by all people. Antidepressant medications can be helpful in treating dysthymia and their effect can be boosted by cognitive-behavioral therapy. All clinicians, regardless of specialty, should inquire about the presence of dysthymia, as identifying it may lead, through treatment, to an improved quality of life.

Adjustment Disorder with Depressed Mood

See *DSM-IV-R* for the criteria for this diagnosis. Whereas the diagnosis of major depressive episode does not require the presence of a precipitating stress, adjustment disorder does. In lay terms this disorder would be referred to as like "being discouraged about something." The depressive reaction can, albeit rarely, be acute and severe with suicide risk. As with dysthymia, most people who are discouraged about something do not seek professional help (although if they were to, could easily meet criteria). The best treatment is any form of psychotherapy that permits talking through the problem to understand its dimensions and improve coping with the precipitating stressor(s).

Substance Abuse Induced Mood Disorder

The common comorbidity of mood disorder and alcohol/drug abuse presents a conundrum. Alcohol and/or substance abuse can cause mood disorders and the converse is also true. One among many ways to tease this out is to ask a depressed patient with a history of alcohol or substance abuse to recall their longest sober or straight period.

If there has been such a period, one asks the patient to recount the weeks and months leading-up to alcohol or drug relapse. If the lead-up period was marked by neuro-vegetative depressive symptoms such as insomnia and diminished appetite, the patient is likely to have primary depressive disorder. If, on the other hand, the lead-up period was not characterized by these types of symptoms, then alcohol or substance abuse disorder is likely the primary psychiatric disorder. This would be a case of alcohol or substance induced mood disorder.

Bipolar Affective Disorders, Types I and II

Type I refers to patients who have had one or more manic episodes. Type II refers to patients with histories of hypomanic but not manic episodes.

Essentially, the distinction between mania and hypomania is that symptoms of hypomania, while bearing some similarities to those of mania, are less severe. This is the reason that hypomanic episodes do not result in the need for hospitalization while mania frequently does. These conditions are characterized by hyper-energized states, which could be likened to a revved-up engine. Not surprisingly, the symptoms of both subtypes (I & II) involve, to one degree or another, reduced need for sleep, and more energy with consequent hyperkinesis, which can lead to an increased goal-directed activity. For example, hypomanic and manic patients may stay up late into the night cleaning house. Additionally, a patient's thinking is rapid (often experienced as "racing thoughts"), mood is elevated or irritable, and speech can be rapid, loud and continuous.

As pointed out above, in mania, these symptoms are more intense and there is increased risk of hypersexuality (with the concomitant risk of sexually dangerous behavior) and excessive spending, which may result in legal problems as the spending may be well beyond the patient's means.

Judgment can be so impaired that patients may put themselves at risk of injury or death. One patient seen in our ED was planning to walk 60 miles barefoot in the middle of a cold winter night as part of a political protest. Nutrition can be ignored. Untreated manic states have resulted in death due to the complications of several days of sleep deprivation and neglected self-care.

Mood elevation can range from mild, as seen in hypomania, to ecstasy that can be seen in mania. Psychotic symptoms can occur in manic states and

Table 4

***DSM-IV-R* Criteria for a Manic Episode**

A. A distinct period of abnormally and persistently elevated, expansive or irritable mood, lasting at least 1 week (or any duration if hospitalization is necessary)

B. During the period of mood disturbance, three (or more) of the following symptoms have persisted (four if the mood is only irritable) and have been present to a significant degree:
   1. inflated self-esteem or grandiosity;
   2. decreased need for sleep (eg, feels rested after only 3 hours of sleep);
   3. more talkative than usual, or pressure to keep talking;
   4. flight of ideas, or subjective experience that thoughts are racing;
   5. distractibility (ie, attention too easily drawn to unimportant or irrelevant external stimuli);
   6. increase in goal-directed activity (at work, at school, or sexually) or psychomotor agitation;
   7. excessive involvement in pleasurable activities that have a high potential for painful consequences (eg, engaging in unrestrained buying sprees, sexual indiscretions, or foolish business investments).

C. The symptoms do not meet criteria for a Mixed Episode.

D. The mood disturbance is sufficiently severe to cause marked impairment in occupational functioning or in usual social activities or relationships with others, or to necessitate hospitalization to prevent harm to self or others, or there are psychotic features.

E. The symptoms are not due to the direct physiological effects of a substance (eg, a drug of abuse, a medication or other treatment) or a general medical condition (eg, hyperthyroidism)

Note: Manic-like episodes that are clearly caused by somatic antidepressant treatment (eg, medication, electroconvulsive therapy, light therapy) should not count toward a diagnosis of bipolar I disorder.

these symptoms are often congruent with the elevated mood. For example, I recall one patient who thought her son was Christ. When told this, the resident as he examined her said, "You must be very proud." This endeared her to him and led to an improvement in treatment compliance.

In mania (less so in hypomania) denial of illness presents the greatest challenge to treatment. Hospitalization often is imposed against the patient's will.

The caveat about ruling out medical/neurological causes of major depression is true as well for mania. As an example, mania induced by steroids is indistinguishable from idiopathic mania.

While it is relatively easy to diagnose a manic state or history of same, eliciting and verifying past history of hypomania is often more challenging. However, doing so is a necessary step in planning treatment for depression. One strategy is to describe to the patient a manic state, then ask the patient if she or he has ever experienced a milder version of the manic state.

Recitation of the treatments of bipolar I and II is beyond the scope of this chapter and is available in several of the reference sources provided at the end of this chapter. Suffice it to say that acute states of mania can be managed by lithium or depakote and, in recent years, treatment with some of the atypical antipsychotics has been shown to be effective. Benzodiazepines have an additional calming effect in the acute stage of mania. Finally, electroconvulsive therapy can be counted upon to lyse mania that is unresponsive to psychotropic agents.

Once mania subsides, long-term maintenance with a mood stabilizer is most often needed. The most common agents used are lithium, Depakote®, and more recently, lamotragine. Rapid cycling is a not uncommon form of bipolar disorder where frequent and rapid onset mood shifts between mania and depression occur. This may be difficult to treat. There is evidence that depakote may be the most effective mood stabilizer for rapid cycling. Psychotherapy has not been shown to be effective in treating acute mania or ameliorating the course of bipolar disorder over time.

Schizoaffective Disorder

This will be discussed below in the section on schizophrenia. Although it is a different illness than schizophrenia, it shares psychotic stigmata.

Anxiety Disorders

There is growing evidence that obsessive-compulsive disorder (OCD), now classified in the *DSM-IV-R* as an anxiety disorder, should be otherwise reclassified, based on the fact that it involves dyregulation of neural circuits involving certain subregions of prefrontal cortex, basal ganglia and thalamus, whereas all the other anxiety disorders are more amygdalocentric in nature. (This is not to say that more anterior brain regions are not involved in the anxiety disorders.) Another way of considering the anxiety disorders is that they are likely related to abnormalities in the neural machinery underlying fear responses. Post-traumatic stress disorder (PTSD) is also thought to involve the hippocampus.

The fear response-related anxiety disorders are panic disorder, with and without agoraphobia, generalized anxiety disorder (GAD), phobic and social anxiety disorders, and PTSD.

It is important to rule out medical/neurological contributants to or causes of anxiety disorder. Hyperthyroidism that can present with anxiety symptoms comes to mind.

When trying to elicit panic and generalized anxiety disorders, I will often explain to a patient that anxiety comes in two forms, one with generally heightened nervousness and the other with episodic outbursts of intense anxiety, manifest variably by rapid breathing, rapid heart rate, diaphoresis and an intense feeling of fear (ie, panic attacks). I add that some people have both versions of anxiety. I then ask the patient which of the forms of anxiety they experience. If they indicate they have had panic attacks, I will ask if agoraphobia is present after explaining what agoraphobia is.

Elicitation of a history of phobias, social anxiety and PTSD is usually straightforward. The diagnosis of PTSD requires a severe trauma and subsequent nightmares, flashbacks, emotional numbing (the subjective sense of diminished emotional reactions), and other symptoms which can be found in the *DSM-IV-R*. Of note is that recent evidence has suggested that ongoing stressful situations can also bring about PTSD symptoms. As to pathophysiology of PTSD, there is growing evidence, primarily form fMRI-based studies, that there is a "bottom up" problem of exaggerated amygdala responsivity and a "top down" problem of diminished ability of specific sets of anterior cingulate neurons to suppress or extinguish fearful responses.

An important caveat is that panic episodes and GAD can be imbedded in major depressive episodes, such that treatment of the depression may resolve the anxiety symptoms. It is also necessary, as is the case for all psychiatric disorders, to inquire about suicidal thoughts.

In eliciting a history of OCD, I usually describe its manifestations and then ask patients if they have had such experiences. The manifestations are either obsessive or compulsive behaviors or both. OCD is thought to be caused by dysregulation in at least two of the five described parallel cortical-striato-thalamico-cortical circuits (motor, oculomotor, dorsolateral prefrontal, lateral orbitofrontal and anterior cingulate), namely the latter two circuits.

As mentioned above, the fear-related anxiety disorders are thought to be amygdalocentric. Interestingly, general anxiety disorder may be related more to dysregulation in circuitry involving the bed nucleus of the stria terminalis.

All of the anxiety disorders have been shown to improve with CBT, psychotropic medications, or both. Formerly, tricyclic antidepressants and in the past two decades SSRIs, have been the mainstays of medication management of the fear-related anxiety disorders, while general anxiety disorder often responds to buspirone. The exposure-based desensitization form of CBT has been shown to be effective for PTSD, phobic and social anxiety disorders and OCD.

Table 5

***DSM-IV-R* Criteria for Schizophrenia**

A. Characteristic Symptoms: Two (or more) of the following, each present for a significant portion of time during a 1-month period (or less if successfully treated):

1. delusions
2. hallucinations
3. disorganized speech (eg, frequent derailment or incoherence)
4. grossly disorganized or catatonic behavior
5. negative symptoms, ie, affective flattening, alogia, or avolition

Note: Only one Criterion A symptom is required if delusions are bizarre or hallucinations consist of a voice keeping up a running commentary on the person's behavior or thoughts, or two or more voices conversing with each other.

B. Social/Occupational Dysfunction: For a significant portion of the time since the onset of the disturbance, one or more major areas of functioning such as work, interpersonal relations, or self-care are markedly below the level achieved prior to the onset (or when the onset is in childhood or adolescence, failure to achieve expected level of interpersonal, academic, or occupational achievement).

C. Duration: Continuous signs of the disturbance persist for at least 6 months. This 6-month period must include at least 1 month of symptoms (or less if successfully treated) that meet Criterion A (ie, active-phase symptoms) and may include periods of prodromal or residual symptoms. During these prodromal or residual periods, the signs of the disturbance may be manifested by only negative symptoms or two or more symptoms listed in Criterion A present in an attenuated form (eg, odd beliefs, unusual perceptual experiences).

D. Schizoaffective and Mood Disorder Exclusion: Schizoaffective Disorder and Mood Disorder with Psychotic Features have been ruled out because either: (1.) no Major Depressive, Manic, or Mixed Episodes have occurred concurrently with the active-phase symptoms; or (2.) if mood episodes have occurred during active-phase symptoms, their total duration has been brief relative to the duration of the active and residual periods.

E. Substance/General Medical Condition Exclusion: The disturbance is not due to the direct physiological effects of a substance (eg, a drug of abuse, a medication) or a general medical condition.

F. Relationship to a Pervasive Developmental Disorder: If there is a history of Autistic Disorder or another Pervasive Developmental Disorder, the additional diagnosis of Schizophrenia is made only if prominent delusions or hallucinations are also present for at least a month (or less if successfully treated).

The terms used in describing psychotic symptoms and manifestations of other psychiatric disorders often appear ambiguous. http://www.abess.com/glossary.html provides clear definitions of these terms.

Schizophrenia and Schizoaffective Disorder

Schizophrenia

This phenotypically heterogeneous disorder, thought to be neurodevelopemental in etiology, involves dysregulation of neural circuits involving certain prefrontal cortical regions (dorsolateral and anterior cingulate), certain midbrain/basal ganglia interconnections (between the ventral tegmental area of Tsai and the nucleus accumbens), hippocampus, inferior parietal lobule (combined supramarginal and angular gyrus), thalamus, cerebellum and parahippocampal gyrus.

Schizophrenia usually unfolds as follows: Over the many years before the first psychotic episode (usually in the late teens or early twenties), these patients are frequently socially ill at ease in one way or another. This may represent an early manifestation of the "negative symptoms" seen in schizophrenia (see below). This is thought to be related to deficiencies in development of certain frontal lobe regions. The first and subsequent psychotic breaks are manifest variably by hallucinations (more likely auditory than visual) and delusions. These later manifestations, designated "positive symptoms" of schizophrenia, are postulated to represent consequences of hyperactivity of dopaminergic neurons which project from the ventral tegmental area of the midbrain to the nucleus accumbens, a ventral component of the basal ganglia. There are also well-documented cognitive deficits in patients with schizophrenia thought to be caused by abnormal neural circuit activity involving the hippocampus, certain regions of prefrontal cortex, and the inferior parietal lobule.

Most commonly, once the first acute psychotic episode has subsided in response to antipsychotic medication, the patient is often left with a variety of negative symptoms such as apathy and abulia. These are thought to reflect the aforementioned neurodevelopmental prefrontal deficits. These, along with subsequent to the first episode outbreaks of positive symptoms, render the patient significantly impaired in day-to-day function. The positive and negative symptoms of schizophrenia are listed in Table 6.

Optimal treatment of schizophrenia includes aggressive treatment of the first psychotic episode, or perhaps ideally identifying at-risk individuals and intervening in some way before the first psychotic break. Once schizophrenia is diagnosed, optimal treatment is provided via the kind of comprehensive services often available at community mental health centers where teams, consisting of case managers, psychotherapists skilled in psychoeducation of patients and their family members, and in CBT, nurses and psychiatrists, are devoted to each patient's care. The best possible medication regimen is identified, often in sequential trials of antipsychotic agents. CBT comes to the assistance of the patient's impaired prefrontal cortical function and case managers work with the patient on day-to-day problems encountered by the patient. In the best of treatment milieus there is a program for supported employment where the patients are mainstreamed into the work force and kept active by vigilant monitoring in the work place.

Table 6

The Positive and Negative Symptoms of Schizophrenia

Positive Symptoms

1. delusions
2. conceptual disorganization
3. hallucinations
4. excitement
5. grandiosity
6. suspiciousness, ideas of persecution
7. hostility

Negative Symptoms

1. blunted affect
2. emotional withdrawal
3. poor rapport
4. passive/apathetic social withdrawal
5. concrete thinking
6. lack of spontaneity and poor flow of conversation
7. stereotyped thinking

Pharmacologic management of schizophrenia remains far from ideal. While the short-term risk of extrapyramidal side effects and long-term risks of tardive dyskinesia have been diminished by the shift in the past decade or so to atypical antipsychotic medications, the latter come with their own significant long-term side effect burdens of heightened risk of diabetes mellitus and cardio- and cerebrovascular disease. These are of particular concern in people with schizophrenia, both because the baseline risk of these diseases is higher than the general populations risk and because of the high rates of smoking among people with schizophrenia. (Of course, the high rate of smoking may account for a significant contribution to the development of cerebro- and cardiovascular disease in this population.)

The commonly used atypical antipsychotics are clozapine, olanzapine, rispiridone, ziprasidone and apipirazole. The first three confer the greatest risk of diabetes mellitus, and cardiovascular and cerebrovascular disease. The latter confer minimal risk but may be ineffective for the symptoms of schizophrenia in many patients. Experimental drugs that target gabergic/glutaminergic cortical systems (proposed relatively recently to be involved in the pathophysiology of schizophrenia) may lead to more effective and less toxic treatment than is currently available.

A patient with a first episode psychosis, especially if there is no premorbid pattern of personality oddness, should be assessed for underlying neurological disease. I recall a 25-year-old patient who was normal premorbidly and who became acutely psychotic. She had no localizing neurological findings on examination. She proved to have colloid cyst of the third ventricle which, when treated surgically, abated her psychotic symptoms.

Schizoaffective Disorder

Simply stated, schizoaffective disorder is characterized longitudinally by episodes of mood disorder (depression, mania or both) with interspersed psychotic symptoms. If a patient becomes psychotic while depressed or manic but has no history of psychotic symptoms when neither manic nor depressed, then the patient does not have schizoaffective disorder. Pharmacologic treatment targets: 1.) the mood disorder episodes when they occur acutely and prevention of relapse once the acute episode has remitted; and 2.) the residual psychotic symptoms. Schizoaffective disorder is associated with a somewhat better prognosis than schizophrenia.

Somatoform Disorders

Table 7 lists the disorders grouped together as the somatoform disorders.

Patients with these disorders complain of, or exhibit, physical symptoms for which no physiologic bases or medical diseases are found despite medical investigations appropriate to the complaints. Three of these disorders—somatization, hypochondriac, and pain disorder (by definition, chronic)—are so diffuse in their presentation that they defy traditional disease models. They rather seem to represent ways of life that engage the health care system with a tenacity that often challenges the patience of health care providers.

Somatization Disorder, Hypochondriasis, Pain Disorder

The *DSM-IV-R* criteria for somatization criteria include several years of behaviors, beginning before age 30, of seeking medical attention for, or being impaired by, at least four pain symptoms (in different locations or involving different bodily functions); at least two different gastrointestinal complaints; at least one sexual complaint; and at least

Table 7

The Somatoform Disorders

1. Somatization
2. Hypochondriasis
3. Chronic pain
4. Conversion (includes non-epileptic seizures)
5. Body dysmorphic disorder
6. Munchausen syndrome
7. Malingering

one pseudoneurological symptom—finally with the proviso that no explanatory diseases are found.

Hypochondriasis is also, by definition, a chronic condition and is characterized by a belief that one is suffering from a terrible, possibly fatal disease, and also carries the proviso that medical investigation reveals no such diseases.

Pain disorder refers to chronic pain for which no medical explanation if found. There may be a history of tissue injury, for example, to the low back. However, in this disorder the pain seems out of proportion to the original tissue injury.

These illnesses or behaviors are in a domain of psychiatric disorders distinct from the disorders considered previously in this chapter: mood disorders, schizophrenia, and so on. These more "traditional" diseases appear to involve neural circuitry dysregulation, related etiologically to genetic and environmental influences. The etiology of somatoform conditions is unknown.

The traditional advice in approaching these patients is to acknowledge sincerely their suffering, do whatever medical work-up and obtain whatever specialty consultations seem reasonable, explain to the patient what disorder they have, and emphasize that the symptoms are "real." Diagnose and treat any comorbid psychiatric conditions such as depressive or anxiety disorder. The care is best coordinated by one physician, such as the patient's primary care provider. Relatively frequent and brief visits often provide the patient with the emotional support needed to endure their suffering.

An important caveat for patients with these disorders is that they also can and do develop known diseases. This requires ongoing clinician vigilance regarding each new symptom.

Conversion Disorder

This disorder, often presenting acutely, is the development of a neurological symptom which is not anatomically possible (eg, stocking and glove anesthesia), or for which no physiological explanation can be found. One of the most common types of conversion disorder symptoms are non-epileptic seizures. Not infrequently, epileptic seizures are concomitantly present. A feature, besides its often acute presentation, that distinguishes conversion disorder from somatization disorder, hypochrondriasis and pain disorder, is that there are usually events or circumstances in the sufferer's current life which the patient has reacted to with a conversion symptom. In other words, some kind of psychological conflict is present. Absent such a conflict, it is very difficult to make a case for conversion disorder. One problem is that seizures that emanate from the frontal lobe or the medial temporal lobe are not uncommonly bizarre in appearance. And one has to face the fact that seizure foci that cause these seizures are not infrequently undetectable by standard EEG or telemetry. In fact, a surface EEG may not register seizure activity even while a patient is in the midst of a temporal or frontal lobe seizure.

This disorder is to be distinguished from dissociative disorders that consist of "spells" that may appear like absence seizures but which actually reflect activation of a mental state of "leaving the scene" in response to stressful situations. These spells occur most frequently in people who have been severely traumatized, usually early in life but occasionally as adults, such as by the emotional trauma of intense combat exposure. Patients who dissociate often have PTSD.

Non-epileptic seizures or other conversion disorder symptoms may develop in the context of comorbid psychiatric disorders such as an anxiety or depressive disorder. These need to be diagnosed and treated, which sometimes will clear up the conversion symptom.

In any case the patient does need to be informed that they have a bonafide medical problem that represents their response to stress. This can often be addressed by cognitive-behavioral therapy targeting stress management, and in some cases physical therapy.

Body Dysmorphic Disorder

This disorder is characterized by a patient's belief that some feature of their appearance, usually involving the face, has rendered them ugly. This belief may be based on a minor blemish or an idea that some normal part of their anatomy like their nose is ugly. Avoiding plastic surgery is one goal of treatment. This disorder is best managed by a mental health professional.

Munchausen Syndrome
This uncommon disorder is manifest by a patient claiming physical symptoms or engaging in self-injurious behaviors in order to invite invasive diagnostic or therapeutic interventions. These patients will go to several hospitals over many months or years to achieve these interventions. I recall such a patient who swallowed open safety pins in order to secure surgical intervention. He died from surgical complications after a decade of this behavior. These patients are not psychotic but they not infrequently abuse drugs or alcohol. The cause of this disorder is not known, nor is any treatment usually effective.

Factitious Disorder
Factitious disorder involves lying in order to assume a sick role. Malingering is lying to achieve a goal such as economic gain. It is often very difficult to know if someone is lying or not.

Personality Disorders
Everyone, of course, has a personality style such as being outgoing or shy, obsessive or lackadaisical, and so on. Some of these styles can be advantageous. For example, a medical student who is not to some degree obsessive in nature may not succeed well in school.

On the other hand, personality disordered people are those whose personality style creates problems in interpersonal relationships. In some of these disorders, it is other people who suffer from the person's behavior. Examples would be the demanding self-entitled nature of many people with narcissistic personalities, the clinging behavior of those with dependant personality disorder and the lying, cheating and criminal behavior of those with antisocial personality disorder.

In some personality disorder, both the patient and often the clinician are challenged. An example would be borderline personality disorder (BPD), symptoms of which include (among other symptoms) cutting behaviors and suicide threats. The cause of personality disorders is unknown except for BPD, which almost invariably is caused by major betrayals early in life in the form of repeated physical and/or sexual trauma. Patients with BPD frequently have co-morbid PTSD.

Some personality disorders do not impact other people or cause suffering for the individual with the disorder. Examples are schizoid and avoidant personality disorder. These people in a sense are "in their own world" and are not necessarily suffering, nor do they often come to medical attention.

The diagnostic criteria of the personality disorders can be found in the *DSM-IV-R*.

The treatment of patients with personality disorder depends upon the disorder being treated. Some examples: narcissistic personality disorder will usually improve with long-term psychodynamic psychotherapy; borderline personality disorder is best treated with dialectic behavior therapy (DBT); and antisocial personality disorder does not respond usually to treatment of any kind.

The non-mental health clinician should become familiar with these disorders as the behaviors of these patients often have impacts on compliance with treatment, and on interactions with the clinician which may be angst-laden.

The Substance-Related Disorders
These disorders are grouped into two divisions: 1.) substance use disorders (either abuse or dependence), and 2.) substance-induced disorders. Covering the latter is beyond the scope of this chapter as there are at least ten such disorders. Suffice it to say that substance abuse can produce symptoms of nearly all psychiatric disorders. When this occurs, treatment of the underlying substance problem and the disorders themselves are usually necessary. Sometimes, however, successful treatment of the substance abuse component will "cure" the disorder induced. In some cases of substance-induced mood disorder, for example, abstinence alone may resolve the mood problem.

In some other substance-induced disorders, such as substance-induced psychotic disorder, the psychotic symptoms most often require targeted treatment such as with antipsychotic medication. In these cases, while certain aspects of the substance abuse problem, such as withdrawal symptoms, may require concomitant treatment of the withdrawal state and the psychotic symptoms, addressing the underlying substance abuse problem, eg, with measures such as Alcoholics Anonymous, can only be brought to bear once the psychotic symptoms are under control.

The Substance Abuse Disorders

The substances that can lead to an abuse and/or dependence are alcohol, amphetamine, caffeine, cannabis, cocaine, hallucinogens, inhalants, nicotine, opioids, phencyclidine, sedatives, hypnotics and anxiolytics. The difference between abuse and dependence is a matter of severity, as measured by the degree of negative impact substance use has on the user's life. Also, substance tolerance and withdrawal are among the symptoms possible with a dependence diagnosis, while this is not the case for substance abuse alone. It should be emphasized, however, that dependence can be diagnosed in the absence of tolerance and withdrawal.

See the *DSM-IV-R* for the diagnostic criteria that distinguish dependence and abuse. The *DSM-IV-R* also elucidates which substances are associated with withdrawal states and which substances are associated with which substance-induced disorders. An example of the latter is that caffeine and nicotine do not produce psychotic symptoms, while all the other substances can (whether by virtue of a withdrawal state or use).

Regarding the pathophysiology of abuse of substances, an important common denominator is that they all work their effects by activating, in one way or another, the mesolimbic dopamine system. More specifically, on the ventral midbrain's dopaminergic neuron projections to the gabergic medium spiny neurons (MSNs) of the nucleus accumbens. The cell bodies of these neurons are aggregated in the ventral midbrain's ventral tegmental area (VTA) of Tsai. Figure 1 illustrates these points.

Activation of these dopaminergic neurons has an inhibitory effect on the gabergic MSNs, the net effect being a disinhibition on widespread downstream targets of the MSNs. This disinhibitory effect is hypothesized to underlie the "high" produced by many substances of abuse, although which specific target(s) are responsible for the "high" is (are) not known. Finally, the MSNs are under the modulatory effects of projections from certain prefrontal cortex regions, the amygdala and the hippocampus. There is some evidence that these modulatory effects may be central to the pathophysiology of substance abuse disorders.

Review of diagnosis and treatment of the vast variety of substance use disorders is beyond the scope of this chapter and are available in standard psychiatry texts such as are listed at chapter's end.

Here are a few miscellaneous but salient facts relating to alcoholism, among the most common of addiction disorders:

1. *Delirium tremens* is a distinct entity from delirium of any other cause. The latter always causes reduced dominant background frequencies (down to 8 Hz or less) as measured by EEG. This is not the case in delirium tremens.

2. *Increased autonomic arousal* occurs in both moderate-to-severe anxiety and in several withdrawal states (eg, from opiods, alcohol and benzodiazepine, to name a few). A distinguishing feature between anxiety and withdrawal states is that the latter cause postural hypotension and the former do not. This can be useful in an ED situation where the history is less than clear.

3. *Wernicki-Korsakoff syndrome* occurs in some cases of alcohol withdrawal. It is characterized by ataxia, bilateral paresis of lateral gaze, and delirium.

4. In postmortem examination of the brains of patients who had Korsakoff psychosis, an illness dominated by disturbances of memory, lesions are found in the mammilary body of the hypothalamus and the anterior and medialdordal nuclei of the thalamus. The mammilary body and anterior thalamic nuclei are members of the Papes circuit. Papes hypothesized that this circuit served emotion, but research in the past few decades has shown that Papes circuit is involved in memory functions.

5. Alcoholic hallucinosis is a disorder that features, in the presence of a clear sensorium, psychotic symptoms (often persecutory hallucinations and

Figure 1

Actions of substances of abuse on VTA's dopaminergic projections to the nucleus accumbens

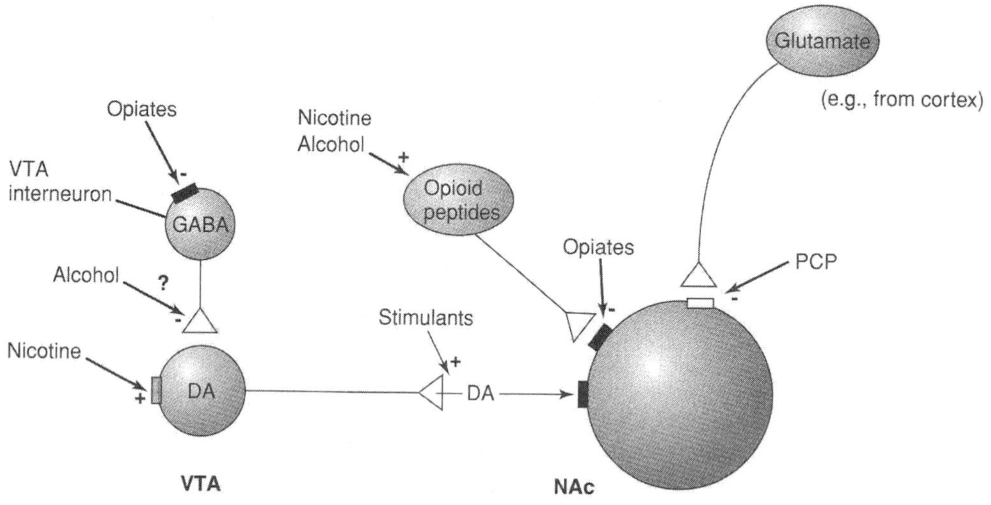

Taken from Nestler EJ, Hyman SE, Malenka, RC. Molecular Neuropharmacology: A Foundation for Clinical Neuroscience. *McGraw-Hill, New York, 2001. Reprinted with permission by the McGraw-Hill Companies.*

delusions). It usually occurs when heavy alcohol consumption is reduced or stopped.

3. Psychiatric Issues in Stroke, Delirium and Dementia

These illnesses can all cause psychiatric symptoms which are indistinguishable from the symptoms caused by "traditional" psychiatric illnesses. Stroke is particularly likely to cause disorders of mood by affecting neural circuits known to be involved in mood regulation. The type of mood disorder often correlates with location of the stroke. If a stroke leads to symptoms of major depressive disorder, it is most commonly a left hemisphere stroke in the anterior frontal lobe. When mania occurs as a consequence of stroke, the lesion is commonly in the right hemisphere. Psychiatric treatment is the same as for idiopathic mood disorder.

Delirium (diffuse reversible neuronal metabolic impairment), such as that due to hypoxia and hyponatremia, usually occurring in hospitalized patients, can cause, in addition to diffuse cognitive impairment, any and all psychiatric symptoms. The latter usually resolve with successful treatment of the cause of the delirium. Until the underlying cause of the delirium is treated, the patient's behavior, such as psychotically driven agitation, may require treatment with antipsychotic agents such as haloperidol. Short-term use of haloperidol is usually safe and effective in these situations. Safety measures such as restraints or net beds may be required.

It should be remembered that psychiatric symptoms may persist for some time after correction of an underlying metabolic abnormality such as hyponatremia. If there is any doubt that delirium, as opposed to a underlying psychiatric disturbance, is the cause of the abnormal behavior, an EEG can be diagnostic. Psychiatric illness does not cause bilateral slowing of dominant background frequency, but delirium always does (not surprising, given the diffuse neuronal metabolic impairment which causes the delirium).

Dementias of any type can, as does delirium, cause any and all psychiatric symptoms. Paranoid psychoses, depressive and anxiety disorders are not uncommon. These can usually be controlled to some extent in the same manner that these disorders are treated in the absence of dementia.

Both delirium, dementia and certain focal neurological lesions (such as in pseudobulbar palsy) can cause emotional lability, one version of which is pathological crying. Thus, these behaviors should not be misconstrued as evidence of depressive disorder.

Mention should also be made in this section that certain focal neurological lesions can cause specific psychiatric symptoms. A good example are the Lillipilutian hallucinations that can be caused by a small ventral midbrain stroke. This syndrome is referred to as peduncular hallucinosis. This symptom can occur in the presence of otherwise clear mentation. Steroids can also cause psychiatric symptoms such as mania, depression or psychosis in the absence of clouded mentation.

4. References

1. Gelder M, Harrison P, Cowen P. *Shorter Oxford Textbook of Psychiatry*. Oxford, England: Oxford University Press; 2006,

   (An excellent, concise overview of the field.)

2. *Kaplan H, Sadock B. Kaplan and Sadock's Comprehensive Textbook of Psychiatry*. 8th edition. Philadelphia: Lippincott Williams & Wilkins; 2004.

   (A comprehensive overview of the field.)

3. Rosenbaum J, Arana G, Hyman S, Labbate F. *Handbook of Psychiatric Drug Therapy*. 5th edition. Philadelphia: Lippincott Williams & Wilkins; 2004.

   (Outstanding overview of this subject.)

4. Capsi A, et al. Influence of life stress on depression: moderation by a polymorphism in the 5-HTT gene. *Science*. 2003; 301(5631):291-293.

   (A seminal study of genetic influences on vulnerability to major depression.)

5. Mayberg HS, et al. Deep brain stimulation for treatment-resistant depression. *Neuron*. 2005, 3;45 (5):651-660.

   (The first, best look at regional brain disturbances in major affective disorder.)

6. *Diagnostic and Statistical Manual of Mental Disorders*. 4th edition. Washington, DC: American Psychiatric Association; 1994.

5. Questions

1. A 23-year-old woman comes for help with what you diagnose to be a major depressive episode. She has no history of hypomanic or manic episodes but her mother has bipolar affective disorder. What influence does the patient's family history have on your treatment recommendations?

A. The family history is irrelevant to your pharmacologic recommendations.

B. You will use aggressive doses of antidepressants.

C. You will be cautious in use of antidepressants out of concern for precipitating hypomania or mania.

D. You will be cautious in use of antidepressants out of concern for precipitating psychosis.

2. Schizoaffective disorder is characterized by:

A. Manic episodes in which patients become psychotic.

B. Depressive episodes in which patients become manic.

C. Mood disorder in patients with a schizoid personality.

D. Psychotic symptoms during intervals between mood disorder episodes.

3. All of the following regions have been implicated in schizophrenia except:

A. Occipital lobe.

B. Prefrontal cortex.

C. Hippocampus.

D. Dopaminergic system.

4. A 37-year-old man is treated for what has been diagnosed as a major depressive episode by an SSRI at maximum recommended dose for six weeks without response. His spouse thinks his depression is in fact worsening as he seems increasingly withdrawn, unmotivated and disinterested in his surroundings. At this point, what avenue would you pursue?

A. Switch to a different antidepressant.

B. Obtain a head CT scan.

C. Augment the current antidepressant with lithium.

D. Refer to a psychotherapist.

5. A 23-year-old woman is seen in the ED because of 24 hours of "spells" of apparent altered states of consciousness. Which of the following would tend to rule out non-epileptic seizures?

A. Normal EEG.

B. Bizarre-appearing spells.

C. Co-existing grand mal seizures.

D. Absence of psychological stressors or symptoms of psychiatric illness.

6. The negative symptoms of schizophrenia include all of the following except:

A. Low motivation.

B. Delusions of nihilism.

C. Paucity of speech.

D. Inactivity.

7. A 45-year-old woman with a history of depressive episodes with psychotic features is admitted to hospital for lumbar disk surgery. Two days postoperatively, she develops persecutory delusions but does not appear depressed. A metabolic screen is normal and she is afebrile. The treatment team is divided on the diagnostic possibilities explaining the delusions. Some believe she has developed another episode of psychiatric disorder while others believe she may have delirium. What diagnostic step could settle the dispute?

A. Minnesota Multiphasic Personality Inventory.

B. EEG.

C. A neurologic examination.

D. Obtain additional information from the patient's family.

8. A 23-year-old woman presents to an ED admitting that she just inflicted lacerations on the volar surface of each wrist immediately after an argument with her boyfriend and has a history of burning her arms with cigarettes when stressed. What is the most likely diagnosis?

A. Dysthymic disorder.

B. Narcissistic personality disorder.

C. Borderline personality disorder.

D. Antisocial personality disorder.

9. The atypical antipsychotic agents with a higher risk of producing lipid abnormalities include all of the following except:

A. Ziprasidone

B. Clozapine

C. Olanzapine

D. Rispiridone

10. An otherwise healthy 45-year-old man is diagnosed with panic disorder. Of the medication and medication types listed, which would likely be most efficacious?

A. Atypical antipsychotics

B. Buspirone

C. SSRIs

D. Antihistaminics

11. A 50-year-old man is hospitalized for a flare of multiple sclerosis which had become progressively disabling over the preceding two months. He indicates his mood has been quite depressed and that his motivation and energy have been low. He says that he is especially despondent first thing in the morning but that his mood lightens as the day progresses. This last comment suggests that he:

A. Has an adjustment disorder with depressed mood.

B. Has bipolar affective disorder.

C. Has major depressive disorder.

D. Is malingering about his mood.

12. A 40-year-old woman complains of a mild chronic feeling of unhappiness although has no abnormalities of sleep or appetite. The most likely diagnosis is:

A. Dysthymia.

B. Adjustment disorder with depressed mood.

C. Schizoid personality.

D. Cyclothymia.

13. Parents of a 15-year-old boy express a concern about him that, throughout his youth, and worsening in adolescence, he has had no close friends, and spends most of his time, while not at school, at home in his room. If these behaviors presage a psychiatric disorder, which one is most likely?

A. Bipolar affective disorder.

B. Panic disorder.

C. Somatization disorder.

D. Schizophrenia.

14. Positive symptoms of schizophrenia include ALL but:

A. Abulia.

B. Delusions of persecution.

C. Hallucinations.

D. Bizarre behavior.

15. A region of the brain recently implicated in major depressive disorder is:

A. Cerebellum.

B. Precuneous gyrus.

C. Subgenual prefrontal cortex.

D. Temporal pole.

16. A 50-year-old man with major depressive illness has only partially responded to an aggressive trial of fluoxetine, an SSRI. Various agents have proven to be effective in augmenting the antidepressant effect of antidepressants, including SSRIs. In order to improve this patient's mood further, all of the following agents would be reasonable to consider as augmenters except for:

A. Benzodiazepines

B. Triiodothyronine (T3)

C. Buspirone

D. Lithium

17. Which of the following personality disorders often respond to dialectic behavior therapy?

A. Dependant personality disorder.

B. Borderline personality disorder.

C. Antisocial personality disorder.

D. Obsessive personality disorder.

18. In interpreting the results of a cognitive examination such as the Mini-Mental Status Examination, it is important to establish:

A. Family history of psychiatric disorders.

B. Age of onset of the patient's illness.

C. General intelligence and grade achieved in school.

D. The nature of any precipitating stressor to the patient's illness episode.

19. Phobia and panic disorder, both of which are manifest by fearful behavior most likely involve which of the following brain regions?

A. Caudate nucleus

B. Cerebellum

C. Superior colliculus

D. Amygdala

20. Seasonal affective disorder is often characterized by all of the following except:

A. Hypersomnia.

B. Carbohydrate craving.

C. Paranoid delusions.

D. Onset of depressed mood in the fall or early winter.

Answers

1. C.
People with first-degree relative history of bipolar affective have a greater risk of developing hypomania than patients without such family history.

2. D.
The description in answer "D" fits the definition of schizoaffective disorder but none of the other answers fit.

3. A.
There is scant evidence for occipital lobe involvement in schizophrenia.

4. B.
The patient's increasing abulia may be due to a frontal lobe tumor, which could be the reason that his depressive symptoms have not responded to treatment and his functioning is worsening.

5. D.
Non-epileptic seizures are nearly invariably in response to stressors or are imbedded in some psychiatric disorder but are not ruled out by normal EEG, bizarre appearance of spells or co-existing grand mal epilepsy.

6. B.
Delusions are considered among the positive symptoms of schizophrenia.

7. B.
An EEG showing bilateral slowing, below 8 Hz, of dominant background brain frequency would be characteristic of delirium.

8. C.
Self-cutting is more indicative of borderline personality disorder than answers A., B. and D.

9. A.
Ziprasidone has a lower risk of producing lipid abnormalities than those listed as answers B., C. and D.

10. C.
The answers A., B. and D. are not used to treat panic disorder.

11. C.
The patient's diurnal mood variation is strong support for a diagnosis of major depressive disorder.

12. A.
Dysthymia is far more likely to explain the patient's complaint than any of the other diagnoses listed.

13. D.
The boy's behavior is a common premorbid pattern of patients who develop schizophrenia.

14. A.
Abulia is among the "negative" symptoms of schizophrenia.

15. C.
As reviewed in this chapter, the subgenual area has been demonstrated in imaging studies to be hyperactive in major depression.

16. A.
While benzodiazepines are used at times to allay the anxiety often present in major depressive episodes, they have not been shown to be effective adjuncts in bringing about remission of depression.

17. B.
Among the disorders listed, only borderline personality disorder has been shown to respond to dialectic behavior therapy.

18. C.
Performance on cognitive tasks is not dependent on A., B. or D., but is influenced significantly by C.

19. D.
Mammalian fear responses have been shown to be amygdala driven.

20. C.
Delusions are not manifestations of seasonal affective disorder.